Emergency Care
as Practiced
at the
Massachusetts
General Hospital

MGH TEXTBOOK OF
emergency medicine

SECOND EDITION

MGH TEXTBOOK OF
emergency medicine

Emergency Care as Practiced at the Massachusetts General Hospital

SECOND EDITION

EDITOR

EARLE W. WILKINS, JR., M.D.

Chief, Emergency Services, and Visiting Surgeon, Massachusetts General Hospital; Clinical Professor of Surgery, Harvard Medical Schol

ASSOCIATE EDITORS

JAMES J. DINEEN, M.D.

Associate Physician, Massachusetts General Hospital; Assistant Professor of Medicine, Harvard Medical School

ASHBY C. MONCURE, M.D.

Visiting Surgeon, Massachusetts General Hospital; Assistant Clinical Professor of Surgery, Harvard Medical School

PETER L. GROSS, M.D.

Associate Chief, Emergency Services, and Assistant Physician, Massachusetts General Hospital; Instructor in Medicine, Harvard Medical School

EDITORIAL ASSOCIATE

CATHERINE P. FITZGERALD, B.A.

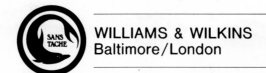

WILLIAMS & WILKINS
Baltimore/London

Copyright ©, 1983
Williams & Wilkins
428 East Preston Street
Baltimore, MD 21202, U.S.A.

Made in the United States of America

Library of Congress Cataloging in Publication Data

Main entry under title:

MGH textbook of emergency medicine.

"Emergency care as practiced at the Massachusetts General Hospital"—P.
Includes index.
1. Emergency medicine. 2. Hospitals—Emergency service. I. Wilkins, Earle W. II. Massachusetts General Hospital. III. Title: M.G.H. textbook of emergency medicine.
[DNLM: 1. Emergency medicine. WB 105 M106]
RC86.7.M49   1983   616'.025   82-8443
ISBN 0–683–09084–4

Composed and printed at the
Waverly Press, Inc.
Mt. Royal and Guilford Aves.
Baltimore, MD 21202, U.S.A.

To the House Staff of the Massachusetts
General Hospital, who have manned the front
lines of the Emergency Ward.

Preface to Second Edition

The first national medical specialty board was recognized in 1917. In September 1979, 62 years later, the American Board of Emergency Medicine (ABEM) became the 23rd specialty board. A resolution adopted by the American Board of Medical Specialties recognized the ABEM as a conjoint board of the American Board of Family Practice, the American Board of Internal Medicine, the American Board of Obstetrics and Gynecology, the American Board of Otolaryngology, the American Board of Pediatrics, the American Board of Psychiatry and Neurology, the American Board of Surgery, the American College of Emergency Physicians, the American Medical Association's Section on Emergency Medicine, and the University Association for Emergency Medicine. Like the American Board of Family Practice, the ABEM is structured by means of "horizontal categorization" rather than the conventional "vertical categorization." Because of this cross-disciplinary framework, Emergency Medicine must be prepared to provide diagnosis and treatment for the entire spectrum of problems cared for by the sponsoring boards. This is a mighty challenge!

The coming-of-age of the specialty of Emergency Medicine has brought added responsibilities. Foremost among these are medical education, the development of standards of care for emergency departments as well as patterns of follow-up care that compensate for the episodic nature of the doctor-patient relationship, the formulation of mutually acceptable working arrangements with other specialties, and research into the common problems that are encountered in this broad field.

This textbook is directed toward the difficult task of education in perhaps the broadest specialty of all. Its contents originally stemmed from lectures presented to participants in the 2-week practical course sponsored by the Department of Continuing Education at the Harvard Medical School and the Massachusetts General Hospital (Emergency Care: An Extended Workshop). This course is now in its 14th year, and the present course director, Dr. Peter L. Gross, has been added as associate editor of this second edition.

Textbook preparation has been an immense task. An attempt has been made to avoid an encyclopedic treatise and to maintain a physically manageable size, while providing an in-depth approach to specific patient problems. The purpose has been to include material covering all aspects of medical care in the emergency department, to help bridge the sometimes difficult transition from emergency department to hospital specialty care, and to provide insights into subsequent diagnosis and therapy that may be affected by decisions made in the first moments of care. A criticism of the first edition was that it was largely written by traditional specialists and not by emergency physicians. Although this is still the case, every effort has been made in the second edition to heed specific suggestions of earlier critics.

The basic format of five sections has been maintained. In section 1, Life Support, a chapter on the treatment of the patient with multisystem trauma has been added, and in section 2, Medicine, chapters have been added on environmental hazards (including hyperthermia, radiation, barotrauma, and bites and stings) and on states of altered consciousness. In addition, Chapter 14, (new Chapter 17) Toxicologic Emergencies, has been reorganized. In section 4, Administration, the two chapters on the Massachusetts General Hospital Emergency Ward have been deleted; teaching hospitals that found this information useful can still refer to the first edition. Chapter 36, Emergency Medical Services Systems, is new, and describes the development and management of the excellent prehospital system of patient care in the city of Boston; this chapter was written by two authorities from the Boston City Hospital, which is the resource hospital for Medic IV, the regional emergency medical services system project. Finally, section 5, Illustrated Techniques, has been expanded, with the continued excellence of principal artist Mrs. Edith Tagrin.

The editors wish to express special gratitude to Ms. Catherine P. Fitzgerald, Editorial Associate, and to Mrs. Jane S. McDermott, who has skillfully handled the entire task—familiar to all editors—of coaxing authors, correlating material, and meeting deadlines.

EARLE W. WILKINS, JR., M.D.

Preface to First Edition

In many large urban centers, the emergency ward has become the focus of a number of medical activities. An emergency ward (1) may function as a 24-hour diagnostic and treatment facility for urgent medical problems, (2) may provide access to hospital admission for acutely and chronically ill patients, (3) may train residents, emergency physicians, and emergency medical technicians, (4) may initiate and participate in municipal emergency medical service systems, and (5) may take the lead in planning hospital response to disasters in the community.

The changing role of the emergency ward has resulted from many unrelated phenomena. Medical education since World War II, with its emphasis on specialization, has led to the disappearance of the general practitioner from the inner city; patients now expect sophisticated treatment in the hospital rather than at home. The postwar population explosion and migration to the city have made a large impact on the metropolitan hospital emergency facility. A dramatic rise in the accident rate has resulted from high-speed driving and the burgeoning use of alcohol and drugs. Increasing longevity has resulted in a new emphasis on emergency problems of the elderly. The effect of these developments is reflected in the census of users of the emergency ward of the Massachusetts General Hospital in the last 25 years, from 15,000 in 1951 to almost 100,000 (including those seen in the walk-in clinic) in 1976.

Until this decade, the response of urban hospitals to the growth in numbers and types of patients had been unplanned and inadequate. Several factors are probably responsible for this. No single method of planning, directing, staffing, or operating an emergency facility had become obviously superior, and therefore, time was required to develop patterns of care and to train innovative medical leadership. In addition, the specific role of the emergency ward was unclear, with the often conflicting purposes of treating the walk-in or "convenience" patient, managing the critically ill or injured patient, and serving as an admissions unit at times of high hospital census. Hospital administrators concerned about financial responsibility and confronted with escalating deficits

from emergency facilities often deliberately delayed improvements to avoid attracting greater numbers of patients. Finally, it has taken an unexpectedly long time for the speciality of emergency medicine to develop and to gain acceptance.

Emergency medicine has, however, now become a recognized career. Training programs are available for both the graduating physician and those already in practice. Medical schools, responding to the stimulus of the University Association for Emergency Medicine, are offering courses in emergency medicine for undergraduates, and some hospitals and medical schools offer residency programs in emergency medicine. The American College of Emergency Physicians is the principal sponsor of a program of continuing education. A board of emergency medicine has not yet been approved. The development of emergency medical services systems nationwide has been led and funded by the Division of Emergency Medical Services of the Department of Health, Education, and Welfare (now DHH).

Despite this improvement, however, a formidable challenge remains. Community hospitals and metropolitan general hospitals must, both individually and collectively, respond to the needs of consumers of medical care by providing a decent physical plant, a carefully trained staff, and a system for rendering care to patients with a wide range of problems. Access to appropriate care must be facilitated so that treatment of trauma or acute illness can begin earlier.

This text is designed to respond to the challenge by providing assistance in the training and continuing education of emergency physicians. It is a survey of methods developed and put into use at a large private metropolitan hospital, the Massachusetts General Hospital. The authors are primarily practitioners in the general hospital who also provide care and teaching in the emergency setting.

The book is divided into five sections. The first section entitled "Life Support" is intended to assemble the physiologic and therapeutic considerations that could apply to resuscitative efforts in the following chapters. The second and third sections treat medical and surgical topics, respectively. The fourth section is devoted to the administrative aspects of an emergency facility. The final section illustrates some of the more common techniques performed in the emergency ward. Selected reading lists at the conclusion of chapters are intended to complement the discussions and are not exhaustive surveys of the literature.

Most of the art work has been the effort of Ms. Edith S. Tagrin, head of the Medical Art Department of the Massachusetts General Hospital. Illustrations for Chapters 18, 19, and 28 were done by Mr. Sidney Rosenthal of Arrco Medical Art and Design, Inc.; Ms. Hedwig Murphy furnished some of the illustrations for Chapter 30. Most of the photographic work was done by the Photography Laboratory of the Massachusetts General Hospital under the direction of Mr. Stanley Bennett.

The editors wish to express their gratitude to all who have spent the long hours and sometimes frustrating moments necessary in coordinating this textbook. Ms. Catherine P. Fitzgerald has been patient, persuasive, and highly competent as chief technical editor and general orchestrator of the entire manuscript, with the able assistance of Ms. Susanna Adams. Mrs. Jane McDermott was instrumental in the organization of the book at the conceptual stage and was extremely helpful in accumulating manuscript. To these three women in particular, I would like to give sincere and everlasting thanks that words are inadequate to express.

EARLE W. WILKINS, JR., M.D.

Contributors

William H. Anderson, M.D.
Chairman, Department of Psychiatry, St. Elizabeth's Hospital; Associate Psychiatrist, Massachusetts General Hospital; Assistant Clinical Professor of Psychiatry, Harvard Medical School

Christos A. Athanasoulis, M.D.
Chief, Section of Vascular Radiology, Massachusetts General Hospital; Professor of Radiology, Harvard Medical School and Massachusetts General Hospital

Ann S. Baker, M.D.
Assistant Physician, Massachusetts General Hospital; Epidemiologist, Consultant in Infectious Diseases, Associate Director of Bacteriology, Massachusetts Eye and Ear Infirmary; Assistant Professor of Medicine, Harvard Medical School

Edward P. Baker, Jr., M.D.
Assistant Visiting Neurosurgeon, Massachusetts General Hospital; Assistant in Surgery, Harvard Medical School

Joseph S. Barr, Jr., M.D.
Chief Amputation Clinic, and Associate Orthopaedic Surgeon, Massachusetts General Hospital; Assistant Clinical Professor of Orthopaedic Surgery, Harvard Medical School

Robert J. Bates, M.D.
Urologist, Holland Community Hospital and Zeeland Community Hospital Holland, Michigan; formerly Assistant in Urology, Massachusetts General Hospital

Barbara R. Bennett, R.N., B.S.N.
Paramedic Nurse Educator, Boston City Hospital

Ronald Benz, M.D.
Director, Pediatric Ambulatory Service, and Associate Pediatrician, Massachusetts General Hospital; Instructor in Pediatrics, Harvard Medical School

Peter C. Block, M.D.
Director, Cardiac Catheterization Laboratory, and Associate Physician, Massachusetts General Hospital; Assistant Professor of Medicine, Harvard Medical School

Andrew G. Bodnar, M.D.
Assistant in Medicine, Massachusetts General Hospital; Instructor of Medicine, Harvard Medical School

Robert D. Brandstetter, M.D.
Clinical and Research Fellow in Medicine, Massachusetts General Hospital; Research Fellow in Medicine, Harvard Medical School

Burton A. Briggs, M.D.
Director, Surgical Intensive Care Unit; Assistant Professor of Pediatrics and Associate Professor of Anesthesiology, Loma Linda University, Loma Linda, California; formerly Assistant in Anesthesia, Massachusetts General Hospital

Frank P. Castronovo, Ph.D.
Radiation Safety Officer, and Radiopharmacologist, Department of Radiology, Massachusetts General Hospital; Assistant Professor in Radiology, Harvard Medical School

David S. Chapin, M.D.
Assistant Gynecologist, Massachusetts General Hospital; Obstetrician-Gynecologist, Brigham & Women's Hospital, Clinical Instructor in Obstetrics and Gynecology, Harvard Medical School

Cecil H. Coggins, M.D.
Clinical Director, Renal Unit, and Associate Physician, Massachusetts General Hospital; Associate Professor of Medicine, Harvard Medical School

Carla B. Cohen, M.D.
Assistant Pediatrician, Massachusetts General Hospital; Instructor in Pediatrics, Harvard Medical School

Rita Colley, R.N.
Formerly Nurse Clinician, Hyperalimentation Unit, Massachusetts General Hospital

David J. Cullen, M.D.
Anesthetist, Massachusetts General Hospital; Associate Professor of Anaesthesia, Harvard Medical School

Gilbert H. Daniels, M.D.
Assistant Physician, Massachusetts General Hospital; Assistant Professor of Medicine, Harvard Medical School

Roman W. DeSanctis, M.D.
Director, Coronary Care Unit, and Physician, Massachusetts General Hospital; Professor of Medicine, Harvard Medical School

James J. Dineen, M.D.
Associate Physician, Massachusetts General Hospital; Assistant Professor of Medicine, Harvard Medical School

R. Bruce Donoff, D.M.D., M.D.
Acting Chief, Department of Oral and Maxillofacial Surgery, and Visiting Oral and Maxillofacial Surgeon, Massachusetts General Hospital; Acting Chairman, Department of Oral and Maxillofacial Surgery, Harvard School of Dental Medicine, and Assistant Professor of Oral and Maxillofacial Surgery, Harvard School of Dental Medicine

Stephen P. Dretler, M.D.
Assistant Urologist, Massachusetts General Hospital; Assistant Professor in Surgery/Urology; Harvard Medical School

Leonard Ellman, M.D.
Associate Physician, Massachusetts General Hospital; Associate Professor of Medicine, Harvard Medical School

A. John Erdmann, III M.D. (Deceased)
Formerly Assistant Surgeon, Massachusetts General Hospital; Assistant Professor of Surgery, Harvard Medical School

Ruth M. Farrisey, R.N., B.Sc., M.P.H.
Associate Director, Department of Nursing, Massachusetts General Hospital

Josef E. Fischer, M.D.
Surgeon-in-Chief, University of Cincinnati Hospital; Christian R. Holmes Professor, Chairman, Department of Surgery, University of Cincinnati Medical Center, Cincinnati, Ohio; formerly Associate Visiting Surgeon, Massachusetts General Hospital and Associate Professor of Surgery, Harvard Medical School

Thomas B. Fitzpatrick, M.D.
Chief, Dermatology Service, Massachusetts General Hospital Edward Wigglesworth Professor of Dermatology, Harvard Medical School

Susan Schmiedel Fox, R.N.
Formerly Triage Nurse, Emergency Ward, Massachusetts General Hospital

Albert R. Frederick, Jr., M.D.
Associate Surgeon in Ophthalmology, Massachusetts Eye and Ear Infirmary, Clinical Instructor in Ophthalmology, Harvard Medical School; Associate Visiting Surgeon of Ophthalmology, Boston University Medical Center

Herbert Freund, M.D.
Senior Lecturer in Surgery, Hadassah Hebrew University, Jerusalem, Israel; formerly Clinical and Research Fellow in Surgery, Massachusetts General Hospital and Research Fellow in Surgery, Harvard Medical School

Peter L. Gross, M.D.
Associate Chief, Emergency Services, and Assistant Physician, Massachusetts General Hospital; Instructor in Medicine, Harvard Medical School

Walter C. Guralnick, D.M.D.
Visiting Oral and Maxillofacial Surgeon, Massachusetts General Hospital; Professor of Oral and Maxillofacial Surgery, Harvard School of Dental Medicine.

Charles A. Hales, M.D.
Associate Director, Pulmonary Unit, and Assistant Physician, Massachusetts General Hospital; Associate Professor of Medicine, Harvard Medical School

Hamilton R. Hayes, M.D.
Director, Emergency Department, Anna Jaques Hospital, Newburyport, Massachusetts; Emergency Department Physician, J.B. Thomas Hospital, Peabody, Massachusetts; formerly Clinical Associate, Massachusetts General Hospital

John M. Head, M.D.
Chief, Surgical Service, Veterans Administration Hospital, White River Junction, Vermont; Professor of Clinical Surgery and Deputy Chairman for Academic Affairs, Department of Surgery, Dartmouth Medical School, Hanover, New Hampshire; formerly Associate Visiting Surgeon, Massachusetts General Hospital and Assistant Clinical Professor of Surgery, Harvard Medical School

John T. Herrin, M.B.B.S.
Chief, Pediatric Nephrology, and Pediatrician, Massachusetts General Hospital; Assistant Pediatrician, Shriners Burns Institute; Assistant Professor of Pediatrics, Harvard Medical School

Eleanor T. Hobbs, M.D.
Staff Emergency Department Physician, Lahey Clinic, Burlington, Massachusetts; formerly Assistant Chief, Emergency Services and Assistant in Medicine, Massachusetts General Hospital and Instructor in Medicine, Harvard Medical School

B. Thomas Hutchinson, M.D.
Surgeon in Ophthalmology, Massachusetts Eye and Ear Infirmary; Assistant Clinical Professor of Ophthalmology, Harvard Medical School

Adolph M. Hutter, Jr., M.D.
Director, Coronary Care Unit, and Associate Physician, Massachusetts General Hospital; Associate Professor of Medicine, Harvard Medical School

Lenworth M. Jacobs, M.D., M.P.H.
Director, Emergency Medical Services, Boston City Hospital; Assistant Professor of Surgery, Boston University Medical Center

Richard A. Johnson, M.D.
Clinical Associate in Dermatology, Massachusetts General Hospital; Clinical Instructor in Dermatology, Harvard Medical School

Robert Arnold Johnson, M.D.
Assistant Physician, Massachusetts General Hospital; Assistant Professor of Medicine, Harvard Medical School

Dorothy H. Kelly, M.D.
Assistant Pediatrician, Massachusetts General Hospital; Assistant Professor of Pediatrics, Harvard Medical School

Sean K. Kennedy, M.D.
Assistant Anesthetist, Massachusetts General Hospital; Instructor in Anaesthesia, Harvard Medical School

Samuel H. Kim, M.D.
Associate Visiting Surgeon, Massachusetts General Hospital; Assistant Clinical Professor of Surgery, Harvard Medical School

Daniel C.-S. Lee, M.D.
Clinical Assistant in Medicine, Massachusetts General Hospital; Instructor in Medicine, Harvard Medical School

Michael B. Lewis, M.D.
Assistant in Surgery, Massachusetts General Hospital; Surgeon and Chief, Division of Plastic Surgery, New England Medical Center Hospital; Instructor in Surgery, Harvard Medical School; Associate Professor in Surgery, Tufts University Medical School

Charles J. McCabe, M.D.
Assistant Chief, Emergency Services, and Assistant in Surgery, Massachusetts General Hospital; Instructor in Surgery, Harvard Medical School

M. Terry McEnany, M.D.
Karl Klassen Professor of Thoracic Surgery; Chief, Division of Thoracic and Cardiovascular Surgery, Ohio State University Hospitals; formerly Assistant Surgeon, Massachusetts General Hospital, and Assistant Professor of Surgery, Harvard Medical School

M. B. Maughan, R.N.
Unit Teacher, Emergency Ward/Overnight Ward, Massachusetts General Hospital

Lawrence G. Miller, M.D.
Clinical and Research Fellow in Medicine, Massachusetts General Hospital; Research Fellow in Medicine, Harvard Medical School

Ashby C. Moncure, M.D.
Visiting Surgeon, Massachusetts General Hospital; Assistant Clinical Professor of Surgery, Harvard Medical School

Edward A. Nardell, M.D.
Pulmonary Consultant, Cambridge Hospital, Cambridge, Massachusetts; Instructor in Medicine, Harvard Medical School; formerly Clinical and Research Fellow in Medicine, Massachusetts General Hospital

Nicholas E. O'Connor, M.D.
Surgeon, Brigham and Women's Hospital; Assistant Professor of Surgery, Harvard Medical School; formerly Chief Resident in Plastic Surgery, Massachusetts General Hospital

Leslie W. Ottinger, M.D.
Visiting Surgeon, Massachusetts General Hospital; Associate Professor of Surgery, Harvard Medical School

Rufus C. Partlow, Jr., M.D.
Associate Surgeon, Massachusetts Eye and Ear Infirmary; Clinical Instructor in Otolaryngology, Harvard Medical School

Joseph L. Perrotto, M.D.
Staff Physician, Norwood Hospital, Norwood, Massachusetts and Sturdy Memorial Hospital Attleboro, Massachusetts; formerly Clinical Assistant in Medicine, Massachusetts General Hospital, and Clinical Instructor in Medicine, Harvard Medical School.

Amy A. Pruitt, M.D.
Assistant in Neurology, Massachusetts General Hospital; Instructor of Neurology, Harvard Medical School

James M. Richter, M.D.
Assistant in Medicine, Massachusetts General Hospital; Instructor in Medicine, Harvard Medical School

James T. Roberts, M.D.
Associate Anesthetist, Massachusetts General Hospital; Instructor in Anaesthesia, Harvard Medical School

Carter R. Rowe, M.D.
Senior Orthopaedic Surgeon, Massachusetts General Hospital

Eric J. Sacknoff, M.D.
Active Staff, Mount Auburn Hospital, Cambridge, Massachusetts; Instructor in Urologic Surgery, Harvard Medical School; formerly Assistant in Urology, Massachusetts General Hospital

Howard S. Schwartz, M.D.
Chief, Emergency Medical Services, St. Louis County Hospital, St. Louis, Missouri

Harvey B. Simon, M.D.
Associate Physician, Massachusetts General Hospital; Assistant Professor of Medicine, Harvard Medical School

Richard J. Smith, M.D.
Chief, Hand Surgery Service, Department of Orthopaedic Surgery, Massachusetts General Hospital; Clinical Professor of Orthopaedic Surgery, Harvard Medical School

George E. Thibault, M.D.
Director, Medical Intensive Care Unit/Coronary Care Unit and Medical Practices Evaluation Unit, Assistant Chief, Department of Medicine, and Associate Physician, Massachusetts General Hospital; Assistant Professor of Medicine, Harvard Medical School

Isabella Tighe, M.B.A.
Assistant Director, Bureau of Medical Services, Maine Department of Human Services, Augusta, Maine; formerly Director of Patient Care Representatives, Massachusetts General Hospital

I. David Todres, M.D.
Director, Pediatric Intensive Care Unit, Anesthetist, and Associate Pediatrician, Massachusetts General Hospital; Associate Professor of Anaesthesia (Pediatrics), Harvard Medical School

Katharine K. Treadway, M.D.
Assistant in Medicine, Massachusetts General Hospital; Instructor in Medicine, Harvard Medical School

Virginia Tritschler, R.N., B.S.
Clinical Nursing Leader, Emergency Ward/Overnight Ward, Massachusetts General Hospital

James M. Vaccarino, J.D.
Vice-president of Johnson and Higgins of Massachusetts, Inc.; formerly Staff Counsel, Massachusetts General Hospital

Arthur C. Waltman, M.D.
Associate Radiologist, Massachusetts General Hospital; Associate Professor of Radiology, Harvard Medical School

James G. Wepsic, M.D.
Assisting Visiting Neurosurgeon, Massachusetts General Hospital; Attending Staff, New England Baptist Hospital

Ernest A. Weymuller, Jr., M.D.
Otolaryngologist-in-Chief, Harborview Medical Center; Associate Professor of Otolaryngology, University of Washington, Seattle, Washington; formerly Associate Surgeon, Massachusetts Eye and Ear Infirmary, Assistant Clinical Professor of Otolaryngology, Harvard Medical School

Earle W. Wilkins, Jr., M.D.
Chief, Emergency Services, and Visiting Surgeon, Massachusetts General Hospital; Clinical Professor of Surgery, Harvard Medical School

Gerri A. Wittrock, B.S.N.
Staff Nurse, Cardiac Surgery, Massachusetts General Hospital; formerly Head Nurse/Clinical Leader, Emergency Ward, Massachusetts General Hospital

Edward R. Wolpow, M.D.
Neurologist and Director of Electromyography Laboratory, Mount Auburn Hospital, Cambridge, Massachusetts; Clinical Associate in Neurology, Massachusetts General Hospital; Assistant Clinical Professor of Neurology, Harvard Medical School

Edwin T. Wyman, Jr., M.D.
Chief, Fracture Service, and Associate Orthopaedic Surgeon, Massachusetts General Hospital; Instructor in Orthopaedics, Harvard Medical School

Bertram Zarins, M.D.
Assistant Orthopaedic Surgeon, Massachusetts General Hospital; Clinical Instructor in Orthopaedic Surgery, Harvard Medical School

Demetrios Zukin, M.D.
Assistant in Pediatrics, Massachusetts General Hospital; Instructor in Pediatrics, Harvard Medical School

Contents

SECTION 1:

Life Support

SECTION 2.

Medicine

SECTION 3.

Surgery

SECTION 4:

Administration

SECTION 5:

Illustrated Techniques

Life Support

CHAPTER 1

Pathophysiologic Principles

HAMILTON R. HAYES, M.D.
BURTON A. BRIGGS, M.D.

In simplest terms, an organism survives by maintaining oxygenation, circulation, and the integrity of its cellular milieu. Each of these elements comprises many interrelated anatomic, physical, and physiologic aspects. To consider the principles involved in detail, they will be separated and discussed as indicated in Table 1.1.

AMBIENT ATMOSPHERE

The pathway leading to oxygenation of peripheral tissues begins with the composition of the inspired air. This becomes important in the clinical setting when the oxygen supply is depleted, as in asphyxiation, or when a toxic gas is added, as in carbon monoxide poisoning; the clinician must remember that room air at sea level contains 21% oxygen and a negligible amount of carbon dioxide. The total and partial pressures of gases are presented in Table 1.2.

PATENCY OF AIRWAY

Possession of thorough knowledge of the anatomy of the respiratory tract and of the skills required to establish and to maintain its patency constitutes one of the cornerstones in the practice of emergency medicine. Establishment of an open airway is the first procedure in most resuscitative exercises. Securing and defending the airway is frequently lifesaving in itself—the definitive resuscitative measure. Conversely, failure to establish an airway will doom any additional measures, however heroic, to defeat.

The airway may become obstructed at several anatomic sites (Fig. 1.1). Foreign bodies such as vomitus or dentures, edema due to anaphylaxis or burns, hematomas, mechanical disruption, and loss of tone of the supporting musculature following depression of the central nervous system all can occlude the passage. Obstruction of the nasopharynx in adults is not critical, but blockage at any point from the oropharynx to the tracheal carina is life-threatening. Patency of the oropharynx is a function of the muscular support of the mandible and of the floor of the mouth. In the obtunded patient, the tongue tends to collapse back and to rest against the posterior wall of the

Table 1.1.
Life-support chain.

Element	Common Derangements
Composition of ambient atmosphere	Oxygen depletion, noxious gases
Patency of airway	Obstruction with foreign body, edema, hematoma
Effective bellows action of thorax	Flail chest, pneumothorax
Ventilation-perfusion ratio	Pulmonary edema, pulmonary embolism, shock lung
Oxygen-carrying capacity of blood	Anemia, carbon monoxide poisoning
Blood volume-intravascular compartment relations	Hemorrhage, burns, shock
Effectiveness of heart as pump	Cardiogenic shock, arrhythmia, pericardial tamponade
Microcirculation and maintenance of blood pressure	Septic shock, anaphylaxis
Cellular chemical milieu	Acidosis, hyperosmolality, electrolyte imbalance, toxins

Table 1.2.
Total and partial pressures of gases.[a]

	Dry Air	Moist Tracheal Air (37°C)	Alveolar Gas	Arterial Blood	Mixed Venous Blood
P_{O_2}	159.1[b]	149.2[b]	104[b]	100	40
P_{CO_2}	0.3	0.3	40	40	46
P_{H_2O}	0.0	47.0	47	47	47
P_{N_2}[c]	600.6	563.5	569	573	573
P total	760.0	760.0	760	760	706

[a] Usual values in a resting, healthy man at sea level (barometric pressure = 760 mm Hg).

[b] This is an approximate value for man breathing air at sea level (760 mm Hg). The total atmospheric pressure at Denver or Salt Lake City is about 640 mm Hg, and the partial pressure of oxygen in inspired and alveolar gases is well below values for man at sea level.

[c] Includes small amounts of rare gases.

(Reprinted by permission, from Comroe JH: *Physiology of Respiration: An Introductory Text*, 2nd Ed., Copyright © 1974 by Year Book Medical Publishers, Inc., Chicago.)

hypopharynx, occluding the airway. Blockage also may occur from edema of the epiglottis in patients with epiglottitis.

The larynx, beneath the epiglottis, is maintained rigidly by several articulated cartilages; it contains the narrowest portion of the upper part of the respiratory tract in the adult, that is, the space between the vocal cords. In a child, however, the narrowest point is distal to the larynx at the level of the cricoid cartilage. The cartilaginous structures of the larynx are subject to contusion and fracture. Distal to the larynx, the airway becomes a cylinder supported by a series of posteriorly incomplete cartilaginous rings; this cylinder bifur-

cates into the mainstem bronchi at the level of the sternal angle of Louis. The physical finding most frequently associated with partial obstruction of the larynx and trachea is stridor.

Details of techniques for establishing and maintaining a patent airway are presented in Chapter 2.

MECHANICS OF RESPIRATION

The thoracic cavity is formed by the muscles, ribs, and parietal pleura of the chest; its floor is the diaphragm, its apex is the first two ribs and the musculature of the neck. Divided by the mediastinum into left and right halves, the thoracic cavity is lined by the parietal pleura. This membrane reflects over the surface of the lungs as the visceral pleura, and forms a smooth interface between the lungs and the chest wall. The elastic recoil of the lungs and chest wall creates a slight negative pressure between the pleural surfaces, which becomes evident if a communication to the atmosphere develops—through penetration of the chest wall or rupture of an emphysematous bleb, for example. If this occurs, air rushes in and the lung collapses away from the chest wall.

With the lungs suspended in this closed space, expansion of the chest wall and contraction of the diaphragm increase the negative pressure. Air is drawn in through the trachea, and the lungs fill. Exhalation can be passive or active—passive by elastic recoil of the thoracic cage and lungs, active by contraction of the abdominal muscles leading to forced elevation of the diaphragm. Trauma to the chest wall that divides individual ribs at two points or causes some combination of two-point rib/sternal disruption produces a flail segment that moves paradoxically with respiration, impairing its efficiency.

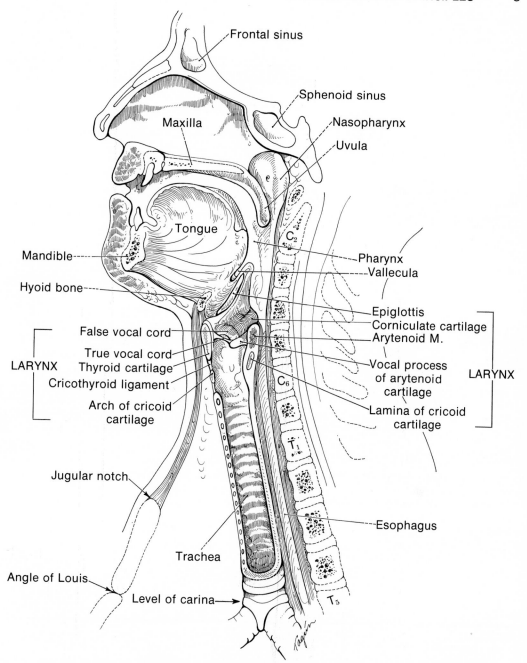

Figure 1.1. Anatomic relations of upper airway.

The active phases of the respiratory cycle require muscular work with expenditure of energy, consumption of oxygen, and tendency to fatigue. In many situations, the work of respiration is increased: exhaling against narrowed airways in asthma or emphysema; breathing with rapid, shallow respirations in severe pneumonia or pulmonary edema; moving noncompliant lungs; or breathing against an elevated diaphragm in the presence of obesity, ileus, pregnancy, or retroperitoneal hematoma. The onset of fatigue and the possibility of respiratory failure may be detected clinically by serial measurements of the vital capacity and of the maximal inspiratory force that the patient can generate. A vital capacity of less than 20 ml/kg of body weight indicates marginal respiratory reserve.

Respiratory efforts are controlled by a center in

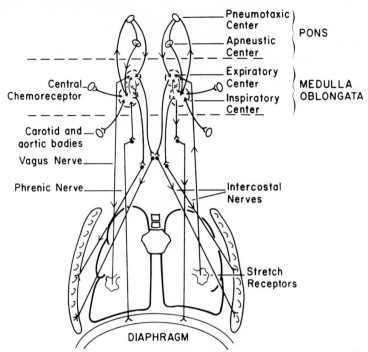

Figure 1.2.   Neural regulation of breathing. (Reproduced by permission, from Thal AP, Wilson RF: Shock. *In* Ravitch MM (Ed), Current Problems in Surgery, September 1965. Copyright © 1965 by Year Book Medical Publishers, Inc., Chicago.)

the medulla oblongata that is stimulated by chemoreceptors in the carotid body, aortic arch, and the medulla itself (Fig. 1.2). In the carotid body and the aortic arch, chemoreceptors are sensitive to changes in partial pressures of oxygen (Po_2) and, to a lesser extent, carbon dioxide (Pco_2). The medullary chemoreceptors are exquisitely sensitive to alterations in pH, which is usually a function of Pco_2. Normally, the hypercapnic stimulus is more significant than the hypoxic drive. However, the hypercapnic drive commonly becomes blunted in the presence of chronic carbon dioxide retention, and breathing in these patients is primarily based on the hypoxic impetus.

The efferent impulses from the respiratory center travel via somatic nerves to the thoracic muscles and through the third to fifth cervical roots via the phrenic nerve to the diaphragm. Consequently, some respiratory activity can be maintained even if the spinal cord is transected at or below the sixth cervical vertebra; its efficacy will depend on the compliance of the lung, the chest wall, and the abdominal cavity. The efferent pathway to the muscles of respiration can be interrupted at many points: in the medulla by drug or hypoxic suppression of the respiratory center, at the level of the cervical portion of the spine or lower motor

Table 1.3.
Causes of acute respiratory failure.

Cause	Clinical Examples
Neurological	
Brainstem respiratory center depression	Anoxia, stroke, drug overdose (narcotics, barbiturates), trauma
Motorneuron, neuromuscular function, anterior horn cells of spine	Trauma, demyelinating diseases, myasthenia gravis, curare, Guillain-Barré, inorganic phosphate poisoning
Respiratory	
Muscle weakness	Muscular dystrophy
Loss of chest wall integrity	Trauma
Airway obstruction Central	Foreign body, tumor, epiglottitis, tracheal stricture
Lower	COPD, asthma
Parenchymal disease, with shunting	CHF, pneumonia, adult respiratory disease syndrome

neuron by trauma, in the anterior horn of the spinal cord by poliomyelitis, or at the neuromuscular junction by curare or inorganic phosphate blockade.

The causes of acute respiratory failure are listed

Table 1.4.
Clinical factors influencing decision to intubate.

Favoring Conservative Management	Inclining Toward Prompt Intubation
Patient's overall condition good, not fatigued, muscle power intact, able to cooperate	Patient fatigued, uncooperative
Cough reflex intact, capable of clearing secretions	Cough reflex inadequate to clear secretions
CO_2 retention: none to slight	Severe or increasing hypercapnia
Acidosis: not present to mild	Acidosis disproportionate to degree of CO_2 retention
Respiratory efforts coordinated	Respiratory efforts becoming disorganized

Table 1.5.
Guidelines for ventilatory support in adults with acute respiratory failure.[a]

Datum	Normal Range	Tracheal Intubation and Ventilation Indicated
Mechanics		
Respiration rate (breaths/min)	12–20	>35
Vital capacity (ml/kg of body weight[b])	65–75	<15
FEV_i (ml/kg of body weight[b])	50–60	<10
Inspiratory force (cm H_2O)	75–100	<25
Oxygenation		
Pao_2 (mm Hg)	100–75 (air)	<70 (on mask oxygen)
$P(A\text{-}aDo_2)^{1.0}$ (mm Hg[c])	25–65	>450
Ventilation		
$Paco_2$ (mm Hg)	35–45	>55[d]
V_D/V_T	0.25–0.40	>0.60

FEV_1 = first sec vital capacity; Pao_2 = arterial partial pressure of oxygen; $P(A\text{-}aDo_2)^{1.0}$ = alveolar-arterial oxygen tension difference during ventilation with 100% oxygen; $Paco_2$ = arterial partial pressure of carbon dioxide; V_D/V_T = ratio of dead space to tidal volume.

[a] The trend of values is of utmost importance. The numerical guidelines should obviously not be adopted to the exclusion of clinical judgment. For example, a vital capacity less than 15 ml/kg may prove sufficient provided the patient can still cough "effectively," if hypoxemia is prevented, and if hypercapnia is not progressive. However, such a patient needs frequent blood-gas analyses, and must be closely observed in a well-equipped, adequately staffed recovery room or intensive care unit.

[b] "Ideal" weight is used if weight appears grossly abnormal.

[c] After 10 min of 100% oxygen.

[d] Except in patients with chronic hypercapnia.

(Modified by permission, from *N Engl J Med* 287: 749, 1972.)

in Table 1.3, and the criteria for its diagnosis and for the decision to intervene are presented in Table 1.4 and 1.5. Depending on the derangement, the type of intervention may be a surgical procedure (such as chest tube insertion), establishment of a secure airway by intubation, administration of oxygen, or mechanical assistance with ventilation. These measures must be coordinated with therapy of the underlying condition whenever possible.

The important concept is as follows: the thorax acts as an elaborate mechanical bellows that ventilates the alveoli, bringing in fresh air and washing out waste products. The common result of failure of the bellows action is carbon dioxide retention. Thus, the arterial partial pressure of carbon dioxide ($Paco_2$) is the indicator of effective alveolar ventilation.

VENTILATION-PERFUSION RATIO

For a given CO_2 production alveolar ventilation determines $Paco_2$. In contrast, the arterial partial pressure of oxygen (Pao_2) is a function of FIO_2 (the fraction of oxygen in inspired air—see below under oxygen transport) and the relation of ventilation to the pulmonary capillary blood flow, that is, the ventilation-perfusion ratio ($\dot{V}/\dot{Q}$). This concept is of paramount importance in understanding the mechanisms underlying hypoxic states. Most types of hypoxia are now thought to be explainable in terms of a disturbance of $\dot{V}/\dot{Q}$ (called shunting), and older concepts such as alveolar capillary diffusion blocks have largely been supplanted.

In an ideal lung, each alveolus would be equally

ventilated and each perialveolar capillary net would receive an equal share of cardiac output from the right ventricle. In this situation, the $\mathring{V}/\mathring{Q}$ would be unity and no difference would exist between partial pressures of arterial and alveolar oxygen ($Pao_2 = PAo_2$). However, this ideal state never exists, even in the healthy person at rest. Normally, there is an oxygen step-down of 9–10 mm Hg from the alveolar space to the artery. This difference (A-aDo$_2$) is attributed to two factors: the anatomic shunt and the effect of gravity on the distribution of blood flow and ventilation (Fig. 1.3). The anatomic shunt is produced by blood flowing through the bronchial, pleural, and thebesian veins. This bypass represents only 1–5% of the cardiac output, but it is a true right-to-left shunt, and slightly reduces the Pao$_2$. More importantly, gravity alters both perfusion and ventilation. The effect is that basal (dependent) zones are hyperperfused and apical (nondependent) segments are somewhat hypoperfused relative to ventilation in each part. Consequently, some blood traverses the dependent zones without being fully oxygenated, while some ventilation of the nondependent zones is wasted.

In many diseases, this shunting is increased. Ventilation or perfusion or both may become strikingly deranged, producing a much greater A-aDo$_2$ (Fig. 1.4). Some conditions increase shunting by exaggerating the normal gravitational effect. In hypovolemia, for example, the apical segments receive an even smaller proportion of right ventricular output. Other processes block ventilation of alveoli without impairing perfusion. Pulmonary edema, pneumonia, atelactasis, and airway obstruction by mucous plugs are typical examples of such wasted perfusion. Alternatively, some states may be characterized by wasted ventilation. This may follow interruption of blood flow to some alveoli because of pulmonary microemboli or destruction of the normal architecture and increase in the dead space to be ventilated because of emphysema.

Discovery of a depressed Pao$_2$ should alert the emergency physician to the existence of a $\mathring{V}/\mathring{Q}$ disturbance. He must treat the hypoxia, but must

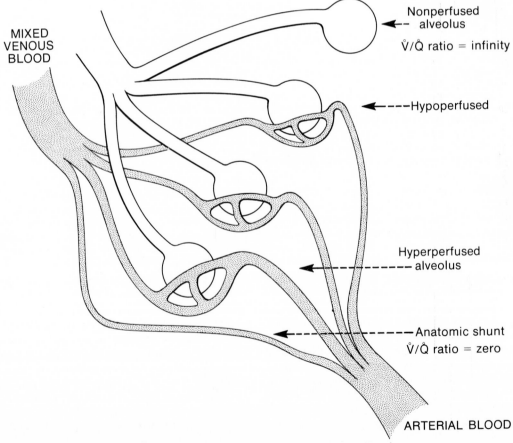

Figure 1.3.   Variation in ventilation-perfusion ratios.

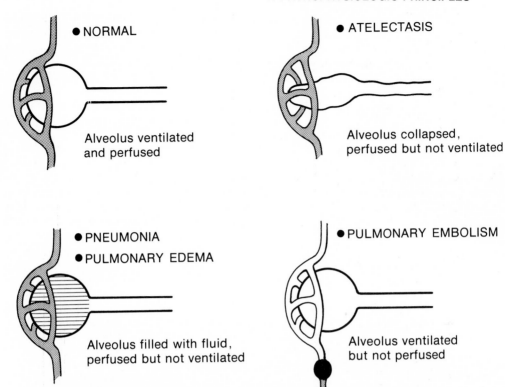

Figure 1.4.   Pathologic causes of increased ventilation-perfusion imbalance.

understand that it is only symptomatic. The primary concern should be to understand the nature of the shunt and to correct its cause.

TRANSPORT OF GASES BY BLOOD

The next major phase in the life-support sequence concerns the transport of oxygen and carbon dioxide by the blood. Ready availability of accurate measurements of these gases in the arterial blood has provided valuable clinical insights, but interpretation requires knowledge of the peculiarities of their carriage in this medium.

Oxygen Transport

Oxygen is transported in the blood in two ways: a minor percentage is physically dissolved in the plasma and in the aqueous component of the red blood cell, and a much greater amount is chemically associated with hemoglobin. Only 0.3 vol% of oxygen can be dissolved in the plasma of a patient breathing room air (F_{IO_2}, 0.21) at sea level. (F_I designates the fractional concentration of an inspired gas; thus, an oxygen concentration of 21% is expressed as 0.21.) Increasing the F_{IO_2} to 1.0 (100% oxygen) only increases the dissolved fraction to 2.0 vol%, which may be important in a marginal state, but is inadequate to sustain life. In

contrast, 20.4 vol% is carried in combination with hemoglobin while breathing room air.

The amount of oxygen combined with hemoglobin is the result of several factors, the principal determinant being the Pa_{O_2}. Oxygen is freely diffusible across the red cell membrane, and the dissolved oxygen is in equilibrium with the oxygen associated with hemoglobin. Therefore, the quantity of hemoglobin-bound oxygen is proportional to the Pa_{O_2}. In practice, the clinician utilizes the Pa_{O_2} values, and the objective of oxygen therapy is to saturate the hemoglobin molecule.

"Saturation" of hemoglobin is spoken of because hemoglobin is a complex protein molecule containing four iron atoms, each of which is a potential binding site for oxygen; one hemoglobin molecule can combine with one to four oxygen molecules. These combining sites interact with oxygen in a characteristic fashion, influencing one another in such a way that the binding of a molecule of oxygen to one site increases the affinity of the remaining sites for additional oxygen molecules.

This facilitative process accounts for the sigmoid shape of the oxygen-hemoglobin dissociation curve (Fig. 1.5). The flat upper range of the curve assures a constant high level of hemoglobin saturation over a wide variation (75–95 mm Hg) of

OXYGEN−HEMOGLOBIN
DISSOCIATION CURVE

BOHR EFFECT ON OXYGEN−HEMOGLOBIN
DISSOCIATION CURVE

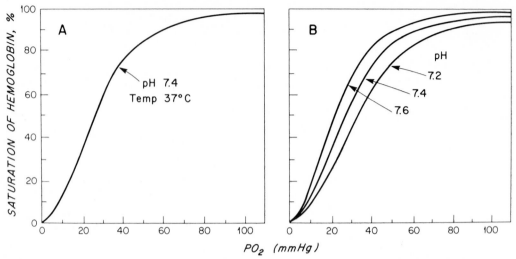

Figure 1.5.   Oxygen-hemoglobin dissociation curves. **(A)** Normal curve. **(B)** Bohr effect.

Pa_{O_2}. However, as the Pa_{O_2} decreases toward values in the venous range, the slope of the curve becomes steeper. In the nearly vertical segment between 60 and 15 mm Hg, a relatively minor decrease in Pa_{O_2} results in a precipitous unloading of oxygen. This is the situation present in the peripheral tissues where it is desirable for hemoglobin to surrender oxygen readily to the cells. In reverse, the contour of the curve permits rapid uptake of oxygen in the rising Pa_{O_2} gradient encountered in the pulmonary capillaries.

The physician must be aware of the implications of the oxygen-hemoglobin dissociation curve, and the clinical objective must be to maintain the Pa_{O_2} of the patient above the upper limit of the steep portion of the curve to prevent cellular hypoxia. A clinically valid objective is maintenance of the Pa_{O_2} above 60 mm Hg.

The oxygen-hemoglobin bond is unusual. Rather than being a full chemical combination (oxidation), it is a loose, reversible association (oxygenation), and it is subject to numerous influences. In addition to Pa_{O_2}, these include pH, temperature, and concentration of 2,3-diphosphoglycerate (2,3-DPG) in the red blood cells.

The lower pH ranges in acidotic environments facilitate release of oxygen from the hemoglobin molecule. Increasing the temperature does the same. Thus, in the relatively hot, acidic milieu of exercising muscle, for example, hemoglobin releases oxygen more readily. Conversely, alkalotic pH values increase the affinity of hemoglobin for oxygen. In the clinical setting, this could become important if an alkalinizing agent such as sodium bicarbonate were administered in excess. Rendering the patient's serum alkalotic would hinder the release of oxygen from hemoglobin and could exacerbate cellular hypoxia. The effect of pH on the oxygen-hemoglobin dissociation curve is known as the Bohr effect (Fig. 1.5B). Acidosis shifts the curve to the right, while alkalosis shifts it to the left.

The organic phosphate 2,3-DPG normally is present within red blood cells, where it competes with oxygen for the binding sites on hemoglobin. Decreased 2,3-DPG levels mean that the hemoglobin has an increased affinity for oxygen and releases it less readily—an effect similar to that of alkalosis. The levels of 2,3-DPG tend to decrease in banked blood, particularly that stored in ACD preservative. The clinician must bear in mind that banked blood more than 5–7 days old may have decreased 2,3-DPG levels, and, consequently, may be a less effective oxygen donor, gram for gram of hemoglobin, than is fresh blood.

Carbon Dioxide Transport

Carriage of carbon dioxide in the blood is in many ways the mirror image of oxygen transport (Fig. 1.6). Carbon dioxide is produced in the tissues as a metabolic byproduct at the fairly constant rate of approximately 200 ml/min (a function of body mass and temperature). Like oxygen, it is carried in the blood both dissolved in plasma and

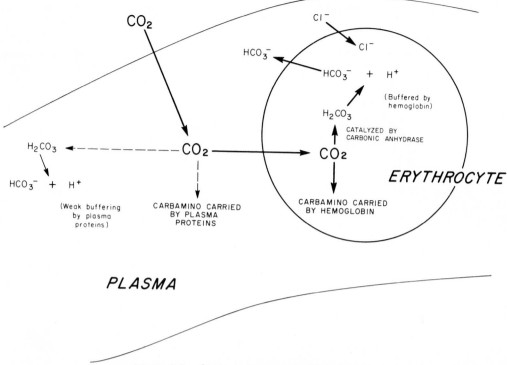

Figure 1.6. Carriage of carbon dioxide in blood.

combined with hemoglobin. The dissolved fraction is larger, since carbon dioxide is 21 times more soluble in water than is oxygen. Unlike oxygen, 60% of the carbon dioxide is carried in another form, bicarbonate.

Only 25–30% of the carbon dioxide is associated with hemoglobin (as carboxyhemoglobin), contrasted with 90% of the oxygen. The hemoglobin binding site for carbon dioxide is not the iron molecule but the amino group, where it is reversibly held in a manner analogous to the binding of oxygen.

The largest amount of transported carbon dioxide is hydrated to form carbonic acid in a reaction within the red blood cell catalyzed by carbonic anhydrase. Carbonic acid in turn yields bicarbonate and hydrogen ions, the former diffusing into the plasma, the latter remaining within the red blood cell where they are buffered by hemoglobin. In the pulmonary capillaries, the process is reversed; carbon dioxide is regenerated and diffused into the alveoli, whence it is exhaled. The rate of carbon dioxide production is influenced by temperature and stress; for most clinical purposes, it is considered constant. As stated previously, the principal determinant of the Pa_{CO_2} is alveolar ventilation.

Mass of Red Blood Cells

Because hemoglobin occupies a central role in the transport of gases, its quantitative aspects are important. When the mass of red blood cells is abnormally small, as in patients with profound anemia, hypoxia may develop despite oxygen supplementation. If significant amounts of hemoglobin are lost, the body must compensate. In an acute condition such as hemorrhage, the response is to increase cardiac output. In the chronic situation, red blood cell production also increases. The physician's task is to estimate the deficit of hemoglobin, to assure saturation of the hemoglobin present, and if necessary, to transfuse blood to a level permitting carriage of adequate amounts of oxygen to the periphery.

Oxygen Therapy and Arterial Blood-Gas Determinations

The ability to increase the percentage of oxygen in the inspired air—the FI_{O_2}—is one of the mainstays of therapeutics. With the wide variety of devices and techniques available, the physician can administer oxygen in concentrations from 21–100%, and there are situations in which administration of 100% oxygen is appropriate. However,

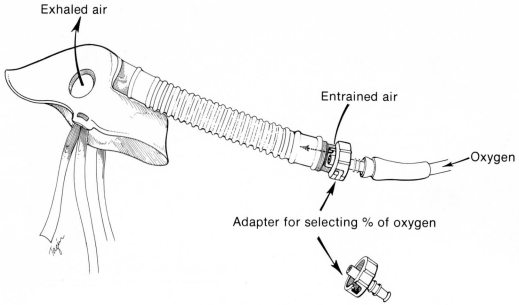

Exhaled air

Entrained air

Oxygen

Adapter for selecting % of oxygen

Figure 1.7.   Venturi mask.

oxygen supplementation is a two-edged sword. Its uncritical use is poor practice, and in some commonly encountered situations, it can be lethal. The classic example of this danger is the unmonitored administration of oxygen to the patient with chronic hypercapnia who is breathing by means of hypoxic drive.

The point to be emphasized regarding oxygen therapy is that oxygen should be regarded as a drug. Like any drug, it should be administered in graded doses tailored to the clinical situation. After a dose has been given, time should be allowed for equilibration to occur, the effects of the dose should be evaluated, and the F_{IO_2} should be modified if necessary.

Two tools available to the emergency physician facilitate this approach to oxygen therapy. These are the venturi mask (Fig. 1.7) and arterial blood-gas determinations. Venturi masks are oxygen-administration face masks designed to employ the venturi principle. In this application, one gas (oxygen) flows at a given rate through a nozzle system specially designed to entrain a known amount of a second gas (air). The masks are available with aperture sizes permitting delivery of a preset percentage of oxygen—typically 24, 28, 35, or 40%. With such a mask, the physician can select with considerable precision the F_{IO_2} appropriate for a particular patient.

For the patient with chronic hypercapnia, the choice of a venturi mask providing 24 or 28% oxygen might permit a slight increase in Pa_{O_2}

Table 1.6.
Relationship of oxygen tension to hemoglobin saturation.

Pa_{O_2}	% Saturation
95	95
70	90
60	85
50	65
30	40

without suppressing the hypoxic drive to breathe. If the patient's initial Pa_{O_2} were between 30 and 40 mm Hg, the oxygen-hemoglobin ratio would be on the steep portion of the dissociation curve. Raising the Pa_{O_2} by only a few millimeters of mercury could significantly enhance hemoglobin saturation. The effect of such therapy must be monitored by obtaining serial arterial blood-gas measurements. With this approach, the clinician should be able to improve oxygen saturation without eliminating the hypoxic drive to ventilate (aiming for a target Pa_{O_2} of 55–60 as a minimum (Table 1.6).

Arterial blood gas determinations usually include measurement of Po_2, pH, Pco_2, and hemoglobin saturation. They permit calculation of base excess or deficit, replace imprecise clinical estimations by providing accurate data about fundamental processes, and represent a major improvement in the data base with which the clinician can work.

The Pa_{O_2} is a function of the F_{IO_2} and $\dot{V}/\dot{Q}$, while the Pa_{CO_2} is principally determined by alveolar ventilation. The pH is a function of a complex interaction between waste-product production and the efficacy of the body's buffering and excretory systems and cannot be estimated clinically with any degree of certainty. However, when measured and considered with the Pa_{O_2} and Pa_{CO_2}, the pH can clarify the patient's current acid-base status, provide insight into the route by which the patient reached that point, and suggest therapeutic options. The arterial blood gas interpretation is considered in more detail later in this chapter.

HEMODYNAMIC FACTORS

Hemodynamic factors include: (1) blood volume-intravascular compartment relations, which determine venous return to the heart; (2) the heart as a pump, which transforms venous return into cardiac output; and (3) the dynamics of the microcirculation, which define peripheral resistance. These elements interact to regulate the arterial blood pressure and tissue perfusion.

Blood Volume—Intravascular Compartment Relations

If the oxyhemoglobin formed in the lungs is to be distributed to the peripheral cells, an effective blood volume must be maintained. The blood volume is effective when the relation between the actual blood volume and the supporting tone of the intravascular compartment results in an adequate filling pressure for the heart. Circulatory collapse with inability to generate acceptable perfusion pressures can occur through loss of intravascular fluid volume, or increase in the size of the vascular space by vasodilation, or failure of the pumping action of the heart.

Neither the blood volume nor the size of the vascular space can be conveniently measured in the clinical setting. However, their relation can be estimated by several techniques, some of which are simple observations on physical examination Jugular venous distension and a positive hepatojugular reflex indicate relative volume overload, and marked postural (orthostatic) hypotension signifies hypovolemia. The usefulness of these clinical observations should not be underestimated, since they frequently yield the same information as do more elaborate and invasive procedures, with less expense, less delay, and fewer complications. In some cases, however, physical findings alone are not adequately informative, and more invasive techniques must be employed.

Central Venous Pressure Determination

Measurement of central venous pressure provides a means for quantitating the fit of the blood volume to the vascular space, and its use has become widespread in recent years. Initially, it was advocated as the definitive technique in many problems of fluid imbalance, but through clinical experience its usefulness and limitations have become clear.

To measure central venous pressure, a hollow catheter is threaded through the venous system until its tip lies in the superior vena cava or in the right atrium (Fig. 1.8). The catheter is then connected to a water manometer, the zero point of which is aligned with the right atrium. Normal values for central venous pressure range up to 12 cm H_2O above the zero reference point. In general, central venous pressure measurement is more helpful for preventing overhydration when values are high and for monitoring a patient's fluid status through serial determinations than for use as an absolute numerical standard.

The procedure for measurement of central venous pressure is straightforward, but it has several potential hazards: sepsis, air embolization, induction of arrhythmias, catheter embolization, hemorrhage from puncture sites, inadvertent arterial puncture, and pneumothorax. Moreover, if correct positioning of the catheter tip is not verified on x-ray film, misleading data can be generated.

The level of the central venous pressure is a function of three variables: the size of the circulating blood volume, the tone of the vasculature, and the effectiveness of the *right* side of the heart (Table 1.7). This last point—that the central venous pressure is a measure only of right-sided cardiac filling pressure—has been realized rather late. Initially, it had been thought that the right and left sides of the heart acted in tandem and that the central venous pressure represented a reliable index of left-sided cardiac competence as well. Only after a large number of patients were transfused into a state of iatrogenic pulmonary edema (despite low central venous pressure values) did the degree of functional dissociation of the two ventricles possible in various disease states become apparent. It has now been proved that a vigorous right ventricular musculature can maintain the central venous pressure in the normal range despite a failing left ventricle. This has prompted development of other means for selectively monitoring left ventricular function, specifically, the pulmonary artery catheter.

Blood volume also influences the central venous

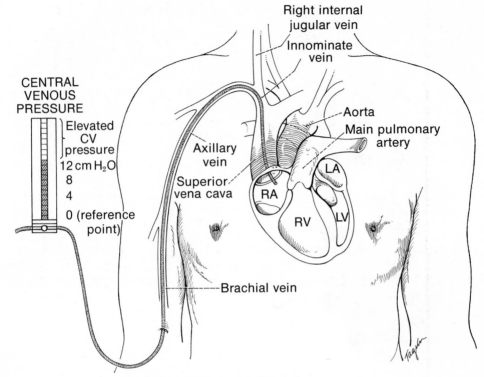

Figure 1.8.   Measurement of central venous pressure.

Table 1.7.
Causes of various central venous pressure readings.

Erroneous reading
  Inaccurate localization of zero point of manometer relative to level of right atrium
  Failure to position catheter tip in central venous circulation (vena cava or right atrium)
  Obstruction of catheter tip by clot
  Coughing, straining, or use of artificial ventilation during measurement
Accurate elevation
  Absolute hypervolemia
  Failure of right side of heart
Accurate depression
  Hypovolemia
  Vigorous pumping of right side of heart
  Loss of tone of venous capacitance vessels

pressure. In the average-sized adult, the intravascular fluid volume approximates 5 liters; it is in equilibrium with a considerably larger reservoir, the interstitial fluid volume, which approximates 10 liters. The forces of the equilibrium are the intravascular hydrostatic pressure, which tends to extrude fluid from the vascular spaces, and the plasma protein oncotic pressure, which tends to retain fluid in the intravascular compartment. Reduction of blood pressure after a blood loss creates a net inward gradient, and a type of autotransfusion of interstitial fluid results. The loss of protein in patients with burns, on the other hand, favors plasma extravasation and further depletion of circulating volume.

The size of the intravascular compartment is the final factor determining the central venous pressure, and it is also subject to wide variation. Alteration in the intravascular volume is largely produced by changes in the venous circulation. The tone of the arterioles creates the *resistance* important in the minute-to-minute regulation of blood pressure. The venules and veins provide a *capacitance* or reservoir function. The venules can contain a greater volume than can the capillary bed; their walls are composed of elastic and muscular tissue that is responsive to many neural, chemical, thermal, and mechanical factors. In its capacitance function, the venous circulation has great adaptive value: it can distend to pool blood and to ameliorate circulatory overload or it can constrict in the presence of hypovolemia.

In patients with left ventricular failure, central venous pressure readings must be interpreted with care. Measurement of central venous pressure is most reliable in the assessment of volume status in patients with normal cardiac function, supplementing the stethoscope, intake-and-output sheet, history, and careful physical examination. It *always* requires thoughtful interpretation.

Cardiac Output

Life depends on uninterrupted perfusion of critical tissues with oxygenated blood. The force behind this flow is the rhythmically contracting heart. The work product of cardiac activity—the volume pumped per minute—is the cardiac output, which must continue without significant interruption for the lifetime of the organism. In addition, the heart must be able to vary its output over a wide range in response to variation in metabolic demands. The average-sized adult at rest has a cardiac output of approximately 5 liters/min. However, in response to exercise, fever, or other stress, this output may have to be increased as much as six-fold. To facilitate comparison between persons of different sizes, another figure, the cardiac index, can be calculated by dividing the cardiac output in liters per minute by the body surface area in square meters (liters/min/m^2). Cardiac output is a complex interaction of two variables, heart rate and stroke volume (Fig. 1.9).

Heart Rate

In the absence of atrioventricular block, the heart rate is determined by the rate of firing of the sinoatrial node, the heart's intrinsic pacemaker. The rate of discharge of the sinoatrial node is in part a function of the decay properties of its membrane potential, but it is subject to significant modification by neural (parasympathetic and sympathetic), hormonal (adrenomedullary and thy-

roid), and physical (temperature) factors. All these modifiers are important physiologically and pathologically, and most also have diagnostic or therapeutic applications or both.

The regulators of heart rate in the autonomic nervous system are the most important modifiers. The resultant rate represents a balance between parasympathetic and sympathetic stimulation of the sinoatrial node. Many of the mechanisms by which the autonomic nervous system controls heart rate are poorly understood. Chemoreceptors in the central nervous system and great vessels monitor the blood gases and pH, and regulate both cardiac output and respiration. In addition, stretch-sensitive baroreceptors in the aortic arch and carotid sinus reflexly tailor the cardiac output to the level of the systemic blood pressure. These baroreceptor reflex arcs slow the heart via the vagal cholinergic fibers in response to hypertension or accelerate it via adrenergic fibers as blood pressure decreases. The vagal arc is frequently employed clinically in carotid sinus massage, and parasympathetic stimulation is blocked when atropine is utilized to treat bradycardia. The sympathetic effect is mimicked when β-adrenergic agents such as isoproterenol are administered to increase heart rate. Endogenous circulating catecholamines also speed the intrinsic pacemaker. At unusually fast or slow rates, cardiac output is largely rate dependent. In adults with heart rates more than 120–140 beats/min, cardiac output decreases because adequate time for diastolic filling is not available. This diminished cardiac output plus the increased cardiac work associated with rapid rates and reduced time in diastole for coronary artery perfusion explains why some persons tolerate tachycardia poorly. Profound bradycardia

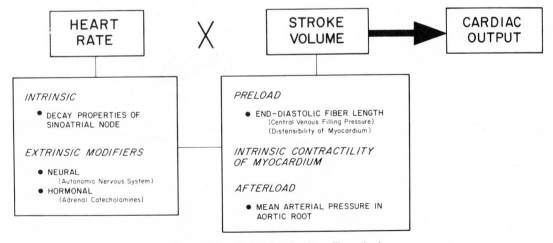

Figure 1.9.   Determinants of cardiac output.

is similarly detrimental and must be treated directly, as with atropine in a patient with an inferior myocardial infarct.

Stroke Volume

The second major determinant of cardiac output is the stroke volume—the amount of blood ejected with each ventricular contraction. While stroke volume is quantitatively less effective than heart rate in varying cardiac output, clinical situations do occur in which the ability to augment stroke volume and to coax a small increase in output can be critical.

The amount of blood the ventricle expels is largely a function of the volume of the ventricle at the end of diastole. This volume determines the length to which the myocardial fibers are stretched, which in turn determines the tension that the muscle will generate during contraction. The presumed explanation is that increased stretch makes more sites on the actin and myosin filaments available for interaction. The force of contraction varies directly with the fiber length over a wide range; stretching beyond the peak range of efficiency in which the normal heart functions, however, results in progressively weaker contraction forces (Fig. 1.10). This relation between the left ventricular end-diastolic fiber length and the tension generated was elaborated by Frank and Starling.

The left ventricular end-diastolic fiber length is determined by the so-called preload of the heart (the pressure in the venae cavae) and by the distensibility of the ventricular walls. The clinician attempts to optimize preload when cautiously administering a trial of volume expansion to the patient with cardiogenic shock. The loss of normal ventricular distensibility (or compliance) that develops on the second or third day after myocardial infarction contributes to impaired cardiac function in this setting.

The intrinsic contractility of the myocardium plays a role in determining the stroke volume as well. Not all of the factors that determine the contractile state are known, but several have been elucidated. The contractile state can be improved by increasing the availability of calcium ions to the contracting proteins and by β-adrenergic stim-

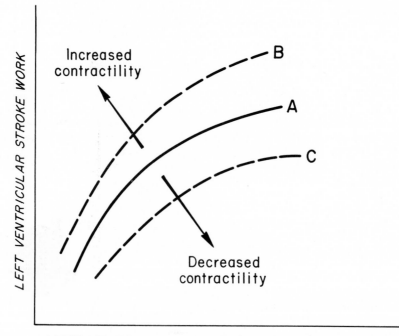

Figure 1.10. Relation of stroke work to end-diastolic fiber length. A family of function curves can be generated for any given left ventricle. Over the greater portion of these curves stroke work varies directly with end-diastolic fiber length. Beyond the optimal range, however, further distention of the chamber decreases the efficiency of the contraction generated. The heart may move to a more effective curve within its family (left shift) under the influence of agents such as digitalis, calcium, and β-adrenergic stimulators. Hypoxia, loss of contractile elements, and depressant drugs shift the heart to a less efficient curve (right shift).

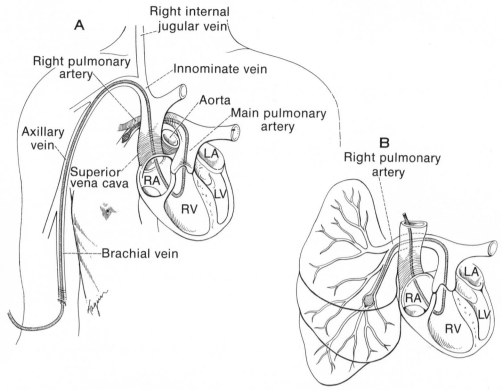

Figure 1.11. Measurement of pulmonary capillary wedge pressure. **(A)** Catheter tip "floating" in right pulmonary artery. **(B)** Catheter tip advanced to "wedge" position; balloon inflated.

ulation—hence the use of calcium and epinephrine during cardiac arrest. Contractility is impaired in ischemia and destroyed through loss of contractile units as in transmural myocardial infarction ("pump failure").

The final determinant of stroke volume is the afterload (the myocardial systolic tension). Afterload is a product of intraventricular pressure, intraventricular volume, and arterial pressure against which blood must be expelled. Although preload and afterload are intimately related, it has become apparent that for any given combination of preload and myocardial contractile state, cardiac function is quite sensitive to changes in afterload.

The intact heart responds to increased afterload with a marked increase in stroke work (to generate higher tension) preventing the ventricular end-diastolic pressure from rising. However, in the damaged heart with impaired inotropic status, increase in afterload results in falling stroke volume and higher end-diastolic ventricular pressures. These concepts have led to the increasing use of vasodilator agents in the treatment of heart failure (see Chapter 7).

Atrioventricular Synchronization

The foregoing has assumed normal intracardiac conduction and an orderly contraction mechanism for the ventricular muscle. However, certain atrioventricular blocks and arrhythmias adversely affect cardiac output. In third-degree (complete) heart block, the atria and the ventricles beat independently. The lack of synchronization means that injection of blood by atrial contraction will fail to optimize the left ventricular end-diastolic volume (preload) and cardiac output will suffer. By eliminating this "atrial kick," atrial fibrillation diminishes output up to 20%. In ventricular fibrillation, the contraction sequence of the ventricular musculature becomes completely disorganized and all effective pumping ceases. The ultimate derangement of cardiac output is, of course, cardiac standstill.

Pulmonary Artery Catheterization

Because it may be critically important to maximize cardiac output in some situations and because the impaired reserve of the diseased heart makes it difficult to improve output without aggravating

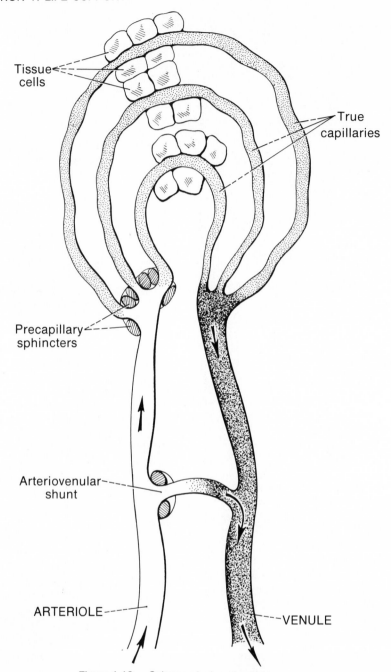

Figure 1.12.   Schema of microcirculation.

failure, the development of better left ventricular monitoring techniques has been desirable. The inaccuracy of central venous pressure as a measurement of left ventricular function was noted previously.

To monitor left ventricular function more accurately, the Swan-Ganz pulmonary artery cathe-

ter has been introduced into clinical practice. This flexible, end-hole, balloon-tipped flotation catheter can be introduced through any vein with central access. It is then floated through the right side of the heart and into one of the branches of the pulmonary arterial tree (Fig. 1.11). To "wedge" the catheter, the balloon is inflated carefully. This

Table 1.8.
Acid-base concepts for the clinician.

Term	Definition
Acid	Any hydrogen ion (H⁺) donor; the more readily the H⁺ is donated (ionized), the stronger the acid.
Base	Any H⁺ acceptor; the more avidly the H⁺ is received, the stronger the base.
pH scale	Scale designed to represent the H⁺ concentration because actual concentrations are unwieldy. True concentrations are minute, and vary widely in different physiologic fluids (for example, gastric secretions vs. pancreatic secretions); the pH varies inversely with the log of the H⁺.
Normal range of pH	7.38–7.42
Acidosis	Condition in which pH values are below 7.38
Alkalosis	Condition in which pH values are above 7.42
Buffer	Compound capable of interacting with added acid or base to dampen change produced in final pH of system

isolates the orifice at the tip of the catheter from the pulmonary arterial pressure. With the balloon inflated, the catheter "sees" the pressure in the pulmonary capillary network; this wedge pressure is thought to be a reasonably accurate reflection of left atrial filling pressure. In the absence of mitral valvular disease, it correlates well with the left ventricular end-diastolic pressure, the preload of the left ventricle. Several important potential complications are associated with use of the pulmonary artery catheter: infection, unrecognized prolonged occlusion of a pulmonary artery with resultant infarction, and ventricular arrhythmia.

Total Peripheral Resistance and Arterial Blood Pressure

Cardiac output is one factor regulating blood pressure; the other one is total peripheral resistance. Because of the importance to the organism of maintaining an effective level of arterial blood pressure and because of the frequency with which its derangements are encountered clinically, this section will examine the factors responsible for peripheral resistance.

As stated earlier, the tone of the venous circulation serves a *capacitance* function, but the peripheral *resistance* is a function of the tone of the precapillary arterioles. These are the terminal divisions of the arterial tree, and contain smooth muscles, receive autonomic innervation, and have both α- and β-cholinergic receptors. The arterioles give rise to two types of vessels: thin-walled true capillaries that are the site of fluid and metabolic exchange and arteriovenular shunts that permit blood to bypass the true capillaries. In both types of vessels, the orifices are guarded by precapillary sphincters (Fig. 1.12).

The capillaries open and close constantly in response to three sets of regulatory influences. These include local factors—the intrinsic rhythmic contraction of the sphincter muscles, hypoxia, acidosis, temperature changes, and locally elaborated vasodilators; neural factors—principally the postganglionic, adrenergic, sympathetic constrictor fibers; and hormonal factors—specifically, adrenomedullary catecholamines, angiotensin, and glucocorticoids.

In the resting state, local regulatory factors predominate. When a major physiologic adaptive change is needed, such as constriction of a vascular bed, neural regulators take effect. The end result of these complex influences is a remarkably dependable and flexible system that can support a minimal level of diastolic pressure sufficient to maintain perfusion of the coronary circulation, shunt blood from a less vital to a more vital vascular bed, and selectively perfuse an organ to match its functional demand. (Cerebral perfusion is a function of mean blood pressure and intracranial pressure.)

The microcirculation becomes a direct concern of the clinician in several situations. During the warm phase of septic shock, for example, it appears that the true capillaries are shut down and the arteriovenular shunts are open. In reflex or high spinal anesthetic shock, the critical derangement is loss of venous tone with increased capacitance, as well as a slight decrease in total peripheral resistance. In cardiogenic shock, considerable reflex and hormonal vasoconstriction may be present, but it may be inadequate to maintain the diastolic pressure at an acceptable level because of the profound reduction in cardiac output.

Many therapeutic agents affecting the microcirculation are available to the clinician, including peripheral vasoconstrictors (α agents), peripheral vasodilators (β agents), dopaminergic stimulators, and corresponding blocking agents. These compounds and the glucocorticoids whose actions on

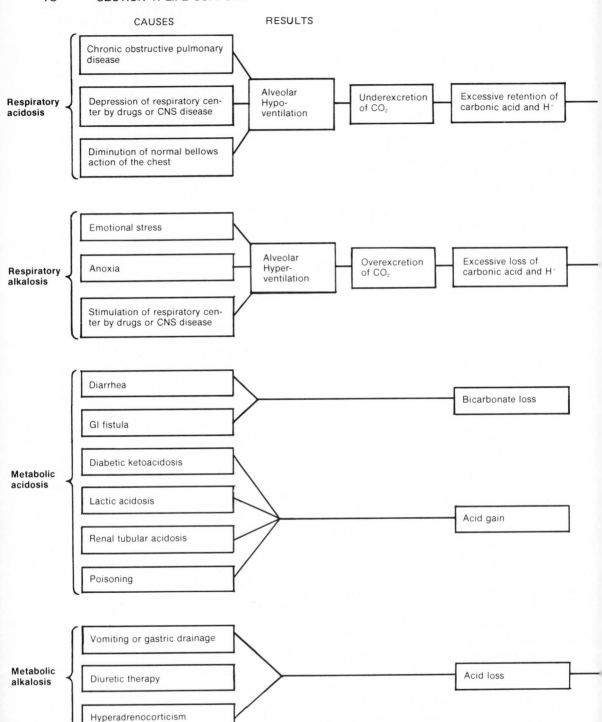

Figure 1.13. Physiologic progression of acid-base problems and compensatory mechanisms. (Used with permission, from *Patient Care*, May 15, 1975. Copyright © 1975, Miller and Fink Corp., Darien, CT. All rights reserved.)

BUFFERING   COMPENSATION

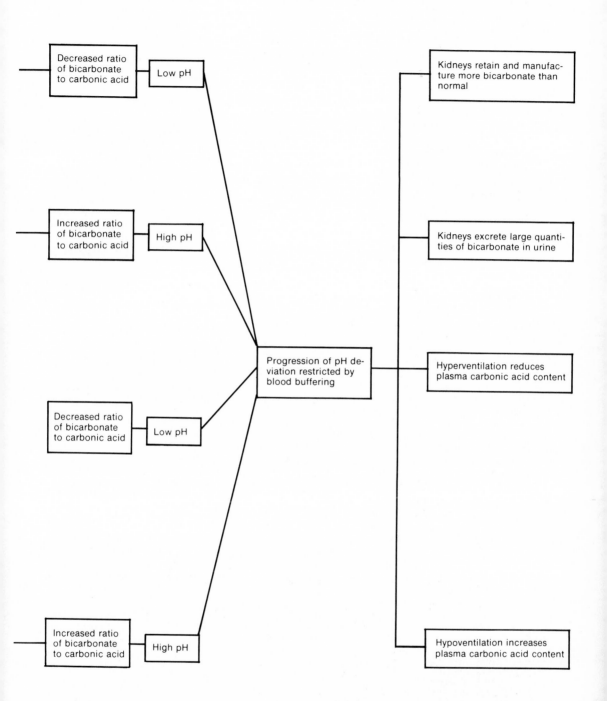

the microvasculature are still incompletely defined are discussed in Chapter 3, pages 48–51.

The blood pressure is the hydrostatic force that carries blood and nutrients to the tissues and re-

moves accumulated waste products; as such, it must be defended to maintain organ perfusion. Faced with hypotension or frank shock, the physician must be able to identify the derangement as

Table 1.9.
Classification of metabolic acid-base disturbances.

Underlying Factor	Mechanism of Acidosis	Anion Gap	Treatment
Hyperchloremic Acidoses			
Diarrhea	Loss of HCO_3^- from intestine (up to 90 mEq/liter)	Normal	Therapy of diarrhea; HCO_3^- if acidosis is severe

Small bowel drainage
  Oral suction from small bowel
  Fistulas
  Surgical drains
	Loss of HCO_3^- from small bowel	Normal	Surgical therapy as required; HCO_3^- administration if acidosis is severe

Ureterosigmoidostomy	Loss of HCO_3^- in exchange for Cl^- in urine draining into sigmoid colon	Normal	HCO_3^- administration; use of ileal loop presently favored surgical therapy
Carbonic anhydrase inhibitors	Partial blockage of renal tubular absorption of HCO_3^-	Normal	Discontinue medication
Proximal renal tubular acidosis	Inability to reabsorb HCO_3^- normally in proximal tubule	Normal	HCO_3^- and K^+ replacement
Distal renal tubular acidosis	Decreased acid secretion in distal tubule	Normal	HCO_3^- and K^+ replacement

Acid administration
  HCl
  NH_4Cl
  Arginine HCl
	Acid load exceeding renal excretory ability	Normal	Discontinue acid administration

High Anion-Gap Acidoses			
Uremia	Decreased renal ability to excrete acid	Elevated	HCO_3^- administration if $[HCO_3^-] < 12$ mEq/liter dialysis
Diabetic ketoacidosis	Increased circulating keto acids	Elevated	Treatment of diabetes; HCO_3^- administration if $[HCO_3^-] < 12$ mEq/liter
Lactic acidosis	Increased lactic acid production	Elevated	HCO_3^- administration; dialysis

Toxic ingestion
  Methyl alcohol
  Ethylene glycol
  Paraldehyde
  Salicylate
	↑ Formic acid
	↑ Oxalic acid
	↑ Acetic acid
	↑ Salicylic acid
	
	plus impaired cellular metabolism and increased production of organic acids
		Elevated	General
			  HCO_3^- administration; dialysis
			Specific
			  Intravenous ethanol for methanol and ethylene glycol intoxication;
			  forced alkaline diuresis for salicylate intoxication

Table 1.9.—*continued*

Underlying Factor	Mechanism of Persistent Alkalosis	Urine [Cl⁻]	Treatment
	Cl-Responsive Alkaloses		
Gastric suction Diuretic administration Villous adenoma of colon Congenital Cl⁻-losing diarrhea; Posthypercapnic alkalosis	Cl⁻ depletion	≤10–20 mEq/liter	NaCl administration
	Cl-Resistant Alkaloses		
Primary hyperaldosteronism Adrenal hyperplasia	Increased distal tubular exchange of Na⁺ for H⁺ and K⁺; ± K⁺ depletion	≥10–20 mEq/liter	Correction of underlying adrenal disorder
Bartter's syndrome	Same as above	≥10–20 mEq/liter	Aldosterone antagonists
Licorice ingestion	Same as above	≥10–20 mEq/liter	Discontinue licorice ingestion
Severe chronic K⁺ depletion	?Impaired tubular reabsorption of Cl⁻	≥10–20 mEq/liter	K⁺ replacement
Rapid HCO₃⁻ administration (especially in renal failure)	HCO₃⁻ administration exceeding renal excretory ability	≥10–20 mEq/liter	Discontinue HCO₃⁻ administration

(Reprinted by permission, from *Hosp Practice, 9:*164, © 1974 by HP Publishing Co., Inc.)

decreased cardiac output hypovolemia or loss of peripheral tone and to correct the abnormality. If tissue perfusion becomes inadequate, cellular hypoxia followed by lactic acidosis and ultimately cell death will result.

CELLULAR MILIEU—ACID-BASE DISTURBANCES

The degree of acidity of the intravascular, interstitial, and intracellular fluids is a key variable carefully regulated by homeostatic mechanisms. With other fundamental factors such as osmolarity and concentrations of certain ions, the pH must be maintained within a narrow range to prevent inactivation of enzyme systems, disruption of membrane integrity, and loss of electrical or contractile function. Acid-base disturbances are commonly encountered in emergency practice; their recognition and prompt correction are imperative and may be lifesaving (Table 1.8).

Water has a hydrogen ion concentration of 10^{-7} mEq/liter (pH 7) and is chemically neutral. The normal pH range of the blood is slightly alkaline (7.38–7.42). Since values significantly outside this range are life-threatening, the pH is defended by a three-tiered series of mechanisms: buffers, pulmonary ventilation, and renal excretory and synthetic capacities.

The metabolic machinery of the human body produces a potentially overwhelming volume of acidic ash. Carbohydrate and fat combustion daily releases 13,000 mEq of carbon dioxide into the circulatory system, and protein and phospholipid metabolism contributes 1 mg/kg/day of nonvolatile organic compounds such as sulfuric, phosphoric, and uric acids. In contrast, alkalosis usually arises by loss of acid, not by overproduction of base (Fig. 1.13). Derangements leading to alkalosis include loss of chloride from gastric suction or diuretic therapy, increased renal excretion of hydrogen ions in patients with primary hyperaldosteronism, and hyperventilation resulting in loss of carbon dioxide. However, alkalosis can also be produced iatrogenically by excess administration of alkali such as bicarbonate.

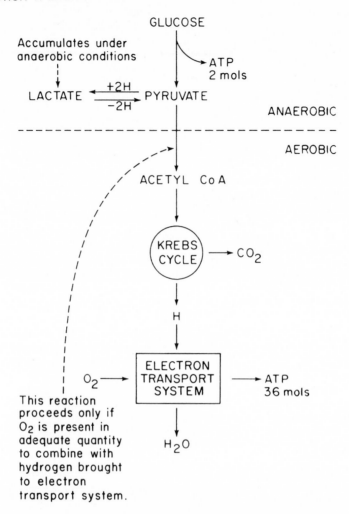

Figure 1.14. Energy production from glucose degradation. (Reproduced by permission, from Thal AP: *Shock*. Copyright © 1971 by Year Book Medical Publishers, Inc., Chicago.)

Buffer Systems

The first line of defense against wide alterations in pH are the blood buffer mechanisms. Several buffers are present in the blood, including plasma proteins, hemoglobin, and organic radicals such as Na^+ and $SO_4^=$. The predominant buffer system, however, is the carbonic acid-bicarbonate combination. Like other buffer systems, it consists of a weak acid in equilibrium with its salt. Added acid combines with the bicarbonate, forcing the reaction toward formation of carbonic acid; hydrogen ions are thereby taken from highly ionized acids and are bound in weakly ionized carbonic acid, minimizing the effect on pH.

$(H^+ + anion^-) + (Na^+ + HCO_3)$
highly ionized   sodium salt of
acid   carbonic acid
                                $H_2CO_3 + Na(anion)$
                     weakly ionized   salt
                     carbonic acid

Two features of the carbonic acid-bicarbonate combination render it uniquely effective in buffering acid loads. First, it is in equilibrium with carbon dioxide, which is continuously being eliminated by the lungs; thus, the acid is constantly being removed. Second, the bicarbonate ion is being regenerated continuously by the kidney as the tubules excrete hydrogen ions of organic acids.

Respiratory Response

The blood buffers are immediately available, but a massive acid load can exhaust them faster than they can be regenerated. At this point, the second tier of response takes effect. The respiratory center senses the change in pH and $Paco_2$ of the blood perfusing it, and resets the rate and depth of respiration appropriately. Metabolic acidosis is offset by hyperventilaton, as in diabetic ketoacidosis, whereas metabolic alkalosis is compensated by hypoventilation and carbon dioxide retention. While less immediately available than the blood buffers, the respiratory response becomes effective within minutes, and is valuable because of its ongoing nature.

Renal Mechanisms

The kidney, in the third response tier, is the slowest to react. However, by reabsorbing or excreting more bicarbonate, it can respond to acidosis or alkalosis over a period of hours to days. Two-thirds of a renal acid load is excreted as ammonium ions and the remainder as free (titratable) hydrogen ions that are exchanged for sodium or potassium ions.

The acid-base regulatory mechanisms are compensatory. In general, they produce only partial correction, bringing the pH back toward the normal range. Rarely does the clinician encounter an uncomplicated situation; primary disturbances with compensatory responses are more common.

A useful aid in understanding acid-base problems is an acid-base map of the kind illustrated in Figure 9.8 (see page 169). This relates pH to $Paco_2$ and bicarbonate values, enabling the clinician to enter any two factors on the plot and to obtain a qualitative description of the type of disturbance present.

A second device for characterizing acidosis is calculation of the anion gap. In this simple calculation, the routine serum electrolyte determination is used to distinguish acidosis with anion gap from acidosis in which the patient is hyperchloremic. To determine whether an anion gap is present, the sodium and potassium cations are totaled and compared with the total of the chloride and bicarbonate anions. (In some clinical laboratories, the carbon dioxide content is substituted for bicarbonate in this calculation.) Normally, the sodium and potassium ions total approximately 140 mEq/liter, and the sum of the chloride ions (110 mEq/liter) and bicarbonate ions (25 mEq/liter) is only 5–12 mEq/liter less. This normal difference represents the electrical "space" occupied by unmeasured anions such as proteins, sulfate, and phosphate. If the cation-anion difference is more than 12–15 mEq/liter, an anion gap is said to exist, and some other unmeasured anion, such as lactate, a keto acid, or salicylate, is present.

In all types of acidosis, the bicarbonate buffer is consumed and the bicarbonate level decreases. This widens the difference between the totals of anions and cations. How the void left by the consumed bicarbonate is filled determines the type of acidosis. In the acidosis seen with anion gap, it is filled, as mentioned, by other anions. In hyperchloremic acidosis, the void is filled by increase in chloride ion concentration. Hyperchloremic acidosis usually follows excessive loss of bicarbonate. It may develop as a result of a diarrheal state, small bowel drainage, carbonic anhydrase inhibitors, and other factors listed in Table 1.9.

The few minutes required for the anion gap calculation are well spent if the results indicate the likelihood of an unrecognized overdose of methanol or salicylate or unappreciated lactic acidosis. The results may point to the need for specific tests such as toxic screening and serum acetone determinations, and may directly influence therapy.

Lactic Acidosis

This common form of metabolic acidosis is encountered in many conditions that result in cellular hypoxia; when present, it should spur the physician's efforts to improve oxygenation of tissues. Lactic acidosis also occurs in a wide variety of incompletely understood states not marked by cellular hypoxia. These include diabetes mellitus, leukemia, hepatic coma, ethanol overdose, glycogen storage diseases, and idiopathic lactic acidosis, as well as vigorous exercise. In most cases, however, lactic acidosis indicates poor tissue perfusion.

The mechanism of development of lactic acidosis is as follows: poor tissue perfusion leads to cellular hypoxia, and this oxygen shortage then denies the cell access to the aerobic tricarboxylic acid (Krebs') cycle as a source of energy-rich phosphates. Normally, in the presence of adequate oxygen a glucose molecule is degraded stepwise through distinct sequences. The first of these, glycolysis, is a ten-step anaerobic pathway that degrades glucose to pyruvate and liberates a *small* amount of energy. Glycolysis is usually a preliminary event, and the pyruvate that is produced enters the much more efficient Krebs' cycle, which completes the process of extracting energy from glucose (Fig. 1.14). Because the Krebs' cycle is oxygen dependent and cannot function in the presence of significant cellular hypoxia, the only source of energy-rich compounds available to the cells in such a situation is the anaerobic glycolytic pathway.

Even the glycolytic route will not function, however, if pyruvate is allowed to accumulate; in such an instance, pyruvate is converted to lactate, a strong organic acid. As lactic acid is produced, plasma buffers are expended, the respiratory center is stimulated by the lower pH of its perfusate, hyperventilation begins, carbon dioxide is eliminated, and if the patient survives long enough, the kidney increases bicarbonate reabsorption. If the buffering and compensatory capacities are overwhelmed by lactate production, the pH of the blood decreases, enzymes cease to function, lysosomes rupture, membranes lose their ability to conduct impulses, and death follows.

Illustrative Examples

Three hypothetical cases illustrate the application of the foregoing concepts.

In the first case, cardiac arrest is followed by successful resuscitation. At the conclusion of the resuscitative effort, the attending physician must treat an intubated patient who is being ventilated by a respirator delivering 100% oxygen (FIO_2, 1.0). The patient has received 2 ampules of bicarbonate and 200 ml of a 5% bicarbonate drip during the extended resuscitative effort. Results of blood-gas determinations are as follows: PaO_2, 265 mm Hg; $PaCO_2$, 65 mm Hg; and pH, 7.25. The acid-base diagram shows that these values describe pure respiratory acidosis. Thus, bicarbonate administration was appropriate, but the respirator setting is incorrect, and the minute ventilation of the respirator should be increased.

In the second case, a patient is seen with florid pulmonary edema, and the usual therapeutic measures are instituted, including administration of morphine. Intermittent positive-pressure breathing with oxygen supplementation is carried out, but increasing drowsiness of the patient makes this treatment difficult. The cardiac monitor then shows frequent ventricular premature beats that persist despite administration of lidocaine by bolus and drip. Arterial blood-gas measurements are belatedly obtained: PaO_2, 48 mm Hg; $PaCO_2$, 75 mm Hg; and pH, 6.97. This represents a profound metabolic (lactic) and respiratory acidosis. Clearly the patient needs to receive bicarbonate and to be intubated and ventilated as well. The ventricular irritability may well be related to the severe acidosis.

The third case is that of a middle-aged man who is first seen in a coma and with an odor of alcohol about him. No history is provided. There are no localizing neurologic signs and no evidence of trauma. A venous blood specimen is drawn, and is sent to the clinical laboratory for determination of blood glucose, blood urea nitrogen, serum electrolyte, and serum acetone levels. The patient is given an ampule of glucose without significant improvement. An arterial sample is sent for blood-gas determinations. The physician measures neither blood glucose (Dextrostix reagent strips) nor acetone levels in the emergency ward.

The blood-gas levels are the first results back: PaO_2, 88 mm Hg; $PaCO_2$, 32 mm Hg; and pH, 7.1. This is metabolic acidosis with compensation. The serum electrolyte results come in next, and show a sodium level of 142 mEq/liter; potassium, 5 mEq/liter; chloride, 98 mEq/liter; and bicarbonate, 10 mEq/liter. The anions total only 108 mEq/liter, the cations 147 mEq/liter, so an anion gap is present. This anion gap (Table 1.9) indicates abnormal amounts of some acidic species, later identified as keto acids by the serum acetone test, which is strongly positive at 1:8 dilution, and by the blood glucose level of 675 mEq/liter.

The first and second cases involved resuscitative efforts. The clinical appearance of the patients was probably similar after arrest. Both had profound acid-base imbalance, and the second patient also had a life-threatening, therapy-resistant arrhythmia. Application of the principles of acid-base chemistry clarified their statuses, and importantly, indicated specific corrective therapeutic measures.

The third case was presented to make a point regarding the information obtainable from certain laboratory values—the blood-gas and serum-electrolyte levels. It was *not* offered as appropriate management of diabetic ketoacidosis (see Chapter 14, pages 290–298).

Suggested Readings

Bear RA, Gribik M: Assessing acid-base imbalances through laboratory parameters. Hosp Pract 9:157–165, 1974

Billingsley JG, Egan DF, Materson BJ, et al: Putting acid-base problems in balance. Patient Care 7:22–46, 1973

Braunwald E: Regulation of the circulation. N Engl J Med 290:1124–1129, 1420–1425, 1974

Fulop M, Horowitz M, Aberman A, et al: Lactic acidosis in pulmonary edema due to left ventricular failure. Ann Intern Med 79:180–186, 1973

Hobbe J: Metabolic acidosis. Am Fam Physician 23:220–227, 1981

Keyes JL: Blood-gases and blood-gas transport. Heart Lung 3:945–954, 1974

Miller WC: Acute respiratory failure. Am Fam Physician 24:176–182, 1981

Pontoppidan H, Geffin B, Lowenstein E: Acute respiratory failure in the adult. N Engl J Med 287:743–752, 1972

Thomas HM III, Lefrak SS, Irwin RS, et al: The oxyhemoglobin dissociation curve in health and disease: Role of 2,3-diphosphoglycerate. Am J Med 57:331–348, 1974

CHAPTER 2

Cardiopulmonary Resuscitation

JAMES T. ROBERTS, M.D.
HAMILTON R. HAYES, M.D.

The ability to resuscitate victims of accident or disease adroitly is the defining skill of emergency medicine. Resuscitation requires coolness under pressure, dexterity in performing physical procedures, understanding of pathophysiology, possession of a large fund of therapeutic knowledge, and the ability to lead a complex team effort. The body of information employed in resuscitation is usually arbitrarily divided into basic and advanced life support. Basic life support (BLS) refers to recognition of cardiopulmonary arrest, simple airway and ventilation techniques, and closed chest massage. Advanced life support (ALS) encompasses more sophisticated airway approaches, drugs, defibrillation, and other specific therapeutic and diagnostic modalities.

This BLS-ALS distinction, while useful, is artificial. In fact, the two are interdependent segments of a therapeutic spectrum. The material to follow will focus on advanced techniques employed in the hospital emergency ward. BLS is well discussed elsewhere, and knowledge of BLS will be assumed for the purposes of this discussion. This is not, however, meant to downplay the importance of BLS. On the contrary, every emergency physician should be trained to the level of a BLS instructor as an absolute minimum. Only through instructing and certifying others, then recertifying at appropriate intervals, can the practitioner maintain the level of technical expertise and the ability to supervise others that are necessary to manage a successful "code."*

THE DECISION TO START CARDIOPULMONARY RESUSCITATION

Before methodology is considered, the process must be addressed by which the physician decides to begin or forego cardiopulmonary resuscitation (CPR). The emergency physician frequently is presented with an apneic, pulseless patient about whom essentially nothing is known. In a matter of seconds, some form of assessment must be carried out and a critical choice must be made. Several factors incline the physician toward starting therapy: his or her instinct to treat; the expectations of the emergency ward staff, the patient's family, and society regarding the capability of the medical profession; and the fear of being misled by initial negative impressions and thus failing to treat a salvageable patient. Balanced against these considerations are the knowledge that only a small percentage of patients who appear dead on arrival will be long-term survivors, the spector of reviving the heart and lungs in a person with irreversible brain damage, a sense of respect for the person's right to death with dignity when the condition is beyond salvation, and an awareness of the cost to family and society of the support systems that are set in motion by the decision to resuscitate.

Given these conflicting impulses, how is the decision to be made? The two fundamental considerations that would compel the physician to begin CPR are (1) the probability of brain viability and (2) the absence of specific medical contraindications. However, these are precisely the two issues that usually are in doubt. Efforts have been made to devise firm criteria that would facilitate decision-making. These guidelines include the following: a period longer than 10 minutes from initial insult to CPR, efficacy of prehospital CPR, presence of underlying disease, advanced age, and other equally arbitrary or unknowable elements. All such criteria are fraught with inaccuracy and subject to so many exceptions that they offer the practitioner little guidance. (For example, in children and in patients suffering from hypothermia or immersion, the time from initial trauma to the start of CPR can be extended significantly.)

---

* "Code" is the local word for the ultimate emergency, cardiac arrest.

What usually happens is this: A patient is brought to the emergency ward with some form of CPR in progress. Information is scant and frequently undependable. In the absence of a gross contraindication such as rigor mortis or marked livedo reticularis, the emergency physician should continue BLS and begin ALS, while attempting to acquire additional information. While the resuscitation proceeds in a graduated manner, witnesses are interviewed and consultation is sought from other staff members. At any point during the process, significant new information (such as a phone call from an attending physician confirming the presence of an underlying terminal illness) may result in a decision to discontinue the effort. As ALS proceeds, the patient's response itself becomes a determining factor.

In the final analysis, the decision to resuscitate is a matter of judgment on the part of the physician on the scene. Unfortunately, at this time no fixed set of medicolegal guidelines exists to aid in that decision. Experience is helpful, but inevitably, some incorrect decisions are made. The tendency and the recommendation is to err on the side of proceeding with resuscitation. If a patient is truly unresponsive, this will become apparent soon enough. If this approach is adopted, unfortunately, some patients with irreversible brain damage will be resuscitated to the point of life support in an intensive care unit. The decision to terminate life support, however, then may be rendered on the basis of a set of much firmer criteria. Studies have shown that the number of long-term survivors with significant brain damage after inappropriately instituted CPR is minimal. Balanced against the certainty of death without resuscitation, this seems to be an acceptable consequence.

CONTROL OF VITAL FUNCTIONS

The initial stages of resuscitation are the most crucial and involve augmentation of both ventilation and circulation when necessary. Respiratory function depends on an intact neural pathway beginning with regulatory centers in the central nervous system and continuing along the phrenic and intercostal nerves to the diaphragm and intercostal muscles, a bellows system within an intact thoracic cage, a patent airway, and functioning alveoli (see Chapter 1, pages 1–7). Respiratory support may be required for a malfunction anywhere in this system.

Establishing the Airway

The first step in CPR is to establish a patent airway (Table 2.1):

(1) First, the unconscious patient should be

Table 2.1.
Five means of establishing an airway.

1. Position the patient's head and neck.
2. Remove foreign body from the mouth or pharynx.
3. Insert a mechanical airway.
4. Intubate.
5. Surgically enter the trachea.

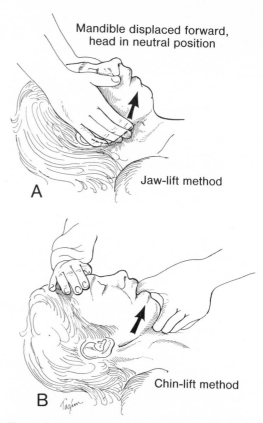

Figure 2.1. Alternate methods to open airway if cervical spine injury is suspected are shown.

placed on his back with the neck extended. This action lifts the tongue from the posterior pharyngeal wall, opening the airway in many cases. *When the possibility of neck injury exists, minimize neck motion.* In such a case, instead of the extended position, the *jaw-thrust maneuver* should be used (Fig. 2.1).

(2) Any obstructing foreign body in the airway should be removed by: (1) a finger sweep of the mouth, (2) four blows to the back, or (3) four manual thrusts to the epigastrium.

(3) If these basic procedures do not open the airway, a mechanical airway is required. Four types are available: oropharyngeal, nasopharyngeal, esophageal obturator airway (EOA), and esophageal gastric tube airway (EGTA).

The *oropharyngeal airway* (Fig. 2.2) is particu-

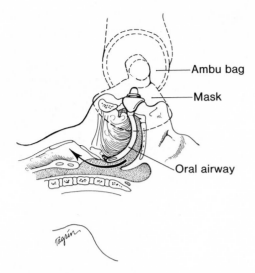

Figure 2.2. Oropharyngeal airway is correctly positioned to permit ventilation.

larly useful in the semiconscious or unconscious patient when the tongue is obstructing air flow. In the conscious patient, it may induce gagging, vomiting, and aspiration.

The *nasopharyngeal airway* is useful when the mouth cannot be opened. It is usually better tolerated in the semiconscious patient than the oropharyngeal airway. Proper lubrication is necessary to prevent epistaxis.

The *EOA* is a cuffed, tubular device occluded distally, open proximally, and perforated with multiple holes at its upper portion. It is attached to a face mask, and it is meant to be inserted blindly into the esophagus, after which the face mask is sealed around the nose and mouth, the cuff inflated, and ventilation begun with an Ambu bag (Fig. 2.3A). Ease of insertion by emergency medical technicians in the field and its ability to provide a reliably secure airway account for its increasing use. Although the EOA may minimize

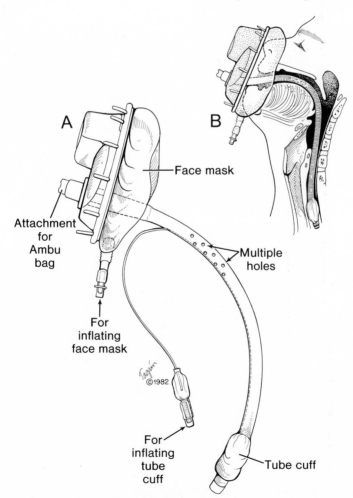

Figure 2.3. The esophageal obturator airway (EOA): **(A)** the structure of the device, **(B)** correctly placed in the esophagus with cuff inflated and mask creating a seal.

gastric dilation from forced bag-mask ventilation (in contrast with the oral airway), serious complications can occur, such as esophageal rupture and inadvertent tracheal cannulation. Proper position is illustrated in Figure 2.3B. Removal of the EOA is almost always accompanied by vomiting. The EGTA, therefore, has a major advantage over the EOA since the stomach contents can be suctioned through the EGTA before removal of the device.

The *EGTA* is similar to the EOA, but the tube has no side holes and air flow is via the nostrils. It has an opening in the distal end of the esophageal portion to permit passage of a No. 16 gastric tube (Fig. 2.4). The technique of insertion of an EGTA is similar to the technique of insertion of an EOA. Both the EOA and EGTA should be used *only in the unconscious patient* and *only as a temporary substitute for endotracheal intubation* (for example,

during transport). Therefore, the EOA and EGTA are seldom used in the emergency ward.

Endotracheal Intubation

Endotracheal intubation should be performed when the airway cannot be secured by the measures previously discussed, when prolonged ventilation is anticipated, or when the trachea needs to be protected from aspiration of gastric contents. The endotracheal tube offers direct access to the airway for ventilation, suction, and even examination with a fiberoptic laryngoscope or bronchoscope. Intubation, however, carries obvious risks as well as benefits.

The technique of endotracheal intubation is illustrated on pages 910–913; however, certain comments about intubation during CPR are in order. CPR must be interrupted for intubation. *The interruption should last no longer than 30 seconds.* The patient should be well oxygenated by bag-mask before intubation attempts whenever possible, and suction with a tonsil-tip aspirater should be immediately available. The physician should select an oral endotracheal tube one size (1 mm) smaller than indicated in Table 2.2. If the tube is too small, it can be changed later under more favorable conditions, but if it is too large, intubation may fail.

For rapid intubation, the patient's head should be in the sniffing position (Fig. 2.5), supported on a small, firm pillow or a rolled sheet. The physician should select a laryngoscope blade with which he or she is familiar, and then sweep the tongue to the left to obtain a visual path with the advancing blade, placing the tip of a curved blade in the vallecula or lifting the epiglottis with the tip of a straight blade. The force vector applied to the laryngoscope at this time is critical because *the force vector that is naturally applied is incorrect.*

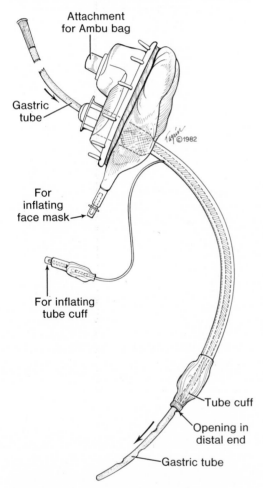

Figure 2.4. The esophageal gastric tube airway (EGTA) has a port permitting insertion of a tube and removal of gastric contents prior to extubation.

Table 2.2.
Recommended sizes for elective endotracheal tubes. Reduce by 1 mm in emergency situations.

Age	Endotracheal Tube Internal Diameter, mm
Newborn	3.0
6 months	3.5
18 months	4.0
3 years	4.5
5 years	5.0
6 years	5.5
8 years	6.0
12 years	6.5
16 years	7.0
Adult (female)	8.0–8.5
Adult (male)	8.5–9.0

This natural, incorrect motion uses the upper teeth as a fulcrum, causing dental injury. The correct force vector, depicted in Figure 2.6, lifts the laryngoscope up and away at a 45-degree angle vector.

The physician should insert and position the endotracheal tube under direct vision so that the upper portion of the cuff lies immediately below the vocal cords. The cuff should be inflated to a seal, and the position of the tube with respect to

the teeth then should be recorded. This allows correct repositioning of the tube if it is inadvertently moved during taping and auscultation.

The epigastrium as well as both axillae should be auscultated after intubation. Listening over the epigastrium detects inadvertent esophageal intubation (gurgling sounds are heard as air is forced into the stomach), whereas listening to both chest walls assures tracheal rather than bronchial intu-

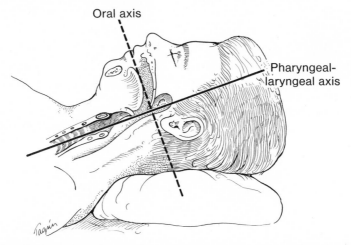

Figure 2.5.   The head is in a neutral position and demonstrates misalignment of oral and pharyngeal-laryngeal axis.

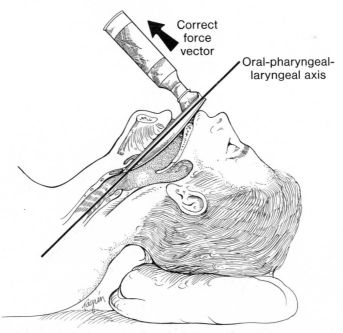

Figure 2.6.   The head is brought forward and extended on the neck aligning axes and facilitating visualization of the glottic opening. *Note* that the vector of the force applied is parallel to the axis of the laryngoscope handle.

bation. In addition to fractured teeth and esophageal intubation, complications include cannulation of a mainstem bronchus, aspiration, trauma to the soft tissues (including hypopharyngeal perforation), and cuff failure.

Other Techniques

On occasion, oral intubation fails. If the airway is patent, bag-mask ventilation with 100% oxygen should be resumed and intubation attempted again, modifying the original technique. If the airway is obstructed and the blockage cannot be promptly cleared (within 30 seconds), transtracheal jet insufflation or cricothyrotomy may be employed. Figure 2.7 schematically represents alternate approaches if intubation fails.

Percutaneous jet insufflation (Fig. 2.8) is a temporary measure to gain up to 10 minutes while a definitive airway is being established by other means. The physician should require no more than 30 seconds to insert a percutaneous tracheal catheter successfully and to begin to insufflate the lungs with 100% oxygen. Ventilation may or may not be possible with this method, particularly if a complete obstruction of the upper airway (preventing expiration) exists. The details of the technique are as follows:

(1) Insert a 12- or 14-gauge plastic Angiocath

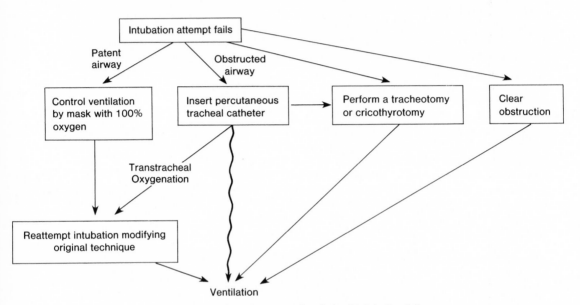

Figure 2.7.   Alternate approaches to try if intubation fails.

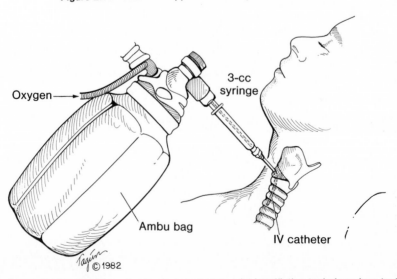

Figure 2.8.   Apparatus for supplying oxygen via percutaneous jet insufflation technique (see text) is shown.

percutaneously into the trachea and withdraw the introducing needle.

(2) Connect the hub of the catheter to the barrel of a 3-cc plastic syringe after removing the plunger.

(3) Insert a No. 8 endotracheal tube adapter into the large end of the syringe barrel.

(4) Connect an Ambu bag or intermittent high-pressure oxygen source, and ventilate or oxygenate the patient.

This may allow temporary oxygenation until more definitive access to the airway is established by cricothyrotomy.

Cricothyrotomy, which is depicted on pages 920–921, is probably a better short-term solution to an airway obstruction than is percutaneous tracheal catheterization. The cricothyrotomy tube should be adapted to an Ambu bag or ventilator. An immediate attempt to perform cricothyrotomy, however, may unnecessarily delay CPR, which is not the case with transtracheal catheter insufflation.

Ventilating the Patient

Once an airway is established by any of the means discussed, the second stage of CPR, ventilation, should begin. The method by which the airway is secured determines the equipment, technique, and complications of ventilation. Spontaneous ventilation is unacceptable in early arrest because tidal volumes may be inadequate despite seemingly normal respiration rates. Ventilation may be supplemented by a variety of means:

(1) *Mouth-to-mouth* ventilation requires no ancillary equipment, but delivers a less than optimal FIO_2 (19–20%).

(2) *Ventilation by bag-mask* with 100% oxygen is the quickest noninvasive method of raising the alveolar FIO_2. Technique is critical. An inexperienced person may force the mask posteriorly onto the patient's face. The correct method (Fig. 2.9) places 10% of effort on applying the mask and 90% on bringing the mandible anteriorly to meet the mask, form a seal, and open the airway. The anterior force is applied to the rami of the mandible. Inadvertent pressure by the fingers on the soft tissue of the neck obstructs rather than facilitates air flow.

(3) *Endotracheal intubation*: improper bag-mask ventilation may cause gastric distention, vomiting, and aspiration, and the patient should be intubated if any of these complications occur. With manual ventilation, accurate assessment of the degree of ventilation is difficult without arterial blood-gas analysis. Adults may initially be hyperventilated for 3–5 breaths with 100% oxygen, then ventilated at a normal rate, that is, 12 breaths/min. The guiding rule is: $0.1 \times$ weight in kilograms

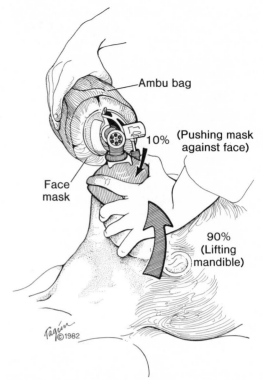

Figure 2.9. Technique of bag-mask ventilation indicates the importance of lifting the mandible to create a seal without occluding the airway.

= minute ventilation in liters (= 583 cc tidal volume at 12 breaths/min in a 70-kg man).

This same minute ventilation may be used to set a mechanical ventilator. Volume ventilators are preferred to pressure-limited ventilators, since the latter may result in hypoventilation when resistance to air flow in the airway is excessive or when intrathoracic pressure is raised, as it is during CPR. There may be significant air leakage with cricothyrotomy, and minute ventilation must be increased proportionately.

CLOSED CHEST CARDIAC MASSAGE

The second concern in resuscitation is circulation, and the cornerstone of circulatory support is closed chest cardiac massage. The technique of closed chest massage is well taught in monographs on BLS, but in practice, certain errors recur with alarming frequency. The emergency physician functions as team captain during the code procedure, and as such, he or she must supervise the actions of other team members who typically rotate the task of compressing the chest. During code exercises, it must never be assumed that the various individuals compressing the chest are equally skilled in performing the technique. Specifically, errors tend to occur in hand placement, the rate and depth of compression, the timing of the compression cycle, and the length of time during which compression is interrupted.

Hand placement is critical. The heel of the hand should rest over the lower one-third of the sternum in adults, the long axis of the heel of the hand in the midline of the sternum. If the hand is placed too far superiorly, the thrusts are ineffective in compressing the ventricles. If placement is too far inferiorly, the liver or spleen may be lacerated by the xiphoid process. Hands placed too far laterally apply force to the costal cartilages and can dislocate them or fracture ribs.

The rate of compression should be 60 beats/ minute in adults, but is frequently very different during an actual resuscitation. Inexperienced rescuers often increase the rate. This allows inadequate time for filling of the ventricular chambers, and consequently reduces cardiac output. Conversely, a rescuer can inadvertently slow the rate, also diminishing cardiac output. The solution to these problems is to encourage personnel to count, preferably with reference to the sweep second hand of a clock.

The timing of the phases of the compression cycle likewise has an important impact on cardiac output. The desired ratio is approximately 50% compressed to 50% relaxed. Sharp jabbing thrusts or a pause in the compressed position should be avoided.

Finally, the ultimate insult to cardiac output is complete cessation of massage. At best, external cardiac compression can generate 30% of normal cardiac output. When compression is interrupted, output drops to zero. Consequently, compression should be continued with interruptions of no more than 5 seconds for diagnostic procedures such as studying the electrocardiogram, or for no more than 15–30 seconds for such procedures as central line placement, intubation, or defibrillation.

In practice, it is often helpful to have someone, usually the physician in charge, rest a hand on the femoral artery during a resuscitation procedure. Constant palpation is the best simple technique to monitor the effectiveness of cardiac compressions. Should the rate or depth of compression change significantly, it will become immediately apparent in the pulse quality. Further, absence of a palpable pulse with seemingly effective compression should alert the physician to the possibility of myocardial rupture or pericardial tamponade.

DRUG THERAPY

Access to the Circulation

After compression, the second critical facet of circulation control is venous cannulation. This provides a secure route for fluid therapy and drug administration. There are pros and cons to selection of venous sites: peripheral veins in the hands, forearms, and lower extremities can be used without interrupting CPR, but central veins—subclavian and jugular—permit delivery of drugs directly to the vicinity of the myocardium and allow central venous pressure measurement. Placement of a central line, however, generally requires interruption of CPR. Once established, central lines are more secure than short peripheral lines in the extremities. The median basilic vein in the antecubital fossa has advantages in that it both permits access to the central circulation with a long catheter and avoids interruption of CPR. When the usual veins are inaccessible to cannulation or when damage to the superior vena caval system is suspected, cannulation of the femoral vein often permits easy access to the central circulation. Nursing care of an indwelling line in the femoral region is a bit more difficult, however, and the infection rate is probably higher.

The type of cannula selected is not critical if the primary purpose of the line is drug administration and the infusion of small amounts of crystalloids. In this case, either basic type of cannula—catheter over the needle or catheter inside the needle—will suffice. If the objective of cannulation is to permit administration of large volumes of fluid, and especially if blood transfusion is indicated, however, multiple short large-bore (14- to 16-gauge) lines should be inserted. In such a case, the catheter over the needle type is appropriate. Administration of blood through long lines is to be discouraged because of the frequency with which these lines become occluded.

The technique of subclavian catheter placement is presented on pages 922–925, but one important point should be stressed. When the catheter inside the needle is used, care must be taken to avoid shearing the catheter on the sharp bevel of the needle and producing a catheter embolus. Withdrawal of the catheter through the needle after it has been advanced should be avoided or done with utmost care. If the catheter is inadvertently sheared off and disappears into the vein, a tourniquet should immediately be placed above the site and an x-ray film obtained at the earliest opportunity to locate the embolized segment.

Two special techniques deserve comment: transtracheal drug administration and surgical cutdown for venous cannulation. It is possible to instill lidocaine hydrochloride, epinephrine, and atropine through an endotracheal tube when a vein cannot be readily cannulated. These drugs are well absorbed across the pulmonary epithelium. Because the pulmonary bed receives virtually 100% of cardiac output and has a vast surface area, drugs sprayed through the endotracheal tube actually have a more rapid onset of action than those given intravenously. Although blood levels achieved by the endotracheal route are eight to ten times lower than those by the intravenous route, the effect on blood pressure and pulse is only two to three times less than that achieved by intravenous medication. Furthermore, the duration of action of drugs sprayed into the pulmonary tree is prolonged relative to the intravenous route. The technique of endotracheal administration is straightforward: drug is sprayed through the endotracheal tube with a spinal needle while the patient is being ventilated. Oil-based medications should not be used. Water is preferred to saline solution as a diluent since it is absorbed faster. Sodium bicarbonate should not be administered by this route because it is irritating to the respiratory epithelium.

The second technique, surgical venous cutdown, may be indicated in addicts, obese patients, persons in profound vascular collapse, and others if adequate access to the circulation cannot be achieved by the percutaneous route. The veins usually cannulated by cutdown are the saphenous (located anterior to the medial malleolus at the ankle) and the basilic (in the distal portion of the upper arm). Although venous cutdown provides a secure line, it is time-consuming and has a higher risk of wound infection. Furthermore, in cardiac arrest, identification of structures becomes more difficult and inadvertent arterial cannulation or nerve damage may occur. Most adults do not require this technique.

Essential Drugs in CPR

Oxygen

The treatment of hypoxemia with oxygen is of primary importance in all resuscitation attempts. With controlled ventilation, 100% oxygen should be used. High-frequency ventilation is currently being evaluated as a substitute for "normal" ventilatory patterns. Its use in the arrest situation remains to be evaluated, but this method looks promising.

Sodium Bicarbonate

The acidosis of cardiac and respiratory arrest has a dual origin. Respiratory arrest causes accumulation of carbon dioxide and the end product of anaerobic metabolism, lactic acid. Both drug therapy and electrical defibrillation of refractory ventricular fibrillation, frequently associated with cardiac arrest, are optimized at a normal arterial pH. Acidosis should be treated by ventilation for the respiratory portion and intravenous sodium bicarbonate for the metabolic portion. The dose of sodium bicarbonate should be calculated from arterial pH and P_{CO_2} measurements. Without the availability of these measurements, the accepted initial emergency dose of sodium bicarbonate is 1 mEq/kg, with one-half of this dose repeated at 10-minute intervals or until results of blood-gas determinations become available. Sodium bicarbonate corrects acidosis but increases Pa_{CO_2} and the carbon dioxide load to the lungs. Excessive administration of sodium bicarbonate may even produce alkalosis (with a resultant shift to the left of the oxygen-hemoglobin dissociation curve), as well as hyperosmolarity and hypernatremia. Finally, CO_2 diffusing across the blood brain barrier may cause CSF acidosis, even at normal blood pH values.

Epinephrine

Epinephrine is frequently administered during resuscitation because of its effects on the heart and peripheral vasculature. The heart responds to epinephrine with an increase in myocardial contractile force and a slight increase in rate (β effect). Excessive epinephrine may produce ventricular fibrillation. If ventricular fibrillation is already present when epinephrine is administered, it may be made coarser. Coarse ventricular fibrillation has a lower threshold for defibrillation, so this is a desirable effect. With ventricular standstill, epinephrine may stimulate return of cardiac activity in the form of bradycardia, fibrillation, or sinus mechanism that should then be treated appropriately.

Catecholamines such as epinephrine, isoproterenol hydrochloride, norepinephrine, and dopamine work best at a pH from 7.35–7.50, so pH correction with sodium bicarbonate is mandatory.

Epinephrine has a biphasic effect on the peripheral vasculature. In low doses, the β effect predominates, resulting in vasodilation. Larger doses stimulate vasoconstriction. As with other vasoconstricting agents, the detrimental side effects of decreased urinary output, metabolic acidosis, and increased left ventricular stroke work must be balanced against the need for improving coronary arterial blood flow. External cardiac massage should be continued when there is any suggestion of inadequate perfusion. The dose of epinephrine is 0.5–1.0 mg (5–10 ml of a 1:10,000 solution) given intravenously every 5 minutes. Alkaline solutions inactivate epinephrine.

Atropine

Atropine is useful for treating sinus bradycardia, atrioventricular block (especially Wenckebach), and ventricular asystole. The initial intravenous dose is 0.5–0.75 mg, repeated up to a total dose of 2.5 mg, or until a suitable (60 beats/minute) rate is achieved. Use of atropine in the presence of myocardial infarction requires extreme caution, since it may increase myocardial oxygen consumption and worsen myocardial ischemia as the heart rate increases. Ventricular tachycardia or fibrillation may occasionally result.

Calcium Chloride

Calcium is not one of the first drugs administered in cardiac arrest except in one situation, hyperkalemic arrest. Potassium ions produce cardiac arrest by raising the threshold potential needed to initiate contraction. Calcium lowers the threshold potential, making it easier to initiate contraction. Calcium potentiates digitalis effects and toxicity, and a clinically valid concept views calcium as "instant digitalis," with essentially the same effects, indications, and contraindications. It, therefore, should be used with caution in patients with hypokalemia or a high digitalis level.

Calcium is a "second-line" drug in refractory electromechanical dissociation, asystole, and fibrillation refractory to countershock. The dosage of calcium required varies widely, but intravenous administration of 5–7 ml/kg of a 10% solution of calcium chloride (2.5–5 ml of a 10% solution). Calcium cannot be administered with bicarbonate and it has the potential to induce bradycardia if administered too rapidly.

DIFIBRILLATION

Electrical countershock is the definitive treatment of ventricular fibrillation. In addition to those physico-chemical elements of the myocardium already mentioned, success of defibrillation depends on the duration of fibrillation, the output of the specific defibrillator, resistance of the skin, paddle size, paddle placement, previous attempts at defibrillation, and the wave form of the defibrillation impulse. Additional factors such as digitalis toxicity may affect the advisability and success of defibrillation.

The appropriate amount of energy to be delivered by a defibrillator has been a subject of considerable debate. The most recent standards for CPR and extracorporeal circulation (1980) have reduced the recommended minimum-delivered energy from 320 joules to 200–300 joules. The object is to achieve defibrillation without inflicting electrical damage to the myocardium. The concept of a "dose" of energy relating to the patient's weight appears to be inaccurate. Only the impedance offered by the chest wall to the passage of current is of concern. The length of the current pathway is relatively constant in most individuals.

Paddle placement is critical to maximize the amount of myocardial tissue traversed by the defibrillating impulse and to avoid high impedance structures such as the sternum. Two variations of paddle position are acceptable (Fig. 2.10.): (1) one paddle placed to the right of the sternum and the other at the cardiac apex, and (2) one paddle on the anterior thorax to the left of the sternum and the other posteriorly directly beneath it. The paddles should be applied with firm pressure, and an effective low-impedance conducting material should be liberally applied. Of the available conducting media, gel pads have the highest impedance.

The electrode surface area is also important. A larger area results in lower impedance. Most paddles in use in the United States have an 8-cm diameter. Studies indicate, however, that a 12-cm diameter is more effective.

Tandem countershock administration may permit successful defibrillation in some cases of refractory ventricular fibrillation. In tandem defibrillation, a pair of shocks are administered at the same energy output setting within seconds of each other. The rationale is that one shock decreases the impedance for conduction through the tissue pathway, enabling higher current to be delivered to the myocardium with the same output setting on the defibrillator.

MANAGEMENT OF DIFFICULT PROBLEMS IN ADVANCED LIFE SUPPORT

Arrhythmia Prophylaxis

The debate over the advisability of instituting antiarrhythmic agents prophylactically in suspected infarction is yet unresolved, but the weight of evidence now supports this approach. The principal cause of death in the immediate period after infarction, whether the infarct is transmural or subendocardial, anterior or posterior, inferior or high lateral, is the development of lethal arrhythmias. Ventricular fibrillation develops in 5–10% of patients with documented myocardial infarction. In 25–50% of these patients, fibrillation occurs in the first 12–24 hours without any classic "warning" arrythmias (premature ventricular contractions that are multifocal, frequent, or paired, or R-on-T phenomena).

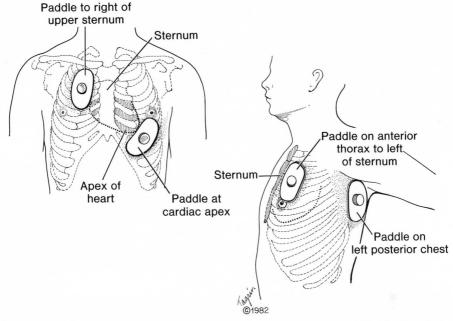

Paddle to right of
upper sternum

Sternum

Paddle on anterior
thorax to left
of sternum

Sternum

Apex of
heart

Paddle at
cardiac apex

Paddle on
left posterior chest

©1982

Figure 2.10.   Acceptable defibrillation paddle placement: **(A)** both paddles are applied to the anterior chest wall; **(B)** paddles are applied anteriorly and posteriorly to the left thorax.

The most basic strategy in preventing myocardial irritability is to maintain adequate oxygenation, optimal pH, and electrolyte balance. Beyond this, data indicate that lidocaine hydrochloride administered early after a suspected infarct is effective in preventing the development of lethal ventricular tachycardia and fibrillation, even though it may not suppress all premature ventricular contractions. Lidocaine should be administered early (in the field if ALS is available) in all cases of suspicious chest pain. A loading dose is required because lidocaine has a wide volume of distribution (90% is initially cleared by the liver). Various dosage schedules have been proposed, but one that is effective is 100–200 mg of lidocaine as a slow bolus followed by an intravenous drip at 2–4 mg/minute. Some authors suggest that the initial bolus should be followed approximately 10 minutes later with a second bolus of 50–100 mg intravenously. There is good documentation that such a regimen will reduce early mortality.

Refractory Ventricular Fibrillation

The pathophysiology of the production of this dysrhythmia is discussed in Chapter 5, pages 80–83. Several points, however, are pertinent to a discussion of electrical defibrillation. Approximately 75% of cases of prehospital cardiac arrest occur via the mechanism of ventricular fibrillation. Untreated ventricular fibrillation deteriorates to asystole in approximately 30 seconds. When defibrillation can be carried out within this 30-second interval, 98% of patients will be successfully defibrillated. If 2 minutes elapse without supportive therapy, the success rate drops to 27%. In this situation, perhaps more than in any other, basic concepts must be recalled: an anoxic, acidotic, or hypothermic heart is difficult or impossible to defibrillate. Establishment of a patent airway, adequate ventilation with 100% oxygen, and administration of sodium bicarbonate are mandatory. When this therapy is combined with administration of epinephrine, 5 ml of a 1:10,000 aqueous solution intravenously every 5 minutes, the amplitude of fibrillatory waves increases and defibrillation becomes more effective.

Several drugs with antiarrhythmic properties are in common clinical use. Two have special value during cardiac arrest and ventricular fibrillation. Lidocaine hydrochloride has little myocardial depressant effects in appropriate therapeutic doses does not alter the total peripheral vascular resistance, and does not produce hypotension. At therapeutic levels, the effect of lidocaine on atrioventricular conduction is minimal. Rarely, particularly in the presence of an inferior myocardial infarct, a second-degree or third-degree block can be precipitated by administration of lidocaine.

After successful defibrillation, a 100-mg bolus of lidocaine should be administered routinely intravenously, followed by an intravenous drip (at 4 mg/minute) to prevent recurrence of fibrillation.

The second important antiarrhythmic drug is bretylium tosylate. Introduced in the 1950s as an antihypertensive agent, bretylium was all but abandoned because of variability of effect and development of tolerance, but was "rediscovered" in the 1960s as an antiarrhythmic drug. It acts systemically via the peripheral adrenergic nerve terminals to decrease vascular resistance, producing orthostatic hypotension. Bretylium also increases the electrical fibrillation threshold of the myocardium in both normal and ischemic tissue. Currently, the approved indication for the drug is the treatment of life-threatening ventricular arrhythmias unresponsive to "first-line" drugs (lidocaine and procainamide).

In an urgent situation, bretylium tosylate can be administered intravenously, 5–10 mg/kg as a rapid bolus. If time permits, however, it should be diluted in 50 ml of normal saline solution and given over 10 minutes. Onset of antiarrhythmic action is rapid when bretylium is given intravenously, and the antiarrhythmic effect of a single dose lasts 6–12 hours. If the arrhythmia is persistent, a second dose may be administered in 1–2 hours. Bretylium exerts a positive inotropic effect on the heart and may potentiate dc defibrillation, but more importantly, it is capable of causing chemical cardioversion of the fibrillating heart, as well as preventing fibrillation. The most common side effect of bretylium is hypotension, but this is not critical with a recumbent patient, and indeed, the decrease in afterload produced by reduction of peripheral vascular resistance may prove beneficial (see Chapter 3, pages 48–49). Bretylium may cause ventricular arrhythmias due to digitalis toxicity to worsen.

Asystole

Asystole may be the initial event of cardiopulmonary collapse, or it may be the end result of a deterioration from ventricular tachycardia through ventricular fibrillation. Asystole implies major myocardial injury or marked metabolic disturbance or both; consequently, it is associated with a high mortality. Therapy for asystole includes the basic steps in resuscitation as detailed previously and specific measures including the intravenous administration of sodium bicarbonate and epinephrine (preferably by a central line) in the doses mentioned earlier. If these drugs are ineffective in restoring a rhythm, calcium chloride, 5 ml of a 10% intravenous solution, may be given slowly. The intravenous line should be cleared of sodium bicarbonate before calcium chloride is injected. If calcium chloride proves ineffective, atro-

pine may be beneficial (this implies that the arrest was occasioned by excessive parasympathetic tone as seen in an inferior myocardial infarct). Atropine should be given in a dose of 0.5–1.0 mg intravenously.

Additional approaches to asystole include intracardiac administration of epinephrine (with the attendant risks of myocardial laceration, coronary artery laceration, and pericardial tamponade) and infusion of isoproterenol hydrochloride, 2 mg in 250 ml of 5% dextrose in water run at 2–4 μg/min. When these pharmacologic measures are unsuccessful, a temporary pacing wire, either transvenous or transthoracic, may capture the ventricle and restore a paced rhythm.

Electromechanical Dissociation

In this situation, there is cardiographic evidence of organized electrical activity in the sinoatrial node and cardiac conducting system, but no discernible ventricular contraction, that is, no audible heart sounds or palpable pulse. Electromechanical dissociation carries a grave prognosis. While not completely understood, it may represent an impairment of the calcium ion transport system, resulting in separation of the electrical impulse from the mechanical action.

Therapy for electromechanical dissociation includes the basic support mentioned previously, intravenous epinephrine, sodium bicarbonate, and calcium chloride. Isoproterenol hydrochloride and military anti-shock trousers (MAST) have also been employed, but with disappointing results. Two treatable conditions may mimic electromechanical dissociation: pericardial tamponade and myocardial rupture. Pericardial tamponade may be determined by pericardiocentesis (see pages 935–937), and removal of a small amount of blood may be lifesaving. When recognized, myocardial rupture has occasionally been successfully treated surgically.

Anticipation and Prevention of Specific Complications

Infarcts in certain locations have the potential for causing specific complications. Anterior myocardial infarcts, which involve the anterior portion of the intraventricular septum, can lead to atrioventricular blocks of the Mobitz II variety. Infarcts occurring more inferiorly in the septum can lead to a variety of fascicular blocks such as the classic right bundle-branch left anterior hemiblock. The possibility of these complications indicates the need for insertion of a prophylactic temporary pacing wire. Early insertion may prevent progression to cardiogenic shock if third-degree heart block develops.

Inferior myocardial infarcts are often associated with a high degree of parasympathetic tone, leading to profound bradycardias and even cardiac arrest. This exaggerated vagal tone should be interrupted with atropine (see pages 33–34).

MONITORING THE CIRCULATION

With ventilation and compression underway, appropriate lines in position, and prophylactic antiarrhythmic agents administered, a measure of control is achieved. Additional data will now become available to guide further therapy.

Cardiac monitoring with an oscilloscope or electrocardiograph should be ongoing. Palpation of the femoral or carotid pulse, as mentioned previously, is useful. A Doppler probe positioned over the radial artery may give greater sensitivity.

Measurement of central venous pressure in a code situation is difficult and often not helpful. In cardiac arrest, there is usually a great functional discrepancy between the left and right ventricles. Central venous pressure measurements, which monitor the right side of the circulation, may produce a misleading impression of cardiac and pulmonary status. Typically, central venous pressure is low; this may lead to fluid administration in a patient bordering on congestive failure.

Pulmonary capillary wedge pressures provide information that clarify this dilemma. In the patient with cardiac arrest, however, it may be practically impossible to insert the Swan-Ganz balloon-tip flotation catheter during external cardiac compression.

An arterial catheter is useful for two reasons. Arterial samples for blood gas determination may be repeatedly obtained and intra-arterial blood pressure may be continuously monitored. Blood pressure readings from extremity cuff placement often does not accurately reflect true pressures in the patient with vasoconstriction or shock. If cannulation of an artery is difficult or time-consuming in the patient with cardiopulmonary arrest, surgical cut-down may be required. The radial artery is the vessel of choice. Thrombosis of more proximal arteries, such as the brachial or femoral, may produce threatening circulatory deprivation to the hand or leg.

ONGOING PATIENT ASSESSMENT

Ongoing monitoring generates data concerning the neurologic and circulatory status of the resuscitated arrest patient. Persisting fixed and dilated pupils, despite restoration of effective oxygenation and circulation, is a worrisome prognostic sign for neurologic recovery. Reassuring signs include the return or persistence of spontaneous respiration and improved muscular tone. The most important hemodynamic sign heralding recovery is the generation of a pulse and measurable blood pressure. A twelve-lead electrocardiogram should be obtained as soon as cardiac rhythm is restored.

Serial arterial blood-gas determinations are essential to monitor blood pH and to guide bicarbonate administration. The effectiveness of oxygenation and ventilation is evident from these determinations. A portable chest roentgenogram provides information on endotracheal tube position, location of the central venous catheter, and diagnostic cardiopulmonary conditions such as pulmonary edema.

COMPLICATIONS OF CPR

As a result of its invasive and often violent nature performed under stressful circumstances, CPR is a process fraught with potential complications. Some, such as rib fractures during chest compression, may be unavoidable. Good technique will minimize others. Awareness of complications is paramount. In particular, pericardial tamponade and tension pneumothorax are potentially lethal conditions which are fully correctable. A successful resuscitation should be followed by a thorough evaluation for complications.

DECISION TO TERMINATE CPR

The decision to stop resuscitative efforts, like the decision to commence CPR, is a matter of clinical judgment. In essence, the indication to stop is a conviction that cerebral death has occurred. The usual signs of cerebral death—deep unconsciousness, absence of spontaneous respiration, absence of brainstem reflexes, and fixed dilated pupils—are ominous but not foolproof indicators in this setting. Cardiac viability is more readily assessed in the clinical situation. Since cerebral viability becomes a moot issue if the heart cannot supply blood to the brain, the decision to terminate CPR ultimately rests on an estimate of the heart's viability.

Cardiovascular unresponsiveness is determined by a clinical trial. The therapeutic measures of BLS and ALS are applied in a timely and appropriate manner and the patient's response is noted. Refractoriness to acceptable CPR over a period deemed reasonable by the attending physician constitutes the indication to terminate.

Although the lack of hard criteria for such a critical decision is indeed troublesome, efforts to establish guidelines have proved unsuccessful and even undesirable. The many exceptions that exist to arbitrary end points can make them unworkable.

CARE AFTER RESUSCITATION

If CPR has been successful, the patient should have continuous cardiac monitoring, sequential arterial blood-gas determinations, frequent monitoring of vital signs, and if indicated, assisted or controlled ventilation. Arrangements should be made to move the patient to an intensive care or coronary care unit for further treatment and monitoring; however, the patient should not be transported unmonitored or in an unstable condition.

The smooth and cooperative performance of CPR by a team of personnel does not happen by chance. There should be time devoted to education, instruction, and practice so that each individual involved knows his or her role. Within the hospital setting and particularly in the emergency ward, this is of paramount importance. In each resuscitative effort, one person must clearly be in charge. A record should be kept of the time that CPR was begun, the medications administered, and the procedures performed. After each resuscitation, it is extremely helpful if the participants discuss the procedure and review any errors in technique or diagnosis, as well as the successes of therapy. The responsibility for improving the results of CPR in this setting rests with the emergency physician, who should initiate personnel training, supervise drills, and conduct review sessions after CPR.

Suggested Readings

Chipman C, Adelman R, Sexton G.: Criteria for cessation of CPR in the emergency department. *Ann Emerg Med 10:*11–17, 1981

Crampton D, MD, High versus low energy defibrillation in cardiac arrest. *Top Emerg Med 3:*69–78, 1981

Goodman SL, Geiderman JM, Bernstein IJ: Prophylactic lidocaine in suspected acute myocardial infarction. *JACEP 8:*221–224, 1979

Kerber RE, Jensen SR, Grayzel, J, et al: Elective cardioversion: Influence of paddle-electrode location and size on success rates and energy requirements. *N Engl J Med 305:*658–662, 1981

Koch-Wesler J: Drug therapy bretylium. *N Engl J Med 300:*473–477, 1979

Lambrew C: To resuscitate or not to resuscitate (editorial). *JACEP 6:*569, 1977

McIntyre KM, Lewis AJ (eds): *Textbook of Advanced Cardiac Life Support American Heart Association,* 1981

Nowak RM, Bodnar TJ, Dronen S: Bretylium tosylate as initial treatment for cardiopulmonary arrest: Randomized comparison with placebo. *Ann Emerg Med 10:*404–407, 1981

Roberts JR, Greenberg MI, Baskin SI: Endotracheal epinephrine in cardiorespiratory collapse. *JACEP 8:*515–519, 1979

Rogove H: Pathophysiology of cardiac arrest. *Top Emerg Med 1:*17–27, 1979

Standards and Guidelines for Cardiopulmonary Resuscitation (CPR) and Emergency Cardiac Care (ECC). *JAMA,* 244:453–509, 1980

Wayne A: The hidden killer—Tension pneumothorax. *Curr Concepts Trauma Care* Fall, 5–8, 1980

CHAPTER 3

Shock

HAMILTON HAYES, M.D.
SEAN KENNEDY, M.D.

Shock, a state characterized by decreased tissue perfusion, may develop during the course of several diverse diseases, and often may be fatal. Although shock may be classified in many ways, for the purposes of this discussion the traditional division into hypovolemic, cardiogenic, and septic varieties will be employed.* Figure 3.1 is a diagrammatic representation of the shock states according to the underlying pathophysiologic derangement.

The clinical presentation of the patient with established shock is characterized by alteration in the sensorium ranging from anxiety to obtundation, weakness or prostration, pallor, diaphoresis, clamminess, tachycardia, thready pulse, hypotension, and tachypnea. The most notable variation is the warm shock sometimes seen early with sepsis.

Hemorrhage, myocardial infarction, sepsis, anaphylaxis, spinal cord injury, and administration of high spinal anesthetics are a few of the many causes of the shock syndrome. Although seemingly unrelated, these processes all affect the microcirculation and the cells lining the capillary beds (see Chapter 1, pages 17–19). Their common impact is to produce diminished perfusion of the capillaries, which deprives the cells of needed oxygen and nutrients, allows accumulation of waste products, and leads to lactic acidosis.

Physiologic Responses

To defend itself against this life-threatening sequence, the body employs several compensatory mechanisms designed to maintain perfusion pressure in the tissues. The initial response is a sympathetic discharge, an outflow of catecholamines that stimulates the heart, increases the rate and force of contraction and improves cardiac output. The afferent arterioles of nonessential vascular beds are simultaneously constricted, raising the peripheral resistance and increasing the intra-arterial pressure. These neurohumoral responses produce the pale, cool clammy skin and rapid, thready pulse characteristic of the shock state. Their principal function is to increase the effective circulating blood volume and, thereby, to maintain the blood pressure at a level adequate to perfuse the coronary and carotid arteries. If sustained, however, this vasoconstricted state itself becomes harmful, leading to sludging of the blood trapped in the capillaries, disseminated intravascular coagulation, and profound acidosis. Ultimately, tissue hypoxia results in loss of cell function and membrane integrity, followed by cell death and organ failure.

In addition to shutting down the nonessential vascular beds, the body compensates for shock by constricting the venous capacitance vessels, reducing the size of the intravascular compartment and transiently increasing right-sided return. In the subacute state, loss of intravascular hydrostatic pressure allows interstitial fluid to return to the intravascular compartment. This shift, constituting an autotransfusion of a cell-free and protein-free solution, occurs at significant rates (up to 1 liter/hour). The clinician further can augment autotransfusion by elevating the legs of the patient, or more effectively, by applying Military Anti-Shock Trousers (MAST, see Therapy, page 43–45). The head-down position should be avoided, however, since it interferes with respiration.

Thus, the body constricts both arterioles and venules to increase the central blood volume, increases the cardiac output to circulate the available blood more rapidly, and draws on interstitial fluid reserves to supplement the total intravascular fluid

---

* Another category of shock, neurogenic shock (shock due to sympathetic blockade and resultant loss of vasomotor tone), is rarely seen as an Emergency Department presentation. Its most common cause is high spinal anesthesia. Therapy consists of fluid replacement and vasopressors as discussed under hypovolemic and cardiogenic shock.

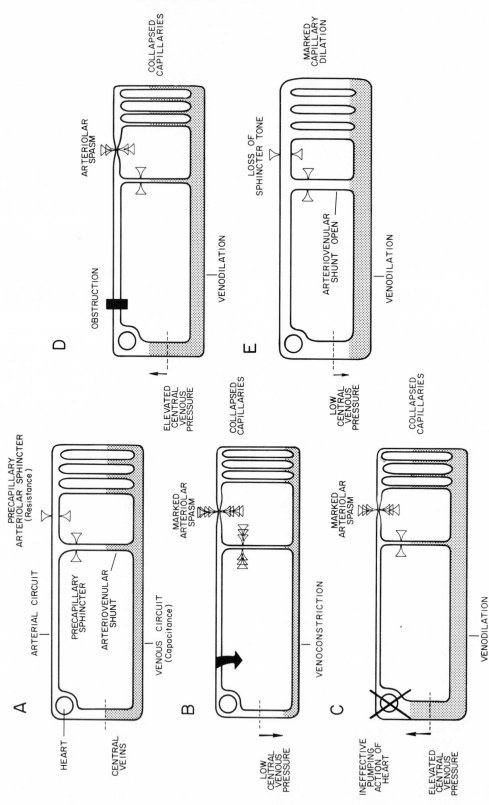

Figure 3.1. Schema of circulatory system: mechanisms of production of shock. **(A)** Normal circulatory system **(B)** Shock due to loss of intravascular volume from hemorrhage, extravasation, anaphylaxis, dehydration or burn **(C)** Cardiogenic shock from myocardial infarction or arrhythmia **(D)** Obstructive shock from pulmonary embolus or pericardial tamponade **(E)** Peripheral shock of septic, anesthetic, or neurogenic origin.

volume. Through these mechanisms, loss of up to 30% of the intravascular fluid can be compensated; however, additional losses or continuing stress at this level for extended periods can lead to rapid deterioration of the clinical status.

HYPOVOLEMIC SHOCK

The classic example of the pattern of derangement and response just described is hypovolemic shock. The fluid lost can be plasma or whole blood with the same effect on circulatory dynamics—or the loss may be more subtle. Dehydration through inadequate fluid intake or excessive sweating, or loss from the stomach or intestine resulting from vomiting or diarrhea can produce significant hypovolemia. Occult blood loss into body cavities, the intestine, or major muscle groups can also lead to shock without overt hemorrhage. Two important clinical objectives, therefore, are recognition of the hypovolemic but compensated patient and detection of occult blood loss in the patient with shock (Table 3.1). The compensated patient whose condition is about to deteriorate can frequently be recognized simply by obtaining orthostatic blood pressure readings (measuring the blood pressure and heart rate with the patient supine and repeating the measurement with the patient seated). Decrease of 10 mm Hg or more in systolic pressure or increase in heart rate of 10 beats/minute or more on assuming the sitting position indicates significant hypovolemia.

Occult bleeding must be sought aggressively. Percussion of the chest for dullness, palpation of the abdomen for rigidity, careful measurement of thigh girths, digital rectal examination and/or nasogastric aspiration with guaiac testing of specimens, paracentesis with peritoneal lavage, and thoracentesis all may be indicated in individual instances.

The clinical laboratory plays a limited but important role in the assessment of the patient with shock. Initial hemoglobin and hematocrit determinations will offer no clues to the magnitude of the blood loss if the process is acute, since hemodilution by the interstitial fluid requires time, but these values serve as valuable baseline information. Arterial blood-gas studies indicate the severity of the acid-base imbalance, and serum lactate levels reflect the degree of anaerobic metabolism. Serum electrolytes and renal function tests provide additional baseline data (it must be remembered that blood in the intestine elevates the blood urea nitrogen level). Typing and crossmatching an appropriate quantity of blood is of utmost importance; Table 3.1 correlates the magnitude of fluid deficit with the clinical status, and may assist in estimating the initial quantity of blood to be ordered.

A valuable adjunct to the treatment of the patient with shock is use of a flow sheet relating laboratory studies, physical data, and therapy to time. Such a chart provides the nursing staff with a convenient, central location for recording information as it is obtained, and it allows the emergency physician and the admitting physician to review at a glance the patient's course in the emergency ward. A sample flow sheet is illustrated in Figure 3.2.

A major aspect of the treatment of patients with shock of any cause is the ongoing monitoring of vital parameters. These observations include vital sign determinations, repeated physical examinations, assessment of the state of the sensorium, hourly monitoring of the urine output via an

Table 3.1.
Correlation of magnitude of volume deficit and clinical presentation.

Approximate Deficit	Decrease in Blood Volume	Shock	
		Degree	Signs
ml	%		
0–500	0–10	None	None
500–1200	10–25	Mild (compensated)	Slight tachycardia
			Postural blood pressure changes
			Mild peripheral vasoconstriction
1200–1800	25–35	Moderate	Thready pulse, 100–120 beats/min
			Blood pressure, 90–100 mm Hg systolic
			Marked vasoconstriction
			Diaphoresis
			Anxiety, restlessness
			Decreased urinary output
1800–2500	35–50	Severe	Thready pulse > 120 beats/min
			Blood pressure < 60 mm Hg systolic
			Marked vasoconstriction
			Marked diaphoresis
			Obtundation
			No urinary output

Patient Assessment

Clinical Observations								Laboratory Values											
Time	Temperature	Pulse	Respirations	Blood Pressure	Mental Status	Urinary Output	Central Venous Pressure	Time	Hgb	Hct	Na^+	K^+	Cl^-	CO_2	BUN	PO_2	PCO_2	pH	Other

Therapy

Volume					Drugs				
Time	Crystalloid	Colloid	Blood Ordered	Blood Administered	Time	Drug	Route	Dose	Rate of Administration

Figure 3.2. Flow sheet used in emergency ward to record data pertaining to patients with shock.

indwelling catheter, evaluation of the pulmonary status via portable chest x-ray films, and monitoring the electrical activity of the heart using a cardioscope. The mental status and urinary output reflect the perfusion of the cerebral cortex and kidney, respectively. In selected patients, the central venous, pulmonary arterial, and the radial artery pressures should be measured since they serve as guides for fluid administration.

Therapy

The measures involved in treating patients with hypovolemic shock include controlling hemorrhage (by direct pressure, tourniquet, MAST, Sengstaken-Blakemore tube, or ligation of bleeders, as examples), establishing and maintaining an airway, assisting ventilation if necessary, supplying oxygen, replacing lost volume, and correcting acid-base or electrolyte disturbances. MAST application and fluid administration are essential therapies for hypovolemic shock and are important in the management of other varieties of shock as well. The role of pressor agents and other vasoactive drugs in the treatment of patients with hemorrhagic shock is always secondary and often is contraindicated.

MAST

An early step in treating hypovolemic shock is the application of MAST (Tables 3.2 and 3.3). MAST has found increasing utilization in the field and in emergency departments in recent years, and now have superseded the G-Suit. MAST is available in several configurations commercially, but is, in essence, a compartmented pneumatic garment designed to be applied to the lower extremities and abdomen. Figure 3.3 illustrates the technique of application. When inflated, the suit applies external compression to the anatomic parts it encircles. In doing so, it produces several benefits: (1) a prompt redistribution of approximately 1 liter of blood from the legs to the central circulation; (2) a reduction in the size of the vascular

Table 3.2.
Indications for the use of MAST.

HYPOVOLEMIC SHOCK ("AUTOTRANSFUSION")
Blood loss (e.g., trauma, gastrointestinal bleeding, leaking abdominal aortic aneurysm, ruptured ectopic pregnancy)

RELATIVE HYPOVOLEMIA
Compression of vascular space (e.g., neurogenic shock, anaphylaxis, drug overdose)

SKELETAL STABILIZATION
(e.g., pelvic or lower extremity fracture)

CONTROL OF HEMORRHAGE IN LOWER EXTREMITIES

Table 3.3.
Contraindications to the use of MAST.

| Absolute |

Pulmonary edema (MAST will increase venous return)

| Relative |

Pregnancy
Suspected splenic injury } May inflate the leg
Dyspnea   chambers only
Head injury   Avoidance of aggravation of cerebral edema

compartment by compression of vessels within the trousers; (3) a tamponading of any bleeding which is ongoing in the parts enclosed; and (4) stabilization of any fractures of the lower extremity which may be present.

The MAST has several benefits in practice: it does not encumber the chest, arms are accessible for intravenous placement, and the pudendal area is left open permitting urethral catheterization and rectal examination. The garments have means of regulating pressure (pop-off valves or gauges), are helpfully color-coded, and have Velcro fasteners for ease of application.

There are however, some disadvantages: once applied, the covered areas become inaccessible to repeat examination. There is some restriction of lung expansion and obvious limitation of movement of the lower extremities.

It is important to note that cyanosis of the feet is expected when the MAST is inflated. This cyanosis is not a reason to remove the garment. Pedal pulses should be palpable, however, since the suit inflates only to 104 mm Hg.

Finally, and of critical importance, the MAST must be deflated carefully. It should never be removed abruptly (and in particular, it should never be cut off), or a precipitous fall in blood pressure will occur. Rather, it should be removed in a stepwise fashion, compartment by compartment, in the reverse order in which it was inflated. MAST is only to be removed in two circumstances: (1) in the operating room where all is in readiness for definitive surgical intervention, or (2) in the emergency room after bleeding has been controlled and the intravascular volume has been repleted. In this latter situation, the deflation is done in a sequential manner with repeated vital signs as each chamber is deflated. If the systolic pressure falls by 5–10 mm Hg at any stage, that compartment should be reinflated and additional fluid administered.

Fluid Administration

The objective of volume expansion is to refill the vascular compartment. This allows the heart

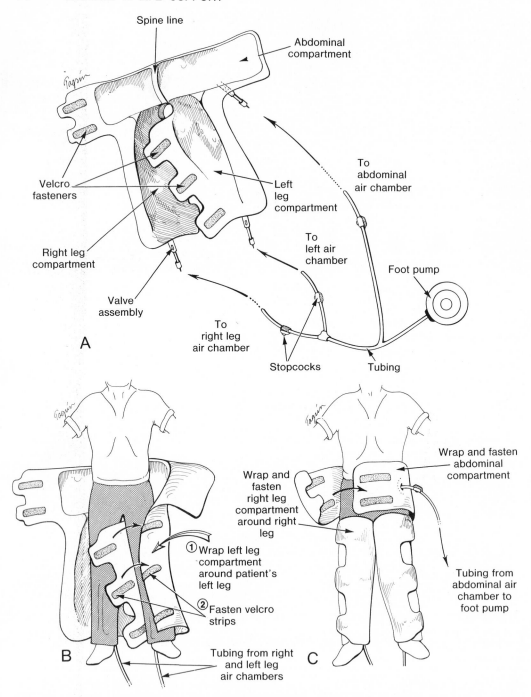

Figure 3.3. **(A)** The garment is opened and spread with the left leg overlying the right, ready to receive the patient. Place patient on garment, supine, with top of abdominal section resting just below the lowest rib. **(B)** Individual compartments are wrapped and secured with Velcro strips, beginning with the left leg, and the tubing is connected to the foot pump. **(C)** After all indicated compartments are closed, the valves are opened and the garment inflated, again beginning with the legs. A pop-off valve or needle gauge regulate the final pressure attained.

to generate adequate cardiac output and to produce enough hydrostatic pressure to perfuse the tissues. The physician has available many types of solutions for fluid therapy, some containing electrolytes only (crystalloids), some containing large molecular weight molecules (colloids), and some containing red blood cells (whole blood or packed cells). The reasons for choosing one fluid instead of another are important, and the choice is governed by the clinical situation.

Two generalizations can be made about fluid replacement therapy: first, any fluid will improve perfusion, at least transiently; and second, only red blood cells carry significant amounts of oxygen. Fluid should be administered via a short, large-bore, indwelling cannula or cannulas; the central venous pressure line should not be used for administration of red blood cells. The amount of fluid administered depends on the clinical presentation of the patient. If the deficit has existed for some time, it is necessary to replenish both the intravascular fluid and some of the interstitial fluid. The rate of administration is governed by the rapidity of the ongoing bleeding and the magnitude of the pre-existing loss.

The central venous pressure as a guide to fluid administration is most dependable in patients with hypovolemic shock without complications. If primary myocardial dysfunction is suspected, central venous pressure readings may be deceptive and pulmonary arterial pressure measurements may be indicated (see Chapter 1, pages 16–17). In all patients, the central venous pressure measurement should be supplemented with repeated auscultation of the chest and serial chest x-ray films during vigorous fluid replacement.

Selection of Replacement Fluid. As noted previously, the selection of a solution for correcting hypovolemia is of considerable importance. It is also the subject of heated debate. Logically, blood lost would be replaced with blood. In practice, however, there are available safer and less expensive solutions which can be used to correct mild to moderate deficits. Asanguineous replacement solutions, crystalloids and colloids, both have had extensive clinical use, but, remarkably, controversy still surrounds their selection.

The debate hinges on which fluid is more likely to produce interstitial pulmonary edema when administered in quantity. Crystalloids, as mentioned, are small molecules, and can rapidly escape from the vascular space into the interstitium to produce peripheral and pulmonary edema. Consequently, their volume-expansion effect is relatively short-lived. Colloids, in contrast, are macromolecular polymers, and leave the circulation less readily. Their presence increases the plasma oncotic pressure which allows them to attract water

from the interstitium, actually producing intravascular volume expansion in an increment above that which is administered. Their large size means that they remain in the circulation longer than the crystalloids.

The reverse of this coin is that when colloids ultimately do escape the circulation, and they do so faster when capillary damage exists, they raise the interstitial oncotic pressure in similar fashion and draw water back into the perivascular spaces. Obviously, if the interstitium in question is the pulmonary interstitium, this can lead to a particularly resistant type of pulmonary edema. There is currently no conclusive evidence that the type of fluid used in volume resuscitation influences the development of pulmonary complications.

Crystalloids. For these reasons, crystalloids are the mainstay of asanguineous fluid replacement therapy. Those commonly employed are normal saline and lactated Ringer's solution. Both are "balanced" (isotonic with the extracellular fluid), and there is no compelling reason to choose one over the other (Table 3.4). The sodium lactate in lactated Ringer's solution does not contribute to lactic acidosis. Crystalloids are nonallergenic, have no potential to produce a hypotensive reaction, and are virus free. They are much less expensive than the colloidal solutions. Glucose-containing solutions should be avoided if concurrent blood transfusions are anticipated.

Colloids. There are currently four colloidal solutions available for clinical use: dextran, hetastarch, plasma protein fraction, and preparations of serum albumin.

Dextran. One of the solutions is a polysaccharide (polymer of glucose) available in two formats—high molecular weight (dextran-70, a 6% solution with an average molecular weight in the 70–75,000 range) and low molecular weight (dextran-40, a 10% solution averaging 40,000). Both dextran preparations offer low cost and effective volume expansion. Dextran-70 remains in the vascular bed 2–3 days and dextran-40 lasts for 12–18 hours. A red-cell and platelet-coating effect occurs, advocated as a beneficial antisludging effect.

However, serious difficulties considerably limit the usefullness of dextran. Dextran can cause anaphylactic reactions, and renal failure has been attributed to its use. Dextran-70 impairs platelet and fibrinogen function, and can cause a bleeding diathesis if more than 1 liter is administered. Obviously, this limits its use as a replacement fluid. Of even more import, dextran can agglutinate red blood cells, making subsequent crossmatching impossible.

Hetastarch. A new colloidal plasma volume expander recently introduced into clinical practice is hetastarch. Hetastarch (Hespan) is an artificial

Table 3.4.
Composition of commonly employed crystalloid solutions.

Solution	Combination	Nonelectrolyte Constituent	gm/100 ml	Cation[a]				Anion[a]	
				Na	K	Ca	Mg	Cl	Bicarbonate as Lactate
0.45% sodium chloride injection, i.e., half-normal saline				77				77	
0.9% sodium chloride, i.e., normal saline (Sodium Chloride Injection, USP)				154				154	
Dextrose in water (Dextrose Injection, USP)	With 5% dextrose	Dextrose	5.0						
Ringer's Lactated Injection, USP				130	4	3		109	28

[a] mEq/liter.

polymer derived from the waxy starch amylopectin and closely resembles glycogen. It has a molecular weight averaging 450,000 and, consequently, provides a long-lasting volume expansion effect (being detectable in the circulation 24–36 hours after administration). It is supplied as a 6% solution in normal saline.

Hetastarch in large volumes alters coagulation, but does not produce clinically significant hemostatic problems in therapeutic doses. Unlike dextran, it does not interfere with subsequent blood typing and crossmatching. Hetastarch is relatively nonallergenic, having a reaction rate similar to that for albumin. It is, however, significantly less expensive than albumin.

At this writing, clinical experience with hetastarch is limited. It seems to be a promising addition to available therapy, but has yet to stand the test of time.

Plasma Protein Fraction. This is a readily prepared plasma derivative, a 5% protein solution containing at least 83% albumin. It includes α- and β-globulins and is essentially plasma with fibrinogen and γ-globulins removed. It is heat treated to inactivate hepatitis virus, and is inexpensive, but it also has a serious disadvantage. Probably due to contained kinins or their precursors, plasma protein fraction can cause hypotensive reactions. Because of this potential complication, it cannot be recommended for the treatment of hypotension.

Serum Albumin. This is available as a 5 or 25% solution. The former is an effective plasma volume expander, the latter is a more potent elevator of plasma oncotic pressure. Both are stabilized and heat treated to kill hepatitis virus. They have a lower incidence of serious allergic reactions, have no deleterious effect upon hemostasis, and do not produce a paradoxical hypotensive effect. Therefore, unlike dextran, the volume of albumin which may be transfused is not restricted. However, the albumin preparations are expensive.

Beyond expense, however, several recent studies have called into question the use of albumin. There is evidence that albumin has a negative inotropic effect, causes excessive salt retention, and alters coagulation such that blood requirements are increased. Nevertheless, albumin has a long track record of clinical effectiveness and safety.

Given this controversy, the following guidelines provide a practical approach to the treatment of hypovolemic shock: (1) establish at least two short, large-bore intravenous lines; (2) obtain blood for typing and crossmatching (in an appropriate number of units for the clinical situation); (3) regard crystalloid as the keystone of therapy, begin an infusion of saline or lactated Ringer's, giving 2–3 liters over the first 20–30 minutes; (4) carefully monitor vital signs and pulmonary status after every 200 ml infused.

If time and facilities permit, place a central line and obtain serial pressure readings. The clinical objective is a systolic blood pressure over 90. If there is an inadequate clinical response to 2–3 liters of crystalloid, 5% albumin may be added in a 1:1 ratio. By this time, whole blood or packed red blood cells should be available to provide oxygen-carrying capacity.

Blood Transfusion. Currently, blood is the only practical solution that transports a significant amount of oxygen, so it is ultimately required in profound blood loss. Traditionally, whole blood was advocated for the treatment of patients with hemorrhagic shock under the compelling logic of matching the fluid administered to the fluid lost. Current practice, however, favors administration of packed red blood cells together with a crystalloid or colloid solution or both. This practice reflects standard blood bank procedure in which drawn blood is immediately fractionated into platelets, plasma, and packed red cells. It reduces the risk of hepatitis by reducing the volume of plasma transfused. Additionally, it prevents microembolization to the lungs by white blood cells and platelets which can aggregate in stored whole blood, and it reduces the possibility of stimulating the host's immunologic system by transfused white blood cells. These objections to whole blood are relative, and whole blood should be used if transfusion is indicated and packed cells are unavailable.

Ideally, adequate time exists or can be gained to permit the patient's blood to be typed and fully crossmatched. If, however, exsanguination or irreversible shock seems imminent, complete matching cannot be accomplished and compromises must be made (Table 3.5). The best choice in the urgent situation is type-specific blood, which is available in minutes and which avoids the incompatibility reactions of the ABO blood group. Type-specific blood is preferable to O-negative (universal donor) blood for several reasons: type O Rh-negative blood is not available in many blood banks, there is an increasing incidence of significant titers of anti-A and anti-B antibodies in O-negative donors, and transfusion of large amounts of type O blood can make subsequent typing and crossmatching of the patient's blood impossible. If type O-negative blood is used, only blood from donors with low titers of anti-A and anti-B antibodies or O-negative packed red blood cells suspended in AB plasma or saline should be transfused.

If 15 minutes more are available, saline cross-matching can be carried out in addition to typing. This permits determination of the Rh factor and detects strong antibodies of the minor blood groups (for example, anti-Kell), avoiding severe reactions.

It is preferable to use the freshest blood possible, since stored blood undergoes many undesirable changes (Table 3.6). Labile coagulation factors degenerate, platelets become nonfunctional, the blood becomes acidic, and 2,3-diphosphoglycerate levels decrease in the red blood cells (see Chapter 1, page 8). Much like lactate, the high citrate

Table 3.5.
Time required for blood typing procedures.

Blood Bank Activity	Time Required
Release O-negative blood (no testing)	1 minute
Issue type specific blood (group and type recipient's blood)	15 minutes
Carry out saline and albumin crossmatches	30 minutes
Finish complete crossmatch (regroup, retype, carry out saline, Coombs, and albumin crossmatches, screen recipient's blood for antibodies)	45 minutes

Table 3.6.
Some potentially deleterious effects of massive transfusion of stored blood.

Volume related
  Transmission of disease
  Immunologic mismatch
  Immunization of recipient

Rate and volume related
  Altered hemoglobin affinity for oxygen
  Coagulation abnormalities
  Acid-base imbalance
  Citrate toxicity
  Hypothermia
  Microembolization
  Impaired red blood cells deformability
  Infusion of plasticizers
  Infusion of denatured proteins
  Infusion of vasoactive substances
  Elevated potassium, phosphate, ammonia levels
  Hemolyzed blood products
  Impaired antibacterial defenses
  Graft-vs.-host reactions
  Toxicity of new additives

(Reprinted by permission, from Collins JA: Problems associated with the massive transfusion of stored blood. *Surgery* 75:274–295, 1974.)

content of preserved blood is metabolized by the liver to bicarbonate once circulation is restored, and this can produce metabolic alkalosis after resuscitation. Banked blood is also hypocalcemic, since citrate binds calcium.

In the case of massive transfusion, a blood warmer should be used to defend the core temperature and the heat-sensitive coagulation mechanism. To avoid platelet washout, 4 platelet packs should be transfused after every 4 units of blood. Fresh frozen plasma, containing clotting factors, should be administered in the ratio of 2 units for every 10 units of packed cells. Calcium gluconate is probably not necessary.

In summary, specific therapy for hypovolemic shock involves control of hemorrhage and administration of appropriate volume expanders. The application of external pneumatic compression devices like the MAST are of value while the volume is being replaced or while the patient is being transported to the operating room. Pressor agents are rarely, if ever, indicated in treating hypovolemic shock. The pharmacologic agents which may occasionally be employed are discussed in the following section.

CARDIOGENIC SHOCK

The second major division of the shock state is cardiogenic shock, in which failure to perfuse tissues adequately is a consequence of impairment of cardiac pumping, not loss of intravascular fluid volume. Impaired pumping ability of the heart may result from destruction of contractile elements, as in myocardial infarction, or from disruption of the normal conduction sequence, as in heart blocks or arrhythmia. The result of these pathologic mechanisms is decreased cardiac output, the fundamental physiologic defect in cardiogenic shock. Thus, in contrast to hypovolemic shock, the central venous pressure and the pulmonary capillary wedge pressure typically are elevated in cardiogenic shock.

While not strictly cardiac, several other disease entities also produce reduction in cardiac output, and the shock that results can be considered with cardiogenic shock. These states include: obstructive processes such as dissecting aortic aneurysm, vena caval occlusion, intracardiac tumors, and valvular heart disease; and restrictive processes such as pericardial tamponade. Attention in this chapter will focus on the most common situation—cardiogenic shock after myocardial infarction as a model for the approach to therapy.

Cardiogenic shock has been defined formally by a set of clinical criteria to facilitate comparison of therapeutic results. These diagnostic criteria include: systolic pressure less than 80 mm Hg; cardiac index less than 2.1 liters/min/m^2; urinary output less than 20 ml/hr; diminished cerebral perfusion as evidenced by confusion or obtundation; and cool, damp, mottled skin characteristic of the low output state. Thus defined, cardiogenic shock is the most lethal variety of shock. It occurs as a complication of 15% of myocardial infarcts, and the resultant mortality ranges from 70–90%. Among patients who fail to respond to the initial conventional measures of treatment and who have no surgically correctable lesion, the mortality approaches 100%. This grim prognosis, which has improved little in the past decade, has spawned the development of specialized investigational units and exploration of many aggressive therapeutic models. These include intra-aortic balloon counter-pulsation, coronary recanalization procedures, acute-phase bypass procedures, and heart transplantation. The role of the emergency physician is to recognize the situation, to institute stabilization measures, and to ensure transport of the patient to the appropriate treatment facility in that hospital or geographic area.

Barring the appearance of arrhythmias or blocks, the development of cardiogenic shock is a function of the location and size of the infarct. Typically, shock occurs when more than 40% of the left ventricular myocardium is involved. Onset of the shock syndrome occurs within the first 24 hours after infarction in 70% of patients and by 72 hours in 90%.

General Principles of Therapy

Basic therapy is the same as for other forms of shock—establishment of an airway, ventilation, oxygenation, relief of pain, correction of acidosis, and positioning the patient. However, derangement of ventilation-perfusion ratios may be exaggerated because of pulmonary edema and microembolization (see Chapter 1, pages 6–8). Scrupulous attention to pulmonary status is even more important in this variety of shock. The cardiac rhythm must, of course, be monitored, since the heart receives the double insult of the initiating infarct and the shock syndrome with poor coronary artery perfusion, hypoxia, and acidosis. These all depress the myocardium further and favor the development of arrhythmias. Specific therapy for cardiogenic shock centers on the objective of increasing cardiac output (see Chapter 1, Section on Cardiac Output). In the Emergency Ward, there are three possible ways to improve cardiac output. First, intravascular volume can be increased modestly to elevate the cardiac preload; this stretches the myocardial fibers at the end of diastole, amplifying left ventricular stroke work. Second, the force of the myocardial contraction can be increased with drugs. Third, the afterload against which the heart must pump can be decreased by lowering the peripheral resistance. In practice, these techniques may be applied in various combinations either simultaneously or sequentially.

Optimize the Preload

Patients in cardiogenic shock are often actually or relatively hypovolemic because of pain-induced reflex vasodilation, reduced oral intake, vomiting, sweating, or drug therapy with nitrates or morphine. In addition, the damaged left ventricle shifts to a different Starling curve (see Chapter 1), one which functions better at filling pressures above normal. Thus, if an adequate stroke volume is to be produced, a fluid push is needed to achieve a pulmonary capillary wedge pressure in the 16- to 20-mm Hg range.

However, the same myocardial dysfunction which puts these patients in shock renders them extremely sensitive to volume overload and makes them prone to the development of pulmonary vascular congestion. Close monitoring of this phase of volume expansion is consequently essential. As noted previously, this is a situation in which central venous pressure measurement is notoriously undependable and, therefore, repeated physical examinations, chest x-rays and the data gained from a Swan-Ganz pulmonary artery catheter and an arterial line are most valuable.

Volume expansion has traditionally been accomplished by the administration of intravenous fluids. Colloids such as low molecular-weight dextran are appropriate, but this would seem to be an ideal indication for 25% salt-poor albumin because a small volume administered produces a potent oncotic effect and proportionately greater intravascular volume expansion.

An alternative approach is the application of MAST. By compressing the lower extremities and the abdomen, the MAST instantly autotransfuses the patient with up to 1 liter of the most physiologic solution possible, his or her own blood. And, unlike the situation with infused fluid, the MAST-induced autotransfusion is rapidly reversible.

Improve the Inotropic State of the Myocardium

If the response to volume expansion is inadequate, pharmacologic agents may be employed. A number of categories of drugs have been advocated for this indication over the years, including vasopressors, digitalis glycosides, sympathomimetic cardiac stimulants, adrenergic blocking agents, and corticosteroids. Protocols have come and gone for the use of various drugs, and the issue remains controversial.

Catecholamines are the drugs most commonly utilized in the treatment of cardiogenic shock. They act by stimulating myocardial and vascular smooth muscle receptors (Table 3.7). Catecholamines are subdivided by the specific receptors they stimulate. These receptor sites are designated α (capable of peripheral vasoconstriction when stimulated), β_1 (cardiac stimulation), and β_2 (peripheral vasodilation). Specific amines have the ability to stimulate one or another receptor with varying degrees of specificity. Methoxamine, for example, is a pure α stimulant, whereas isoproterenol is strictly a β agent. Most drugs affect different receptors quantitatively in varying degrees with cardiac and peripheral effects occurring in inverse proportion. The potent cardiac stimulants are also potent arrhythmogenic agents.

Dopamine is exceptional in its ability to contort itself into shapes fitting a number of receptor sites, including unique (dopaminergic) splanchnic and renal bed vasodilating receptors.

It is important to understand that the use of sympathetic amines in the immediate postinfarct period is a double-edged sword: the drugs may be beneficial in maintaining blood pressure at a level adequate to perfuse the coronary arteries in the tissues, but this improved perfusion may be obtained at the expense of increased myocardial oxygen consumption and extension of the infarct.

α **Agents.** Pure or predominantly α drugs such as methoxamine and phenylephrine, once the keystone of shock therapy, rarely are used to treat cardiogenic shock. The peripheral vasoconstriction they produce may elevate the blood pressure, but it does so at the expense of increased cardiac work, and actually decreases cardiac output, impairing tissue perfusion. These pressors may have limited utility as stopgap measures to maintain coronary artery circulation while other modalities are readied (e.g., the intra-aortic balloon pump), and they may be indicated for the treatment of neurogenic shock. In general, however, the agents listed in the following sections are more appropriate in this setting.

Mixed Agents. Drugs with both α- and β-stimulating properties have been used widely in the therapy of shock states. Included in this group are epinephrine (discussed in Chapter 2, page 33), norepinephrine, and dopamine.

Norepinephrine is a potent α- and weaker β-stimulant which constricts both venous capacitance vessels and arteriolar resistance vessels, and also stimulates the heart. The net result is that cardiac output either remains the same or is de-

Table 3.7.
Some sympathomimetic amines commonly used in shoch.

Drug	Usual IV Dosage[a]	Adrenergic Effects		Arrhythmogenic Potential	Comments
		α	β (Cardiac)		
Norepinephrine (Levophed)	2–8 μgm/min	Small dosages Moderate Large dosages Marked	Minimal Moderate	Moderate	Despite β-adrenergic effects, may cause reflex slowing of heart rate because of increase in blood pressure
Epinephrine (Adrenalin)	1–4 μgm/min	Small dosages Minimal Large dosages Moderate	Moderate Marked	Marked	May cause tremor and anxiety
Dopamine (Intropin)	2–10 μgm/kg/min	Small dosages Minimal Large dosages Marked	Minimal Moderate	Moderate to marked	Exhibits a unique "dopaminergic" effect increasing renal blood flow at dosages of <6 μgm/kg/min; may cause nausea and vomiting
Metaraminol (Aramine)	8–15 μgm/kg/min	Small dosages Minimal Large dosages Moderate	Minimal Moderate	Moderate	Appears to act in part by activating release of endogenous catecholamines
Isoproterenol (Isuprel)	0.5–4 μgm/min	Pure β-receptor stimulation		Marked	May cause tremor and anxiety
Methoxamine (Vasoxyl)	8–15 μgm/kg/min	Pure α-receptor stimulation		None	Of particular value in shock patients who have good cardiac function and low peripheral resistance
Phenylephrine (Neo-synephrine)	5–20 μgm/min	Predominantly α-receptor stimulation		None	
Dobutamine (Dobutrex)	2.5–10.0 μgm/kg/min	Predominantly stimulates myocardial β-receptors responsible for inotropy		Minimal	Minimal chronotropic and peripheral vasoconstrictor effects; especially useful in cardiogenic shock

[a] The usual objective of therapy is to raise the systolic pressure to 90–100 mm Hg; larger or smaller dosages may be required in any given case.

Modified by permission, from DeSanctis RW: In: Rubenstein E, Federman DD (eds): *Scientific American Medicine.* New York, Scientific American, 1980.

creased slightly and that mean arterial blood pressure is increased. By stimulating the heart and supporting diastolic blood pressure, norepinephrine enhances coronary artery perfusion. Thus, it differs from the pure α agents in improving coronary blood flow as well as increasing cardiac work. Administration of norepinephrine leads to a decrease in myocardial lactate production, reflecting the improved perfusion. Renal, splanchnic, skeletomuscular, and cutaneous blood flow are all decreased, but cerebral perfusion is augmented. Norepinephrine may be administered in hemorrhagic shock and is indicated in cardiogenic shock characterized by profound hypotension. The therapeutic objective is to produce a blood pressure in the 80- to 100-mm Hg range, not to restore the pressure to its preinfarction level. In general, however, better understanding of the underlying pathophysiology of cardiogenic shock has resulted in a decreasing reliance on norepinephrine in favor of vasodilating drugs to reduce afterload.

Dopamine is another mixed agent which has the unique property, mentioned previously, of dilating mesenteric and renal beds, thereby protecting the kidneys. This increases its utility. Dopamine is remarkably dose dependent in its effects. At low dose ranges (1–2 μgm/kg/min), the dopaminergic (renal and mesenteric dilatation) effect is seen without cardiac stimulation or pressor response. In intermediate dose ranges (2–10 μgm/kg/min), dopamine's β (cardiac stimulant) effect predominates. In this regard, dopamine is less potent than isoproterenol and dobutamine, but it does increase cardiac output. At progressively higher infusion rates, (10–20 μgm/kg/min), the α-stimulating effect of dopamine becomes more prominent, producing peripheral vasoconstriction (even to the point of reversing the dopaminergic effect at rates above 20 μgm/kg/min). At these high levels, there is also a corresponding increase in the cardiac stimulating effect.

In practice, the infusion is begun in the 2- to 5-μgm/kg/min range and increased cautiously, noting response of blood pressure and urine output. The principal limitations to dopamine's use are its tendency to produce undesirable tachycardias and the propensity to excessive vasoconstriction at high dosage levels. Dopamine is inactivated in alkaline solutions and it should not be administered in the same line as sodium bicarbonate. Dopamine works partly by release of endogenous catecholamines and may be less reliable in patients who are depleted of this substance (as in a patient previously treated with reserpine).

Pure β Agents. Isoproterenol is a pure β-stimulant that increases the heart rate and the strength of myocardial contraction while producing considerable peripheral vasodilatation. This seemingly desirable combination produces some unfortunate results. The peripheral vasodilation is nonselective; blood flow to nonessential organs, such as the skin and skeletal muscles, increases. This occurs partly at the expense of the renal circulation, the proportion of cardiac output that reaches the kidneys decreasing. Moreover, as vasodilation lowers the diastolic pressure, coronary artery perfusion suffers, and myocardial lactate production increases. In effect then, isoproterenol stimulates the heart while simultaneously diminishing the myocardial blood supply. The main indication for its use is the shock syndrome with only mild hypotension; in this situation, it can be administered alone or with another pressor agent to coax and increase cardiac output. All β drugs have a strong potential to produce arrhythmias.

The newest catecholamine to be approved for use in cardiogenic shock, dobutamine has unique and attractive features. It is primarily a potent β_1 (inotropic) stimulant, on a par with isoproterenol in this regard. However, it has much less ability to dilate the periphery, hence there is virtually no reflex tachycardia with its use (when administered in 2.5- to 10-μgm/kg/min range). Furthermore, dobutamine has essentially no α (peripheral vasoconstrictive) effect, and a low potential for arrhythmia production. Thus, as a selective inotropic agent capable of raising cardiac output and blood pressure, it appears to be the drug of choice in treating cardiogenic shock.

Digitalis Glycosides. Other than catecholamines, the drugs which are useful in cardiogenic shock are few. Digitalis glycosides have been demonstrated to have little utility in the acute phase of cardiogenic shock. Indeed, awareness of the potential for digitalis toxicity is an important factor. However, survivors of the cardiogenic shock state are likely to require digitalization in subacute and chronic phases.

Reduction of the Afterload

As noted in Chapter 1 (pages 13–17), the cardiac output is in large measure dependent on the afterload of the heart when the heart has sustained injury. Consequently, after the preload has been optimized and efforts have been made to improve the inotropic status of the heart, the remaining variable which can be manipulated is the afterload. The damaged heart appears to be exquisitely sensitive to alterations in the afterload. Consequently, various vasodilators, alone or in combination with sympathetic amines, have been employed in treating hypotension in the setting of myocardial damage. This is done in an effort to decrease vascular impedance, promote ventricular emptying, and thereby lower filling pressure of the heart.

Sodium Nitroprusside. The obvious concern in this regard is to avoid further lowering of the blood pressure and reduce tissue perfusion. Because of its rapid onset and rapid inactivation, the vasodilator of choice in cardiogenic shock is presently sodium nitroprusside. If doses are titrated properly, it is often possible to improve tissue perfusion, to enhance cardiac output enough to offset the reduction in total peripheral resistance, and to maintain systemic blood pressure without triggering reflex tachycardia.

Sodium nitroprusside is unstable when in solution; it must be constituted at the time of its use by mixing 50 mg of powder with 250–1000 ml of D5W. Having done that, it must be shielded from the light during infusion by wrapping the bottle and tubing with some opaque material, usually aluminum foil. To ensure accuracy of its delivery, it is best administered with an infusion pump.

Vasodilator therapy is particularly effective in treating cardiogenic shock with an element of congestive failure. In this situation, venodilatation reduces right heart return and enhances ventricular emptying. In doing so, it drops the left ventricular end-diastolic pressure and alleviates pulmonary congestion.

In the difficult clinical situation of simultaneously developing hypotension and congestive failure (in the postinfarct state), the combination of dobutamine and nitroprusside, each used as described previously, offers a logical and sometimes effective approach.

Other Modalities

The effectiveness of corticosteroids remains unproved in cardiogenic shock. They are recommended as vasodilators but other agents are considerably more effective for this indication; and, certainly, more potent cardiac stimulants exist. Whether corticosteroids stabilize cellular organelles is unclear. Advocates suggest their use prophylactically asserting that some percentage of the population may be subclinically adrenally deficient and, therefore, unable to meet the stress of an acute illness. In this regard, a single bolus of 40–50 mg/kg of hydrocortisone intravenously may be administered.

Invasive approaches available for treating cardiogenic shock include the intra-aortic balloon pump primarily used in supporting a patient with a surgically reparable cause of shock, such as ruptured chordae tendineae or intraventricular septal defects, in the preoperative period. Efforts have been made to reopen occluded coronary arteries mechanically or with drugs such as streptokinase. Advocates of performing coronary artery bypass grafts in the acute postinfarct stage have demonstrated some improvement in survival statistics. All of these procedures deserve further exploration and hold some promise, but at this time, are experimental and their use should be confined to specialized centers. Cardiogenic shock remains a potentially lethal condition.

SEPTIC SHOCK

The third major type of shock is septic shock, in which hypoperfusion of tissues results from the action of bacterial toxins on the circulatory system. Until recently, bacteremic shock was virtually synonymous with gram-negative sepsis, and was seen principally in newborns, women after septic abortions, the elderly, and the debilitated. Several factors have modified this epidemiologic pattern: intravenous drug abuse has increased, and with it, the introduction of unusual organisms into the circulation of addicts; the increased availability of legal, professionally performed abortions has reduced the frequency of sepsis after this procedure; and progress in treating previously fatal disorders has increased the number of compromised hosts in the general population. Compromised hosts include patients receiving cancer chemotherapy, corticosteroids, and other immunosuppressive drugs, patients who have had splenectomy, and patients with advanced or debilitating disease such as cirrhosis, nephrosis, diabetes, and severe burns. In persons with impaired defenses, usually innocuous agents such as *Candida albicans* can become deadly pathogens. Furthermore, the intensive use of potent antibiotics in clinical care has resulted in the development of drug-resistant bacterial strains in the hospital setting. Venipuncture, venous and arterial cannulation, and indwelling prosthetic devices give these organisms access to the circulation.

Although the epidemiologic and microbiologic aspects of septic shock have changed, the mortality remains high, ranging from 50–80% in reported series. In part, this reflects the nature of the population at risk and, in part, the refractoriness of the disease process itself.

The pathophysiologic development of bacteremic shock is complex and incompletely elucidated. Two hemodynamic phases occur. Initially, peripheral resistance falls, heart rate and cardiac output rise (but not enough to offset the drop in total peripheral resistance), and the blood pressure cannot be maintained. In this hyperdynamic or warm stage, the skin is pink and dry, and the patient is likely to be alkalotic, secondary to hyperventilation. Later, peripheral vasoconstriction develops and the cardiac output falls. The patient then assumes the classic picture of shock with cool clammy skin, cyanosis, and the development of lactic acidosis.

The tendency toward hypotension is further exacerbated by impaired capillary integrity and the loss of fluid from the vascular compartment to the interstitium.

The mechanism appears to be the following: a septic focus or blood-borne bacterial infection releases lipopolysaccharide endotoxins into the circulation. These activate factors in the coagulation and complement sequences which generate vasoactive kinins and trigger the intrinsic coagulation system. Consequently, the clinical picture of decreased total peripheral resistance, increased capillary permeability, and disseminated intravascular coagulation with fibrinolysis occur. The activation of the complement cascade further increases capillary permeability and impairs antibody function. The switchover from vasodilation to vasoconstriction may correspond to an early rise in the vasodilating prostaglandin E_2 and a subsequent appearance of the vasoconstricting prostaglandin $F_{2\alpha}$. As a further insult, myocardial function falters several hours into the septic shock syndrome with a rising left ventricular end-diastolic pressure. This deterioration occurs in association with shifts in calcium ion, but the bacterial endotoxins responsible for the development of septic shock may themselves be injurious to the myocardium.

Therapy

The general therapeutic measures discussed for hypovolemic and cardiogenic shock—establishment of an airway, oxygenation, ventilation, monitoring, correction of acidosis, volume expansion, and administration of vasoactive agents as needed to maintain coronary and cerebral perfusion—apply to septic shock as well. The efficacy of corticosteroids remains controversial. Specific therapy for bacteremic shock involves antibiotic administration and surgical intervention when indicated (for example, drainage of an abscess or removal of an obstruction).

Pretreatment Assessment

The choice of an antibiotic presents problems since the urgency of the patient's condition frequently demands institution of therapy before the causative organism can be cultured and identified. The emergency physician in this situation has two responsibilities. First, one must ensure that all appropriate specimens are correctly obtained and processed for microbiologic evaluation. Second, one must elicit whatever history is available, carry out a thorough physical examination, order those laboratory studies yielding immediate results, and formulate an estimate regarding the identity of the causative organism.

The patient's prognosis correlates with his cardiac output. If the cardiac output is greater than 3½ liters/min, survival rates are greater than 60%. If the cardiac output is less than 3.0 liters/min, mortality approaches 100%.

Typical specimens for culture include serial blood samples, urine, sputum, cerebrospinal fluid, and purulent aspirates or drainage. The classic history in patients with septic shock includes a shaking chill leading to prostration. However, to aid in identifying the organism, the physician must seek a description of antecedent symptoms such as cough or dysuria, or history of underlying disease, drug abuse, alcohol consumption, medications taken, and recent medical instrumentation or surgical procedures. Family interviews, hospital chart reviews, and consultation with other physicians who have treated the patient may provide valuable data. In general, the answers to two questions are sought: Is the patient in any way a compromised host? Are there sufficient clues to localize the inciting infectious process?

The problem for the emergency physician in selecting initial therapy may be less difficult than for the physician dealing with hospitalized patients. The latter is more likely to encounter the unusual or antibiotic-resistant organisms common in the hospital setting. However, it must be reiterated that there are drug addicts and compromised hosts in the population who may be seen in the emergency ward with infections caused by atypical organisms.

Physical examination must be detailed. Inspection of the skin may reveal telltale needle tracks, septic emboli, abscesses, or characteristic eruptions such as those seen in ecthyma gangrenosum caused by *Pseudomonas*. Nuchal rigidity, tenderness of the costovertebral angle, lymphadenopathy, auscultatory evidence of pneumonia or pleural effusions, and localized abdominal tenderness, guarding, or masses are some of the critical observations on physical examination.

Important laboratory studies whose results are rapidly available include a complete blood count, routine urinalysis, and Gram stains of the urine (unspun), cerebrospinal fluid, sputum, and purulent discharges. Chest x-ray films, abdominal x-ray films, or other specialized radiologic studies may also aid in localizing the infectious process.

Of particular importance is the Gram stain because it offers the only real opportunity to identify specific organisms definitively before receiving culture results. Although their results will not be available immediately, a battery of coagulation studies should be ordered.

Table 3.8.
Bacteremia: Common initiating infections and probable pathogens.

Anatomic Site and Condition	Pathogens Likely in Unmodified Host	Possible Complicating Factors	Additional Organisms to Be Considered in Compromised Host
Respiratory tract			
Pneumonia	*Hemophilus influenzae* (children <6 years; adults with chronic obstructive pulmonary disease)	Pneumococcus Aspiration, alcoholism	*Escherichia coli*, Bacteroides, Klebsiella-Enterobacter-Serratia, oral flora
	Staphylococcus aureus (especially after influenza) Group A streptococci	Nosocomial infection (tracheostomy, ventilatory assistance)	*Pseudomonas aeruginosa*, Klebsiella-Enterobacter-Serratia, Herellea species, *E. coli*
Pulmonary abscess	Bacteroides Fusospirochetes Anaerobic streptococci } after aspiration		
	Klebsiella S. aureus } progression from necrotizing pneumonia		
Empyema	Bacteroides Fusospirochetes Anaerobic streptococci } after aspiration		
	Intestinal flora (progression from subdiaphragmatic process)		
Central nervous system			
Meningitis	Pneumococcus (direct extension from otitis or sinusitis; bacteremia from lung) Meningococcus *H. influenzae* (6 months to 6 years) *E. coli* and other enteric gram-negative organisms (newborns)	Immunosuppression, debilitation, neurosurgical procedure, head trauma	Gram-negative bacilli, staphylococcus, streptococcus
Peritoneal cavity			
Peritonitis of intestinal origin (appendicitis, diverticulitis)	*Bacteroides fragilis* *E. coli*		
Intraperitoneal abscess	Proteus species Other gram-negative bacilli Enterococcus (aerobic group D streptococcus)		

Site / Disease	Organisms	Predisposing factors	Organisms in special circumstances
Biliary tree and liver			
Cholangitis	E. coli		
Cholecystitis	Proteus species Klebsiella-Enterobacter-Serratia		
Urinary tract			
Acute pyelonephritis	E. coli Enterococcus Proteus mirabilis Other Proteus species Other gram-negative organisms (Citrobacter, Enterobacter, Klebsiella)	Recurrent, treated urinary tract infection, instrumentation	E. coli, Klebsiella-Enterobacter-Serratia, Proteus species, P. aeruginosa, enterococcus
Genitalia			
Pelvic inflammatory disease	Neisseria gonorrhoeae Intestinal flora (Bacteroides, E. coli, groups A, B, and C streptococci)	Instrumentation, abortion, postpartum sepsis	Bacteroides species, clostridia, anaerobic streptococci
Urethritis	N. gonorrhoeae		
Toxic shock syndrome	S. aureus	Prolonged use of super absorbent tampon	
Bones and joints			
Septic arthritis	N. gonorrhoeae Meningococcus S. aureus Pneumococcus Streptococcus	Pediatric age group Debilitation, drug addiction	H. influenzae Gram-negative bacilli
Osteomyelitis	S. aureus	Drug addiction	Pseudomonas
Skin and subcutaneous tissues	S. aureus Group A steptococci	Traumatic and surgical wounds Immunosuppression, burns	Gram-negative bacilli, clostridia, anaerobic streptococci Gram-negative bacilli, P. aeruginosa, Herellea species, Serratia
Cardiovascular system			
Acute bacterial endocarditis	S. aureus Enterococcus	Drug addiction	Gram-negative bacilli
Other		Venous cutdown, indwelling catheter, intracardiac pacemaker	S. aureus, Streptococcus epidermidis, P. aeruginosa, Herellea species, Serratia

While it is true that it is urgent to institute antibiotic therapy, it is also true that the interval between presentation and institution of treatment may represent the only chance to obtain meaningful bacteriologic specimens. The correctness of the initial choice of antibiotic may determine the patient's chance of survival.

With this protocol and knowledge of local patterns of infection, the emergency physician should be able to categorize the patient with sepsis into one of three groups: those in whom no specific organ or organ system can be implicated as the likely source of sepsis; those in whom involvement of a specific organ or organ system (for example, the urinary tract) is likely, but no causative pathogen can be identified; and those in whom a particular bacterium can be identified with some degree of certainty, usually by means of a Gram stain. Patients in the first group, which fortunately is small, must be treated with antibiotics chosen to cover a wide spectrum, while for patients in the third group, a specific antibiotic can be matched to the suspected pathogen. It is the large group in the middle that poses the greatest intellectual challenge. Knowing the likely localization allows the spectrum of possible antibiotics to be narrowed considerably, but the physician must choose carefully to cover both the most common causative pathogens for a given site and the important unusual organisms.

Choice of Antibiotic

Several general statements can be made regarding the choice of an antibiotic in septic shock. The antibiotic should be bactericidal when possible, it should be administered intravenously, due regard must be given to allergies of the patient and to the specific toxicities of the drugs used, and the maintenance dose must be tailored to renal function in those drugs excreted by the kidneys.

Specific recommendations regarding choice of antibiotic therapy are based on two factors: knowledge of the pathogens likely to invade via a specific portal (Table 3.8), and knowledge of the typical patterns of antibiotic sensitivities of those pathogens (see Table 11.2).

When no insight to the likely pathogen can be gained, however, a broad spectrum regimen, such as a semisynthetic penicillin plus an aminoglycoside in full dosage should be begun (see Chapter 11, page 245).

Role of Surgery

Septic shock is usually associated with a high degree of septicemia, which is frequently produced by pus under pressure. Clearly, early surgical consultation and intervention are mandatory if such a situation is suggested. For example, drainage of an obstructed, infected gallbladder is the definitive therapeutic measure, and will do more for the well-being of the patient than any antibiotic available.

Corticosteroids

Their effectiveness remains unproved and their use is controversial. The Food and Drug Administration recently has removed septic shock as an indication for the use of methylprednisone sodium succinate (Solu-Medrol).

Anaerobic Infections

With improved culture techniques, it has become apparent that anaerobic organisms, which are normal inhabitants of the mouth and pharynx, the intestine, and the female reproductive system, can be recovered from some infections associated with septic shock. With proper technique, anaerobic bacteria can be cultured from the "sterile" pus often recovered from intra-abdominal, tuboovarian, and pulmonary abscesses. Studies have shown that infections associated with contamination by the fecal, oral, or vaginal flora are likely to be the results of both aerobes and anaerobes. The number of anaerobes in the intestine is large. Currently, attention is focused on bacteroids (*Bacteroides fragilis* from the intestine), clostridial species, and anaerobic cocci (peptostreptococci and peptococci). The question of colonization versus infection has not been fully resolved. However, in the treatment of potentially life-threatening infections derived from contamination by intestinal, vaginal, or oral flora, it would seem prudent to assume the anaerobes are pathogens and to administer the proper antimicrobial agents. Most anaerobes in the oral cavity are penicillin-sensitive. Therefore, penicillin should be included in the coverage of sepsis due to empyema or pulmonary abscess. The intestinal and pelvic anaerobes, however, are best treated with chloramphenicol or clindamycin, both of which are effective but have significant side effects.

For specific information regarding the collection of specimens, the organisms likely to invade a particular organ system, and antibiotic recommendations and dosage schedules, the reader is referred to Chapter 11.

SHOCK LUNG

As more patients were resuscitated successfully from the acute phase of various shock states, it became apparent that many had severe and often fatal pulmonary complications. Known as shock lung, the adult respiratory distress syndrome, post-perfusion lung, Da Nang lung, and by other descriptive phrases, this syndrome of pulmonary involvement is seen in many clinical settings. It was reported associated with hypovolemic or septic shock, but an identical syndrome has been described associated with nonthoracic trauma (particularly to the head), cardiopulmonary bypass procedures, massive blood transfusions, respirator-assisted ventilation, aspiration pneumonia, pancreatitis, and other states.

The onset of shock lung is heralded by increase in tracheobronchial secretions, tachypnea, and cyanosis. Laboratory investigations reveal an arterial partial pressure of oxygen (PaO_2) that is decreasing and an arterial partial pressure of carbon dioxide ($PaCO_2$) that initially may be low and that then may begin to rise as the patient's condition becomes decompensated. Metabolic acidosis alone followed by both respiratory and metabolic acidosis frequently occurs. Pulmonary function studies at the bedside show decreased tidal volume and reduced pulmonary compliance requiring increased inspiratory pressure to maintain a given tidal volume.

No single cause of shock lung has been identified. Numerous factors have been implicated, and it is likely that the syndrome represents a final convergent pathway of several insults, including injury to the central nervous system, aspiration, disseminated intravascular coagulation, microembolization, fat embolization, and infection.

The pathophysiologic sequence leading to shock lung has not been clearly delineated, in part because of the paucity of observations regarding the early phases. Loss of integrity of the pulmonary endothelium, diminished plasma oncotic pressure, increased hydrostatic pressure with escape of protein into the alveolar spaces, and decreased surfactant activity have been observed. Increased affinity of the interstitial collagen for sodium apparently occurs, contributing to interstitial edema. A consistent finding fairly early in the process is an increase in pulmonary vascular resistance occurring at the distal end of the pulmonary capillaries or in the pulmonary veins. Pathologic findings vary with the stage of the process. Shock lung is characterized by interstitial edema followed by alveolar edema, atelectasis, microthrombosis, hemorrhage, and consolidation.

Recommendations regarding prevention and therapy are nonspecific at present. Careful transfusion to avoid overhydration, filtration of blood products to prevent microembolization, maintenance of long-term oxygen administration at the minimal effective fractional concentration (FIO_2 less than 0.5 if possible), and good pulmonary toilet are all reasonable suggestions. Intubation and assisted ventilation utilizing intermittent positive-pressure breathing and positive end-expiratory pressure may be indicated as well, and maintenance of the plasma oncotic pressure through judicious administration of albumin and diuretics may also be beneficial. More definitive therapy awaits improved knowledge of the underlying pathophysiologic mechanisms.

Suggested Readings

Baxter CR, Canizaro PC, Carrico CJ, et al: Fluid resuscitation of hemorrhagic shock. *Postgrad Med* 48:95–99, 1970

Bednarek J, Matsumoto T: Diagnosing and treating shock lung. *Hosp Physician* 10:66–73, 1974

Braunwald E: Vasodilator therapy—A physiologic approach to the treatment of heart failure (editorial). *N Engl J Med* 297:331–332, 1977

Collins JA: Problems associated with the massive transfusion of stored blood. *Surgery* 75:274–295, 1974

Dahn MS, Lucas CE, Ledgerwood AM, et al: Negative inotropic effect of albumin resuscitation for shock. *Surgery* 86:235–241, 1979

Dauber JH: Medical emergencies (section on shock), in Boedeker EC, Dauber JH (eds): *Manual of Medical Therapeutics*, Ed 21. Boston, Little, Brown, 1974, pp. 409–417

Goldberg LI: Dopamine—clinical uses of an endogenous catecholamine. *N Engl J Med* 291:707–710, 1974

Gorbach SL, Bartlett JG: Anaerobic infections. *N Engl J Med* 290:1177–1184, 1237–1245, 1289–1294, 1974

Holzer J, Karliner JS, O'Rourke RA, et al: Effectiveness of dopamine in patients with cardiogenic shock. *Am J Cardiol* 32:79–84, 1973

Huss P, Miller J, Unverferth DV, et al: The new inotropic drug, dobutamine. *Heart Lung* 10:121–126, 1981

Johnson SD, Lucas CE, Gerrick SJ, et al: Altered coagulation after albumin supplements for treatment of oligemic shock. *Arch Surg* 114:379–383, 1979

Kamada RO, Smith JR: Editorial: The phenomenon of respiratory failure in shock: The genesis of "shock lung." *Am Heart J* 83:1–4, 1972

Kones RJ: The catecholamines: Reappraisal of their use for acute myocardial infarction and the low cardiac output syndromes. *Crit Care Med* 1:203–220, 1973

Lucas CE, Ledgerwood AM, Higgins RF: Impaired salt water excretion after albumin resuscitation for hypovolemic shock. *Surgery* 86:544–549, 1979

Moellering RC, Jr, Rosenblatt JE, Finegold SM, et al: Infectious Disease Workshop: Seminar on Gram-negative infections. Kenilworth, NJ, Schering Corporation

Moss G: Shock lung: A disorder of the central nervous system? *Hosp Pract* 9:77–86, 1974

Rahal JJ, Jr: Bacteremia, in Conn HF (ed): *Current Therapy*. Philadelphia, WB Saunders, 1974, pp. 5–10

Reichgott MJ, Melmon KL: Should corticosteroids be used in shock? *Med Clin North Am* 57:1211–1223, 1973

Sheagren JN: Septic shock and corticosteroids. *N Engl J Med* 305:456–457, 1981

Shoemaker WC: Pattern of pulmonary hemodynamic and functional changes in shock. *Crit Care Med* 2:200–210, 1974

Tarazi RC: Sympathomimetic agents in the treatment of shock. *Ann Intern Med* 81:364–371, 1974

Weaver DW, Ledgerwood AM, Lucas CE, et al: Pulmonary effects of albumin resuscitation for severe hypovolemic shock. *Arch Surg* 113:387–391, 1978

Winslow EJ, Loeb HS, Rahimtoola SH, et al: Hemodynamic studies and results of therapy in 50 patients with bacteremic shock. *Am J Med* 54:421–432, 1973

CHAPTER 4

Initial Evaluation and Treatment of the Trauma Patient

CHARLES J. McCABE, M.D.

GENERAL CONSIDERATIONS

Trauma is a major cause of morbidity and mortality in the United States. It is estimated that more than 10 million disabling accidents occur each year, with a resultant cost of over $60 billion in insurance and hospital fees. Trauma is the leading cause of death in persons less than 40 years old, and is the fourth leading cause of death in all age groups. Motor vehicle accidents are responsible for the majority of deaths, followed by falls, homicides, suicides, and burns. Recognition of the seriousness of the problem has led to an intense effort to improve treatment of the trauma victim.

The ultimate outcome after trauma depends on three variables: (1) the severity of the injury; (2) the interval between occurrence of the injury and institution of therapy; and (3) the quality of care delivered. The severity of the injury cannot be easily altered by current methods of prevention, and most effort has been expended in improving the other two variables.

The Emergency Medical Services Systems Act of 1973 (Public Law 93–154) provided the impetus for implementation of municipal and regional emergency services to improve medical care of the trauma victim. The organization of transportation services, the training of emergency medical technicians and paramedics, and the use of radio communication all grew rapidly in the 1970s. Radio communication between trained paramedics and "medical control" hospitals has improved the results of immediate resuscitation efforts in the field. Experience in Viet Nam documented the lower mortality rate associated with more rapid transportation and immediate delivery of emergency services (Table 4.1), and studies also have documented the decreased mortality rate seen with more rapid transportation in civilian injuries. Helicopter transportation also has been implemented to decrease time in transit.

The Committee on Trauma of the American College of Surgeons has established guidelines and recommendations for the regional categorization of hospitals into three levels on the basis of their capabilities for treating trauma patients (Table 4.2). The differences between the levels consist of the immediate availability of (1) facilities (emergency ward, operating rooms, intensive care unit, cardiopulmonary bypass capability); (2) diagnostic capabilities (angiography, computed tomography); and (3) personnel (surgical specialists, anesthesiologists, medical specialists, registered nurses, and physician's assistants). The committee also has recommended the field categorization of patients on the basis of severity of injury (Table 4.3). Ideally, triage should match the various levels of injury to the level of hospital capability, and in fact, improved care and survival have been shown with this approach.

Injury Scores

Refinements in the estimation of injury severity have been recommended. Improved characterization of the severity of injury is required for the appropriate use of available facilities, for the prediction of outcome, and for evaluation of the quality of emergency medical care.

The severity of injury is estimated first at the scene, usually by medical personnel who are not physicians. Reliable data are easily obtained by means of the triage index (Table 4.4). This index is based on functional variables of the central nervous system, the cardiovascular system, and the respiratory system; points are given depending on the degree of dysfunction. The Glasgow Coma Score (GCS) is used to estimate central nervous system involvement and then is converted to a trauma score. The total score of the three systems

Table 4.1.

Historical correspondence of mortality rates with transportation times to a medical facility.

	Mortality Rate %	Transportation Time (hr)
World War I	5.8	12–15
Korea	2.4	4–6
Viet Nam	1.7	1–4

Table 4.2.

Hospital categorization on the basis of trauma treatment capability.

Level I
>500 beds
Metropolitan area
>1000 cases of trauma per year
Trauma training program and research
Trauma service
Full-time support services and staff

Level II
Similar to level I, but with lack of full-time staff
  specialists and research/training program

Level III
100–200 beds
Community area
Lack of full-time (in-hospital) staff specialists

Table 4.3.

Field categorization of trauma patients.

Category I
Combined systems injury
Bleeding open fractures
Uncontrolled hemorrhage
Severe maxillofacial injuries
Severe head, neck, and upper respiratory tract
  injuries
Unstable chest injuries
Pelvic fractures
Blunt abdominal trauma with hypotension and/or
  penetrating abdominal injuries
Severe neurologic injuries

Category II
Open or closed fractures
Soft-tissue injuries, stabilized bleeding
Multiple rib fractures without flail segment
Blunt abdominal trauma without hypotension
Transient loss of consciousness

Category III
Uncomplicated fractures
No hypovolemia or hypotension
No neurologic injury
No abdominal injuries
Moderate soft-tissue injuries
Chest injuries without respiratory distress

Modified with permission from *Bull Am Col Surg* 65:28, 1980.

provides accurate assessment of the patient's condition at the scene and appropriate matching of trauma victims with available resources.

Table 4.5 shows another method of scoring injuries, in which each injury is categorized by body area and severity. The three highest scores are squared and then added to give the "injury severity score." This score provides a numerical description of the overall severity of the injury for patients with multiple trauma, and has been shown to correlate well with survival.

Trauma Team

To provide efficient, organized care in the emergency ward, a well-trained medical team is essential. This should include surgeons, anesthesiologists, nurses, and paramedical personnel. A team leader should be designated and should be responsible for the patient's overall treatment and for the direction of the team's activity. Each member of the group should have a designated responsibility and sufficient experience to optimize patient care.

Priorities

All clothing must be removed and vital signs obtained immediately. Results will establish the rapidity with which subsequent diagnosis and therapy must proceed.

Three conditions will cause death within minutes if they are not recognized and corrected rapidly. They are: (1) airway obstruction or inadequate ventilation; (2) hemorrhage; and (3) cardiac arrest and circulatory insufficiency. The initial goal in the treatment of the trauma victim is to obtain control of the airway and ventilation and to replace intravascular volume. Once this is accomplished, further assessment, diagnosis, and therapy may be carried out.

Airway

The airway should be given the highest priority and immediate attention. Any evidence of a compromised airway or inadequate ventilation requires rapid correction. In patients with acute trauma, the most common causes of inadequate ventilation are upper airway obstruction and altered chest wall mechanics. Upper airway obstruction usually is caused by maxillofacial injuries, the tongue, dentures, other foreign bodies, or direct laryngeal or tracheal trauma. Treatment consists of clearing the oropharynx of any obstructing agent and proper positioning of the chin and jaw (see Chapter 2, pages 28–30); this normally provides a patent airway. Altered chest wall mechanics result from tension pneumothorax, hemothorax, flail chest, or an open sucking wound. Appro-

Table 4.4.
Trauma scale (on Triage index) (Boston EMS System).

I. Blood pressure
    Enter blood pressure: _____   Score: _____
    Systolic pressure:_____
        90+ = 2
    70–89   = 3
    50–69   = 4
     1–49   = 1
    None   = 0
Capillary return   Score: _____
    Normal   = 2
    Delayed = 1
    None   = 0
Respiration rate
    Enter rate per minute: _____   Score: _____
        36+ = 2
    25–35   = 3
    10–24   = 4
     1–9   = 1
    None   = 0
Respiratory effort   Score: _____
    Normal   = 1
    Shallow   = 0
    Retractive = 0

II. Glascow Coma Score (GCS)
        Eye opening   Score: _____
    Spontaneous = 4
    To voice   = 3
    To pain   = 2
    None   = 1
Verbal response   Score: _____
    Oriented   = 5
    Confused   = 4
    Inappropriate words   = 3
    Incomprehensible words   = 2
    None   = 1
Motor response   Score: _____
    Obeys command   = 6
    Localizes pain   = 5
    Withdrawal (pain stimulus) = 4
    Flexion (pain stimulus)   = 3
    Extension (pain stimulus)   = 2
    None   = 1

III. Convert GCS score to trauma score as follows:

Total GCS	Trauma Score	
14–15	5	
11–13	4	
8–10	3	Score: _____
5–7	2	
3–4	1	

IV. Add trauma score to scores from section I to get a final score from 1–16. Higher scores indicate a better
     prognosis.
        FINAL SCORE: _____

Table 4.5.
Injury severity score.[a]

Score	Soft Tissue	Head and Neck	Chest	Abdomen	Extremities and Pelvis
1	Aches all over Minor lacerations, contusions, abrasions (first aid, simple closure) All first-degree burns	Head trauma—dizziness, headache, no loss of consciousness Whiplash without findings Eye abrasions, contusions, retinal hemorrhage Tooth fractures, dislocations	Muscle ache Chest wall stiffness	Muscle ache Seat-belt abrasions	Minor sprains Digit fracture, dislocation
2	Extensive contusions, abrasions Lacerations up to 10 cm long Second- and third-degree burns over 10–20% of body surface area	Head trauma ± skull fracture, patient unconscious up to 15 min, no amnesia Skull fracture, undisplaced Facial bone fracture, undisplaced Eye lacerations Disfiguring facial lacerations Whiplash with x-ray findings	Rib/sternal fracture Major chest wall contusions without respiratory embarrassment Clavicular fracture	Major contusions	Compound digit fracture Long-bone fracture, undisplaced Pelvic fracture, undisplaced Sprains of major joints Tendon laceration of hand
3	Multiple extensive contusions, abrasions Lacerations >10 cm long Second- and third-degree burns over 20–30% of body surface area	Head trauma ± skull fracture, patient unconscious more than 15 min, no severe neurologic signs, amnesia up to 3 hr Skull fracture, displaced Eye loss Facial bone fracture, displaced Orbital bone fracture Cervical spine fracture without cord trauma	Ribs, multiple fractures Hemothorax Pneumothorax Diaphragm rupture Pulmonary contusion	Contusion of abdominal organs Extraperitoneal bladder rupture Retroperitoneal hemorrhage Ureteral avulsion Urethral laceration Thoracic, lumbar, sacral spine fracture without cord trauma	Long-bone fracture, displaced or compound Hand/foot fractures, multiple Pelvic fracture, displaced Major joints, dislocated Digits, multiple amputations Major vessels of extremities, lacerated
4	Lacerations with hemorrhage Second- and third-degree burns over 30–50% of body surface area	Head trauma ± skull fracture, patient unconscious more than 15 min, abnormal neurologic signs, amnesia 3–12 hr Skull fracture, compound	Open wounds Flail chest Pneumomediastinum Myocardial contusion without circulatory embarrassment	Minor intra-abdominal lacerations Ruptured spleen Traumatized kidney Pancreatic tail laceration Intraperitoneal bladder rupture Avulsion of genitalia Thoracic, lumbar, sacral spine fracture with cord trauma	Long-bone fracture, multiple closed Amputated limb
5	Second- and third-degree burns over >50% of body surface area	Head trauma ± skull fracture, patient unconscious more than 24 hr, amnesia >12 hr, intracranial hemorrhage and signs of increased intracranial pressure Cervical spine fracture with cord fracture Major obstruction of airway	Major respiratory compromise Tracheobronchial laceration Hemomediastinum Aortic laceration Myocardial rupture with circulatory embarrassment	Intra-abdominal lacerated vessels Major organ laceration (exclude spleen, kidney, ureter)	Long-bone fracture, multiple open

[a] Add the squares of the scores for the three most severely injured areas (maximum score, 75).   Modified from Committee on Medical Aspects of Automotive Safety. *JAMA 215:*277, 1971.

priate management of these problems usually will relieve the respiratory difficulty.

If any doubt exists as to the adequacy of ventilation, an endotracheal airway should be established and artificial ventilation begun. Normally, this can be accomplished by orotracheal or nasotracheal intubation. Tracheotomy is rarely required, but in cases of oropharyngeal or tracheal trauma, a direct tracheal airway may be necessary. This is most easily and rapidly accomplished by means of cricothyrotomy (see Illustrated Techniques, page 920–921). A classic tracheotomy is too time-consuming if performed correctly, and too bloody if performed as an emergency procedure.

In the unconscious patient, tracheal intubation clearly is indicated, but care must be taken since a cervical cord injury may also exist. Rigid laryngoscopy, which would extend the neck, is precluded, and the airway is best established by "blind" nasotracheal intubation. Fiberscopic laryngoscopy is a newer technique which permits intubation without neck extension but requires an experienced anesthesiologist.

Bleeding

Hemorrhage commonly results from major trauma and may result in serious cardiovascular compromise. Ongoing external hemorrhage is usually obvious, and is controlled best by direct pressure rather than by a proximal tourniquet. Internal hemorrhage is occult, but the site is identifiable by means of several techniques: chest x-ray films will identify intrathoracic hemorrhage, abdominal lavage will reveal intra-abdominal sources of hemorrhage, and examination of the extremities for fractures and hematomas will identify blood loss in these areas. The retroperitoneum is the only site where bleeding is difficult to document and to quantitate, and massive blood loss may occur, usually associated with pelvic fractures and urologic injuries. Intracerebral injuries are never the site of exsanguinating hemorrhage, and should not be implicated as a source of blood loss or as a cause of hypotension.

Therapy requires rapid establishment of adequate intravenous routes with 14-gauge catheters and replacement of both the volume deficit and any ongoing loss. Ringer's lactated solution is initially administered. After 2 liters are given, however, blood replacement is required. Clotting factors also must be replaced by administration of fresh-frozen plasma and platelets; 2 units of fresh-frozen plasma and 10 units of platelets are given for every 10 units of blood administered. Albumin

is used only when fresh-frozen plasma is not available. The rate of infusion varies from situation to situation. Initially, the infusate is run quickly enough to obtain a systolic blood pressure of approximately 100 mm Hg, and then continued at a rate to maintain stable vital signs and a reasonable urinary output.

Autotransfusion devices have been successful in elective vascular and cardiac surgery. In the trauma victim, in whom hemorrhage is the most common cause of hypovolemic shock, a method of acute blood replacement using the patient's blood would be most advantageous. Methods are currently available for use in the treatment of hemothorax resulting from chest trauma. These methods are simple to use.

Cardiac Arrest

The immediate causes of death after trauma are mechanical, obstructive, or related to volume. Recovery is often possible if the cause of cardiac arrest is recognized and rapidly reversed. Perfusion and oxygenation must be maintained in the interim by artificial means to prevent cerebral and myocardial damage. The most common causes of shock and arrest are: (1) hemorrhage; (2) cardiac arrhythmias, contusion, infarction, or pericardial tamponade; and (3) tension pneumothorax. A full resuscitative effort is required, including vigorous volume replacement with type 0-negative blood and temporary mechanical circulatory assistance. Where 0-negative blood is required, it should be from donors with low titers of anti-A and anti-B antibodies.

Complete Physical Examination

Once the three conditions that have been discussed are controlled or excluded, complete physical examination is performed in a rapid but meticulous manner. The patient is examined from head to foot, both dorsally and ventrally. Posterior wounds and sites of missile exit will be missed otherwise. The examination should be conducted as follows:

(1) Head—examine for cranial defects or wounds, blood in the auditory canal, maxillofacial fractures, and intraoral or ophthalmic injuries.

(2) Neck—of prime attention here is the cervical portion of the spinal cord. All patients should be considered to have a cervical spine injury until it is proved otherwise. The neck must be auscultated for the presence of carotid bruits and palpated for crepitation.

(3) Chest—ensure bilateral expansion and observe for flail segment or an open wound; examine

for bilateral equal breath sounds and for a tracheal shift.

(4) Abdomen—examine for penetrating wounds, distention, bowel sounds, and tenderness.

(5) Pelvis—palpate the pelvic rami and the iliac wings; perform a rectal examination; examine the urethral meatus.

(6) Extremities—examine carefully for fractures and neurovascular injury.

(7) Back—examine for posterior injuries and flank hematomas; thoracic and lumbar spine injuries must be excluded.

A brief history often may be obtained during examination. Use of the AMPLE mnemonic will provide all the information necessary:

Allergies;

Medication;

Previous diseases;

Last meal eaten;

Events leading to trauma.

It is absolutely necessary to obtain information concerning allergies from the patient or a relative. Antibiotics commonly are administered to the injured patient, and an anaphylactic reaction will compound the trauma problem. Similarly, information concerning any medication that the patient might be taking is important, since use of digoxin, coumadin (sodium warfarin), corticosteroids, or medicine to relieve angina would all affect the care of the patient. The "P" in AMPLE is to remind the physician to obtain a history of any previous disease process. A trauma victim with coronary artery disease or asthma may require special monitoring or drug therapy. A history of diabetes and insulin use would be invaluable. The "L" stands for the last meal eaten. If the patient ate recently, a full stomach should be expected, in which case aspiration must be guarded against if anesthesia is necessary. The "E" stands for events leading to the accident. If the patient had a transient ischemic attack or an anginal episode leading to the accident, this would be of crucial importance.

Technical Procedures

Diagnosis and therapy must often proceed simultaneously. The customary technical procedures are:

(1) Intubate and establish an adequate airway as necessary.

(2) Establish an intravenous access. Large-gauge catheters need to be put in place both above and below the diaphragm. Obviously, a vena caval injury superior or inferior to the heart will lead to extravasation of administered fluids; placement of intravenous lines both above and below the diaphragm partially circumvents this problem. A saphenous vein cutdown at the ankle often provides rapid and useful venous access. Two to four lines are usually necessary. A central venous pressure line is not safely placed in the initial emergency setting, and does not allow rapid infusion rates. These lines should be inserted when the procedure can be performed safely and with a minimal likelihood of complications.

(3) Monitor the urinary output. A Foley catheter often is necessary, but is contraindicated in the presence of urethral injury. The cardinal signs of urethral injury are:

(a) Full distended bladder;

(b) Inability to void;

(c) Blood at the urethral meatus (if no blood is initially present, milking the urethra will often reveal the injury);

(d) "Floating" prostate (on rectal examination, the prostate will not be palpated in its normal position).

In these patients, evaluation should include a urethrogram, a cystogram, and an intravenous pyelogram; suprapubic drainage should then be established.

(4) Insert chest tubes as necessary. Multiple injuries are often associated with chest trauma; although intrathoracic injury initially may not be obvious, delayed hemorrhage and pneumothorax may occur. If operation is necessary for some other reason in a patient with penetrating injuries to the chest, chest tubes should be inserted in the appropriate side to prevent occult blood loss or development of pneumothorax during the operative procedure.

(5) Insert a nasogastric tube.

(6) Type and crossmatch blood, determine a baseline hematocrit level and blood chemistry studies.

(7) Peritoneal lavage should be done as necessary (see Illustrative Technique, page 946–948).

(8) Antibiotics and tetanus prophylaxis administered when indicated.

Shock After Trauma

There are few primary causes of severe circulatory insufficiency after trauma. The major causes are:

(1) Hemorrhage.

(2) Cardiac dysfunction, which may be caused by arrhythmias, myocardial contusion or infarction, or pericardial tamponade.

(3) Tension pneumothorax, which results in decreased filling of the heart and altered respiratory

mechanics, followed by severe cardiovascular compromise.

(4) Spinal cord injuries, which may result in loss of peripheral vasomotor tone and severe hypotension. Before shock from spinal cord injury is diagnosed, the other causes of hypotension must be excluded.

A useful device in the treatment of shock in the trauma victim is the pneumatic "anti-shock" garment (PASG, G-suit, MAST). This provides external tamponade of abdominal or pelvic hemorrhage and splints long-bone fractures. In addition, it causes autotransfusion of an estimated 1–1.5 liters of venous blood. The garment is used beneficially in patients unresponsive to the normal treatment of hypovolemic shock, and it should be used when a patient in unstable condition requires transport for an extended period. It is particularly useful for patients with a ruptured abdominal aortic aneurysm who require transport. In such a case, the garment is left inflated until anesthesia is completed in the operating room.

INITIAL ASSESSMENT OF REGIONAL INJURY

Abdominal Trauma

Abdominal trauma may be divided into two broad categories: penetrating and nonpenetrating injuries. Penetrating injuries are most commonly the result of a stab or a gunshot wound. Blunt injuries occur secondary to falls, motor vehicle accidents, altercations, and blasts. The extent of injury and the organs damaged depend on the mechanism of injury.

Penetrating Abdominal Injuries

Gunshot Wounds. The handgun has replaced the knife as the most common cause of penetrating abdominal injury. It is important to recognize that a high abdominal injury may have penetrated the thoracic cavity, and that a low thoracic injury may have penetrated the abdominal space. The path that a bullet may follow is totally variable, as is the number of organs injured in its path. The management of gunshot wounds of the abdomen is fairly straightforward; all these injuries require exploration. Even tangential wounds that traverse the abdominal wall may require exploration, depending on the velocity of the missile. It also must be remembered that any penetrating injury of the abdominal space that results in severe hypotension usually is associated with an arterial or venous injury to a major blood vessel. Adequate intravascular access and volume replacement should be

anticipated. Whenever a patient with this type of injury is taken to the operating room, the need for intrathoracic access must be anticipated and the patient should be "prepped" from the suprasternal notch to midthighs.

Knife Injuries. Knife injuries are deceptive, and the extent of injury usually is not recognized easily. The maxim that all knife injuries that penetrate the peritoneum require abdominal exploration recently has been challenged, and two methods of managing abdominal stab wounds currently exist.

The first method is careful clinical observation of the patient by one examiner, with serial hematocrit measurements. The abdomen is examined frequently for tenderness or pain. If the abdominal findings remain normal and the patient remains asymptomatic, no further procedures are performed and the patient is discharged after 24–36 hours. If signs and symptoms of peritoneal injury develop at any time during the period of observation, exploratory operation is performed.

The second method of management is based on the concept that if the peritoneal space has been penetrated, exploration is mandatory. This method, which depends on the ability to prove peritoneal penetration, may involve several diagnostic techniques.

(1) Kidney-ureter-bladder and upright films of the abdominal space—free air under the diaphragm will indicate peritoneal injury.

(2) Local exploration of the wound.

(3) Sinograms—unfortunately, this technique is not totally accurate since false-negative results may occur. In addition, once dye has been injected in the subcutaneous space, it causes a severe inflammatory reaction and may mimic peritoneal injury.

(4) Peritoneal lavage—this has commonly been used to evaluate blunt abdominal trauma, and is now becoming more frequently used in penetrating injuries. Contraindications to peritoneal lavage include:

(a) Full bladder;

(b) Pregnancy;

(c) Previous abdominal surgery and abdominal incisions (usually a contraindication)—adhesions around the incision and the absence of a free peritoneal space may lead to false-positive results or to damage of vital intraperitoneal structures.

(d) Clear-cut indications for abdominal exploration—if the patient clearly needs to undergo abdominal exploration, the time spent on peritoneal lavage is wasted.

If peritoneal penetration cannot be proved with these techniques, the patient should be observed and discharged at an appropriate time. The combination of local exploration of the wound with peritoneal lavage has been highly successful in screening patients for abdominal exploration.

Nonpenetrating Abdominal Injuries

Clinical evaluation of blunt abdominal trauma can be very difficult. For example, fractured ribs and soft-tissue injuries often evoke pain that extends to the abdomen. Patients with blunt abdominal trauma are even more difficult to evaluate if they have suffered neurologic injuries and are unconscious.

When obvious peritoneal signs are present, abdominal exploration is required. If examination is equivocal or if the patient is unconscious, however, peritoneal lavage often plays a role in evaluation of the abdomen. Peritoneal lavage permits rapid formulation of a diagnosis and treatment plan, and minimizes both delays and the number of blood transfusions. If a patient requires anesthesia for some other reason, such as treatment of neurologic or peripheral trauma, and if the status of the abdominal space is unclear, peritoneal lavage may be used to exclude the abdomen as a source of future problems.

Pelvic fractures often are associated with abdominal injuries, and can be the source of massive blood loss. Clinical diagnosis may be difficult, and a routine pelvic x-ray examination is recommended. Urethral and bladder injuries must always be suspected and contrast studies (urethrogram, cystogram) performed. Application of a G-suit and the use of angiography are helpful in controlling massive hemorrhage.

Chest Trauma

Thoracic injuries, like abdominal injuries, are separated into two categories, penetrating and nonpenetrating, and the causes of these injuries are similar to those of abdominal trauma. The vital organs of ventilation and cardiac function in the chest make severe injuries to this area life threatening. Any injury to the chest should be considered potentially lethal until proved otherwise. Initial evaluation should proceed as previously outlined. The most important diagnostic study is an immediate chest x-ray film, portable if necessary. The clinical diagnosis of pneumothorax, hemothorax, or rib fracture is often difficult in the trauma setting. Chest x-ray examination will reveal the major pathologic process rapidly and should be performed early.

Chest Wall. Soft-tissue damage may occur, but treatment is usually not difficult. Large chest wall defects, however, may result in an open pneumothorax and dysfunctional breathing. The wound is often apparent because of a loud sucking noise as air moves through the chest wall defect. Stabilization is accomplished by covering the defect with a petrolatum gauze or sterile dressing and then placing a chest tube to relieve the pneumothorax.

Rib fractures often are associated with blunt injuries and may cause pain and muscle splinting. Former techniques of rib splinting and taping often resulted in atelectasis and pneumonitis, and no longer are used. If pain is minimal, oral analgesics are normally sufficient. If pain is severe, regional blockade of the intercostal nerves is often beneficial in totally relieving symptoms. Pneumothorax may be a component of rib fractures and commonly requires chest tube insertion. When multiple ribs are fractured in two or more locations, the patient may have a flail segment, resulting in paradoxical motion of the injured segment with respiration. This may lead to contusion or atelectasis of the underlying lung and perhaps pneumonitis. Therapy depends on the degree of respiratory compromise. Immediate prehospital care may be provided by laying the patient on the affected side to decrease the paradoxical motion of the chest wall. Hospital admission is necessary to provide vigorous chest physical therapy, endotracheal suction, and analgesics. If severe respiratory compromise occurs, as evidenced by an elevated Pa_{CO_2} and a decreasing Pa_{O_2} or by the development of pneumonia, endotracheal intubation and intermittent positive-pressure breathing are necessary. This will help prevent atelectasis and pneumonitis while the rib fractures stabilize.

The clavicle and scapula are often fractured. Depending on the location of the clavicular fracture, vascular injury or damage to the brachial plexus may also occur. Hemothorax on the side of a proximal clavicular fracture should lead to the suspicion of a subclavian artery injury.

The first rib has been used as a hallmark of the severity of chest injury. If it is fractured, it should provide a good estimation of the force of injury. Fractures of the first rib are often associated with mediastinal and great-vessel injuries and a high index of suspicion should be raised if a first rib fracture is present. Arch aortography is the definitive diagnostic procedure.

Pulmonary Injuries. Contusions of the lung from blunt injury and pneumothorax from penetrating injury or fractured ribs are common. The contusion may not cause any respiratory compromise unless severe, and then may require intubation and ventilation until the process resolves. Pneumothorax after trauma is usually managed by chest tube insertion. Tension pneumothorax resulting in a shift of the mediastinal structures and cardiac compromise requires rapid therapy. Placement of a large needle into the chest cavity will relieve the tension and create an open pneumothorax. This then will allow more elective chest tube insertion.

Penetrating injuries normally result in pneumothorax, but if mediastinal structures are injured, the patient will be seen with cardiovascular compromise. Bleeding from intercostal arteries may also result in severe blood loss. Parenchymal lung hemorrhages may be self-limiting.

Trachea and Bronchi. Direct tracheal and laryngeal injuries usually result from either blunt force applied to the neck or penetrating injuries. Severe respiratory compromise often results, and the patency of the airway is always in jeopardy. Air commonly will be present in the soft tissues of the neck as evidenced by x-ray examination or by crepitation. A tracheal airway may need to be established quickly by means of cricothyrotomy. If more time is available, tracheotomy may be performed. Direct laryngeal and tracheal repair then is often possible.

Bronchial tears usually result from deceleration forces. The mainstem bronchus may be partly or completely torn from the trachea. This results in pneumomediastinum or a total pneumothorax that may progress to tension pneumothorax. The injury often is evidenced after chest tube insertion by a large air leak and by the inability to expand the lung fully. The diagnosis is confirmed by bronchoscopic examination. Direct, immediate repair is usually successful.

Esophagus. The esophagus is fairly well protected in the chest from the forces of blunt trauma, but tears may occur. If penetrating injury is suspected to have traversed the esophagus, vigorous examination with contrast studies and endoscopy is necessary. Esophageal injury is one of the possible causes of air in the mediastinum and neck.

Aorta. Aortic tears occur most commonly after high-speed motor vehicle accidents. They commonly result in acute aortic rupture and instantaneous death. If the injury is only partially through the aortic wall or if immediate tamponade of the injury by the surrounding mediastinal structures occurs, the situation is still life-threatening. Rupture can occur at any time, and a rapid workup is necessary. A widened mediastinum is often apparent on chest x-ray films, and an aortogram is necessary to provide both clear-cut diagnosis and to identify the site of the tear. The most common location of aortic disruption is at the ligamentum arteriosum, with the second most common site

being the ascending aorta just above the aortic valve.

Penetrating injuries that damage the aorta or great vessels result in massive hemorrhage and severe cardiovascular compromise.

Diaphragm. The diaphragm may be injured by any penetrating object. Penetrating injuries to the chest or abdomen may involve both body spaces, and the physician must be aware of this possibility. Blunt injuries, usually from motor vehicle accidents, may result in tears of the diaphragm with herniation of abdominal contents into the chest. These injuries most often occur on the left side of the diaphragm, although right-sided diaphragmatic injuries and herniations are possible. Chest x-ray examination will usually suggest the possibility of diaphragmatic injury.

Myocardium. Cardiac contusions commonly result from blunt trauma, but rarely cause cardiovascular compromise. The possibility of pericardial tamponade after blunt myocardial injury requires a high index of suspicion. As a result of increasingly rapid transportation from the scene of the accident, more patients with myocardial rupture secondary to blunt trauma are now reaching hospital facilities, and this injury should be suspected in patients with cardiovascular compromise and distended neck veins. Pericardiocentesis and the removal of very small quantities of blood may be both diagnostic and therapeutic.

Penetrating injuries can damage any vascular structure. The diagnosis is suspected by the location of the wound and the presence of cardiovascular compromise. Pericardial tamponade after blunt or penetrating injury requires rapid therapy. Initial management may include pericardiocentesis, but emergency thoracotomy is more frequently necessary.

Thoracotomy in the emergency ward is a dramatic event requiring experienced personnel. The goals should be specific: (1) relieve pericardial tamponade, and (2) control exsanguinating hemorrhage. Indications for emergency thoracotomy are limited:

(1) Any penetrating pericardial or left-chest injury that results in cardiovascular compromise.

(2) Exsanguination from the chest. The patient may be suffering from shock, and chest x-ray examination will reveal extensive hemothorax. Placement of a chest tube may result in exsanguinating hemorrhage, and immediate control is absolutely necessary.

(3) Control of intra-abdominal hemorrhage. This technique has been used often, but the results of clamping the thoracic aorta to control intra-abdominal hemorrhage have been poor.

Neurologic Injuries

Injuries to the brain, spinal cord, and peripheral nervous system are seen after both penetrating and blunt trauma, and in fact, neurologic injuries are the most common cause of death in patients with multiple injuries. The accumulation of a very small amount of blood in the closed cranial vault can lead to a rapid increase in intracranial pressure. Subdural and epidural hematomas usually cause lateralizing signs and require rapid recognition and operation. Cerebral contusions also cause severe neurologic symptoms and increased intracranial pressure. The use of computed tomography has made rapid and accurate differentiation and diagnosis of these entities possible.

Neurologic injury should be suspected in all trauma patients, particularly if the patient is unconscious. Rigid precautions should be taken to prevent flexion and extension of the neck and spinal cord in transport. If intubation is necessary, a nasotracheal tube is the optimal choice, since laryngoscopy is precluded unless x-ray films reveal no cervical spine injury. The cervical and thoracolumbar portions of the spine should be stabilized until fractures are excluded. If neurologic injury is the primary problem, fluid infusions should be kept minimal to prevent increase in intracranial pressure and the patient should undergo immediate neurosurgical evaluation. Initial attempts to decrease intracranial pressure with mannitol and dexamethasone (Decadron) are helpful. However, mannitol may compound the problem by decreasing the brain size and, therefore, increasing the intracranial space, thus allowing expansion of bleeding. Immediate placement of burr holes is sometimes necessary in the emergency ward, although always preferably accomplished in the operating room.

Arterial Injuries

Major vascular injury may occur centrally or peripherally. Central arterial or venous injury (chest or abdominal vascular system) usually results in massive hemorrhage with hypotension and hypovolemia. Any patient with penetrating abdominal or thoracic injury and shock should be examined for major vascular disruption. Early fluid replacement with blood and rapid surgical intervention are necessary. Peripheral vascular lesions may occur after penetrating injuries, and commonly are associated with blunt injuries resulting in fractures and dislocations. Arterial injury should be suspected when the following signs are present:

(1) penetrating injury along the course of a major vascular structure;

(2) excessive hemorrhage or expanding hematoma;

(3) distal ischemia;

(4) bruit over the course of a vessel;

(5) lack of distal pulses;

(6) displaced fractures.

In the diagnosis of arterial injury, peripheral pulses should be sought carefully. Plethysmography and determination of the presence or absence of Doppler signals are also helpful measures. An arteriogram is often necessary to exclude arterial injury.

Knee injuries and fractures of the femur are commonly associated with popliteal artery disruptions or thromboses. Peripheral ischemia is often profound, and arterial vasospasm secondary to the fracture may delay diagnosis and therapy. Ischemia distal to a fracture site should be assumed to be the result of arterial disruption until proved otherwise.

Amputation injuries may lead to severe hemorrhage, and tourniquet control just above the level of amputation is often necessary. Clamping of arterial vessels in the base of the wound is not recommended.

Burns

Thermal injuries commonly cause severe tissue destruction and cardiorespiratory insufficiency. Initial treatment must focus on the immediate causes of death: hypovolemia: and inadequate ventilation. Vigorous fluid resuscitation and intubation are required early, with careful monitoring of urinary output. Escharotomy occasionally is necessary over the thorax for deep burns interfering with expansion of the chest. The possibility of associated injuries must be considered.

Orthopaedic Injuries

The most commonly injured system in the body is the bony skeleton. Injury may be isolated or it may be associated with other visceral injuries. Bony injuries usually have a low priority in the treatment of patients with multiple injuries, since they are rarely life-threatening. However, bleeding from fracture sites can be massive and shock may result, particularly with pelvic fractures. With all orthopaedic injuries, continuity of blood vessels and nerves must be assured. Initial treatment requires splinting of the fracture to prevent further injury.

Suggested Readings

Baker CC, Oppenheimer L, Stephens B, et al: Epidemiology of trauma deaths. *Am J Surg 140*:144–150, 1980

Baker SP, O'Neill B, Haddon W Jr, et al: The injury severity score: a method for describing patients with multiple injuries and evaluating emergency care. *J Trauma 14:*187–196, 1974

Boyd DR: A symposium on the Illinois Trauma Program: A systems approach to the care of the critically injured. *J Trauma 13:*275–290, 1973

Boyd DR, Micik SH, Lambrew CT, et al: Medical control and accountability of emergency medical systems. *IEEE Trans Vehic Technol 28:*249–262, 1979

Brawley RK, Hauer RJ: Autotransfusion seminar. *Surgery 84:*693–732, 1978

Bulletin of American College of Surgeons: Trauma Appendices. *65:*9–35, February, 1980

Champion HR, Sacco WJ, Hannan DS, et al: Assessment of injury severity. The Triage Index. *Crit Care Med 8:*201–208, 1980

Committee on Medical Aspects of Automotive Safety, American Medical Association: Rating the severity of tissue damage. I. The Abbreviated Scale. *JAMA 215:*277–280, 1971

Cornell WP, Ebert PA, Zuidema GD: X-ray diagnosis of penetrating wounds of the abdomen. *J Surg Res 5:*142, 1965

Flint LM, Brown A, Richardson D, et al: Definitive control of bleeding from severe pelvic fractures. *Ann Surg 189:*709–716, 1979

Galbraith TA, Oraskovich MR, Heimbach DM, et al: The role of peritoneal lavage in the management of stab wounds of the abdomen. *Am J Surg 140:*60–64, 1980

Hale HW: Symposium on blunt abdominal trauma. *Contemp Surg 16:*39–52, 1977

Hardaway RM III: Viet Nam wound analysis. *J Trauma 18:*635–643, 1978

Jorgens ME: Peritoneal lavage. *Am J Surg 133:*365–369, 1977

Moore EE, Moore JB, Gallaway AC, et al: Post-injury thoracotomy in the emergency department: a critical evaluation. *Surgery 86:*588–599, 1979

Moore EE, Moore JB: Mandatory laparotomy for GSW penetrating the abdomen. *Am J Surg 140:* 647, 1980

Nance FC, Wennar MH, Johnson LW, et al: Surgical judgment in the management of penetrating wounds of the abdomen. *Ann Surg 179:*639–646, 1974

O'Donnell TF, Brewster DC, Darling RC, et al: Arterial injuries associated with fractures and/or dislocations of the knee. *J Trauma 17:*275–284, 1977

Olsen WR, Redman HC, Hildrett DH: Quantitative peritoneal lavage in blunt abdominal trauma. *Arch Surg 104:*536, 1972

Parvin S, Smith DE, Asher WM: Effectiveness of peritoneal lavage in blunt abdominal trauma. *Ann Surg 181:*255–261, 1975

Patton AS, Guyton SW, Lawson DW, et al: Treatment of severe atrial injuries. *Am J Surg 141:*465–471, 1981

Richardson JD, McElvein RB, Trinkle JK: First rib fracture: a hallmark of severe trauma. *Ann Surg 181:*251–254, 1975

Sacco WJ, Champion HR, Carnazzo AJ: Trauma Score. *Curr Concepts Trauma Care*, Spring, 9–11, 1981

Sheely CH, Mattox KL, Eall AC: Management of acute cervical tracheal trauma. *Am J Surg 128:*805–808, 1974

Waters JM, Wells CH: The effects of a modern emergency care system in reducing automobile crash deaths. *J Trauma 13:*645–647, 1973

Weems WL: Management of genitourinary injuries in patients with pelvic fractures. *Ann Surg 189:*717–722, 1979

West G, Trunkey DD, Lim RC: Systems of trauma care. *Ann Surg 114:*455–460, 1979

Williams JB, Silver DG, Laws HL: Successful management of heart rupture from blunt trauma. *J Trauma 21:*534–537, 1981

Yarbrough DR: A guide to the immediate care of the injured patient. *Hosp Med 2:*8–16, 1975

Medicine

CHAPTER 5

Cardiology: Arrhythmias

GEORGE E. THIBAULT, M.D.
ROMAN W. DeSANCTIS, M.D.

Editor's note: In contradistinction to other topics, cardiology is arbitrarily divided into three sections—Chapters 5, 6 and 7—stressing three distinct aspects of the subject. Additional coverage of cardiac entities is available in Section 1 (Life Support) and in Chapter 21 (Cardiovascular Emergencies).

It is essential to remember that cardiac rhythm disturbances do not occur in isolation—they occur in a particular patient whose age, previous therapy, and coexisting cardiac and noncardiac diseases are important determinants of how well the arrhythmia is tolerated and of the urgency and appropriateness of treatment. The diagnosis and the treatment of an arrhythmia, which are only the first steps in the total evaluation of the patient's condition, should raise several important questions: Why did the arrhythmia occur? Does the patient have heart disease, and if so, what kind? What other diagnoses may be suggested or modified by the rhythm disturbance? What additional diagnos-

tic or therapeutic measures should be instituted to elucidate causes further and to prevent recurrences?

To treat cardiac arrhythmias successfully in the emergency ward, the physician must understand the normal anatomy and physiology of the cardiac pacemaking and conducting systems and the ways in which they can be deranged, he must know what methods are available for accurate diagnosis of the rhythm disturbance, and finally, he must select the correct therapy for restoring normal rhythm.

ANATOMY AND PHYSIOLOGY

Any cardiac cell that can spontaneously depolarize, reach its threshold potential, and discharge without the aid of another stimulus is capable of acting as a cardiac pacemaker cell. This property is known as *automaticity*, and is possessed by specialized cells in several locations in the heart, such as the sinus (sinoatrial) node, the atrioventricular (AV) node and junction, and the His-

Purkinje system. At any given time, the cells with the fastest rate of spontaneous diastolic depolarization constitute the dominant pacemaker, and suppress the formation of impulses in cells with slower discharge rates. This dominant-pacemaker function is usually served by the sinus node, a collection of cells and fibrous tissue located at the junction of the superior vena cava and the right atrium. Since it is a superficial structure, it is easily affected by pericardial inflammation, resulting in the atrial arrhythmias common in patients with pericarditis. The artery to the sinus node courses directly through it, and pressure within the artery may help regulate the discharge rate of the pacemaker cells; this artery is a proximal branch of the right coronary artery in 55% of patients and of the left circumflex coronary artery in the remainder. The impulse generated in the sinus node is propagated through the atria along at least three loosely organized internodal bundles that terminate in the AV node.

The AV node is located near the junction of the interatrial and interventricular septa; its slow conduction time limits the number of impulses that can reach the ventricle and provides a delay between atrial systole and ventricular systole that facilitates proper ventricular filling. The artery to the AV node comes from the right coronary artery in 90% of patients and from the left circumflex coronary artery in the remainder.

From the AV node, the impulse is conducted down the bundle of His, which soon divides into a thin right branch coursing into the right ventricle and a thicker left branch entering the left ventricle. The left bundle branch divides into anterior and posterior segments. Hence, there are three major divisions or fascicles—the right bundle branch and the anterior and posterior divisions of the left bundle branch. The blood supply to the bundle branches is primarily from septal branches of the left anterior descending coronary artery.

Throughout its course, the propagation of the impulse depends on its reaching cells that are *excitable*, that is, capable of being depolarized. A cell that is not excitable is *refractory*. The *refractory period* is the time needed for a depolarized cell to recover so that it can discharge again in response to a stimulus. The normal electrical sequence, therefore, depends on coordination of automaticity, conduction velocities, excitability, and refractoriness. Disorders of cardiac rhythm result from abnormalities in these functions that occur individually or in combination. For example, atrial tachycardia with block represents a combination of enhanced atrial automaticity and depressed AV conduction. Furthermore, each of these properties

may be altered by physiologic events (for example, electrolyte changes or alteration in sympathetic or parasympathetic tone), pathologic processes (for example, ischemia, infarction, fibrosis, or inflammation), or drugs.

CONSEQUENCES OF ARRHYTHMIAS

The ability of a patient to tolerate an arrhythmia depends on the nature of the arrhythmia, its duration, the vigor of the heart, and the patient's general health. Certain principles may be applied in understanding the consequences of arrhythmias:

(1) **Rate tolerance.** The normal heart tolerates a wide range of rates without decompensation. In healthy persons, a satisfactory cardiac output can be maintained with heart rates in excess of 170 beats/min or as low as 40 beats/min. Tachycardia, however, shortens diastole, and also increases myocardial oxygen consumption considerably. Two important events occur during diastole—ventricular filling and coronary artery perfusion. For these reasons, sustained tachycardia is tolerated poorly by patients dependent on long diastolic periods for ventricular filling, such as those with mitral stenosis, and by patients who cannot tolerate increased myocardial oxygen consumption and decreased coronary artery perfusion, such as those with angina pectoris or acute myocardial infarction.

Bradycardia is tolerated poorly by patients with relatively fixed stroke volumes, such as those with aortic valvular disease or a failing left ventricle. A bradycardic rhythm may cause no problems until a stress such as fever or increased activity requires increased cardiac output. The ability to tolerate either tachycardia or bradycardia is directly related to the functional state of the heart, primarily the left ventricle; this point is fundamental in deciding on the urgency with which an arrhythmia should be terminated in any given patient.

(2) **Atrial transport.** Atrial contraction at the end of diastole completes ventricular filling before the ventricle contracts, and may be responsible for 10–30% of the cardiac output. This atrial transport function is more important in diseased hearts than it is in healthy hearts, and is particularly needed in patients with hypertrophic or noncompliant left ventricles, such as patients with aortic stenosis, idiopathic hypertrophic subaortic stenosis, hypertensive heart disease, and some patients with coronary artery disease. Loss of this atrial "kick" may be important in the deterioration of hemodynamic status that can result from atrial fibrillation, ventricular tachycardia, or complete heart block.

(3) **Arrhythmias resulting in other more serious**

arrhythmias. Because of hemodynamic deterioration and underlying heart disease—particularly ischemic heart disease—it is common for one arrhythmia to give way to another, which further jeopardizes the patient's condition. For example, the rapid heart rate of paroxysmal atrial tachycardia may cause coronary ischemia which, in turn, can precipitate ventricular tachycardia or ventricular fibrillation. Bradyarrhythmias such as complete heart block may result in either asystole or ventricular fibrillation. The prevention of such a sequence is one of the strongest reasons for the prompt treatment of arrhythmias, particularly in elderly patients and in those with coronary artery disease.

GENERAL PRINCIPLES IN DIAGNOSIS OF ARRHYTHMIAS

Three sources of information are available to the physician in diagnosing an arrhythmia: the history, physical examination, and electrocardiogram.

History

As much information as possible should be gathered regarding the patient's drug history, known cardiac diagnoses, and any previous arrhythmias and response to therapy. Being alert to the possibility of digitalis toxicity, electrolyte disorders (particularly hypokalemia in patients receiving diuretics), and previous adverse drug reactions may help in both diagnosis and choice of therapy. In a patient who has had recurrent arrhythmias, such as paroxysmal supraventricular tachycardias, it is useful to know which therapeutic maneuvers or drugs have or have not been effective. The duration of the rhythm disturbance, possible precipitating events, and the patient's report of symptoms such as angina, dyspnea, or syncope are all important in guiding therapy.

Physical Examination

Awareness of the patient's state of perfusion as indicated by blood pressure, skin color and temperature, mental status, and urinary output is essential to establish how well the arrhythmia is being tolerated and how urgently intervention is required. If the patient has no pulse and is unconscious, a precordial thump followed by "blind" defibrillation is indicated. If the patient has a rapid heart rate (150 beats/min or more) and evidence of severely decreased perfusion, immediate cardioversion also may be required even before establishing a definitive diagnosis. If the patient is not in such a state of hemodynamic collapse, more

time can be taken for a careful physical examination before therapy.

Inspection of the jugular veins can yield information about atrial activity and the presence or absence of AV dissociation. With practice, the physician can recognize the normal "a" waves (P waves on the electrocardiogram) caused by atrial contraction and their relation to the normal "v" waves of ventricular contraction (QRS interval). Two "a" waves per ventricular systole suggest 2:1 heart block. Large intermittent cannon "a" waves are diagnostic of AV dissociation, which suggest either complete heart block or ventricular tachycardia with an independent atrial rhythm. Cannon waves result from the backward pressure generated by the atrium contracting against a tricuspid valve closed by simultaneous ventricular contraction. Occasionally, the rapid flutter waves (300 waves/min) of atrial flutter can be seen in the neck. An "irregularly irregular" pulse and absence of "a" waves suggest atrial fibrillation.

Cardiac auscultation may provide additional diagnostic information. Variability of the first heart sound suggests either atrial fibrillation, a changing P-R interval, or some type of AV dissociation. Wide splitting of both the first and second sounds and gallop sounds, which may be variable in intensity and timing, strongly suggests ventricular tachyarrhythmia. Auscultation is also important for the identification of murmurs, gallops, or rubs that may enable more accurate diagnosis of the underlying heart disease. Knowing that the patient has mitral or aortic valvular disease or a dilated, failing heart is important in predicting how well a rhythm disturbance is likely to be tolerated.

AV dissociation, which usually occurs in ventricular tachycardia, often can be recognized more readily from physical examination than from the electrocardiogram. When the atria and ventricles beat asynchronously, there is a veritable cacophony on auscultation, with variation in the intensity and splitting of the heart sounds and intermittent gallop sounds. Inconstant cannon waves are seen in the jugular veins, and there is beat-to-beat variation in the systolic blood pressure. All these findings are due to the random relation of the atrial and ventricular contractions. In contrast, the heart sounds in arrhythmias in which the atria and ventricles beat synchronously—as in paroxysmal atrial tachycardia—are similar to each other, and there are no beat-to-beat variations in heart sounds, the jugular veins, or systemic blood pressure.

In the remainder of the physical examination, the physician should establish whether there is evidence of left or right ventricular failure (rales, jugular venous distention, hepatomegaly, or peripheral edema), and should look for coexisting diseases that may have precipitated the arrhythmia, such as pneumonia, pulmonary embolic disease, or thyrotoxicosis.

Electrocardiogram

Electrocardiographic examination is crucial in the diagnosis of an arrhythmia, and it must be approached systematically. The physician should ask four key questions:

(1) Is there evidence of atrial activity represented by P waves or flutter waves?

(2) Is the QRS complex, representing ventricular depolarization, normal or wide (more than 0.12 second), fast or slow, regular or irregular?

(3) Is there any relation between the P waves and the QRS complex?

(4) Are there premature beats or pauses that need to be explained?

Atrial Activity

In the standard electrocardiogram, atrial activity is represented by the P waves, usually best seen in the inferior leads (II, III, and aVF) or right precordial leads (V_1 and V_2). Additional right precordial leads such as V_3R and V_4R may be helpful. Modification of the lead system sometimes may reveal atrial activity not seen with the standard leads. One such modification is the CR system, in which the right arm electrode is used as the indifferent electrode and the left arm electrode is used as an exploring precordial electrode while the electrocardiogram is recorded from lead I.

If these leads are not sufficient to define atrial activity, other means must be used. An esophageal electrode may be placed behind the left atrium by passing it down the esophagus a distance of 32–36 cm from the nares. This then can be connected to the exploring V electrode by an insulated wire with an alligator clamp at each end, the electrocardiogram being recorded from the V lead. Because this procedure is often uncomfortable for the patient, it may be difficult to perform.

A right atrial electrocardiogram can be recorded directly by means of a central venous pressure line, the tip of which is positioned in the right atrium. The line is filled with a 10% solution of sodium bicarbonate, and an external metal needle is connected by alligator clips to the V electrode. In many instances, this salt bridge will provide an interpretable atrial electrocardiogram recorded from the V lead. Finally, a definitive atrial electrocardiogram can usually be obtained by passing a pacemaker electrode transvenously into the right atrium and connecting the external tip of the wire to the V lead with alligator clips (Fig. 5.1). This can be done at the bedside with virtually no risk to the patient.

QRS Complex

The width of the QRS complex represents the amount of time required for the depolarizing electrical impulse to travel from the V mode throughout the ventricle. Normally, the QRS width is less than 0.12 second because the impulse travels along the left and right bundles, which are high-speed conduction tissue. A QRS width less than 0.12 second represents a rhythm starting above the ventricle and having access to a normal conduction system via the AV node, that is, a supraventricular rhythm. If the QRS complex is wider than normal, three possibilities exist: (1) the impulse may start within the ventricle, and thus not have access to the conduction system; (2) the conduction system may be permanently interrupted, that is, the patient may have left or right bundle-branch block; or (3) there may be a temporary dysfunction of the conduction system resulting in aberrant conduction. Such aberrant conduction may occur if a demand is made on the system to conduct too

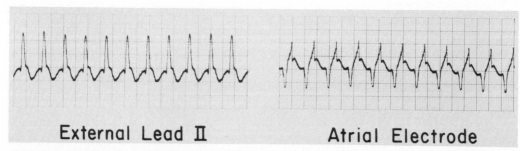

External Lead II   **Atrial Electrode**

Figure 5.1. Use of atrial electrode to diagnose arrhythmia. External electrocardiogram reveals a regular tachycardia at 160 beats/min with narrow QRS complexes and no discernible atrial activity. The atrial electrode reveals regular atrial activity with 1:1 relation between P waves and QRS complexes. The diagnosis of paroxysmal atrial tachycardia can now be made and appropriate therapy instituted. (Reproduced by permission, from *Circulation*, Vol. 43, No. 5, © 1971, The American Heart Association.)

Table 5.1.
Differential electrocardiographic features of tachycardia with wide QRS complexes.

Differential Feature	SVT with Aberrant Conduction	Ventricular Tachycardia
Atrioventricular dissociation on electrocardiogram and physical examination	No	Often (diagnostic if present) (about 20% have retrograde atrial activity and therefore do not show AV dissociation)
Capture or fusion beats or both	No	Often (diagnostic if present)
QRS structure	Commonly right bundle-branch block, especially with RSR' in V_1 (R' usually > R)	Less often right bundle-branch block, rarely with RSR' in V_1 (R > R')
Initial 0.04-sec vector of QRS complex	Identical with normally conducted beats	Different from normally conducted beats
Rate	150–240 beats/min	120–250 beats/min
Regularity	Usually regular (unless atrial fibrillation or supraventricular tachycardia with variable block)	May have slight variation in cycle length (0.02–0.03 sec)
Response to carotid sinus pressure	May slow or revert to normal sinus rhythm	No response
Relation to prior electrocardiographic events	Structure may resemble preexisting bundle-branch block or previous aberrantly conducted premature beats	Structure may resemble previous ventricular premature beats

many beats per minute (rate related) or to handle a premature beat before it has recovered from the previous beat. The distinction between supraventricular tachycardia with aberrant conduction and ventricular tachycardia can be difficult. The following considerations are helpful (Table 5.1):

(1) AV dissociation. AV dissociation refers to that situation in which atrial and ventricular complexes are independent of each other. If a tachycardia originates in the atrium, the ventricular response bears a constant relation to atrial activity. However, if the tachycardia is ventricular, the atria often but not always depolarize independently at an entirely different and usually slower rate; the exception to this is the occasional case of ventricular tachycardia with constant retrograde atrial activation. Electrocardiographic evidence of AV dissociation is the strongest indication of a ventricular tachycardia (Fig. 5.2). As previously mentioned, physical findings of AV dissociation, such as cannon waves in the jugular veins and variable heart sounds, may provide additional clues.

(2) Capture or fusion beats. If the atria are beating independently of the ventricles and there is normal AV nodal function, occasionally a supraventricular impulse may be timed such that it finds the ventricle vulnerable. This results in an entirely normal and usually premature QRS complex in the midst of the widened complexes (a capture beat) or in a complex intermediate in width and configuration between the normal and abnormal complexes (a fusion beat or Dressler beat). Capture or fusion beats are further evidence that a tachycardia is ventricular. They usually

occur when the ventricular ectopic rate is relatively slow, thus allowing enough time for the AV node to recover sufficiently to conduct a sinus impulse.

(3) Structure of the QRS complex. Since the refractory period of the right bundle is normally longer than that of the left, aberrant ventricular conduction usually assumes the pattern of right bundle-branch block. Unfortunately, rhythms arising in the left ventricle also have a right bundle-branch block configuration. A right bundle-branch block pattern due to ventricular origin of the heart is more likely to be monophasic or if bi- or tri-phasic (RR' or RSR'), the R wave is of greater amplitude than the R'. With aberrant conduction, an RSR' pattern is more common and the R' wave is usually of greater amplitude than the R.

Additional information may be obtained from analysis of the first 0.04-second vector of the QRS complex. This portion is usually unaffected by aberration, that it, it is in the same direction as it is in the patient's normally conducted beats. It is different from that of the normal beats, the tachycardia is likely to be ventricular. To determine the direction of this vector accurately, it is necessary to examine the QRS complex in all the standard leads.

(4) Rate, regularity, and response to carotid sinus pressure. There is considerable overlap in rate between ventricular and supraventricular rhythms, but ventricular tachycardia rarely exceeds 200 beats/min. There is more likely to be slight variation in the R-R interval (0.02–0.03 second) with ventricular tachycardia, whereas su-

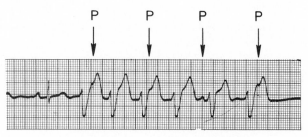

Figure 5.2. Ventricular tachycardia. This 6-beat aberrant tachycardia can be diagnosed as ventricular in origin because of electrocardiographic evidence of AV dissociation. Sinus P waves that continue through the tachycardia indicate that the atrium is beating independently of the ventricle.

praventricular tachycardia is more likely to be absolutely regular, with the exception of atrial fibrillation, which is characterized by total irregularity. A decrease in rate or conversion to sinus rhythm with carotid sinus pressure is diagnostic of a supraventricular origin (Fig. 5.3). (Technique is described on page 99).

(5) Relation to previous electrocardiographic events. Review of the patient's past electrocardiograms may provide diagnostic information. If the patient has had previous ventricular premature beats of identical configuration or has had similar aberrantly conducted supraventricular beats, the arrhythmia is likely to be related to these events.

Premature Beats and Pauses

The electrocardiogram must be analyzed for premature beats and pauses. Once the regular pattern of atrial and ventricular activation has been identified, it is possible to recognize beats that occur earlier than expected; these usually indicate increased automaticity of another pacemaker focus. It is also important to appreciate the failure of a beat to occur on time, which usually indicates delay within the conduction system or a disturbance of impulse formation within the dominant pacemaker. Premature beats and pauses often accompany each other, as is the case with either a ventricular premature beat followed by a compensatory pause or a nonconducted atrial premature beat.

DIAGNOSIS AND TREATMENT OF SPECIFIC ARRHYTHMIAS

We prefer to consider the recognition and treatment of cardiac rhythm disturbances according to features that are easily distinguished on the electrocardiogram. Three fundamental electrocardiographic characteristics form the basis of this approach: the heart rate, the regularity of the QRS complexes, and the width of the QRS complexes. This approach is schematically represented in Figure 5.4.

Tachycardias

Tachycardias are rhythms with rates more than 100 beats/min.

Regular Tachycardias with Narrow QRS Complexes

These constitute the most common group of rhythm disturbances. The narrow QRS complex indicates that the arrhythmia originated above the bifurcation of the bundle of His; hence, these are all supraventricular. The differential diagnosis is among *sinus tachycardia*, *paroxysmal supraventricular (atrial or junctional) tachycardia, atrial flutter*, and *nonparoxysmal junctional tachycardia*. Although junctional rhythms have been referred to as nodal rhythms, recent studies indicate that the AV node has little spontaneous automaticity and that most such rhythms arise in sites distal to the AV node but proximal to the bifurcation of the bundle of His—hence the term "junctional."

Sinus Tachycardia. This is not a true cardiac arrhythmia, but is merely an acceleration of the normal discharge rate of the sinus node. Sinus tachycardia is invariably secondary to a condition that is driving the heart at a faster rate.

In patients with sinus tachycardia, the heart rate rarely exceeds 150 beats/min, except in infants and children and in adults engaging in maximal physical exertion. There may be slight irregularity due to sinus arrhythmia, although at rapid heart rates, sinus arrhythmia is usually not present.

One of the problems in diagnosing sinus tachycardia lies in the fact that the P wave may be incorporated into the T wave of the preceding beat. A constant hump often subtly inscribed in the T wave may indicate the P wave. Also, comparison of prior electrocardiograms at slower rates may reveal more peaked T waves resulting from a combination of P and T waves. Carotid sinus pressure may produce enough slowing to dissociate the P wave from the T wave. Slowing is always gradual, and the heart usually resumes its prior rate on release of carotid sinus pressure. If premature beats are present, the sinus P wave may appear in the beat after the compensatory pause. If the P wave can be dissociated from the previous T wave, its axis will be normal—approximately +60 degrees.

With rare exceptions, treatment of sinus tachycardia is not directed at the rhythm itself. Rather, a careful search should be made for the underlying cause, and this should be appropriately managed.

Common causes include fever, sepsis, congestive heart failure, hypovolemia, hypoxemia, anemia, pulmonary embolism, thyrotoxicosis, anxiety, and drugs that accelerate the heart rate. Digitalis glycosides are indicated *only* if the sinus tachycardia is secondary to congestive heart failure.

One exception regarding therapy is sinus tachycardia in the presence of angina pectoris or acute myocardial infarction. Since the heart rate is a major determinant of myocardial oxygen consumption, slowing it may be important in the

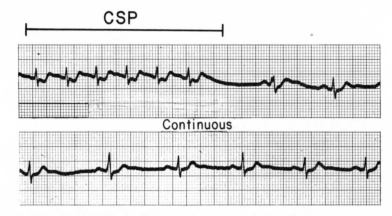

Figure 5.3. Paroxysmal atrial tachycardia converting to normal sinus rhythm with carotid sinus pressure. Initially there is a regular tachycardia at 140 beats/min with narrow QRS complexes and no clear atrial activity. With carotid sinus pressure, the rhythm changes abruptly—initially a pause, then a junctional escape beat, then return of normal sinus rhythm with gradual increase in rate as sinus node "warms up."

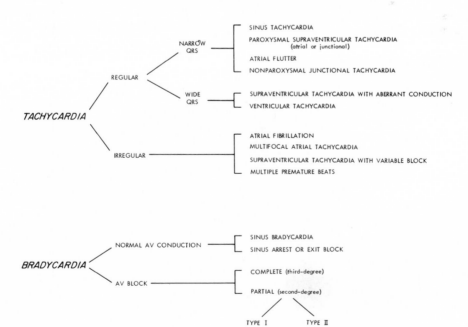

Figure 5.4. Arrhythmia flow sheet based on electrocardiographic features.

patient with myocardial ischemia. Angina may be relieved by slowing the heart rate with carotid sinus pressure. Slowing of sinus tachycardia may also abolish the ischemic pain of myocardial infarction, and may even limit the size of the necrotic area. Propranolol (Inderal), 1–5 mg intravenously to a maximum of 0.1 mg/kg of body weight, may be administered for this purpose if the sinus tachycardia is not associated with congestive heart failure. *Propranolol is contraindicated when congestive heart failure is present.* Caution should be exercised in administering intravenous propranolol to any patient with electrocardiographic evidence of an acute myocardial infarction. In general, we prefer to have a pulmonary artery line in place to monitor the pulmonary capillary wedge pressure and cardiac output before administering intravenous propranolol to patients with an acute myocardial infarction.

Paroxysmal Supraventricular Tachycardia. The term "paroxysmal supraventicular tachycardia" (SVT) includes paroxysmal tachycardia of both atrial and junctional origin, since in practice these are indistinguishable. The heart rate is usually between 150 and 200 beats/min, but it occasion-

ally may be faster, especially in infants and patients with Wolff-Parkinson-White syndrome.

These tachyarrhythmias are usually characterized by abrupt onset and termination, and the history often suggests the diagnosis. They tend to recur, and may occur in young persons without heart disease. Some patients experience polyuria concomitantly.

There are at least four types of paroxysmal supraventricular tachycardia and sometimes distinctions can be made based on the location and morphology of the P wave. The most common mechanism is a re-entry mechanism involving the AV node. In these cases, the P wave is usually invisible as it is buried in the QRS complex. If the P wave is visible, it is inverted in leads II, III and F, and is seen immediately after the QRS complex (Fig. 5.5). If the tachycardia is due to a re-entry mechanism involving an accessory pathway (see below), the P wave always follows the QRS complex and is retrograde. If the tachycardia is due to sinus node or atrial re-entry, the P wave will precede the QRS complex and usually will be of normal or nearly normal configuration. Finally, the tachycardia may be due to enhanced automa-

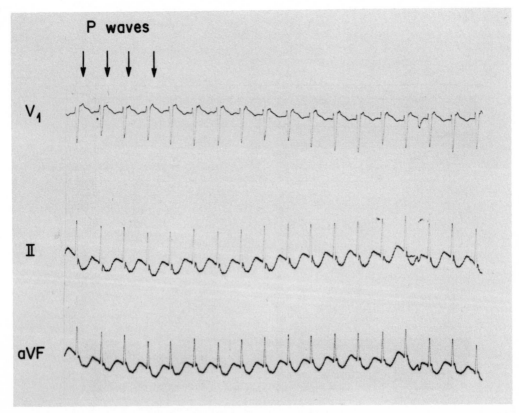

Figure 5.5.   Paroxysmal atrial tachycardia. This is a regular tachycardia at 180 beats/min with narrow QRS complexes. P waves at rate of 180 waves/min can be seen in lead V_1.

ticity of an ectopic pacemaker. In these cases, the P wave precedes the QRS complex and its morphology is variable depending on the site of the ectopic focus. SVTs due to this last mechanism may not have the abrupt onset or termination that is characteristic of those that occur by any of the re-entry mechanisms.

On physical examination, the heart sounds are uniform. In some cases, the atria and ventricles may contract simultaneously, causing constant cannon waves in the jugular veins. The response to carotid sinus pressure is often diagnostic, since abrupt cessation of the rhythm may be seen. Sinus rhythm returns after a pause, which sometimes is interrupted by junctional escape beats while the sinus "warms up" (Fig. 5.3). The tachycardia is characteristically regular, although it may be irregular for the first few beats. If the beginning of the arrhythmia is recorded, an atrial or junctional premature beat will be seen initiating the tachycardia. Once sinus rhythm is restored, sporadic atrial or junctional premature beats may provide further diagnostic clues. On application of carotid sinus pressure, a small number of patients have some degree of AV block rather than reversion to normal sinus rhythm. This should arouse suspicion of digitalis toxicity, which is present in about 75% of such patients (see below).

Initial treatment includes measures to increase vagal tone, such as carotid sinus pressure, Valsalva's maneuver, or induction of gagging. Vagal tone can be increased pharmacologically with edrophonium chloride (Tensilon), 5–10 mg intravenously. Its effect peaks in 1–3 minutes, and is dissipated in 10–15 minutes. Some patients experience nausea, cramps, or increased salivation. Administration of this drug to digitalized patients must be very cautious, because of an increased risk of profound bradycardia. Atropine sulfate, 0.5–1.0 mg, should be ready for immediate intravenous administration if an excessive vagal reaction develops. If conversion has not occurred by the time the effect of edrophonium chloride peaks, the maneuvers to increase vagal tone should be repeated.

If all of these measures are unsuccessful, a rapid-acting intravenous digitalis glycoside should be administered. We prefer digoxin (Lanoxin), 0.5 mg, Lanatoside C (Cedilanid), 0.8 mg, or ouabain, 0.5 mg, which may be administered alternatively. Digoxin begins to exert its effect in 15–30 minutes. Vagal stimulation should be repeated if conversion has not occurred by this time, since the digitalis glycosides further enhance vagal tone and may increase responsiveness to these maneuvers. If digoxin and vagal maneuvers are unsuccessful, ver-

apamil is the drug of choice. It is particularly effective for the cessation of re-entry arrhythmias involving the AV node, and some clinicians now may argue that it is the first drug of choice in these cases. The intravenous dose is 0.075 to 0.15 mg/kg (5–10 mg total dose in an average sized adult) given over 2–3 minutes. It has its peak effect within 10 minutes, and a repeat dose may be given if necessary in 30 minutes. Verapamil should be used with caution (if at all) in the presence of hypotension, severely depressed left ventricular function, or known conduction system disease. Elderly patients may be more prone to its adverse effects, particularly its bradycardic response.

Propranolol is another useful drug for the treatment of paroxysmal SVTs provided that the patient has neither severe hypotension nor a history of severe congestive heart failure or bronchospastic pulmonary disease. Propranolol may be administered intravenously in 1-mg increments every 5 minutes until either conversion is achieved or a total dose of 0.1 mg/kg (5–10 mg) is administered. Electrocardiographic monitoring and frequent determinations of blood pressure must accompany administration of propranolol, since profound bradycardia and hypotension may develop. Intravenous propranolol should never be given in close proximity to intravenous verapamil because of the risk of profound bradycardia and/or profound dysgenesis of ventricular function.

If the arrhythmia is still refractory, vasopressor agents may be administered to selected patients. Because of the risk of an adverse reaction to an excessive rise in blood pressure, this therapy should be reserved for young patients with healthy hearts and with relative hypotension accompanying the arrhythmia. The agent may be administered as an intravenous bolus (for example, phenylephrine [Neo-Synephrine], 0.5–1.5 mg, or methoxamine hydrochloride [Vasoxyl], 5–10 mg) or as a continuous intravenous infusion (for example, metaraminol [Aramine], 100 mg in 500 ml of 5% dextrose in water), titrating the infusion rate against the blood pressure. The goal is to return the blood pressure to a normal range or to slightly above normal, for example, approximately 150/90 mm Hg or 150/100 mm Hg. Drug administration must be stopped immediately on conversion or if blood pressure becomes excessively elevated. Blood pressure must be monitored carefully, and an intravenous α-adrenergic antagonist such as phentolamine (Regitine), 1–3 mg, must be available to counteract a potentially dangerous blood pressure elevation. A common consequence of excessive blood pressure response is severe occipital headache. Fatal intracerebral hemorrhage has resulted from the overzealous use of vasopressor agents.

In addition to the aforementioned drugs, intravenous lidocaine (Xylocaine) has been successful in a small number of patients. Intravenous phenytoin (Dilantin) may also be administered, but its effectiveness may be restricted to patients, with digitalis toxicity, especially when paroxysmal atrial tachycardia is accompanied by AV block. Rarely either quinidine sulfate or procainamide may be useful in treating these arrhythmias, particularly if they are associated with a pre-excitation syndrome (see below).

If these interventions have failed, and the patient is not tolerating the arrhythmia, either synchronized direct-current countershock or rapid atrial stimulation (see pages 79–80) is likely to be successful. It is unusual, however, to have to apply either of these measures.

Once conversion to sinus rhythm has been achieved, consideration must be given to prescribing an antiarrhythmic agent to prevent recurrences. The decision should be based on the frequency of the attacks and the severity of associated symptoms. The agents most likely to be successful in long-term prophylaxis are digoxin, 0.25 mg daily, or propranolol, 20–30 mg four times a day, or both. Quinidine, 200–300 mg four times a day, may also be effective as may procainamide or disopyramide. It is important to caution the patient about the possible role that caffeine, nicotine, sympathomimetic drugs, and other stimulants may play in the initiation of paroxysmal SVT.

Atrial Flutter. This arrhythmia, which tends to occur in patients with heart disease, is usually episodic. Atrial flutter is due to regular atrial depolarization at a rate of 250–300 beats/min. Since in most situations the AV node cannot conduct impulses at this rate, a physiologic 2:1 AV block results, in which the ventricular response is approximately 150 beats/min (Fig. 5.6A). In infants, 1:1 conduction can occur. *Any absolutely regular SVT at a rate of 150 beats/min should raise the suspicion of atrial flutter.* The response to carotid sinus pressure may be characteristic in that it results in a stepwise decrease in rate caused by increasing degrees of AV block (usually from 2:1 to 4:1) without a change in the underlying atrial mechanism. Atrial activity can be seen on the electrocardiogram at a rate of approximately 300 beats/min appearing as "sawtooth" deflections in the inferior leads or as positive deflections in the right precordial leads (Fig. 5.6B). When atrial activity cannot be clearly distinguished in the baseline electrocardiogram or after carotid sinus pressure, edrophonium chloride, 5–10 mg intravenously, may cause transient AV block and allow identification of flutter waves. If this fails, a right atrial electrocardiogram usually permits clear definition of atrial activity.

The drugs of choice for conversion or control of heart rate or both in patients with atrial flutter are the digitalis glycosides, verapamil, or propranolol alone or in combination. Digoxin can be administered in an initial bolus of 0.5 mg intravenously. Digoxin may result either in the establishment of a higher degree of AV block, or may cause conversion to sinus rhythm. Verapamil (5–10 mg in-

A. V₁

B. LEAD II

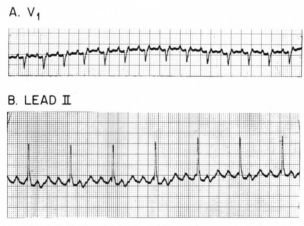

Figure 5.6. Atrial flutter. **(A)** Atrial rate is 300 beats/min and ventricular rate is 150 beats/min; there is a physiologic 2:1 AV block. This is the most common presentation of atrial flutter: a regular tachycardia at 150 beats/min with narrow QRS complexes. Note that flutter waves are positive in lead V₁. **(B)** Electrocardiogram from different patient, which illustrates atrial flutter with 4:1 AV block. This occurred in a fully digitalized patient in whom digitalis caused a higher degree of AV block. Atrial rate is 280 beats/min, and ventricular rate is 70 beats/min with narrow QRS complexes. Note that flutter waves are negative "sawtooth" deflections in lead II.

travenously) has its sole effect on AV conduction, so it may result in a beneficial slowing of the ventricular response, but will not convert atrial flutter to sinus rhythm. Propranolol can be administered intravenously at the rate of 1 mg/min every 3–5 minutes until conversion has been achieved, the heart rate has been slowed, or a total dose of 0.1 mg/kg has been given. As noted above, intravenous propranolol should not be given in close proximity to intravenous verapamil.

If conversion to sinus rhythm does not occur with initial drug administration, we prefer to convert the arrhythmia electrically. Atrial flutter is extraordinarily responsive to electrical cardioversion, and can usually be terminated with low energy levels, for example, 20–100 joules. Cardioversion is safe with the small amounts of digitalis glycosides that have been recommended, but it becomes risky if larger quantities have been given as is often necessary to control the ventricular response. Hence, we prefer to cardiovert early in the course of atrial flutter.

In refractory cases and when digitalis excess is suspected, rapid atrial stimulation may be success-

ful in converting the rhythm (Fig. 5.7). A transvenous electrode is placed in the right atrium, and the position is confirmed electrocardiographically and radiographically. The atrium is stimulated initially at a rate of 150 impulses/min with sufficient current (usually about 5 milliamperes) to capture it or to interrupt the flutter waves. The rate and amperage may be progressively increased to 1200 impulses/min and 25 milliamperes, respectively, if necessary. The pacemaker must be turned off after several seconds of pacing at each increment to determine whether the rhythm has been altered. In 40–50% of patients, sinus rhythm is restored. In 25%, atrial flutter is converted to atrial fibrillation, which may then spontaneously revert to sinus rhythm; even if it does not, however, the heart rate can be controlled more easily with digitalis glycosides than is the case with atrial flutter. Atrial fibrillation cannot be converted by rapid atrial stimulation.

Occasionally, a patient is tolerating atrial flutter sufficiently well to allow a more leisurely approach in which case one can slowly digitalize the patient over 24 or 48 hours (with or without adjunctive

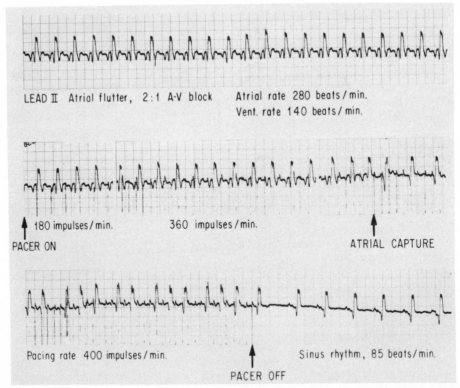

LEAD II Atrial flutter, 2:1 A-V block   Atrial rate 280 beats/min.
Vent. rate 140 beats/min.

180 impulses/min.   360 impulses/min.   ATRIAL CAPTURE
PACER ON

Pacing rate 400 impulses/min.   Sinus rhythm, 85 beats/min.
PACER OFF

Figure 5.7. Rapid atrial pacing to convert atrial flutter. Top panel shows classic atrial flutter with negative atrial depolarization at rate of 280 beats/min (flutter waves) in lead II and with regular ventricular response of 140 beats/min. Rate of atrial pacemaker was increased progressively until atrium was captured, and sinus rhythm returned with cessation of pacing. (Reproduced by permission, from *Circulation*, Vol. 43, No. 5, © 1971, The American Heart Association.)

therapy with propranolol or verapamil). If control of the ventricular response is achieved in this way, but the patient remains in atrial flutter, then an attempt can be made to convert the patient pharmacologically with an agent such as quinidine sulfate. There is a small risk of acceleration of the ventricular response with the addition of quinidine and patients need to be hospitalized and closely monitored if this approach is to be taken.

Once conversion has occurred, it is wise to leave the pacing electrode in the atrium for a period of observation so that it is available for the diagnosis or treatment of any subsequent arrhythmias. Long-term oral administration of digoxin and an agent such as quinidine sulfate, 200–300 mg every 6 hours, may be helpful in preventing recurrences.

Nonparoxysmal Junctional Tachycardia. This arrhythmia is due to gradual acceleration of the junctional pacemaker, and is distinguished from the paroxysmal SVTs by its gradual onset and termination and its slower rate, which rarely exceeds 140–150 beats/min. It occurs most commonly in patients with digitalis toxicity or acute inferior myocardial infarction, and may also be seen after cardiac operations (particularly mitral valve replacement) and in patients with inflammation in the region of the AV node due to acute rheumatic or viral myocarditis or bacterial endocarditis. The electrocardiogram reveals regular QRS complexes of normal width with absent or retrograde atrial activity. Carotid sinus pressure usually evokes no response. Constant cannon waves may be seen in the jugular veins.

Nonparoxysmal junctional tachycardia is usually well tolerated, and rarely requires therapy other than withholding digitalis if digitalis excess is the cause. Correction of hypokalemia is also important. This arrhythmia is usually unresponsive to conventional antiarrhythmic drugs, and its presence should stimulate a search for a possible underlying cause. Occasionally a patient with severely impaired ventricular function may not tolerate this rhythm because of a fall in cardiac output due to the loss of atrial systole. In these cases, overdrive atrial pacing may be necessary to restore physiologic atrial and ventricular synchrony.

Regular Tachycardias with Wide QRS Complexes

These are among the most challenging of all the arrhythmias because the differential diagnosis lies between a *SVT with aberrant conduction and ventricular tachycardia*. The principles followed in making this differentiation have already been detailed (Table 5.1). It should be stressed that, if the condition of a patient with such an arrhythmia is hemodynamically compromised, the treatment of choice is cardioversion, whether the arrhythmia is ventricular or supraventricular. The only possible exception is the patient in whom digitalis toxicity is suspected.

SVT with Aberrant Conduction. Treatment is that of the particular supraventricular rhythm disturbance. The presence of aberrantly conducted ventricular complexes does not influence the choice of therapy. The hemodynamic status of these patients is usually more stable than that of a patient with ventricular tachycardia at a similar rate and, thus, there usually is time to employ drug therapy safely.

Ventricular Tachycardia. This type of tachycardia is diagnosed by electrocardiographic evidence of AV dissociation (Fig. 5.2) and by findings on physical examination such as cannon waves and variable heart sounds and blood pressure. Physical findings of AV dissociation are absent in ventricular tachycardia if either atrial fibrillation or 1:1 retrograde activation of the atria by the ventricles is present. Ventricular tachycardia almost always is associated with underlying heart disease, which is often ischemic; a small number of patients, however, may have isolated or recurrent ventricular tachycardia without any other evidence of heart disease.

Cardioversion is the treatment of choice in the presence of significant hemodynamic compromise, and the decision whether to perform cardioversion must be made quickly at the bedside. Some patients are obviously moribund when first seen, in which case cardioversion should be performed immediately. Others tolerate the arrhythmia reasonably well. Cardioversion should usually be undertaken if any of the following complications are pesent: (1) a systolic blood pressure of 90 mm Hg or less; (2) poor peripheral perfusion indicated by cool, clammy, mottled extremities, mental obtundation, and oliguria; (3) congestive heart failure manifested by dyspnea, orthopnea, pulmonary edema, or a considerably elevated systemic venous pressure; and (4) ischemic myocardial pain. Once again, the only relative contraindication to cardioversion in patients with ventricular tachycardia is digitalis toxicity (see pages 94–95). Cardioversion is successful in more than 90% of patients, and can usually be accomplished with a low energy level from 50–100 joules. A firm thump delivered to the precordium with a clenched fist may deliver enough energy to cardiovert this rhythm in some instances. This technique (thump version) should be tried once the diagnosis has been made and while preparing for cardioversion, but should not persist with repeated attempts once ready to cardiovert electrically.

In less urgent situations and when ventricular tachycardia recurs after initial conversion, pharmacologic therapy is indicated. Lidocaine is the first agent of choice because of its efficacy and relative safety. An initial intravenous bolus, 1–2 mg/kg, should be administered to achieve a therapeutic level in the blood rapidly (2–5 μg/ml). Additional boluses of 1 mg/kg can be administered every 5–10 minutes until either conversion has occurred or a maximum of 5 mg/kg has been administered. The most common toxic effects are central nervous system reactions such as drowsiness, dysarthria, tinnitus, bizarre behavior, and seizures. After conversion, further ventricular ectopy can usually be suppressed by a constant intravenous infusion of lidocaine, 20–55 μg/kg/min, which is about 1–4 mg/min in an average-sized adult. Lidocaine has little depressant effect on myocardial contractility and on conduction time, although isolated cases of sinoatrial and AV block have been reported after lidocaine therapy. The drug is quickly metabolized, primarily in the liver, and toxic levels may be more rapidly achieved in the presence of severe hepatic disease or congestive heart failure.

Lidocaine may be ineffective in 10–20% of patients, and procainamide (Pronestyl) is the next drug of choice. Although there is slightly greater risk of hypotension with intravenous use of this drug, it usually can be administered safely in 100-mg increments every 5 minutes to a total dose of 1 gm or until a toxic reaction or abolition of the arrhythmia occurs. Blood pressure must be carefully monitored during intravenous administration of procainamide, and the electrocardiogram must be watched closely for evidence of AV or intraventricular block, since procainamide can prolong conduction times. Therapeutic levels of the drug are between 4 and 8 μg/ml; above these levels, significant prolongation of QRS complexes and of Q-T intervals is likely. Since the drug is rapidly metabolized and excreted by the kidney, oral or intramuscular doses should be repeated at 3-hour intervals to maintain a therapeutic level. Usually, 250–500 mg every 3–4 hours provides adequate suppression of further ventricular ectopic activity.

In cases of stubborn ventricular irritability unresponsive to intravenous lidocaine, an intravenous infusion of procainamide, 20–40 μg/kg/min (1–4 mg/min), may be effective in suppressing the ectopy. When given in this manner, procainamide should be administered by means of a constant infusion pump.

A third drug for the treatment of recurrent or resistant ventricular tachycardia is bretylium. It may be given as a single intravenous dose of 5 mg/kg over 10 minutes. Since bretylium initially causes release of stored catecholamines from nerve terminals, there may be an initial hypertensive response, and it also has been reported to cause an initial exacerbation of ventricular ectopy in such patients. Though the drug may lower immediately the ventricular fibrillation threshold, its effect in suppressing ventricular ectopy may not be seen for 20 minutes to 2 hours. The major side effect of the drug is hypotension due to peripheral vasodilatation. In some cases, this may be profound and may require rapid volume infusion or administration of α-adrenergic agents. For this reason, patients should always be in the supine position when given the drug. There also may be an increased risk of exacerbating ventricular ectopy if bretylium is administered to patients with digitalis intoxication. In some cases of refractory ventricular tachycardia, continuous infusion with bretylium (1–2 mg/min) is necessary for control of these arrhythmias.

Another drug is phenytoin. This is more likely to be successful—and may be the drug of choice—if the arrhythmia is induced by digitalis. It is not very effective in terminating ventricular tachycardia that is not due to digitalis excess. Phenytoin may safely be administered intravenously in 100-mg increments every 5 minutes until a total of 1 gm has been given, the arrhythmia has been controlled, or side effects have developed. It has little myocardial depressant effect, and causes little or no depression of conduction times, although hypotension, arrhythmias, and respiratory arrest have been reported during rapid intravenous administration. The therapeutic level in the blood is 10–18 μg/ml; above this level, neurologic toxic reactions develop, such as nystagmus, ataxia, and somnolence. Phenytoin is caustic, and when administered intravenously, it should be delivered through a central line or into a peripheral line with a rapidly running solution of 5% dextrose in water. It should not be administered intramuscularly because of erratic absorption. Once a therapeutic blood level has been achieved, it usually can be maintained with oral doses of 300–400 mg daily.

Intravenous propranolol also may be administered, either alone or in conjunction with one or more of the aforementioned agents. Like phenytoin, it appears to be more effective if the ventricular tachycardia is digitalis induced. The intravenous dose is 1 mg every 5 minutes up to either 0.1 mg/kg, cessation of the arrhythmia, or tolerance. Major limitations are its considerable myocardial depressant effect and its potential for inducing bronchospasm. Antiarrhythmic blood levels usually can be maintained with a total dose of 80–240 mg daily in 4–6 divided doses.

Quinidine may also be useful in suppressing recurrent ventricular arrhythmias, but because its intravenous administration has been associated with severe hypotensive reactions, it plays little role in the management of the acute arrhythmia. Therapeutic blood levels can usually be maintained with doses of 200–400 mg orally or intramuscularly every 6 hours. It has now been well shown that in some cases, quinidine actually may exacerbate ventricular ectopy. This phenomenon in part may be mediated by quinidine's capacity for prolonging the QT interval, though its does not correlate entirely with that phenomenon. It is likely that this potential for exacerbating ventricular ectopy is also true of other antiarrhythmic agents, and it should be considered as a possible cause for refractory or worsening ventricular ectopy in the face of escalating numbers and doses of antiarrhythmic therapy.

A particular malignant form of ventricular tachycardia with a characteristic morphology has been named "Torsade de pointe", a name chosen to reflect the turning of the QSR axis during the tachycardia. This form of ventricular tachycardia has been particularly associated with situations that prolong the QT interval (such as quinidine therapy), underlying bradyarrhythmias, or acute ischemia or inflammation.

To suppress refractory ventricular irritability, the aforementioned drugs may be administered in combination; at present such therapy in the acute situation is largely empirical.

If drug therapy fails to prevent recurrence of ventricular tachycardia, *overdrive pacing* of either the right atrium or the right ventricle may be successful in suppressing an ectopic pacemaker (Fig. 5.8). Pacing is more likely to be successful if the patient's normal heart rate is slow. Suppression is usually achieved with pacing rates between 90 and 120 impulses/min. In patients with coronary artery disease, pacing at such rates may be tolerated poorly because of the concomitant increase in oxygen consumption, and ischemic pain or a paradoxical increase in ventricular irritability may result.

Every effort must be made to identify and to treat the factors contributing to the genesis and propagation of ventricular tachycardia. The importance of recognizing digitalis excess has already been mentioned. The serum potassium level should be brought to the upper range of normal (4.5–5.0 mEq/liter) by an intravenous infusion of potassium chloride, 10–20 mEq/hr. Hypoxemia

A.

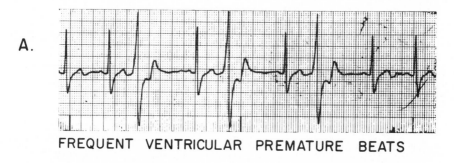

FREQUENT VENTRICULAR PREMATURE BEATS

B.

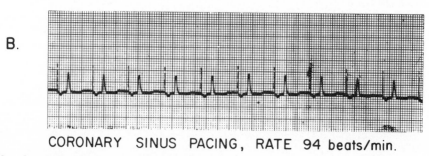

CORONARY SINUS PACING, RATE 94 beats/min.

Figure 5.8.   Overdrive pacing for suppression of ventricular ectopic beats. **(A)** Ventricular bigeminy in patient with history of recurrent ventricular tachycardia resistant to pharmacologic suppression. **(B)** Ventricular ectopic activity has been eliminated by instituting coronary sinus (atrial) pacing at 94 impulses/min. (Reproduced by permission, from *Circulation*, Vol. 43, No. 5, © 1971, The American Heart Association.)

should be corrected, and any exogenous source of β-adrenergic stimulation should be withdrawn. The possible role of intracardiac mechanical factors should also be kept in mind. A central venous pressure catheter that has migrated into the right ventricle or a pacing electrode or Swan-Ganz pulmonary artery catheter in the right ventricle may be responsible for persistent or recurrent ventricular tachycardia that is particularly resistant to therapy.

Ventricular Flutter and Fibrillation. Ventricular flutter is a prefibrillatory rhythm in which there is still regular ventricular electrical activity at rates of 200–300 beats/min, but there is little or no effective mechanical activity. Ventricular fibrillation represents totally chaotic ventricular electrical activity with no cardiac output (Fig. 5.9). Both of these rhythms are medical emergencies requiring immediate electrical conversion. Ventricular fibrillation is likely to recur, particularly in the patient with ischemic heart disease. Therefore, once the heart is successfully defibrillated, immediate attention must be given to correction of underlying causes and to institution of prophylactic antiarrhythmic therapy with lidocaine or procainamide or both.

Irregular Tachycardias with Narrow or Wide QRS Complexes

Only rarely is a very irregular tachycardia exclusively ventricular. With an irregular tachycardia, widening of the QRS complex is due to either aberrant conduction or ventricular ectopic beats in the presence of another rhythm. Whether the QRS complexes are wide or narrow, the differential diagnosis of an irregular tachycardia is among *atrial fibrillation, multifocal atrial tachycardia, SVT with varying degrees of AV block,* and *multiple premature beats of atrial, junctional,* or *ventricular origin.*

Atrial Fibrillation. This is usually easily recognized by its irregularly irregular ventricular response and the undulating baseline between QRS complexes (Fig. 5.10). There is no organized atrial activity. At very fast rates, the ventricular response

is less irregular than at slow rates. The fibrillatory waves in the baseline may be almost inapparent ("fine" atrial fibrillation) or may be several millimeters in amplitude ("coarse" atrial fibrillation). Fine fibrillatory waves are seen more commonly in ischemic or hypertensive heart disease, and coarse waves are more common in rheumatic mitral valvular disease. Carotid sinus pressure characteristically results in gradual slowing of the ventricular response without affecting the atrial mechanism or degree of irregularity.

Atrial fibrillation may occur with either narrow or wide QRS complexes. Wide complexes are uniformly present if right or left bundle-branch block accompanies the atrial fibrillation. When wide complexes are present intermittently, the distinction must be made between an occasional aberrantly conducted beat and coexisting ventricular premature beats. This can be done by recognizing the *Ashman phenomenon*, that is, that an aberrantly conducted beat often ends a short cycle (R-R interval) that has followed a long cycle (Fig. 5.11). These aberrantly conducted beats almost invariably exhibit a right bundle-branch block pattern. The ventricular origin of wide beats is favored by the absence of the Ashman phenomenon, the presence of a left bundle-branch block pattern, or a difference between the initial 0.04-second vector of the normal and abnormal beats. In addition, ventricular premature beats are likely to have a nearly constant coupling interval with the preceding normal beats and are likely to be followed by a pause. The distinction between aberrancy and ventricular ectopy may be important in deciding whether a patient with atrial fibrillation requires more digitalis or is already showing signs of digitalis excess.

Atrial fibrillation usually occurs in patients with heart disease, and it should stimulate attempts to determine the underlying condition. Arteriosclerotic and hypertensive heart diseases are the most common causes, but rheumatic heart disease always must be considered, particularly mitral stenosis or regurgitation or both. Cardiomyopathy, pericarditis, and certain noncardiac diseases, such

MONITOR LEAD

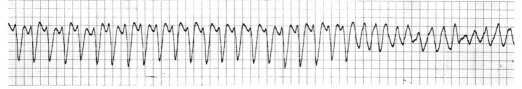

Figure 5.9. Ventricular fibrillation. Ventricular tachycardia at 155 beats/min degenerates into ventricular fibrillation with chaotic, disorganized ventricular rhythm.

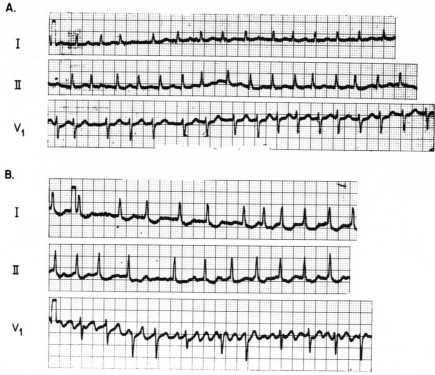

Figure 5.10. Atrial fibrillation **(A)** Irregularly irregular ventricular response with narrow QRS complexes and no clearly definable atrial activity. This is "fine" atrial fibrillation with rapid ventricular response. **(B)** QRS complexes are narrow and are irregularly irregular. Atrial activity is seen in lead V₁ as irregular fibrillatory waves bearing no constant relation to QRS complexes. This is "coarse" atrial fibrillation with rapid ventricular response.

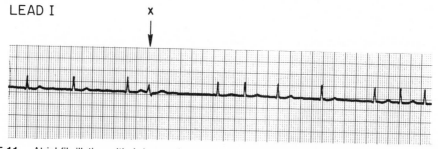

Figure 5.11. Atrial fibrillation with Ashman phenomenon. The ventricular activity is irregularly irregular with no discernible atrial activity. One beat (marked "X") is broader than other complexes and has terminal S wave. This beat concludes shortest R-R interval on strip and follows one of longest intervals. This sequence of long interval followed by short interval favors aberrant conduction (often with right bundle-branch block pattern) as shown here. This type of aberrant conduction seen in atrial fibrillation is known as the Ashman phenomenon.

as pulmonary embolism, pneumonia, chronic obstructive pulmonary disease, and thyrotoxicosis, are also possible underlying causes. A small number of patients have *paroxysmal* atrial fibrillation without other evidence of heart disease. These patients are often young, and the onset of fibrillation may be correlated with stress or the use of alcohol or other stimulants. A smaller group of patients may have chronic atrial fibrillation in the absence of any obvious heart disease; this is "lone" atrial fibrillation, and is probably a form of sick sinus syndrome (see below).

Digitalis glycosides are the drugs of choice for rate control. Large amounts may be needed, particularly in patients who have atrial fibrillation of recent onset, who previously have not been receiving digitalis, or who are acutely ill. The shorter-acting digitalis preparations offer little advantage over digoxin, and the physician should be familiar with this preparation, which can be used in both acute and chronic situations. In the patient who has not been receiving a digitalis preparation, initial doses of 0.5–0.75 mg of digoxin may be administered intravenously; in the patient who has previously received digitalis, 0.125 or 0.25 mg is the proper dose if the ventricular rate is rapid. Intravenous digoxin begins to exert its effect in 15–30 minutes, and its peak effect occurs in 1½–4 hours. Additional digoxin may be administered every 2–4 hours in increments of 0.125 or 0.25 mg as needed for rate control. Sometimes up to 2 mg is necessary in the first 24 hours. If the heart rate is refractory to digitalis, intravenous propranolol in 1-mg increments may be administered if no contraindications are present; the total dose must not exceed 0.1 mg/kg.

The calcium channel blocking agent verapamil is another agent which is effective for control of the ventricular response to atrial fibrillation. It exerts its electrophysiologic effects solely on the AV node. It may be administered in an intravenous dose of 5–10 mg and it usually will exert its slowing effect in 10 minutes. Its main side effects are hypotension and depression of ventricular function. In some instances, it may cause profound bradycardia, particularly in elderly patients with underlying conduction system disease or prior administration of β-adrenergic blocking drugs. Though it has the advantage over digoxin of being more rapidly acting and more specific in its site of action, its duration of action is shorter (30–60 min) and it usually will not obviate the need to give digitalis glycosides. For that reason, digoxin has remained the drug of choice in our opinion, with the use of verapamil as adjunctive therapy to gain additional control of the ventricular response while waiting to get the patient fully digitalized.

"Adequate" control of heart rate usually means a ventricular response of 70–90 beats/min. However, a rapid ventricular response in a patient with atrial fibrillation may be partly a physiologic response to hypoxemia, fever, hypovolemia, congestive heart failure, or other stimuli. Thus, measures to correct these problems should be instituted while administering digoxin or propranolol or both.

In most patients with rapid atrial fibrillation, the heart rate is slowed with the measures just mentioned, but atrial fibrillation continues. In about 15–20% of patients with new onset of atrial fibrillation, conversion to sinus rhythm occurs with digitalis, verapamil, propranolol, or simply the passage of time. In another small percentage, the hemodynamic status may deteriorate because of the rapid rate and loss of atrial transport, and these patients should be considered for early emergency cardioversion. If the patient is unresponsive to therapy, it is best to perform cardioversion early, since the risk of this procedure is substantially increased if it is performed after large doses of digitalis have been administered. Cardioversion has been successful in restoring sinus rhythm at least transiently in about 90% of patients with atrial fibrillation.

Some patients with atrial fibrillation have bradycardia rather than tachycardia. In this situation, digitalis toxicity or intrinsic conduction system disease should be suspected, and digitalis and other drugs that further depress AV conduction should be administered very cautiously, if at all. Digitalis toxicity is particularly likely if the patient has either a slow but regular ventricular rate (indicating a junctional rhythm, Fig. 5.12) or frequent ventricular premature beats or both. Rarely, pervenous ventricular pacing is required to accelerate the heart rate.

Multifocal Atrial Tachycardia. This condition is easily confused with atrial fibrillation. It is similar in rate and irregularity, but is distinguished by the presence of organized atrial activity. Characteristically, P waves of three or more configurations occur at varying P-P intervals with variation in P-R intervals as well (Fig. 5.13). The arrhythmia is usually unresponsive to carotid sinus pressure, although some degree of AV block may be induced. It occurs most commonly in elderly patients with acute or chronic respiratory disease.

Treatment is primarily that of the underlying causative respiratory and metabolic abnormalities. The most serious error in the management of this arrhythmia is administration of increasing doses of digitalis glycosides for rate control in the belief that the rhythm is atrial fibrillation. Although it does not appear that the rhythm itself is often due to digitalis toxicity, it does not respond to digitalis, and digitalis toxicity may readily result. If congestive heart failure is present, however, digitalis may be indicated. Antiarrhythmic agents do not suppress multifocal atrial tachycardia satisfactorily, and efforts must be directed at correcting hypoxemia, hypokalemia, and acid-base disorders. The arrhythmia is associated with a high mortality of 40–50%, primarily because of the critical condition of the patients in whom it is seen.

Wandering atrial pacemaker is a variant of the same rhythm disturbance in that varying P-wave structures are seen, but at a slower rate. Unlike multifocal atrial tachycardia, this rhythm may occur in the absence of cardiac or systemic disease, and is usually benign.

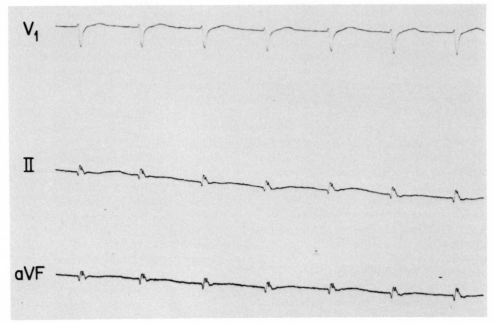

Figure 5.12. Accelerated junctional rhythm due to digitalis toxicity. There is no discernible atrial activity and there is a regular ventricular rate of 70 beats/min with narrow QRS complexes. The patient had been in atrial fibrillation, and increasing doses of digitalis had been given to control ventricular response. This "regularized" rhythm resulted and is due to acceleration of the junctional pacemaker. Atrial mechanism is still atrial fibrillation, and an irregularly irregular ventricular response returned when digitalis was withheld.

Lead II

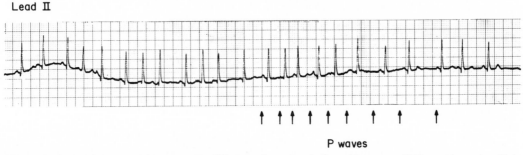

P waves

Figure 5.13. Multifocal atrial tachycardia. This is an irregular rhythm with narrow QRS complexes in which every QRS complex is preceded by a P wave. There are, however, several different P-wave morphologies and P-R intervals; this indicates that impulses arise from several different foci in atrium.

SVT with Varying Degrees of AV Block. If the AV node permits every second, third, or fourth beat to be transmitted from the atrium to the ventricle at different times, an arrhythmia that ordinarily might be a regular SVT, such as atrial flutter or paroxysmal SVT, becomes manifested as an irregular ventricular response. The diagnosis depends on identification of atrial activity, as well as appreciation of a recurrent pattern to the irregularity rather than the irregular irregularity of atrial fibrillation or multifocal atrial tachycardia.

Treatment is that of the particular supraventricular arrhythmia; however, either digitalis toxicity or intrinsic AV nodal disease may be present in patients with variable AV block. Atrial tachycardia with AV block must be presumed to be due to digitalis toxicity whenever it occurs in a patient known to be receiving a digitalis preparation.

Multiple Premature Beats. These may simulate a tachyarrhythmia, and may produce similar hemodynamic consequences if they diminish the number of mechanically effective beats.

Atrial or Junctional Premature Beats. These premature beats usually have QRS complexes similar to or only slightly different from the QRS complexes of the sinus beats. If they are preceded by upright P waves in leads II, III, and aVF, they are presumed to be atrial; if there is no identifiable atrial activity or if there are P waves preceding or following the QRS complex that are inverted in leads II, III, and aVF, they are presumed to be junctional. Atrial and junctional premature beats that retrogradely depolarize the atrium characteristically reset the sinus pacemaker. Therefore, the interval from the premature beat to the next normally conducted beat is usually approximately equal to the normal R-R interval, that is, there is no compensatory pause.

Atrial and junctional premature beats are benign, and rarely require treatment. They may, however, indicate the potential development of a more serious supraventricular arrhythmia, such as atrial fibrillation, atrial flutter, or paroxysmal SVT. When multiple atrial or junctional premature beats occur in a patient with a history of sustained or recurrent supraventricular arrhythmia, prophylactic suppression with drugs such as quinidine or propranolol may be indicated.

Ventricular Premature Beats. These beats, which have wide, sometimes bizarre QRS complexes, must be distinguished from supraventricular premature beats with aberrant conduction. In addition to the absence of preceding atrial activity and the presence of the morphologic features of the QRS complex listed in Table 5.1, ventricular premature beats usually are followed by a compensatory pause, and the resultant interval from the premature beat to the subsequent conducted beat exceeds the normal R-R interval (Fig. 5.14). The interval from the preceding conducted beat to the subsequent conducted beat equals *two* normal R-R intervals. Occasionally, a ventricular premature beat is timed in such a way that the next conducted beat occurs exactly when it should, without a pause. Such a premature beat is said to be *interpolated*, occurring between two normally conducted beats.

Ventricular premature beats are of two types: re-entrant and parasystolic. Re-entry results from delay in the passage of a normally conducted impulse through an area of the ventricle; delay may be caused by ischemia, fibrosis, inflammation, or other factors. When the impulse finally traverses the area of retarded conduction, it finds the ventricle repolarized, and it is discharged prematurely. In contrast, parasystole is caused by the repetitive discharge of a so-called protected focus in one of the ventricles, which captures the ventricles whenever it finds them susceptible. Most ventricular premature beats are due to re-entry.

The coupling interval between a re-entrant ventricular premature beat and the preceding normal beat is usually constant, and intervals that vary up to 0.06–0.08 second are still considered "fixed." When no constant coupling intervals occur and the beats are clearly ventricular, parasystole should be suspected. This diagnosis is confirmed by examining a long rhythm strip and finding that the intervals between ectopic beats are whole-number multiples of a common interval. An additional feature of parasystole is that fusion beats are common. Fusion beats have a configuration intermediate between that of ectopic beats and normally conducted beats.

Ventricular premature beats originating in the left ventricle usually display a pattern of right bundle-branch block, and those originating in the right ventricle usually exhibit a left bundle-branch block configuration. They are the most common form of cardiac rhythm disturbance, and although they do not necessarily indicate heart disease, they are more common in such patients, particularly those with coronary artery disease. The decision as to whether treatment is required depends on the presence or absence of symptoms, the setting in which they occur, and the presence or absence of certain features that suggest the possibility of a more serious condition. In general, ventricular premature beats should be suppressed if any of the following is fulfilled, alone or in combination: (1) the patient is symptomatic, with palpitations, light-headedness, or syncope presumably related to more serious ventricular arrhythmias triggered by the premature beats; (2) there is evidence of active myocardial ischemia or infarction as indicated by ischemic chest pain or electrocardiographic

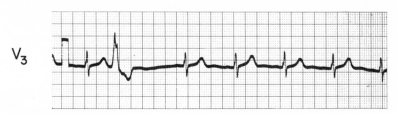

Figure 5.14.   Ventricular premature beat. An isolated ventricular premature beat is recorded. There is a full compensatory pause. QRS complex of premature beat has left bundle-branch block pattern.

changes or both; (3) digitalis toxicity is suspected; or (4) the premature beats occur sequentially, arise from more than one focus, fall close to or on the T wave of the preceding beat, or are very frequent (usually more than 5–10 beats/min).

The drugs used to suppress ventricular premature beats are the same as those discussed for ventricular tachycardia—lidocaine, procainamide, bretylium, phenytoin, propranolol, and quinidine—and attention must be given to the possible role of hypokalemia, hypoxemia, drugs, or mechanical factors in predisposing the heart to ventricular irritability.

Bradycardias

Rhythms with rates less than 60 beats/min are classified as bradycardias. The differential diagnosis is less complex than with the tachyarrhythmias, but the same principles are followed—identification of atrial and ventricular activity and determination of their relation. These rhythm disturbances involve *dysfunction of the sinus or AV node.*

Sinus Bradycardia

In sinus bradycardia, there is a normal 1:1 relation between P waves and QRS complexes; only the rate is slow. Sinus bradycardia may indicate dysfunction of the sinus node, or it may be a normal, physiologic arrhythmia, especially in well-trained athletes. It also may be drug induced, particularly by propranolol or other β-adrenergic blockers, and it may be seen in states of heightened vagal tone and in patients with hypothyroidism.

Sinus bradycardia usually does not require treatment, unless the slow rate is associated with hypotension, congestive heart failure, or symptoms. If treatment is required, atropine sulfate, 0.5–1.0 mg intravenously, or isoproterenol (Isuprel), 1–2 μg/min intravenously, is the agent of choice. Rarely, transvenous pacing may be required if the bradycardia is profound or refractory to these medications.

Sinus Arrest or Exit Block

In sinus arrest or exit block, P waves are either absent or only intermittent. If present, each P wave is followed by a QRS complex, but long pauses may be ended by QRS complexes without P waves (*junctional escape beats,* Fig. 5.15). Isolated pauses simulating sinus arrest may be caused by *nonconducted atrial premature beats.* These can be diagnosed by appreciating some deformity in the T wave preceding the pause. This deformity results from superimposition of a premature P wave on a normal T wave.

The indication for treating sinus arrest or exit block is the same as that for treating sinus bradycardia. Likewise, treatment is the same, except that sinus arrest or exit block is more often resistant to drug therapy, and if the patient is symptomatic, transvenous pacing is more likely to be required.

AV Block

First-degree AV block is present if the P-R interval is prolonged beyond 0.20 second but all P waves are followed by a QRS complex. In second- and third-degree AV block, there are more P waves than QRS complexes. In second-degree block, some P waves are conducted to the ventricles and some are not. This degree of heart block, which is described by the ratio of P waves to QRS complexes (for example, 2:1, 3:2, or 4:3), can be divided into type I (Wenckebach-Mobitz I) and type II (Mobitz II). In type I, the P-R intervals of the conducted beats become progressively longer

LEAD II

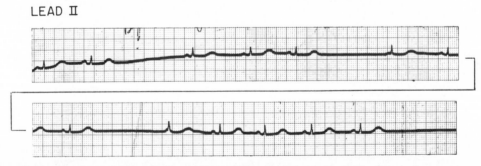

Figure 5.15.   Sinus arrest. Sinus rhythm is present with slight sinus arrhythmia. There are several pauses lasting approximately 2 seconds in which no P waves are seen. Two pauses are ended by narrow (supraventricular) complexes that are not preceded by P waves, and then a sinus beat follows. Pauses are due to sinus arrest, and some pauses are terminated by junctional escape beats. If patient's condition is symptomatic during pauses, a pacemaker is indicated.

until a P wave is not conducted (Fig. 5.16). In type II, the P-R intervals of the conducted beats are constant; blocked beats occur without progressive prolongation of the P-R interval (Fig. 5.17). To some extent, these two types of block correspond to disorders at different levels of the conducting system. Type I block usually occurs in the AV node and type II in the more distal His-Purkinje system. The features of these two types of block are summarized in Table 5.2.

In contrast with second-degree block, third-degree block is characterized by total absence of any relation between P waves and QRS complexes (Fig. 5.18). P waves are seen to march through the QRS complexes—sometimes in front of, some-

times buried in, and sometimes following them. The QRS complexes, which are usually regularly spaced, may be relatively narrow, indicating a junctional origin of the subsidiary escape pacemaker, or they may be very wide and clearly ventricular. If the pacemaker is junctional, the ventricular rate may be 40–60 beats/min, a rate that is tolerated well. In contrast, a ventricular escape focus usually has a slower rate (20–40 beats/min), and is more likely to result in symptoms that are due to decreased cardiac output.

In third-degree block, physical findings of AV dissociation are present. Intermittent cannon waves are seen in the jugular veins, and there is variability of the first heart sound and of the

LEAD II

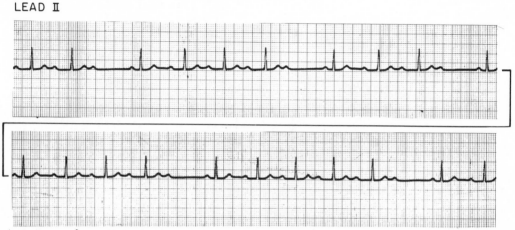

Figure 5.16. Type I (Wenckebach-Mobitz I) second-degree AV block. There is regular atrial activity at 72 beats/min. P-R interval becomes progressively prolonged, and every fourth, fifth, or sixth P wave is not conducted to ventricle. QRS complexes are narrow, and R-R interval becomes progressively shorter before each pause.

LEAD V₁

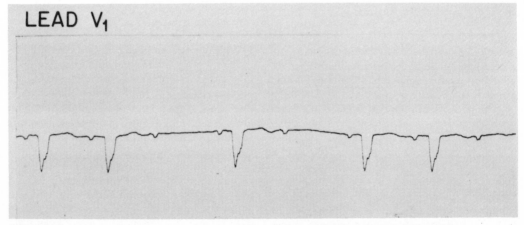

Figure 5.17. Type II (Mobitz II) second-degree AV block. P-R interval is constant at 0.18 second, and every second or third P wave is not conducted, which results in periods of 3:2 and 2:1 AV block. QRS complex has left bundle-branch block pattern, indicating disease of His-Purkinje system. Atrial rate is regular at 80 beats/min.

Table 5.2.
Differential electrocardiographic features of atrioventricular block.

Differential Feature	Type I (Wenckebach-Mobitz I)	Type II (Mobitz II)
P-R interval	Progressively prolonged in conducted beats, never normal	Constant in conducted beats, may be normal
QRS complex of conducted beats	Usually normal	Often prolonged, bundle-branch block or hemiblock frequent
Time course	Often transient, sudden asystole rare	More likely chronic, definite risk of sudden asystole
Ventricular rate if complete heart block occurs	Usually 40–50 beats/min because of effective junctional pacemaker	Very slow (ventricular pacemaker) or asystole
Response to drug therapy	Conduction usually improves with atropine or isoproterenol	Poor response
Associated conditions	Digitalis toxicity, inferior myocardial infarction, inflammatory condition involving the atrioventricular node	Anterior myocardial infarction, chronic conduction system disease
Level of conduction abnormality	Atrioventricular node	His-Purkinje system

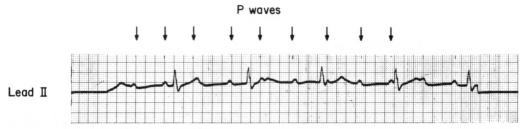

P waves

Lead II

Figure 5.18.   Complete heart block. There is no constant relation between P waves and QRS complexes. Atrial rate is 88 beats/min and ventricular escape rate is 39 beats/min. Nonconducted P waves distort T waves as they march through QRS complexes. This rhythm is an indication for a temporary pacemaker.

systemic blood pressure corresponding to the beat-to-beat changes in the relation of atrial and ventricular systole.

Complete heart block is often preceded by block in two of the three fascicles of the bundle branches. Bifascicular block may be manifested by any of the following patterns: (1) complete left bundle-branch block; (2) right bundle-branch block with block of the left anterior fascicle of the left bundle, giving an electrocardiographic pattern of right bundle-branch block with left axis deviation; (3) right bundle-branch block with block of the left posterior division of the left bundle, giving a pattern of right bundle-branch block with considerable right axis deviation. Right bundle-branch block with left anterior fascicular hemiblock is 10–20 times more common than right bundle-branch block with left posterior hemiblock.

Syncope (Adams-Stokes attacks) in patients with heart block usually is due to profound bradycardia or asystole, but can also be secondary to recurrent ventricular tachycardia or ventricular fibrillation (Fig. 5.19). At slow heart rates, the

ventricles tend to repolarize less uniformly, and ventricular tachycardia or fibrillation may result. *Whether symptoms are due to asystole or recurrent ventricular arrhythmias, the treatment of choice is acceleration of the heart rate by transvenous ventricular pacing.* This intervention in the emergency ward may be lifesaving.

When Adams-Stokes attacks are caused by recurrent ventricular arrhythmias, the tendency is to administer antiarrhythmic drugs. These may aggravate rather than improve the situation, however, since they suppress the automaticity of the lower escape foci, and they are contraindicated in therapy for complete heart block *unless* the ventricles are electrically paced.

Lesser degrees of heart block do not necessarily require emergency therapy; treatment is dictated by the patient's symptoms and by the setting in which heart block occurs (see page 93 for discussion of heart block in the presence of myocardial infarction).

Type I second-degree AV block is more likely to be transient and to respond to pharmacologic

MONITOR LEAD

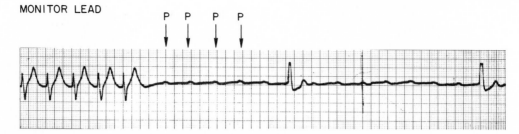

Figure 5.19. Complete heart block. Initially there is a regular tachycardia at 105 beats/min, and then there is sudden loss of ventricular activity with continuation of atrial activity at 105 beats/min. There is a slow, irregular ventricular escape pacemaker at about 15 beats/min. This sudden development of complete heart block was associated with syncope (Adams-Stokes attack).

therapy (atropine sulfate or isoproterenol) than is type II. In any patient with type I block known to be receiving a digitalis preparation, digitalis toxicity should be suspected. Temporary pacing is indicated for type I block only in the presence of hypotension, congestive heart failure, or severe ventricular irritability. Prophylactic pacing is not indicated.

In contrast, patients with type II second-degree AV block are much more likely to have a chronic disorder of AV conduction and at some time to have symptomatic bradycardia. Many also have coexisting bundle-branch block. All patients with type II block should receive a temporary transvenous pacemaker, and most require permanent pacing.

An additional therapeutic dilemma is posed by the patient with chronic bifascicular disease without AV block. It has been our practice to place temporary pacemakers in these patients only if they have had symptoms (syncope or presyncope) or if monitoring reveals intermittent second- or third-degree AV block. In an acute medical or surgical emergency, patients with first-degree AV block and bifascicular block of unknown duration should probably also receive a temporary pacemaker; subsequent monitoring or further studies of the AV conduction may then help determine whether permanent pacing is indicated.

Arrhythmias in Special Situations

Myocardial Infarction

At least 90% of patients with acute myocardial infarction seen in the hospital experience some disturbance of cardiac rhythm, which usually occurs soon after infarction. For example, the likelihood of ventricular fibrillation is estimated to be 15 times greater in the first 4 hours after the onset of infarction than in the next 8, and 25 times greater than in the 12–24 hours after infarction. Arrhythmias are also more likely to occur in pa-

tients with severe left ventricular dysfunction due to the infarct.

Table 5.3 summarizes the incidence of arrhythmias in four series of hospitalized patients with acute myocardial infarction. These arrhythmias are managed in generally the same way as in patients without infarction. However, it is even more important to treat tachyarrhythmias and ventricular ectopy promptly, because the increased oxygen consumption caused by the tachycardia may increase the size of the infarct, and ischemic myocardium is more unstable electrically and more susceptible to the development of life-threatening arrhythmias.

Several specific circumstances should be considered:

(1) Bradycardia in the patient with inferior myocardial infarction must be considered. For many reasons, bradycardia is likely to develop in patients with inferior myocardial infarction; these reasons include compromise of circulation to the sinus and AV nodal arteries and increased vagal tone. Recent studies have questioned whether such bradycardia should be treated to prevent electrical and hemodynamic deterioration, and have suggested that bradycardia is not itself dangerous and even may be desirable. When bradycardia occurs with hypotension, however, as it frequently does in the early phase of infarction, the heart rate should be accelerated. Bradycardia should also be treated when congestive heart failure or significant ventricular irritability is present.

When heightened vagal tone is the apparent cause (as suggested by hypotension coexisting with diaphoresis, cool and mottled extremities, nausea, vomiting, tenesmus, or tracheal burning) and the situation is not urgent, atropine sulfate is the drug of choice, 0.4–0.6 mg intravenously every 10–15 minutes until vagal manifestations have been reversed or a total of 2 mg has been administered. The most serious complication of atropine therapy is potentially hazardous tachycardia from an ex-

Table 5.3.
Arrhythmias in patients with acute myocardial infarction.[a]

Rhythm[b]	Average Incidence	Range
	%	
Ventricular		
Extrasystoles	90	45–100
Tachycardia	23	6–30[c]
Fibrillation	5	2–10
Supraventricular		
Sinus tachycardia	35	30–43
Atrial and nodal tachycardia	8	4–11
Atrial fibrillation	11	7–16
Atrial flutter	4	2–5
Sinus bradycardia	18	11–26
Atrioventricular block		
Second degree	7	4–10
Third degree	7	4–10

[a] Based on four series totaling 791 patients (Julian et al., Kimball and Killip, Lown et al., and Meltzer and Kitchell).

[b] Many patients have more than one rhythm disturbance.

[c] Many series do not distinguish between ventricular tachycardia (rate > 100 beats/min) and accelerated idioventricular rhythm (rate < 100 beats/min). In our experience, about 8–10% of patients have ventricular tachycardia and 10–15% have accelerated idioventricular rhythm.

cessive dose. Atropine sulfate also may cause urinary retention, and it may cause a toxic reaction of the central nervous system manifested in its most severe form as an agitated, hallucinatory psychosis that may last for days. Because these complications are more common in elderly patients, we rarely administer more than 1 mg to patients over 65 years old.

In more urgent situations, isoproterenol or epinephrine, 1–3 μg/min, can be administered as a continuous intravenous infusion. These drugs must be used with caution because they increase myocardial oxygen demands considerably and may extend the area of myocardial ischemia or infarction. They should be used only until a temporary pacemaker can be placed.

The most reliable means of accelerating the heart rate is temporary transvenous pacing, which should be undertaken if the bradycardia is not quickly responsive to pharmacologic therapy or if complications of drug therapy occur. Pacing may be done from the right atrium if AV nodal function is normal—thus preserving the benefit of atrial

transport—or from the right ventricle if AV block is present.

(2) Ventricular premature beats deserve special consideration. In patients with acute myocardial infarction, all ventricular premature beats should be suppressed because of the risk of ventricular fibrillation. Since up to 50% of instances of ventricular fibrillation in acute infarction occur without premonitory ventricular ectopy, it has been argued that prophylactic antiarrhythmic agents should be used. In several studies testing this hypothesis with procainamide, quinidine, or lidocaine, a decrease in serious ventricular arrhythmias has been seen, but no change in survival in the setting of a coronary care unit. Nonetheless, it has been our practice routinely to administer intravenous lidocaine prophylactically (50- to 100-mg bolus followed by 1–3 mg/min) in all patients in whom an acute MI is definitely present or in whom the suspicion is high. The rationale for this is that even though the patient is likely to be resuscitated successfully from ventricular tachycardia or fibrillation, the occurrence of such an arrhythmia is likely to have an adverse effect in a number of other ways such as the size of the infarct, the perfusion of other organs, and the patient's psyche. It, therefore, seems the most prudent course to prevent these arrhythmias if at all possible. Prophylactic drugs should not be administered to patients with second- or third-degree AV block unless a pacemaker is in place.

If patients have ventricular ectopy after initiation of lidocaine therapy, the first step would be to give another bolus of 50–75 mg of lidocaine and increase the infusion rate by 1 mg/min (provided there are no signs of lidocaine toxicity). If there is still ventricular ectopy present after realizing an infusion rate of 4 mg/min (or signs of lidocaine toxicity), then either procainamide or bretylium should be added, as outlined in the previous section on the treatment of ventricular arrhythmias.

(3) AV conduction abnormalities are another consideration. Inferior myocardial infarction may be associated with transient abnormalities of AV conduction, such as first-degree block, type I second-degree block, and rarely, third-degree block. These abnormalities, which are due to either increased vagal tone or reversible ischemia of the AV node, are usually transient and do not appear to alter prognosis. Atropine sulfate may reverse the component of AV block that is due to vagotonia. Ventricular pacing is not recommended unless hypotension, congestive heart failure, or ventricular irritability exist in the presence of bradycardia. Even third-degree block may be well tolerated, since the junctional pacemaker usually pro-

vides an adequate heart rate, but pacing is indicated if the escape rate is inadequate.

Anterior infarction, on the other hand, may be associated with bundle-branch block and higher degrees of AV block that carry a grave prognosis. This prognosis is dictated by the fact that conduction abnormalities in anterior infarction usually indicate a large area of myocardial damage, and consequently, coincident severe ventricular failure is common. Some deaths, however, are related to sudden asystole due to the failure of an escape junctional or ventricular pacemaker to emerge when heart block develops. For this reason, temporary ventricular pacing is indicated in any patient with anterior infarction and complete heart block. We also insert a prophylactic transvenous pacemaker in any patient with anterior infarction and evidence of *new* bundle-branch block or with type II second-degree AV block. Although prophylactic pacing has not yet been shown to alter survival in these patients, it can be accomplished at low risk, and it may avoid the need for emergency pacemaker placement. It also may provide a smoother hemodynamic transition with the onset of heart block. Because of the risk of competition with conducted or premature beats, ventricular pacing in patients with myocardial infarction should always be of the demand type.

(4) Accelerated idioventricular rhythm also demands attention. This is a slow ventricular rhythm with a rate between 60 and 100 beats/min, which results from a combination of acceleration of an ectopic ventricular pacemaker and slowing of the rate of the sinus node (Fig. 5.20). It occurs most commonly in inferior myocardial infarction, and usually appears as an end-diastolic rhythm lasting from 4–30 beats. It is generally well tolerated, and appears to be benign. Occasionally, it may herald or be accompanied by other more serious ventricular arrhythmias requiring treatment. If the rhythm is well tolerated and is unaccompanied by other more serious ventricular ectopy, therapy is not needed. If suppression is required, increasing the sinus rate with atropine sulfate or pacing may be successful, but frequently, active suppression with the drugs used to treat ventricular ectopy may be necessary.

Digitalis Toxicity

Between 20 and 30% of hospitalized patients who have been receiving digitalis may have digitalis toxicity. Virtually every known rhythm disturbance can result from this complication; Table 5.4 lists the incidence of various arrhythmias in four series of patients. These arrhythmias are a manifestation of the ability of digitalis to increase automaticity and to decrease conduction.

Treatment of these arrhythmias is similar to that when they occur in the absence of digitalis toxicity, with a few notable exceptions. Administration of digitalis glycosides should be stopped immediately. In some instances, it may be difficult to be sure of the role of digitalis, but if there is any suspicion at all, digitalis should be withheld. Atrial tachycardia with block (Fig. 5.21) is perhaps the most difficult rhythm to judge in this regard; it is often secondary to digitalis intoxication; but if it is not due to digitalis excess it will often respond to digitalis therapy.

Potassium deficiency commonly precipitates or aggravates the arrhythmic manifestations of digitalis toxicity, and potassium replacement is of prime importance in therapy. If the serum potassium level is low, potassium should be infused intravenously at a rate of 10–20 mEq/hr to raise the serum level to 4.5–5.0 mEq/liter. The one toxic manifestation of digitalis that should not be treated aggressively with potassium is AV block (except paroxysmal atrial tachycardia with block), since it may be aggravated by elevating potassium

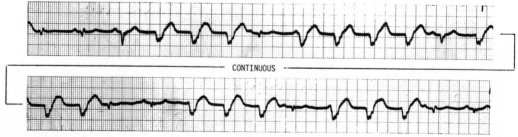

Figure 5.20.   Idioventricular rhythm. This patient had recent inferior-wall myocardial infarction. There is an accelerated ventricular pacemaker with rate of 85 beats/min, which is slightly faster than sinus rate. The two pacemakers are competing, and the patient alternates between sinus rhythm and idioventricular rhythm. Ventricular origin of rhythm is confirmed by the fusion beat, which initiates first period of idioventricular rhythm. This rhythm is usually benign and does not require treatment unless patient's hemodynamic status is compromised or unless rhythm accelerates to ventricular tachycardia.

Table 5.4.
Arrhythmias as manifestations of digitalis toxicity.[a]

Rhythm[b]	Average Incidence	Range
	%	
Ventricular premature beats (often multifocal)	63	47–85
Second- or third-degree atrioventricular block	21	11–40
Nonparoxysmal junctional tachycardia	17	6–30
Junctional escape rhythm (usually with atrial fibrillation)	16	5–35
Atrial tachycardia (with or without block)	10	6–12
Ventricular tachycardia	10	4–18
Atrial flutter or fibrillation	7	6–13
Sinus arrest or exit block	4	3–5

[a] Based on four series totaling 392 patients (Beller et al., Chung, Resnekov [1970], and Rios et al.).

[b] Many patients have more than one rhythm disturbance.

levels to above normal. Even in this case, however, potassium replacement is indicated if the serum potassium is low.

In the presence of digitalis toxicity, ventricular premature beats and ventricular tachycardia are ominous and must be treated promptly. Phenytoin is the drug of choice (Table 5.5). Lidocaine is also effective, and propranolol may be successful in the absence of overt congestive heart failure. Procainamide also may be effective if the other agents fail, though rarely is this necessary unless the patient has a pre-existing tendency to serum ventricular arrhythmias. Quinidine should be used with great caution (if at all) in this setting because of its well-documented capacity for elevating the serum digoxin level. Worsening of ventricular ectopy in the setting of digitalis toxicity also has been reported following the administration of bretylium.

Cardioversion usually is contraindicated in the presence of digitalis toxicity because of the risk of precipitating an even more serious arrhythmia. In rare instances, cardioversion may be necessary to convert a tachycardia, in which case the risk can

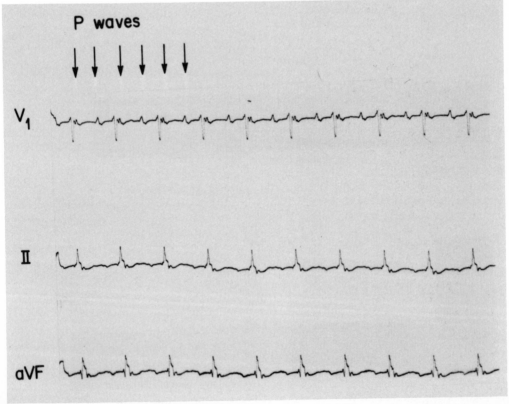

Figure 5.21.   Atrial tachycardia with 2:1 AV block. Atrial rate is 200 beats/min and ventricular rate is 100 beats/min. Nonconducted P wave is apparent in initial portion of each ST segment. This rhythm should be presumed to be due to digitalis toxicity.

Table 5.5.
Agents commonly administered intravenously for emergency treatment of arrhythmias.

Drug	Dosage	Indications	Complications
Atropine sulfate	0.5–1.0 mg initially, not to exceed 2.0 mg total	Symptomatic sinus bradycardia or atrioventricular block	Tachycardia Central nervous system toxicity Urinary retention
Digoxin	0.25–0.50 mg initially, with 0.125–0.25 mg increments to total of 1.0–2.0 mg	Rate control in rapid atrial fibrillation Rate control in atrial flutter (do not exceed 0.75 mg if cardioversion indicated) Conversion of paroxysmal SVT (in absence of atrioventricular block)	Ventricular arrhythmias Atrioventricular block
Phenytoin sodium (Dilantin)	100 mg every 5 min, not to exceed 1 gm total	Ventricular arrhythmias in presence of digitalis toxicity Refractory ventricular arrhythmias when lidocaine and procainamide ineffective SVT due to digitalis toxicity	Hypotension Bradycardia Central nervous system toxicity
Lidocaine (Xylocaine)	50- to 100-mg bolus followed by 1–4 mg/min continuous infusion	Ventricular arrhythmias (treatment of choice) Refractory paroxysmal SVT (occasionally successful)	Central nervous system toxicity Heart block or sinus arrest (rare)
Procainamide	100 mg every 5 min, not to exceed 1 gm total; 1–4 µg/min continuous infusion	Ventricular arrhythmias refractory to lidocaine Refractory SVT (rarely)	Hypotension Congestive heart failure Heart block
Propranolol	1 mg every 5 min, not to exceed 10 mg total	Rate control in atrial fibrillation or atrial flutter refractory to digitalis Conversion of paroxysmal SVT or atrial flutter Ventricular arrhythmias refractory to other agents	Congestive heart failure Hypotension Bradycardia Bronchospasm
Verapamil	5–10 mg iv over 3 min, may repeat in 30 min	Conversion of paroxysmal SVT Rate control in AF and atrial flutter	Hypotension Congestive heart failure Bradycardia
Bretylium	300 mg iv over 5–10 min, rarely continuous infusion 1–2 mg/min	Refractory ventricular arrhythmias	Hypotension Rarely worsening of ventricular ectopy

be lessened by prior administration of phenytoin or lidocaine.

Other agents, such as magnesium and ethylenediaminetetraacetic acid (EDTA), have also been used to treat digitalis toxicity, but conventional antiarrhythmic therapy and correction of metabolic abnormalities usually suffice. The administration of digoxin-specific antibodies to reverse the effects of digitalis directly appears promising, particularly in instances of massive overdose.

Pacemaker-Related Arrhythmias

In patients with fixed-rate ventricular pacemakers and preservation of normal sinus and AV nodal function, there is a potential for competition between the intrinsic pacemaker and the artificial pacemaker. Although such competition rarely provokes serious ventricular arrhythmias, it may do so in the presence of ischemia or ectopic beats. With the increasing use of demand pacemakers, this is now seldom a problem.

Demand pacemakers are of two types: "R wave inhibited," in which no pacemaker spike is seen if the ventricle is spontaneously depolarizing at a rate faster than the preset rate of the pacemaker, and "R wave synchronous," in which each spontaneously occurring QRS complex discharges the pacemaker and is deformed by a pacemaker spike. Both types pace the heart when the heart rate falls below the preset rate of the unit.

The R-wave inhibited pacemaker has the advantage that it permits interpretation of structural changes in the QRS complex, ST segment, and T wave in normally conducted beats, as in cases of suspected myocardial infarction. Its disadvantage is that it may be difficult to differentiate between a nonfunctioning pacemaker and one that is appropriately suppressed by a faster intrinsic heart rate. Slowing the heart rate with carotid sinus pressure may enable paced beats to emerge, and many recent models can be converted temporarily to a fixed rate by applying a magnet directly over the unit.

Since the R-wave synchronous pacemaker shows a pacemaker spike in each QRS complex, its function can be assessed easily. Its major disadvantage is that the QRS complex is deformed by the pacemaker artifact, making it difficult to detect any change in the QRS complex, ST segment, or T wave. The location of the pacemaker spike must be scrutinized to determine whether it initiates or follows the beginning of the QRS complex, thus indicating if the beat is paced or spontaneous. If the patient has spontaneous tachycardia, it may appear to be pacemaker induced unless this fact is appreciated. Additionally, all demand pacemakers have a refractory period that is usually about 400 msec, during which they will not sense a beat and will not discharge. In the presence of a spontaneous tachyarrhythmia, this can create a confusing electrocardiographic tracing in which there are conducted beats with pacemaker spikes, normally conducted beats without a pacemaker artifact, and perhaps paced beats as well. These must be analyzed carefully, and they do not necessarily indicate pacemaker failure.

Pacemaker failure is usually manifested by slowing of the paced rate, failure to sense spontaneous beats (hence converting a demand pacemaker to a fixed mode), or failure to capture the ventricle (Fig. 5.22). Older models may accelerate when failure occurs, causing ventricular tachycardia. It is important to identify the type of pacemaker either from the patient's identification card or from the radiographic appearance of the unit and to obtain detailed information from the manufacturer regarding the features of the particular device.

A. Lead II

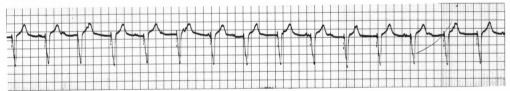

B. Lead II

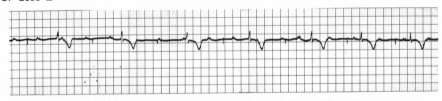

Figure 5.22. Ventricular pacemaker with pacemaker failure. **(A)** A demand ventricular pacemaker is firing at 72 beats/min with 1:1 capture of ventricle. Atrial rate is 95 beats/min and P waves march through QRS complexes without being conducted to ventricle (complete heart block is present). This is a right ventricular endocardial pacemaker, and paced beats have left bundle-branch block pattern. **(B)** In same patient, pacemaker rate is still 72 beats/min, but none of paced beats now results in ventricular depolarization. Atrial rate is still 95 beats/min, and there is junctional escape rhythm at about 40 beats/min. This is pacemaker failure, which was due to perforation of right ventricle by pacemaker wire.

Wolff-Parkinson-White Syndrome and other Pre-Excitation Syndromes

Patients with this syndrome or a variant have one or more anomalous conduction pathways that bypass all or a portion of the normal AV junctional system. When conduction occurs through the by-pass tract, the electrocardiogram has the characteristic features of a *short P-R interval*, a Δ-*wave*, and a *wide QRS complex* (Fig. 5.23). Three types are distinguished on the basis of the orientation of the Δ-wave: (1) type A, in which the Δ-wave is anteriorly directed and is positive in leads V_1 and V_6, creating a pattern that resembles right bundle-branch block; (2) type B, in which the Δ-wave is posteriorly directed and is negative in lead V_1 and positive in Lead V_6, creating a pattern that resembles left bundle-branch block; and (3) type C, which includes patients who are not easily classified as having type A or type B. In other forms of pre-excitation syndrome due to other types of bypass pathways, the P-R interval may be shortened without change in the QRS complex, or there may be a wide QRS complex with Δ-wave without P-R interval shortening.

Patients with Wolff-Parkinson-White syndrome may have normal conduction patterns at some times and abnormal patterns at other times. During abnormal conduction, QRS patterns may simulate those in myocardial infarction. These may be repolarization abnormalities simulating ischemia.

The availability of two or more pathways for conduction from the atria to the ventricles creates a situation in which a *re-entry* or *reciprocating tachycardia* may occur. The most common manifestation of this is paroxysmal SVT. The QRS complexes are usually normal during such a tachycardia, indicating antegrade conduction through normal pathways and retrograde conduction through the anomalous pathway. If P waves are visible, they will follow the QRS complex and be of retrograde fashion (i.e., inverted in leads II, III and F). Treatment of this arrhythmia is similar to that described previously, with the exception that the rate may be more rapid in patients with Wolff-Parkinson-White syndrome, and the tachycardia may be more resistant to therapy. Digoxin is often effective because of its effect on AV conduction, but it does not affect conduction in the bypass pathway. Propranolol, other β-adrenergic blocking drugs, and verapamil also have been found effective. Quinidine and procainamide have been particularly effective in many difficult cases because they have been shown to affect conduction in the bypass tract. Because of symptomatic recurrences, many of these patients require long-term antiarrhythmic prophylaxis, at times with several agents. A small number may require either permanent pacing or resection of the anomalous pathway. A number of new drugs are being investigated for treatment of refractory supraventricular arrhythmias in these patients, but these have not yet been released for use.

Atrial fibrillation also is seen in patients with Wolff-Parkinson-White syndrome. It is particularly dangerous in these patients because conduction of impulses to the ventricle may be by means of the rapidly conducting bypass pathway rather than through the AV node. Ventricular rates up to 300 beats/min may occur, and may precipitate hemodynamic collapse, although young patients may tolerate such rates remarkably well. The QRS complexes are aberrant because of antegrade conduction in the anomalous pathway. Digitalis and verapamil are successful in slowing the ventricular response, and may in fact result in a faster ventricular rate. This is the one situation in which both digitalis and verapamil are *contraindicated* for the control of the ventricular response in atrial fibrillation. Lidocaine, procainamide, quinidine, and cardioversion are the treatments of choice.

Sick Sinus Syndrome

This is not a single arrhythmia, but a group of arrhythmias. It deserves special mention because the treatment of a given arrhythmia in this context may be slightly different from its treatment if it occurred alone. The sick sinus syndrome usually occurs in elderly patients, who often have no other evidence of heart disease. These patients may have periods of sinus bradycardia or sinus arrest that frequently are punctuated by atrial tachyarrhythmias (bradycardia-tachycardia syndrome). There is also a high associated incidence of AV nodal and His-Purkinje dysfunction. The spectrum of tachyarrhythmias is wide, including paroxysmal atrial fibrillation, atrial flutter, atrial tachycardia, and multifocal atrial tachycardia.

In patients with sick sinus syndrome who have an atrial tachyarrhythmia, profound symptomatic bradycardia may develop on termination of the arrhythmia; this may occur either spontaneously or with therapy. Such a possibility may be indicated by a history of syncopal episodes or by evidence of sinus or AV nodal dysfunction on previous electrocardiograms. Negatively chronotropic agents, especially propranolol and verapamil must be used with great caution in these patients. Cardioversion may be risky because of the likelihood that there will be no spontaneous sinus activity after conversion. If cardioversion is

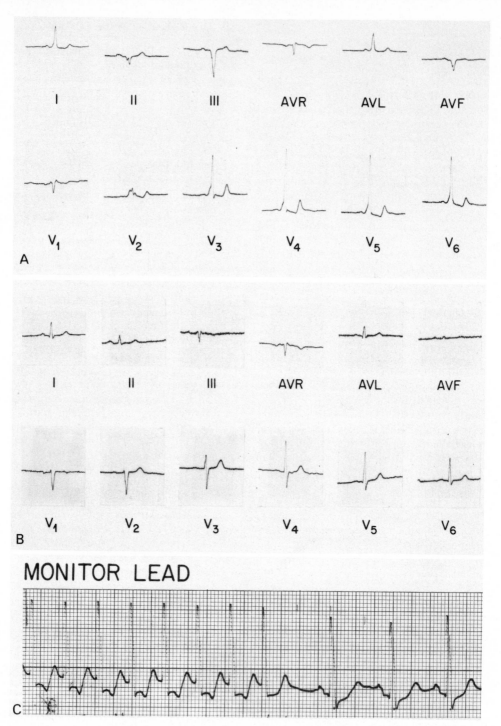

Figure 5.23. Type A Wolff-Parkinson-White syndrome. **(A)** Classic findings of Wolff-Parkinson-White syndrome are illustrated in this electrocardiogram from patient with recurrent paroxysmal atrial tachycardia. P-R interval is 0.12 second and there is a Δ-wave that is anteriorly and superiorly directed. QRS complex in leads II, III, and aVF has "pseudoinfarct" pattern. Abnormal conduction pattern was intermittent, and there were no inferior Q waves when conduction pattern was normal. **(B)** Electrocardiogram from same patient. Conduction pattern is now normal and Wolff-Parkinson-White syndrome cannot be diagnosed. **(C)** Monitor lead from same patient showing brief run of paroxysmal atrial tachycardia at 180 beats/min. Note narrow QRS complex and normal conduction pattern during this episode. This is true in about 85% of cases of SVT with Wolff-Parkinson-White syndrome, and indicates that antegrade conduction is through the AV node (normal pathway) and that retrograde conduction uses the anomalous pathway, thus completing the re-entry cycle.

98

required, a prophylactic temporary pacing catheter should be used.

Special Procedures in Diagnosis and Treatment of Arrhythmias

Carotid Sinus Pressure

This important technique is used in the differential diagnosis and therapy of many atrial tachyarrhythmias, and lack of response can frequently be ascribed to its faulty application. The following steps are recommended:

(1) Attach an electrocardiographic monitor with the ability to record the rhythm. Insert an intravenous line, and have equipment for emergency defibrillation and pacing at hand.

(2) In elderly patients, auscultate the carotid arteries for evidence of a stenotic bruit. If one is heard, do not apply carotid sinus pressure.

(3) Extend the patient's neck as much as possible, using a small pillow or some folded towels placed behind the neck and shoulders. Rotate the patient's head slightly away from the side to be compressed. These maneuvers expose the carotid sinus maximally.

(4) Locate the area of the carotid sinus, which is at the carotid bifurcation just below the angle of the jaw. The carotid sinus is usually at the point of maximal palpable carotid pulsation.

(5) Apply light pressure first. If there is no response or no adverse effect, more pressure—enough to cause the patient slight discomfort—may be applied. Firm pressure should be exerted for 5–10 seconds and released immediately on evidence of a change in rhythm. If there is no effect, pressure may be reapplied, especially after edrophonium chloride or digitalis has been administered to increase vagal tone.

(6) If pressure on one side is ineffective, exert pressure on the opposite side. At no time should bilateral carotid sinus pressure be applied. Usually, compression of the right carotid sinus is more likely to prove successful in terminating an arrhythmia.

Intracardiac Electrode Placement

This is an extremely important procedure that has several applications. Placement of an electrode in the right atrium to record activity enables diagnosis of complicated or obscure tachyarrhythmias. Right ventricular placement for pacing may be lifesaving in patients with complete heart block or other profound bradycardias. Rapid atrial or ventricular pacing may also be applied therapeutically to suppress ventricular ectopic activity or to convert a supraventricular tachyarrhythmia.

The preferred approach for temporary pervenous electrode placement is via the subclavian or internal jugular vein by direct percutaneous puncture. Many flexible, semifloating pacemakers are available that may be passed through a large polyethylene intravenous catheter. The position of the electrode can be monitored with either an electrocardiograph (Fig. 5.24) or a fluoroscope. When only electrocardiographic monitoring is used, the electrode should be advanced slowly into the atrium, and the point at which ventricular potentials are first recorded should be noted. The electrode should then be advanced 2–4 cm more into the right ventricle. Except in the most emergent of situations, we prefer to place the electrode under fluoroscopic guidance to assure the optimal and most stable pacing position.

The electrode usually can be positioned in the atrium from either the right or left venous system. Stable ventricular positioning, however, is often better achieved from the left side. The tip of the electrode should be directed slightly downward and fixed in the trabeculae carneae of the right ventricle so that it does not float freely with each contraction. It usually is possible to find an area with a pacing threshold of 1–2 milliamperes that will accurately sense spontaneous ventricular depolarization. The optimal pacing rate for each patient must be determined individually. Rates of 90–100 impulses/min usually maximize cardiac output if congestive heart failure or hypotension is the indication for pacemaker placement, although lower rates often are desirable in patients with ischemia or if the electrode has been placed for prophylactic purposes.

The diaphragm may be paced with right atrial pacing; pacing of the diaphragm or of the intercostal muscles with ventricular pacing may indicate perforation of the ventricular wall or may result from excessive current. If the pacemaker wire has perforated the ventricle, it usually malfunctions, that is, it fails to capture or sense or both. This is successfully managed by withdrawing the pacemaker until pacing is restored, and there is rarely sufficient bleeding to cause cardiac tamponade. Rarely, perforation of the ventricular septum also may occur. This results in pacing of the left ventricle, which is indicated by a right bundle-branch block pattern on the electrocardiogram and a widely but physiologically split second sound. Right ventricular pacing results in a left bundle-branch block pattern and single or paradoxically split second sound.

Electrode placement may also be achieved via the femoral veins, or brachiocephalic system. In extreme emergencies, transthoracic pacing may be

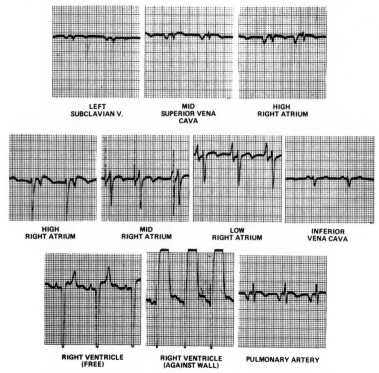

Figure 5.24. Electrocardiographic monitoring of electrode placement. With external end of pacemaker attached to lead V of electrocardiograph by means of alligator clip, tracings can be recorded for various locations to guide in bedside pacemaker placement. Of particular importance are large atrial deflections obtained with electrode in atrium and large intracavitary QRS complex (similar to aVR) with electrode in ventricle. Injury current is obtained with electrode against right ventricular wall (optimal position for ventricular pacing). (Reproduced by permission, from the *New England Journal of Medicine*, Vol. 287, p. 651, 1972.)

achieved by direct cardiac puncture and insertion of a pacing needle or a special electrode. This maneuver may be lifesaving in some situations, and may provide time to institute more stable measures in others.

Cardioversion

A distinction must be made between emergency cardioversion in the case of circulatory arrest and semielective or elective cardioversion of an arrhythmia that has been resistant to therapy but that the patient is tolerating reasonably well. In treating circulatory arrest, the physician is treating either ventricular fibrillation or an unknown rhythm disturbance in a pulseless patient. Cardioversion should be applied at maximal energy (400 joules), without premedication or synchronization. In the case of an elective conversion, there is usually time to premedicate the patient. Intravenous diazepam (Valium), 5–10 mg, is both effective and safe. We also frequently use sodium methohexital (Brevital), a short-acting barbiturate administered by an anesthetist in doses up to 1 mg/kg. Equipment must be available for tracheal in-

tubation, and an anesthesiologist should be present. Synchronized direct-current cardioversion is preferred to minimize the risk of serious ventricular arrhythmias. Cardioversion should initially be attempted with an energy level of 25–50 joules, and increments of 50–100 joules should be employed until cardioversion has been achieved or a level of 300–400 joules has been reached. Some arrhythmias, such as atrial flutter, are more likely to be converted at low energy levels. If digitalis toxicity is suspected as causing the arrhythmia, it is particularly important to begin with extremely low energy levels (5–10 joules), and lidocaine, 2–4 mg/min, should be infused prophylactically. The same precautions apply if the patient has had an acute myocardial infarction. Since serum enzyme levels may be elevated after cardioversion, their subsequent interpretation in diagnosing acute myocardial infarction may be difficult.

Suggested Readings

Arrhythmias: General

Cranefield PF, Wit AL, Hoffman BF: Genesis of cardiac arrhythmias. *Circulation 47:*190–204, 1973

Harvey WP, Ronan JA, Jr: Bedside diagnosis of arrhythmias. *Prog Cardiovasc Dis 8:*419–445, 1966

Marriott HJL, Sandler IA: Criteria, old and new, for differentiating between ectopic ventricular beats and aberrant ventricular conduction in the presence of atrial fibrillation. *Prog Cardiovasc Dis 9:*18–28, 1966

Schamroth L: How to approach an arrhythmia. *Circulation 47:*420–426, 1973

Tachyarrhythmias: Supraventricular

Antman EM, Stone PH, Muller JE, et al: Calcium channel blocking agents in the treatment of cardiovascular disorder. Part I. Basic and clinical electrophysiologic effects. *Ann Intern Med 93:*875–885, 1981

Josephson ME: Paroxysmal SVT: An electrophysiologic approach. *Am J Cardiol 41:*1123–1126, 1978

Pittman DE, Makar JS, Kooros KS, et al: Rapid atrial stimulation: Successful method of conversion of atrial flutter and atrial tachycardia. *Am J Cardiol 32:*700–706, 1973

Rosen KM: Junctional tachycardias: Mechanisms, diagnosis, differential diagnosis and management. *Circulation 47:* 654–664, 1973

Shine KI, Kastor JA, Yurchak PM: Multifocal atrial tachycardia: Clinical and electrocardiographic features in 32 patients. *N Engl J Med 279:*344–349, 1968

Ticzon AR, Whalen RW: Refractory supraventricular tachycardias. *Circulation 47:*642–653, 1973

Tachyarrhythmias: Ventricular

Bigger JT, Schmidt DH, Kutt H: Relationship between the plasma level of diphenylhydantoin sodium and its cardiac antiarrhythmic effects. *Circulation 38:*363–374, 1968

Collinsworth KA, Kalman SM, Harrison DC: The clinical pharmacology of lidocaine as an antiarrhythmic drug. *Circulation 50:*1217–1230, 1974

DeSanctis RW, Kastor JA: Rapid intracardiac pacing for treatment of recurrent ventricular tachyarrhythmias in the absence of heart block. *Am Heart J 76:*168–172, 1968

Giardina EV, Heissenbuttel RH, Bigger JT: Intermittent intravenous procainamide to treat ventricular arrhythmias: Correlation of plasma concentration with effect on arrhythmia, electrocardiogram, and blood pressure. *Ann Intern Med 78:*183–193, 1973

Koch-Weser J: Drug therapy: Bretylium. *N Engl J Med 300:*473–477, 1979

Pick A, Langendorf R: Parasystole and its variants. *Med Clin North Am 60:*125–147, 1976

Rothfeld EL, Zucker IR, Parsonnet V, et al: Idioventricular rhythm in acute myocardial infarction. *Circulation 37:* 203–209, 1968

Smith WM, Gallagher JJ: "Les Torsades de pointes": An unusual ventricular antirhythm. *Ann Intern Med 93:*578–584, 1980

Willerson JT, Yurchak PM, DeSanctis RW: Ventricular tachycardia. *Cardiovasc Clin 2:*69–86, 1970

Bradyarrhythmias

Kastor JA: Atrioventricular block. *N Engl J Med 292:* 462–465, 572–574, 1975

Rosenbaum MB, Elizari MV, Lazzari JO: The Hemiblocks: New Concepts of Intraventricular Conduction Based on Human Anatomical, Physiological, and Clinical Studies. Oldsmar, FL, Tampa Tracings, 1970

Arrhythmias in Special Situations: Myocardial Infarction

Dhurandhar RW, Macmillan RL, Brown KW: Primary ventricular fibrillation complicating acute myocardial infarction. *Am J Cardiol 27:*347–351, 1971

Julian DG, Valentine PA, Miller GG: Disturbances of rate, rhythm, and conduction in acute myocardial infarction: A prospective study of 100 consecutive unselected patients with the aid of electrocardiographic monitoring. *Am J Med 37:*915–927, 1964

Kimball JT, Killip T: Aggressive treatment of arrhythmias in acute myocardial infarction: Procedures and results. *Prog Cardiovasc Dis 10:*483–504, 1968

Koch-Weser J, Klein SW, Foo-Canto LL, et al: Antiarrhythmic prophylaxis with procainamide in acute myocardial infarction. *N Engl J Med 281:*1253–1260, 1969

Lown B, Klein MD, Hershberg PI: Coronary and precoronary care. *Am J Med 46:*705–724, 1969

Meltzer LE, Kitchell JB: The incidence of arrhythmias associated with acute myocardial infarction. *Prog Cardiovasc Dis 9:*50–63, 1966

Nimetz AA, Shubrooks SJ, Jr, Hutter AM, Jr, et al: The significance of bundle-branch block during acute myocardial infarction. *Am Heart J 90:*439–444, 1975

Norris RM: Heart block in posterior and anterior myocardial infarction. *Br Heart J 31:*352–356, 1969

Arrhythmias in Special Situations: Digitalis Toxicity

Beller GA, Smith TW, Abelmann WH, et al: Digitalis intoxication, a prospective clinical study with serum level correlations. *N Engl J Med 284:*989–997, 1971

Chung EK: *Digitalis Intoxication.* Baltimore, Williams & Wilkins, 1969

Resnekov L: Prevalence diagnosis and treatment of digitalis-induced dysrhythmias. In Sandoe E, Flensted-Jensen E, Olesen KH (Eds): *Symposium on Cardiac Arrhythmias.* Sodertalje, Sweden, AB Astra, 1970

Rios JC, Dziok CA, Ali NA: Digitalis-induced arrhythmias: Recognition and management. *Cardiovasc Clin 2:*261–279, 1970

Arrhythmias in Special Situations: Pacemaker-Related Arrhythmias

Castellanos A, Jr, Lemberg L: Pacemaker arrhythmias and electrocardiographic recognition of pacemaker. *Circulation 47:*1382–1391, 1973

Walter WH, III, Wenger NK: Radiographic identification of commonly used implanted pacemakers. *N Engl J Med 281:*1230–1231, 1969

Arrhythmias in Special Situations: Wolff-Parkinson-White Syndrome

Narula OS: Wolff-Parkinson-White syndrome: A review. *Circulation 47:*872–887, 1973

Arrhythmias in Special Situations: Sick Sinus Syndrome

Rubenstein JJ, Schulman CL, Yurchak PM, et al: Clinical spectrum of the sick sinus syndrome. *Circulation 46:*5–13, 1972

Special Procedures

DeSanctis RW: Diagnostic and therapeutic uses of atrial pacing. *Circulation 43:*748–761, 1971

Lown B: Electrical reversion of cardiac arrhythmias. *Br Heart J 29:*469–489, 1967

Resnekov L: Present status of electroversion in management of cardiac dysrhythmias. *Circulation 47:*1356–1363, 1973

CHAPTER 6

Cardiology: Unstable Angina and Acute Myocardial Infarction

ADOLPH M. HUTTER, Jr., M.D.
ANDREW G. BODNAR, M.D.

DIAGNOSIS OF ISCHEMIC CARDIAC PAIN

The accurate and expeditious evaluation of chest pain is one of the most important responsibilities of the physician in the emergency ward. Many patients whose chest pain ultimately proves to have been noncardiac are mislabeled as suffering from angina. Too frequently, the misdiagnosis is the result of an inadequate history or physical examination. Although a full discussion of the differential diagnosis of chest pain is beyond the scope of this chapter, we will mention those conditions most commonly confused with angina. Chest trauma, aortic dissection, and pulmonary embolism are fully discussed elsewhere (see Chapters 22, 21, and 9). Esophageal spasm may cause substernal, squeezing pain closely resembling angina pectoris. Pain from this source tends to occur in the supine position, especially after a big meal, and it may be relieved by antacids. The fact that the pain may also be relieved by nitroglycerin (Orlando and Bozymski, 1973) increases the confusion with coronary ischemia.

Chest wall pain due to costochondritis is classically exacerbated by chest movement, especially deep breathing and coughing. It is associated with tenderness over the costochondral joints along the sternal border or the inferior edge of the rib cage. This condition, however, is frequently overlooked because the examining physician fails to ask the proper questions or to palpate each costochondral junction looking specifically for tenderness.

Pericarditis may be confusing since it is commonly associated with sternal or parasternal chest pain that can extend to the neck or shoulder, although it rarely extends down the arm. Careful questioning usually elucidates the sharpness of the pain intensified by deep inspiration, the recumbent position (especially left lateral decubitus), coughing, deep breathing, and even swallowing. Relief of pain is noted on sitting up or holding one's breath. A pericardial friction rub confirms the diagnosis; this is a scratchy, superficial sound that occasionally has a coarse, leathery quality. There may be one to three components (ventricular systole and diastole and atrial systole). The pericardial rub usually is best heard to the left of the lower part of the sternum with the patient leaning forward, but sometimes is heard only in the supine position. During auscultation, the patient should hold his breath in various phases of respiration, since the rub sometimes is best heard in expiration and sometimes in inspiration. The rub may be evanescent, and may not be audible a few hours later. The electrocardiogram may reveal diffuse elevation of the ST segments with upright T waves early in the course of pericarditis. Later, the T waves invert after the ST segments return to baseline. This contrasts with ST-segment elevations due to coronary ischemia, which frequently have concurrent T-wave inversion. However, differentiation between the ST-segment and T-wave changes of pericarditis and those of ischemia, particularly "hyperacute" ischemic changes with upright T waves, can be difficult. A clue to the diagnosis of pericarditis is a depressed P-R interval, which is often overlooked because of its association with elevated ST segments (Spodick, 1974). This phenomenon (Fig. 6.1) is best seen in the inferior leads (II, III, and aVF) and occasionally in the apical leads (V_5 and V_6), and is not a feature of coronary ischemia. Since late pericarditis may occur after myocardial infarction (Dressler's syndrome) or an open-heart operation (postpericardiotomy syndrome), this possibility should

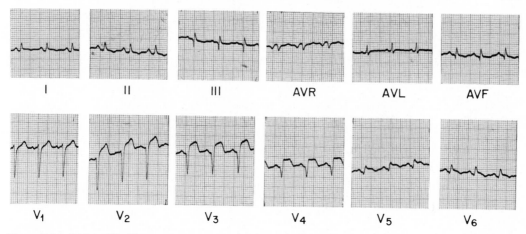

Figure 6.1.   Pericarditis. Electrocardiogram of patient with acute anterior myocardial infarction. P-R interval is depressed relative to T-P interval in leads I, II, V₅, and V₆ with reciprocal P-R elevation in AVR. This finding suggests pericarditis, but is often overlooked because of the ST-segment elevation.

be considered in patients with return of chest pain after either of these events.

Even a careful history and physical examination may not result in accurate differentiation among the various possible causes of chest pain, particularly in patients who complain of more than one type of pain or who have multiple potential sources. Correct determination that the pain is of ischemic cardiac origin is crucial to the subsequent diagnostic and therapeutic plan. The misdiagnosis of severe or unstable angina pectoris made on the basis of an inadequate history may lead to unindicated coronary angiography, which may nevertheless demonstrate obstructive coronary lesions. The resultant choices between medical and surgical therapy and decisions to restrict the patient's activity obviously will be inappropriate for the patient who has only costochondritis or esophageal spasm and in whom the finding of coronary artery disease is, in fact, only incidental.

Proof that chest pain is due to myocardial ischemia can be established by recording an electrocardiogram, examining the patient, and monitoring hemodynamic performance *during* pain. Physical examination during such episodes may reveal tachycardia, elevated systemic blood pressure, transient paradoxical splitting of the second heart sound, the appearance or intensification of a fourth heart sound, and occasionally, a third heart sound (S₃ gallop) or a murmur indicating mitral regurgitation due to papillary muscle dysfunction. Hemodynamic findings may include a rise in left ventricular filling pressure as reflected by the pulmonary capillary wedge pressure measured with a Swan-Ganz catheter. Although hemodynamic monitoring is not routine, especially in the emer-

gency ward, the emergency physician should make every attempt to record an electrocardiogram and to examine the patient during pain to establish with certainty that the pain in question is angina.

Electrocardiographic abnormalities that occur during anginal pain usually return to baseline when the pain abates. The most common electrocardiographic abnormality during pain is transient depression of ST segments (Fig. 6.2), although ST segments may be elevated in Prinzmetal's angina. Sometimes, only T-wave inversions appear, and occasionally, previously inverted T waves become upright during pain ("pseudonormalization" of T waves), as seen in Figure 6.3. In addition to helping establish the cardiac origin of pain, the fluctuating electrocardiographic abnormalities indicate the area of heart involved and, to some degree, the amount of myocardium jeopardized. Table 6.1 correlates the area of myocardium and the coronary artery usually involved with the electrocardiographic leads showing ischemic changes. For example, transient marked depression of ST segments over the entire anterior precordium (leads V₂ to V₆) as well as over the inferior surface (leads II, III, and aVF) probably indicates that a large area of myocardium is at risk from the ischemic episode. Another example is ST-segment depression over the anterior surface in a patient with recurrent pain after an old inferior myocardial infarction, indicating that a second coronary artery is involved.

The prognosis for patients with coronary artery disease and the decisions for medical or surgical therapy are best correlated with the amount of myocardium put at ischemic risk by coronary obstructive lesions and the state of left ventricular

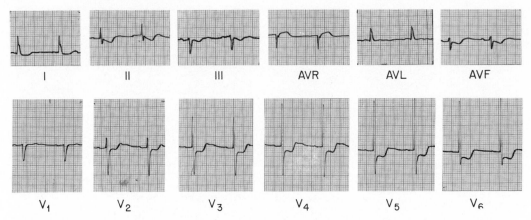

Figure 6.2. Subendocardial ischemia during chest pain. ST-segment depression in leads V_2 through V_5 begins with marked J point depression and ends with sharp "squaring" of the ST-T junction, giving a horizontal ST-segment depression characteristic of subendocardial ischemia. Lesser but similar changes are seen in leads II, III and aVF. This electrocardiogram indicates ischemia of the anteroseptal, anterior, apical, and inferior surfaces of the heart.

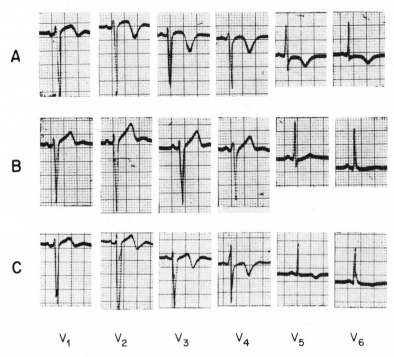

Figure 6.3. "Pseudonormalization" of abnormal T waves during angina. **(A)** Baseline electrocardiogram shows recent anteroseptal infarction. **(B)** During angina, T waves become upright and appear more "normal." **(C)** After pain, T waves revert to baseline. These changes indicate that the anterior wall is the location of the ischemia and that, therefore, there must still be live muscle in the area of the recent anteroseptal infarction.

function (European Coronary Surgical Group, 1980; Hutter, 1980; Takaro et al., 1976). Documentation of transient ST-segment and T-wave changes during pain is important not only to establish the anginal cause of pain, but also to identify patients with a large amount of live myo-

cardium at ischemic risk. If such patients are otherwise suitable candidates, they should be considered for coronary angiography.

In the variant of angina pectoris sometimes called Prinzmetal's angina, ST-segment elevation rather than ST-segment depression is seen during

Table 6.1.
Correlation between location of ischemic changes on electrocardiogram and involved myocardial region.

Electrocardiographic Leads	Myocardial Region	Coronary Artery
II, III, aVF	Inferior	RCA
V_1, V_2 (reciprocal changes)	Posterior	RCA
V_2–V_4	Anteroseptal	Left anterior descending branch of LCA
V_3–V_5	Anterior	Left anterior descending branch of LCA
I, aVL	High lateral	Circumflex marginal or diagonal branch of LCA
V_5–V_6	Apical	Usually left anterior descending branch of LCA; can be posterior descending branch of RCA

RCA = right coronary artery; LCA = left coronary artery.

pain, with resolution to baseline after relief of pain (Prinzmetal et al., 1959; Pasternak et al., 1979) (Fig. 6.4). The diagnosis cannot be made until subsequent electrocardiograms prove that the ST segments have returned to baseline *without* evolution of a myocardial infarction. Characteristically, the pain occurs at rest, often at similar times during the day. Some patients may also have exertional pain. Arrhythmias are common during pain, and include ventricular premature beats, ventricular tachycardia, ventricular fibrillation, atrioventricular block, sinus bradycardia, sinoatrial exit block, and supraventricular tachyarrhythmia.

UNSTABLE ANGINA PECTORIS

The syndrome of unstable angina pectoris is in the "gray zone" between stable angina on the one hand and acute myocardial infarction and perhaps sudden death on the other. It is best divided into three main groups. First, in patients with previously stable angina, the frequency, severity, or duration of pain may increase considerably. Pain is brought on with less and less stress, even occurring at rest, and it becomes more and more resistant to relief from nitrates. This crescendo pattern occurs in the absence of precipitating factors such as anemia, arrhythmias, or thyrotoxicosis. Second, in patients without previous angina, pain begins abruptly and demonstrates the same rapidly progressive pattern usually in the course of days or weeks. Third, in some patients, a prolonged episode of coronary pain develops that suggests myocardial infarction but without electrocardiographic or enzymatic evidence of infarction.

Once unstable angina is diagnosed, the patient should be hospitalized, preferably in a coronary care unit. Hospitalization is necessary to stabilize the patient's condition, to exclude the diagnosis of myocardial infarction, to institute prompt medical therapy, and to consider further diagnostic studies, including coronary angiography in order to decide between continued medical treatment and surgical

therapy. Once myocardial infarction has been ruled out and the patient's condition is stabilized on medical therapy, coronary angiography can be carried out as safely as in patients with stable angina (National Cooperative Study Group, 1976).

The medical treatment of angina pectoris should be instituted promptly and aggressively. Adequate sedation can usually be achieved with oxazepam (Serax), diazepam (Valium), or chlordiazepoxide hydrochloride (Librium). When pain cannot be controlled with other measures, morphine sulfate, 2–5 mg intravenously, is preferable to other analgesics.

β-adrenergic blocking agents and nitrates are the mainstays of medical therapy, the general aim of which is to improve the relationship between myocardial oxygen and its supply. β-blocking agents diminish myocardial oxygen demand by reducing heart rate, blood pressure, and the rate of rise of ventricular pressure. In the absence of contraindications such as evident congestive heart failure or history of bronchospasm, they should be started immediately and increased until adequate physiologic levels are reached, as indicated by a resting heart rate of 50–60 beats/min (Nies and Shand, 1975). Propranolol hydrochloride (Inderal) is the most commonly used β-adrenergic blocking agent in the United States. Oral dosage ranges from 40 mg/day to as high as 800 mg/day in two to four divided doses. When the oral route is unavailable or when more immediate onset of action is desired, propranolol can be given intravenously. Increments of 0.5 mg can be given every 5 minutes until an appropriate physiologic effect is achieved. Usually, 0.05 mg/kg is a reasonable total initial dose, but some patients require more. A maintenance dose, usually equal to the initial dose, can be administered as an intravenous drip. Intravenous doses are usually 5–10% of the oral dose. Although there are reliable assays for blood levels of propranolol, they usually do not measure the active metabolite, 4-hydroxypropranolol, and

Baseline

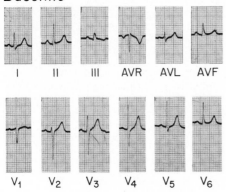

During pain

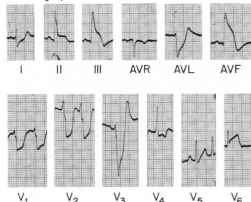

5 minutes after pain

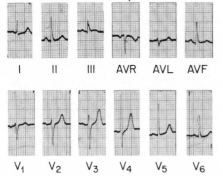

Figure 6.4. Prinzmetal's angina. During pain, marked ST-segment elevation is seen in leads II, III, AVF, and V₆ with reciprocal ST-segment depression in leads AVL, V₁, V₂, and V₃ indicating inferoposteroapical epicardial injury current. After pain, ST segments return to baseline without subsequent evolution to myocardial infarction.

they are not generally as effective a guide as the monitoring of physiologic parameters such as blood pressure and heart rate. Propranolol is generally contraindicated in patients with left ventricular failure, high-grade atrioventricular block, or hypotension. In addition, by blocking β-adrenergic receptors in the bronchial tree, propranolol can precipitate bronchial spasm. Patients who have resting bradycardia must be carefully monitored for additional slowing after administration of propranolol. Other β-adrenergic blocking agents currently approved in the United States include metoprolol tartrate (Lopressor), which is relatively cardioselective and therefore less likely to induce bronchospasm; nadolol (Corgard), a nonselective β-adrenergic blocking agent that requires administration only once a day because of its longer duration of action; timolol (Blocadren), a nonselective agent; and atenolol (Tenormin), a cardioselective agent that also can be given once a day. Atenolol, nadolol, and timolol are less lipophilic than propranolol and metoprolol, and therefore may be associated with fewer central nervous system side effects (Frishman, 1981).

Nitrates, which may cause reflex tachycardia when administered alone, are used effectively in conjunction with β-adrenergic blocking agents. When the drugs are given concurrently, control of both heart rate (50–60 beats/min) and blood pressure (100–120 mm Hg systolic, depending on the individual) can usually be achieved. The primary effect of the nitrates is thought to be venodilation, which results in diminished venous return to the heart and, thus, in a decreased preload. Nitrates also cause some dilation of the arterioles, resulting in decreased afterload and lower blood pressure. They also dilate coronary arteries, and there is evidence that they increase circulation through collaterals between major coronary arteries (Goldstein et al., 1974). The patient with active unstable angina and adequate blood pressure should be treated in the emergency ward with nitroglycerin, 0.3 or 0.4 mg sublingually. If the blood pressure is well maintained, the dose can be repeated every 5 minutes. If pain persists after three doses, however, morphine sulfate should be given. Once pain is controlled, longer-term treatment may be started with isosorbide dinitrate, 5–20 mg every 2–3 hours sublingually, as permitted by blood pressure. If pain is not relieved, intravenous nitroglycerin can be administered as a constant infusion, starting with 15–20 μg/min and increasing to as high as 400 μg/min (Armstrong et al., 1980). Because of the potential for hypotension, patients receiving intravenous nitroglycerin should be monitored with continuous intra-arterial pressure monitoring and, in most cases, a pulmonary arterial line to measure left ventricular filling pressure. Because of these requirements, intravenous nitrate administration usually is deferred until the patient has left the emergency ward.

The less acutely ill patient may be treated with isosorbide dinitrate, 10–80 mg every 4 hours orally (Thadani et al., 1980). Nitroglycerin ointment, when applied to the skin in 1- to 3-inch ribbons of extruded paste, has a duration of action of up to 6 hours and can be used effectively, particularly for extended nighttime protection (Reichek et al., 1974). Headache, the most frequent limiting side effect of nitrate therapy, may be ameliorated in some patients by switching from oral to cutaneous administration. Isosorbide dinitrate capsules (Isordil Tembids) have an extended antianginal effect and result in improved exercise tolerance for as long as 6 hours (Lee et al., 1976), but have variable absorption and therefore should not be used in an unstable situation. In addition to headache, hypotension may be a limiting factor in administration of nitrates. This is particularly true in elderly patients with attenuated autonomic nervous system responses and in patients who are volume depleted because of concurrent administration of diuretics or inappropriate dilation related to a recent myocardial infarction. Thus, fluids may have to be administered to patients with large nitrate requirements who are hypotensive with a low left ventricular filling pressure. Patients whose nitrate regimen has been started on an outpatient basis should be given a test dose of nitroglycerin sublingually to ensure that they will not experience an unacceptable decrease in blood pressure.

Calcium antagonists, a class of agents recently introduced to general use in the United States, are likely to attain a position of major importance in the treatment of ischemic heart disease. Nifedipine (Procardia) was the first of these drugs approved by the Food and Drug Administration for oral use. In addition to its effectiveness in the treatment of coronary spasm (Antman et al., 1980), this medication appears to be effective in the treatment of angina pectoris resulting from fixed coronary artery obstruction (Moskowitz et al., 1979). It dilates coronary and peripheral arterioles and can lower the blood pressure. Oral dosage of nifedipine is 10 mg three to four times a day, which may be increased to as high as 40 mg four times a day. Nifedipine is also effective when given intravenously or sublingually, but insufficient experience with these routes precludes recommendation for routine use in the emergency ward. Verapamil (Isoptin) recently has been approved in the United States. It has antianginal effects similar to those of Nifedipine and is, in addition, highly effective in the treatment of supraventricular tachyarrhythmias which involve the A-V node. It is available for both intravenous and oral use, with oral doses ranging from 240–480 mg/day. Diltiazem, another calcium antagonist, has not yet been approved for use in the United States.

Patients with continuing pain in the setting of persistent elevation of blood pressure may benefit from blood pressure (afterload) reduction. Although all of the antianginal treatments previously described have hypotensive potential, hypertension that persists even in the face of treatment with the medications discussed should be aggressively managed. In most cases, treatment with diuretics or other specific antihypertensive agents will suffice. For those patients requiring immediate blood pressure reduction in an ischemic setting, intravenous infusion of a hypotensive agent closely titrated to blood pressure is preferable to a "bolus" that may result in uncontrolled hypotension and exacerbation of the ischemia. If sublingual or intravenous nitroglycerin is insufficient to control blood pressure, sodium nitroprusside may be added 20–50 μg/min intravenously (Miller et al., 1975; Palmer and Lasseter, 1975). Except in the most serious emergency during which pressure may be continuously monitored manually, intra-arterial pressure monitoring should be a prerequisite to the administration of this medication. In addition, since sodium nitroprusside may unfavorably affect the coronary circulation in the ischemic heart (Chiariello et al., 1976), it should be added to a nitrate regimen already increased to a high level.

When left ventricular failure is evident and may be contributing to unstable angina, digitalis glycosides and diuretics may relieve pain by reducing left ventricular volume, transmural pressure, and therefore, myocardial oxygen consumption. Except in this setting, digitalis has no role in the therapy for unstable angina, since it may increase peripheral vascular resistance, myocardial oxygen consumption, and therefore, ischemia.

The treatment of arrhythmias is discussed in Chapter 5, but it should be emphasized here that achievement of normal sinus rhythm is more urgent in patients with ongoing coronary ischemic pain, whether due to unstable angina or acute myocardial infarction. By increasing myocardial oxygen consumption, persistent, rapid atrial fibrillation or paroxysmal atrial tachycardia may result in progression of unstable angina to myocardial infarction or extension of an existent myocardial infarct. Thus, prompt cardioversion of such patients to normal sinus rhythm is recommended. Similarly, use of a temporary pacemaker or appropriate pharmacologic therapy for the various bradyarrhythmias is more urgent in the patient with ongoing ischemia in whom a normal heart rate is essential for maintenance of adequate cardiac output and coronary perfusion.

Ongoing coronary pain despite a maximal medical program can often be managed with intra-aortic balloon counterpulsation (Gold et al., 1973; Levine et al., 1978). By deflating just before systole, the balloon reduces the pressure against which the left ventricle must empty (afterload). In addition, it reduces left ventricular end-diastolic pressure (preload) and, therefore, left ventricular size and wall tension. Both of these effects reduce myocardial oxygen consumption. By inflating in diastole, the balloon transiently increases diastolic pressure and improves coronary artery blood flow. In patients whose condition is very unstable, we have found the intra-aortic balloon useful not only in relieving pain but also in enhancing the safety of coronary angiographic examination and operation (Levine et al., 1978). Although intra-aortic balloon counterpulsation is not used in the emergency ward and is not available in many hospitals, knowledge of its efficacy and indications is necessary so that the physician can either mobilize the appropriate resources within the hospital or transfer the patient to an institution with the proper equipment.

ACUTE MYOCARDIAL INFARCTION

In the emergency ward, a careful history, a competent physical examination, and evaluation of the electrocardiogram form the basis for a diagnosis of acute myocardial infarction. The patient's complaint is usually chest pain, often with extension to the neck or arm, commonly accompanied by sweating, nausea, shortness of breath, and pallor. If the patient has pre-existent angina, the pain is frequently reminiscent of the usual pain, but is more intense and unremitting. Many patients have symptoms that are not classic. Elderly patients, in particular, are frequently seen without pain after the sudden onset of dyspnea or worsening of congestive heart failure (Pathy, 1967). If the history continues to suggest prolonged ischemia or infarction after consideration of the other possible causes of chest pain, the patient should be admitted and myocardial infarction ruled out, even in the presence of a normal electrocardiogram.

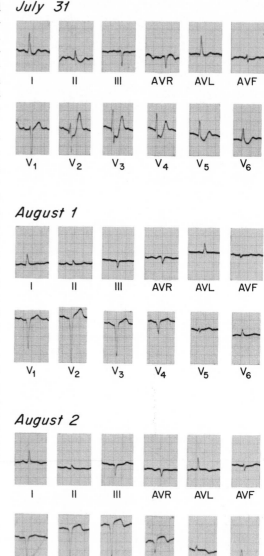

Figure 6.5. Evolution of anteroseptal myocardial infarction. "Hyperacute" tall T waves associated with depressed ST segments may be seen in the first few hours (July 31). Later, T-wave inversion and ST-segment elevation occur in association with loss of R wave and development of Q waves in leads V_1 through V_4 (August 1 and 2).

Figure 6.5 depicts the electrocardiographic evolution of acute myocardial infarction. The electrocardiogram may be diagnostic in the emergency ward if pathologic Q waves are seen with ST-segment elevation and T-wave inversion. These findings may also indicate an old myocardial infarct with ventricular aneurysm, but the burden of proof is on the person who claims the changes are old. The location of Q waves indicates the location of the infarct, the coronary artery involved, and, to some degree, the extent of damage (Table 6.1). In a true posterior infarction, Q waves are not seen on the standard electrocardiogram; rather, reciprocal changes occur in leads V_1 and V_2 with tall, broad R waves (more than 0.04 second), depressed ST segments, and upright T waves. The Q waves would be seen in lead V_{10} placed behind the heart on the left posterior region of the chest.

Since the amount of muscle still in jeopardy as well as the amount already infarcted, is extremely important in determining the patient's ultimate course, other leads should be studied for evidence of additional areas of compromise. For example, a patient with classic inferior myocardial infarction with Q waves and elevated ST segments in leads II, III, and aVF may also have ST-segment depression in leads V_3 and V_4 indicating anterior subendocardial ischemia. A second electrocardiogram recorded only a few hours later may show the evolving inferior myocardial infarction, but no longer may show any anterior changes. Nevertheless, the patient probably has two-vessel disease (right coronary artery and left anterior descending branch of the left coronary artery) rather than single-vessel, right coronary artery disease. This observation is important and should be documented, since it may indicate a need for subsequent coronary angiographic examination.

The diagnosis of acute ischemia and myocardial infarction can be made in the presence of right bundle-branch block (RBBB) since only the terminal part of the QRS complex is involved with this conduction defect, causing an R′ in lead V_1 and a broad, slurred S wave in lead I. Thus, pathologic Q waves (more than 0.04 second) can still be read in any lead (Fig. 6.6). In left bundle-branch block (LBBB), on the other hand, the initial as well as the terminal portions of the QRS complex are abnormal, and therefore it is often taught that infarction cannot be read in the presence of LBBB. There are two important exceptions to this rule. First, in LBBB an R wave is normally present in leads II, III, and aVF even in the presence of considerable left axis deviation, in which case lead II has an RS configuration. The occurrence of Q waves in leads II, III, and aVF, therefore, permits diagnosis of inferior myocardial infarction in the presence of LBBB (Fig. 6.7).

Second, anteroseptal infarction can also be determined in the presence of LBBB, although not by the usual poor anterior R-wave progression since this is a normal feature of LBBB. In LBBB, the ventricular septum, which normally depolarizes from left to right, depolarizes from right to

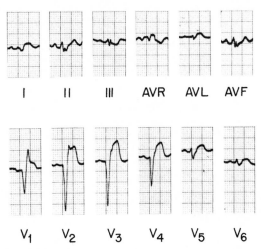

Figure 6.6. Acute anteroseptal myocardial infarction and right bundle-branch block (RBBB). Q-wave and ST-segment elevation is clearly seen in leads V_1 through V_3 in presence of complete RBBB. The latter is indicated by the tall terminal R′ in lead V_1 and 0.16-second duration of QRS complex.

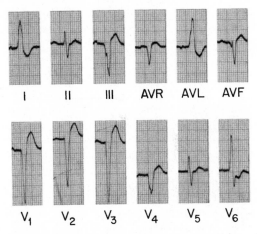

Figure 6.7. Old inferior myocardial infarction in presence of left bundle-branch block (LBBB). QRS-complex duration of 0.12-second, initial positive deflection of QRS in leads I and AVL, and poor R-wave progression in leads V_1 through V_1 are all features of LBBB. Q waves in leads III and AVF indicate inferior myocardial infarction since an R wave is normally present in leads II, III, and AVF in LBBB, even if there is marked left axis deviation. (Lead V_2 was taken at one-half standardization.)

left. This results in an initial positive deflection of the QRS complex in leads I and aVL, which "look at" the free left ventricular wall from the left shoulder. In an anteroseptal infarct, the initial septal forces are lost, and the second forces, which are right ventricular and therefore directed to the right, initiate the QRS complex, resulting in Q

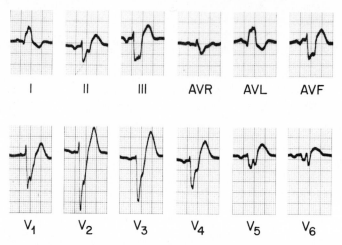

I   II   III   AVR   AVL   AVF

V₁   V₂   V₃   V₄   V₅   V₆

Figure 6.8. Septal myocardial infarction in left bundle-branch block (LBBB). Q waves in leads I and AVL indicate septal (and, therefore, anteroseptal) infarction in presence of LBBB.

waves in leads I and aVL. Thus, new Q waves in leads I and aVL in a patient with LBBB indicate a septal infarct (Fig. 6.8).

Acute injury currents can also be read in the presence of LBBB. The repolarization changes of uncomplicated LBBB consist of downsloping ST segments and asymmetric T-wave inversion in those leads with a positive QRS complex (leads I, aVL, V_5, and V_6). Reciprocal changes of upsloping ST segments and upright T waves are seen in those leads with a negative QRS complex (leads V_1 to V_3). Therefore, elevation of ST segments in a lead with an upright QRS complex may indicate epicardial injury (Fig. 6.9), and depression of ST segments in a lead with a negative QRS complex may indicate subendocardial injury.

Another important aspect in diagnosing myocardial infarction is knowledge of serial myocardial enzyme levels. In patients without classically evolving Q waves, the differentiation between unstable angina and myocardial infarction greatly depends on valid interpretation of enzyme levels.

In such patients, three sets of enzyme determinations should be performed within the first 24 hours, since levels can peak and then decrease to normal within this time. It is precisely for those patients with only ST-segment and T-wave changes that this more subtle knowledge of the enzyme curve is needed. In institutions where it is available, an assay for CK-MB, the myocardium-specific subtype of creatine kinase, should be performed with each set of cardiac enzyme determinations (Roberts and Sobel, 1978). Since the creatinine phosphokinase level or serum glutamic oxaloacetic transaminase level or both can be elevated with intramuscular injections, it is impor-

tant to avoid this method of drug administration and to use subcutaneous or intravenous routes in such patients.

Physical examination during acute myocardial infarction may reveal those phenomena associated with angina pectoris, namely, tachycardia, elevated systemic blood pressure, transient paradoxical splitting of the second heart sound, and appearance or exacerbation of a fourth heart sound. More significant left ventricular failure may be indicated by a third heart sound (S_3 gallop), congestive rales, or hypotension. Murmurs indicating mitral regurgitation due to papillary muscle dysfunction are relatively frequent, occurring in more than 70% of patients with inferior myocardial infarction and in more than 50% with anterior myocardial infarction under ideal conditions for auscultation (Heikkilä, 1967). The murmur frequently is missed unless the patient is examined in the left lateral decubitus position with full expiration in a quiet room, with the diaphragm of the stethoscope placed directly over the apex. This murmur is usually of auscultatory interest only, and the mitral regurgitation is of no hemodynamic significance. Occasionally, however, regurgitation may be severe, requiring aggressive therapy. Papillary muscle rupture occurs in only about 1% of patients with acute myocardial infarction, and usually is indicated by abrupt onset of a harsh systolic murmur at the apex, with extension to the axilla or to the left sternal border. These patients are almost always critically ill with severe pulmonary edema or cardiogenic shock or both. With both severe papillary muscle dysfunction and papillary muscle rupture, acute congestive heart failure is left sided, with pulmonary edema and a loud S_3

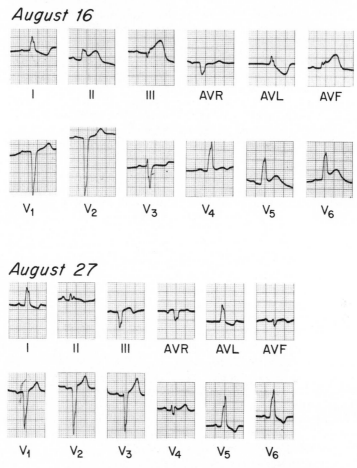

Figure 6.9.   Acute inferoapical injury in LBBB. ST-segment elevation in leads II, III, AVF, V_5, and V_6 indicates epicardial injury current (August 16) since ST segments should be downsloping in leads with a positive QRS complex in LBBB. ST segments return to baseline on August 27.

gallop. The murmur may be absent in the presence of profound hypotension. Right-heart catheterization with a Swan-Ganz catheter reveals a high pulmonary capillary wedge pressure with tall V waves.

Rupture of the ventricular septum is another mechanical complication of myocardial infarction associated with a systolic murmur. The murmur is usually loud, diamond-shaped, and holosystolic, beginning just before the first heart sound and best heard at the left sternal border. A systolic thrill is usually felt. In contrast with the clinical appearance of pulmonary edema associated with acute mitral regurgitation, rupture of the ventricular septum overloads the right ventricle, causing the clinical findings of severe right-sided congestive heart failure with less pulmonary congestion. Since some patients may have both papillary muscle dysfunction and a ruptured ventricular septum, any patient with acute myocardial infarction who

has a new systolic murmur and whose hemodynamic status is unstable should undergo right-heart catheterization. Blood samples should be obtained from the right atrium, right ventricle, and pulmonary arteries to determine the presence of an oxygen step-up. The pulmonary capillary wedge pressure should be determined with a Swan-Ganz catheter, and the tracing should be inspected for tall V waves.

Pericarditis may occur early in the course of transmural acute myocardial infarction, resulting in pain that can be misinterpreted as ongoing ischemic pain. Since the implications differ greatly, careful examination for a pericardial friction rub and determination as to whether the pain changes with change in position are important. If the pain is exacerbated by a deep breath and is either relieved or made worse by sitting up, it is more likely to be pericarditis, even in the absence of a pericardial friction rub. In questionable cases, a short-term trial with an effective anti-inflammatory agent such as indomethacin, 25 mg every 6 hours for 2 or 3 days, is sometimes helpful.

The treatment of acute myocardial infarction has changed significantly in the past few years, many studies having indicated that the size of infarction may be reduced by techniques designed to lessen myocardial oxygen consumption while maintaining adequate coronary artery perfusion pressure (Maroko and Braunwald, 1973; Maroko et al., 1971).

Sublingual nitroglycerin acts primarily as a venodilator reducing preload (left ventricular filling pressure) (Gold et al., 1972; Williams et al., 1975). Intravenous nitroglycerin has a greater effect on arteriolar dilation, decreasing afterload (peripheral resistance) (Epstein et al., 1975; Flaherty et al., 1975; Williams et al., 1975); it reduces the area of ST-segment elevation and presumably myocardial injury after coronary artery ligation in dogs (Epstein et al., 1975) and after myocardial infarction in human beings (Borer et al., 1975; Come et al., 1975; Flaherty et al., 1975). When the nitroglycerin-induced increase in heart rate and decrease in blood pressure are prevented in dogs by phenylephrine hydrochloride or methoxamine hydrochloride (α-adrenergic agonists causing peripheral vasoconstriction with no direct cardiac action), the favorable effect of nitroglycerin can be enhanced. In man, this enhancement is seen primarily in patients without heart failure. In patients with heart failure, nitroglycerin alone can reduce the area of ST-segment elevation; addition of phenylephrine partly reverses this effect. In the emergency ward, sublingual nitroglycerin or sublingual isosorbide dinitrate or both should be administered with careful measurement of blood pressure before and after administration. Since an adequate nitrate effect can be achieved via this route, there is, in general, no indication for intravenous nitrates in the emergency ward.

Intravenous administration of propranolol hydrochloride may also limit eventual infarct size (Maroko et al., 1971; Mueller and Ayers, 1977). Propranolol reduces oxygen consumption by decreasing contractility, arterial blood pressure, and heart rate. In patients with adequate blood pressure and no evidence of congestive heart failure, the initial intravenous dose is 0.05 mg/kg given in increments of 0.5 mg every 5–10 minutes. The maintenance intravenous dose ranges from 1–3 mg every 4–6 hours, but most patients should be able to take propranolol orally once their condition has become stabilized. The patient should be closely observed for evidence of congestive heart failure,

an unacceptably slow heart rate, or hypotension. As a general rule, patients with evidence of significant anterior wall injury should be monitored with a Swan-Ganz pulmonary artery line during administration of propranolol to ensure that the additive myocardial depressant effects of the evolving infarction and the medication do not combine to precipitate frank congestive heart failure.

Intra-aortic balloon counterpulsation reduces afterload and preload, and at the same time, increases coronary artery perfusion pressure by augmenting diastolic blood pressure. The device can now be inserted percutaneously (Subramanian et al., 1980), and thus, it may in rare cases be considered part of the emergency ward armamentarium. Although balloon counterpulsation can relieve pain and stabilize hemodynamics, studies performed on patients with or without congestive heart failure soon after myocardial infarction have thus far failed to demonstrate long-term benefit (Leinbach et al., 1978; O'Rourke et al., 1981). Thus, with rare exception, this mode of early intervention is reserved for patients who may be expected to benefit from nearly immediate operative intervention, but who require short-term stabilization before operation.

Nitroprusside has both strong venodilating (preload) and arteriolar (afterload) actions and can be administered effectively to patients with persistent elevation of blood pressure, especially when it is associated with a high left ventricular filling pressure. For the reasons noted previously, when nitroprusside is administered in the presence of acute ischemia or infarction, we prefer to treat the patient concurrently with nitroglycerin in the hope of maintaining coronary circulation through the collateral channels.

There is promising early evidence that intracoronary thrombolysis with infusion of streptokinase into the occluded coronary artery preferably within 3 hours after the onset of symptoms may result in diminution of infarct size (Ganz et al., 1981). This procedure, which may in some cases be combined with percutaneous transluminal coronary angioplasty, is in the earliest phases of investigation and is not recommended as routine therapy. Nevertheless, in situations in which it is to be used, the decision must be made shortly after the patient's arrival in the emergency ward, and thus, the emergency physician must be familiar with the available facilities and individuals to notify.

Such aggressive forms of therapy are clearly unnecessary and inappropriate in most patients with an uncomplicated infarction and adequate blood pressure and heart rate. Such patients should be treated in the emergency ward with the classic regimen consisting of pain relief and sedation; usually this is best accomplished with morphine sulfate, oxygen delivered through a nasal cannula, close monitoring of the heart rate, rhythm, and blood pressure, and expeditious transportation to the coronary care unit. In addition, because "warning arrhythmias" are an unpredictable precursor of disastrous ventricular arrhythmias, and because prophylactic administration of lidocaine hydrochloride (Xylocaine) has been shown to diminish the frequency of primary ventricular fibrillation (Lie et al., 1974; Wyman and Hammersmith, 1974), we routinely infuse lidocaine prophylactically for the first 24–48 hours after acute myocardial infarction. An effective regimen requires a loading dose of 50–75 mg of lidocaine as an intravenous bolus, followed by an infusion of 1–4 mg/min. Administration of a second bolus of 50 mg approximately 20 minutes after the first dose may be required to maintain adequate levels (Greenblatt et al., 1976). Doses should be reduced in the elderly, in patients with hepatic dysfunction, and in patients with incipient circulatory collapse.

For patients with continuing ischemic pain or congestive heart failure in whom aggressive therapy is appropriate, the emergency physician should make immediate arrangements for insertion of an intra-arterial cannula for constant monitoring of the arterial blood pressure and of a Swan-Ganz arterial catheter for measurement of left ventricular filling pressure. The fact that most emergency wards are not equipped with such monitoring capabilities reinforces the need for avoiding delay in transporting the patient to the appropriate unit. In an emergency situation, when hemodynamically active medications such as nitroprusside, nitroglycerin, and propranolol are administered without the appropriate monitoring devices, counteracting agents should be immediately available. Such agents would include an intravenous solution of isoproterenol or epinephrine to combat the effect of propranolol and a pure α-adrenergic agonist such as phenylephrine hydrochloride to negate the effects on blood pressure of nitroprusside or nitroglycerin.

Hypotension complicating acute myocardial infarction may be related to easily reversible causes or may presage a truly ominous syndrome, cardiogenic shock. Examples of easily reversible causes are considerable sinus bradycardia in a patient with inferior myocardial infarction treatable with

atropine, isoproterenol, or a temporary pacing wire, and rapid paroxysmal atrial tachycardia treatable with cardioversion and appropriate antiarrhythmic drugs. The treatment of bradycardia in the absence of symptoms, ventricular premature beats, or hypotension remains controversial. We usually withhold treatment in this setting to avoid unnecessary and perhaps dangerous stimulation (Epstein et al., 1975). When atropine is given, the minimum dose should be 0.4 mg intravenously to avoid the paradoxical slowing that has been reported at lower doses. The maximum dose should be 1.0 mg to avoid the sinus tachycardia occasionally seen with higher doses. Loss of a properly timed atrial contraction may cause significant diminution in cardiac output in patients with impaired myocardial function, and restoration of atrioventricular synchrony by cardioversion, atrial pacing, or atrioventricular sequential pacing may improve both cardiac output and blood pressure. The appearance of a bifascicular conduction system disturbance, including LBBB or RBBB with either left anterior or posterior hemiblock, may herald imminent progression to complete atrioventricular block. Most patients who die with this complication have extensive anterior infarction and ventricular failure. A small number of patients have relatively well-preserved left ventricular function and thus will benefit from the prompt prophylactic insertion of a temporary transvenous right ventricular pacing wire at the time of the appearance of bifascicular block (Hindman et al., 1978).

Another promptly reversible but often unrecognized cause of hypotension in myocardial infarction is relative hypovolemia due to excessive diuresis or inappropriate peripheral vasodilation. The classic example is the patient with pulmonary edema who has received a potent diuretic such as furosemide that has prompted considerable diuresis with subsequent hypotension. Such a patient may have a low intravascular volume at a time (even up to 24 hours) when interstitial edema is still present, either seen on the chest x-ray film or manifested as congestive rales.

Right ventricular infarction, usually associated with infarction of the inferior left ventricular wall, may result in systemic hypotension in the absence of severe left ventricular dysfunction. The failure of the right ventricle in this setting results in insufficient left-sided filling pressure and, thus, reduced cardiac output (Isner and Roberts, 1978; Lorell et al., 1979). Unlike in the case of left ventricular failure, hypotension from this cause responds to volume expansion.

Knowledge of the left ventricular filling pressure

attained with a Swan-Ganz catheter allows appropriate volume replacement, preferably with a colloid such as albumin that stays in the intravascular space rather than one such as saline that also goes into the extravascular, extracellular (interstitial) space. Knowledge of the left ventricular filling pressure is sometimes not readily obtainable. In such a situation, rapid administration (at least within 10 minutes) of 200 ml of 5% dextrose in water may be helpful. The pulse and blood pressure should be measured every 3 or 4 minutes; if the pulse rate slows and the blood pressure rises with the fluid challenge, good evidence of hypovolemia is obtained and longer-term replacement therapy can then be instituted. If no beneficial effect is seen, even with a repeated challenge, the need for volume replacement must be seriously questioned. We recommend 5% dextrose in water administered rapidly because it moves into the intracellular space quickly, thus challenging the intravascular compartment only briefly and with relative safety. Another cause of hypovolemia that is being recognized more often is inappropriate peripheral vasodilation in patients with acute infarction. Although we have noted this more frequently in inferior and posterior myocardial infarctions, perhaps related to stimulation of the vagal afferent or efferent nerves, it also occurs in anterior myocardial infarctions. Here again, knowledge of the left ventricular filling pressure or a challenge with 5% dextrose in water will allow appropriate decisions concerning volume replacement. In the patients seen so far, peripheral vasodilation has resolved after 24–72 hours.

Severe hypotension not due to arrhythmias or hypovolemia may indicate cardiogenic shock with its ominous prognosis. In patients with cardiogenic shock, systolic blood pressure is usually less than 90 mm Hg, or 50 mm Hg lower than former levels, and is accompanied by signs of peripheral vasoconstriction, a urinary output less than 20 ml/hr, and mental obtundation. Pulmonary congestion may or may not occur. The characteristic hemodynamic findings are a cardiac index less than 2 liters/min/m^2, a mean arterial pressure less than 60 mm Hg, and a pulmonary capillary wedge pressure more than 20 mm Hg. A vicious cycle ensues, with low cardiac output causing low arterial blood pressure leading to reduced coronary artery perfusion resulting in further reduction of cardiac output, and so on. The goal of therapy is to support the blood pressure at a level sufficient to maintain both peripheral circulation and coronary artery perfusion pressure (trying to achieve a mean arterial pressure of about 70 mm Hg) in such a way that myocardial oxygen consumption does not increase. This poses a problem since agents such as epinephrine, isoproterenol, and norepinephrine increase myocardial oxygen consumption by their central β-adrenergic action, and yet this direct stimulation of the heart is usually essential to maintain overall circulation. Pure α-adrenergic agents such as phenylephrine hydrochloride and methoxamine hydrochloride are usually ineffective in patients with cardiogenic shock. Probably the best supporting pharmacologic agent currently in clinical use is norepinephrine, 2–30 μg/min intravenously. This agent has both an α action (peripheral vasoconstriction) and central β action (increased cardiac contractility), but the former is stronger; an acceptable compromise results in which the peripheral circulation, the central coronary artery perfusion pressure, and the myocardium are supported. Dobutamine, a recently introduced synthetic catecholamine, improves cardiac output and lowers left ventricular filling pressure in patients with evolving myocardial infarction without significantly accelerating heart rate or precipitating arrhythmias (Gillespie et al, 1975; Goldstein et al, 1980). Except in the treatment of atrial tachyarrhythmias, digitalis has no role in the emergency ward therapy of heart failure from acute myocardial infarction.

The most effective therapeutic device in the management of cardiogenic shock is intra-aortic balloon counterpulsation (Dunkman et al, 1972). As mentioned previously, by deflating in systole, the balloon reduces the afterload and preload, decreasing myocardial oxygen consumption, and by filling in diastole, it augments the central diastolic aortic pressure, increasing coronary artery perfusion pressure. The intra-aortic balloon is now established as an effective device that allows subsequent coronary angiographic examination and operation in suitable candidates. The ideal patient is a young person with no previous infarct and with a normal-sized heart in whom balloon support is initiated within 24 hours of acute infarction. Other favorable indications include a murmur signaling a possibly treatable mechanical complication or angina indicating viable but ischemic myocardium. The poorest candidate is the older patient with multiple previous infarcts and a large heart with no evidence of a surgically correctable mechanical lesion, such as a ventricular septal defect, severe mitral regurgitation, or a large, discrete aneurysm. It is useful to keep these guidelines in mind, because the best results in cardiogenic shock are obtained with early use of the balloon, and the decision for or against such therapy is often made in the emergency ward.

Suggested Readings

Armstrong PW, Armstrong JA, Marks GS: Pharmacokinetic-hemodynamic studies of intravenous nitroglycerin in congestive heart failure. *Circulation 62:*160–166, 1980

Antman E, Muller J, Goldberg S, et al: Nifedipine therapy for coronary-artery spasm. *N Engl J Med 302:*1269–1273, 1980

Borer JS, Redwood DR, Levitt B, et al: Reduction in myocardial ischemia with nitroglycerin or nitroglycerin plus phenylephrine administered during acute myocardial infarction. *N Engl J Med 293:*1008–1012, 1975

Chiariello M, Gold HK, Leinbach RC, et al: Comparison between the effects of nitroprusside and nitroglycerin on ischemic injury during acute myocardial infarction. *Circulation 54:*766–773, 1976

Come PC, Flaherty JT, Baird MG, et al: Reversal by phenylephrine of the beneficial effects of intravenous nitroglycerin in patients with acute myocardial infarction. *N Engl J Med 293:*1003–1007, 1975

Dunkman WB, Leinbach RC, Buckley MJ, et al: Clinical and hemodynamic results of intraaortic balloon pumping and surgery for cardiogenic shock. *Circulation 46:*465–477, 1972

Epstein SE, Kent KM, Goldstein RE, et al: Reduction of ischemic injury by nitroglycerin during acute myocardial infarction. *N Engl J Med 292:*29–35, 1975

European Coronary Surgical Group: Prospective randomized study of coronary artery bypass surgery in stable angina pectoris. *Lancet 2:*491–495, 1980

Flaherty JT, Reid PR, Kelly DT, et al: Intravenous nitroglycerin in acute myocardial infarction. *Circulation 51:*132–139, 1975

Frishman WH: Drug therapy: β-adrenoceptor antagonists: New drugs and new indications. *N Engl J Med 305:*500–506, 1981

Ganz W, Buchbinder N, Marcus H, et al: Intracoronary thrombolysis in evolving myocardial infarction. *Am Heart J 101:*4–13, 1981

Gillespie TA, Ambos HD, Sobel BE, et al: Effects of dobutamine in patients with acute myocardial infarction. *Am J Cardiol 39:*588–594, 1975

Gold HK, Leinbach RC, Sanders CA: Use of sublingual nitroglycerin in congestive failure following acute myocardial infarction. *Circulation 46:*839–845, 1972

Gold HK, Leinbach RC, Sanders CA, et al: Intraaortic balloon pumping for control of recurrent myocardial ischemia. *Circulation 47:*1197–1203, 1973

Goldstein RA, Passamani ER, Roberts R: A comparison of digoxin and dobutamine in patients with acute infarction and cardiac failure. *N Engl J Med 303:*846–850, 1980

Goldstein RE, Stinson EB, Scherer JL, et al: Intraoperative coronary collateral function in patients with coronary occlusive disease: nitroglycerin responsiveness and angiographic correlations. *Circulation 49:*298–308, 1974

Greenblatt DJ, Bolognini V, Koch-Weser J, et al: Pharmacokinetic approach to the clinical use of lidocaine intravenously. *JAMA 236:*273–277, 1976

Heikkilä J: Mitral incompetence complicating acute myocardial infarction. *Br Heart J 29:*162–169, 1967

Hindman MC, Wagner GS, JaRo M, et al: The clinical significance of bundle branch block complicating acute myocardial infarction. 1. Clinical characteristics, hospital mortality, and one-year follow-up. *Circulation 58:*679–688, 1978

Hutter AM, Jr: Is there a main left equivalent? *Circulation 62:*207–211, 1980

Isner JM, Roberts WC: Right ventricular infarction complicating left ventricular infarction secondary to coronary heart disease. *Am J Cardiol 42:*885–894, 1978

Lee G, Mason DT, Amsterdam EA, et al: Improved exercise tolerance for six hours following isosorbide dinitrate capsules in patients with ischemic heart disease. (Abstract) *Am J Cardiol 37:*150, 1976

Leinbach RC, Gold HK, Harper RW, et al: Early intraaortic balloon pumping for anterior myocardial infarction without shock. *Circulation 58:*204–210, 1978

Levine FH, Gold HK, Leinbach RC, et al: Management of acute myocardial ischemia with intraaortic balloon pumping and coronary artery bypass surgery. *Circulation 58 (Suppl):* 69–72, 1978

Lie KI, Wellens HJ, Van Capelle FJ, et al: Lidocaine in the prevention of primary ventricular fibrillation: a double-blind randomized study of 212 consecutive patients. *N Engl J Med 291:*1324–1326, 1974

Lorell B, Leinbach RC, Pohost GM, et al: Right ventricular infarction. *Am J Cardiol 43:*465–471, 1979

Maroko PR, Braunwald E: Modification of myocardial infarction size after coronary occlusion. *Ann Intern Med 79:*720–733, 1973

Maroko PR, Kjekshus JK, Sobel BE, et al: Factors influencing infarct size following experimental coronary artery occlusions. *Circulation 43:*67–82, 1971

Miller RR, Vismara LA, Zelis R, et al: Clinical use of sodium nitroprusside in chronic ischemic heart disease: Effects on peripheral vascular resistance and venous tone and on ventricular volume, pump and mechanical performance. *Circulation 51:*328–336, 1975

Moskowitz RM, Piccini PA, Nacarelli GV, et al: Nifedipine therapy for stable angina pectoris: preliminary results of effects on angina frequency and treadmill exercise response. *Am J Cardiol 44:*811–816, 1979

Mueller HS, Ayers SM: The role of propranolol in the treatment of acute myocardial infarction. *Prog Cardiovasc Dis 19:*405–412, 1977

National Cooperative Study Group to Compare Medical and Surgical Therapy: Unstable Angina Pectoris I. Report of protocol and patient population. *Am J Cardiol 37:*896–902, 1976

Nies AS, Shand DG: Clinical pharmacology of propranolol. *Circulation 52:*6–15, 1975

Orlando RC, Bozymski EM: Clinical and manometric effects of nitroglycerin in diffuse esophageal spasm. *N Engl J Med 289:*23–25, 1973

O'Rourke MF, Norris RM, Campbell TJ, et al: Randomized controlled trial of intraaortic balloon counterpulsation in early myocardial infarction with acute heart failure. *Am J Cardiol 47:*815–820, 1981

Palmer RF, Lasseter KC: Drug therapy: Sodium nitroprusside. *N Engl J Med 292:*294–297, 1975

Pasternak RC, Hutter AM Jr, DeSanctis RW, et al: Variant angina: Clinical spectrum and results of medical and surgical therapy. *J Thorac Cardiovasc Surg 78:*614–622, 1979

Pathy MS: Clinical presentation of myocardial infarction in the elderly. *Br Heart J 29:*190–199, 1967

Prinzmetal M, Kennamer R, Merliss R, et al: Angina pectoris. I. A variant form of angina pectoris: Preliminary report. *Am J Med 27:*375–388, 1959

Reichek N Goldstein RE, Redwood DR, et al: Sustained effects of nitroglycerin ointment in patients with angina pectoris. *Circulation 50:*348–352, 1974

Roberts R, Sobel BE: Creatinine kinase isoenzymes in the

assessment of heart disease. *Am Heart J 95:*521–528, 1978

Spodick DH: Electrocardiogram in acute pericarditis: Distributions of morphologic and axial changes by stages. *Am J Cardiol 33:*470–474, 1974

Subramanian VA, Goldstein JJ, Sos TA, et al: Preliminary clinical experience with percutaneous intra-aortic balloon pumping. *Circulation 62 (Suppl I):*123–129, 1980

Takaro T, Hultgren HN, Lipton MJ, et al: The Virginia Cooperative Randomized Study of Surgery for Coronary Arterial Occlusive Disease. II. Subgroup with significant left main lesions. *Circulation 54 (Suppl III):*107–117, 1976

Thadani U, Fung HL, Darke AC, et al: Oral isosorbide dinitrate in the treatment of angina pectoris: dose response relationship and duration of action during acute therapy. *Circulation 62:*491–502, 1980

Williams DO, Amsterdam EA, Mason DT: Hemodynamic effects of nitroglycerin in acute myocardial infarction: Decrease in ventricular preload at the expense of cardiac output. *Circulation 51:*421–427, 1975

Wyman MG, Hammersmith L: Comprehensive treatment plan for the prevention of primary ventricular fibrillation in acute myocardial infarction. *Am J Cardiol 33:*661–667, 1974

CHAPTER 7

Cardiology: Heart Failure

ROBERT ARNOLD JOHNSON, M.D.
DANIEL CHIA-SEN LEE, M.D.

DEFINITION AND CAUSES OF HEART FAILURE

Confusion regarding use of the term "heart failure" is a persistent and common problem in medical practice. Introductory courses for medical students and textbooks of cardiovascular medicine usually offer the following definition: heart failure is an inability of the heart to supply blood in an amount adequate for the metabolic needs of the tissues. Although this definition may seem attractive at first, it loses its appeal when it becomes necessary to decide whether an individual patient does or does not have heart failure. How is the clinician to recognize a disparity between blood supply and the metabolic needs of the tissues? It is cumbersome and often impractical to measure the blood supply (cardiac output), to say nothing of the "metabolic needs." It is insufficient to reply that the disparity between supply and needs is measured by a pathologic increase in the systemic arterial-mixed venous oxygen content difference, because the term heart failure may be applied in certain circumstances when the systemic arterial-mixed venous oxygen content difference is actually decreased rather than increased (for example, thyrotoxicosis, systemic arteriovenous fistula, Paget's disease, or anemia).

An alternative approach is suggested by examination of the behavior of clinicians themselves, who use the term most consistently when referring to a syndrome comprising a constellation of clinical findings determined by an increase in the mean pressure of one or both atria. Thus, *left heart failure (LHF)* may be defined as an abnormal increase in the mean left atrial pressure (above 12 mm Hg), *right heart failure (RHF)* as an abnormal increase in mean right atrial pressure (above 5–6 mm Hg or, expressed in more familiar terms, 7–8 cm H$_2$O), and *combined* or *bi-sided heart failure*

(BHF) as abnormal elevations of both atrial pressures. The manifestations of LHF are those of pulmonary venous congestion, and the manifestations of RHF are those of systemic venous congestion.

Several observations concerning these definitions are noteworthy. First, no statement is made about the contractile state of the ventricular myocardium by the term left heart failure or right heart failure. Having made a diagnosis of heart failure, the clinician must determine the contributions of myocardial and nonmyocardial factors to the elevation of atrial pressure. Heart failure, as defined here, does not necessarily imply that ventricular myocardial performance is impaired. For example, in patients with mitral stenosis, obstruction of the mitral valve results in elevation of left atrial pressure; this may be appropriately termed heart failure, yet left ventricular function is usually normal. Second, no statement is made regarding the cardiac output, which may be high, normal, or low, depending on the cause of heart failure. Third, this view of heart failure encourages the clinician from the outset to consider separately those therapeutic maneuvers aimed at treating the consequences of elevated atrial pressure and those aimed at treating the underlying cause.

The causes of LHF or BHF may be grouped into four categories on the basis of left ventricular diastolic pressure (LVDP), left ventricular diastolic volume (LVDV), and left ventricular ejection fraction (LVEF), as shown in Table 7.1. The causes of isolated RHF may be grouped analogously.

Causes of Left Heart Failure

In *isolated left atrial overload*, LVDP and LVDV are normal or diminished, and LVEF is normal or nearly normal. The causes are listed in Table 7.2.

Table 7.1.
Categories of left- and bi-sided heart failure (LHF and BHF).

	LVDP	LVDV	LVEF
Isolated left atrial overload	normal, ↓	normal, ↓	>0.40
Depressed left ventricular compliance	↑	normal, ↓	>0.40
Left ventricular volume overload	↑	↑	>0.40
Depressed LVEF	↑	↑	<0.40

Table 7.2.
Causes of isolated left atrial overload.

Mitral valve stenosis
    Rheumatic
    Congenital
    Infective endocarditis
    Libman-Sacks endocarditis
    Atrial myxoma
    Left atrial thrombus
Metastatic tumor to left atrium
Cor triatriatum
Mitral regurgitation (some cases)
Tachycardias
Ventriculoatrial conduction

Rheumatic mitral stenosis is the prototype, but it is not always a discrete example. The LVEF is 0.40 or less in approximately 15% of patients with mitral stenosis, for instance; the LVDP and LVDV may be elevated in such cases. In addition, we sometimes see patients with mitral stenosis whose LVEF exceeds 0.40 and whose LVDV is normal, but whose LVDP is elevated. These patients have abnormal left ventricular compliance in addition to mitral stenosis; they have not been described clearly in the literature. Patients with mitral stenosis, therefore, may have LHF from more than one category listed in Table 7.1, and the same is true of some patients with other cardiac disorders. Even so, in most patients, the cardiac defect causing heart failure does so by only one of these general mechanisms, and in those in whom more than one is involved, one usually predominates. In addition, when more than one general mechanism is involved, analysis of LHF in terms of category helps define how much improvement is likely if a proposed operation or treatment affects only one of the responsible mechanisms.

The category of *depressed left ventricular compliance* is characterized by an elevated LVDP despite a normal or nearly normal LVDV and LVEF. The causes are listed in Table 7.3. Many other causes of depressed left ventricular compliance exist, but those listed are the ones that may be severe enough to produce LHF. (The term left ventricular compliance is used here in the general sense of volume compliance [end-diastolic pressure-volume relationship], not in the more specific

Table 7.3.
Causes of left heart failure resulting from depressed left ventricular compliance.

Isolated or relatively isolated left ventricular abnormality
    Hypertrophic cardiomyopathy, including the hypertension-induced form (which may be concentric)
    Left ventricular hypertrophy from valvular, subvalvular, or supravalvular aortic stenosis or coarctation of the aorta
    Endomyocardial disease (some cases)
    Hypoplastic left heart syndrome

Biventricular abnormality
    Pericardial tamponade
    Constrictive pericarditis
    Effusive-constrictive pericarditis
    Mediastinal hematoma or tumor
    Nonhypertrophic nondilated cardiomyopathy
        Amyloid heart disease
        Endomyocardial disease (some cases)
        Metastatic tumor

sense of left ventricular muscle compliance.) Some patients in whom LHF results from valvular aortic stenosis, for example, are in this category. In these patients, left ventricular hypertrophy exists in sufficient degree to maintain a normal or nearly normal LVEF, and hence a normal or nearly normal LVDV, but the cost is enough hypertrophy-induced reduction in ventricular compliance to produce an elevated LVDP.

The causes of *left ventricular volume overload* are listed in Table 7.4. In this category, the LVDP and LVDV are both increased, but the LVEF exceeds 0.40. Patients with aortic regurgitation provide typical examples, as do patients in whom heart failure results from a systemic arteriovenous fistula. To categorize these diseases in this way does not mean that their continued presence does not cause some degree of myocardial disease. It simply means that the physician may deduce from the coexistence of a substantially increased LVDV and an LVEF exceeding 0.40 that the predominant mechanism of LHF or BHF is the volume load itself: a treatment that relieves the volume load will relieve the heart failure, even if the LVEF remains moderately depressed (0.40–0.60).

Table 7.5 lists the causes of a substantially *depressed LVEF*. The LVEF can be severely reduced by either of two means: a disease that directly affects the left ventricular myocardium, or a disease that greatly magnifies left ventricular afterload. In the latter case (valvular aortic stenosis, for example), relief of the high afterload causes the LVEF to rise to a value exceeding 0.40. If permanent left ventricular disease results from the high-afterload state, it is seldom severe enough to produce an LVEF of less than 0.40 once the high afterload is eliminated. Cardiac diseases may coexist, of course. Severe aortic stenosis and a disease directly affecting the left ventricular myocardium, such as myocardial infarction or dilated cardiomyopathy, may be present in the same patient, and the clinician cannot know from the depressed LVEF which disease is its cause. A new technique for distinguishing the effect of impaired contractility from that of high afterload, based on end-systolic force-volume relations, may provide a solution for this dilemma (Gunther and Grossman, 1979). Diseases that cause an LVEF of less than 0.40 as a consequence of ventricular impairment are more common than those that have their effect as a consequence of high afterload.

Special Problem of Heart Failure in Coronary Artery Disease

It has become clear in recent years that coronary artery disease may cause heart failure by several different mechanisms and that distinction among these may have important therapeutic implications.

Table 7.4.
Causes of left ventricular volume overload.

Aortic regurgitation (most cases)
Mitral regurgitation (most cases)[a]
Transposition of the great arteries
Left-to-right shunt at the great-arterial or ventricular level
Systemic high-output states[b]
    Anemia
    Systemic arteriovenous fistula
    Beriberi
    Hydatiform mole
    Hepatic hemangiomatosis
    Renal cell carcinoma
    Paget's disease of bone
    Carcinoid syndrome

[a] Many patients exist in whom the LVEF is <0.40, but most of these patients may have a dilated cardiomyopathy syndrome.

[b] Of the many causes of elevated cardiac output, these are the ones that are in themselves known to be capable of producing LHF or BHF.

Table 7.5.
Causes of a substantially depressed LVEF.

Disease of the left ventricular myocardium
    Cardiomyopathy syndrome resulting from atherosclerotic coronary artery disease (multiple infarctions)
    Large, single myocardial infarction
        Remote (left ventricular aneurysm)
        Acute
    Dilated cardiomyopathy without atherosclerotic coronary artery disease
        Idiopathic
        Alcoholic
        Acute myocarditis
        Peripartum
        Hypophosphatemia
        Drugs (e.g., phenothiazines and adriamycin)
        Other[a]
    Chronic aortic regurgitation (some cases)
    Chronic mitral regurgitation (some cases, especially if examined after mitral valve replacement)

Extreme elevation of left ventricular afterload
    Valvular aortic stenosis (some cases)
    Coarctation of the aorta (severe, in infancy)
    Severe systemic hypertension

[a] At least 57 others causes of dilated cardiomyopathy, (including the various causes of acute myocarditis) exist in addition to those listed. These are enumerated and referenced in Table 25.5 of Johnson RA, Palacios I. Dilated cardiomyopathy and nonhypertrophic nondilated cardiomyopathy. In: Johnson RA, Haber E, Austen WG, (Eds). The Practice of Cardiology. Boston: Little Brown. 1980:637–640.

Acute myocardial infarction is a common cause of acute LHF. The infarct may be large enough to cause significant depression of the overall LVEF, both by virtue of the amount of ventricular mass removed from contraction and by its outward bulging (dyskinesis) during systole. A corollary of this is that the probability of heart failure in a first myocardial infarction depends on the size of the infarct. Anterior myocardial infarctions are usually larger than inferior myocardial infarctions— hence the clinical observation that it is common for heart failure to complicate an anterior myocardial infarction, but that it is uncommon for heart failure to complicate an inferior myocardial infarction unless there are associated mechanical complications, unrecognized old infarcts, concomitant areas of ischemia, or right ventricular infarction. In addition to the depressed ejection fraction produced by acute infarction, there may be a mechanical complication with ensuing heart failure. These consist of rupture of the ventricular septum, leading to a left-to-right shunt, and infarction or rupture of a papillary muscle, causing mitral regurgitation.

Cardiomyopathy syndrome due to coronary artery disease occurs because of multiple and widespread abnormalities of left ventricular wall motion produced by multiple infarctions. These patients may have chronic heart failure punctuated by acute exacerbations that are produced by a precipitating factor (see page 121) or by new infarction or ischemia, and may constitute the majority of patients in whom chronic heart failure results from coronary artery disease. If the patient is diabetic, neither infarction nor other manifestations of coronary artery disease are necessarily apparent in the presence of the cardiomyopathy syndrome. However, in an elderly and nondiabetic population, the syndrome seldom exists in patients who do not have manifestations of coronary artery disease (Boucher et al.). A similar clinical presentation may be produced by a large, isolated *ventricular aneurysm* (or scar), with the important difference that aneurysms, existing in a single and discrete location, are potentially resectable. Resection can ameliorate heart failure by augmenting the LVEF and reducing the LVDV and wall stress. Without performing contrast left ventriculography, the physician may find it difficult to distinguish between a ventricular aneurysm and cardiomyopathy syndrome. Occasionally, a *ventricular septal defect* or severe *mitral regurgitation*, as a consequence of myocardial infarction, is a relatively isolated cause of chronic LHF. These are also important to identify as lesions potentially correctable by operation. Unfortunately, mitral regurgitation in coronary disease is more commonly associated with severe depression of the LVEF—a much less optimistic situation from a surgical standpoint.

Acute LHF may occasionally be a predominant clinical manifestation of *transient ischemia* with or without accompanying angina. In most patients, this is probably due to involvement of a large amount of jeopardized myocardium in the ischemic process, although there may be rare cases of severe, transient mitral regurgitation secondary to ischemia of a papillary muscle. The role of surgical revascularization in these patients may be much greater than in patients in whom heart failure complicates multiple infarctions.

Causes of Right Heart Failure

These may be organized similarly to the causes of LHF (Table 7.6). The right ventricle behaves somewhat differently from the left ventricle in that

Table 7.6.
Causes of right heart failure (RHF).

Isolated right atrial overload
  Tricuspid stenosis
  Right atrial myxoma
  Rapid supraventricular arrhythmia

Depressed right ventricular compliance
  Pericardial tamponade
  Constrictive pericarditis
  Effusive-constrictive pericarditis
  Mediastinal hematoma or tumor
  Nonhypertrophic nondilated cardiomyopathy (Table 7.3)

Right ventricular volume overload
  Tricuspid regurgitation
  Pulmonary regurgitation
  Left-to-right shunt at atrial level (late stage)
  High-output states (Table 7.4)

Depressed right ventricular ejection fraction resulting from disease of right ventricular myocardium
  Cardiomyopathies
  Right ventricular infarction
  Ebstein's anomaly

Depressed right ventricular ejection fraction resulting from elevated right ventricular afterload
  Increased pulmonary vascular resistance secondary to:
    Left heart failure
    Pulmonary emboli
    Intrinsic lung disease
    Chronic obstructive airways disease with carbon dioxide retention and hypoxemia
    Primary pulmonary vascular disease
  Acute right ventricular outflow tract obstruction

pressure loads are tolerated poorly, except in congenital lesions in which marked right ventricular hypertrophy has time to develop. Elevations of pulmonary vascular resistance in the adult commonly result in RHF, where a comparable change in systemic vascular resistance would not result in LHF. The most common reason for elevated pulmonary vascular resistance in the adult is elevation of left atrial pressure—thus the clinical maxim, "The most common cause of right heart failure is left heart failure." However, only some patients with LHF have elevated pulmonary vascular resistance, so LHF is commonly isolated. A passive increase in mean pulmonary arterial pressure caused by a rise in left atrial pressure should be distinguished from a rise in pulmonary vascular resistance caused by a rise in left atrial pressure. The latter, apparently a reactive phenomenon in only some patients, results in a disproportionate rise in pulmonary arterial pressure, and commonly results in RHF. The former usually does not cause RHF unless there is associated impairment of right ventricular function or a volume load.

Elevated right atrial pressures result in systemic venous congestion, defined clinically by an elevated jugular venous pressure. Obstruction of the superior vena cava, which is most commonly caused by tumor or expanding aortic aneurysm, also results in jugular venous distention and must be differentiated from RHF. Evaluation of the jugular veins is sometimes difficult. The top of the venous column, which is usually best seen in the external jugular veins, must be visualized and then compared with the level of the right atrium, which is estimated by assuming the sternal angle to lie 5 cm above the right atrium in the supine or semirecumbent patient. The position of the patient's head and torso must be adjusted so that the top of the venous column is visible. In some patients, an unusual neck configuration or obesity makes identification of the jugular veins difficult or impossible; in other patients, the configuration of the sternum and thoracic cage may make the assumed relation between sternal angle and right atrium questionable. In such instances, direct measurement of the right atrial or central venous pressure may be necessary before a diagnosis of RHF is confirmed or excluded.

Precipitating Factors of Heart Failure

In many of the diseases listed in Tables 7.2–7.6, the patient's condition is often "compensated," that is, atrial pressures are normal or only mildly elevated, until a precipitating event results in a rise in one or both atrial pressures. These events (Table 7.7) do not in themselves usually cause heart failure, but when superimposed on underlying heart disease, they may "tip the scales." Special mention should be made of pulmonary emboli, which, in addition to being a primary cause of isolated RHF when they are massive or multiple, may precipitate LHF in patients who have underlying left heart disease. The mechanism is uncertain, but possibly involves the increased cardiac output due to the hypoxemia caused by pulmonary embolism.

In addition to the precipitating factors listed in Table 7.7, there are two conditions that may be severe enough in themselves to cause heart failure or that may do so when superimposed on other heart disease; these are *infective endocarditis*, which may be surprisingly occult, especially in the el-

Table 7.7.
Precipitating factors of heart failure.

States resulting in increased cardiac output:
  Pregnancy
  Hypoxia
  Hepatic disease
  Infection
  Anemia
  Dietary salt excess
  Fluid overload
  Fever
  Renal failure
  Heat
  Acute abdominal disease (e.g., intestinal infarction, pancreatitis)
  Acute minor pulmonary thromboembolism
  Thyrotoxicosis
  Emotional stress
  Obesity
  Hyperosmolality of serum (combined with renal failure)
  Indomethacin or phenylbutazone administration
  Other high-output states (Table 7.4)
Negative inotropic agents such as β-adrenergic blockers, calcium antagonists, and disopyramide
Tachyarrhythmia
Bradyarrhythmia
Poorly controlled hypertension
Poor compliance with medical regimen

derly, and *ruptured chordae tendineae* with varying degrees of mitral regurgitation.

MANIFESTATIONS AND DIAGNOSIS OF LEFT HEART FAILURE

The manifestations of LHF may be divided into two categories—those secondary to elevated left atrial pressure and those related to the specific underlying cause. Most of the following discussion will be concerned with the former.

Changes in Pulmonary Function

The consequences of increased left atrial pressure are respiratory. The degree to which pulmonary physiology is altered depends on the degree and chronicity of the left atrial pressure elevation. Chronicity is a factor because of the ability of the pulmonary interstitial lymphatic system to increase lymphatic drainage with time, thus preventing alveolar pulmonary edema at relatively high left atrial pressures. Pulmonary capillary hydrostatic pressure, which is primarily determined by left atrial pressure, and capillary oncotic pressure have long been considered the major forces involved in the formation of pulmonary edema. It is now known, however, that pulmonary interstitial hydrostatic pressure, interstitial oncotic pressure, the capacity of interstitial lymphatics, alveolar pressure, and alveolar surface tension may all play a role in determining the transfer of fluid from pulmonary capillaries to interstitial and alveolar spaces. The interaction of these forces has been reviewed by Robin et al. (1973). Despite the many factors involved, the relationship of the clinical manifestations of LHF to the absolute elevation of left atrial pressure is surprisingly consistent. Thus, dyspnea usually may be correlated with a left atrial pressure more than 20 mm Hg, and "radiologic" interstitial edema may be correlated with a left atrial pressure of 20–35 mm Hg; radiologic alveolar edema usually does not develop until left atrial pressure exceeds 30 mm Hg.

The symptoms of LHF are correlated with characteristic abnormalities in whole lung physiology. The pressure-volume relationship of the lung shifts in the direction of increasing lung stiffness, thereby increasing the work of breathing; this is probably the major factor in the subjective sensation of dyspnea. A second cause of ventilatory impairment in many patients is increased airway resistance, which is presumably due to bronchial edema and venous vascular congestion; when this is severe, wheezing may result.

Gas exchange may be altered in three ways. First, interstitial edema causes ventilation-perfusion mismatching; this results in a widened alveolar-arterial oxygen tension difference and hypoxemia (decreased arterial Po_2) when the patient is breathing room air or relatively low concentrations of oxygen. The widened alveolar-arterial oxygen tension difference and hypoxemia disappear when the fraction of oxygen in inspired gas approaches 1.0 ($Fio_2 = 1.0$). Second, alveolar edema is associated with intrapulmonary right-to-left shunting, defined as an alveolar-arterial oxygen tension difference that persists when the Fio_2 equals 1.0. Third, if the work of breathing is severely increased, alveolar hypoventilation may occur. Alveolar hypoventilation is defined as an increase in arterial Pco_2 accompanied by hypoxemia. It is particularly likely to develop if the patient becomes fatigued or obtunded.

Radiologic Manifestations

It is appropriate to discuss the chest x-ray findings in LHF before discussing other clinical features, because the plain film of the chest is the central and most important tool in the diagnosis of LHF. The diagnosis of LHF is primarily a radiologic diagnosis. Normally, in the upright position, pulmonary blood flow is greater to the lung bases than to the lung apices. This can be seen on the plain chest film by comparing the caliber of the vessels, particularly the veins, of the lower lung zones with the caliber of the vessels of the upper lung zones. In the early 1960s, Simon reported that patients with elevated left atrial pressure have *redistribution of pulmonary blood flow to the upper zones*, so the caliber of upper zone vessels becomes equal to, or greater than, the caliber of lower zone vessels; this is true regardless of the cause of left atrial pressure elevation. Redistribution occurs because interstitial edema is more severe in lower lung fields as a result of the combined effects of gravity and elevated mean left atrial pressure; the microvasculature is consequently compressed, and blood flow is shunted upward. It is important to realize that radiologic interstitial and alveolar edema are nonspecific and occur in a wide variety of circumstances. The specific hallmark of LHF is upper zone flow redistribution (Figs. 7.1–7.5).

There are at least three situations in which caution need be exercised in interpreting upper zone flow redistribution. First, some patients with emphysema have pulmonary parenchymal loss that is much greater in the lower zones. Consequently, the pulmonary vascular resistance is higher in the lower zones and blood flow to the apices increases, thus simulating the pattern of LHF. The clue that emphysema, rather than LHF, may be the cause of flow redistribution consists of the concomitant presence of hyperinflation, especially depressed diaphragms, and basilar rarefaction. In the absence of these stigmata, upper zone flow redistribution can usually be attributed to LHF, even if the patient also has chronic obstructive airways disease. Second, chest films taken with the patient supine may not reveal flow redistribution, since its occurrence depends on the effect of gravity on the upright lung. Finally, there may be chronic loss of vascular definition by interstitial scarring, making it difficult to interpret vessel size. This is particularly likely to occur in elderly patients, and also occurs in several diseases producing interstitial pulmonary fibrosis.

As mentioned previously, *interstitial pulmonary edema* occurs when the left atrial pressure is elevated above 20 mm Hg. The radiologic pattern of interstitial edema consists of varying combinations of septal, perivascular, and subpleural edema. Septal edema is manifested by Kerley A or B lines. Kerley A lines, which represent edematous interlobular septa in the upper lung fields, are straight, nonbranching lines 3–10 cm long that often run diagonally toward the hilus (Figs. 7.2 and 7.4). Kerley B lines (Figs. 7.1 and 7.3) are shorter, nonbranching lines seen at the periphery of the lower lung fields, extending to and perpendicular

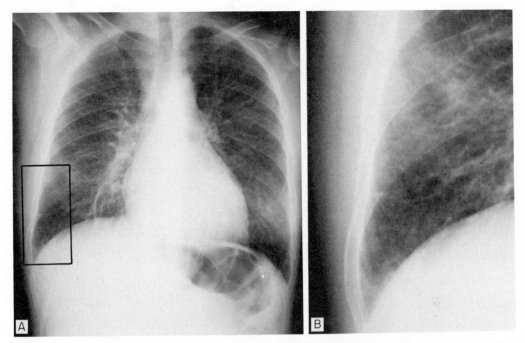

Figure 7.1. **(A)** Prominence of upper zone vessels and loss of vascular definition in lower zone vessels (flow redistribution) in 51-year-old patient with myocardial infarction. There are also Kerley B lines at periphery of bases. **(B)** Enlargement of area outlined in **(A).**

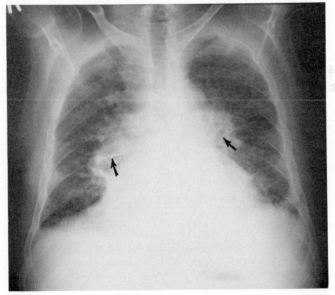

Figure 7.2. Upper zone blood flow redistribution and marked interstitial edema. Note complete loss of vascular definition in lower zones. Blurring of central vascular definition gives impression of hilar enlargement. Kerley A lines are present (*arrows*). There is peripheral haze in lower and midpulmonary zones.

to the pleural surface. Another pattern of interstitial edema, peripheral haze, may also represent septal edema; it may consist of short, crisscross lines in the basilar regions (Kerley C lines), or it may have a peripheral honeycomb or reticular appearance (Figs. 7.2 and 7.3). Perivascular edema is manifested both as central (hilar) haze and as loss of definition of lower zone vessels (Figs. 7.1

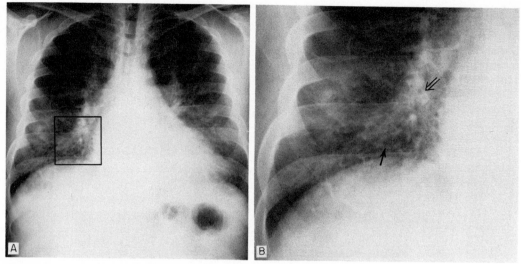

Figure 7.3. **(A)** Upper zone flow redistribution and interstitial edema in 44-year-old man with multiple myocardial infarcts. **(B)** Enlargement of area outlined in **(A)**. Note peribronchial "cuffing" (*upper arrow*) with edema and peripheral haze (*lower arrow*). There are also Kerley B lines.

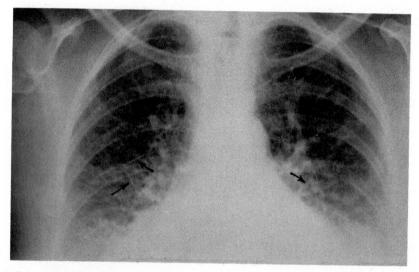

Figure 7.4.   Upper zone flow redistribution and pulmonary edema. Note Kerley A lines (*arrows*).

and 7.2). Hilar haze (loss of definition of central vessels) often results in a general impression of hilar enlargement (Fig. 7.2). Subpleural edema is indicated by a sharp pleural margin associated with poorly defined density extending into the underlying lung. Interstitial edema is also seen in the form of peribronchial "cuffing" when airways are viewed in cross-section on chest films (Figs. 7.3 and 7.5).

Alveolar edema occurs when left atrial pressure is elevated above 30 mm Hg, and is manifested by frank pulmonary opacification. The distribution of edema may be the typical central "batwing" pattern (Fig. 7.5), may be diffuse (Fig. 7.6), or may be asymmetric (even unilateral). Opacification is usually homogeneous, but occasionally resembles miliary densities, nodules, or patchy bronchopneumonia.

The relation of interstitial and alveolar edema to left atrial pressure may be modified by several factors. First, it may be affected by alterations in serum oncotic pressure. At a low serum albumin level, radiologic edema may occur at a relatively low left atrial pressure, and in the extreme, a very low serum albumin level may cause pulmonary edema when the left atrial pressure is in the normal range. Second, a left atrial pressure exceeding 35 mm Hg may be manifested only by interstitial edema if the elevation of left atrial pressure has been long-standing, because of an expanded capacity of the interstitial lymphatic system. Third, there may be a lag of several hours before the appearance of radiologic pulmonary edema when the elevation of left atrial pressure occurs acutely, for example, in acute myocardial infarction. Conversely, when left atrial pressure is acutely lowered with therapy, the chest film may continue to show edema for several hours.

These modifications of the relation of radiologic findings to left atrial pressure should not obscure the central clinical point, however; they are the exceptions that prove the rule. In general, respiratory distress due to LHF is associated with typical radiologic features. If a patient with respira-

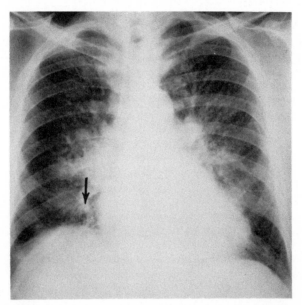

Figure 7.5. Upper zone flow redistribution and alveolar edema in central "batwing" distribution. Note peribronchial "cuffing" (*arrow*).

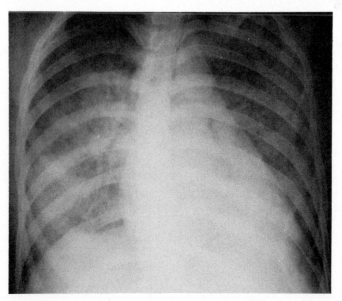

Figure 7.6. Diffuse alveolar edema in patient with mean pulmonary capillary wedge pressure of 40 mm Hg because of ruptured papillary muscle leading to acute mitral regurgitation.

tory distress does not manifest upper zone flow redistribution and interstitial or alveolar edema on a chest film taken near the time of distress, the diagnosis of LHF as the cause of the respiratory distress should be suspect, and another cause of respiratory distress should be sought.

Small *pleural effusions* may be due to isolated LHF, but large pleural effusions due to heart failure are almost always associated with combined RHF and LHF. Isolated RHF is seldom a cause of pleural effusion. Pleural effusion due to heart failure is often bilateral; when unilateral, it usually occurs on the right (the reason for this is unknown). There are useful corollaries of these statements. When only LHF is present (jugular venous pressure less than 7 cm H_2O), a large pleural effusion should not be attributed to heart failure, and another cause should be sought, such as pulmonary infarction. This is also the case when pleural effusion is isolated to the left side of the thorax.

Clinical Syndrome of Left Heart Failure and Acute Pulmonary Edema

Symptoms of LHF are determined by the degree and, to a lesser extent, by the duration of left atrial pressure elevation, and may be viewed as reflecting various points along a spectrum of left atrial pressures ranging from nearly normal to extremely elevated. At one end of the spectrum are patients who are asymptomatic at rest, but who have dyspnea with effort or awakening them at night. When due to LHF, these complaints correspond to left atrial pressures that range from normal to moderately elevated at rest (10–25 mm Hg), but which become substantially elevated (more than 25 mm Hg) with exercise or with mobilization of systemic interstitial fluid from the lower extremities while lying down. In the middle of the spectrum are patients with resting left atrial pressures of 20–30 mm Hg who may complain of dyspnea with recumbency or mild effort or who may have a common complication of chronic LHF, bacterial pneumonia. At the extreme of the spectrum are patients with left atrial pressures of 35 mm Hg or more, whose condition is a medical emergency— the syndrome of acute pulmonary edema.

The clinical characteristics of acute pulmonary edema are among the most dramatic in medicine. It is often difficult for the clinician to contain his or her anxiety at the sight of a terrified patient, sitting bolt upright, refusing to assume even a semirecumbent position, desperate with the anxiety of air hunger, straining every muscle of respiration, and profusely diaphoretic. The pink, frothy fluid spewed from the mouth and nose of some patients with pulmonary edema adds a further awesome note to this scene.

The *history* provides information relevant to the cause of pulmonary edema in almost every case, although it may have to be obtained from family members, since the patient is often too distressed to answer questions. Information may be specific, for example, a history of known valvular disease, a history of severe retrosternal chest pain preceding or accompanying the respiratory distress, or a history suggesting a recent precipitating factor (pneumonia, pulmonary embolus, febrile illness, poor drug compliance, and so on) superimposed on known cardiac disease. In the absence of specific historical clues, general information may be derived from analysis of the mode of onset of acute respiratory distress. When pulmonary edema complicates cardiomyopathy syndrome due to coronary artery disease, other cardiomyopathy syndromes, aortic insufficiency, or rheumatic mitral regurgitation, it is almost always preceded by milder, chronic symptoms of LHF. Pulmonary edema without preceding symptoms suggests ruptured chordae tendineae, acute myocardial infarction, or prolonged ischemia. In a third group, there may be preceding mild dyspnea on effort—seemingly insignificant—until the abrupt occurrence of pulmonary edema. This occurs in mitral stenosis when the pulmonary vascular resistance is normal, especially if precipitated by the new onset of rapid atrial fibrillation; it also occurs in aortic stenosis.

Three pitfalls are to be avoided in interpreting the history. The first is overemphasis on the role of dietary salt "indiscretion" in precipitating pulmonary edema. Although increased sodium ingestion may lead to pulmonary edema as a complication of severe valvular disease, multiple myocardial infarctions, large ventricular aneurysms, or cardiomyopathy, it is often incorrectly assigned a role in the absence of these conditions. As a consequence, more relevant etiologic factors may be overlooked, such as painless myocardial infarction, transient ischemia, transient arrhythmias, or ruptured chordae tendineae. The second pitfall is the assumption that a history generally consistent with coronary artery disease is an adequate explanation for pulmonary edema. This is not the case. LHF may complicate coronary artery disease for a variety of reasons, as discussed previously; attempts should be made to determine which of these is most likely in a given patient. Third, preceding respiratory symptoms of chronic or subacute heart failure and even dyspnea at rest accompanying frank pulmonary edema may occasionally be obscure in elderly patients. These patients are sometimes unable to give an interpretable history themselves, and relatives may tell the clinician only that the patient "just hasn't been doing well" recently, as evidenced by change in mental status, anorexia, insomnia, cough, and decreased activity.

The *physical examination* in acute pulmonary edema is usually dominated by the general appearance of an extremely dyspneic patient with rapid, shallow respirations and a variable degree of central cyanosis. Exceptions are those elderly patients just mentioned, who may not assume the typical upright posture or complain of dyspnea and who are often obtunded, but who usually exhibit rapid, shallow breathing nonetheless. Also, patients with cardiogenic shock—severe LHF associated with extreme reduction in cardiac output—may not appear typically dyspneic because of obtundation.

Except in patients with cardiogenic shock, blood pressure is either normal or high. Elevated blood pressure is commonly associated with acute pulmonary edema, presumably because of outpouring of endogenous catecholamines resulting from respiratory distress; this does not imply an independent hypertensive state, even when the degree of elevation is considerable. On the other hand, when hypertension is severe (diastolic pressure more than 120 mm Hg), it is sometimes difficult to know whether the situation represents malignant hypertension complicated by pulmonary edema or pulmonary edema that has led to hypertension. Examination of the ocular fundi is important in this situation, since the absence of typical funduscopic findings of severe hypertension argues strongly against malignant hypertension. Unfortunately, this is often complicated by morphine-induced miosis. The absence of electrocardiographic indications of left ventricular hypertrophy also argues against a primary hypertensive state.

The cardiac rhythm is usually sinus tachycardia, although frequent exceptions occur because the rhythm is in large part determined by the nature of the underlying heart disease. For example, atrial fibrillation is common in chronic mitral valvular disease, heart failure complicating acute myocardial infarction, and cardiomyopathy, but is rare in isolated aortic valvular disease. Also, a primary rhythm disturbance superimposed on underlying heart disease may have been the precipitating factor for pulmonary edema; such rhythm disturbances include rapid supraventricular arrhythmias, ventricular tachycardia, marked sinus bradycardia with inadequate escape rhythm, and high-grade atrioventricular block.

Examination of the chest often reveals loud inspiratory and expiratory rales diffusely distributed from lung bases to apices, which completely obscure the heart sounds. Rales may be accompanied by severe expiratory wheezing. In less dramatic situations, rales may extend only part way up from the bases and may be only fine, moist crackling sounds in mid and late inspiration. In patients who have had chronic left atrial hypertension, there often is rather severe respiratory distress due to interstitial pulmonary edema when no rales are audible, although there may be wheezing. Also, other causes of severe respiratory distress may produce diffuse rales that may be indistinguishable from the rales of cardiac pulmonary edema (see Differential Diagnosis of Acute Cardiac Pulmonary Edema, pages 134–137). Unwarranted emphasis on either the presence or absence of rales constitutes one of the most common reasons for misdiagnosis of LHF.

Physical signs of pleural effusion may be present if there is coexistent RHF. The jugular venous pressure in acute pulmonary edema also depends on the presence of coexistent RHF, which in turn depends on the specific nature of the underlying heart disease (see Causes of Right Heart Failure, pages 120–121). LHF and pulmonary edema in themselves are commonly unassociated with RHF, the absence of elevated jugular venous pressure does not argue against LHF as a cause of respiratory distress.

The findings on cardiac examination are determined by the nature of the left heart disease. On initial examination, cardiac findings are often completely obscured by respiratory distress, rales, and wheezing. It is important to re-examine the patient frequently as he begins to improve following the institution of therapy. This is true even in the emergency ward, since the specific causes of pulmonary edema that have special therapeutic implications should be recognized as soon as possible so that appropriate management plans may be initiated. The patient should also be examined carefully for possible precipitating factors of pulmonary edema.

The *electrocardiogram* reveals the rhythm abnormalities previously discussed. In addition, it contains important information concerning etiologic diagnosis, such as left ventricular hypertrophy in chronic pressure or volume loads, multiple infarct patterns in cardiomyopathy syndrome due to coronary artery disease, and ST-segment elevations in acute infarction or ventricular aneurysm. Patients with pulmonary edema virtually never have completely normal electrocardiograms. If the patient has sinus rhythm, special attention should be paid to P-wave morphology. Left atrial enlargement, indicated by terminal P-wave negativity in lead V_1 exceeding 0.03 mm·sec (Fig. 7.7),

A

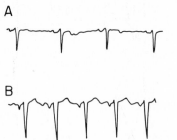

B

Figure 7.7. Comparison of P waves in lead V_1 in **(A)** normal patient and in **(B)** patient with cardiomyopathy with left atrial enlargement. Electrocardiographic left atrial enlargement is determined by terminal P-wave negativity in lead V_1 (exceeding 0.03 mm sec).

is common in patients with elevated left atrial pressure of any cause; its absence should place the diagnosis of acute pulmonary edema in doubt. This electrocardiographic sign seems to depend more on left atrial pressure than on left atrial size, since it may develop rapidly and subsequently diminish in patients in whom left atrial pressure rises acutely and later falls with therapy.

Abnormalities of gas exchange in LHF were discussed previously. Arterial hypoxemia, as measured by arterial blood-gas samples, is present in interstitial pulmonary edema because of ventilation-perfusion mismatching. Arterial Pco_2 is usually modestly decreased because of hyperventilation produced by the decreased Po_2. In alveolar edema, arterial Po_2 is depressed both by ventilation-perfusion mismatching and by intrapulmonary right-to-left shunting; arterial Pco_2 may be mildly decreased or normal. In extremely severe pulmonary edema, particularly in the elderly, fatigued, or obtunded patient, arterial Pco_2 may be elevated—sometimes markedly so, causing severe respiratory acidosis. If the cause of pulmonary edema is also a cause of critically low cardiac output, metabolic (lactic) acidosis may be present. Results of *other laboratory tests* also may be abnormal. Elevations in serum glutamic oxaloacetic transaminase and lactate dehydrogenase of hepatic origin are common in patients with pulmonary edema, especially in the presence of associated low cardiac output or RHF, and they cannot alone be taken as evidence of myocardial infarction. Also, the white blood cell count is often elevated because of demargination of the normally marginated pool of intravascular leukocytes; this does not by itself constitute evidence of infection.

MANAGEMENT OF PULMONARY EDEMA

The number of causes of LHF (Tables 7.2–7.5) may seem imposing at first glance. Fortunately, many of the measures utilized in the treatment of pulmonary edema (Table 7.8) are applicable regardless of cause. These include measures to improve oxygenation, to reduce anxiety, and to decrease venous return, as well as therapy for precipitating factors. Measures taken to improve the LVEF are somewhat more specific in that they apply to causes of LHF that involve depression of the ejection fraction, an abnormal volume load, or a chronic pressure load. Diseases in these categories are the most common causes of acute pulmonary edema seen in the emergency ward: acute myocardial infarction, cardiomyopathy syndrome due to coronary artery disease, cardiomyopathy of the elderly, hypertension, severe aortic stenosis, aortic insufficiency, and mitral regurgitation. From the standpoint of emergency therapy, they may be approached similarly, although there are special problems, particularly if the patient has acute myocardial infarction or aortic stenosis.

Initial Evaluation and Institution of Therapy

On arrival at the emergency ward, the patient should be placed in a "trunk-up" position—a position the patient usually insists on anyway. Humidified *oxygen* should immediately be administered by face mask at a high flow rate. Nasal prongs are inadequate. If there is a possibility that the patient has chronic carbon dioxide retention due to chronic obstructive airways disease, a mask delivering a controlled 24% oxygen should be utilized. Acute carbon dioxide retention due to pulmonary edema does not contraindicate high-flow oxygen therapy so long as the patient is observed carefully for increasing obtundation.

The awesome anxiety of patients with acute pulmonary edema is frequently contagious to inexperienced medical personnel. It is important that a series of steps be instituted quickly, efficiently, and methodically by a team that minimally should consist of an experienced physician and nurse; several of these steps can be accomplished nearly simultaneously.

Vital signs must be measured immediately and at frequent intervals. An adequate intravenous cannula must be secured at the outset; in severely ill patients it should extend into the thorax (with care that it not reach the right ventricle, where it may stimulate ventricular tachycardia). A central line is preferred because it is a means by which intravenous norepinephrine can be safely administered should severe hypotension subsequently develop. In addition, it is important to estimate the right atrial pressure; although this may be done reliably in most patients by inspection of the jug-

Table 7.8.
Therapy for cardiac pulmonary edema.

Useful in Emergency Ward	Useful in Intensive Care Unit and Occasionally in Special Circumstances[a]
Improve oxygenation	
Increase F_{IO_2} by face mask	PEEP
Aminophylline for bronchospasm	
Controlled positive-pressure ventilation	
Treat anxiety	
Morphine	
Decrease left atrial pressure	
Decrease venous return (left ventricular preload)	
Morphine	Dialysis
Nitrates	
Diuretic	
Tourniquets	
Phlebotomy	
Improve LVEF	
Increase contractility	
Digitalis	Other inotropic agents
Morphine	β-adrenergic stimulants
	Calcium
	Amrinone
Decrease left ventricular afterload	
Morphine	Nitroprusside
	α-adrenergic blocking agents
	Nitrates
	Intra-aortic counterpulsation
	Angiotensin converting enzyme inhibitors (e.g., captopril)
Treat precipitating factors (Table 7.7)	

F_{IO_2} = fractional concentration of inspired oxygen; PEEP = positive end-expiratory pressure; LVEF = left ventricular ejection fraction.
[a] If pulmonary capillary wedge pressure and systemic blood pressure are being monitored, or with certain causes of heart failure.

ular veins, obesity or respiratory distress can make visualization of the top of the jugular venous column uncertain, and in these patients the central venous line allows a more accurate measurement. In patients in whom development of hypotension seems unlikely or in whom antecubital veins cannot be cannulated, a shorter cannula in a peripheral vein may suffice. A scalp-vein needle is never adequate because the incidence of cardiac arrest is substantial in patients with pulmonary edema, and these needles are seldom secure under such circumstances. Central intravenous lines usually must be inserted in an antecubital vein in patients with pulmonary edema because the distress and upright posture of the patient make cannulation of the subclavian or jugular vein dangerous. Blood samples for determination of blood urea nitrogen, electrolytes, and a complete blood cell count can be drawn when the intravenous cannula is placed.

A short history should be taken from the patient, a brief examination conducted, and an electrocardiogram recorded. Electrocardiographic monitoring of the heart rhythm should be instituted. If the diagnosis of cardiac pulmonary edema is secure, *morphine* should be administered. A sample should be drawn for arterial blood-gas determinations, and determinations should be repeated at intervals varying with the patient's progress.

Certain *arrhythmias* may require immediate therapy. Frequent ventricular extrasystoles should be suppressed with intravenous lidocaine. Ventricular tachycardia must be quickly converted by either drug therapy or electrical cardioversion. Rapid atrial fibrillation is discussed subsequently.

A portable chest film should be obtained as soon as feasible. If relatives or other persons who know the patient have accompanied the patient to the hospital, a brief account of the patient's history should be taken from them; this is often necessary because patient distress prevents elicitation of a reliable history. It is especially important to obtain an accurate history of recent medications.

Specific Therapy

Table 7.8 lists therapeutic measures for pulmonary edema according to general mechanism. In the left column are listed those measures appropriately used in the emergency ward; in the right column are listed a variety of measures that may be appropriate following transfer to the intensive care unit, if monitoring of pulmonary capillary wedge pressure and on-line measurement of systemic blood pressure are instituted, or if certain specific causes of heart failure are present.

Aside from oxygen, the most efficacious agent in most instances of pulmonary edema is *morphine sulfate*. The prinicpal mechanism of action seems to be an increase in systemic venous capacitance (venodilation), which results in reduction of systemic venous return and consequent lowering of left atrial pressure. Other actions of morphine may also be important: anxiety is reduced; systemic arteriolar resistance is reduced, which reduces left ventricular pressure load, thereby increasing systolic ejection fraction; and a modest inotropic action may occur (indirectly, through stimulation of sympathoadrenal discharge). Morphine should be given intravenously; 5–10 mg is given slowly, and may be repeated at 15-minute intervals. Absorption from subcutaneous and intramuscular injections may be unpredictable in patients with peripheral vasoconstriction; if an initial dose is given by either of these routes and is not effective, it is common to find that delayed absorption concomitant with subsequent intravenous doses produces profound obtundation and respiratory depression. Morphine antagonists (nalorphine or naloxone hydrochloride) should be available. Significant pulmonary disease, hepatic failure, severe kyphoscoliosis, and myxedema are relative contraindications to morphine administration. It must be given cautiously when systolic blood pressure is reduced, since arterial hypotension may be exacerbated, and it must be withheld in the presence of shock. If the diagnosis of cardiac pulmonary edema is certain and if there is severe respiratory distress, morphine should not be withheld while awaiting the results of arterial blood-gas determinations on the theory that an elevated Pco_2 would constitute a contraindication. On the other hand, morphine should not be administered to significantly obtunded patients, except in preparation for rapid endotracheal intubation and controlled ventilation.

The *rapidly acting diuretics*, furosemide and ethacrynic acid, are often administered intravenously in the treatment of pulmonary edema. Furosemide not only induces diuresis but also lowers left atrial pressure by systemic venodilation before diuresis begins. Urinary flow begins to increase 10–30 minutes after intravenous administration of furosemide, and diuresis peaks at 60 minutes. Lesch et al. (1968) have compared intravenous ethacrynic acid with a mercurial diuretic; they found that ethacrynic acid induced more extensive early diuresis, but not a more extensive total diuresis. In their study, no correlation was found between degree of clinical improvement and extent of diuresis; this seems predictable, given the number of different mechanisms by which left atrial pressure may be elevated and given that the most common of these, coronary artery disease, may cause an elevated left atrial pressure by several different mechanisms. The administration of a rapidly acting diuretic is appropriate in most patients with pulmonary edema, although these agents must be given with caution or withheld in patients with hypotension until the pulmonary capillary wedge pressure can be monitored.

In patients with pulmonary edema due to acute myocardial infarction or aortic stenosis, hypotension or shock may develop following overexuberant diuresis with these powerful diuretics. Furosemide is given in an initial dose of 40 mg intravenously; an additional dose of 40–120 mg may be given if the patient is known to have had chronic heart failure, but it should be remembered that large doses have occasionally caused ototoxic reactions, including deafness. The usual intravenous dose of ethacrynic acid is 50 mg. Occasionally, the addition of another diuretic, such as chlorothiazide, 250–500 mg intravenously, facilitates diuresis in patients who do not respond sufficiently to maximal doses of either furosemide or ethacrynic acid.

The diuretic response to furosemide and ethacrynic acid is accompanied by an increase in potassium excretion. It is important that serum electrolyte levels be checked at frequent intervals and that potassium replacement be instituted promptly; this is particularly true if hypokalemia due to previous diuretic therapy exists at the outset. Hypokalemia may induce ventricular tachyarrhythmias and occasionally atrioventricular block. The likelihood of these rhythm disturbances is further increased by the coexistence of digitalis administration and hypokalemia, but it should be emphasized that hypokalemia may cause arrhythmias even in the absence of digitalis. This is especially so in patients with pulmonary edema, because other factors related to production of ventricular arrhythmias are often present: hypoxia, acidosis, and high levels of endogenous catecholamines. If the cause of pulmonary edema is myocardial disease or coronary artery disease or if the cardiac output is depressed, the probability of ventricular arrhythmias is increased further. Hypokalemia must also be avoided in patients with severe hepatic disease, since it may precipitate hepatic encephalopathy. Furosemide and ethacrynic acid may produce severe hyperuricemia, especially when repeated intravenous doses are given for several days, and gout may result. Hyponatremia may also occur, but is usually a consequence of large-dose diuretic therapy in patients with chronic heart failure associated with low cardiac output.

Digitalis has a secondary role in the treatment of most patients with acute pulmonary edema. It is unclear whether digitalis benefits patients with LHF due to acute myocardial infarction; reported studies are conflicting. Reasoning from the standpoint of known determinants of myocardial oxygen consumption (state of contractility, wall tension, and heart rate) also proves inconclusive: on the one hand, the inotropic effect of digitalis tends to increase myocardial oxygen consumption, thus increasing the extent of ischemia or infarction; on the other hand, if the inotropic effect were sufficient to reduce left ventricular chamber radius enough to lower wall tension (wall tension is related to chamber radius by the law of Laplace: tension = pressure × radius), the overall effect might be reduction in extent of ischemia or infarction. Thus, ambivalence regarding the use of digitalis in acute myocardial infarction is understandable. If digitalis is used, loading and maintenance doses should probably be somewhat smaller than usual, since these patients may be particularly susceptible to digitalis-related arrhythmias.

Digitalis has been of uncertain efficacy in patients with LHF complicating chronically depressed left ventricular performance due to cardiomyopathy or to cardiomyopathy syndrome caused by coronary artery disease. In a study of acute digitalization in this group of patients, Cohn et al. (1975) were unable to demonstrate hemodynamic benefit. However, a recent study at the Massachusetts General Hospital demonstrated a sustained beneficial clinical response to digoxin in a subset of outpatients with heart failure and sinus rhythm. The responders were characterized by more severe and more chronic heart failure, greater depression of the LVEF, greater left ventricular dilation, and the uniform presence of an audible third heart sound (Lee et al.). The usefulness of the third heart sound as a predictor of response to digoxin remains to be corroborated.

Digitalis has not been found to be of benefit in patients with mitral stenosis and sinus rhythm. In contrast, it may be lifesaving in patients with mitral stenosis and pulmonary edema that has been precipitated by rapid atrial fibrillation. Left atrial pressure rises rapidly as a consequence of increasing heart rate in mitral stenosis; in such patients, digitalis is administered not because of its inotropic property but because of its ability to slow atrioventricular conduction and thereby limit the ventricular response to atrial fibrillation. Rapid atrial fibrillation may precipitate pulmonary edema in other types of heart disease as well, and constitutes a strong indication for use of digitalis in the emergency ward, although in some circumstances the arrhythmia is best treated with immediate cardioversion. Clinical observation suggests that digitalis is also beneficial in heart failure due to congenital or acquired defects that cause a left ventricular volume or pressure load. This is most striking in infants with ventricular septal defect or patent ductus arteriosus, but also seems true (although less dramatically so) of patients with aortic or mitral regurgitation, coarctation of the aorta, aortic stenosis, and systemic hypertension. In asymmetric septal hypertrophy with outflow tract obstruction (idiopathic hypertrophic subaortic stenosis), however, left atrial pressure may actually rise with digitalization, because increased contractility leads to more severe outflow obstruction in this disease.

In the emergency treatment of patients with acute pulmonary edema, digoxin is the digitalis preparation of choice. The onset of action following intravenous administration occurs at 15–30 minutes, and the peak effect occurs at 1½–5 hours. Although intravenous ouabain has a more rapid onset of action and might be theoretically preferable in treating rapid atrial fibrillation, this advantage is offset by the increased familiarity of most clinicians with digoxin. Familiarity with the drug preparation is particularly important in the use of digitalis because the ratio of toxic to therapeutic levels is low. Furthermore, the physician selecting the preparation in the emergency ward must consider whether the physician assuming responsibility for the subsequent care of the patient is familiar with the preparation employed, since the latter must supervise the transition from intravenous to oral dosage.

Rapid atrial fibrillation in a patient not previously taking digitalis is treated with an initial intravenous digoxin dose of 0.75 mg. Subsequently, incremental intravenous doses of 0.25 mg are administered every 45–60 minutes until the ventricular rate begins to slow; this is followed by 0.125-mg increments at 2- or 5-hour intervals until the desired heart rate is achieved. If the patient had been previously taking a maintenance dose of digitalis, an initial intravenous digoxin dose of 0.25 mg is given, and this dose is repeated at 45- to 60-minute intervals until the ventricular rate begins to decrease. The rate of ventricular response to atrial fibrillation can be utilized as an index of adequacy of digoxin dosage in most patients. However, caution must be exercised in patients with accelerated atrioventricular conduction associated with shock, infection, or fever, in which case repeated increments of digoxin may eventually result in "digitoxic" arrhythmias before the ventricular response to atrial fibrillation is controlled. This is more commonly a problem in treating a rapid ventricular rate due to atrial flutter than in treating a rapid ventricular rate due to atrial fibrillation. When digitalis toxicity is suspected, but further slowing of the ventricular response is needed, either propranolol hydrochloride or verapamil, a calcium antagonist introduced recently for intravenous use, can be useful in producing further atrioventricular block. However, the known negative inotropic effect of propranolol and a potentially similar effect of verapamil limit their use to patients who do not have severe depression of LVEF.

In undigitalized patients with pulmonary edema and sinus rhythm, the initial intravenous digoxin dose is 0.5 mg; the remainder of the loading dose, for a total of 0.75–1.0 mg, is spread over the first 24 hours. The half-life of digoxin in patients with normal renal function is 36 hours; it is extended if the glomerular filtration rate is reduced. Considerations of the half-life, however, lead to alterations in the maintenance dose, not to alterations in the initial dose in the emergency ward, unless the patient was previously taking digitalis. Patients in sinus rhythm who have been receiving a maintenance dose of digitalis should not be treated with additional digoxin in the emergency ward unless there is evidence that the maintenance dose had been inadequate; the development of pulmonary edema in itself does not constitute such evidence. The inotropic effect of digitalis is proportional to the serum level (more directly, to the myocardial tissue level). Digoxin should not be "pushed" with the misconception that there is a threshold "digitalizing dose" below which contractility will not increase; if inotropic benefit is to be achieved at all, it may be seen to some degree even with low doses.

Increased peripheral vascular resistance has been seen in the clinical setting with both intravenous ouabain and digoxin, and untoward rises in arterial blood pressure may result. Consequently, it is probably best to administer intravenous digoxin slowly over several minutes rather than as a bolus injection. Emergency physicians should be familiar with the arrhythmias that may occur as a consequence of digitalis toxicity (see Table 7.12). The most common extracardiac toxic manifestations of digoxin therapy seen in the emergency ward are nausea and vomiting. Rarely, digitalis overdose has caused acute hyperkalemia (see Digitalis Toxicity, page 141).

In addition to morphine and diuretics, there are *other measures to reduce venous return* (Table 7.8). Tourniquets may be placed on three extremities at a time and rotated every 15–20 minutes; they should be tightened sufficiently to occlude venous, but not arterial, flow. Devices that automatically inflate and deflate blood pressure cuffs placed on the extremities are now widely employed instead of tourniquets. Cuffs should be inflated to a level lower than arterial pressure but higher than venous pressure. Although venous occlusive devices are a time-honored therapy for acute pulmonary edema, little evidence supports their efficacy. Habak et al. (1974) were unable to demonstrate significant lowering of pulmonary capillary wedge pressure with inflated cuffs, but in none of their patients was the pulmonary capillary wedge pressure at pulmonary edema levels. Inflated cuffs or tourniquets should be used with caution or withheld if the patient has severe peripheral arterial occlusive disease.

If pulmonary edema fails to subside within 20–30 minutes of the institution of therapy, a favorable response, which is occasionally dramatic, is sometimes brought about by withdrawal of 100–500 cc of blood by phlebotomy. If the skin is carefully prepared and sterile collection systems are used, the blood withdrawn may later be given back in the form of packed red blood cells. As with diuretics, phlebotomy or tourniquets must be used cautiously when pulmonary edema has developed in the presence of a normal blood volume, that is, when it has not been preceded by chronic heart failure. This is most common in patients with acute myocardial infarction and in some patients with aortic stenosis. Neither tourniquets nor phlebotomy should be used if the patient is hypotensive.

Intravenous, sublingual, and cutaneous nitrates (nitroprusside, nitroglycerin, nitroglycerin ointment, and isosorbide dinitrate) lower venous return and have been used to treat heart failure. Initial experience with the use of sublingual nitroglycerin in patients with acute pulmonary edema suggests that one or two 0.3-mg tablets seldom have any effect (Bussman and Schupp, 1978). Administration of 0.3 mg, blood pressure measurement 5 minutes later, administration of 0.6 mg, another blood pressure measurement in 5 minutes, and subsequent doses of 0.6 mg every 10 minutes until improvement occurs or until the systolic blood pressure reaches 100–110 mm Hg is a regimen more likely to be of benefit. Nitrates in any form should not be given if the initial systolic blood pressure is less than 100 mm Hg. Regardless of the initial systolic blood pressure, intravenous nitrates are best reserved for use in the intensive care unit after institution of on-line monitoring of at least the systemic arterial pressure. Because of a rapid venodilating effect, nitrates should be used even more cautiously in diseases such as critical aortic stenosis, in which maintenance of adequate stroke volume depends on a high left ventricular filling pressure. If nitrate-induced hypotension (systolic pressure less than 90 mm Hg) occurs, it can usually be reversed by leg elevation and cautious infusion of phenylephrine, 10–100 $\mu g/min$, through a central intravenous line. Patients with intractable heart failure may also be treated in the intensive care unit with reduction of blood volume by dialysis.

Treatment to *improve the LVEF by improving contractility* primarily consists in administration of digitalis. Other inotropic agents (dopamine, epinephrine, norepinephrine, isoproterenol, calcium, and possibly amrinone) are reserved for patients with LHF associated with significant hypotension and shock. Reservations concerning digitalis in patients with acute myocardial infarction, which are based on a potential increase in infarct size, apply to an even larger extent to these more powerful inotropic agents. Occasionally, patients with hypotension associated with valvular disease, especially aortic stenosis, may require support with one or more of these drugs in the emergency ward so that emergency catheterization and valve replacement can then be performed. Currently, dopamine is probably the best drug for this purpose because increased contractility is combined with maintenance of total peripheral vascular resistance, while visceral (including renal) blood flow is preserved or increased.

Except for administration of morphine and lowering blood pressure in patients with pulmonary edema associated with accelerated or malignant hypertension, measures to *improve the LVEF by decreasing ventricular afterload* are best reserved for use in the intensive care unit after institution of on-line monitoring of pulmonary and systemic arterial pressures. These measures consist mainly in reduction of systemic vascular resistance by adrenergic blocking agents, arterial vasodilators, and intravenous or sublingual nitrates. In selected critically ill patients with acute myocardial infarction or valvular disease (excluding aortic insufficiency), intra-aortic counterpulsation provides hemodynamic support through catheterization and possibly operation. In patients with critical aortic stenosis, emergency valve replacement is occasionally mandatory.

In all patients with pulmonary edema, attention should be directed toward *identifying potential precipitating factors* (Table 7.7), so that prompt treatment may be instituted. In particular, fever may have to be reduced with salicylates, acetaminophen, or a cooling blanket.

Controlled Ventilation

It is helpful to think of acute pulmonary edema primarily as a respiratory disorder. Arterial blood-gas levels should be determined frequently until there is no doubt that the patient's condition is improving. If respiratory acidosis is severe (pH less than 7.15) and does not rapidly improve or if arterial Po_2 is lower than 50 mm Hg with initial therapy, including oxygen by face mask, endotracheal intubation should be performed and controlled positive-pressure ventilation instituted. The decision whether to institute controlled ventilation is often difficult. Endotracheal intubation is not without its hazards, particularly if performed by unskilled personnel. It should be performed before severe respiratory acidosis or hypoxemia leads to ventricular fibrillation, asystole, or severe hypotension. Medical personnel skilled in intubation should be present so that the patient may be appropriately sedated or paralyzed and intubation safely and rapidly performed. Endotracheal intubation during a cardiac arrest is more difficult, and the occurrence of a cardiac arrest significantly decreases the probability of survival. Ventricular fibrillation may be impossible to convert to sinus rhythm in severely hypoxemic patients, and the incidence of asystolic arrest, which has an even worse prognosis, is high. Myocardial function, which may be impaired at the outset, is worsened by severe acidosis and hypoxemia. Furthermore, hypoxemia increases myocardial oxygen consumption. If acute myocardial infarction is present, infarct size may be increased if hypoxemia persists. Patients with severe respiratory distress due to pulmonary edema who are not significantly obtunded or hypotensive require morphine; it should not be withheld for fear of inducing hypoventilation. If severe hypoventilation should occur following administration of morphine—

and it occasionally does—endotracheal intubation should be performed and controlled ventilation instituted.

Controlled ventilation may initially be applied with a pressure-cycled respirator, but as soon as it is practicable, a volume-cycled respirator should be substituted because patients with pulmonary edema often have erratic and unpredictable tidal volumes on pressure-cycled respirators. It is important that large tidal volumes (600–1000 cc) be ensured so that subsegmental atelectasis, which often complicates respiratory failure of any cause and which further worsens gas exchange, is prevented. Positive-pressure ventilation reduces venous return. As with other measures that reduce venous return, care must be taken that undue hypotension does not ensue.

Occasionally, gas exchange remains critically impaired even after controlled ventilation with a volume-cycled respirator is instituted. Improvement may be brought about by keeping the end-expiratory pressure positive by 5–10 cm H_2O (continuous positive-pressure ventilation). This technique is now extensively utilized in intensive care units.

Acidemia

Acidemia (blood pH less than 7.36) is common in acute pulmonary edema, and may be due to respiratory acidosis or metabolic acidosis or both. Severe respiratory acidosis (pH less than 7.15–7.20; Pco_2 more than 65–75 mm Hg) necessitates institution of controlled ventilation. Metabolic (lactic) acidosis usually does not require specific therapy; bicarbonate need not be administered unless acidemia is extremely severe, in which case shock is usually present. There is hazard in administering the sodium load incumbent on bicarbonate therapy to patients who can ill-afford further expansion of the extracellular fluid compartment. Patients with severe metabolic acidosis associated with cardiogenic shock (pH less than 7.10–7.15) may require bicarbonate, but controlled ventilation is also usually required in these patients, which partly alleviates the consequences of the exogenous sodium load.

DIFFERENTIAL DIAGNOSIS OF ACUTE CARDIAC PULMONARY EDEMA

The causes of acute respiratory distress are listed in Table 7.9. *Acute bronchitis with bronchospasm* is not usually a diagnostic problem in younger patients with atopic asthma and in patients with obvious exposure to noxious fumes, including smoke, but differentiating it from acute pulmonary edema is an extremely difficult and common problem in older patients with asthmatic bronchitis. Oxygen should be administered at an Fio_2 of 0.24 until initial blood-gas determinations exclude carbon dioxide retention. Until a diagnosis is made, morphine should be withheld, but aminophylline may be helpful. Aminophylline must be used with extreme caution; an initial intravenous dose of 4–6 mg/kg followed by a continuous infusion of 0.5–1.0 mg/kg/hr yields a therapeutic serum theophylline level between 10 and 20 μg/ml. In most patients with heart failure, the lower infusion rate suffices to maintain therapeutic levels.

Pulmonary emboli are also a common source of diagnostic confusion, both as a cause of respiratory distress in themselves and as a precipitating cause of pulmonary edema when there is underlying left heart disease. In the former situation, the plain chest film does not show cardiac pulmonary edema, and the electrocardiogram does not show left atrial enlargement. In the latter situation, treatment should proceed as for pulmonary edema, and the diagnosis of pulmonary emboli should be made by appropriate means subsequently.

Widespread pneumonitis (bacterial, viral, or a noninfectious inflammatory state) and *pneumonia superimposed on chronic pulmonary disease* are also common causes of acute respiratory distress. Some patients with pneumonia and hypoxemia may precipitously become more distressed, in which case cardiac pulmonary edema is mimicked further. In addition, acute bronchospasm may develop. The approach to treatment of these patients is similar to that described for acute bronchitis; it is particularly important to withhold morphine and to avoid the induction of hypovolemia with diuretics.

Patients with bronchitis, pulmonary emboli, and pneumonia may sometimes have chest x-ray findings that do not allow confident exclusion of cardiac pulmonary edema. Conversely, the radiographic findings in cardiac pulmonary edema are sometimes not distinctive enough to allow confident confirmation of the diagnosis. In these patients, specific treatment for cardiac pulmonary edema, especially administration of morphine and diuretics, may have to be deferred in the emergency ward and await direct measurement of the pulmonary capillary wedge pressure in the intensive care unit.

With widespread application of the bedside technique for measurement of pulmonary capillary wedge pressure in intensive care units, it has become apparent that there are many causes of radiologic pulmonary edema and acute respiratory

Table 7.9.
Causes of acute respiratory distress.

Cardiac pulmonary edema (resulting from elevation of left atrial pressure, see Tables 7.2–7.5)

Noncardiac pulmonary edema
  Increased negativity of intrathoracic pressure
    Upper airway obstruction
      Laryngospasm after attempted intubation
      Epiglottitis/Croup
      Suffocation
      Hanging
    Unilateral pulmonary edema after reexpansion of collapsed lung or after rapid thoracentesis
  Increased alveolocapillary membrane permeability
    Infectious pneumonia—bacterial, viral, parasitic
    Inhaled toxins

Beryllium salts	Oxygen in high concentration
Boron	Ozone
Cadmium salts	Phosgene
Carbon monoxide	Polyvinyl derivatives
Chlorine	Rocket propellants
Diethyl sulfate	Smoke
Hydrogen fluoride	Teflon fumes
Hydrogen sulfide	Toluene
Metallic chloride salts	Toluidine compounds
Methyl bromide	Turpentine
Nitrogen dioxide	Xylene

    Circulating foreign substances
      Snake venom
      Bacterial endotoxins (in bacteremia)
    Aspiration of gastric contents
    Aspiration of baby powder
    Acute radiation pneumonitis
    Drowning
    Disseminated intravascular coagulation
    Hereditary angioneurotic edema (histamine mediated)
    Idiopathic capillary leak syndrome
    Immunologic or idiosyncratic
      Hypersensitivity pneumonitis
      Leukoagglutinin (transfusion reaction)
      Systemic lupus erythematosus and other vasculitides
    Drug-induced

Busulfan	Hydralazine
Colchicine	Hydrochlorothiazide
Cyclophosphamide	Methotrexate
Dextran 40	Nitrofurantoin
Diphenhydramine hydrochloride	Radiographic contrast material
Ethchlorvynol (intravenous)	Salicylates
Fluorescein	Sulfonamides
Hexamethonium	

  Lymphatic insufficiency
    After lung transplantation
    Lymphangitic carcinomatosis
    Fibrosing lymphangitis (e.g., silicosis)
  Unknown or incompletely understood
    High altitude
    Uremia
    Neurogenic (intracranial hypertension or postictal)
    Pulmonary embolism (fat, air, amniotic fluid, or thrombus)
    Overdose
      Opium alkaloids, including meperidine (Demerol)

Table 7.9. *continued*
Causes of acute respiratory distress.

Cardiac pulmonary edema (resulting from elevation of left atrial pressure, see Tables 7.2–7.5)
    Methadone
    Propoxyphene hydrochloride (Darvon)
    Pentobarbital
    Chloral hydrate
    Methaqualone
  Postcardioversion
  Postanesthesia
  Postcardiopulmonary bypass
  Recovery from diabetic ketoacidosis
  Hepatic failure
  Pancreatitis
  Closed chest trauma
  Nonthoracic trauma

Causes not associated with pulmonary edema
  Acute massive pulmonary thromboembolism
  Atopic asthmatic bronchitis
  Asthmatic bronchitis superimposed on chronic airways disease or on chronic restrictive pulmonary disease
  Upper airway obstruction (laryngeal or tracheal)
  Pneumothorax
  Hypovolemic or septic shock
  Transient reversible restrictive pulmonary disease
  Dyskinetic respiratory muscles

---

distress other than heart failure. These are listed in Table 7.9 as causes of *noncardiac pulmonary edema*. Opium alkaloid overdose has been recognized for many years as a cause of pulmonary edema and represents a common emergency ward problem. The treatment of these patients will not be discussed here except to mention that general measures for treating impaired gas exchange are the cornerstone of therapy. Except when the cause is obvious, as in opium alkaloid overdose, the diagnosis of noncardiac pulmonary edema is usually made outside the emergency ward after measurement of pulmonary capillary wedge pressure.

The differential diagnosis of acute cardiac pulmonary edema constitutes one of the most difficult and challenging problems in clinical medicine. There are several guidelines that are helpful:

(1) Do not be intimidated into making a diagnosis. It is often better to proceed initially with a diagnosis of acute respiratory distress of uncertain cause than to start therapy for a specific cause that turns out later to be nonexistent.

(2) The end result of all causes of respiratory distress is impaired gas exchange. Give oxygen by face mask; if there is concern that the patient may have chronic hypercapnia due to pulmonary disease, give low-flow oxygen by a mask delivering a controlled F_{IO_2} of 0.24—a little oxygen may go a long way. If possible, use a positive-pressure device. If the patient has bronchospasm, cautiously give intravenous aminophylline. If severe hypoxemia persists despite face-mask oxygen therapy, if severe respiratory acidosis exists, or if the patient is severely obtunded, initiate controlled ventilation.

(3) If the diagnosis of cardiac pulmonary edema is uncertain, withhold morphine unless it has been decided that endotracheal intubation is imminent regardless.

(4) Do not equate the presence of diffuse rales with the diagnosis of cardiac pulmonary edema. The most powerful diagnostic evidence of cardiac pulmonary edema, other than a measured pulmonary capillary wedge pressure, is provided by chest x-ray examination.

(5) Almost all patients with cardiac pulmonary edema have some clue that implicates the heart, although the nature of the clue depends on the type of heart disease present (ischemic chest pain, myocardial infarction on the electrocardiogram, cardiac enlargement, gallops, murmurs, and so on). Electrocardiographic evidence of left atrial enlargement is a common, although not invariable, manifestation of virtually all forms of left heart disease severe enough to be associated with elevated left atrial pressure. Be reluctant to diagnose cardiac pulmonary edema in the absence of at least one of these clues. Old age by itself does not constitute such a clue. Beware of the temptation to hear gallops; they are easy to "manufacture"

when the physician wants desperately to solve a diagnostic dilemma. This rule cannot be inverted; it is obvious that patients with heart disease may suffer from causes of acute respiratory distress other than pulmonary edema.

SOME SELECTED ASPECTS OF HEART FAILURE

Left Heart Failure With a Normal Heart Size on Chest X-Ray Film

Clinicians sometimes tend to think that LHF and cardiomegaly are inseparable except in mitral stenosis. This is not the case, however. Causes of LHF with a normal-sized heart include the diseases listed in Table 7.3. Other causes include some instances of acute myocardial infarction, LHF associated with transient ischemia, some instances of acute mitral regurgitation, and the diseases listed in Table 7.2.

Recognition of Critical Aortic Stenosis

Most patients with LHF due to aortic stenosis improve with therapy and may subsequently undergo cardiac catheterization and aortic valve replacement. Occasionally, however, patients with critical aortic stenosis have pulmonary edema or cardiogenic shock that is unresponsive to therapy. These patients are at great risk for sudden cardiac arrest (any of the three types: electromechanical dissociation, ventricular fibrillation, or asystole), and often cannot be resuscitated. It is important that they be recognized early, since aortic valve replacement even in these critically ill patients is lifesaving. Although the mortality of an emergency operation is high, it is acceptable given the dismal prognosis otherwise. Recognition is occasionally complicated by absence of the characteristic murmur and carotid pulse abnormality when the cardiac output is critically depressed; aortic valvular calcification on the plain chest film may be the only clue in such cases. A high index of suspicion is necessary; the physician should consider aortic stenosis in all patients with LHF of inapparent cause, especially in the elderly. Carotid pulses must be carefully examined for even a hint of upstroke plateau or thrill. Evidence for left ventricular hypertrophy should be sought on the electrocardiogram and in the examination of the apical impulse (sustained). The characteristic harsh, grunting, systolic murmur may only be heard in the subclavicular area, in the neck, or at the cardiac apex. High-quality chest films should be obtained as soon as possible, including a lateral view, so that the presence or absence of valvular calcification may be evaluated.

Right Heart Failure With Hypotension

RHF associated with hypotension may eventually complicate many of the causes of left heart disease, cor pulmonale due to chronic lung disease, primary pulmonary hypertension, Eisenmenger's syndrome, and pulmonic stenosis. It is also characteristic of acute right ventricular infarction. However, special mention should be made of two relatively common causes of this syndrome that have distinct therapeutic implications in the emergency ward: massive pulmonary emboli and pericardial tamponade. *Pulmonary embolic disease* has already been discussed as a precipitating factor of pulmonary edema and as a problem in the differential diagnosis of acute respiratory distress. Acute cor pulmonale, which is still another complication of pulmonary embolization, is even more ominous, and occurs when embolization is massive; its clinical features consist of the abrupt onset of intense dyspnea, cyanosis varying from mild to profound, elevation of the jugular venous pressure, and in some cases, extreme agitation. A right ventricular impulse is often palpable. The intensity of pulmonic closure is increased, although sometimes less so initially than hours or days subsequently. Systolic or continuous murmurs along either sternal edge occasionally are audible. Electrocardiographic abnormalities are common when embolization is massive (Stein et al., 1975). Syncope is a frequent initial manifestation. Small movements of the central clot, sometimes brought about by external cardiac massage, may result in resumption of consciousness and return of the systemic arterial blood pressure toward normal (Johnson and Harrist, 1977). Immediate therapy with intravenous heparin is mandatory as soon as the diagnosis is reasonably secure. Pulmonary angiography, performed on an emergency basis, usually is indicated to confirm the diagnosis. If the patient survives the initial few minutes of hypotension, the most common cause of subsequent death is a recurrent embolus; hence, pulmonary embolectomy is only rarely advisable in the management of massive pulmonary embolism.

Pericardial tamponade as a cause of hypotension is exceedingly important to recognize, since pericardiocentesis is often lifesaving. Pericardial effusion may result from any form of acute pericarditis, but the most common causes are acute benign pericarditis (idiopathic or viral), neoplasm metastatic to the pericardium, uremia, rupture of a myocardial infarct, and dissection of the aorta. When the amount of pericardial fluid reaches a critical level, ventricular filling is impaired, diastolic pressures in all chambers become equal, and stroke volume decreases. The amount of fluid needed to initiate this sequence depends on the rapidity of fluid formation—less is required if fluid appears rapidly. In a sense, combined heart failure is present because left atrial pressure and right atrial pressure are equal; however, RHF—manifested by elevated jugular venous pressure—is more evident. Left atrial pressure is normally higher than right atrial pressure; thus, elevation of both atrial pressures to the same level represents a more striking abnormality on the right side of the circulation. The key feature of pericardial tamponade is paradox in the arterial pulse (decrease of more than 10 mm Hg in systolic blood pressure with inspiration). This can usually be detected by palpation of the femoral pulses, although systolic blood pressure in both phases of respiration should be measured carefully. This sign is often impossible to detect if the rhythm is atrial fibrillation, but is virtually always present if there is sinus rhythm and frank hypotension. Kussmaul's sign—rise in the mean jugular venous pressure with inspiration—is often absent in patients with pericardial tamponade, as contrasted with patients with constrictive pericarditis, in whom it is usually present. The tip-off to the diagnosis of tamponade often consists of: (1) noticing that a right ventricular impulse is absent and that physiologic splitting of S_2 is preserved despite elevation of the jugular venous pressure; or (2) finding that neither ventricular impulse is palpable on examination despite an increase in cardiac silhouette on the plain chest film. Once the diagnosis is suspected, arterial paradox should be sought. The presence of pericardial fluid is confirmed by means of echocardiography or right atrial cineangiography. The presence of pericardial fluid does not ensure that tamponade is the cause of hypotension—if arterial paradox is absent, pericardial fluid and hypotension are unlikely to be related.

The treatment for pericardial tamponade is pericardiocentesis, which should be performed in the operating room by a thoracic surgeon if the condition of the patient permits. However, if shock is too severe to allow time or transport, pericardiocentesis should be performed in the emergency ward (see Chapter 21, pages 464–466). Pericardiocentesis may pose a special hazard in patients with uremic pericarditis; it is possible that these patients should undergo partial pericardiectomy as initial treatment of tamponade.

Situations Requiring Cautious Administration of Diuretics

Although intravenous diuretics have become a cornerstone in the treatment of pulmonary edema,

the clinician should remember that improvement usually precedes the onset of diuresis and does not correlate with the extent of diuresis. In addition, situations exist in which diuretics must be given with caution or withheld. Patients with critical *aortic stenosis* may be dependent on high left ventricular filling pressures to maintain an adequate stroke volume; excessive diuresis may occasionally lead to a critical reduction in cardiac output and sudden death. Acute pulmonary edema complicating *acute myocardial infarction* may exist despite a normal total blood volume. It has been recognized in recent years that a small number of patients with cardiogenic shock due to myocardial infarction are hypovolemic because of overly aggressive use of diuretics and respond to fluid administration. *Elderly patients with left ventricular disease*, especially those with reduced left ventricular compliance associated with hypertrophy, often tolerate extensive diuresis poorly. Similarly, diuresis in patients with reduced ventricular compliance due to cardiac constriction (*pericardial tamponade* or *constrictive pericarditis*) may lead to severe hypotension. Diuresis is sometimes associated with precipitation of hepatic failure in patients with *severe liver disease*, especially if it is accompanied by the development of hypokalemia and metabolic alkalosis.

Electrical Cardioversion in Patients With Supraventricular Tachyarrhythmias

Patients with rapid supraventricular tachyarrhythmias (ventricular rate more than 150 beats/min resulting from atrial fibrillation, paroxysmal atrial tachycardia, or atrioventricular junctional tachycardia) associated with LHF are usually treated as they would be if heart failure were not present. In the absence of a severely depressed LVEF, intravenous verapamil may prove to be an excellent drug for converting reentrant supraventricular tachyarrhythmias.

If significant hypotension is present or if initial therapy fails to alleviate pulmonary edema, electrical cardioversion should be performed in the emergency ward with a synchronized direct-current cardioverter. This is particularly true if atrial fibrillation is known to be of recent onset; cardioversion is a less appropriate therapy if atrial fibrillation is chronic, in which case sinus rhythm is unlikely to be maintained and the rapid ventricular response is more likely to be secondary to hemodynamic compromise or to underdigitalization. Intravenous diazepam may be used to induce sedation and amnesia for electrical cardioversion, although blood pressure must be carefully monitored since hypotension is occasionally produced or exacerbated. Electrical cardioversion is hazardous if excessive digitalis levels are present because intractable ventricular fibrillation may be produced.

Misdiagnosis of Right Heart Failure as the Cause of Ankle Edema

Since the emergency ward is a source of primary medical care in some communities, emergency physicians may have to evaluate bilateral edema of the lower extremities. Ankle edema is correctly attributed to RHF only if the jugular venous pressure is elevated. The misdiagnosis of RHF is frequent; most patients with ankle edema do not have heart failure. Far more common causes are bilateral chronic venous insufficiency of the lower extremities, occlusive disease of the pelvic veins, and prolonged dependency of the lower extremities in obese or disabled patients; in some instances, an explanation cannot be found. Less commonly, edema is discovered to be due to hepatic disease, renal disease, or another systemic cause.

Subacute and Chronic Heart Failure: Decisions in the Emergency Ward

The most obvious reasons for which patients with heart failure are seen in the emergency ward is treatment of acute pulmonary edema. However, in recent years, the emergency ward has been used increasingly as a source of primary medical care. Physicians in the emergency ward must frequently make decisions with respect to the diagnosis and management of heart failure that has become manifest in forms milder than acute pulmonary edema that do not represent true medical emergencies. When the condition is severe, the diagnosis of heart failure is usually not difficult. However, when heart failure is mild, diagnosis may be elusive. Formalization of the process whereby clinicians establish the presence of LHF helps avoid both underdiagnosis and overdiagnosis of the condition. Table 7.10 shows one possible set of criteria for diagnosis of LHF. When these criteria are not met, but LHF is suspected nevertheless, the physician should consider measuring the pulmonary capillary wedge pressure, or if circumstances are appropriate, he or she should institute a "therapeutic trial" for heart failure. If the latter route is chosen, the physician should have clear endpoints for declaring the trial either a success or a failure; otherwise, the patient might be committed to a protracted course of therapy, the risk of which could exceed its benefit.

Patients with heart failure of any stage of severity require ongoing primary medical care—there

Table 7.10.
Criteria of left heart failure.

Event	Points for Diagnosis[a]
Chest x-ray film	
Alveolar edema	4
Interstitial edema	3
Upper zone flow redistribution	2
Causal relationship	
Third heart sound	3
Presence of known potential cause of heart failure	2
Cardiothoracic ratio > 0.50	2
Dyspnea	
Rest dyspnea or orthopnea	2
Paroxysmal nocturnal dyspnea	2
Dyspnea on exertion	1
Evidence that heart failure is bi-sided (JVP > 7 cm H_2O)	2
Other	
Pulmonary crackles (posttusive)	1
P-wave negativity in V1 > 0.03 mm-sec	1
Heart rate (sinus)	
> 90	1
> 100	2

JVP = mean jugular venous pressure.

[a] Six points or more are required for diagnosis. Only one event each can be counted from the chest x-ray film, causal relationship, dyspnea, or "other" categories.

Reproduced by permission from Johnson RA: Heart Failure. In: The Practice of Cardiology. Johnson RA, Haber E, Austen WG (Eds). Boston, Little, Brown & Co. 1980; pages 31–95.

is no substitute for the primary care physician. Heart failure always means severe cardiac impairment; "a little heart failure" is a euphemism. Most patients must be carefully evaluated to establish a cause, even when symptoms are mild, because the natural history of some forms of heart disease is unrelated to the severity of accompanying left atrial hypertension (for example, the high incidence of sudden death in aortic stenosis once symptoms develop). Also, therapy for some causes of heart failure must be specific (valve replacement in valvular disease, β-adrenergic blockade in asymmetric septal hypertrophy with obstruction, and so on). These causes of heart failure are often unrecognized on initial evaluation; they may become suspected only during follow-up evaluation, at which time cardiologic consultation may be obtained. In addition, treatment of patients with chronic heart failure due to the most common causes—cardiomyopathy syndrome due to coronary artery disease, cardiomyopathy of the elderly, and other cardiomyopathy syndromes—is often the most complicated. Since the incidence of embolization is high, anticoagulants may be appropriate. Arrhythmias, commonly the result of digitalis, must be prevented. Diuretic therapy must be carefully monitored, and hypokalemia must be avoided. Vasodilator therapy can benefit patients in whom heart failure persists despite vigorous treatment with digitalis and diuretics, but its use is also associated with potentially adverse effects (Table 7.11). Neither systematic evaluation nor systematic management can be provided by erratic visits to an emergency ward. When patients who have not had the care of a primary physician come to an emergency ward with mild or chronic LHF, they must be referred to a primary care physician for subsequent follow-up care.

A corollary of this problem involves decisions regarding hospital admission for patients not previously followed up by a physician. Patients with dyspnea at rest, even without frank pulmonary edema, should be admitted to the hospital for evaluation, initiation of therapy, and observation. In addition, the following guidelines may prove useful criteria for admission:

(1) When the cause or suspected cause would in itself be grounds for admission. Such causes include acute myocardial infarction, heart failure due to coronary disease when it is accompanied by unstable angina (new onset of angina at rest, accelerating frequency of angina, or prolonged angina), and aortic stenosis. Patients with heart failure suspected to be due to aortic stenosis should always be admitted to the hospital because management is difficult and because they require early evaluation for surgical intervention.

(2) When symptoms have progressed in the course of several days or when their progression is uncertain.

(3) When there is a suspected precipitating factor such as pulmonary embolus, arrhythmia, pneumonia, or urinary tract infection. The course of heart failure in these patients is usually too uncertain to allow outpatient management, even if the precipitating factor in itself does not necessitate hospital admission.

(4) When there is RHF of any cause in a patient not previously evaluated. RHF always has serious implications. It is not a complication of left heart disease unless LHF is severe and accompanied by elevated pulmonary vascular resistance, rapid atrial fibrillation, or significant right ventricular functional impairment. The other causes of RHF (Table 7.6) are serious in themselves and necessitate careful evaluation because treatment must often be directed specifically toward the cause and must not be limited to management of the symptomatic consequences of elevated right atrial pressure.

Having made the decision to admit a patient who has heart failure, but who does not yet have pulmonary edema, the emergency physician often must decide whether intensive or routine care is necessary. In general, intensive care should be provided whenever hemodynamic or electrical instability exists or is anticipated as a result of the underlying disease or its treatment, or whenever the progression of heart failure appears unrelenting despite initiation of treatment in the emergency ward. Pulmonary arterial catheterization should be considered in the following situations:

(1) When the diagnosis of heart failure remains in doubt and the choice of one among several divergent therapeutic courses hinges on establishing an accurate diagnosis.

(2) When the regulation of treatment is difficult without the aid of precise and easily accessible hemodynamic measurements.

(3) When hemodynamic studies may help establish the cause of heart failure (for example, acute mitral regurgitation or ventricular septal rupture). As soon as the decision to provide hemodynamic monitoring is made, arrangements to secure facilities and personnel to implement the decision should be started.

Treatment begun in the emergency ward must

Table 7.11.
Commonly used nonparenteral vasodilator regimens and their side effects.

Regimen	Side Effects
Hydralazine hydrochloride, 25–100 mg every 6 hr,	Nausea, vomiting, and lupus syndrome (at high doses)
plus	
nitrates (usually oral isosorbide dinitrate, 20–40 mg every 4 hr)	Headache
Prazosin, 1–7 mg every 8 hr	Postural hypotension, drowsiness, depression, nausea, vomiting, and rarely, an idiosyncratic first-dose hypotensive response

not be disrupted in the transition from the emergency to the inpatient ward and from the emergency to the primary physician. In addition, the appropriateness of each mode of treatment must be reassessed frequently, since heart failure and the side effects of its treatment often fluctuate.

Digitalis Toxicity: Diagnosis and Treatment

Heart failure is the most frequent reason for digitalis therapy, hence familiarity with the diagnosis and treatment of digitalis toxicity is vital to physicians who take care of heart-failure patients. Manifestations of digitalis toxicity can be divided into cardiac and extracardiac categories; in turn, cardiac manifestations can be divided generally into rhythm disturbances resulting from increased automaticity and those resulting from decreased conduction (Table 7.12). Patients with a higher risk of digitalis toxicity include those with diminished renal function (when digoxin is used), diminished hepatic function (when digitoxin is used), electrolyte disturbance (hypokalemia, hypomagnesemia, or hypercalcemia), acute myocardial infarction, acute or chronic pulmonary disease, hypothyroidism, and recently instituted quinidine therapy. Treatment for digitalis intoxication (including inadvertent or intentional overdose) comprises antiarrhythmic agents such as phenytoin and lidocaine hydrochloride to decrease au-

tomaticity, atropine to facilitate atrioventricular conduction, and temporary transvenous ventricular pacing to support the heart rate. Dialysis and oral cholestyramine have been employed to promote excretion of the drug with limited success. In the near future, antibody fragments that bind specifically to digitalis and hence reverse its toxic effects may become more widely available; this represents a revolutionary approach to the treatment of digitalis toxicity.

Suggested Readings

Baxley WA, Kennedy JW, Field B, et al: Hemodynamics in ruptured chordae tendineae and chronic rheumatic mitral regurgitation. *Circulation* 48:1288-1294, 1973

Boucher CA, Fallon JT, Johnson RA, et al: Cardiomyopathic syndrome caused by coronary artery disease III: Prospectives clinicopathologic study of its prevalence among patients with clinically unexplained chronic heart failure. *Br Heart J 41:* 613-620, 1979

Brody W, Criley JM: Intermittent severe mitral regurgitation: Hemodynamic studies in a patient with recurrent acute left-sided heart failure. *N Engl J Med* 283:673-676, 1970

Bussmann W, Schupp D: Effect of sublingual nitroglycerin in emergency treatment of severe pulmonary edema. *Am J Cardiol* 41:931-936, 1978

Cohn K, Selzer A, Kersh ES, et al: Variability of hemodynamic responses to acute digitalization in chronic cardiac failure due to cardiomyopathy and coronary artery disease. *Am J Cardiol* 35:461-468, 1975

Dikshit K, Vyden JK, Forrester JS, et al: Renal and extrarenal hemodynamic effects of furosemide in congestive heart failure after acute myocardial infarction. *N Engl J Med* 288:1087-1090, 1973

Fulop M, Horowitz M, Aberman A, et al: Lactic acidosis in pulmonary edema due to left ventricular failure. *Ann Intern Med* 79:180-186, 1973

Gunther S, Grossman W: Determinants of ventricular function in pressure-overload hypertrophy in man. *Circulation* 59:679-688, 1979

Habak PA, Mark AL, Kioschos JM, et al: Effectiveness of congesting cuffs ("rotating tourniquets") in patients with left heart failure. *Circulation* 50:366-371, 1974

Hutter AM, Jr, DeSanctis RW, Nathan MJ, et al: Aortic valve surgery as an emergency procedure. *Circulation* 41:623-627, 1970

Johnson RA: Heart Failure. In: *The Practice of Cardiology.* Johnson RA, Haber E, Austen WG (Eds). Boston, Little, Brown & Co. 1980, pp. 31-95

Johnson RA, Harrist TJ: Collapse and cyanosis in a 45-year-old man. *N Engl J Med* 296:33-40, 1977

Lee DCS, Johnson RA, Bingham JB, et al: Heart failure in outpatients: A randomized trial of digoxin versus placebo. *N Engl J Med* 306:669-705, 1982

Lesch M, Caranasos GJ, Mulholland JH, et al: Controlled study comparing ethacrynic acid to mercaptomerin in the treatment of acute pulmonary edema. *N Engl J Med* 279:115-122, 1968

Meszaros WT: Lung changes in left heart failure. *Circulation* 47:859-871, 1973

Miller GAH, Kirklin JW, Swan HJC: Myocardial function and left ventricular volumes in acquired valvular insufficiency. *Circulation* 31:374-384, 1965

Robin ED, Cross CE, Zelis R: Pulmonary edema. *N Engl J*

Table 7.12.
Manifestations of digitalis toxicity.

Gastrointestinal symptoms
  Nausea
  Vomiting
  Anorexia

Neurologic symptoms
  Visual disturbances
  Headache
  Confusion
  Delirium

Cardiac rhythm disturbances
  Increased automaticity
    Ectopic rhythms at atrial, junctional, or ventricular level
    Nonparoxysmal junctional tachycardia
    Atrioventricular dissociation
  Decreased conduction (especially atrioventricular conduction)
    Sinoatrial exit block or sinus arrest
    Paroxysmal atrial tachycardia with or without atrioventricular block
    Atrial fibrillation with slow ventricular response
    Second- or third-degree atrioventricular block

Med 288:239–246, 292–304, 1973

Simon M: The pulmonary vessels: Their hemodynamic evaluation using routine radiographs. *Radiol Clin North Am* 1:363–376, 1963

Singh S, Newmark K, Ishikawa I, et al: Pericardiectomy in uremia: The treatment of choice for cardiac tamponade in chronic renal failure. *JAMA* 228:1132–1135, 1974

Smith TW: Digitalis glycosides. *N Engl J Med* 288:719–722, 942–946, 1973

Stein PD, Dalen JE, McIntyre KM, et al: The electrocardiogram in acute pulmonary embolism. *Prog Cardiovasc Dis* 17:247–257, 1975

Yatteau RF, Peter RH, Behar VS, et al: Ischemic cardiomyopathy: The myopathy of coronary artery disease. Natural history and results of medical versus surgical treatment. *Am J Cardiol* 34:520–525, 1974

CHAPTER 8

Management of Hypertensive Emergencies

CECIL H. COGGINS, M.D.
KATHARINE K. TREADWAY, M.D.

Hypertension is epidemic, with elevated blood pressure existing in more than 15% of the adult population of the United States. The percentage is higher among blacks and in the older age groups, and it is still higher if borderline hypertension is included.

Even mild degrees of blood pressure elevation increase the risk of cardiovascular disease and death from cerebral thrombosis or hemorrhage, heart failure, myocardial infarction, and renal failure. Effective treatment decreases the death rate toward normal; however, only about one-half of the hypertensive patients in the population have been discovered, and in only a small minority of these is hypertension satisfactorily controlled.

It is therefore not surprising that the emergency physician is often challenged with hypertensive crises. These crises may be the malignant culmination of prolonged essential hypertension, of hypertension secondary to other disease (Table 8.1), or they may represent the major manifestation of a new illness. Even moderate hypertension may constitute an emergency when it is superimposed on arterial bleeding, aortic dissection, or severe heart failure. This chapter will discuss the diagnosis and management of the hypertensive crisis.

HYPERTENSIVE EMERGENCIES

The key to successful management of a hypertensive emergency is prompt recognition and initiation of treatment, the goal being rapid reduction of blood pressure within minutes to hours. Usually this requires that treatment be started after only a brief evaluation. Table 8.2 lists the situations considered to represent hypertensive emergencies. These conditions are discussed below.

Malignant Hypertension

Malignant hypertension is defined as severe hypertension diastolic blood pressure usually greater than 130–140 mm Hg with grade IV Keith-Wagener retinopathy (papilledema, hemorrhages, and exudates). Patients with a similar elevation of blood pressure and grade III retinopathy (hemorrhages and exudates without papilledema) are considered to have accelerated hypertension. These conditions represent a continuum, and both are associated with diffuse arteriolitis and fibrinoid necrosis.

Malignant hypertension usually occurs in the setting of poorly controlled essential hypertension, although it may occur in young patients, particularly black males, without a known history of hypertension. It also may occur with some forms of secondary hypertension, namely, pheochromocytoma and renovascular hypertension, as well as in association with acute or chronic renal failure. Patients most commonly have headache and visual complaints. They may or may not have encephalopathy, and they also may have signs of chronic hypertension such as left ventricular hypertrophy, congestive heart failure, or other atherosclerotic disease. Less commonly, patients are entirely asymptomatic. Prompt treatment is mandatory. Untreated, the patient's condition may progress rapidly to coma, convulsions, and death, with survival of less than 1% at the end of 1 year. Recent statistics suggest that with proper treatment more than 75% are alive at 1 year.

Hypertensive Encephalopathy

Encephalopathy usually occurs as an acute or subacute depression of central nervous system function in the setting of severely elevated blood pressure. Patients usually have symptoms ranging from confusion to coma, with or without associated headache and nausea. It is important to note that in patients without a history of hypertension (as in patients with acute renal failure or eclampsia) encephalopathy may occur with diastolic blood pressure from 95–120 mm Hg. Hypertensive encephalopathy must be distinguished from other central nervous system catastrophes (Table 8.3). Significantly elevated diastolic blood pressure, evidence of chronic hypertension, hypertensive retinopathy, and lack of focal neurologic signs, as well as prompt (usually within several minutes) clearing of central nervous system symptoms with effective therapy usually will establish the diagnosis.

Eclampsia

Preeclampsia is characterized by acute vasospasm and sodium retention in a previously healthy woman during the third trimester of pregnancy. Manifested by hypertension, edema, and proteinuria, preeclampsia puts the patient at great risk for progression to eclampsia, with convulsions, coma, and frequently, renal failure. It is most likely to occur in women who have never borne children before, women over 35 years old, patients carrying multiple fetuses, and patients with hydatidiform moles. It should be remembered that blood pressure is normally somewhat lower than usual during the second and third trimesters of pregnancy (often averaging 100–90/50–60 mm Hg) and that a rapid rise in blood pressure to 160/100 mm Hg may be severe enough to cause encephalopathy. These patients also must be distinguished from those who have a history of hypertension. The latter patients usually have hypertension before the third trimester and do not have accompanying edema or proteinuria. Eclampsia is ordinarily an indication to terminate the pregnancy, but extreme elevations of blood pressure require immediate pharmacologic control.

Catecholamine Crisis

Catecholamine crisis may occur associated with tumor, drug use, or withdrawal of antihypertensive

Table 8.1.
Hypertension classified by cause.

Essential hypertension—not associated with defined disease; more than 90% of hypertensive patients

Secondary hypertension—less than 10% of hypertensive patients
  Coarctation of aorta
  Renal disease
    Parenchymal
    Vascular
  Adrenal disease
    Medulla or chromaffin cells—pheochromocytoma
    Cortex
      Cushing's syndrome
      Primary hyperaldosteronism
      Other mineralocorticoid excess
  Toxemia of pregnancy
  Central nervous system disease
  Hypertension associated with contraceptive pills

Table 8.3.
Differential diagnosis of hypertensive encephalopathy.

Uremic encephalopathy
Encephalopathy secondary to metabolic derangements
Subarachnoid hemorrhage
Intracerebral hemorrhage
Cerebrovascular accident
Subdural hemorrhage
Head injury
Intracranial mass
Postictal state
Encephalitis
Cerebral vasculitis

Table 8.2.
Hypertensive emergencies.

Malignant hypertension	
Hypertensive encephalopathy	
Eclampsia	
Catecholamine excess secondary to	pheochromocytoma
	monoamine oxidase inhibitors
	clonidine hydrochloride withdrawal
Severe hypertension associated with	acute left ventricular failure
	myocardial infarction
	acute aortic dissection
	intracranial hemorrhage
	acute glomerulonephritis

medication. In a patient with pheochromocytoma, extreme hypertension may accompany the release of catecholamines from epinephrine- or norepinephrine-secreting chromaffin tumors in the adrenal medulla or in the abdomen. The diagnosis should be suspected in any patient with a history of episodic headache, palpitation, tremors, sweating and tachycardia associated with elevated blood pressure, and the condition should not be mistakenly diagnosed as an anxiety attack.

In these patients, hypertension may be either labile or sustained. Patients with pheochromocytoma are usually thin and frequently exhibit a decrease in blood pressure when standing, unlike most patients with essential hypertension. Patients who have pheochromocytoma and episodic blood pressure elevation often do not have the cardiac enlargement and retinopathy that would be expected with sustained hypertension of a similar degree. Signs of chronic hypertension may be present, however, in those patients with sustained hypertension.

A catecholamine crisis may also result from intake of catecholamine precursors or analogues by a person whose ability to metabolize such compounds is impaired. Such impairment results from the use of antidepressant monoamine oxidase inhibitors (Table 8.4). Catecholamine precursors include tryamine, which is naturally found in foods such as aged cheese and Chianti wine, and amphetamine or ephedrine, which may be found in cold preparations and cough medicines. In ad-

Table 8.4.
Significant nonproprietary and proprietary names.

Nonproprietary Name	Proprietary Name
Monoamine oxidase inhibitors	
Isocarboxazid	Marplan
Nialamide	Niamid
Pargyline hydrochloride	Eutonyl
Phenelzine dihydrogen sulfate	Nardil
Tranylcypromine sulfate	Parnate
Other	
Clonidine hydrochloride	Catapres
Diazoxide	Hyperstat
Furosemide	Lasix
Hydralazine hydrochloride	Apresoline
Methyldopa	Aldomet
Sodium nitroprusside	Nipride
Phenoxybenzamine hydrochloride	Dibenzyline
Phentolamine	Regitine
Propranolol hydrochloride	Inderal
Reserpine	Serpasil
Trimethaphan camsylate	Arfonad

dition, the extreme elevations of blood pressure that have been reported to occur after abrupt withdrawal of the antihypertensive drug clonidine hydrochloride in many respects resemble a catecholamine crisis.

Complicated Hypertension

Even when hypertension is not itself an immediate threat to life, it may demand emergency treatment when combined with another illness such as acute left ventricular failure, myocardial ischemia or infarction, acute aortic dissection, or intracranial hemorrhage. In these settings, severe hypertension usually exacerbates the underlying condition, and in the case of aortic dissection or intracranial hemorrhage, even modest degrees of hypertension may become life-threatening. These conditions require special treatment considerations, which are discussed on pages 149–150; their clinical appearance and approaches to diagnosis are described in other chapters of this text.

PHARMACOLOGIC AGENTS

Although several potent, rapidly acting antihypertensive drugs are now available, the physician will treat hypertensive emergencies most effectively by becoming expert in the use of a few agents. Almost all hypertensive emergencies can be managed with one of two primary drugs (diazoxide and nitroprusside), two ancillary drugs (propranolol hydrochloride and furosemide), and special purpose drugs for pheochromocytoma and aortic dissection.

Diazoxide

Diazoxide is a benzothiadiazide compound structurally related to the thiazide diuretics, but with a sodium-retaining effect rather than a diuretic effect.

Action

The primary action of diazoxide is to relax arteriolar smooth muscle, thus reducing peripheral resistance. It has little effect on capacitance vessels (veins) and no direct cardiac effect. The onset of action is within 1 minute. Peak action is in 5–10 minutes and the duration is 3–18 hours. A sympathetic reflex response to the lower blood pressure produces increased heart rate, cardiac index, and cardiac work. Sympathetic or ganglionic blocking agents such as propranolol or guanethidine may therefore have a synergistic effect by blocking this reflex response. Diazoxide is highly bound to plasma proteins. The antihypertensive effect results from the unbound fraction and hence is poorly correlated with total serum levels. In patients with uremia, the drug is less completely bound and more slowly excreted, so required doses may be reduced. In the pregnant patient, the relaxant effect on smooth muscle may arrest labor, and the patient may require oxytocin to resume uterine contractions.

Administration

An average dose of diazoxide is 300 mg (5 mg/kg) injected in 10 or 15 seconds through an already established large-bore intravenous line. Pressure will begin to decrease within 2–5 minutes. Although it is generally believed that rapid injection is essential to ensure that some of the drug will not be bound to the circulating albumin, recent studies have demonstrated efficacy with 100–150 mg repeated after 5 minutes if response is inadequate. Slow intravenous infusion at 20 mg/min is also effective, producing a response within 20 minutes. Blood pressure should be measured every 5 minutes for the first 30 minutes and less frequently thereafter. If the effect in 30 minutes is insufficient, the dose may be repeated. Smaller amounts may be given with proportionately smaller effects. Caution should be used if another antihypertensive drug has already been administered, because in this circumstance blood pressure may decrease to subnormal levels after administration of a standard dose of diazoxide. Volume depletion or β-blockade will also enhance the effect of diazoxide.

Side Effects

Salt and water retention regularly occurs after use of diazoxide. Furosemide, 40 mg intravenously may be given either initially or with each successive dose, unless volume depletion is present. Hyperglycemia occurs, but rarely requires treatment unless diazoxide is given repeatedly over 2–3 days. Hyperuricemia and hyperlipidemia also may occur. If blood pressure decreases to undesirable levels, the patient's head should be lowered and the legs may be raised.

Sodium Nitroprusside

The action of sodium nitroprusside in reducing blood pressure has been apparent since 1929, but no stable commercial preparation became available until recently.

Action

Sodium nitroprusside acts by direct dilation of vascular smooth muscle. This not only reduces peripheral resistance but by diminishing venous tone (increasing capacitance), it also reduces cardiac filling pressure. Therefore, blood pressure decreases with little change in cardiac output. In addition, reflex tachycardia does not occur. There is little direct effect on the heart itself. The different cardiovascular effects of sodium nitroprusside and diazoxide are apparent in Figure 8.1. Sodium nitroprusside is in large part metabolized to cyanide in the red blood cells; the cyanide reacts with thiosulfate in the liver to form thiocyanate. Thiocyanate, in turn, is excreted by the kidneys. In hepatic failure, therefore, cyanide may accumulate and in renal failure or with infusions lasting 2 or more days, toxic levels of thiocyanate may occur.

Administration

Administered by constant intravenous infusion, sodium nitroprusside has an immediate effect proportionate to the infusion rate and lasting only as long as the infusion continues. It therefore requires minute-to-minute titration and constant attention in the emergency ward or intensive care setting. When available, constant infusion pumps aid in precise regulation of administration and arterial lines aid in monitoring pressure. One vial (50 mg) is dissolved in 500 ml of 5% dextrose in water, and the bottle is covered with aluminum or a paper bag because of sensitivity to light. An initial infusion of 0.5 μg/kg/min (35 μg/min or 0.35 ml/min for a 70-kg patient) should be given and the rate adjusted for adequate control. Different individuals may require from 0.5–8.0 μg/kg/min, with an average dose of 3 μg/kg/min.

Side Effects

Nausea, sweating, or apprehension initially may be noted, but usually diminishes with time. The main disadvantage is not the presence of side effects, but rather the extreme potency of the drug, which requires very close attention to blood pressure and infusion rate. If thiocyanate in the blood rises to toxic levels, muscular weakness, delirium, or coma may develop. In patients at risk, thiocyanate levels should be monitored and infusion discontinued if possible when levels exceed 10 mg/100 ml. If necessary, thiocyanate may be removed by dialysis. One instance of methemoglobinemia occurring on the fourth day of infusion has been reported.

Trimethaphan Camsylate

Trimethaphan camsylate is a ganglionic blocking agent that causes inhibition of both adrenergic and cholinergic ganglia. This accounts for both its

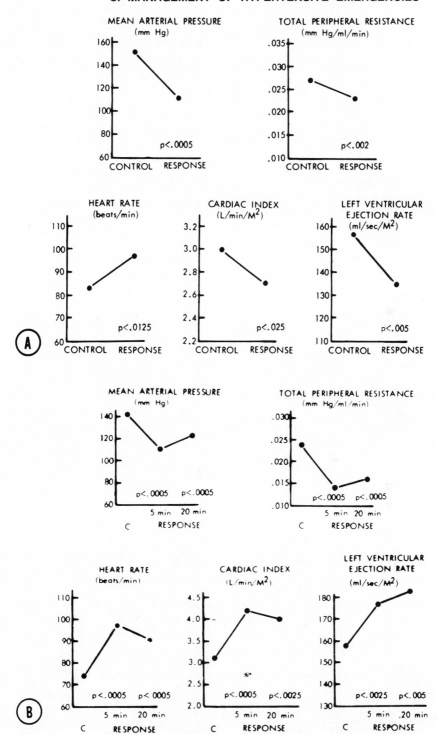

Figure 8.1. **(A)** Hemodynamic effects of sodium nitroprusside (7 patients). Each point represents the average for each hemodynamic function before (*control*) and after (*response*) treatment with the intravenously administered hypotensive agent. The probability statistic represents the p value by paired data analysis. **(B)** Hemodynamic effects of diazoxide (9 patients). C = control. (Reproduced by permission, from Bhatia SK, Frohlich ED: Hemodynamic comparison of agents used in hypertensive emergencies. *Am Heart J* 85:367–373, 1973.)

efficacy and its numerous side effects. Adrenergic blockade causes vasodilation and subsequent reduction in blood pressure; it also reduces systolic ejection velocity and cardiac output. Anticholinergic action may cause urinary retention, hypomotility of the intestine with development of ileus or gastric retention, and blurred vision. Respiratory paralysis has been reported.

Administration is by constant intravenous infusion; 500 mg is mixed in 500 ml of 5% dextrose in water and given as an initial dose of 0.5–1.0 mg/min. The dose is then titrated to achieve desired pressure. Elevation of the head at 45 degrees will enhance the antihypertensive effect.

Because trimethaphan camsylate is extremely potent, its use requires constant monitoring, preferably with an arterial line. Tachyphylaxis is common, and usually occurs within 48–72 hours.

Phentolamine

Phentolamine is a pure α-adrenergic blocking agent used specifically for treatment of catecholamine crisis. It is given as a 5–10 mg intravenous bolus. The effect is immediate and lasts approximately 15 minutes, so constant intravenous infusion is used to continue the effect. Phentolamine may cause tachyarrhythmias or angina. Phenoxybenzamine, a long-acting α-adrenergic blocking agent may be given orally after initial treatment with phentolamine.

MANAGEMENT

Does An Emergency Exist?

When the patient is not outwardly critically ill or in extreme distress, the most difficult decision is whether to use potent rapidly acting intravenous hypertensive drugs or to use slower drugs that can be incorporated later into the chronic treatment program. The physician must estimate the threat to the patient posed by several hours or a day of continued, severe hypertension. In general, severe hypertension associated with any of the following requires rapid (within minutes) lowering of blood pressure: grade III or IV retinopathy with or without symptoms of encephalopathy, eclampsia, aortic dissection, acute myocardial ischemia or infarction, or intracranial hemorrhage.

Evaluation of the Patient

Although severe hypertension requires consideration of correctable secondary causes and often a series of laboratory studies, initial therapy in a hypertensive emergency must begin after the briefest evaluation. The only benign conditions in the differential diagnosis of severe hypertension are anxiety attacks and defective blood pressure measuring equipment, including undersized cuffs applied to obese patients.

History

The physician should determine the following: Is there a history of hypertension? Is the patient taking any medication, including diuretics, antihypertensive drugs, monoamine oxidase inhibitors, or birth control pills? Have there been episodes of palpitation, pallor, sweating, and headache that would suggest pheochromocytoma? Has dyspnea, orthopnea, angina pectoris, or papilledema been noted? In a patient suspected of having hypertensive encephalopathy, a careful history of the symptoms and the course of onset is especially important.

Physical Examination

Immediate examination should include determination of blood pressure in both arms and evaluation of the heart, lungs, and neck veins for evidence of congestive failure; examination of the optic fundi for retinopathy or papilledema, and determination of all pulses, especially if aortic dissection is suspected. The examiner also should look briefly for café au lait spots and neurofibromas that may accompany pheochromocytoma, and should perform a rapid neurologic examination, including determination of mental status.

An electrocadiogram should be obtained, an intravenous line of at least 18-gauge tubing established, the patient's head elevated at a 45-degree angle, and arrangements made for admission to the hospital. A chest x-ray film is usually obtained, but treatment should not be delayed by a slow trip through the radiology department.

Treatment

General Considerations

The selection of appropriate therapy will be simplified by taking into consideration the following:

(1) Urgency—Patients with malignant hypertension, encephalopathy, or complicated hypertension require immediate control with rapidly acting antihypertensive agents. In the asymptomatic patient with accelerated hypertension, the condition may be controlled in the course of hours.

(2) Blood presure goal—Except in patients previously normotensive (such as children or patients with eclampsia or acute renal failure) and patients with aortic dissection, the initial goal of treatment

is not to achieve completely normal blood pressure. Patients with chronic hypertension often have thickened arterial walls and atherosclerosis, so perfusion to vital organs may be compromised by normal pressures. In general, in the previously hypertensive patient the immediate blood pressure goal is 180–160/110–100 mm Hg. In the patient who was previously normotensive, the goal is 140/90 mm Hg or lower. In the presence of aortic dissection, despite a history of hypertension, the blood pressure goal is usually approximately 100–110/60 mm Hg to prevent further dissection. In the patient with myocardial ischemia or infarction, the physician must weigh the need to lower the blood pressure for reduction of myocardial work against the need to maintain adequate coronary perfusion.

(3) Hemodynamic stability—Because of its relatively long duration of action, diazoxide is ideal for patients with uncomplicated hypertensive emergencies. In situations that may become potentially unstable, such as myocardial infarction, pulmonary edema, or intracranial hemorrhage, more precise control is necessary, and sodium nitroprusside is preferred.

Uncomplicated Hypertension—Specific Recommendations

In uncomplicated hypertensive emergencies, the primary circulatory abnormality is increased peripheral resistance. In this circumstance, the ideal emergency drug would be one with a predominant action of reducing resistance, rapid onset of action, and relatively few side effects. Diazoxide and sodium nitroprusside approach this ideal, although neither is perfect.

In general, except in catecholamine crisis, uncomplicated hypertensive emergencies are best treated with diazoxide because of its ease of administration and proved efficacy. In complicated hypertensive emergencies, sodium nitroprusside is preferred because of its lack of reflex cardiac stimulation and its potency and short duration of action, which allows precise control in hemodynamically unstable situations. Recommendations for treatment of hypertensive emergencies are summarized in Tables 8.5 and 8.6.

Complicated Hypertension—Specific Recommendations

Pulmonary Edema. Patients with pulmonary edema frequently have extreme hypertension. Initial management should be directed at specific treatment of the pulmonary edema (diuretics, morphine, oxygen and so on). Occasionally, pulmo-

nary congestion does not resolve with standard measures and blood pressure remains elevated. In such cases, sodium nitroprusside is the drug of choice.

Acute Myocardial Ischemia. Similarly, sodium nitroprusside is the drug of choice in acute myocardial ischemia complicated by severe hypertension. It allows gradual, precise reduction of blood pressure without increasing ischemia. Intravenous nitroglycerin also may be useful in the patient with hypertension and ongoing ischemia. Used alone, it is inadequate to control severe hypertension. If hypertension is less severe and the patient's condition is hemodynamically stable, nitrates and propranolol hydrochloride may be tried initially.

Aortic Dissection. The treatment of aortic dissection is aimed at reducing the forces that propagate the dissection—elevated pressure and velocity of systolic ejection. This is achieved by a combination of propranolol hydrochloride and sodium nitroprusside. Propranolol is given first as a 0.5-mg intravenous test dose, followed in 5 minutes by 1-mg intravenously which is repeated every 5 minutes until the heart rate is between 60 and 70 beats/min or until a total dose of 0.15 mg/kg has been attained. Nitroprusside is then given to lower pressure to approximately 100/60 min Hg. During this time, arrangements should be made either to have the patient evaluated by a cardiologist and a cardiac surgeon or to transfer the patient immediately to a facility in which aortic angiography and cardiac surgery can be performed. If the patient has congestive heart failure or a history of significant pulmonary disease or asthma, propranolol is hazardous and the drug of next choice is trimethaphan camsylate. Trimethaphan may be given by intravenous infusion, 0.5–1.0 mg/min, and titrated until the desired pressure is reached. As a ganglionic blocking agent, it both lowers blood pressure through vasodilation and reduces systolic ejection velocity and cardiac output, so it may be used alone. In the patient with aortic dissection, its effect is enhanced by elevating the patient 45 degrees. Like sodium nitroprusside, it is an extremely potent antihypertensive agent and requires constant monitoring to avoid profound hypotension.

Intracranial Hemorrhage. While severe hypertension may precede intracranial hemorrhage, it may also be secondary to increased intracranial pressure, and thus it may fluctuate in response to measures that reduce intracranial pressure. In such a situation, sodium nitroprusside is the drug of choice if monitoring is available. Intracranial hemorrhage has not been shown to benefit from blood pressure control; thus, pressure should be lowered

Table 8.5.
Drug considerations in the treatment of hypertensive emergencies.

	Route and Dosage	Time Course			Mechanism of Action	Side Effects	Disadvantages	Advantages
		Onset	Peak	Duration				
General								
Diazoxide	IV push: 300 mg (5 mg/kg), 150 mg, or infusion	1–2 min	2–4 min	4–12 hours	Direct arterial vasodilation	Reflex tachycardia, sodium retention, hyperglycemia, vomiting, uterine atony	Hypotension, painful extravasation	Prompt effect, potent, continuous infusion not required, constant monitoring not required
Sodium nitroprusside	IV infusion: 50 mg in 500 ml D$_5$W—begin at 25–50 µg/min and titrate ↑	<1 min	1–2 min	2–5 min	Direct smooth muscle relaxation (arterial and venous)	Nausea, restlessness, hypotension, thiocyanate toxicity after prolonged use	Constant monitoring required, extreme photosensitivity	Precise control, ↓ both preload and afterload
Special Purpose								
Trimethaphan camsylate	IV infusion; 500 mg in 500 ml D$_5$W—begin at 0.5–1.0 mg/min and titrate ↑	1–2 min	2–5 min	10 min	Ganglionic blockade	Ganglionic blockade, urinary retention, ileus, cycloplegia, respiratory arrest	Tachyphylaxis, constant monitoring required	Potent, precise control
Propranolol hydrochloride	0.5 mg IV test dose, then 1 mg IV q 5 min until pulse < 70 or total 0.15 mg/kg	<1 min	1–2 min	2–6 hours	β-blockade	Bradycardia, ↓ atrioventricular conduction, bronchospasm, myocardial depression		
Phentolamine	IV bolus 5–10 mg followed by IV infusion of 1.5–2 µgm/kg/min	<1 min		5–30 min	α-adrenergic blockade	Tachyarrhythmias, angina, palpitation		Use only in circumstances of catecholamine excess

IV = intravenous; D$_5$W = 5% dextrose in water.

Table 8.6.
Specific pharmacologic recommendations.[a]

Syndrome	Drugs of Choice	Drugs to Be Avoided
Malignant hypertension	Diazoxide or Sodium nitroprusside	
Hypertensive encephalopathy	Diazoxide or sodium nitroprusside	Reserpine, methyldopa
Eclampsia	Diazoxide	
Excess catecholamines	Phentolamine followed by propranolol hydrochloride or sodium nitroprusside	Propranolol hydrochloride in the absence of α-blockade
Hypertension complicated by:		
Acute left ventricular failure	Sodium nitroprusside	
Intracranial hemorrhage	Sodium nitroprusside	Reserpine, methyldopa, diazoxide
Aortic dissection	Sodium nitroprusside and propranolol hydrochloride or trimethaphan camsylate	Diazoxide, hydralazine
Aortic ischemia or infarction	Sodium nitroprusside	Diazoxide, hydralazine

[a] These recommendations are based on known benefits and hazards and may not be universally applicable.

Table 8.7.
Other drugs that may be useful in hypertensive emergencies.

Drug	Action	Administration	Onset	Duration
Hydralazine hydrochloride	Arteriole dilation, increase in cardiac output, possible increase in cardiac work, preservation of renal blood flow Good in combination with propranolol, especially for chronic use	10–50 mg intravenously	15 min	4–6 hours
Methyldopa	Reduction in sympathetic tone If acute emergency is not present, parenteral use may lay groundwork for later oral methyldopa therapy	250–500 mg intravenously	2 hours	8–10 hours
Reserpine	Reduction in sympathetic tone, central nervous system depression	1–5 mg intramuscularly	2 hours	8–24 hours or more

carefully to about 20–30% below the original systolic pressure. Any drug that may depress central nervous system function such as reserpine or methyldopa should be avoided.

Catecholamine Crisis. Because catecholamine crisis occurs secondary to a sudden excess of catecholamines, whether endogenous or exogenous, treatment is aimed at blocking both α- and β-adrenergic effects. To avoid an increase in peripheral resistance and thus further pressure elevation, the physician must achieve α-blockade first. This is accomplished with the α-blocking agent, phentolamine, 1–10 mg as an intravenous bolus every 5 minutes until pressure is lowered. This then may be followed by intravenous propranolol hydrochloride as previously described. Sodium nitroprusside is also effective, and if there is any doubt about the diagnosis, it is the preferred agent.

Eclampsia. Whereas the treatment of eclampsia remains controversial, most authors agree that severe hypertension should be treated with either diazoxide or sodium nitroprusside in the same manner as in any patient with uncomplicated hypertension. Although magnesium sulfate has been used for years, and is effective in controlling neuromuscular irritability, it is not an effective antihypertensive agent in the presence of severely elevated blood pressure. Diazoxide is effective, although it will decrease uterine contractions and may cause hyperbilirubinemia and hyperglycemia in the newborn. These side effects are not contraindications to its use in the eclamptic patient. Sodium nitroprusside is also safe and effective. Special care must be taken to avoid intravascular volume depletion since eclamptic patients are frequently hypovolemic despite peripheral edema. A central venous pressure line usually is recommended. Stabilization of the patient's condition with subsequent rapid delivery is the treatment of choice.

Other Drug Therapy

We have emphasized the usefulness of diazoxide and sodium nitroprusside in most hypertensive emergencies. This should not imply that these are the *only* drugs useful in such emergencies. Table 8.7 contains a list of other frequently used drugs. It is likely, however, that the emergency physician who is thoroughly experienced with the actions of two drugs will treat hypertensive crises more effectively than one who has passing familiarity with a large number.

We have not included the newer antihypertensive agents such as minoxidil, captopril, and nifedipine because experience is limited regarding appropriate use in hypertension crises. Undoubtedly, at least some of these agents will prove useful in the acute management of the severely hypertensive patient.

Once blood pressure is under control, treatment has only begun. An oral regimen of therapy should be started if possible even as the emergency program is in progress. Diuretics are almost universally useful as a foundation of therapy, and propranolol hydrochloride also has a place in most current programs, so emergency use of these drugs is a good start. Methyldopa, clonidine hydrochloride, hydralazine hydrochloride, or other drugs as best fit the patient's needs are then added. A search for correctable causes of secondary hypertension should be instituted—the extent of the search depending on the age and clinical characteristics of the patient.

Suggested Readings

Berglund G, Andersson O, Wilhelmsen L: Prevalence of primary and secondary hypertension: Studies in a random population sample. *Br Med J* 2:554–556, 1976

Chiariello M, Gold HK, Leinbach RC, et al: Comparison between the effects of nitroprusside and nitroglycerin on ischemic injury during acute myocardial infarction. *Circulation* 54:766–773, 1976

Cohn JN, and Burke LP: Nitroprusside. *Ann Intern Med* 91:752, 1979

Finnerty FA: Treatment of hypertensive emergencies. *Heart Lung* 10:275, Mar–Apr 1981

Goldberg LI: Current therapy of hypertension: A pharmacologic approach. *Am J Med* 58:489–494, 1975

Grossman SH, and Gunnels JC: Recognition and treatment of hypertensive emergencies. *Cardiovasc Clin* 3:47, 1981

Guiha NH, Cohn JN, and Mikulic E, et al: Treatment of refractory heart failure with infusion of nitroprusside. *N Engl J Med* 291:587–592, 1974

Kaplan NH: Hypertensive crises. In: *Clinical Hypertension.* 2nd ed., Williams & Wilkins, Baltimore, 1976

Keith TA: Hypertension crisis, recognition and management. *JAMA* 237:1570–1577, 1977

Koch-Weser J: Drug therapy: Diazoxide. *N Engl J Med* 294:1271–1274, 1976

Langfeld SB: Hypertension: Deficient care of the medically served. *Ann Intern Med* 78:19–23, 1973

Mukherjee D, Feldman MS, and Helfant RH: Nitroprusside therapy: Treatment of hypertensive patients with recurrent resting chest pain, ST-segment elevation, and ventricular arrhythmias. *JAMA* 235:2406–2409, 1976

National Center for Health Statistics: National Health Survey: Hypertension and Hypertensive Heart Disease in Adults, U.S. 1960–62. Vital and Health Statistics Series 11, No. 13. US Department of Health, Education, and Welfare, May 1966

Palmer RF, Lasseter KC: Drug therapy: Sodium nitroprusside. *N Engl J Med* 292:294–297, 1975

Ram CVS, and Kaplan N: Individual titration of diazoxide dosage in the treatment of severe hypertension. *Am J Cardiol* 43:627, 1979

Sheps SG, and Kirkpatrick RA: Hypertension. *Mayo Clin Proc* 50:709–720, 1975

Slater EE, and DeSanctis RW: The clinical recognition of dissecting aortic aneurysm. *Am J Med* 60:625, 1976.

Wheat MR, Jr, and Palmer RF: Dissecting aneurysms of the aorta, in Sabiston DC, Jr, Spencer FC (Eds): *Gibbon's Surgery of the Chest*, ed 3. Philadelphia, WB Saunders, 1976, pp. 913–933

CHAPTER 9

Pulmonary Emergencies

CHARLES A. HALES, M.D.
ROBERT D. BRANDSTETTER, M.D.
LAWRENCE G. MILLER, M.D.
EDWARD A. NARDELL, M.D.

Editor's Note: Like many other specialties, pulmonary medicine has some aspects that have surgical overtones. Some of these are discussed in Chapter 22 (Thoracic Emergencies). Pulmonary edema is discussed in Chapter 8 (Cardiology: Heart Failure).

PULMONARY EMBOLISM

Definition

A frequently unrecognized emergency medical problem, pulmonary embolism is the result of clot or other particulate matter lodging in the pulmonary vascular bed. Annual incidence in the United States probably exceeds 500,000, but as many as two-thirds go undiagnosed. Subsequent mortality is 30–40%, primarily the result of recurrent embolism. However, when the diagnosis is established by lung scanning or pulmonary angiography and anticoagulant therapy is administered, the mortality is 8–9%.

Natural History

Pulmonary embolism is usually the consequence of clot from the deep venous system, known as deep venous thrombosis (DVT). DVT usually begins in the lower extremities, although occasionally clots form in pelvic veins and rarely in veins of the upper extremities. Most thrombi originate in the soleus veins of the calf, often at sites of decreased flow such as valve cusps or bifurcations. The majority of calf thrombi resolve spontaneously; if embolism to the lung occurs, clinical manifestations may be absent. About 20–30% of clots propagate to the iliofemoral venous system, and an additional 10–20% of all DVT begin in proximal veins without prior calf involvement.

Iliofemoral thromboses appear to be the source of most clinically apparent pulmonary emboli.

Once in the pulmonary circulation, large clots may lodge at the bifurcation of the pulmonary and lobar arteries, causing hemodynamic compromise. Smaller clots continue distally to arterioles or capillaries. Lower lobes are more often involved than upper lobes, and emboli are usually multiple. Only about 10% of emboli cause infarction, probably because of collateral flow between the bronchial and pulmonary circulations. Infarction is more common in patients with pre-existent cardiopulmonary disease.

Factors predisposing to pulmonary emboli include (1) history of prior embolism; (2) factors promoting stasis such as bed rest or inactivity; (3) endothelial damage such as operation on a lower extremity; (4) hypercoagulability such as antithrombin III deficiency.

Clinical Manifestations

Autopsy series showing wide prevalence of pulmonary emboli suggest that many emboli are silent. When they are clinically apparent, symptoms and signs depend on the size of the embolic material. Small to medium emboli lodge in segmental or more distal branches of the pulmonary artery. Symptoms are usually pulmonary, including dyspnea, chest pain, and cough. Tachypnea and tachycardia are present in most patients. Mild fever below 102.2°F (39°C) is common, but wheezing occurs in less than 5% of patients. If infarction occurs, hemoptysis, pleuritic pain, and a pleural rub may be present (Tables 9.1 and 9.2).

Massive pulmonary emboli occur in lobar arteries or the pulmonary artery, with predominantly cardiovascular findings.

Table 9.1.
Frequency of symptoms of pulmonary embolism in 160 patients.

Symptom	Percent
Dyspnea	81
Pleuritic pain	72
Apprehension	59
Cough	54
Hemoptysis	34
Sweats	26
Syncope	14

(Modified by permission, from Sasahara AA, et al: The urokinase pulmonary embolism trial: A national cooperative study. *Circulation 47* and *48* (suppl 2):1–108, 1973, © The American Heart Association, Inc.)

Table 9.2.
Frequency of physical signs of pulmonary embolism in 160 patients.

Sign	Percent
Respiration rate > 16/min	88
Rales	53
Elevated S$_2$P	53
Pulse rate > 100/min	43
S$_3$-S$_4$ gallop	34
Diaphoresis	34
Thrombophlebitis	33
Edema	23
Murmur	23
Cyanosis	18

(Modified by permission, from Sasahara AA, et al: The urokinase pulmonary embolism trial: A national cooperative study. *Circulation 47* and *48* (suppl 2):1–108, 1973, © The American Heart Association, Inc.)

Symptoms include syncope, chest pain, and dyspnea, and the following signs of right ventricular dysfunction may be present: right ventricular heave, increased pulmonary component of the second heart sound (S$_2$P), , right ventricular S$_3$ gallop, jugular venous distention, and tricuspid regurgitant murmur. Systemic hypotension almost always signifies elevated right ventricular pressure.

In patients in whom pulmonary embolism is suspected, a history or findings of DVT should be sought. Whereas DVT will not be clinically evident in most patients, a history of calf or leg pain, signs of unilateral edema, and increased calf warmth or tenderness combined with the respiratory presentation should heighten the suspicion of pulmonary embolus and focus the diagnostic approach. It must be remembered, however, that the diagnosis of DVT is difficult on clinical grounds alone since DVT is often silent and since it is not the only cause of pain, tenderness, and swelling in the leg. Noninvasive studies of the legs with impedance plethysmography aid greatly in documenting proximal DVT but are less useful in documenting DVT of the calf veins. Calf veins, though, are rarely the source of symptomatic pulmonary emboli. Venography provides the definitive diagnosis of DVT although it is more uncomfortable for the patient and carries a low risk of resultant phlebitis. In patients with smaller pulmonary emboli, the differential diagnosis includes hyperventilation, asthma, congestive heart failure, pleurodynia, and serositis. If infarction is present, clinical findings may resemble pneumonia, bronchial obstruction by mucus or tumor, or pleural effusion of various causes.

In summary, signs and symptoms of pulmonary embolism are nonspecific. Vigilance is required to suspect the diagnosis and to initiate further evaluation.

Laboratory Evaluation

Noninvasive laboratory findings may further suggest, but rarely confirm, the diagnosis of pulmonary embolism. Nonspecific findings include leukocytosis, elevated erythrocyte sedimentation rate, and abnormal serum lactate dehydrogenase (LDH) or serum glutamic oxaloacetic transaminase (SGOT) level with normal bilirubin level. Fibrin degradation products are more common in the serum of patients with pulmonary emboli, but are nondiagnostic. However, absence of these products and soluble fibrin complexes makes the diagnosis unlikely.

Arterial blood-gas studies usually reveal hypoxemia, hypocapnia, and respiratory alkalosis. Massive pulmonary embolus with hypotension and respiratory collapse may lead to hypercapnia and combined respiratory and metabolic acidosis.

The Pao$_2$ is less than 90 mm Hg in almost all patients with pulmonary embolism, and less than 80 mm Hg in 90% of these patients; the average is 60–65 mm Hg. However, Pao$_2$ must be interpreted with caution, since the normal level varies with age and position. Formulas for estimating Pao$_2$ are:

Pao$_2$ (seated) = 104.2 − (0.27 × age in years)
Pao$_2$ (supine) = 103.5 − (0.42 × age in years)
Further, measured Pao$_2$ must be corrected for Paco$_2$, since the two coexist in alveolar gas: for every millimeter of mercury increase in Paco$_2$, Pao$_2$ decreases the same amount. Therefore, a patient with a Pao$_2$ of 100 mm Hg and a Paco$_2$ of 20 mm Hg may be relatively hypoxemic, since

correction to a Pa_{CO_2} of 40 mm Hg yields a Pa_{O_2} of 80 mm Hg. This is especially important given the frequency of hypocapnia in pulmonary embolism.

Hypoxemia may be detected up to 14 days after embolism, and is due mainly to ventilation-perfusion inequalities, with a small proportion due to shunt. Since hypoxemia is common in other diseases, it remains suggestive but nonspecific for pulmonary embolism.

The electrocardiogram is often abnormal in patients with small to medium pulmonary emboli, but findings are nonspecific, including ST-segment and T-wave changes. In the presence of massive pulmonary embolism, findings of right ventricular dysfunction are more common, including right axis deviation, right bundle-branch block, and the classic $S_1Q_3T_3$ pattern.

Even without infarction, radiographic abnormalities occur in most patients with pulmonary emboli (Table 9.3). These include elevation of a hemidiaphragm, atelectasis, and effusion (Figure 9.1). An infarct classically appears as a pleural-based infiltrate with a convex margin directed toward the heart. Effusions are usually small and unilateral. Blood is present in over half, and white blood cell count and differential vary widely.

Perfusion lung scanning is performed by injection of radioisotope-labeled albumin macroaggregates or microspheres. Scanning is sensitive; negative findings virtually exclude pulmonary embolism. Positive results, however, are nonspecific. Since pulmonary arterioles constrict in response to hypoxia, perfusion defects, especially if nonsegmental, may be secondary to a ventilatory abnormality and not to obstruction of flow caused by an embolism. Findings also may be abnormal in patients with atelectasis, asthma, chronic airways obstruction, or other causes of regional hypoventilation.

Ventilation scans may be used to increase the specificity of perfusion scans, although sensitivity is not altered. Ventilation scans are especially valuable when there is no infiltrate apparent on the chest film (Figs. 9.2 and 9.3). Recent evidence indicates that pulmonary embolism can be diagnosed on the basis of scans alone in some cases: (1) normal findings exclude pulmonary embolism; (2) multiple segmental or lobar perfusion defects ventilating normally make the diagnosis likely; and (3) multiple nonsegmental or subsegmental perfusion defects ventilating abnormally make the diagnosis unlikely. When scans are coupled with strong clinical evidence of DVT, and invasive or noninvasive documentation of DVT, further studies can be avoided.

Many patients have nonspecific abnormalities requiring the use of pulmonary angiography to diagnose pulmonary embolism. Angiography, the definitive diagnostic technique in this desease, is performed by injecting radioactive contrast dye into a branch of the pulmonary artery after percutaneous catheterization, which is usually transfemoral. The catheter should be advanced at least to the main pulmonary artery and preferably selectively to the left or right pulmonary arteries to achieve good dye concentration in the pulmonary vessels. A positive result consists of a filling defect or sharp cutoff of small vessels (Fig. 9.4). Selective injection with magnification views increases sensitivity. Negative findings appear to exclude pulmonary embolism, and follow-up studies show the risk of embolization in these patients to be extremely low. Mortality from the procedure is less than 0.4%; death occurs in patients with markedly elevated pulmonary pressure. Morbidity occurs in about 4% and is usually related to catheter insertion.

Table 9.3.
Frequency of chest radiologic abnormalities before heparin infusion in 128 patients.

Finding	Patients	
	No.	%
Lung parenchyma	60[a]	47
Consolidation	53	41
Atelectasis	26	20
Other	2	2
Pleural effusion	36	28
Diaphragmatic elevation	52	41
Pulmonary vessels	50[a]	39
Distention of proximal pulmonary arteries	30	23
Focal oligemia	19	15
Pulmonary arterial hypertension	4	3
Pulmonary venous hypertension	4	3
Other	3	2

[a] Number of patients with at least one radiologic finding of that subgroup.
(Modified by permission, from Sasahara AA, et al: The urokinase pulmonary embolism trial: A national cooperative study. *Circulation 47* and *48* (suppl 2):1–108, 1973, © The American Heart Association, Inc.)

Treatment

An accepted principle in the treatment of pulmonary embolism is the prompt use of anticoagulants, either heparin or thrombolytic agents. The objective of heparin therapy is to prevent further thrombosis in the lower extremities and recurrent

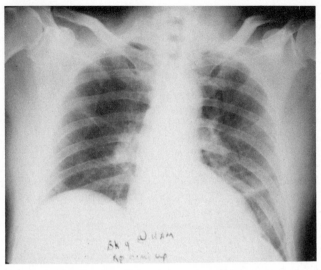

Figure 9.1. Posteroanterior chest x-ray film shows bilateral atelectasis, elevated right diaphragmatic leaf, and diminution of lung markings on right.

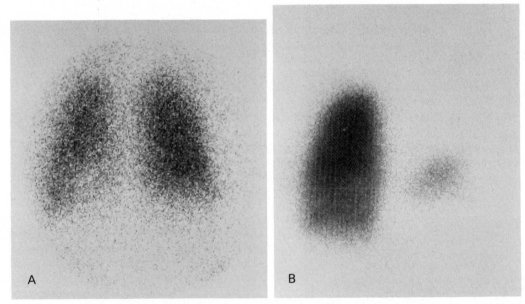

A   B

Figure 9.2. **(A)** Ventilation and **(B)** perfusion combined lung scan (posterior view, same patient as in Fig. 9.1) shows normal ventilation in right lung but almost complete absence of blood flow, except for minimal perfusion in middle lobe.

embolism, allowing endogenous fibrinolytic mechanisms to dissolve existing thrombi. Heparin combines with antithrombin III, leading to rapid inactivation of thrombin.

Constant intravenous infusion of heparin appears to cause fewer hemorrhagic complications than intermittent infusion. A bolus of 5000 units should be followed by approximately 1000 units/hour in most patients; doses should be decreased

if a bleeding tendency or renal or hepatic disease is present. Heparin requirements may decrease after 1–2 days of therapy, perhaps as a result of platelet activation and release of other factors. An activated partial thromboplastin time of 1½–2½ times the control value should be maintained. Lower levels may allow recurrent thromboembolism, whereas higher levels increase risk of bleeding.

Hemorrhage is the major complication of heparin therapy, occurring in about 5% of patients. Heparin may also cause thrombocytopenia, especially with bovine preparations; this is rarely clinically significant. Contraindications to heparin administration include intracranial and other causes of severe bleeding. A known bleeding diathesis and recent operation are relative contraindications. Heparin should not be administered subcutaneously or intramuscularly because of erratic absorption and local hematoma. Sodium warfarin should not be given in the acute situation because of its delayed onset of action.

Thrombolytic therapy is approved for massive pulmonary emboli. On angiographic examination, these are seen as filling defects in two or more

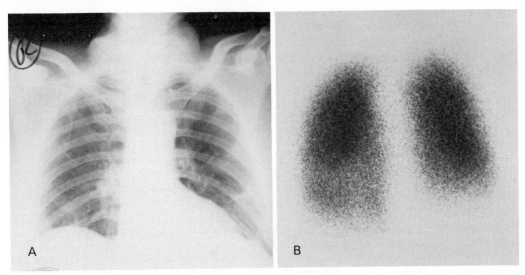

Figure 9.3. **(A)** Posteroanterior chest x-ray film 2 weeks later reveals minimal atelectasis in left lower lobe. **(B)** Posterior perfusion scan shows return of right lung perfusion.

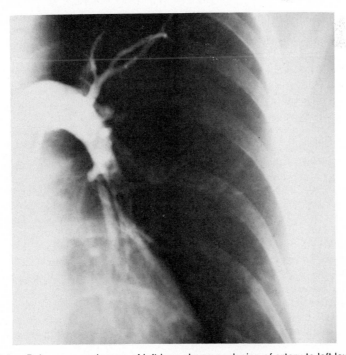

Figure 9.4.   Pulmonary angiogram of left lung shows occlusion of artery to left lower lobe.

lobar vessels. In the clinical setting, they are defined as emboli causing hemodynamic instability. The objective of thrombolytic agents is to accelerate and to potentiate clot lysis, as well as to prevent further thrombosis. Although no clear reduction in mortality has been shown in comparison with heparin, thrombolytic therapy may allow improved pulmonary function after recovery. If thrombolytic therapy is administered carefully, the risk of bleeding may not be greater than with heparin. Contraindications include intracranial bleeding or a strong possibility thereof, or other causes of major bleeding. Relative contraindications are recent operation or trauma.

Two thrombolytic agents are available: urokinase and streptokinase. Urokinase is extremely expensive and thus is seldom used. Streptokinase increases conversion of plasminogen to plasmin. It is antigenic in humans, cross-reacting with anti-streptococcal antibodies. Therefore, a loading dose must be given to bind these antibodies, 250,000 units over 30 minutes in most patients. This is followed by infusion of 100,000 units/hour for 24 hours. No test of the clotting system correlates with thrombolytic effect. Nonetheless, thrombin time or activated partial thromboplastin time should be determined after about 4 hours to ensure the presence of a thrombolytic state. If either test is prolonged, the fixed dose should be continued. If results are normal, the presence of excess antibodies should be determined and the dose adjusted.

Bleeding complications do not correlate with clotting parameters, but rather with invasive procedures. Patients in whom thrombolytic therapy is considered should have procedures performed in distal vessels if possible. If significant bleeding occurs, streptokinase administration should be stopped and whole blood given. Rarely, ϵ-aminocaproic acid is required to reverse the thrombolytic state. As many as one-third of patients treated with streptokinase have mild fever as a result, and a smaller number have allergic reactions, usually manifested by urticaria, itching, or flushing.

If anticoagulant therapy is strongly contraindicated, if septic emboli occur, or if emboli recur despite adequate anticoagulant therapy, an inferior vena cava interruption procedure should be performed to prevent further embolization from leg or pelvic veins. An open surgical procedure appears preferable if the patient's condition allows. Ligation of the inferior vena cava may result in serious morbidity and mortality, and should be reserved for septic emboli or recurrent small emboli causing pulmonary hypertension. Clipping the inferior vena cava is tolerated better by the patient and is preferable in situations in which a few small clots traversing the clip are acceptable. In patients unable to tolerate operations, transvenously placed filters serve the same function. The Kimray-Greenfield filter appears to become occluded less frequently than the Mobin-Uddin umbrella and to produce fewer postphlebitic symptoms in the legs.

The usefulness of embolectomy for massive pulmonary embolus is uncertain, and in part depends on the immediate availability of a cardiopulmonary bypass pump team. Mortality is extremely high, 57% in emergency procedures and 25% in moderately urgent procedures. Randomized comparison with thrombolytic therapy has not been performed.

Other Types of Thromboembolic Disease

Upper extremity thrombosis is uncommon, although it is more frequent in hospitalized patients as a result of cannulation of veins in the upper extremities. Whether pulmonary emboli occur is uncertain, but treatment should be similar to that for DVT in the lower extremities.

Septic emboli usually occur in patients with bacterial endocarditis (for example, tricuspid or left-sided bacterial endocarditis with ventricular septal defect) or septic thrombophlebitis. Diagnosis is based on a chest film showing multiple migratory infiltrates, and therapy consists of antibiotics and removal of septic veins.

The fat embolism syndrome remains poorly defined. It is most often seen after trauma, usually a fracture of a lower entremity. Clinical findings of embolization occur several days after trauma, and often progress to the adult respiratory distress syndrome. Therapy may include corticosteroids but not anticoagulants.

Amniotic fluid embolism occurs after childbirth as a result of infusion of fluid into endocervical veins. It is more common in older, multiparous patients and after complicated labor. Findings are similar to those seen with other types of pulmonary embolism, except that hypotension is common and prognosis is extremely poor. Therapy is supportive.

ASTHMA

Asthma is characterized by increased responsiveness of the trachea and bronchi to various stimuli. This responsiveness is manifested by widespread narrowing of the airways that improves either spontaneously or as a result of therapy. Attacks are of variable duration, and between attacks, pulmonary function is relatively normal and patients are asymptomatic.

Pathophysiologic Mechanisms

The cause of asthma is unknown, although asthmatic patients have been shown to have increased bronchial reactivity to acetylcholine, histamine, serotonin, and nonspecific irritants such as air pollution and dusts. They may also exhibit bronchospasm with exposure to cold air, vigorous exercise, psychologic stress, bronchial infection, or pulmonary edema.

Persons with hypersensitivity to inhaled allergens constitute one large subgroup of asthmatic patients. These atopic patients have IgE antibodies against antigens in the environment, and inhalation of these antigens elicits a series of reactions resulting in bronchospasm. This type of asthma is termed extrinsic asthma, and is associated with other allergic phenomena such as eczema and allergic rhinitis. The second major subgroup comprises those patients with asthma unassociated with the immunologic finding of extrinsic asthma. These patients have not been shown to have antigen-antibody reactions associated with the asthma attacks.

Extrinsic asthma is believed to be an allergic reaction of immediate hypersensitivity. An antigen in the environment enters the body and induces production of IgE antibodies by previously sensitized cells. Once released, the IgE antibodies are bound to the surface of pulmonary mast cells and basophils. When further exposure to the antigen occurs, the antigen interacts with the IgE molecules on the surface of these cells, evoking a series of reactions that result in bronchoconstriction and increased bronchial secretions. As shown in Figure 9.5, antigen bridging of the IgE molecules bound to the mast cell membrane initiates a sequence of biochemical events that result in influx of calcium into the cell, release of the stored mediators histamine and eosinophil chemotactic factor of anaphylaxis (ECF-A), and generation and release of the lipid slow-reacting substance of anaphylaxis (SRS-A), now known to be leukotrienes.

Release of the mediators of bronchoconstriction is modified by intracellular levels of cyclic adenosine monophosphate (cAMP) and cyclic guanosine 3',5'-monophosphate (cGMP). The enzyme systems regulating the levels of these molecules are in turn modified by various drugs. The reaction sequences and pharmacologic modifiers are shown in Figure 9.6 and Table 9.4, respectively.

After release from the mast cell, histamine and SRS-A act directly on the bronchiole to cause bronchoconstriction. As in the mast cell, intracellular levels of cAMP and cGMP in the bronchial smooth muscle are associated with modifications of the bronchoconstrictor response. High levels of cAMP effect decreased mediator release and high levels of cGMP effect increased mediator release; the opposite is true with low levels of cAMP or cGMP. Furthermore, the same pharmacologic agents that modify adenylate cyclase, phosphodiesterase, and guanylate cyclase in the mast cell modify their reactions in the bronchial smooth muscle (Fig. 9.7).

ECF-A results in the accumulation of eosinophils in an area of anaphylaxis. Eosinophils are phagocytic and contain the enzyme arylsulfatase, which can inactivate SRS-A. However, their role in the asthmatic patient has not been clearly defined.

Other factors, such as vagal tone, may also contribute to bronchospasm. Vagal tone is an important regulator of bronchial muscle tone. Bron-

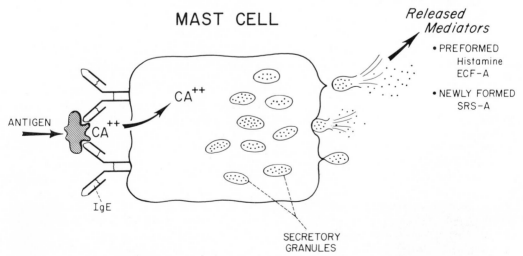

Figure 9.5. Release of mediators of bronchoconstriction.

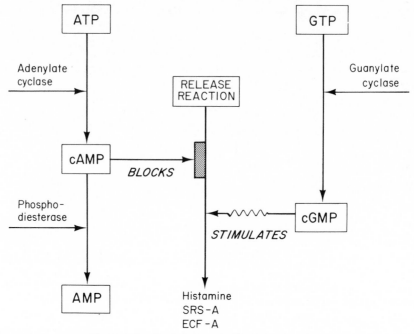

Figure 9.6   Control of mast cell release reaction.

Table 9.4.

Pharmacologic modifiers of enzyme systems regulating levels of cAMP and cGMP.

Adenylate cyclase
  Activators
    β-sympathomimetic agents
      Epinephrine
      Metaproterenol
      Isoproterenol
      Terbutaline sulfate (β-2)
      Isoetharine
      Salbutamol (Albuterol, β-2)
    Corticosteroids
Phosphodiesterase
  Inhibitors
    Xanthines (eg, aminophylline)
Guanylate cyclase
  Activators
    Cholinergic agents
      Acetylcholine
      Methacholine
    Calcium
  Inhibitors
    Anticholinergic agents
      Atropine and analogues

chial muscle tone is increased by cGMP, which is produced from guanosine 5′-triphosphate (GTP) in the presence of guanylate cyclase. This enzymatic reaction is enhanced by acetylcholine. Thus, an increase in vagal tone, because of the associated release of acetylcholine, can increase bronchial muscle tone and, therefore, airway obstruction. Many factors, including anxiety, modify vagal tone. This may at least partly account for bronchospasm associated with anxiety in some asthmatic patients. Anticholinergic drugs such as atropine and its congeners reduce bronchospasm in these individuals.

The vagus nerve also may play a role in antigen-antibody induced asthma through a reflex arc. The mediators released from pulmonary mast cells as a result of the antigen-antibody reaction not only can cause bronchoconstriction directly but also can cause stimulation of vagal irritant receptors in the lung, resulting in a reflex arc with vagal efferent bronchoconstriction.

Other factors that act directly on the bronchi or on the nervous system include bronchial infection, nonspecific irritants such as air pollution, cold air, coughing, laughing, sleep, exercise, and hyperventilation. IgA deficiency has also been associated with an increased incidence of asthma, although not in every case. The reason for this association is unknown.

Clinical Aspects

Signs and Symptoms

An acute exacerbation of asthma (Table 9.5) usually responds to inhaled or oral bronchodilators or removal of the initiating factor. Some attacks, however, persist. The patient frequently

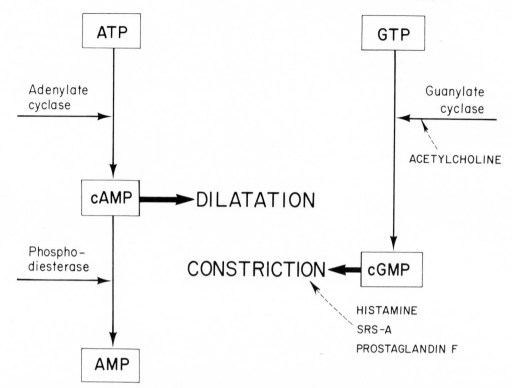

Figure 9.7.   Control of bronchial smooth muscle tone. Activators and inhibitors of depicted enzymes are same as those of mast cell enzymes (Table 9.4). There is a nonspecific relation between changes in cAMP and cGMP and release of mediators. Direct cause-and-effect mechanism has not been elucidated.

Table 9.5.
Indications of severe asthma.

PEFR < 100 liters/min
Pulsus paradoxus
Pao$_2$ on room air < 50 mm Hg
Paco$_2$ > 40 mm Hg
Central cyanosis
Gross overinflation on chest X-Ray
Heart rate > 130 beats/min
Disturbance of consciousness
Sternocleidomastoid retraction
Pneumothorax/pneumomediastinum

PEFR = peak expiratory flow rate.

seeks medical attention only after he has tried his usual medications, which have failed to ameliorate the acute attack of wheezing, coughing, and dyspnea. In fact, usually the symptoms have progressively worsened over several days. This has been termed status asthmaticus.

The patient appears tired and anxious, and is trying hard to breathe, using accessory muscles of respiration. In the presence of high negative inspiratory pressures, pulsus paradoxus may occur and usually indicates severe asthma. Use of the accessory muscles also correlates with moderately severe asthma with a forced expiratory volume in 1

second (FEV$_1$) less than 1 liter, and a peak expiratory flow rate (PEFR) of less than 100 liters/min. Diffuse wheezing is heard unless there is severe obstruction with greatly diminished air flow. Despite the obvious physical findings, it is difficult to assess the degree of obstruction and alveolar hypoventilation on physical examination. Therefore, specific measurements of pulmonary function and arterial blood gases are of value in quantifying the severity of the attack and for following the therapeutic response.

Diagnostic Studies

Diagnostic and therapeutic measures frequently must be performed simultaneously in the very ill patient (Table 9.6), but for convenience they are discussed separately in this chapter. It is important to establish the diagnosis of asthma and the severity of the attack. The sputum of these patients contains eosinophils that can be identified by means of a Wright's stain or a wet mount. The Gram stain is not recommended for this purpose because it may be difficult to distinguish eosinophils from other polymorphonuclear leukocytes with this preparation. Charcot-Leyden crystals (crystallized granules liberated by eosinophils),

Table 9.6.
Regimen for status asthmaticus.

Diagnostic Measures	Therapeutic Measures
1. Vital signs (including pulsus paradoxus)	1. Quiet room
2. Flow rates (peak flow or FEV_1)	2. Rehydration
3. Arterial blood-gas levels	3. Supplemental oxygen
4. Gram stain and Wright's stain of sputum	4. Epinephrine or terbutaline subcutaneously, or inhaled isoproterenol
5. Sputum culture	
6. Chest x-ray film	5. Aminophylline intravenously
7. Total eosinophil count	6. Corticosteroids if Nos. 1–5 unsuccessful in first 2 hours
8. Serum aminophylline level (if indicated)	7. Antibiotics (if indicated)

Curschmann spirals (mucus and other debris in the form of bronchiolar casts), and Creola bodies (compact clusters of columnar epithelial cells, often with cilia that are still beating) also are seen in the sputum. The eosinophil count in the blood is often elevated; if it is not, it may suggest the presence of infection.

Arterial blood-gas determinations are important to assess impairment of gas exchange, and simple pulmonary function tests (FEV_1, peak flow) to evaluate the degree of obstruction. These studies not only indicate the severity of disease but also provide baseline information with which to evaluate response to therapy. With a mild attack the PaO_2 may be normal or reduced because of ventilation-perfusion inequality and right-to-left shunting of blood, but the $PaCO_2$ may be low (less than 40 mm Hg) because of hyperventilation of the alveoli. With increasing obstruction the patient is no longer able to hyperventilate and the $PaCO_2$ becomes normal. In the presence of a severe asthmatic attack, a normal $PaCO_2$ frequently indicates deterioration and is a good criterion for hospitalization. With further deterioration, alveolar hypoventilation occurs, with a $PaCO_2$ greater than 40 mm Hg. At this point, close monitoring is warranted, and intubation with mechanical ventilation must be considered.

Other diagnostic measures, such as a chest x-ray film, electrocardiogram, and Gram stains and cultures, also are indicated to evaluate possible etiologic factors.

Treatment

Therapy is primarily directed at the causes of airway obstruction. Bronchoconstriction due to spasm of the smooth muscle, mucosal edema due to inflammation, and the presence of viscous, inspissated secretions in the bronchial lumina must be corrected.

Since bronchoconstriction is reduced by cAMP in the smooth muscle cells, pharmacologic agents that increase cAMP are effective in decreasing bronchial smooth muscle tone. Therefore, *β-sym-pathomimetic drugs* and *xanthine derivatives* are the agents of choice. Table 9.7 lists pertinent data for the commonly used drugs. Because all of these agents, even the β-2 agents, cause cardiac irritability, especially in the presence of hypoxia, it is important to know the type and amount of medication taken by the patient before seeking emergency care since this may modify the initial dose. Recent evidence has shown that sequentially inhaled agents such as isoproterenol or metaproterenol result in excellent bronchodilation with minimal side effects. In the administration of inhaled bronchodilators, intermittent positive-pressure breathing (IPPB) has no advantage over simple hand-held nebulizers and canisters, and may increase morbidity. Additional evidence has shown that subcutaneous epinephrine (1:1000), 0.5 ml, represents optimal initial catecholamine therapy, as demonstrated in improvement of PEFR, with no significant change in heart rate or pulse as compared with lower doses. In the presence of cardiac irritability, β-sympathomimetic agents with more β-2 activity (affecting bronchial smooth muscle receptors) than β-1 activity (affecting cardiac muscle receptors) may be preferable, for example, terbutaline sulfate or salbutamol (albuterol). The onset of action of β-sympathomimetic drugs does not occur for 5–10 minutes, and effects may not peak for 30 or more minutes. Serial measurement of PEFR can demonstrate continued bronchodilation in responsive patients up to 40 minutes after initial treatment. Such careful monitoring thereby can dictate prudent repeated administration of these sympathomimetic agents.

The pulse rate should be monitored when any bronchodilator is administered; despite the sympathomimetic effect of the drug, it usually remains stable or decreases as bronchospasm is relieved, with obstruction and hypoxemia being corrected. Although serum theophylline determinations are helpful in monitoring aminophylline therapy, they are rarely readily available. Instead, it is common to administer sufficient intravenous aminophylline to induce at least mild tachycardia so that some

Table 9.7.
Medications for status asthmaticus.

Medication	Route of Administration	Dosage	Side Effects
		70 kg	
β-sympathomimetic agents			
Epinephrine			
Aqueous 1:1000	Subcutaneous	0.3 ml (0.2–0.5 ml) every 15–20 min	All β-sympathomimetic agents:
Terbutaline sulfate	Subcutaneous	0.25 mg (0.2–0.5 mg) every 30–45 min	CNS stimulation
			Anxiety, restlessness
			Insomnia
			Headache
			Tremor
Isoproterenol 1:200	Aerosol	0.5 ml in 1.5 ml saline every 4–6 hr or 1 puff from inhaler every 20 min 5 times	Cardiac
			Tachycardia
			Arrhythmias
			Hypertension
Isoetharine, 1%, and phenylephrine, 0.25% (Bronkosol)	Aerosol	0.5 ml in 1.5 ml saline every 4–6 hr	
Salbutamol	Aerosol	1–2 puffs (90–180 μg) every 4 hr	
Xanthine derivatives			
Aminophylline	Intravenous	5–7 mg/kg over 20 min if no theophylline has been given, and 0.6 mg/kg/hr in adult smokers younger than 50, or 0.4 mg/kg/hr for otherwise healthy adults and adults older than 50, or 0.2 mg/kg/hr for adults with cardiac decompensation or hepatic dysfunction	CNS stimulation
			Anxiety, restlessness
			Insomnia
			Tremor
			Seizures
			Cardiac
			Tachycardia
			Arrhythmias
			Vascular
			Peripheral vasodilation
			CNS vasoconstriction
			Renal
			Diuresis
			Gastrointestinal
			Nausea, vomiting
Corticosteroids			
Methylprednisolone sodium succinate or equivalent	Intravenous	80–100 mg every 4–6 hr	Short-term
			Electrolyte disturbances
			Hypokalemia
			Hypochloremia
			Metabolic alkalosis
			Hyperglycemia
			Fluid retention
			Gastrointestinal upset
			CNS stimulation
			Nervousness
			Insomnia
			Seizures
			Psychosis
			Possible exacerbation of ulcer disease
			Long-term
			Infection
			Peptic ulcer
			Myopathy
			Osteoporosis

CNS = central nervous system.

physiologic effect of the drug is noted. The side effects and toxicity of aminophylline have been appreciated over the past few years, and further modification of initial and maintenance doses has been recommended (page 163).

On occasion, after administration of a bronchodilator, flow rates improve, but the Pa_{O_2} decreases. Normally, in regions of the lung with a low PA_{O_2} because of decreased ventilation, reflex vasoconstriction occurs that shunts blood away from the area. This vasoconstrictive response to regional hypoxia can be overcome by the vasodilating effect of these drugs; perfusion of these areas results in a decreased ventilation-perfusion ratio and increased right-to-left shunting of blood, causing increased hypoxemia. The decrease in Pa_{O_2}, however, is usually not clinically significant.

Corticosteroids are of significant value in the treatment of status asthmaticus, although their effect may be delayed. They exert a facilitating or permissive effect on adrenergic receptors, thus increasing the bronchodilating effect of the β-sympathomimetic agents. Also, their anti-inflammatory action reduces mucosal inflammation.

Although the effects of corticosteroids may not be evident for 6–24 hours, it is appropriate to administer them early and in high doses, for example, methylprednisolone sodium succinate, 100 mg intravenously every 4–6 hours. There is little evidence that short courses of high doses exacerbate ulcer disease or tuberculosis. The most common error in the management of status asthmaticus is not excessive administration of corticosteroids, but rather "too little, too late." It is better to start administration in the first hours of a poorly reversible attack since it can be stopped abruptly even after 3–4 days with no fear of adrenal suppression.

The clinical effect of corticosteroids is correlated with the decrease in eosinophils in the peripheral blood. Serial eosinophil counts over a few days will document the effect of the drug or the patient's resistance. If there are still more than 50 eosinophils/mm^3 after 48 hours of corticosteroids, the dose should be doubled.

Inhalant corticosteroids, such as beclomethasone and triamcinolone acetonide, which are not absorbed, tend to be of little value in the treatment of status asthmaticus since they are poorly distributed to the lung. Parenteral corticosteroids should be given initially, with a change to oral corticosteroids as the patient's condition improves. Inhalant corticosteroids should be given only to patients whose condition is stable to reduce symptoms unrelieved by xanthine derivatives and β-sympathomimetic agents.

Removal of bronchial secretions is facilitated by *rehydration* and pulmonary toilet. The signs of dehydration include dry skin, "tenting" of the skin, dry mucous membranes, and postural hypotension. The specific gravity of the urine is elevated, and the blood urea nitrogen level may also be increased. The patient with status asthmaticus is commonly dehydrated, and it may be necessary to restore fluids intravenously if he is too dyspneic to drink adequate amounts of fluid. Although ultrasonic mist with distilled water provides rehydration, it may induce bronchospasm and worsen the asthma attack. Nothing is to be gained from overhydration, and only replacement of the amount of body fluid lost is necessary.

Hypoxia may be relieved with uncontrolled *oxygen* administration, preferably by nasal cannula since face masks are poorly tolerated. Oxygen therapy also results in reduction of arrhythmias and right heart strain due to hypoxic pulmonary vasoconstriction.

In the patient with asthma uncomplicated by another condition, administration of oxygen presents no problems since the Pa_{CO_2} is still a potent stimulus to breathing. Even as the patient tires and the Pa_{CO_2} increases, oxygen administration offers little hazard since the carbon dioxide stimulus is still present, although the patient is simply too weak to respond to it. It is possible that a high Pa_{O_2} will slightly dampen the ventilatory drive of a patient who is retaining carbon dioxide, and for this reason, supplemental oxygen is usually given only to raise the Pa_{O_2} to between 50 and 60 mm Hg, at which level most persons still have a hypoxic drive, but have had reversal of the hypoxic pulmonary vasoconstriction. If it is unclear whether the acute wheezing episode is superimposed on chronic obstructive pulmonary disease such as bronchitis or emphysema, carbon dioxide retention demands judicious use of supplemental oxygen since chronic carbon dioxide retention may in fact be present.

Carbon dioxide retention is partly relieved by oral and aerosol bronchodilators and pulmonary toilet. Chest physical therapy (percussion) is often helpful in promoting pulmonary toilet as the patient recovers from the acute attack. Dyspnea is often too severe initially for the patient to tolerate physical therapy.

The decision to intubate is based on clinical findings. The response of patients to hypoxia and hypercapnia is variable. Inability to raise the Pa_{O_2} to 50 mm Hg with supplemental oxygen or the presence of a Pa_{CO_2} above 40 mm Hg is usually ominous and demands close monitoring with strong consideration of intubation.

Blood-gas levels should be determined at the onset of management if the initial PEFR is less than 100 liters/min so that the degree of impairment can be assessed, the patient's progress followed, and appropriate therapy administered. For example, rapid deterioration may indicate that the patient will soon require intubation, and thus the procedure can be performed under optimal conditions.

Infection, which is usually respiratory, frequently precipitates the asthmatic attack. Gram stains and cultures are required, and if the infection appears to be bacterial, broad-spectrum *antibiotics* are given until the specific antibiotic sensitivities are known. Some clinicians advise starting therapy for respiratory tract infection in all patients with status asthmaticus. Tetracycline or ampicillin is most commonly given unless the Gram stain of the sputum suggests organisms resistant to these drugs, such as staphylococci or *pseudomonas.*

Several measures commonly employed for the treatment of asthma are of questionable value. An expectorant—either glyceryl guaiacolate or potassium iodide—frequently is prescribed. These have been shown to increase mucus production in animals, but whether increased mucus production results in mobilization of secretions or further bronchial plugging has yet to be determined.

Sedatives are also frequently prescribed for the tired patient who is unable to sleep because of cough, dyspnea, and anxiety. Sedatives, antitussive agents, tranquilizers, and antihistamines all may cause respiratory depression, and are contraindicated in patients with status asthmaticus and compromised ventilation. The patient's anxiety usually resolves as breathing improves. If intubation and mechanical ventilation are performed, however, adequate sedation is warranted for the patient to be comfortable.

In the United States, atropine has not been used to treat status asthmaticus for many years because of the fear that excessive drying of bronchial secretions increases inspissation. However, atropine and its analogues do act as bronchodilators by inhibiting the effect of acetylcholine released by the vagus nerve. Atropine has been used successfully in the United Kingdom and holds promise as valuable adjunctive therapy.

Several drugs used to treat chronic asthma and allergies have little or no role in the therapy for status asthmaticus. These drugs include cromolyn sodium (sodium cromoglycate), which stabilizes the membrane of the mast cell, but has no direct bronchodilating effect; inhalant corticosteroids, which are less effective than parenteral and oral corticosteroids and which are not recommended for severely ill patients; and antihistamines, which may, in fact, cause respiratory depression and drying of bronchial secretions. Use of nonsteroidal anti-inflammatory agents in the treatment of chronic asthma remains speculative. The mechanism by which certain drugs such as motrin and aspirin inhibit prostaglandin and thromboxane formation with subsequent influence on bronchodilation or bronchoconstriction in certain responsive asthmatic patients is under investigation. The fear remains in many patients that they may be allergic to aspirin and that the aspirin will worsen rather than help the asthma.

Since anxiety can increase or even cause bronchospasm, placing the patient in a quiet room may be helpful. Flowers, kapok, and feather pillows, as well as other possible allergens, should not be allowed in the room. Likewise, cigarette smoking should be forbidden for the patient and his visitors.

Hospitalization and Outpatient Regimen

When a patient is treated for status asthmaticus in an emergency ward, a decision must be made whether to admit him. If the attack has not subsided after 2–3 hours of therapy, the patient should be hospitalized. Furthermore, a bronchospastic, anxious patient with hypoxia and a normal $Paco_2$ who is unable to hyperventilate should be admitted for observation and continued intensive therapy. Other considerations, such as the ability of the patient to take medications as prescribed, the home situation (especially if this is an aggravating factor), and a history of severe, prolonged attacks, must be considered before discharging the patient.

When the condition of the hospitalized patient improves, he should begin to receive medications orally. The usual regimen is prednisone, 40 mg/day for 5 days followed by tapering of the dosage by 10 mg/day; aminophylline, 200 mg four times a day; metaproterenol sulfate (Alupent), 20 mg three times a day, or terbutaline, 2.5 mg three times a day, or salbutamol, 90–180 μg every 4–6 hours (1–2 puffs); and a 1% solution of isoetharine, 0.5 ml in 2 ml of saline administered via nebulizer. This must be tailored to meet the patient's needs and ability to tolerate the side effects.

The outpatient regimen must also be individualized. The usual order of initiating medications is: (1) a β-sympathomimetic agent given either by inhalation or as a tablet or in conjunction; (2) an aminophylline preparation; (3) an inhalant corticosteroid (beclomethasone); and (4) an oral corticosteroid given at the lowest dose possible and preferably every other day. Inhaled beclomethasone is best given after administration of an inhaled β-sympathomimetic agent to ensure the best dispersal of this agent, which only works topically. In patients who have been receiving long-term prednisone therapy, treatment cannot be abruptly changed to beclomethasone without danger of hypoadrenalism.

Acute exacerbations should be treated aggressively with antibiotics and oral corticosteroids. The patient should be educated to note early changes in the production or color of sputum, increased wheezing, and dyspnea in order to institute vigorous therapy early.

ACUTE DECOMPENSATION OF CHRONIC RESPIRATORY FAILURE

As long as cigarette smoking and air pollution persist, chronic bronchitis and emphysema will continue to cause illness and death. Although it is often useful to separate these diseases because of their distinct pathologies and for the purpose of therapy and prognosis, in the end stage—when respiratory failure most often occurs—their differences are less apparent and their treatment is usually similar. Thus they will be considered in this section as one syndrome best described by their common physiologic defect, chronic airways obstruction (CAO).

Whereas the complications of chronic bronchitis and emphysema are many, their common natural course is the progressive loss of pulmonary function punctuated by episodes of acute respiratory failure. Despite an apparent inability to prevent or to cure the underlying disease processes, advances have been made in the outpatient management of CAO. Early empirical antibiotic treatment of bronchitis flare-ups and yearly immunizations against influenza, which are standard procedures in most chest clinics, may prevent acute decompensation. Use of home and portable equipment for delivery of low-flow oxygen clearly diminishes the discomfort of daily activities for many hypoxemic patients and restores some to gainful employment. In the hypoxic patient, life expectancy is also increased by low-flow oxygen. In the treatment of patients with severe bronchospasm, new and improved bronchodilator drugs have made a major impact.

Despite the best in outpatient management, acute decompensation of chronic respiratory failure still occurs. The purpose of this section is to review the pathophysiology and treatment of such decompensation and to emphasize its differences from the treatment of acute respiratory failure uncomplicated by underlying obstructive lung disease. Although intubation and assisted ventilation sometimes are required in the management of decompensated chronic respiratory failure, they should be necessary only after conservative measures have failed, since their results are usually much poorer and their complications more frequent than in patients without prior pulmonary disease. The explanation for this distinction lies in the pathophysiology of chronic hypercapnia, an understanding of which has led to reliance on continuous low-flow oxygen as the mainstay of therapy for acute decompensation. Before therapeutic guidelines are detailed, it is important to review the pathophysiologic principles relevant to carbon dioxide retention, acid-base regulation, respiratory control, and oxygen transport as they apply to chronic respiratory failure.

Carbon Dioxide Retention

Carbon dioxide is both a waste product of aerobic metabolism and a vital participant in acid-base homeostasis. Although it is artificial to separate these interrelated roles, carbon dioxide is considered here as a potentially toxic byproduct, the elimination of which is a major function of the respiratory system. Whenever an excretory organ is obstructed, the result is retention of the product to be excreted. Thus, it is not surprising that carbon dioxide retention can result from chronic bronchitis and emphysema, since airways obstruction is their fundamental physiologic aberration. The unanswered question is why some patients with comparably obstructed airways retain carbon dioxide while others do not. Several theories have been advanced, but none is totally satisfactory.

One factor agreed to be important to the development and treatment of carbon dioxide retention is the work of breathing. Although expiration is normally a passive process, breathing against obstructed airways requires energy and can account for a large part of resting oxygen consumption and carbon dioxide production in the severely obstructed patient.

The Pa_{CO_2} is determined not only by the volume of air moving in and out of the alveoli each minute but also by the amount of carbon dioxide produced and, in the steady state, excreted each minute, as expressed by the following equation in which 0.863 is a constant:

$$Pa_{CO_2} = \frac{CO_2 \text{ production (or excretion)}}{\text{alveolar ventilation}} \times 0.863$$

Normally, carbon dioxide production is relatively constant and Pa_{CO_2} is a reciprocal function of alveolar ventilation. As alveolar ventilation increases, Pa_{CO_2} decreases. With severe airways obstruction, however, the work required to increase ventilation results in an increase in carbon dioxide production and renders the added ventilation less effective in lowering Pa_{CO_2}. The oxygen required to increase ventilation, moreover, is no longer available for use by other tissues. Chronic hypercapnia therefore may be thought of as a physiologic compromise that conserves oxygen for nonventilatory use and that at the same time minimizes carbon dioxide production. In the steady state, carbon dioxide excretion again equals carbon dioxide production, but at a higher total body content of carbon dioxide. Higher tissue, venous, and alveolar P_{CO_2} allows more carbon dioxide to be eliminated per breath and, thus, fewer breaths per minute to maintain the balance of production and excretion. Patients with chronic respiratory failure live for long periods in this compensated state until factors such as excessive bronchial secretions and bronchospasm further increase the work of breathing, upset the equilibrated state, and cause acute carbon dioxide retention. Most effective therapeutic modalities such as bronchodilators, antibiotics, and chest physical therapy work by decreasing airway resistance, lowering the work of breathing and restoring equilibrium. Mechanical ventilation also helps relieve the work of breathing, although it acts primarily in the inspiratory phase, leaving expiratory work for the patient.

If carbon dioxide is a potentially noxious byproduct, how do patients with chronic respiratory failure tolerate such excessive amounts? The answer is the slow rate with which chronic hypercapnia develops. The toxicity of rapidly developing or extremely high levels of carbon dioxide can be thought of as both pharmacologic and physical.

Pharmacologic Effects of Carbon Dioxide Retention

The pharmacologic effects of carbon dioxide retention are closely related to its role in acid-base chemistry. Carbon dioxide is normally transported from tissues to the lungs largely as bicarbonate ion formed by the reaction of dissolved carbon dioxide with water:

dissolved
$$CO_2 + H_2O \rightleftharpoons H_2CO_3 \rightleftharpoons H^+ + HCO_3^-$$
carbonic
anhydrase

The reaction occurs extremely rapidly in the presence of carbonic anhydrase found in red blood cells; it also occurs more slowly in the absence of this enzyme. Since hydrogen ions are formed in the process, carbon dioxide is potentially a weak acid. Normally the hydrogen ions are buffered by hemoglobin and plasma proteins, which allows the reaction to go to the right. When bicarbonate reaches the pulmonary capillary bed, the process is reversed and carbon dioxide is eliminated as a gas. Smaller amounts of carbon dioxide are transported as carbamino compounds, carbonic acid, and dissolved carbon dioxide.

With acute carbon dioxide retention, hydrogen ions are produced in excess of blood buffering capacity and acidemia results. The mechanisms that exist to minimize pH change in acute and chronic hypercapnia are discussed on pages (168–170).

The signs and symptoms of carbon dioxide toxicity due to acidosis or due to direct effects of carbon dioxide so overlap with the manifestations of hypoxemia that it is unrealistic to separate them. Restlessness, tachycardia, confusion, diaphoresis, jerking tremor, headache, and various degrees of stupor are nonspecific and may not even be present despite severe hypoxemia or hypercapnia. The diagnosis of acute respiratory failure must be based on arterial blood-gas determinations.

Physical Effects of Carbon Dioxide Retention

Dalton's law states that the pressure exerted by each component of a gas mixture is independent of the other gases in the mixture and that the total pressure exerted is the sum of the individual gas pressures. Because alveoli are in contact with atmospheric pressure via the airways, total alveolar gas pressure is considered atmospheric. Since water vapor and nitrogen pressures vary relatively little, carbon dioxide shares the alveolar space with only one other variable gas, oxygen, as expressed in the simplified alveolar gas equation. For convenience the readily obtained Pa_{CO_2} is substituted for PA_{CO_2} since the two values are usually almost identical:

$$PA_{O_2} = \text{inspired } P_{O_2} - \frac{Pa_{CO_2}}{R}$$

If equal amounts of oxygen and carbon dioxide are exchanged, R, the respiratory quotient, equals 1 and the relationship is reciprocal; that is, PA_{O_2} must decrease 1 mm Hg for each 1 mm Hg rise in Pa_{CO_2} since total gas pressure does not change. When R is the usual 0.8, as it is when 200 ml of carbon dioxide is produced for each 250 ml of oxygen taken up per minute, the decrease in PA_{O_2} for a given increase in Pa_{CO_2} is even greater. Unlike the case with P_{CO_2}, a gradient always exists between alveolar and arterial Po_2. The Pao_2 will therefore follow the change in PAo_2, but will be lower.

Using these facts, McNicol and Campbell theorized that in untreated patients with respiratory failure the rise in $PAco_2$ would displace enough oxygen from the alveoli that life-threatening hypoxemia (Pao_2 less than 25 mm Hg) would result before the $Paco_2$ would reach dangerous levels ($Paco_2$ greater than 80 mm Hg, pH less than 7.20). Patients with a $Paco_2$ much higher than 80 mm Hg, therefore, must have been supported by prior oxygen therapy to allow the $Paco_2$ to rise to that level without lethal hypoxemia.

The prediction of McNicol and Campbell proved true in a large series of previously untreated patients with decompensation of known chronic respiratory failure. They found that whereas most patients had a $Paco_2$ between 60 and 80 mm Hg and a pH between 7.22 and 7.44, the majority had a Pao_2 between 25 and 40 mm Hg. The body normally has large carbon dioxide stores and appears to tolerate $Paco_2$ increases of this magnitude relatively well, especially when they develop slowly, allowing the body's buffer systems to minimize pH shifts. Oxygen stores, however, are small, and severe hypoxemia like that observed by McNicol and Campbell can rapidly lead to tissue injury. These data, therefore, not only illustrate the physical consequences of carbon dioxide retention but also emphasize that it is usually hypoxemia, not hypercapnia in itself, that is life threatening to the CAO patients with acute respiratory failure who is seen in the emergency ward. Oxygen therapy in this setting, therefore, is paramount and is considered on pages 172–174.

Acid-Base Regulation in Acute and Chronic Hypercapnia

Carbon dioxide retention results in $[H^+]$ increase through the hydration reaction. Multiple buffer systems interact, however, to minimize pH changes due to respiratory or metabolic causes. The understanding of these complex acid-base interactions is greatly simplified by the belief that changes in one buffer pair—carbonic acid and its conjugate base, bicarbonate—are representative of changes in all other buffer systems with which the pair are in equilibrium. The physicochemical relationship of the three variable components of the carbonic acid system, pH, $Paco_2$, and $[HCO_3^-]$, is given by the Henderson-Hasselbalch equation, in which α is the solubility coefficient for carbon dioxide and

pK is a constant:

$$pH = pK + \log \frac{[HCO_3^-]}{\alpha \cdot Paco_2}$$

The equation states that when $Paco_2$ is elevated, pH will decrease unless $[HCO_3^-]$ rises by an amount proportional to the rise in $Paco_2$. When hypercapnia is acute, the readily available sources for buffering hydrogen ions and for elevating $[HCO_3^-]$ are easily depleted and pH falls. In the first 24 hours after the onset of hypercapnia, buffering of excess hydrogen ions is almost entirely due to cellular proteins. The hydrogen ions enter the blood and tissue cells in exchange for potassium and sodium ions, and chloride enters in exchange for biocarbonate:

dissolved
$$CO_2 + H_2O \rightleftharpoons H_2CO_3 \rightleftharpoons H^+ + HCO_3^-$$

$$HCO_3^- \leftarrow \text{cellular} \rightarrow K^+$$
$$\text{protein}$$
$$Cl^- \rightarrow \text{buffers} \rightarrow Na^+$$

The net result of the limited cellular buffering of acute hypercapnia is only a small increase in the calculated $[HCO_3^-]$ and a relatively large decrease in pH.

When hypercapnia is prolonged, $[HCO_3^-]$ increases to levels well above that achievable in the first 24 hours, raising pH toward normal and replenishing cellular buffers depleted during the acute period. Increased renal retention of bicarbonate accounts for most of the improved pH regulation, although hydrogen is also eliminated in the urine as ammonium and other titratable acids. For electrochemical balance, chloride is excreted as bicarbonate is retained.

Because acute and chronic respiratory acidosis usually require distinct therapies, their differentiation is important. Acid-base diagrams like that proposed by Goldberg et al. (Fig. 9.8) are helpful in the rapid interpretation of arterial blood-gas findings. According to the diagram, a patient with a $Paco_2$ of 80 mm Hg has acute respiratory acidosis if the pH is between 7.14 and 7.18, chronic respiratory acidosis if the pH is between 7.24 and 7.32, and acute decompensation of a chronic respiratory acidosis if the pH is between the bands, that is, 7.18–7.24.

At the bedside it is helpful to estimate the change in hydrogen ion concentration ($\Delta[H^+]$) expected for a change in $Paco_2$ ($\Delta Paco_2$) by use of the following two relationships:
Acute respiratory acidosis:

$$\Delta[H^+] = 0.8 \times \Delta Paco_2$$

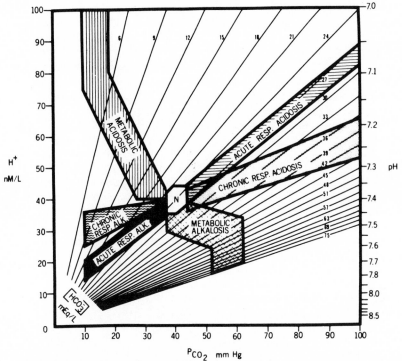

Figure 9.8. Acid-base diagram. *Shaded areas* represent the normal response anticipated for P_{CO_2}, [HCO_3^-], and pH or [H^+] for each of the six simple acid-base disturbances. Numbered lines are bicarbonate isopleths in milliequivalents per liter. (Reproduced by permission, from *JAMA 233:*269–275, © 1973, by The American Medical Association.)

Chronic respiratory acidosis:

$$\Delta[H^+] = 0.3 \times \Delta P_{aCO_2}$$

The substitution of [H^+] for pH eliminates the logarithm and allows use of a linear relationship. Hydrogen ion concentration can be estimated by its coincidental relationship with pH whereby the two decimal digits of the pH are numerically similar to and vary reciprocally with the [H^+] expressed in nanomoles per liter within the clinically important pH range of 7.10–7.50:

pH	[H^+]
7.10	70 nmol/liter
7.20	60 nmol/liter
7.30	50 nmol/liter
7.40	40 nmol/liter
7.50	30 nmol/liter

Problem: Do the following arterial blood-gas data—pH 7.35; P_{CO_2}, 60 mm Hg; P_{O_2}, 40 mm Hg—represent acute or chronic respiratory acidosis?

Solution: Consult an acid-base diagram (Fig. 9.8) or use the bedside estimate as just outlined:

$$\Delta P_{aCO_2} = 60 \text{ mm Hg} - 40 \text{ mm Hg (normal)} = 20 \text{ mm Hg}$$

If this is a chronic condition, the [H^+] increase is predicted by

$$\Delta[H^+] = 0.3 \times \Delta P_{aCO_2}$$
$$= 0.3 \times 20$$
$$= 6 \text{ nmol/liter}$$

Predicted [H^+] = 40 nmol/liter (normal) + 6 nmol/liter = 46 nmol/liter. Using the reciprocal [H^+]-pH relationship:

[H^+]	pH
40 nmol/liter	7.40
46 nmol/liter	7.34

An increase in [H^+] of 6 nmol/liter equals a decrease in pH of 0.06 unit.

The measured pH, 7.35, is close to the 7.34 predicted for chronic respiratory acidosis. If hypercapnia were acute, a much greater decrease in pH would be predicted:

$$\Delta[H^+] = 0.8 \times \Delta P_{aCO_2}$$
$$= 0.8 \times 20$$
$$= 16 \text{ nmol/liter}$$

Predicted [H^+] = 40 nmol/liter + 16 nmol/liter

= 56 nmol/liter. Using the reciprocal [H$^+$] - pH relationship:

$$\frac{[H^+]}{56 \text{ nmol/liter}} = \frac{pH}{7.24}$$

The measured pH 7.35 was not nearly so low as would be predicted in acute respiratory acidosis. In this example, there has evidently been time for both cellular and renal mechanisms to modify the change in pH.

A pH of 7.30 in the same example would be compatible with either decompensated chronic respiratory acidosis or acute respiratory acidosis prior to maximal renal compensation.

This problem illustrates the use of acid-base diagrams and bedside formulas in the diagnosis of hypercapnia as acute, chronic, or acute superimposed on chronic. Aside from ease, the advantage of using an acid-base diagram over using the bedside approximations is that the diagrams provide a range of biologic variation whereas the regression equations do not. Without some guide to normal variance, there is no way at the bedside to predict whether a given acid-base permutation is explainable by a single disturbance or whether multiple disturbances are more likely. It must be remembered that patients with acute respiratory distress, especially the elderly and those with multisystem disease, frequently have more than one acid-base disturbance. The diagnoses suggested by the acid-base diagram are meaningful only in the context of a careful history and physical examination in which causes of nonrespiratory acidosis and alkalosis are sought. Diuretic therapy resulting in hypochloremic hypokalemic metabolic alkalosis is probably the most common concomitant disturbance. Lactic acidosis is much less common in patients with respiratory failure, occurring in the setting of severe hypoxemia combined with impaired circulation due to peripheral vascular disease or congestive heart failure. Serum electrolyte determinations are therefore a vital part of acid-base assessment. Not only do they reveal the presence of hypokalemia or hypochloremia but also the calculation of an elevated unmeasured anion (see Chapter 1) may provide the only readily available clue to lactic acidosis. A serum lactic acid determination is confirmatory.

In the clinical setting, Kettel et al. plotted the pH and PaCO$_2$ values obtained before, during, and after 87 consecutive episodes of acute ventilatory failure in patients with CAO. The confidence bands in Figure 9.9 are similar to those in the complete acid-base diagram (Fig. 9.8). As expected, most values 24 or more hours before acute decompensation (Fig. 9.9A) fell within the chronic

hypercapnia band and returned there after successful treatment (Fig. 9.9C). A PaCO$_2$ of 65 mm Hg or more was usually associated with an abnormal pH even in the chronic state. During the acute episodes, most values were between the acute and chronic bands (Fig. 9.9B). The extremely high PaCO$_2$ values achieved by some patients indicate that they had been supported with prior oxygen therapy (see page 174).

In addition to confirming the usefulness of the acid-base diagram, the above data suggest rational goals in the treatment of patients with CAO. The findings before and after the acute episodes indicate that no purpose is served by correcting pH or PaCO$_2$ in acute respiratory decompensation beyond what the patient can achieve in the chronic well-compensated state.

Chronic Hypercapnia and Control of Respiration

The pH of the blood is regulated less well in response to an acute change in PaCO$_2$ and relatively better when hypercapnia is sustained. The pH of the brain interstitial fluid as reflected in the cerebrospinal fluid is normally slightly lower than that of blood and even better protected against chronic PaCO$_2$ elevation, which suggests that pH may be critical to the brain's complex functions. Carbon dioxide retained in respiratory failure crosses the blood-brain barrier readily and produces acidosis. As in the blood, pH regulation in the brain appears to be due to bicarbonate accumulation. Although initial cellular buffering is ineffective in preventing brain acidosis in acute hypercapnia, within hours of the onset of an elevated PaCO$_2$ the bicarbonate level in the cerebrospinal fluid begins to increase, which results in a pH closer to normal than that of the blood in chronic hypercapnia. Some of the bicarbonate increase appears to be due to endogenous production, while another portion enters the cerebrospinal fluid from the circulation.

These findings would be no more than physiologic curiosities to all but the neuroscientist were it not for the presence of the [H$^+$]-sensitive respiratory center within the brain substance. The elevated brain bicarbonate level in chronic hypercapnia minimizes the [H$^+$] change resulting from further increases in PaCO$_2$ and therefore lessens the respiratory center output for a given PaCO$_2$ stimulus. In the clinical setting this is seen as a flattened carbon dioxide ventilatory response curve when such patients are tested.

The carotid bodies sense the oxygen tension of the arterial blood and ordinarily begin to respond with a strong ventilatory stimulus when a PaO$_2$ of

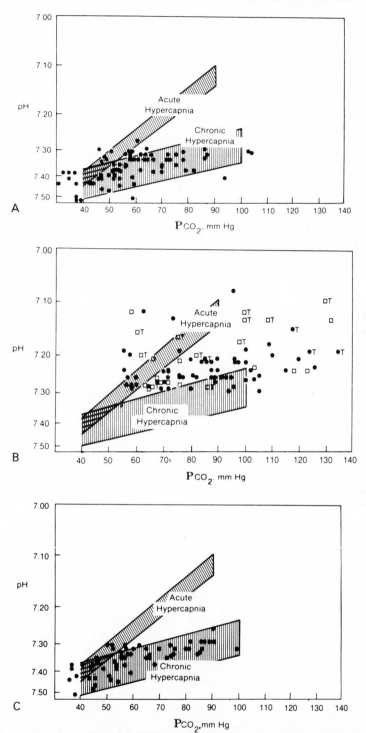

Figure 9.9.   Acid-base values observed in CAO patients before, during, and after acute respiratory decompensation. Shaded areas are similar to those in right upper quadrant of Figure 9.8. **(A)** Arterial blood-gas values 24 hours or more before 87 episodes of acute respiratory decompensation. **(B)** Arterial blood-gas values during acute respiratory decompensation at time of lowest observed pH. Episodes of acute respiratory acidosis from which patient survived (●) and episodes that resulted in death (□) are shown. *T* identifies episodes in which tracheal intubation was used with mechanically assisted ventilation. **(C)** Arterial blood-gas values after acute respiratory decompensation. Values shown are those observed closest to normal pH. (Reproduced by permission, from *JAMA 217*:1503–1508, © 1971, by the American Medical Association.)

50 mm Hg or less occurs. Although this response to hypoxia usually plays a minor role in respiratory control in healthy persons, because of diminished Pa_{CO_2} responsiveness, patients with chronic hypercapnia often rely on the hypoxic drive to ventilate. Relief of the hypoxic drive by uncontrolled oxygen therapy may lead to acute ventilatory depression with marked carbon dioxide retention and acidosis. Use of controlled oxygen therapy, however, can provide adequate oxygen delivery to tissues with only insignificant increases in Pa_{CO_2}.

Controlled Oxygen Therapy

Patients with chronic respiratory failure often live productive lives with moderate degrees of hypoxemia without need of oxygen therapy. When hypoxemia becomes severe either acutely or gradually, symptoms may develop and supplemental oxygen is indicated. As in hypercapnia, the symptoms and signs of hypoxemia are nonspecific, and its accurate assessment depends on measurement of arterial oxygen tension. Cyanosis, which is thought to require 5 gm of reduced hemoglobin per 100 ml, is particularly unreliable as an index of hypoxemia, occurring at lower oxygen tensions in severe anemia and at higher oxygen tensions when peripheral blood flow is impaired, which allows greater oxygen extraction.

An adequate oxygen supply to tissues depends not only on the Pa_{O_2} but also on adequate amounts of hemoglobin capable of carrying oxygen and on sufficient cardiac output and local circulation to deliver it to the tissues.

Figure 9.10 depicts the oxygen-hemoglobin dissociation curve. The x-axis expresses hemoglobin saturation. The next scale to the left, which assumes a normal hemoglobin concentration of 15 gm/100 ml, gives the oxygen content of the blood. Based on a normal cardiac output of 5 liters/min, the next scale estimates oxygen supply to tissues. Finally, since tissues cannot extract the last 20% of oxygen from the blood, the scale furthest to the left predicts the oxygen actually available to tissues at a given Pa_{O_2}. Since the healthy person at rest requires at least 200 ml of oxygen per minute, the lowest tolerable level of hemoglobin saturation is estimated at 40% (P_{O_2}, 25 mm Hg). This would prove inadequate, however, in the presence of increased metabolic demands, severe anemia, congestive heart failure, or impaired peripheral circulation.

Fortunately, the remarkable properties of the hemoglobin molecule make therapy for hypoxemia relatively easy. The oxygen-hemoglobin dissociation curve is steep in its unsaturated portion, so small increases in Pa_{O_2} result in relatively large increases in saturation and, therefore, in oxygen content and supply to the tissues. A 15 mm Hg

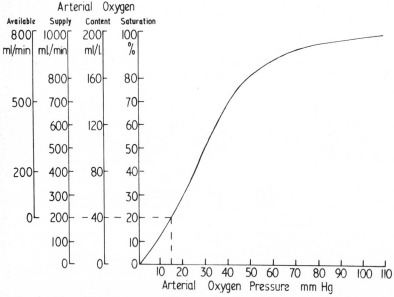

Figure 9.10. Oxygen-hemoglobin dissociation curve and oxygen supply. Vertical scale labeled *Content* assumes a normal hemoglobin level of 15 gm/100 ml. Oxygen *supply* to tissues is calculated on the basis of a normal cardiac output of 5 liters/min. *Available* oxygen assumes that tissues are unable to extract the last 20% of oxygen from hemoglobin. (Reproduced by permission, from Campbell EJM: The J. Burns Amberson Lecture: The management of acute respiratory failure in chronic bronchitis and emphysema. *Am Rev Respir Dis* 96:626–639, 1967.)

increase in PaO_2—from 25 to 40 mm Hg, for example—results in almost a 2½-fold increase in available oxygen. This can often be achieved with only a small increase in inspired oxygen from 21% (ambient air) to 28%. Since the flat (saturated) portion of the curve is reached at about a PaO_2 of 50 mm Hg, further increases in PaO_2 result in relatively small increases in hemoglobin saturation. Oxygen tensions higher than 50 or 60 mm Hg, therefore, result in little benefit and risk dampening the hypoxic stimulus to ventilate on which patients with CAO often depend. In clinical practice, the point at which severe hypoventilation limits oxygen therapy is highly variable and requires a cautious trial-and-error approach monitored by arterial blood-gas determinations 15–20 minutes after each adjustment in oxygen flow. Because of the physiologic considerations just discussed, oxygen therapy should always begin with the lowest controllable concentration and should progress in small increments to higher concentrations. A satisfactory goal is a PaO_2 between 50 and 60 mm Hg, which should be adequate for tissues as estimated by the patient's cerebral function, for example, and which should also result in little increase in $PaCO_2$ or in a stable, tolerable increase as monitored by serial arterial blood-gas determinations.

Adequate oxygen administration is important for yet another reason. Unlike systemic arterioles, which dilate in the presence of tissue hypoxia to permit increased blood flow, the arterioles of the pulmonary vascular tree constrict with alveolar hypoxia, allowing the normal lung to regulate its regional balance of perfusion and ventilation. Were blood flow to continue to a region of the lung where alveoli are underventilated and therefore hypoxic, a low ventilation/perfusion $(\dot{V}/\dot{Q})$ area would exist and contribute to systemic hypoxemia. Local pulmonary vasoconstriction tends to restore the balance between perfusion and ventilation, thus reducing hypoxemia. The design of the pulmonary circulation is such that constriction of as much as half of the pulmonary vasculature normally does not result in a significant increase in pulmonary arterial pressure since the remaining pulmonary vessels may dilate and closed vessels may open. When alveolar hypoxia is generalized, however, most of the pulmonary vasculature is constricted and pulmonary arterial pressure rises. This results in increased work for the right side of the heart, which is normally thin walled and ill equipped to handle a pressure load. Prolonged widespread alveolar hypoxia such as in severe chronic bronchitis can lead to right heart failure (cor pulmonale). Consequently, the treatment of heart failure of this type should be directed primarily not at the heart itself but at the elevated pulmonary arterial pressure and the responsible alveolar hypoxia.

Providing a PAO_2 of 60 mm Hg or more assures minimal pulmonary vasoconstriction. In practice, since alveolar gas tensions are not readily obtainable and since a large alveolar-arterial gradient is known to exist in patients with CAO, a PaO_2 of 50 mm Hg is considered a reasonable goal in preventing reactive pulmonary hypertension. Again the clinician may be faced with the delicate balance between providing enough oxygen to prevent tissue hypoxia and pulmonary vasoconstriction while not suppressing ventilation. Unless the patient is ill enough to require a pulmonary artery catheter to measure right-sided pressure, the clinician must rely on empirical guidelines such as those just presented and, in the long term, on the signs and symptoms of right-sided heart failure.

Careful control of oxygen administration is difficult to achieve with nasal prongs or with face masks whose oxygen delivery rate varies with the patient's ventilation. Development of the venturi mask (see Fig. 1.7), which delivers a predetermined mixture of oxygen and room air regardless of the patient's ventilation, has made controlled oxygen therapy much safer. It must be properly worn, of course, and has the disadvantage of not permitting eating or talking when in place. Such masks are available to deliver 24, 28, 35, and 40% oxygen.

Therapeutic Approach

The previous discussion provides background for the recommendations that follow:

(1) When the patient is apneic or nearly apneic, immediate intubation and mechanical ventilation are indicated.

(2) When spontaneous ventilation is present, arterial blood-gas levels should be determined and oxygen therapy begun with a 24% venturi mask.

(3) The patient's response to therapy must be monitored with serial arterial blood-gas determinations, especially 15–20 minutes after each change in oxygenation or ventilation. Since the time required to obtain results from the blood-gas laboratory may be substantial, it is good practice to return the patient to previously established safe levels of oxygenation or ventilation after arterial blood samples are taken at the new settings. If the values are satisfactory, the new settings can be reestablished.

(4) If the patient has a history or physical signs of long-standing obstructive airways disease or if initial arterial blood-gas levels suggest chronic or

acute-on-chronic respiratory acidosis, a Pa_{O_2} of 50 to 60 mm Hg should be the goal. A mild increase in Pa_{CO_2} is acceptable if it does not produce severe acidosis or clinical signs of carbon dioxide toxicity. An acid-base diagram (Fig. 9.8) or the bedside approximations presented on page 169 are recommended to help interpret the pH and Pa_{CO_2}.

(5) Bicarbonate, 44 mEq at a time by slow intravenous infusion, is required if the pH is less than 7.20 or if it is clearly due to nonrespiratory causes. The pH, serum electrolyte values, and calculated unmeasured anions (anion gap) should be monitored.

(6) Intubation and mechanical ventilation are indicated when: (a) adequate oxygenation cannot be provided without severe carbon dioxide retention and acidosis; and/or (b) there is pharmacologic ventilatory depression or mechanical interference with chest wall function.

There should be nothing in the medical history such as end-stage associated illness or recurrent intractable respiratory failure that raises ethical questions as to the appropriateness of intubation.

(7) The cause of decompensation must be sought and treated. A history of gradual decline with increasing sputum and dyspnea is most common and suggests infection as the cause. More acute failure may also be due to infection, but acute pulmonary embolism, heart failure, and pneumothorax are also considerations. Unless a Gram stain of sputum reveals a predominance of a single organism, a broad-spectrum antibiotic such as tetracycline or ampicillin should be given since *Hemophilus influenzae* is commonly recovered from the sputum of patients with CAO.

(8) Bronchodilators may improve ventilation and reduce the work of breathing. Intravenous aminophylline has the advantage of rapid control, and it can be monitored in some hospitals by serum theophylline levels. It may also provide central respiratory stimulation that may help counteract the ventilatory depression due to oxygen therapy. The intravenous dosage recommended for asthmatic patients (Table 9.7) may require modification for patients with CAO, who are often older and more subject to central nervous system complications and cardiac arrhythmias resulting from aminophylline therapy.

Systemic and topical β-adrenergic drugs act synergistically with aminophylline and should be given to patients in whom an added bronchodilator effect is needed. Inhaled β-2 selective sympathomimetic agents such as albuterol and metaproterenol are extremely useful in patients with CAO who are subject to atrial arrhythmias since the effective dose by aerosol is much less than that required by the oral route. More details on bronchodilators and on corticosteroids that are occasionally required for resistant bronchospasm in patients with CAO may be found on page 163.

(9) Frequent chest physical therapy plays an important role in helping CAO patients clear secretions. Neither physical therapy nor regular side-to-side repositioning of patients should be neglected because of mechanical ventilation, intravenous catheters, or cardiac monitors. Oxygen therapy should not be discontinued during physical therapy or tracheal suction.

(10) Corticosteroids administered intravenously in divided doses over the course of the day have also been shown to hasten recovery of flow rates in decompensation of CAO not due to asthma.

Complications and Special Considerations

(1) Once oxygen therapy is begun, it should be continuous. Because carbon dioxide stores are much greater than oxygen stores in the body, an elevated Pa_{CO_2} due to oxygen therapy stays elevated for several minutes after decrease in alveolar, arterial, and tissue P_{O_2} on discontinuance of supplemental oxygen. The elevated Pa_{CO_2} continues to displace oxygen from the alveolus after the inspired oxygen fraction is lowered and may result in hypoxemia more severe than before treatment.

Whereas venturi masks provide better oxygen control during the initial treatment period, when the patient's condition becomes stabilized, low-flow oxygen by nasal prongs has the advantage of allowing unimpaired eating and speech without interruption of oxygen therapy. Since there is no way of knowing the exact fraction of inspired oxygen delivered with nasal prongs, safe flow must be established by trial and error, with administration of 1 liter/min initially.

(2) The role of IPPB has been the subject of much recent controversy. It has no advantage over hand-held nebulizers and canisters in the delivery of topical bronchodilator drugs. IPPB with saline solution alone seems to have no proved benefit. Pneumothorax, bronchospasm, and infection are common in patients with CAO and may be aggravated by IPPB. The use of IPPB without added oxygen in patients receiving oxygen is another setting for deleterious hypoxemia due to intermittent oxygen therapy. Conversely, the use of high oxygen concentrations with IPPB may lead to hypoventilation after therapy in patients with chronic respiratory failure.

(3) Dehydration and overhydration are important considerations. Dehydration causes thick tenacious sputum, whereas overhydration or left ventricular heart failure can interfere with oxygen

transport, decrease lung compliance, and increase the work of breathing.

While humidification of inspired gases appears essential to normal mucociliary clearance when the nasopharynx is bypassed by intubation or tracheostomy, the role of high humidity and ultrasonic nebulization of water outside these limited circumstances is controversial. Ultrasonic nebulizers carry large quantities of moisture to the nasopharynx, although only a small amount reaches the bronchial tree. What beneficial or harmful effects increased inspired moisture has in patients with CAO is uncertain. Some authorities believe that mucus consistency depends more on systemic hydration than on moisture added via the bronchus. Breathing humidified gases does minimize insensible fluid losses through the respiratory tract. Replacement fluids therefore must be appropriately reduced when fluid balance is critical.

The roles of diuretics and digoxin in treating respiratory failure complicated by left heart failure are discussed in Chapter 7.

(4) Hypokalemia and hypochloremia secondary to chronic acidosis or diuretic therapy should be treated by parenteral or intravenous administration of potassium chloride. The hypokalemic hypochloremic metabolic alkalosis so often seen in patients with CAO further diminishes the central drive to ventilate and can result in fatal alkalosis if mechanical hyperventilation with subsequent acute respiratory alkalosis is superimposed.

(5) CAO patients at high risk from pulmonary embolus—especially those with polycythemia, congestive heart failure, or peripheral venous disease—are candidates for prophylactic anticoagulation.

(6) When patients with severe hypercapnia require mechanical ventilation, care must be taken not to lower $PaCO_2$ too quickly, causing systemic and central nervous system alkalosis. The bicarbonate accumulation resulting from chronic hypercapnia requires adequate chloride and sufficient time (hours to days) to be eliminated by the kidneys. During that period, arterial pH may not represent central nervous system pH since the blood-brain barrier blocks bicarbonate flux. Importantly, cerebral perfusion is considerably reduced in response to central nervous system alkalosis induced by overventilation. Hypoxic brain damage has resulted from overventilation under these circumstances.

Prognosis

Bates suggested that the progression of obstructive airways disease as determined by pulmonary function tests occurs rather independently of acute

exacerbations of bronchitis. For the individual CAO patient, however, each episode of acute respiratory failure represents a potential life-threatening situation. The data of Kettel et al. (Fig. 9.9B) correlate the patients surviving the acute episode (shaded symbols) with type of therapy and degree of acidosis. Among the patients who responded to conservative management or who were not intubated for medical or humanitarian reasons, the survival rate was 87.5%. Only a small number of patients were intubated—presumably, the sickest who were still judged as salvageable. Their survival rate was only 20%. Thus, although this type of investigation cannot be done as a controlled study, the results suggest that when patients with CAO do not respond to conservative management, the prognosis with intubation and assisted ventilation is grim.

Conclusions

Acute respiratory failure in patients with chronic hypercapnia differs in several respects from acute respiratory failure in the absence of chronic pulmonary disease. Obstructed airways increase the work of breathing and, in some patients, lead to carbon dioxide retention. Carbon dioxide is well tolerated when it accumulates slowly, but causes acidosis when the increase is rapid or in excess of cellular buffering. Carbon dioxide increase also worsens hypoxemia by displacing oxygen from the alveolus. Chronic hypercapnia blunts the normal ventilatory carbon dioxide response and leads to dependence on the hypoxic response mediated by the carotid bodies. Low-flow oxygen therapy is the basis of conservative management of acute respiratory decompensation, together with methods to reduce the work of breathing. Intubation and mechanical ventilation should be reserved for patients whose medical history and current status suggest a reasonable chance for survival and who fail to respond to conservative management.

Suggested Readings

Pulmonary Embolism

Cheely R: The role of noninvasive tests versus pulmonary angiography in the diagnosis of pulmonary embolism. *Am J Med 70*:17–22, 1981

Genton E: Thrombolytic therapy of pulmonary thromboembolism. *Prog Cardiovasc Dis 21*:333–341, 1979

Sharma GVRK, Sasahara AA: Diagnosis and treatment of pulmonary embolism. *Med Clin North Am 63*:239–250, 1979

Asthma

Austen KF, Lichtenstein LM (Eds): *Asthma: Physiology, Immunopharmacology, and Treatment.* New York, Academic Press, 1973

Banner AS, et al: Arrhythmogenic effects of orally administered bronchodilators. *Arch Intern Med 139*:434–437,
1979

Brandstetter RD, Gotz VP, Mar DD: Identifying the acutely ill
patient with asthma. *South Med J 74*:713–715, 1981

Brandstetter RD, Gotz VP, Mar DD: Optimal dosing of epinephrine in acute asthma. *Am J Hosp Pharm 37*:1326–
1328, 1980

Franklin W: Treatment of severe asthma. *N Engl J Med
290*:1469–1471, 1974

Hodson ME, Batten JC, Clarke SW, et al: Beclomethasone
dipropionate aerosol in asthma: Transfer of steroid-depend-
ent asthmatic patients from oral prednisone to beclomethasone dipropionate aerosol. *Am Rev Respir Dis 110*:403–
408, 1974

Kanetzky MS, Brandstetter RD, Meyer RC, et al: Acute
asthma. Part I. Comparison of the immediate effects of six
different modes of therapy. *Am J Med Sci 267*:213–223,
1974

Kordansky D, Adkinson NF, Norman PS, et al: Asthma improved by nonsteroidal anti-inflammatory drugs. *Ann Intern
Med 88*:508–511, 1978

Scoggin CH, Salm SA, Petty TL: Status asthmaticus: A nine-
year experience. *JAMA 238*:1158–1162, 1977

Shim C, Williams MH: Bronchial response to oral versus
aerosol metaproterenol in asthma. *Ann Intern Med 93*:428–
431, 1980

Strauss RH, McFadden EK, Ingram RH, et al: Enhancement
of exercise-induced asthma by cold air. *N Engl J Med
297*:743–747, 1977

Van Arsdel P, Glennon HP: Drug therapy in the management
of asthma. *Ann Intern Med 87*:68–74, 1977

Webb-Johnson DC, Andrews JL: Bronchodilator therapy. I
and II. *N Engl J Med 297*:476–482, 758–764, 1977

Weinberger MM, Hendeles L, Arens R: Clinical pharmacology
of drugs used for asthma. *Pediatr Clin North Am 28*:47–75,
1981

Weinberger MM, Hendeles L, Arens R: Pharmacologic management of reversible obstructive airways disease. *Med
Clin North Am 65*:579–613, 1981

Westerman DE, Benatar SR, Potgierter PD, et al: Identification
of the high-risk asthmatic patient. *Am J Med 66*:565–572,
1979

Williams MH: Life-threatening asthma. *Arch Intern Med
140*:1604–1605, 1980

Acute Decompensation of Chronic Respiratory Failure

Albert RK, Martin TR, Lewis SW: Controlled clinical trial of
methylprednisolone in patients with chronic bronchitis and
acute respiratory insufficiency. *Ann Intern Med 92*:753–
758, 1980

Bates DV: The fate of the chronic bronchitic: A report of the
ten-year follow-up in the Canadian Department of
Veteran's Affairs coordinated study of chronic bronchitis.
Am Rev Respir Dis 108:1043–1065, 1973

Brackett NC, Jr, Cohen JJ, Schwartz WB: Carbon dioxide
titration curve of normal man: Effect of increasing degrees
of acute hypercapnia on acid-base equilibrium. *N Engl J
Med 272*:6–12, 1965

Brackett NC, Jr, Wingo CF, Muren O, et al: Acid-base
response to chronic hypercapnia in man. *N Engl J Med
280*:124–130, 1969

Campbell EJM: The J. Burns Amberson Lecture: The
management of acute respiratory failure in chronic
bronchitis and emphysema. *Am Rev Respir Dis 96*:626–
639, 1967

Goldberg M, Green SB, Moss ML, et al: Computer-based
instruction and diagnoses of acid-base disorders: A
systematic approach. *JAMA 223*:269–275, 1973

Kassirer JP, Bleich HL: Rapid estimation of plasma carbon
dioxide tension from pH and total carbon dioxide content.
N Engl J Med 272:1067–1068, 1965

Kettel LJ, Diener CF, Morse JO, et al: Treatment of acute
respiratory acidosis in chronic obstructive lung disease.
JAMA 217:1503–1508, 1971

McNicol MW, Campbell EJM: Severity of respiratory failure:
Arterial blood-gases in untreated patients. *Lancet 1*:336–
338, 1965

CHAPTER 10

Environmental Hazards

PETER L. GROSS, M.D.
ELEANOR T. HOBBS, M.D.
FRANK P. CASTRONOVO, PH.D.
ANN S. BAKER, M.D.

Editor's note: This chapter, new to the second edition, represents an innovative addition to the medical section which has otherwise been arranged by traditional specialty. Much of the material in this topically wide-ranging treatise on man and his environment was not included in the first edition. Some is supplementary to other discussions: smoke inhalation in Chapter 22 (Cardiothoracic Emergencies), carbon monoxide poisoning in Chapter 17 (Toxicologic Emergencies) as well as in Chapter 22, infections resulting from bites in Chapter 11 (Infectious Diseases in the Emergency Ward). At least one topic related to environmental hazards appears elsewhere: frostbite in Chapter 28 (Thermal Injuries).

The emergency physician is often the key first responder in the diagnosis, treatment, and disposition of patients with medical emergencies related to environment hazards. This chapter focuses on selected environmental emergencies, including temperature disorders, drowning, carbon monoxide poisoning, smoke inhalation, barotrauma, radiation exposure, and bites and stings.

Although these emergencies are vastly different in terms of pathophysiology and treatment, their common denominator is the need for accurate diagnosis and often definitive initial therapy beginning in the emergency ward.

TEMPERATURE DISORDERS

Heat-Related Illness

Three heat-related illnesses are seen in the emergency ward. Heat cramps and heat exhaustion are relatively common conditions with little morbid-ity, but heat stroke is a catastrophic medical emergency with high mortality, accounting for approximately 4000 deaths annually in the United States. Whereas 80% of deaths occur in persons above the age of 50 years, there is still an appreciable mortality in young, otherwise healthy individuals. Survival depends on rapid diagnosis and initiation of definitive treatment, since morbidity and mortality from heat stroke correlate with the magnitude and duration of hyperpyrexia.

Physiology: Regulation of Heat Stress

Body temperature reflects the balance of physiologic heat production and the rate of heat loss modulated by the body's thermostat in the hypothalamus and mediated through complex reflex changes involving the cardiovascular and central nervous systems. Figure 10.1 summarizes this interaction. The body can gain heat when the environment is warmer than body temperature or when physiologic responses that help dissipate heat are impaired. Increased heat production from metabolism can also occur, and combinations of these three variables can result in illness.

Increased body temperature may be dissipated by (1) evaporative heat loss secondary to sweating or (2) changes in cardiac output associated with peripheral vasodilation that result in heat loss from the body surface by radiation, conduction, or convection. Only 5% of body heat loss occurs through the warming of urine, feces, or inspired air, whereas 30% is via the sweat mechanism and 65% by convection, conduction, or radiation.

As environmental temperatures approach body temperature, nonevaporative heat loss from the body surface is reduced as the gradient between body temperature and the environment is reduced. When high ambient humidity occurs with high

177

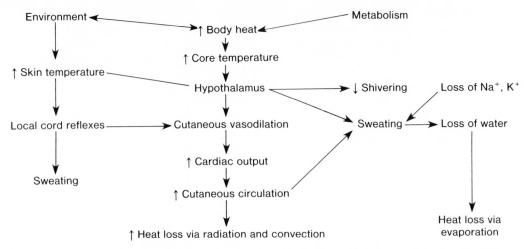

Figure 10.1. Physiologic response to heat stress. (Reproduced by permission from Stine RJ: Heat Illness. *JACEP 8:*154–160, 1979).

environmental temperatures, evaporative heat loss becomes reduced as well. Other factors that may contribute to diminished heat dissipation are listed in Table 10.1. Anticholinergic drugs may impair peripheral heat loss, propranolol hydrochloride may diminish normal cardiac responses, and the hypothalamus can be affected by phenothiazine derivatives. Amphetamines and hallucinogens may cause increased heat production.

Acclimatization to heat stress occurs after exposure on a regular basis over time. Myocardial efficiency improves, as does the sweat mechanism, which can elaborate higher volumes with better sodium preservation. Plasma volume may expand and may be maintained in the face of heat stress, improving circulatory competence and heat dissipation.

Minor Heat-Related Illness

Heat Cramps. Painful contractions in peripheral skeletal or abdominal muscles characterize heat cramps, which may occur in temperate ambient environments or with extremes of high temperature and humidity. The hallmark is strenuous exercise, usually without acclimatization or training.

Although serum electrolyte levels are usually normal, the pathophysiology appears to involve sweat-related sodium depletion from tissues accompanied by enhanced muscle contractility, perhaps mediated by alkalosis and changes in calcium concentration. On clinical examination, patients have normal body temperatures with muscle cramps and a preserved sweat mechanism. Therapy involves reassurance, rest in a cool environment, and oral intake of fluids. Only rarely is

Table 10.1.
Factors in heat-related illness.

Increased Heat Production
  Exercise, exertion
  Infection (febrile state)
  Agitation
  Drugs
      Amphetamines
      LSD
  Hyperthyroidism
Impaired Heat Dissipation
  Lack of acclimatization
  High ambient temperature
  High ambient humidity
  Obesity
  Heavy clothing
  Dehydration
  Cardiovascular disease
  Extremes of age
  Drugs
      Phenothiazines, anticholinergics, diuretics, propranolol hydrochloride
  Sweat gland dysfunction

Modified by permission from Stine RJ: Heat illness. *JACEP 8:*154–160, 1979.

parenteral fluid administration necessary. Salt tablets have been advocated as a preventive measure, but gradual acclimatization, graded exercise, and maintenance of body hydration are usually sufficient.

Heat Exhaustion. Heat exhaustion or heat prostration is the most frequent heat-related illness, occurring during environmental conditions of high ambient temperature and humidity in unacclimatized persons who often have some contributing element of impaired heat dissipation. This illness may be relatively sudden, as in the "parade-ground faint," although commonly there is a pro-dromal period of 10–30 minutes. The patient feels weak, dizzy, sweaty, or nauseated, and may vomit, faint, or complain of headache. Muscle cramps may be associated, and the patient appears ashen, tachypneic, and profusely diaphoretic with clinical findings that may resemble vagotonia except that the heart rate is usually elevated. Body temperature is normal, but when associated with extremes of ambient temperature or muscular exercise it may be elevated slightly to 101.5°F (38.6°C). Acute respiratory alkalosis is related to hyperventilation and is reflected in arterial blood-gas studies. Most often, serum electrolyte levels are normal, although hyponatremia or hypernatremia can occur related to prolonged exposure and loss of varying proportions of salt and water. Hemoconcentration is seen occasionally.

The pathophysiology of heat exhaustion is incompletely understood. Beller and Boyd (1975) have suggested that the exaggerated ventilatory response derives from temperature-stimulated increases in respiration rate and tidal volume, and results in a hyperventilation-induced faint with a vasovagal-like associated syndrome. Others have suggested that changes in tissue levels of sodium and chloride ions and water play a role, though measurable serum electrolyte abnormalities are the exception.

Treatment requires reassurance, a cool environment, and rehydration. Patients with mild heat exhaustion can be given oral fluids, whereas patients with more severe cases require parenteral rehydration with saline solution. Removal of the patient from the environmental conditions and rehydration in a cool environment cause symptoms to abate completely over 1–2 hours in most cases. In older patients, the emergency physician must be alert to other organ system stress that may develop secondary to heat prostration, such as myocardial ischemia.

Heat Stroke

In contrast to heat cramps and heat exhaustion, heat stroke is an uncommon condition but a true medical emergency. Heat stroke is characterized by thermoregulatory failure after exposure to high environmental temperatures and humidity. The cardinal features are hyperpyrexia of 106°F (41.1°C) or higher, central nervous system disturbance (stupor, seizures, or coma), and absence of sweating or anhidrosis.

Anhidrosis is more common in "classical" heat stroke. In most series, sweating is absent in almost 90% of patients. Younger patients with

"exertional" heat stroke in the setting of strenuous exercise may have preserved sweating; this has been reported in up to 50% of patients in some series. The features distinguishing classical from exertional heat stroke are summarized in Table 10.2, but overlap does occur.

Factors predisposing to heat stroke include both environmental conditions and heat regulation difficulties, either impaired dissipation or increased production. The pathophysiology, however, is incompletely understood. Four possible mechanisms have been suggested, and it is likely that interaction of all four may contribute to this catastrophic condition in the proper environmental setting.

Since cessation of sweating occurs in many patients, some have suggested that sweat gland fatigue or failure causes a relatively sudden lack of evaporative heat loss capability with resultant hyperpyrexia. However, not all patients with heat stroke have associated anhidrosis, which has led others to postulate a hypothalamic temperature-regulating dysfunction. Certain drugs, such as phenothiazines, have been reported to produce hyperpyrexia in this way. Cellular effects at the extremes of hyperpyrexia may be a contributing factor, since certain enzyme systems and permeability effects depend on the careful maintenance of cellular environmental temperature, pH, and solutes. At extremes of temperature, intracellular system failure may lead to cell, tissue, and organ system dysfunction. Finally, cardiovascular responses to hyperpyrexia may be inadequate leading to sudden development of heat stroke. Increase in heart rate and cardiac output occurs in response to heat stress, along with peripheral vasodilation to hasten

Table 10.2.
Heat Stroke: clinical presentation.

	Classical Heat Stroke	Exertional Heat Stroke
Age	Older	Younger
Activity level	Sedentary life style	Strenuous exercise
Health	Underlying disease is common; patient may be taking medication affecting temperature regulation.	Good
Prodrome	Lasts hours to days	Brief or absent
Anhidrosis	Seen in 90%	Seen in 50–90%

heat loss from the body surface area. If cardiac responses are limited by underlying disease and medications, heat stress will be poorly tolerated. In addition, physiologic studies have shown that heat stress at the extreme can contribute to markedly increased pulmonary vascular resistance with resultant right-sided cardiac failure, diminished cardiac output, and sudden lack of peripheral heat loss through radiation, conduction, or convection.

In contrast to heat stroke, anesthesia-induced hyperthermia or malignant hyperpyrexia appears to be a hypermetabolic state of increased heat production generated by intense muscular contraction caused by a calcium transport abnormality at the level of the sarcoplasmic reticulum. This phenomenon, which can be familial, occurs in approximately 1 in every 10,000–20,000 procedures, and is heralded by intense muscular rigidity after succinylcholine administration in the setting of inhalation anesthesia. Anesthesia must be stopped, and dantrolene sodium has been shown to be effective. Although muscular exercise may be a factor in heat stroke, such a muscle level defect has not been shown to be a factor.

The pathophysiologic effects of heat stroke often first become manifest with central nervous system alterations. Loss of consciousness occurs in 70% of patients and generalized seizures in 60%. Prodromes of headache, dizziness, faintness, and confusion also may occur. Coma may last as long as 24 hours and then resolve without neurologic residual, but consciousness usually returns as the patient's temperature is brought to normal. The cerebellum is particularly sensitive to heat stress, and cerebellar ataxia may be a residual effect. Pathologic studies reveal diffuse edema of brain substance that is usually associated with petechial hemorrhage and Purkinje cell degeneration.

Hematologic effects occur in up to 20% of heat stroke victims. In more severe cases, disseminated intravascular coagulation may develop secondary to thermal injury to vascular endothelium and thermal destruction of platelets. Hemolysis also may occur. Reduction of temperature is the first priority in treating disseminated intravascular coagulation, but heparin has also been used (see Chapter 13).

Clowes and O'Donnell (1974) have described two hemodynamic states in heat stroke. Both have relatively low total peripheral vascular resistance with peripheral vasodilation. More common is the hyperdynamic state with adequate blood pressure, tachycardia, a wide pulse pressure, and hot, dry, erythematous skin. These patients have an elevated cardiac index, and are often young, with

exertional heat stroke. Severe volume depletion is less common; in such circumstances, the patient has a hypodynamic circulatory state with diminished cardiac output, high pulmonary arterial pressure and hot, dry, but ashen skin. More elderly patients may be hypovolemic from insensitive fluid losses or concurrent diuretic therapy, and often are seen with a hypodynamic circulatory state and associated organ hypoperfusion.

Other organ system effects seen in heat stroke include myocardial injury with occasional infarction, skeletal muscle injury with resultant rhabdomyolysis, and hepatocellular injury manifested by mild to moderate liver function abnormality (rarely of clinical significance). Acute tubular necrosis may occur in 10–35% of heat stroke victims. In addition to thermal injury to renal parenchyma, other causes include hypotension with hypoperfusion and rhabdomyolysis with pigment-induced injury. Heat injury may induce polyuria secondary to tubular injury in the absence of acute renal failure.

Since morbidity and mortality in heat stroke correlate with the degree and duration of hyperpyrexia, the first priority in therapy is to lower body temperature. For the emergency physician, the second priority is to assess organ system injury and to institute appropriate therapy.

There should be little difficulty distinguishing heat stroke from other heat-related illnesses (Table 10.3) during a heat wave. However, in less severe extremes of atmospheric conditions, the physician must consider the differential diagnosis of the febrile patient with altered mental status. The extreme of temperature elevation in adult heat stroke patients may be highly suggestive of this diagnosis, but is by no means an absolute indication. If the circumstances seem to favor heat stroke, the first priority should be temperature control, with brief deferral of diagnostic studies while the temperature is lowered.

In the comatose patient, the airway should be secured, a suitable intravenous cannula placed, and the temperature lowered, preferably in an ice bath with continuous monitoring of core temperature via a rectal probe thermometer. In the absence of an ice bath, the patient may be placed on a cooling blanket with ice packed around him. Profound shivering may occur, with subsequent temperature rebound secondary to skeletal muscle activity. Chlorpromazine, 25–100 mg intravenously, usually controls shivering.

Control of the airway is important both for adequate oxygenation and for protection from aspiration, since severe vomiting occasionally oc-

Table 10.3.
Heat syndromes.

	Clinical Manifestations	Temperature	Sweat Mechanism	Central Nervous System Findings	Pathophysiology	Therapy
Heat cramps	Muscle cramps	Normal	Normal	Normal	Salt and fluid losses	Stop exercise Oral fluids
Heat exhaustion	Weakness Faintness	Normal to 101.5°F (38.6°C)	Diaphoretic	Normal	Salt and fluid losses Hyperventilation	Cool room Oral or intravenous fluids
Heat stroke	Stupor or sudden loss of consciousness	≥106°F (41.1°C)	Absent 50–90%	Coma Seizure Confusion	Unknown	Ice bath Maintain airway Support circulation

curs during the cooling process. The patient should be removed from the bath when body temperature reaches 101°F (38.3°C), since cooling to normal temperature often is followed by an overshoot to subnormal levels. This phenomenon may be more common in the elderly.

Consciousness may return with restoration of temperature, but coma may persist. Persistent seizures should be controlled with intravenous phenytoin or alternative drugs, since uncontrolled seizure activity may contribute both to endogenous heat production with temperature elevation and to skeletal muscle injury with consequent rhabdomyolysis.

After body temperature is lowered, organ system function should be assessed in terms of end-organ injury to the cardiovascular, hematologic, renal, and central nervous systems. Baseline renal function and coagulation parameters should be determined and the patient's hemodynamic state stabilized. A pulmonary artery line is often placed in the emergency ward or on transfer to an intensive care unit.

In most patients with exertional heat stroke, volume deficits are not severe and 1–2 liters of crystalloid over the first 2–4 hours with appropriate physiologic monitoring may be sufficient. Occasionally, volume deficits are greater, or cardiac disease with ventricular failure is limiting. Vasopressors are rarely necessary, but when they are required, pure or predominantly α-adrenergic agents should be avoided, since peripheral and splanchnic vasoconstriction may limit heat loss from the periphery, further compromising renal function. If volume expansion does not rapidly improve hemodynamics and a sympathomimetic agent is added, dopamine in low to moderate doses may be tried.

Prolonged temperatures in excess of 106°F (41.1°C), azotemia, hyperkalemia, and protracted coma are associated with poor prognosis. In the absence of these features, aggressive assessment and therapy in the emergency ward should produce a satisfactory outcome.

Hypothermia

As in heat-related illness, the successful management of hypothermia begins in the emergency ward with rapid recognition and the institution of appropriate therapy. Hypothermia, defined as a core temperature less than 95°F (35°C) can develop in a variety of circumstances. Recreational activities with exposure, sometimes complicated by injury or immersion, are the most common precipitants in otherwise healthy individuals. Hypothermia also occurs with medical illness, such as drug overdose with exposure, central nervous system dysfunction related to stroke or spinal cord injury, and metabolic and endocrine disorders such as diabetic ketoacidosis, hypothyroidism, and hypopituitarism. Persons addicted to alcohol can be particularly prone to hypothermia, which is usually caused by exposure and which is invariably associated with complications of alcohol abuse such as trauma, pancreatitis, seizures, or infection.

The management of hypothermia is controversial and therapeutic strategy depends first on an understanding of the physiologic consequences of hypothermia.

Pathophysiology

Decrease in core temperature results in a complex series of physiologic responses that attempt both to conserve heat and to increase heat production. These responses are modulated by the temperature-regulating center in the hypothalamus. Reflex cardiovascular and central nervous system responses are necessary to maintain normothermia. In the presence of low environmental temperatures, excess heat loss and diminished heat production result in clinical hypothermia.

Heat loss can occur by conduction, convection, or radiation from the body surface. Conductive heat loss increases dramatically in the setting of water immersion, where heat loss may be 30 times more rapid than in air of comparable temperature.

Conservation of body temperature involves (1) vasoconstriction in the periphery to decrease heat loss, and (2) increased heat production in the skeletal muscles. Increased heat production occurs most rapidly via the shivering response, which generates heat, central vasodilation, and delivery of warmed blood to the core circulation. The endogenous catechol response and other neuroendocrine responses play a role in heat production, but at a slightly slower pace.

As body temperature is lowered to 95°F (35°C), heart rate, cardiac output and respiration rate actually increase, and the metabolic rate may be three to six times the basal rate in an effort to increase heat production in response to hypothermic stress. The patient is usually conscious and shivering. However, as temperature declines further, the metabolic rate decreases. At a body temperature of 90°F (32.2°C), heart rate, cardiac output, and respiration rate also are decreased and the shivering response may be lost at temperatures from 86–91°F (30–32.8°C). Confusion, stupor, or coma may develop at this stage, and in the field,

hypothermia-induced altered judgment and associated fatigue, incoordination, weakness, and hallucinosis often lead to further exposure and severe consequences.

At temperatures approximating 86°F (30°C), muscular rigidity occurs and the basal metabolic rate may be 50% of normal. Respiration is depressed and hypoxemia results. Cardiac depression causes decreased cardiac output with associated bradyarrhythmias, conduction disturbances, and hypotension. Sinus bradycardia may give way to atrial fibrillation with a slow ventricular response and associated J waves or Osborne waves that are characteristic of the hypothermic effect on conduction (Fig. 10.2). As hypothermia progresses, absolute and relative refractory periods are prolonged and the rate of spontaneous cardiac depolarization slows. Myocardial irritability increases with hypothermia, and ventricular fibrillation becomes a major risk at about 82.4°F (28°C), particularly when the patient is moved or handled, since the cold heart is sensitive to such activity.

At a temperature of 77°F (25°C) major respiratory depression occurs. Hypothermia also causes bronchorrhea and depression of cough, which become manifest at temperatures from 86–95° F (30–35°C), and aspiration pneumonitis can develop.

Arterial blood-gas measurements must be corrected for hypothermia. Blood samples drawn from hypothermic patients but analyzed under standard conditions at 98.6°F (37°C) are subject to considerable error. The PaO_2 and the $PaCO_2$ will be falsely elevated, and the patient will appear more acidotic than is actually the case. The emergency physician must note the temperature of the patient when the arterial blood sample is drawn. With this information, the blood-gas laboratory can correct the results for temperature effects using Severinghaus' nomogram.

Hypothermia may induce diuresis due to the effects of cold on renal tubules, and at extremes of hypothermia with hypotension and organ system hypoperfusion, acute tubular necrosis may develop. Hemoconcentration occurs with intravascular sludging, and disseminated intravascular coagulation may be seen. As temperature lowers, cerebral blood flow diminishes and pupils dilate.

Either hyperglycemia or hypoglycemia may occur. Hypoglycemia may be a feature in the alcoholic population, resulting from a relatively malnourished nutritional state and the diminished hepatic glyconeogenesis seen in both hypothermia and alcoholism. Shivering may utilize glucose stores and contribute to hypoglycemia as well. Hyperglycemia occurs because severe hypothermia affects intermediary metabolism, blocks in-

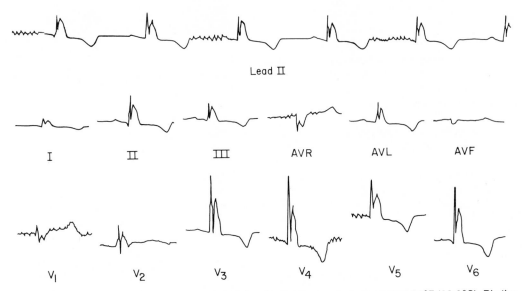

Lead II

I II III AVR AVL AVF

V₁ V₂ V₃ V₄ V₅ V₆

Figure 10.2. Electrocardiogram taken on admission. Rectal temperature was below 90°F (32.2°C). Rhythm is sinus bradycardia at 40 beats/min. PR, QRS, and QT intervals are prolonged and a prominent "J" deflection is seen in most leads. Intermittent oscillations of the baseline are identified in lead II. (Reproduced by permission from Trevine A, et al: *Arch Intern Med 127:*472, 1971)

sulin release, and diminishes peripheral glucose utilization. Blood glucose levels ranging from 300–400 mg/100 ml are not uncommon, but do not require insulin administration. These levels normalize as rewarming reverses the altered physiology.

In hypothermia, acidosis is caused by a combination of respiratory depression and consequent carbon dioxide retention and by lactate accumulation as circulatory failure ensues with hypotension and tissue hypoperfusion. Muscle activity with shivering may add to accumulation of lactate, which is less efficiently metabolized by the liver in the setting of hypothermia. Metabolic and respiratory acidosis added to hypoxemia increase the risk of cardiac arrhythmias, with asystole occurring at temperatures of 68–77°F (20–25°C), sometimes preceding respiratory arrest.

Clinical Features

Environmental temperatures need not be dramatically low for hypothermia to develop, particularly in the elderly or immobilized patient and in those with acute illness or injury superimposed on pituitary or thyroid dysfunction.

Hypothermia should be suspected in the stuporous patient with cold skin, slow pulse rate, low blood pressure, diminished deep tendon reflexes, and shivering, and in the comatose patient with these features and muscular rigidity instead of shivering. Edema may also be a prominent feature

with immersion or long-duration hypothermia. Whereas there is often a history of exposure or immersion to guide the emergency physician, the condition still may be unrecognized and the diagnosis delayed, since most clinical thermometers do not read below 94°F (34.4°C). Frostbite is occasionally the initial clue, although its treatment should be secondary to rewarming of the patient.

The emergency physician not only must be aware of the possibility of hypothermia but also must modify the usual criteria for attempting resuscitation. In the most extreme situation, the patient may appear dead, with muscular rigidity, dilated pupils, barely discernible or absent pulse and respiration, and unobtainable blood pressure. However, recovery without significant sequelae has occurred despite prolonged cardiopulmonary arrest. Patients with asystole of 2 hours' duration or persistent fibrillation lasting 2–3 hours have survived with continous cardiopulmonary resuscitation (CPR) and rewarming efforts. If the patient has been rewarmed to more than 95°F (35°C) without restoration of cardiorespiratory function, resuscitative efforts should be halted.

Evaluation and Treatment

Temperature should be monitored accurately preferably with a rectal probe thermocouple providing continous readings. In the stuporous or comatose patient, initial evaluation should include careful inspection for trauma that may have precipitated the exposure or followed a hypothermic state. All hypothermic patients should have cardiac monitoring, and patients should be handled very carefully because of the risk of ventricular arrhythmias or arrest. Arterial blood-gas samples should clearly indicate the patient's temperature so that appropriate corrections can be made. Initial laboratory studies should include renal function tests, and determination of blood glucose, electrolytes, and parameters for disseminated intravascular coagulation. Liver function and amylase tests should also be performed, particularly if there is evidence or history of chronic alcohol abuse.

Correction of acidosis in the setting of hypothermia requires judicious use of sodium bicarbonate. Respiratory acidosis improves with restoration of ventilation, and to some extent, rewarming reverses metabolic acidosis as circulation is reestablished and normal metabolism returns. However, severe acidosis with cardiopulmonary arrest requires sodium bicarbonate. Extremes of acidosis and temperature make the heart resistant to many cardiac medications and maneuvers. Sympathomimetic amines have little effect below a pH of 7.15, and if ventricular fibrillation is present, electrical defibrillation may not be effective. It is worthwhile to try defibrillation or cardioversion initially when the cardiac rhythm indicates such methods. If this is unsuccessful, further efforts should await rewarming of the patient.

Volume requirements vary. Patients with rapid-onset hypothermia after an immersion accident of relatively short duration may have minimal volume needs, and blood pressure and organ perfusion often respond to rewarming alone. However, patients with hypothermia of longer duration or underlying cardiac disease have extensive volume requirements. Third spacing of volume often occurs, and invasive physiologic monitoring is required as the transition from emergency ward to intensive care unit occurs. Placement of a central venous pressure or pulmonary artery line, however, may be associated with a risk of ventricular ectopy as the cold ventricle is stimulated by these lines. Ideally, initial temperature resuscitation should be underway before these lines are placed.

Rewarming therapy continues to be controversial. In passive external rewarming, the patient is moved from the cold environment, protected from further heat loss by blankets, and allowed to warm slowly by the body's normal metabolism. Active external rewarming involves the use of warming blankets or a heated bath, whereas active core rewarming attempts to warm the central circulation with techniques such as hemodialysis, perito-

neal dialysis, heated intravenous fluids, and cardiopulmonary bypass.

Although all these methods have been used, no well-controlled randomized study has evaluated these techniques and their application. Passive external rewarming is a slow process, but for patients with mild hypothermia with a temperature higher than 95°F (35°C) without hemodynamic compromise, this may be sufficient. Opponents of active external rewarming argue that peripheral vasodilation may worsen hypotension and shock as the hypothermic heart and central circulation fail to meet the needs of the periphery. This type of rewarming has also been associated with "core temperature afterdrop," a phenomenon in which the core temperature decreases as the central circulation receives cold peripheral blood.

The emergency physician should evaluate each patient carefully in an effort to apply the most appropriate therapy available. In the emergency ward, peritoneal dialysis is an easily instituted core rewarming technique. Dialysate tubing can be heated with a blood-warming coil, or dialysate bottles heated to 113°F (45°C) can be used. Intravenous crystalloid, colloid, and blood products should also be warmed to 104°F (40°C) before administration, and heated inspired oxygen with a temperature from 107.6–114.8°F (42–46°C) at the mouth can be applied via face mask or endotracheal tube, providing some central rewarming. Gastric lavage with warmed saline solution as an initial measure has the disadvantage of requiring a nasogastric tube, which may initiate ventricular ectopy. In extreme, resistant cases, open chest CPR with the mediastinum bathed in warmed physiologic saline has been tried, but this invasive approach is not likely to be necessary when other core rewarming techniques are available.

In cases of severe hypothermia in which the temperature is less than 86°F (30°C) or in the presence of cardiopulmonary arrest, active core rewarming is probably the most rational approach. In peritoneal dialysis, for example, potassium-free 1.5% dialysate can be rapidly instilled and removed, providing a significant improvement in temperature in six to eight exchanges. Adjunctive to this approach can be the use of heated intravenous fluids and heated oxygen at the airway while CPR is continued. These methods can be applied easily in the average emergency ward, whereas hemodialysis and cardiopulmonary bypass require more preparation and may not be available in some hospitals.

When hemodynamics are stable and hypothermia is not severe (temperature from 90–95°F

[32.2–35°C]), a combination of core rewarming (heated intravenous fluids and heated oxygen mask) and active external rewarming (warming blankets) may be acceptable unless cardiac rhythm abnormalities develop, temperature decreases, or hypotension worsens.

When the patient's hemodynamic condition is stable and temperature is improved, complete assessment and treatment of other organ system dysfunction or injury can take place, with particular attention to frostbite injury, trauma, pneumonia, pancreatitis, and underlying diseases that may have precipitated or contributed to the hypothermic state.

DROWNING AND NEAR DROWNING

At least 8000 drownings and many additional near drownings occur annually in the United States. About 40% of deaths occur in children less than 4 years old.

Drowning is defined as asphyxia and death resulting from submersion in fluid; near drowning is survival for at least 24 hours after asphyxia due to submersion. Two other types of submersion injury are immersion hypothermia, which may occur with or without drowning, and the rare "immersion syndrome," in which ventricular fibrillation is precipitated by a sudden plunge into cold water. Some individuals, particularly young children, may be transiently protected from cerebral hypoxia by an active diving reflex, in which immersion in cold water produces bradycardia and intense vasoconstriction of all but coronary and cerebral blood vessels, temporarily preserving blood flow to the heart and brain despite the absence of respiration.

Pathophysiology

Two types of pathophysiology have been observed in drownings. In 10–20% of victims, "dry drowning" occurs, in which laryngospasm results in asphyxia and the glottis relaxes only after respiratory efforts have ceased; thus, no fluid is aspirated. In most cases, however, "wet drowning" occurs, in which variable amounts of fluid are aspirated. "Secondary drowning" refers broadly to the development of respiratory distress syndrome following survival after submersion; this may begin from 1–72 hours later.

The immediate result of submersion is asphyxia: Po_2 rapidly decreases, Pco_2 increases, and a combined metabolic and respiratory acidosis develops. Although much has been made of the differences between fresh and salt water drownings, only rarely is enough fluid aspirated to cause clinically significant volume or electrolyte abnormalities. When fresh water is aspirated, the hypotonic fluid is quickly absorbed through the pulmonary capillary membrane, resulting in a washout of lung surfactant and subsequent alveolar collapse, intrapulmonary shunting, and hypoxemia. Since salt water is hypertonic to plasma, when it is aspirated the osmotic gradient favors transudation of fluid into the alveoli, leading to pulmonary edema, intrapulmonary shunting, and hypoxemia. Hypertonic fluid also causes direct damage to the pulmonary capillary membrane with resultant leakage of plasma proteins into alveoli. Impurities and particulate matter such as mud, sewage, detergents, chlorine, or vomitus may be aspirated along with the water, and add to the pulmonary insult. Despite the different mechanisms of pulmonary injury, the net result is ventilation-perfusion mismatch, intrapulmonary shunting, and hypoxemia.

In the rare case in which a large amount of fresh water is aspirated (more than 22 ml/kg), the metabolic abnormalities that may occur include decrease in serum sodium, chloride, calcium, and magnesium levels; volume overload; intravascular hemolysis leading to hyperkalemia, hemoglobinemia, and hemoglobinuria with potential hemoglobinuric renal failure; and disseminated intravascular coagulation. With salt water aspiration, hemoconcentration and hypovolemia may be seen, especially if a large volume of water has also been swallowed and absorbed through the gastrointestinal tract.

Aside from direct pulmonary damage from fluid aspiration and occasional metabolic abnormalities, the effects of drowning and near drowning on the heart, kidneys, and brain are those of anoxia. The two most important prognostic factors for survival with good neurologic function are the duration of the anoxic episode (length of submersion plus time until effective CPR is begun) and the temperature of the water. In warm water submersion, several factors indicate a poor prognosis: submersion for more than 5 minutes, no CPR for 10 minutes, a pH less than 7.10 on arrival at the hospital, a continuing need for CPR in the emergency ward, the presence of deep coma, and especially the presence of fixed dilated pupils. The profound protective effect of hypothermia on brain function is being increasingly appreciated, and the same prognostic factors cannot be applied to submersion in cold water. Many instances of full neurologic recovery after submersion in cold water for 20–40 minutes now have been reported, even when fixed dilated pupils were present on admission. Thus, vigorous attempts at resuscitation and rewarming are warranted in victims of cold water submersion, even when it is prolonged.

Treatment

Emergency treatment should begin with mouth-to-mouth resuscitation as soon as the rescuer reaches the victim, even before removal from the water. If a neck injury is suspected, the cervical spine should be immobilized. CPR and advanced life support, if available, should be instituted at the scene and continued en route. On arrival in the emergency ward, vital signs should be checked, including an accurate temperature measurement and determination of pupil size. If the patient is in cardiopulmonary arrest, the usual advanced life support protocol should be instituted, with the addition of rewarming if hypothermia is present (Table 10.4).

The indications for endotracheal intubation in a victim of near drowning who has regained spontaneous respiration include coma with inability to protect the airway, the presence of copious secretions or gross aspiration of particulate matter, and

Table 10.4.
Steps in treatment of near drowning.

Establish airway, breathing, and circulation (cardio-pulmonary resuscitation, advanced life support)
Check for hypothermia; if present, begin rewarming
Perform appropriate laboratory tests
    Complete blood cell count
    Blood urea nitrogen, creatinine, calcium, and magnesium determinations
    Electrolyte determinations
    Arterial blood-gas determinations
    Prothrombin time
    Partial thromboplastin time
    Urinalysis
    Electrocardiogram
Place nasogastric tube
Obtain chest x-ray film
Perform adjunctive pulmonary therapy[a]
    Ventilation with positive end-expiratory pressure
    Bronchodilation with aminophylline, inhaled or parenteral β-adrenergic agents
    Chest physical therapy and suction
    Bronchoscopy for gross aspiration of particulate matter
Correct fluid and electrolyte abnormalities
Place Foley catheter if indicated
Consider early transfer for intensive cerebral resuscitation
Admit and observe any patient with a significant episode of submersion and aspiration

[a] Prophylactic administration of antibiotics and corticosteroids usually not indicated.

an arterial P_{CO_2} over 45 mm Hg or an arterial P_{O_2} under 80–90 mm Hg on 40% oxygen by mask. Intubated patients should be maintained on a volume ventilator with positive end-expiratory pressure (the amount titrated for each patient); if the patient has spontaneous respiration, intermittent mandatory ventilation with continuous positive airway pressure may be tried, adjusting the F_{IO_2} to maintain an adequate arterial P_{O_2}. In awake, cooperative patients with borderline blood-gas levels, continuous positive airway pressure with a tight-fitting mask may be tried in an attempt to avoid intubation. A nasogastric tube should be placed, since often a large amount of water and air has been swallowed, further compromising ventilation. Blood samples should be obtained for a complete blood cell count, platelet count, and determination of electrolytes, blood urea nitrogen, creatinine, calcium, magnesium, prothrombin time, and partial thromboplastin time. The urine should be tested for hemoglobin. A chest x-ray film should be obtained, with the realization that in 25% of patients with significant pulmonary problems, the initial chest x-ray film is normal. Most patients have radiographic evidence of perihilar or generalized pulmonary edema in the early hours, which later evolves to focal areas of atelectasis or infiltrates.

Once the airway and adequate ventilation are assured, adjunctive therapy to improve gas exchange further should be instituted. This includes standard doses of aminophylline and inhaled or parenteral β-adrenergic agents to treat bronchospasm, chest physical therapy, and suction. When aspiration of particulate matter such as vomitus or mud is suspected, early bronchoscopy should be considered. Prophylactic administration of antibiotics or corticosteroids is not generally considered beneficial in the treatment of the pulmonary complications of near drowning.

An integral part of assessment and treatment is consideration of possible predisposing factors such as a cervical spine injury, alcohol or drug intoxication, seizure disorder, arrhythmia, suicide attempt, or child abuse. The prognosis for meaningful recovery after near drowning has improved in recent years because of the increased availability of centers equipped to carry out intensive cerebral resuscitative measures such as intracranial pressure monitoring, controlled hypothermia, administration of barbiturates, mannitol, and corticosteroids, and careful fluid management to maximize intracranial perfusion pressure. The emergency physician should consider early transfer to such a unit if it seems indicated.

Since it often takes hours for the pulmonary complications of fluid aspiration to develop, all of the patients who have had a significant episode of submersion and aspiration should be observed for at least 24 hours.

BAROTRAUMA AND DECOMPRESSION SICKNESS

With the increasing popularity of scuba diving as a sport, diving-related emergencies will be more frequently encountered by the emergency physician. In sport scuba, the diver breathes air from a pressurized tank through a regulator that delivers air at the ambient pressure, which depends on the depth of the dive.

To understand the causes and treatment of medical problems related to scuba diving, the emergency physician should be familiar with certain principles of physics concerning gases and pressure. The pressure at sea level is 760 mm Hg, which is defined as 1 atmosphere (atm). Each 33 feet of sea water (fsw) exerts 1 additional atm, so the pressure at a depth of 33 feet is 2 atm, and at 66 feet it is 3 atm. Boyle's law states: "at a constant temperature, the volume of a given mass of gas is inversely proportional to its pressure", that is, $PV = K$, where K is a constant. Dalton's law states: "in a mixture of gases, the pressure exerted by each gas is the same as it would exert if it alone occupied the same volume, and the total pressure is the sum of the partial pressures of the component gases." As ambient pressure increases, the partial pressures of the component gases increase proportionately although their percentage in the gas mixture remains constant. For example, at sea level, the partial pressure of oxygen is 160 mm Hg (0.21×760 mm Hg). When air is breathed at 2 atm (33 fsw), the partial pressure of oxygen is 319 mm Hg (0.21×1520 mm Hg), and so on. Henry's law states: "at a given temperature, the amount of gas dissolved in a solvent is proportional to the pressure of the gas in equilibrium with the solvent." These laws form the basis of diving physiology and an understanding of diving emergencies.

Barotrauma

Barotrauma, the most common medical problem of divers, refers to injuries that result from changes in ambient pressure. Because of their water content, body tissues are relatively incompressible, but air-filled spaces such as the middle ear, sinuses, respiratory tract, and to some extent the gastrointestinal tract are compressible and behave according to Boyle's law ($PV = K$). During descent, as ambient pressure increases, unventilated air spaces such as the middle ear and sinuses are "squeezed" unless pressure in these spaces is equilibrated with ambient pressure. Divers are usually able to "equilibrate" by using various maneuvers to open the Eustachian tubes. If pressure is not equilibrated, the diver experiences ear pain, followed by edema, hemorrhage into the middle ear, and ultimately, rupture of the tympanic membrane, a syndrome referred to as "middle ear squeeze." Otoscopic examination usually shows erythema of the tympanic membrane, and in more severe cases, gross hemorrhage or rupture. Treatment includes a systemic decongestant such as pseudoephedrine hydrochloride, 30–60 mg every 6 hours, nasal decongestant drops, and avoidance of further diving until symptoms have abated and the patient can easily equilibrate. Some physicians recommend prophylactic antibiotics to prevent bacterial otitis media. Patients with a ruptured tympanic membrane should be referred to an otolaryngologist for follow-up treatment.

A rarer injury that can occur during descent, usually as a result of a Valsalva's maneuver, is rupture of the round window, resulting in vertigo, tinnitus, and neurosensory hearing loss. When decompression sickness does not appear to be a likely cause of these symptoms, an otologic cause should be suspected. Treatment of round window rupture includes bed rest with the head elevated, avoidance of straining and noseblowing, and referral for evaluation by an otolaryngologist. Some other forms of barotrauma of descent are "sinus squeeze" and "dental squeeze," which is usually associated with air pockets from recent dental work.

Barotrauma of ascent occurs when air spaces in the body expand as ambient pressure decreases. The most serious situation is pulmonary barotrauma. Overdistention of the lung with subsequent rupture can occur with a pressure gradient of 80 mm Hg across the lung. Normally, a scuba diver prevents the development of such a gradient by continuously exhaling on ascent. If a diver holds his breath during ascent, or if there is air trapped in the lungs because of pulmonary disease, the lung may rupture. There are four clinical presentations of lung rupture, which can occur singly or in combination, and which are usually apparent immediately on surfacing from a dive. Pneumothorax may result from rupture of the visceral pleura, and presents with typical symptoms. Subcutaneous emphysema may occur as air tracks up the mediastinum into the neck or rarely into the pericardium. Symptoms may include hoarseness, dysphagia, dyspnea, syncope, and shock; physical examination and radiologic evaluation confirm the presence of subcutaneous and mediastinal air. Pulmonary tissue damage itself is manifested by cough, hemoptysis, and dyspnea as a result of widespread alveolar rupture. Finally, air embolism occurs when air dissects into the pulmonary veins and is embolized into the systemic circulation, causing vascular obstruction and infarction. Although any organ may be affected, the two most serious syndromes are cerebral air embolism, which presents as stroke, and coronary embolism with the typical symptoms of a myocardial infarction.

Treatment of suspected air embolism includes placing the victim on the left side with the head about 30 degrees lower than the feet, administration of 100% oxygen by mask without positive pressure, and as rapid transport as possible to a hyperbaric chamber for definitive treatment. Information about the location of the nearest hyperbaric chamber can be obtained by calling Brooks Air Force Base in San Antonio, Texas, (512) 536–3281. If air transport is required, it is important that the patient be kept at an ambient pressure as close to 1 atm as possible by use of a low-flying or specially pressurized aircraft. Hyperbaric therapy has several effects. It reduces the size of emboli, which allows their distal movement and speeds their resolution. The use of 100% oxygen at 2.5 atm speeds the diffusion of inert nitrogen from the emboli, further enhancing their resolution. Therapy in a hyperbaric chamber needs to be managed by someone familiar with the appropriate treatment schedules. Adjunctive measures for cerebral resuscitation, such as controlled hypothermia, corticosteroids, and mannitol, may be initiated in cases of severe cerebral air embolism.

Treatment of other forms of pulmonary barotrauma depend on the severity of symptoms. The patient should receive 100% oxygen by mask, since this will speed the diffusion of inert nitrogen from the abnormal gas pockets. Positive pressure should not be used since it may force additional gas into tissues. Pneumothorax may require catheter drainage or tube thoracostomy. Other general supportive measures should be instituted as necessary.

Decompression Sickness

Decompression sickness, commonly known as bends, is caused by bubble formation within tissues and blood vessels, occurring under conditions of supersaturation. Gas that has been dissolved in tissue during a period of increased ambient pressure according to Henry's law, will come out of solution and may form bubbles when ambient pressure is decreased, that is, during ascent. Since the oxygen in air is constantly being metabolized, it is with inert nitrogen that the problem of supersaturation arises. The amount of nitrogen dissolved in body tissues during a dive depends on both time and pressure, in other words, the length and depth of the dive. The U.S. Navy Standard Air Decompression Tables, which should be familiar to all divers, establish guidelines for the depth and duration of a dive or series of dives, which, if observed, will prevent decompression sickness in most divers. However, even with strict adherence to the guidelines, some divers will be afflicted.

Decompression sickness is often divided into two categories based on clinical manifestations. Type I decompression sickness refers to skin or joint symptoms, so-called skin-only or pain-only bends. Type II decompression sickness refers to critical organ involvement such as the central nervous system and lungs.

Symptoms of decompression sickness may occur during ascent, particularly if ascent is at a rate of more than 60 feet/min, but they more commonly begin shortly after surfacing and evolve gradually over a period of several hours. Joint pain is a common symptom of decompression sickness. Shoulders, elbows, and any recently injured joint, such as a sprained ankle, are the most commonly affected in sport scuba. The pain usually is described as a steady ache or boring pain, the joint appears normal, range of motion is preserved, and x-ray films are unrevealing. Cutaneous symptoms include itching and burning, and the skin characteristically appears mottled.

Central nervous system involvement can be in either the spinal cord or the brain. Spinal cord ischemia is thought to be caused by bubbles in the venous vertebral plexus, leading to stasis, obstruction to blood flow, and edema. The white matter of the cord, especially thoracic, upper lumbar, and lower cervical segments, most commonly is affected. The usual symptoms are transient back pain followed by lower extremity paresthesias, weakness, ataxia, and finally, urinary retention and paralysis. Brain involvement may present as a typical stroke or with subtle manifestations such as vertigo, which can be difficult to differentiate from barotrauma. Pulmonary symptoms, which divers often refer to as "chokes," are thought to be caused by widespread obstruction to pulmonary blood flow by bubbles. These patients have dyspnea, chest pain, and other signs and symptoms of acutely increased pulmonary arterial pressure. Initially, it may be impossible to differentiate between chokes and pulmonary barotrauma.

The initial treatment of type II decompression sickness is the same as that for suspected air embolism, which is fortunate, since early in the course of illness it may be difficult to distinguish the two. The patient should be positioned on the left side with the head 30 degrees lower than the feet, 100% oxygen should be administered by mask, and arrangements should be made for transport to the nearest available hyperbaric chamber for recompression therapy. If air transport is necessary, it must be accomplished with as little decrease in ambient pressure as possible. Cardiopulmonary and circulatory support may be required. The importance of recompression therapy cannot be overemphasized, even when treatment has been delayed or a chamber is several hours away. Patients may show improvement even when neurologic deficits have been present for as long as 24 hours. When the diagnosis of decompression sickness is under consideration, it is always safer to initiate recompression therapy.

Although type I decompression sickness with only joint pain is less of an emergency, it should also be treated with recompression therapy. Skin-only bends can be treated without recompression, but the patient and physician should be alert to the possible development of more serious symptoms over the ensuing few hours.

SMOKE INHALATION

Pulmonary complications of smoke inhalation are usually associated with body burns, but may occur in isolation. It is estimated that about one-half of the deaths due to fire are attributable to the effects of smoke inhalation.

Pathophysiology

Six mechanisms of respiratory compromise may be seen in victims of fire. (1) Early death due to asphyxia may occur as a result of breathing smoke—a gas with a variably reduced concentration of oxygen and increased concentrations of carbon dioxide and carbon monoxide. (2) Upper airway obstruction may develop within hours of exposure, as heat and noxious particulate matter and gases incite pharyngeal and laryngeal edema. (3) Circumferential thoracic burns can produce severe ventilatory restriction that must be relieved by escharotomies. (4) Carbon monoxide poisoning frequently is associated with smoke inhalation and contributes to morbidity. (5) Inhalation injury,

which in its narrower sense refers to the occurrence of either chemical tracheobronchitis or injury to small airways and alveoli as a result of exposure to smoke, may lead to progressive respiratory compromise. This serves as a substrate for (6) late pulmonary infection, which is often the cause of death in burn victims.

Three components of smoke account for different aspects of pulmonary pathophysiology, and are present to varying degrees in different fires. (1) Heat and steam cause direct thermal injury that is usually confined to the supraglottic region, and produces pharyngeal and laryngeal edema, erythema, and blistering. (2) Particles consisting of carbonaceous material coated with organic acids and aldehydes damage the tracheobronchial mucosa. (3) Among the products of combustion and pyrolysis are gases such as chlorine, phosgene, nitrogen dioxide, sulfur dioxide, ammonia, and hydrochloric acid, which cause a marked inflammatory response in the lung. Pulmonary capillary permeability increases, with leakage of protein-rich fluid into the alveoli and loss of lung surfactant resulting in pulmonary edema, focal atelectasis, and intrapulmonary shunting.

Clinical Features

Certain historical factors suggest that a victim is at high risk for having sustained a significant inhalation injury. Patients exposed to smoke in a closed space, patients with impaired ability to protect themselves (infants, elderly, infirm, drug- or alcohol-intoxicated individuals and those with head injuries or loss of consciousness), and patients with previous lung disease must be considered at high risk. Certain types of smoke and fumes are especially noxious, particularly those liberated by the burning or thermal degradation of polyvinyl chloride, which is present in plastics, telephone and electrical cables, and much upholstery.

The patient may complain of a sore throat or substernal burning (a prominent symptom in fires involving polyvinyl chloride). Hoarseness or stridor indicates upper airway edema and the potential for obstruction. Burns about the face and neck, a singed mustache, or singed nasal hairs frequently are associated with inhalation injury. Positive findings on physical examination include tachypnea, and tachycardia; erythema, edema, and blistering of the orophyarynx; and wheezing, rales, and cough producing carbonaceous sputum. It is important to remember that in some patients with normal initial examination results, significant inhalation injuries may evolve.

Certain laboratory and diagnostic tests are helpful in evaluating the presence, extent, and anatomic level of an inhalation injury. Early blood-gas measurements with the patient breathing room air can be falsely reassuring—showing mild to moderate hypoxemia or even a normal Pao_2. The $Paco_2$ is usually low, but may be normal or high. The calculation of an alveolar-arterial oxygen gradient on room air ($PAo_2 = Pao_2$ where $PAo_2 = 150 - [1.25 \times Pco_2]$ and Pao_2 is that measured) reflects intrapulmonary shunting and increases the sensitivity of room-air arterial blood-gas determinations. A normal gradient is about 8 mm Hg; a gradient of higher than 28 mm Hg has been found to correlate well with inhalation injury documented by other means (Petroff et al., 1976). The initial carboxyhemoglobin level is probably a better indicator of the severity of exposure than initial room-air arterial blood-gas studies. Measurement of the alveolar-arterial gradient on an Fio_2 of 1 increases the sensitivity of blood-gas determinations even further. A Pao_2 less than 250 mm Hg on 100% oxygen or a gradient that increases over time is highly predictive of significant pulmonary injury (Luce et al., 1976).

Initial chest x-ray findings are usually normal, but within 24–48 hours, pulmonary edema and focal atelectasis or infiltrates may be seen. Three additional diagnostic techniques have been used to evaluate further the presence and extent of pulmonary injury. (1) Fiberoptic bronchoscopy, which can be performed transnasally at the bedside under local anesthesia, is helpful in assessing both upper and lower airway injury; positive findings include mucosal erythema, edema, ulceration, and hemorrhage, the presence of carbonaceous sputum, and bronchorrhea. (2) Xenon[133] ventilation lung scanning has been advocated to assess the presence of injury to small airways and alveoli; positive results show a delay in clearance or an inequality of clearance of the isotope from the lungs. False-negative results may occur when the scan is obtained within 1–2 hours of exposure, since it often takes several hours for the pulmonary reaction to develop. False-positive results are seen in patients with pre-existent obstructive lung disease (Agee et al., 1976). (3) The most useful pulmonary function test in the assessment of pulmonary injury is analysis of the maximum expiratory flow volume curve. An expiratory flow rate at 50% of vital capacity, which is less than 50% of predicted, correlates highly with other evidence of pulmonary injury (Petroff et al., 1976). Analysis of the curve can also be used to follow response to therapy. Conventional spirometric measurements may be abnormal, but are less specific.

Treatment

Treatment begins with immediate attention to the upper airway. Experts differ on the timing of intubation in patients whose airway initially is patent but who have signs of upper airway injury and who are at risk for later obstruction. Some favor early prophylactic intubation; others favor waiting until signs of early obstruction develop. Definite indications for intubation are upper airway obstruction, impaired consciousness with inability to protect the airway, elevated $Paco_2$, and hypoxia despite supplemental oxygen. Nasotracheal intubation is the preferred method; tracheotomy should be avoided, especially in patients with body burns. If a patient who is to be transferred for definitive care has evidence of upper airway injury, it is preferable to intubate the patient before transport (after consultation with the receiving facility). All patients, intubated or not, initially should receive as high a concentration of humidified oxygen as can be achieved to treat potential carbon monoxide poisoning. Ventilated patients should be maintained on positive end-expiratory pressure or continuous positive airway pressure to prevent terminal airway closure. Patients should be encouraged to cough and breathe deeply; suctioning is to be avoided unless absolutely necessary, since it adds to the potential for infection. Therapeutic bronchoscopy may be helpful in patients with copious bronchorrhea and carbonaceous sputum. Bronchodilators such as aminophylline and β-adrenergic agents are useful in treating associated bronchospasm. The current consensus is that neither prophylactic antibiotics nor prophylactic corticosteroids are indicated in the management of inhalation injuries; corticosteroids may actually increase morbidity and mortality (Moylan, 1978). Adjunctive measures include placement of a nasogastric tube, prophylactic use of cimetidine to protect against gastric ulceration, and avoidance of fluid overload.

The decision regarding need for admission and length of observation can be difficult; some guidelines are presented in Table 10.5, but within this framework, each case needs to be individualized.

CARBON MONOXIDE POISONING

Acute carbon monoxide poisoning accounts for about 3500 deaths per year in the United States, and contributes to morbidity and mortality in an unknown number of victims of burns and smoke inhalation.

Table 10.5.
Protocol for management of victims of smoke inhalation.

All Patients

History: risk factors and symptoms
Physical examination: vital signs, body burns, special attention to nasal, oropharyngeal, and chest exams
Categorization:
  Trivial exposure: Very low-risk history, no symptoms or signs of inhalation, normal vital signs; short emergency ward observation and discharge
  Mild exposure: Some risk by history, minimal if any symptoms, normal physical examination, possible mild tachycardia
    Room-air, arterial blood gas, and carboxyhemoglobin levels
    Humidified 100% oxygen by facemask
    Electrocardiogram (especially if suspicious of elevated carboxyhemoglobin level)
    Chest x-ray examination
    Observe on oxygen for 4–6 hours from time of exposure; if no signs or symptoms develop and arterial blood-gas and carboxyhemoglobin levels satisfactory, discharge with warning about possible late complications
    If signs or symptoms develop, patient is moved to next category
  Moderate exposure: Moderate-risk history; symptoms or signs such as singed nasal hairs, carbonaceous sputum, cough, tachypnea, tachycardia, wheezing
    Arterial blood-gas and carboxyhemoglobin levels, 100% humidified oxygen, electrocardiogram, chest x-ray examination
    Admit and observe, follow arterial blood-gas levels, perform physical examination, obtain chest x-ray film
    Perform pulmonary toilet
    Brochodilators as needed
    Consider further diagnostic workup to assess extent of injury: alveolar-arterial gradient, fiberoptic bronchoscopy, $Xenon_{133}$ scanning, maximum expiratory flow-volume curve analysis
  Severe exposure: High-risk history, multiple signs and symptoms of upper or lower airway injury
    Assess need for intubation
    Arterial blood-gas and carboxyhemoglobin levels, 100% humidified oxygen, electrocardiogram, chest x-ray examination
    Volume ventilator with positive end-expiratory pressure
    Bronchodilators as needed
    Nasogastric tube, cimetidine
    Consider further diagnostic modalities as above

Pathophysiology

Because carbon monoxide is a colorless, odorless, nonirritating gas, it has been called a "silent killer." It is produced by the incomplete combustion of organic materials, and is present in most fires, motor vehicle exhaust, and many factories. With an affinity for hemoglobin about 240 times that of oxygen, carbon monoxide rapidly binds to hemoglobin, forming carboxyhemoglobin. As carboxyhemoglobin levels rise, oxygen-carrying hemoglobin decreases proportionately, thus impairing oxygen transport. In addition, carboxyhemoglobin shifts the oxyhemoglobin dissociation curve to the left, so the oxygen that is bound to hemoglobin is less readily released to the tissues. At the cellular level, utilization of oxygen is impaired as carbon monoxide binds to the iron-containing molecules of the cytochrome system. Organs with the most active cellular metabolism, such as heart and brain, are the most susceptible to injury.

Clinical Features

The symptoms of carbon monoxide poisoning are those of hypoxia, which are nonspecific. At low levels of carboxyhemoglobin, the only symptom may be dyspnea on exertion or tightness across the head. With levels from 20–30%, patients complain increasingly of headache, nausea, fatigue, dyspnea, dizziness, and dimmed vision. As the carboxyhemoglobin level rises, these symptoms become more pronounced and the patient may experience vomiting, confusion, and syncope. Finally, loss of consciousness, seizures, and respiratory arrest develop (Table 10.6). Patients with coronary artery disease may have angina or arrhythmias even at low carboxyhemoglobin levels.

It is important to remember that the carboxyhemoglobin level measured in the emergency ward may be considerably lower than the patient's peak carboxyhemoglobin level if sufficient time has elapsed since exposure or if oxygen has been administered at the scene or during transport. It is the peak level that carries prognostic significance, so it should be estimated if possible.

On physical examination, the patient usually is tachycardiac and may be tachypneic. The classic cherry-red hue of the lips and skin is not a reliable sign; more often, the patient will appear pale. Because of the nonspecific and protean manifestations of carbon monoxide poisoning, the physician must maintain a high index of suspicion to avoid missing the diagnosis. Some unusual presentations include multiple family members with the simultaneous onset of what appears to be food poisoning or gastroenteritis, patients who appear intoxicated, and firefighters with angina. Carbon monoxide poisoning should always be assumed in victims of smoke inhalation and in patients with major body burns. Treatment should be started presumptively with a high concentration of oxygen while awaiting the results of blood-gas and carboxyhemoglobin determinations. Blood-gas studies usually show a normal Pa_{O_2}, a low Pa_{CO_2}, and a lower pH than would be predicted by the Pa_{CO_2}, that is, a combined respiratory alkalosis and metabolic acidosis. In most hospital laboratories, the oxyhemoglobin saturation reported with the blood-gas analysis is calculated from the Pa_{O_2}, and

is, thus, grossly incorrect in the presence of an elevated carboxyhemoglobin level. An electrocardiogram should be obtained and may show ischemic changes or ventricular arrhythmias even when the patient has no cardiac symptoms.

Treatment

Oxygen is the mainstay of treatment. The two major decisions to be made are (1) which patients to intubate, and (2) when to employ hyperbaric oxygen therapy. The use of hyperbaric oxygen therapy (see page 188) has two major benefits. First, it greatly speeds the rate of carbon monoxide elimination, reducing the half-time for carboxyhemoglobin from 5–6 hours on room air to about 25 minutes on 100% oxygen at 3 atm (Table 10.7). Second, breathing 100% oxygen at 2.5–3 atm results in a dissolved oxygen content in plasma of 5.6–6.9 vol%, which is approximately the amount of oxygen extracted by the body under normal conditions (the normal arteriovenous oxygen content difference is 5–6 vol%). When a chamber is readily available, patients with carboxyhemoglobin levels over 25–30% should be treated with hyperbaric oxygen (Kindwall, 1977). When a chamber is not readily available, awake, cooperative patients with a carboxyhemoglobin level less than 40% can be treated with 100% oxygen by mask. Patients who are comatose, uncooperative, or hypoventilating, or who have a carboxyhemoglobin level over 40% require intubation and ventilation on 100% oxygen. Coma or a carboxyhemoglobin level over 40% indicates the need for transfer to a facility with a hyperbaric chamber, if available within a reasonable transfer time. Regardless of the method of oxygen administration, treatment should be continued until carboxyhemoglobin levels are less than 10%.

In addition to administration of oxygen, an attempt should be made to reduce oxygen demand by keeping the patient quietly at rest, with cardiac monitoring. In severe cases, further measures to reduce oxygen demand and to decrease cerebral edema have been advocated, including controlled hypothermia, corticosteroids, and fluid restriction.

Complications of carbon monoxide poisoning include late neuropsychiatric sequelae, and rarely, rhabdomyolysis with or without myoglobinuric

Table 10.6.
Manifestations of carbon monoxide poisoning.

Carboxyhemoglobin Level, %	Symptoms[a]
≤10	Usually none; dyspnea on extreme exertion
11–20	Band-like or throbbing headache, dyspnea on moderate exertion
21–30	More severe headache, throbbing temples, dyspnea on mild exertion, nausea
31–40	All symptoms of previous level, plus visual dimming, dizziness, irritability, vomiting, tachycardia
41–50	All symptoms of previous levels plus tachypnea, dyspnea at rest, syncope
>50	Coma, seizures, cardiorespiratory depression

[a] Patients with coronary artery disease may have angina at any level.

Table 10.7.
Half-life of carboxyhemoglobin.

F_{IO_2}	Pa_{O_2}, mm Hg	Carboxyhemoglobin half-time	Dissolved oxygen, vol %
0.21 (room air)	160	5–6 hours	0.3
1.0 at 1 atm (sea level)	760	80 min	2.09
1.0 at 3 atm (hyperbaric chamber)	2280	25 min	6.9

renal failure as a result of either pressure myonecrosis or generalized muscle hypoxia.

RADIATION ACCIDENTS

Basic Concepts

The primary purpose of this section is to provide the necessary information for treatment, at the emergency ward level, of accident victims who may be contaminated with radioactive materials or who may have been exposed to high levels of radiation. Accidental radiation exposure may occur outside the hospital (as a result of a transportation or industrial accident, or use of atomic weapons, for example) or within the hospital in situations in which radiation is utilized (as in the use of radiopharmaceuticals, radiotherapy, diagnostic x-rays, and so on). The emergency ward team should be well versed in the protocol for treating victims of a radiation accident. Realistic understanding of the biologic risks to themselves when treating these patients is also a necessity.

When radiation interacts with tissue, the atoms of the tissue become ionized. Ionization occurs when an orbital electron absorbs enough energy from radiation to escape all orbits around the atomic nucleus. The resultant "ion pair" consists of a free electron ("−" charge) and the ionized atom ("+" charge). Machines are one source of ionizing radiation (x-rays, γ-rays, electrons, and so on); radionuclide decay is another (β-particles, x-rays, and γ-rays, for example). Nuclear reactors and cyclotrons generate more potent forms of ionizing radiation, such as neutrons and protons.

The number of ion pairs produced is a function of the intensity of the radiation interacting with the tissue. The greater the number of ion pairs produced, the greater the potential for biologic damage. The unit of biologic absorbed dose is the rad (Table 10.8). When corrections are made relative to the biologic effectiveness of the radiation in question (quality factor), the resultant unit is the rem: rem = (rad) (quality factor). The quality factor for β-particles, x-rays, and γ-rays equals 1; for neutrons and protons, it is approximately 10. Therefore, a 10-rad dose of γ-rays equals 10 rem, and a 10-rad dose of neutrons equals 100 rem. A more common unit is the millirem (mrem) or millirad (mrad), which is 0.001 times the value of the rem and rad, respectively. To put these units into perspective, consider that the average whole-body dose from background radiation (natural and man-made) in the United States is approximately 200 mrem/year, a round-trip flight between Boston and London results in a whole-body dose of approximately 5 mrem, and a routine anteroposterior chest x-ray examination results in an entrance skin dose of approximately 20 mrem.

Persons who work with radiation are considered "occupationally exposed," and are permitted radiation exposure above that produced by background. The maximum permissible dose is the amount of ionizing radiation established by au-

Table 10.8.

Ionizing radiation current nomenclature.

The recent adoption of special names and abbreviations for some units of the Systeme d'Unites International (SI) for use in the field of ionizing radiation follow:

$$Gy = Gray = SI \text{ unit for absorbed dose.}$$
$$Sv = Sievert = SI \text{ unit for dose equivalent.}$$
$$Bq = Bequerel = SI \text{ unit for activity.}$$

To convert from one set of units to another, the following relationships are utilized:

$$1 \text{ rad} = 0.01 \text{ Gy} = 10 \text{ mGy} = 1 \text{ cGy}$$
$$1 \text{ rem} = 0.01 \text{ Sv} = 10 \text{ mSv} = 1 \text{ cSv}$$
$$1 \text{ curie} = 3.7 \times 10^{10} \text{ Bq; } 1 \text{ Bq} = 1 \text{ dps (disintegrations per second)}$$

Table 10.9.

Maximum permissible doses of ionizing radiation per year (in adults).

Organ	Dose, mrem	
	Occupationally Exposed Persons	General Public
Whole body (including gonads, lens of eye, red bone marrow)	5000	500
Forearms, hands, feet, and ankles	75,000	7500
Skin of whole body	30,000	3000

Table 10.10.
Acute radiation syndrome: classification.

Category	Whole-Body Dose, rem	Signs and Symptoms		Prognosis
		Early	Definitive	
Subclinical	≤200	Mild nausea and vomiting lasting 24 hours or less; lymphocytes > 1500/mm³	Usually asymptomatic to minimum prodromal symptoms; depression of neutrophils and platelets by week 4–5 at higher part of dose range	Essentially 100% survival in healthy adults; evidence of some damage at higher part of dose range
Hematopoietic (mild form)	200–400	Intermittent nausea and vomiting in nearly all patients for 2–4+ days; lymphocytes > 1000/mm³	Maximum hematopoietic depression at 3 weeks	Recovery in 5–6 weeks; complete recovery in 4–6 months
Hematopoietic (severe form)	400–600[a]	Severe hematopoietic complications; mild evidence of gastrointestinal damage on upper dose range	Severe neutrophil and platelet depression in 3–5 weeks; evidence of infection and hemorrhage may appear	Zero to 100% mortality in untreated cases; requires bone marrow transplants and other supportive measures; rarely fatal with adequate replacement therapy
Gastrointestinal	600–1000	Severe prodromal symptoms of nausea, vomiting, and diarrhea; difficult management of patient; lymphocytes < 500/mm³	Some recovery, then return of severe diarrhea with blood and electrolyte loss; severe neutrophil and platelet depression by day 10 or earlier; hemorrhage and infection within 1–3 weeks	High mortality even among those given functional replacement therapy; progression to shock and death in 10–14 days; effectiveness of bone marrow therapy not yet evaluated
Central nervous system	≥1000	Severe, intractable nausea and vomiting; central nervous system symptoms; burning sensation at exposure and confusion; lymphocytes essentially lacking	Partial recovery, then progressive confusion and shock; central nervous system damage	100% mortality likely independent of therapy given; death in 14–36 hours; marrow therapy trial indicated

[a] The human whole-body LD$_{50}$ at 60 days is approximately 400–500 rem.

thorities below which there is no reasonable expectation of risk to human health. Table 10.9 lists maximum permissible doses for the general public and for occupationally exposed individuals as a function of organ type. The greater the radiosensitivity of an organ, the less its maximum permissible dose.

Radiation can be detected and measured with suitable equipment. The most common instrument for this purpose in the emergency ward is a portable survey meter with an end-window Geiger-Müller (GM) probe to differentiate between particulate radiation (α- and β-particles) and photons (x-rays and γ-rays). Particulate radiation is not usually detected when internally deposited, whereas photons are able to traverse the tissue layers for subsequent detection. The meter should read directly in mrem units over a wide range, and it should be calibrated periodically to ensure its accuracy. It should be used to monitor patients, personnel, and spaces within the emergency ward.

The Radiation Accident

A radiation accident that qualifies for rapid medical treatment is defined as any unforeseen, unplanned, or unexpected event that causes acute-whole or partial-body radiation exposure with or without radioactive contamination. The radiation dose is usually large enough to result in injury, and when the individual is contaminated (internally or externally or both), rapid removal of the radioactive material is of primary importance.

Radiation accidents, therefore, can be divided into three basic categories: (1) single external radiation exposure; (2) contamination, either internal or external, with radioactive material; (3) exposure to external radiation plus contamination with radioactive material.

External exposure to radiation produces clinical symptoms only if the dose is sufficient to produce such a response. Exposure to a high dose of radiation over a period up to 24 hours is termed acute exposure.

Acute whole-body radiation affects all systems and organs of the body. The pattern of biologic response is dictated by the intensity of the exposure and is termed acute radiation syndrome. Since all organs and biologic systems are not equally sensitive to ionizing radiation, the syndrome is presented clinically in order of increasing severity by the following categories: (1) subclinical (200 rem or less); (2) hematopoietic syndrome: (a) mild (200–400 rem), (b) severe (400–600 rem); (3) gastrointestinal syndrome (600–1000 rem); (4) central nervous system syndrome (1000 rem or more).

Biologic effects common to all four categories include nausea and vomiting, malaise, and fatigue; increased temperature; and hematologic changes. Table 10.10 lists categories of acute radiation syndrome as a function of increasing whole-body radiation exposure.

The clinical management of acute radiation syndrome is a function of the type and extent of the clinical problems, for example, biologic and physiologic responses. Hospitalization is considered essential if the whole-body dose exceeds 100 rem. After a potentially lethal dose of radiation, the primary reason for hospitalization is to limit infection. Adequate fluid and electrolyte replacement is essential for the management of vomiting and diarrhea. If the possibility exists for rapid spread of infection (as evidenced by prolonged granulocytopenia), it may be necessary to administer antibiotics before identification of the organism and sensitivity studies. Hemorrhage will result from trauma, gastrointestinal denudation, or thrombocytopenia. Transfusions of whole blood or platelets or both may be indicated in the presence of severe anemia and thrombocytopenia.

Since 1945, the literature has reported several radiation accidents that have resulted in injury to

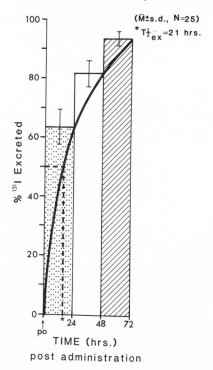

I Cumulative Urinary Excretion

Figure 10.3. ^{131}I cumulative urinary excretion.

individuals. The following is a brief description of one serious accident resulting from a large acute external radiation exposure:

Pittsburgh, Pennsylvania, October 14, 1967: Three technicians employed by the Gulf Research Development Company were accidentally exposed to a high-energy electron beam while attempting to repair the cooling system of a Van de Graaff generator. Because of failure of the safety system, the machine was on without the knowledge of the operators. One hour after exposure, the three men suffered nausea, which they interpreted as a symptom of influenza. However, it soon became evident that they were victims of radiation sickness. One man had received an estimated dose of 6000 rad on his hands and 600 rad on the rest of the body. His life was saved with a marrow transplant from his identical twin. However, gangrene developed in his hands, and seven fingers had to be amputated. The other two men received whole-body doses of 300 R and 100 rad, respectively. They suffered only mild radiation sickness and went back to work a few weeks after the accident.

It must be emphasized that individuals exposed to external radiation are usually not "radioactive." Rarely, natural body atoms, such as sodium and phosphorus, may become radioactive if the human body absorbs a significant dose of neutron radiation.

Contamination is defined as the deposition of radioactive material (radionuclides) where the material is not desired and where its presence may be harmful. Radioactive contamination of the body may be either internal or external. The severity of the accident is a function of the type of radionuclide, its physical properties (half-life and decay

Table 10.11.
On-site radiation accident checklist.

1. Provide emergency medical care immediately for serious injuries and preserve vital functions. Minor injuries can wait until after initial radiation survey has been completed.
2. Remove accident victim from contaminated radiation area. For assisting personnel, individual doses up to 100 rem may be permitted for lifesaving purposes, or up to 25 rem for less urgent purposes. Teams may be used in relays to remove injured persons from areas of very high radiation.
3. Survey victim for surface contamination levels.
4. Obtain smears of nasal mucus. Do this before the victim showers.
5. Remove contaminated clothes and replace with clean coveralls or wrap victim in blanket. Take victim to an area where skin can be decontaminated or a shower can be taken.
6. Decontaminate skin. Remove all transferable contamination if possible by cleansing contaminated skin areas and showering the accident victim.
7. Cover contaminated wounds with sterile dressings before and after decontamination.
8. Alert hospital and call for ambulance service as soon as it is determined that it is needed.
9. Identify radionuclide(s) involved, and if possible, ascertain the chemical form, solubility, and presumed particle size.
10. Send radiation dosimeters of involved personnel for processing.
11. Get complete history of accident, especially as it relates to the activities of the victim. Where was he? What was he doing? Exit path? Symptoms?
12. Evaluate possibility of penetrating radiation exposure.
13. Advise victim on collection of all excreta. Provide containers. Save other contaminated materials in appropriate leak-proof containers.
14. Be sure someone has assumed responsibility for management of the accident area. Is radiation safety assistance needed? Who will request it? From whom?
15. Report initial responses of assisting personnel and evaluation of situation to plant manager.
16. Obtain names of supervisory and health physics personnel who will remain on call in case additional information is needed.
17. Take victim to hospital if injuries require surgical care not available at plant or if further medical or dosimetric evaluation and treatment are required.
18. Take precautions to prevent spread of contamination during transport and movement of victim. Have transport vehicles, attendants, and equipment checked for residual radioactive contamination before release from hospital area.
19. If environmental contamination outside the scene of the accident has occurred, notify public health authorities.
20. Advise family or next of kin about extent of injuries and exposure. Plant management personnel and medical department personnel should agree on proper procedure.
21. Send bioassay specimens for analysis of radioactive content under the supervision of a safety officer. Specify who will receive results.

Table 10.12.
Emergency ward checklist.[a]

1. When did the accident occur? What were the circumstances, and what were the most likely pathways for exposure? How much radioactive material is potentially involved?
2. What injuries occurred? What potential medical problems may be present besides radionuclide contamination?
3. Are toxic or corrosive chemicals involved in addition to radionuclides? Has any treatment been given for chemical exposure?
4. What radionuclides now contaminate the patient? Where? What are the radiation measurements at the surface?
5. What information is available about the chemistry of the compounds containing the radionuclides? Are they soluble or insoluble? Is there any information about probable particle size?
6. What radioactivity measurements have been made at the site of the accident, for example, air monitoring, smears, fixed radiation monitoring, nasal smear counts, and skin contamination levels?
7. What decontamination efforts, if any, have been attempted? With what success?
8. Have any therapeutic measures such as administration of blocking agents or isotopic dilution agents been attempted?
9. Was the victim also exposed to penetrating radiation? If so, what has been learned from processing personal dosimeters, such as film badges, thermoluminescent dosimetry badges, or pocket ionization chambers? If not yet known, when is the information expected?
10. Has clothing removed at the site of the accident been saved in case the contamination on it is needed for radiation energy spectrum analysis and particle-size studies?
11. What excreta have been collected? Where are the samples? What analyses are planned? When will they be performed?

[a] In industrial accidents, the best information is usually obtained from plant personnel, such as the health physicist or occupational physician familiar with the plant and with accident details.

Table 10.13.
Guidelines for patient management after completion of initial emergency procedures.

1. If there is radionuclide contamination, all exposed persons must be surveyed and decontaminated before additional patient management. If this step is neglected, personnel whose duty is to care for patients may become so contaminated themselves as to be rendered ineffective. Proper protective clothing must be available.
2. In performing decontamination procedures, personnel should wear coveralls or a scrub suit, shoe covers, gloves, cap, and respiratory mask as indicated by initial survey.
   Ambulatory patients:
   Spread sheet of paper for patient to stand on. Have patient disrobe, putting clothing in suitable container (bag or wastebasket, for example) for later survey. Perform nose, mouth, and ear wipes. Have patient take shower, resurvey, and repeat procedure until patient is "clean."
   Nonambulatory patient:
   Place patient on sheet and remove clothing. Save clothing as above for later survey. Wash patient, resurvey, and repeat procedure until patient is clean.
3. If there is evidence of massive exposure to external radiation, and if large numbers of persons are involved, perform triage. It may be necessary to limit any extensive medical care to moribund patients in order to use available facilities to care for patients whose lives may be saved. Dose estimates of more than 2000 rem for external radiation or more than 2000 rem/hr for radionuclide contamination indicate that little help can be offered. In such instances, contamination of treatment personnel may become a major problem.
4. Put patient in bed, obtain a detailed history, and perform a brief physical examination.
5. Obtain a routine blood cell count. If there has been neutron exposure, obtain an additional 20-ml sample of venous blood.
6. Hospitalize patients with severe nausea and vomiting.
7. No specific therapy is indicated for acute radiation injury within the first few days after exposure.
8. Patients with a dose estimate of less than 100 rads of external radiation do not require major emergency care.
9. Patients who have received only external exposure to α-, β-, γ-, and x-radiation are not radioactive.
10. Patients who have been exposed to neutron radiation are slightly radioactive, but are not hazardous to personnel caring for them.
11. Patients contaminated with radionuclides present a hazard to emergency personnel. The degree of hazard depends on the level and type of contamination.

emissions), and its chemical form. External contamination may involve parts of the body such as skin or hair, or may be primarily confined to clothing. Internal contamination results when radioactive material enters the body in one of the following ways: (1) inhalation—breathing radioactive dust, aerosol, and gas; (2) ingestion—drinking contaminated liquids, eating contaminated foods, and transferring radioactivity to the mouth by touch; (3) absorption—radioactive material may be absorbed through the intact skin or through a wound.

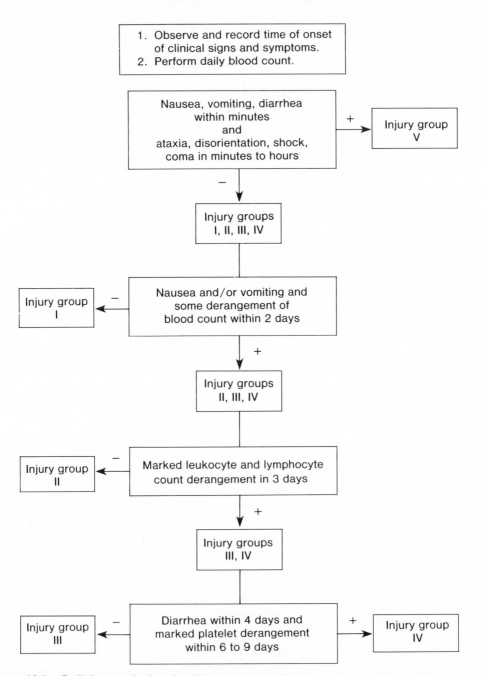

Figure 10.4.   Preliminary evaluation of radiation injury with differentiation into patient groups. (Reproduced by permission from Thoma GE Jr, Wald N: The diagnosis and management of radiation injury. *J. Occup Med* 1:421–447, 1959).

Table 10.14.
Correlation of patient groups with clinical manifestations of radiation injury.

Patient Group	Clinical Manifestations
I	Mostly asymptomatic—occasional minimal prodromal symptoms
II	Mild form of acute radiation syndrome—transient prodromal nausea and vomiting, mild laboratory and clinical evidence of hematopoietic derangement
III	A serious course—severe hematopoietic complications, and some evidence of gastrointestinal damage in upper half of group
IV	Accelerated form of acute radiation syndrome—gastrointestinal complications dominate clinical presentation, severity of hematopoietic complications is related to time after exposure
V	Fulminating course with marked central nervous system impairment

The chemical form of the radionuclide determines the excretion pattern of the compound. For example, more than 70% of orally administered sodium iodide I^{131} is excreted in the urine within 48 hours, with a half-time of 21 hours (fig. 10.3). Identification of the radionuclide and its chemical form will assist in predicting the biologic behavior of the radioactive material.

If the patient is contaminated, he or she is radioactive and represents a radiation source until decontaminated. Emergency ward personnel, by increasing their distance from a source of radiation, lower their exposure for a given period. The physical principle that serves as a basis for dose reduction relative to distance is called the "inverse square law." The inverse square law relationship allows calculation of dose rates at any distance from a point source by application of the following equation:

$$I_2 = I_1 \left(\frac{X_1^2}{X_2^2} \right)$$

where I_2 = dose rates at distance X_2 and I_1 = dose rates at distance X_1.

Example:

800 rem/hr is measured at 20 cm. Find the dose rate at 80 cm.

$$(800) \left(\frac{(20)^2}{(80)^2} \right) = (800) \left(\frac{400}{6400} \right) = 50 \ rem/hr$$

If the above equation is used for an extended source of radiation, such as a radioactive patient, it will give a good approximation of the dose rate.

The following is a brief description of an accident that resulted in internal contamination from the inhalation of radioactive material:

A worker inhaled airborne particles containing what must have been a relatively soluble compound of curium 244 (Cm^{244}) during removal of dry, solid, contaminated waste from a decontamination chamber. Filter papers used to smear the vestibules of his nose removed 0.016 μCi (micro-Curie) from the left nostril and 0.011 μCi from the right. His nasal cavity was irrigated with isotonic saline solution, and external skin contamination was removed by swabbing. His lungs were chelated 2.5 hours after the incident with 4 ml of a 25% solution of trisodium diethylenetriaminepentaacetate (DTPA) with a nebulizer. Blood samples were taken for radioassay before and after treatment with DTPA. A cathartic was given to hasten passage of the radioactive material through the gastrointestinal tract. About 4.5 hours after

Table 10.15.
Patient information that should be readily available to the treatment team.

Name of patient, employer, employee number

Physical injuries and treatment

Skin surface contamination
  Location
  Dose rate and/or count rate measurements initially
    and after decontamination
  Decontamination methods and agents used

Internal contamination
  Radionuclide—chemical form, probable solubility,
    and possible particle character
  Suspected route of contamination
  Nasal smear counts
  Wound counts
  Whole-body counts
  Bioassay samples already collected
  Treatment

External exposure to penetrating radiation
  Precise location and position of patient relative to
    source of radiation at time of exposure
  Exact time and duration of exposure
  Was dosimeter being worn? Where? What type?
  Has dosimeter been collected? By whom? Where
    is it now?
  Symptoms—type and time of occurrence
  Other dosimetric studies underway
  Treatment

Name and telephone number of company health physicist or physician for additional information the incident, 0.014 μCi of Cm^{244} was found by measuring the radioactive emissions from the worker's chest. Subsequent measurements showed that the amount of Cm^{244} rapidly decreased to 0.005 μCi within 4 days.

Emergency Treatment

Table 10.11 is a checklist of on-site emergency actions after radiation exposure. The sequence of these actions will vary with different accident conditions. Table 10.12 lists questions intended to provide useful medical information once the patient arrives in the emergency ward.

An individual may be seen in the emergency ward for one or more of the following: (1) acute radiation syndrome; (2) local radiation injury; (3) local traumatic injury with radionuclide contamination; (4) internal radionuclide contamination

without evident injury. The primary goals of the emergency ward team are to remove from the victim any further sources of exposure (decontamination) and to provide initial treatment for injuries. If contamination with radioactive material is present, decontamination procedures must be vigorously followed to avoid needless and serious spread of radioactive material throughout the hospital. After completion of initial emergency procedures, the team concentrates on additional patient management (Table 10.13).

The primary objective of the diagnostic workup is to determine whether biologically significant radiation exposure is present. If evidence is found, the next objective is to determine the immediate and anticipated biologic damage. As an aid in evaluation of the nature and seriousness of a ra-

Table 10.16.
Decontamination room supplies.

Coveralls or surgical scrub suits
Plastic aprons
Surgical caps
Plastic or rubber gloves
Sterile surgical gloves
Sterile suture sets with additional sterile scissors (2), forceps (4), scalpel (1), and hemostats (6)
Sterile irrigation sets
Sterile applicators and miscellaneous dressings
Long patient gowns or coveralls, socks
Plastic shoe covers
Large towels
Ribbed or nonskid plastic sheets
Safety razor with extra blades and aerosol shaving soap
Bandage scissors (2)
Large plastic or cloth bags for collection of contaminated clothing
Respirators (prefit for team personnel)
Radiation tags
"Do Not Enter" signs for radiation area
Personal dosimeters (self-reading ionization chambers, 200 mR and 20 R levels) and dosimetry badges
    (thermoluminescent type)
Masking tape, 2 inches wide
Labeled containers for collecting urine and fecal specimens
Blankets
Adhesive labels and tags for labeling tissue and contaminated material
Tissue specimen bottles (with formalin if freezing facilities are unavailable)
Felt-tipped pens (black for noncontaminated materials, red for contaminated materials).
Notebooks, paper, pencils
Portable radiation survey meters, both low-range (up to 25 mrem/hr) and high-range (up to 500 rem/hr)
Portable alpha scintillation detector
Large roll 36-inch-wide absorbent (blotter-type) paper or wrapping paper as used in stores (tear-off dispensers
    are available)
Specific decontamination supplies, with instructions on their use, in a separate labeled box
    Detergents
    Titanium dioxide (abrasive)
    Potassium permanganate (and sodium acid sulfite to remove stain)
    Household bleach (5% sodium hypochlorite)
Fiberboard barrels or steel drums with tight-fitting tops for disposal of contaminated clothing and other
    contaminated items

Table 10.17.
Decontamination guidelines for protection of hospital personnel and facilities.

1. Personnel should wear surgical scrub suits or gowns, surgical caps, and rubber gloves. Gloves can be surgical, household, or industrial, depending on their use.
2. The team leader must be able to recognize the rare instance when masks, respirators, or airpacks may be needed because of high levels of α- or β-radionuclides.
3. Rubber or plastic shoe covers are desirable. Those persons performing the actual decontamination with water should wear plastic or rubber laboratory aprons. Temporary shoe covers for dry areas can be improvised from brown paper bags held on with adhesive or masking tape.
4. Unless a special filter system is available for use during decontamination, air conditioning and forced-air heating systems should be turned off so that radioactive particles are not carried into ducts or other rooms.
5. Floors should be protected with a disposable covering both to reduce "tracking" by providing a cleaner surface and to aid cleanup. The covering should be changed when significant contamination is present. Brown paper rolls (36-inch-wide, 60-lb weight) are ideal where water is not used. Ribbed or nonskid plastic sheets are useful where spillage of liquids is a problem.
6. All contaminated clothing should be carefully placed in plastic or paper bags to reduce secondary contamination of area.
7. Splashing of solutions used in decontamination should be avoided.
8. Patients and potentially contaminated personnel should move to clean areas only after survey shows satisfactory decontamination.
9. All persons and property passing between contaminated and clean areas must be surveyed and regulated by monitoring teams.
10. Supplies should be passed through monitoring stations from clean areas to contaminated areas. Reverse flow must not occur unless supplies are monitored and found clean.
11. All persons on the decontamination team must be trained to radiologic monitoring and decontamination techniques. Persons not on the team should be excluded from the work area.
12. Fiberboard or steel drums with tight-fitting tops should be available for disposal of contaminated materials. Labels describing the contents should be affixed so that proper disposal can be carried out without reopening the drums. Lids should be taped to the drums with masking or other sealing tape.
13. All personnel in the decontamination area should have personal dosimeters (pocket ionization chambers, film badges, or thermoluminescent dosimeters). Personnel should be rotated after a dose of 5 rem (or less if possible).
14. Entry of individuals who are not part of the team, including family, visitors, and administrative personnel, should be restricted.

Table 10.18.
Detergent preparations used in decontamination of skin and wounds.

Aqueous preparations
  Soap and water
  Abrasive soap and water
  Commercial detergents (10% active ingredients): Tide, Dreft, Alconox, HemoSol
  Chelating agent (1% versene solution) with or without detergent
Waterless preparations
  Cornmeal and commercial powdered detergent in equal parts made into a watery paste and used without additional water (scrub with brush, remove with cotton or soft tissues)
  Waterless mechanics' hand cream, used without additional water (scrub with brush, remove with cotton or soft tissues)
  Homogenized cream of 8% carboxymethylcellulose, 3% commercial powdered detergent, 1% versene, and 88% distilled water, used without additional water (scrub with brush, remove with cotton or soft tissues)

diation accident, Figure 10.4 illustrates the extent of injury in patient groups up to 6–9 days after radiation exposure. Clinical manifestations are correlated with patient groups in Table 10.14.

Decontamination

If the radiation accident occurred where there is an in-house physician or health physicist, this individual will often be able to provide specific information concerning the incident. Each patient should be identified with as much information as possible before decontamination is begun (Table 10.15). If a survey meter is immediately available, radiation monitoring should be accomplished. Decontamination room supplies are listed in Table 10.16.

Once the patient is ready for decontamination, procedures should be followed to minimize the radiation hazard to personnel and hospital facilities (Table 10.17). Removal of gross contamination is the recommended initial step in patient decontamination, and may be accomplished by removal of contaminated clothing, washing or removal of contaminated hair, and decontamination of wounds. Patients suspected of contamination should be washed as soon as possible. Useful detergent preparations, in order of increasing strength, are listed in Table 10.18. An intermediate stage in decontamination should include further local decontamination of any wounds and support measures such as first aid. Swabs of body orifices should be obtained to determine whether internal contamination is present. More definitive surgical decontamination and other additional treatment might then be necessary.

If radioactive contamination is internal, removal may be accelerated by a number of therapies. Radioactive material that has entered the gastrointestinal tract may be removed by administration of an emetic. To reduce tissue uptake, the emergency team may give large quantities of a stable isotope to cause "isotope dilution" or "metabolic blocking." An example of the latter is administration of stable potassium iodide to block the thyroidal uptake of radioactive iodine isotopes. An increase of fluids will promote rapid turnover and excretion of tritium (^{3}H) if the label is distributed throughout the body as tritiated water. Chelating agents form inactive complexes with certain metal ions that will accelerate the rate of renal excretion of certain radionuclides. They must be administered during the first 24–48 hours for optimum effect, and not all radioactive metals are sensitive to this therapy. A major disadvantage is the nephrotoxic effect of these agents. Bioassay procedures, including the collection of feces, urine, and sputum and the subsequent determination of radionuclide identity and content, as well as in vivo imaging or counting procedures, will assist the clinician in following the biologic release pattern of these radionuclides.

In summary, the medical treatment of a radioactive accident victim can only be a success if the radiation treatment team is properly instructed. Appropriate use of hospital emergency space should be emphasized, along with methods of isolation, containment of contamination, adequate patient decontamination procedures, the cleaning of wounds, and the care of patients who have internal contamination with radioactive material. In addition, emergency ward personnel must be aware of the biologic risks when exposed to radiation, and must understand basic radiation protection procedures, including the use of radiation detection instruments to monitor patients, personnel, and emergency ward spaces.

BITES AND STINGS

More than 500,000 animal bites are reported yearly in the United States and dog bites constitute the largest group (Table 10.19). There are about 90 million dogs and cats in the United States, while the human population is only about 2.5 times that, at approximately 220 million. The human victim is usually a 7- to 9-year-old boy, often teasing or playing with the dog. The biting dog is usually 6- to 12-months old, is often female, and is usually a working dog, such as a boxer, collie, German shepherd, Great Dane, or Saint Bernard, or a sporting dog, such as a pointer, setter, or retriever. Hounds are relatively safe.

The evaluation and treatment of all bites includes a careful history, including the type of animal, the site of the bite, and the geographic setting. Hand wounds and puncture wounds most often become infected. Most bites should be cultured and a Gram stain prepared; they should then be washed, irrigated well, and left open. Selection of an antibiotic depends on the bite history and Gram stain results. Most patients with deep cat bites, deep cat scratches, and sutured wounds should be treated with penicillin or tetracycline because of the increased incidence of *Pasteurella multocida* infection. Tetanus immune status should be evaluated, and rabies immunization should be considered.

Human bites and monkey bites deserve special mention, since 30% become infected with aerobic or anaerobic mouth organisms. Anaerobic infection may spread through the metacarpophalangeal space and cause severe damage. The same procedure as for other animals bites should be followed, that is, culture and Gram stain, thorough washing, and wide dissection. Wounds should be left open

Table 10.19.
Massachusetts Bite Summary, 1979.

Dog	11,356
Cat	423
Hamster	75
Rat	64
Rabbit	45
Gerbil	37
Squirrel	30
Horse	26
Skunk	21
Raccoon	20
Snake	9
Chipmunk	8
Guinea pig	8
Total	12,122

if possible, especially hand wounds. Patients with human bites should be treated with penicillin for 7–10 days. Clenched-fist injuries should be evaluated by a hand surgeon.

Disease Caused by Pasteurella Multocida

A common organism infecting bite wounds is *P. multocida*. Disease due to this organism now is diagnosed more frequently; thus, its presence in the nasopharynx in 50% of dogs and 75% of cats is of public health importance.

Most infections in humans fall into one of three clinical patterns:

(1) The most common pattern is that of local infection with adenitis after a dog or cat bite or scratch. In patients with a cat bite, this then may progress to tenosynovitis or osteomyelitis due to inoculation of the organism into the periosteum by the long, sharp tooth of the animal. Canine teeth are more blunt and less likely to penetrate the periosteum.

(2) Chronic pulmonary infection, in which *P. multocida* may occur as the primary pathogen or in association with other organisms. Bacteria may enter through the respiratory tract by inhalation of barn dust or infectious droplets sprayed by the sneeze of an animal. In such cases, the bacteria probably colonize the respiratory tract and lie dormant in the patient with chronic lung disease. Acute infection occurs only after trauma to the bronchial tree. Bronchiectasis, emphysema, peritonsillar abscess, and sinusitis have all been described with this organism.

(3) Systemic infection with bacteremia or meningitis may occur.

P. multocida is a small gram-negative ovoid bacillus that grows well on blood agar but not on gram-negative media, such as MacConkey agar. Because of its superficial resemblance to *Hemophilus influenzae* and Neisseria organisms, respiratory tract and central nervous system infections with *P. multocida* initially may be misdiagnosed. Failure of growth on routine gram-negative media is an important clue.

Treament of the patient with presumptive *P. multocida* infection (that is, any patient with a deep cat bite or scratch or a deep dog bite) should include careful washing and an attempt to leave the wound open. The antibiotic of choice is penicillin, 8–10 days orally, with careful follow-up of the wound. Ampicillin, tetracycline, and cephalosporins are alternatives. Oxacillin and erythromycin are less active, but still are beneficial, whereas clindamycin is least active.

Plague

Infection with *Yersinia pestis* usually results from a flea bite. Urban plague from *Y. pestis* occurs today as an important cycle only in devastated cities such as in Vietnam. Sylvatic plague is the major cycle in the United States, and the major endemic area is the Southwest. The infected flea vector enters a community of susceptible rodents, such as ground squirrels, prairie dogs, marmots, wood rats, and rabbits, and transmits the bacteria. Mortality is high and transmission to humans has increased recently, as has been documented in states such as New Mexico, California, Arizona, Colorado, and Utah.

Human plague most often occurs when an individual in a rural area is bitten by an infected flea. Infection also may occur while handling the carcasses of small mammals or by transfer of the vector from a domestic pet. In addition, direct skin contact with an infected mammal (as when skinning rabbits) may also result in infection.

Y. pestis is a gram-negative bacillus that grows well in ordinary broth and agar. Bacteria usually are transmitted by the rat flea from the infected rodent. Immune rodents and humans maintain the organism in local vesicles. In less resistant hosts, spread occurs to lymph nodes and the blood stream.

The incubation period is 2–6 days. Tender lymphadenitis and a local bubo then develop. Systemic onset is abrupt, with high fever. Bacteremia and shock then occur in 3–5 days.

Diagnosis is made by Gram stain and culture of the aspirate of a bubo and by blood culture. Other means include inoculation of the organism into mice or guinea pigs. Finally, acute and convalescent sera may be obtained.

All patients with plague should be isolated for the first 48 hours until secondary plague pneumonia can be ruled out. Lymph nodes should not be incised and drained until the patient has been treated with antibiotics. Streptomycin is the preferred agent, 30 mg/kg/day intramuscularly in two divided doses for 10 days. Alternative antibiotics include tetracycline and chloramphenicol.

Patients with plague pneumonia should be isolated, and all contacts should be quarantined and treated with tetracycline for 10 days.

Tularemia

Tularemia has been reported from every state, but four states (Arkansas, Louisiana, Oklahoma, and Texas) have had higher rates of infection with *Francisella tularensis*, a gram-negative pleomorphic coccobacillus. Although the peak seasonal incidence varies with the geographic area, tick-borne tularemia is generally most common in summer, whereas in winter, contact with wild mammals (mainly rabbits during the hunting season) is the most frequent cause of disease.

Although infection with *F. tularensis* has been proved in at least 100 different species of mammal, wild rodents, especially cottontail rabbits, are the principal reservoir. Since transovarial passage occurs in ticks, ticks may serve as both reservoir and vector.

Three main types of human infection occur:

(1) Cutaneous lesions (ulceroglandular)—this form is most common, and often occurs either after skinning or dressing rabbits or deer or after a tick bite. Tularemia is an occupational hazard for hunters, butchers, and sheepshearers, and felt hat manufacturers.

The typical lesion is macular and pruritic, and ulcerates within 2 days. Regional lymph nodes then enlarge, become tender, and drain, accompanied by high fever from 104–106°F (40–41.1°C). The tick bite is not always easy to find. A recent episode occurred in a 5-year-old boy from the Massachusetts coast with fever and occipital lymphadenopathy. After a long search, repeated, careful scalp examination revealed an engorged tick. High tularemia agglutination titers were later found.

(2) Tularemic pneumonia—this form is much less common, but may occur after inhalation of large amounts of infected particles, such as in a patient who skinned and eviscerated six rabbits. An outbreak of tularemic pneumonia occurred in a family on Martha's Vineyard in August 1978 who were vacationing in a cottage where mice were found inside and rabbits and ticks outside. The final premise was that dogs may have mangled the infected rabbits, then transmitted the bacteria via aerosol of saliva in the cottage.

(3) Typhoidal tularemia—this form occurs after ingestion of raw or improperly cooked meat. Symptoms include abdominal pain, diarrhea, fever, and bacteremia. A recent case report described a man in New Mexico who cooked prairie dog meat for only 2 hours.

Tularemia is diagnosed mainly by a history of rabbit or tick exposure. Specific cysteine-dextrose blood agar is required for growth of the organism, but because laboratory propagation is potentially hazardous, culture is not routinely considered. When cultured, the organism may require 10 days for growth. Diagnosis may be confirmed by a fluorescent antibody test or by development of an elevated serum antibody titer within a week of 1:640 or greater.

Streptomycin, 30–40 mg/kg for 3 days, then 20 mg/kg/day is the antibiotic of choice. Tetracycline may be used alternatively.

Rocky Mountain Spotted Fever

Another infection transmitted by ticks is Rocky Mountain spotted fever. There are two principal vectors in the United States. *Dermacentor andersoni*, the wood tick, is distributed in the Rocky Mountain states and is active in the spring and early summer. *D. variabilis*, the dog tick, is mainly found in the eastern half of the United States, especially in the southern portion, extending from Oklahoma to Tennessee, and northeast to Long Island and southern New England.

The clinical syndrome includes severe headache, then myalgia, followed by a maculopapular rash 2–3 days later. The rash typically starts on the wrists and ankles, extends to palms and soles, and then becomes central. If allowed to progress without treatment, the rash may become petechial.

Complement fixation, indirect fluorescent antibody, indirect hemagglutination, latex agglutination, and microagglutination studies are now available. These tests are more specific and more sensitive than the Weil-Felix reaction.

Treatment for presumptive Rocky Mountain spotted fever is with chloramphenicol 2–3 gm/day or tetracycline, 2 gm/day for 10–14 days in adults.

Babesiosis

Babesiosis, a disease caused by the intracellular red blood cell parasite, *Babesia microti*, is also transmitted by ticks. Risk increases in patients with T-lymphocyte depression or after splenectomy, but several cases have occurred in normal hosts. The clinical syndrome of babesiosis includes fever, myalgia, and hemolytic anemia. Diagnosis is made by observation of the intracellular red blood cell parasite on a Giemsa-stained smear. The tetrads may be confused with the findings in falciparum malaria, but Babesia-infected red blood cells do not have pigment granules. Antibody titers are also helpful in making the diagnosis.

Treatment is based on symptoms in the normal host. In splenectomized patients, exchange transfusions have been helpful.

Rat-Bite Fever

Two bacteria that may cause disease after a rat bite are *Streptobacillus moniliformis* and *Spirillum*

Table 10.20.
Rate-bite fever.

	Streptobacillar fever	Spirillar fever
Organism	*Streptobacillus moniliformis*	*Spirillum minus*
Epidemiology	Bite, food	Bite
Incubation	<1 week	1–3 weeks
Bite site	Prompt healing	Initial healing followed by reactivation of bite site at time of diagnosis
Rash	+	+
Arthralgia	+	−
Diagnosis	Culture, titer	Smear, dark field
Treatment	Penicillin × 10 days (1–2 gm/day)	Penicillin × 10 days (1–2 gm/day)

minus. Table 10.20 illustrates the differences between the two diseases.

Cat-Scratch Disease

The cause of cat-scratch disease is unknown. The chlamydia-lymphogranuloma group has been incriminated. Disease results from trauma, often from a cat scratch, less often from a dog or cat bite or a monkey scratch, and sometimes from a scratch from a rose thorn or porcupine quill. The syndrome usually occurs in the early spring, and it is usually a young kitten that transmits the disease. Cats act only as vectors; they do not become ill themselves.

The incubation period is 3–10 days, and the primary lesion is a tender papule. Lymphadenopathy then develops within 5 days to 2 months, and is usually unilateral. The lymph node is tender, with erythema over the skin. About 20% of nodes drain. Systemic symptoms may include headache, fever, and malaise. Rarely, encephalitis or oculoglandular disease (Parinaud's syndrome) may develop.

The diagnosis of cat-scratch disease is made by a history of contact with cats or kittens, evidence of a primary lesion, regional lymphadenopathy, and a positive skin test. The antigen for the skin test is difficult to obtain, however.

Treatment is supportive. Suppurative nodes should be aspirated for diagnostic and therapeutic purposes.

Rabies

The most notorious viral disease caused by an animal bite is rabies. The epidemiology has changed in the past few years, and now, nonimmune dogs account for only 16% of cases, whereas sylvatic animals, such as skunks, foxes, bats, and raccoons, account for more than 80% in the United States. Skunks, raccoons, red and gray foxes, bats, and domestic dogs represent the greatest potential danger; rodents, such as squirrels and hamsters, are probably inconsequential.

Live virus is introduced into nerve tissue at the time of the bite. The virus persists 96 hours at the site, and then spreads to the central nervous system. It replicates in gray matter, and then spreads along autonomic nerves to the salivary glands, adrenal glands, and heart. The incubation period varies with the site of the bite from 10 days to as long as 1 year.

Clinical features include a prodromal period of 1–4 days, followed by high fever, headache, and malaise. Paresthesias at the site of inoculation occur in 80% of patients. The rest of the sequence of events includes agitation, hyperesthesia, dysphagia, paralysis, and death.

The fluorescent antibody method for the viral antigen is the most rapid and sensitive means of diagnosis. Brain biopsy of the animal is also useful.

Pre-exposure prophylaxis is important for spelunkers, veterinarians, and virologists. Human diploid cell vaccine should be given, and the neutralizing antibody titer should be followed.

In postexposure prophylaxis, the following questions should be considered:

(1) What is the status of animal rabies in the locale where the exposure took place?

(2) Was the attack provoked or unprovoked?

(3) Of what species was the animal?

(4) What was the state of health of the animal?

Most animals transmit rabies virus in saliva only a few days before becoming ill themselves (dog and skunk, 5 days; fox, 3 days; cat, 1 day). Bats, however, may harbor the virus for many months.

The physician should regard the skunk, fox, raccoon, and bat as rabid, and should treat patients with bites from these animals with both human diploid cell vaccine and human rabies immune globulin (Tables 10.21 and 10.22). Healthy domestic dogs and cats should be observed.

Treatment of rabies includes the following:

(1) The most important step is to scrub the

Table 10.21.

Rabies Postexposure Prophylaxis Guide (Adapted from *Morbidity and Mortality Weekly Reports*, Center for Disease Control, USPHS, Atlanta, June 13, 1980)

General Measures and Comments:

All bites and wounds should immediately be thoroughly cleansed with soap and water.[a] If vaccine treatment is indicated, both rabies immune globulin (RIG) and human diploid cell rabies vaccine (HDCV) should be given as soon as possible, regardless of interval after exposure. (The administration of RIG is the more urgent procedure. If HDCV is not immediately available, start RIG and give HDCV as soon as it is obtained.) If either RIG or HDCV is unavailable, substitute antirabies serum equine (ARS) and/or duck embryo vaccine (DEV), respectively. Do not exceed recommended RIG or ARS dose. Common local reactions to DEV do not contraindicate continued treatment. Vaccine use should be discontinued if tests of animal tissues for rabies antigen, using fluorescent reagents, are negative.

Animal Species	Condition of Animal at Time of Attack	Treatment of Exposed Person
Household pets Dogs and cats	Healthy and available for 10 days of observation	None unless animal develops rabies. At first sign of rabies in animal, treat patient with RIG and HDCV. Symptomatic animal should be killed and tested as soon as possible.
	Rabid or suspect Unknown (escaped)	RIG and HDCV Consult public health officials. If treatment indicated, give RIG and HDCV.
Wild animals Skunks, bats, foxes, coyotes, raccoons, bobcats, other carnivores	Regard as rabid unless proved negative by laboratory tests. If available, animal should be killed and tested as soon as possible.	RIG and HDCV
Other animals Livestock, rodents, lagomorphs (e.g., rabbits, hares)	Consider individually. Local and state public health officials should be consulted on the need for prophylaxis. Bites by the following almost never call for antirabies prophylaxis: squirrels, hamsters, guinea pigs, gerbils, chipmunks, rats, mice, and other rodents, rabbits, and hares.	

[a] Although copious washing is more important than the type of solution used, I recommend following soap and water with 70% alcohol, which is rabicidal (S.A.P.).

(Reprinted with permission from *Hospital Practice*, November 1980, p. 71, from Plotkin, SA: Rabies vaccination in the 1980s. pp. 65–72).

wound *vigorously* with a brush and soap. Rinse well, then perform a second scrub with green soap or alcohol.

(2) Active immunization is accomplished with either duck embryo vaccine or the new human diploid cell vaccine (Merieux Institute, Inc., Table 10.23). If human vaccine is unavailable, duck embryo vaccine is given in a dosage schedule of 23 doses: 2 doses of 1 ml each for 7 days, followed by 1 ml for 7 days, followed by 2 booster doses. There are rare severe reactions to duck embryo vaccine; however, the major disadvantages are that it is less potent and it must be given over a prolonged period. Pain at the site, itching, and myalgia also occur frequently. These symptoms can be over-come by administration of diphenhydramine hydrochloride (Benadryl) or acetylsalicylic acid or both before injection. Corticosteroids should be avoided during vaccine administration. It is important to measure the antibody titers 30–40 days after the start of treatment with duck embryo vaccine. The mouse inhibition titer should be 1:5 or greater; the rapid fluorescent focus inhibition titer should be $\geq 1:16$ or greater.

Human diploid cell vaccine is more potent than duck embryo vaccine, and thus, fewer doses are needed. The dosage schedule is usually 1, 3, 7, 14, 30, and 90 days, and there are no known side effects. The indications for use of human diploid cell vaccine are (1) bite by an animal known to be

Table 10.22.
Dosage schedules for human diploid cell vaccine and duck embryo vaccine.
POSTEXPOSURE: Postexposure rabies prophylaxis for persons exposed to rabies consists of the immediate, thorough cleansing of all wounds with soap and water, administration of rabies immune globulin (RIG) or, if RIG is not available, antirabies serum, equine (ARS), and the initiation of either HDCV or DEV, according to the following schedule.[a]

Rabies Vaccine	No. of 1-ml doses	Route of Administration	Intervals between Doses	If No Antibody Response to Primary Series, Give:[b]
HDCV	5[c]	Intramuscular	Doses to be given on days 0, 3, 7, 14, and 28[d]	An additional booster dose[d]
DEV	23	Subcutaneous	21 daily doses followed by a booster on day 31 and another on day 41[d] or 2 daily doses in the first 7 days, followed by 7 daily doses. Then 1 booster on day 24, and another on day 34[d]	3 doses of HDCV at weekly intervals[d]

(Reproduced with permission from *Morbidity and Mortality Weekly Report*, June 13, 1980, Vol. 29, no. 3, p. 280, Atlanta, Center for Disease Control.)

[a] The postexposure regimen is greatly modified for someone with previously demonstrated rabies antibody.

[b] If no antibody response is documented after the recommended additional booster dose(s), consult the state health department or CDC.

[c] The World Health Organization recommends a 6th dose 90 days after the 1st dose.

[d] Serum for rabies antibody testing should be collected 2–3 weeks after the last dose.

Table 10.23.
Rabies prophylaxis information.

Local or state laboratory
Center for Disease Control
1600 Clifton Road
Atlanta, GA 30333
(404) 329–3644 (any hour)
Merieux Institute, Inc.
(1) (800) 327–2842

rabid, (2) lack of antibody formation to duck embryo vaccine, and (3) allergy to duck embryo vaccine.

(3) Finally, it is important to immunize passively the patient following a potentially rabid bite. Human rabies immune globulin should be given immediately—50% around the site of the bite and 50% in the thigh or the arm. The dosage is 15–40 of IU/kg. Passive immunization results in the early appearance of antibody, but also inhibits the development of the active antibody from the human diploid cell or duck embryo vaccine; this is the reason for prolonged dosage of the vaccines. Although rabies has been regarded as uniformly fatal, several patients now have survived with prolonged cardiorespiratory support. An aggres-

sive approach in the patient with known rabies infection certainly merits the effort.

Simian Herpes B Virus

Simian herpes B virus is found in old world monkeys, especially rhesus and cynomolgus species. Infection occurs mainly by a bite, and less commonly after inhalation of monkey saliva or contact with infected monkey cell cultures. A vesicular lesion develops at the wound site, with progressive lymphangitis and fever. Confusion, reduced tendon reflexes in lower extremities, and respiratory paralysis may follow.

Diagnosis depends on viral isolation or intranuclear inclusion bodies in lymph nodes or brain biopsy from patient or animal, or a rise in neutralizing antibody titer to simian herpes B virus in the patient's blood. Treatment is supportive.

Orf (Contagious Ecthyma)

Orf is an endemic viral disease of sheep and goats. The disease in humans is contracted through direct cutaneous transmission. A nodular, vesicular, or pustular lesion develops at the site of contact; regional lymphadenopathy follows, and the lesions may progress to diffuse vesiculopapular rash.

Diagnosis is made by a complement fixation

titer more than 1:8 or isolation of virus on bovine kidney cell culture. Treatment is supportive.

Snake Bites

The two major poisonous snakes in the Americas are the pit viper and the coral snake. The coral snake belongs to the family Elapidae (Table 10.24). The remainder of all poisonous snakes in this hemisphere belong to the family Viperidae. The subfamily of pit vipers includes the rattlesnake, water moccasin, and copperhead. There are about 7000 poisonous snake bites reported in the United States annually. The largest number occur in the Southwestern and Gulf states.

Two poisonous snakes are native to New England. The northern copperhead, also called the highland moccasin, is pink or reddish brown, and is marked with large barrels of chestnut brown resembling dumbbells or hourglasses. The bite is painful but rarely fatal. The timber rattler is dark brown with chevrons of black and brown. The horny rattle on the tail buzzes when the snake is disturbed.

The degree of toxicity of a snake bite depends on the potency of the venom, the amount injected, the size and condition of the snake, and the size of the person bitten. There are instant clinical manifestations of the pit viper bite. Pain occurs at the site of the bite, as well as a wheal with local edema, numbness, and within moments, ecchymosis and painful lymphadenopathy. Nausea, vomiting, sweating, fever, drowsiness, and slurred speech may then develop. Bleeding of the gums and hematemesis are common hemorrhagic manifestations.

For proper treatment, it is extremely important to establish that the bite is from a poisonous snake. The patient should have distinct fang punctures and immediate local pain, followed by edema and

Table 10.24.
Classification of selected poisonous reptiles.

Lizards
  Family Helodermatidae: Gila monster: Mexico, Southwest United States—venom is a local irritant and neurotoxic
Snakes
  Family Colubridae: Most are harmless
  Family Elapidae: North American coral snake—neurotoxic
  Family Hydroplidae: Water snakes—venoms act on skeletal muscles
  Family Viperidae: Subfamily Crotalidae (pit viper). All dangerous snakes (except coral snakes) in the Americas belong to this group, for example, rattlesnakes, water moccasins, and copperheads.

discoloration within 30 minutes. It is helpful to inspect the snake, since those that are poisonous may be differentiated from those that are not by the presence of fangs and the shape of the pupils (Fig. 10.5).

The limb should be immobilized and a tourniquet applied proximal to the wound. The tourniquet should be released for 90 seconds every 15 minutes. The physician should make two longitudinal incisions through the fang marks and apply suction intermittently for the first hour. An attempt should be made to neutralize the venom with immune serum. Emergency information and specific immune serum can be obtained from the Oklahoma City Poison Control Center (1–405–271–5454, 24 hours a day). A photograph of snakes common to a specific geographic area is important for all emergency wards.

Polyvalent pit viper antivenom can be used for all American snakes except the coral snake. If possible, it should be administered within 1 hour of the bite, and the patient should first undergo skin testing for hypersensitivity. The dosage is usually about 5 vials in 500 ml of normal saline solution over 30 minutes. Prophylactic antimicrobial therapy and tetanus prophylaxis are recommended for deep bites. Supportive treatment, including hospitalization and careful evaluation of the baseline hematocrit, platelet count, and prothrombin time, is important. Finally, surgical decompression is rarely necessary.

Spider Bites

Emergency physicians should be aware of two spiders in particular, the black widow and the brown recluse. The black widow spider, *Lactrodectus mactans*, may be found in basements and backyards all over the United States, especially in the South and in western Ohio. The female is venomous and aggressive. The spider is jet black and globular, with a red mark shaped like an hourglass on the abdomen. The venom causes central and peripheral nervous system excitement, autonomic activity, muscle spasms, hypertension, and vasoconstriction.

Sharp pain occurs at the site of the bite, followed by cramping pain locally within about an hour, which spreads to the extremities and the trunk. Severe abdominal pain may occur, causing a board-like abdomen that is rigid but not tender. This is an important differentiating point on examination. A fatal outcome is rare. Treatment is usually supportive only; Antivenin may be needed in children or the elderly.

The brown recluse, *Loxosceles reclusus*, prefers

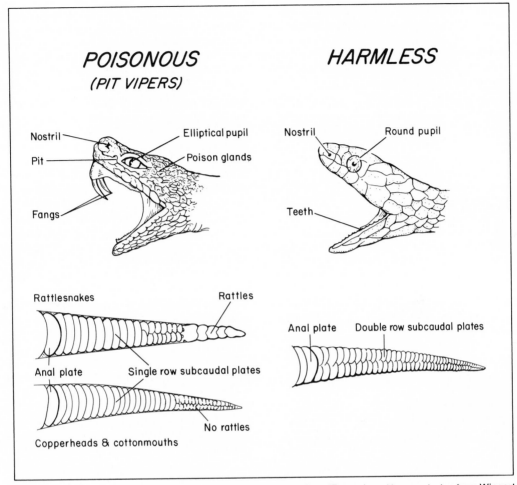

POISONOUS
(PIT VIPERS)

HARMLESS

Nostril — Elliptical pupil

Pit —

— Poison glands

Fangs —

Nostril — Round pupil

Teeth —

Rattlesnakes — Rattles

Anal plate — Single row subcaudal plates

Copperheads & cottonmouths — No rattles

Anal plate — Double row subcaudal plates

Figure 10.5. Ways to differentiate poisonous from harmless snakes. (Reproduced by permission from Wingert WA, et al: *A Quick Handbook on Snake Bites*, Resident and Staff Physician. May 1977, p.56).

dark, undisturbed places like old sofas and old fur coats. Commonly found in the Missouri valley, it is 0.5-inch long and 0.25-inch wide with a dark-brown, violin-shaped marking on the thorax. The brown recluse never attacks unless threatened. After the bite, there is immediate local pain. Extensive extravasation of blood may occur at the site in the next 24 hours. A generalized rash may appear over the body. The area of the bite may become deeply ulcerated, with ulceration extending down to the muscles. Treatment is supportive; there is no antiserum available. Several surgeons suggest early excision of the bite site to prevent severe ulceration.

Scorpion Stings

There are about 650 species of scorpions, approximately 40 of which are found in the United States. Most of these are not venomous. The ven-omous scorpions belong to the family Buthidae. Particularly dangerous species include *Centruroides sculpturatus* and *Centruroides gertschi*, which are found in the southwestern United States.

The clinical symptoms of a scorpion sting are localized numbness at the site of the sting, and rarely, high blood pressure and respiratory impairment.

Therapy includes immersion of the limb in cold water and a tourniquet about the limb, as well as treatment of symptoms. Antivenom is available by calling Arizona State Antivenom Laboratory at (602) 965–3116.

Hymenoptera Stings

Twice as many persons die in the United States from Hymenoptera stings as from snake bites. Hymenoptera include bees, wasps, hornets, and fire ants.

The emergency physician should be able to recognize four prominent members of the order Hymenoptera: the bumblebee (*1*); the honeybee, with a barbed stinger, fuzzy body, and brown, blunt abdomen (*2*); the white-faced hornet (*3*); and the yellow jacket, which has a black shiny thorax with long antennae (*4*) (Fig. 10.6). Hymenoptera venoms contain histamines and other vasoactive substances. These are hemolytic and neurotoxic, in addition to being effective hypersensitizing agents.

The clinical syndrome after a sting includes sharp pain, a local wheal, erythema, and intense itching and edema. In the 1% of the population who are hypersensitive, a single sting may produce serious anaphylaxis with urticaria, nausea, abdominal pain, dypsnea, edema of the face and glottis, hypertension, and death.

Treatment requires removal of the venom sac and washing of the area, followed by local supportive care such as cool compresses. The allergic patient may need 0.3–0.5 ml of epinephrine (1:1000) injected subcutaneously.

The major factor in the consideration of insect stings is prevention. Desensitization with venom rather than with whole-body extract is now possible. The hypersensitive patient should have available an insect sting kit, such as that made by Hollister-Stier, containing medihaler epinephrine and chlorpheniramine maleate (Chlortrimeton).

Marine Diseases

Erysipeloid

Erysipeloid is an acute infection of traumatized skin, usually occurring in fishermen, butchers, and those handling raw fish, poultry, or meat produce. *Erysipelothrix rhusiopathiae* is a gram-positive bacillus found in the mouth of fish, swine, and poultry.

After a bite, the initial symptom is burning pain at the site, followed by a warm, tender, raised, violaceous, or wine-colored area often associated with lymphangitis. As infection advances, the central lesion clears.

The antibiotic of choice is oral penicillin (1–2

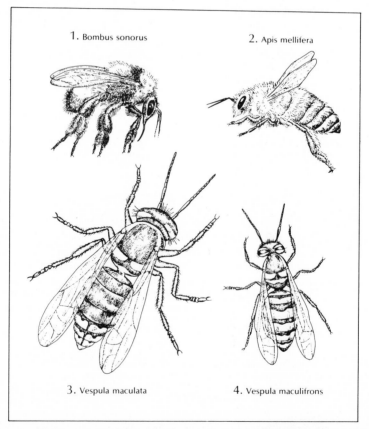

1. Bombus sonorus

2. Apis mellifera

3. Vespula maculata

4. Vespula maculifrons

Figure 10.6.   Four prominent members of the order Hymenoptera that cause many anaphylactic reactions are the bumblebee (1), honeybee (2), white-faced hornet (3), and yellow jacket (4). (Reprinted with permission from, Lichtenstein LM: Anaphylactic reactions to insect stings: A new approach, *Hosp Pract* 69, 1975).

gm/day) for 10 days, with immobilization and soaking of the limb for 2–3 days.

Seal Bite

Normally, seal bite is on the finger of a trainer or a seal hunter, thus the term "seal finger" or "Spaek finger." The etiologic agent is unclear; the Canadian government is now subsidizing a study in an attempt to isolate the organism.

The incubation period is 4–8 days, followed by throbbing pain, erythema, and swelling of the joint proximal to the bite. Untreated, Spaek finger produces cellulitis and progressive arthritis. The treatment before antibiotics was amputation of the affected finger to relieve the severe pain and deformity. Tetracycline, 500 mg orally four times a day for 10 days, is now the antibiotic of choice. It is also helpful to immobilize and elevate the finger, as well as soak it several times a day.

Jellyfish Sting

Venom is discharged from nematocysts in the tentacles of the larger jellyfish. Stings are characterized by instant burning pain where the tentacles contact the skin, followed by the development of a red, elevated, linear lesion. In more severe cases, the victim experiences nausea, vomiting, abdominal and generalized muscular cramps, and difficulty in breathing. Stings of the sea wasps *Chironex fleckeri* and Chiropsalmus are extremely severe.

On-site resuscitation takes first priority. Weak solutions of acetic acid (or vinegar) then will inactivate the penetrating nematocysts.

Suggested Readings

Heat-Related Illness
Beller GA, Boyd AE: Heat stroke. *Milit Med 140:*464–467, 1975
Clowes GHA, O'Donnell TF: Heat Stroke. *N Engl J Med 291:*564–567, 1974
Gottschalk PG, Thomas JE: Heat Stroke. *Mayo Clin Proc 41:*470–482, 1966
Knochel JP: Environmental heat illness—an eclectic review. *Arch Intern Med 133:*841–864, 1974
Stine RJ: Heat illness. *JACEP 8:*154–160, 1979
Wheeler M: Heat stroke in the elderly. *Med Clin North Am 60:*1289–1296, 1976

Hypothermia
Kelman GR, Nunn JF: Nomograms for correction of blood Po₂, Pco₂, pH, and base excess for time and temperature. *J Appl Physiol 21:*1484–1490, 1966
Reuler JB: Hypothermia: Pathophysiology, clinical settings and management. *Ann Intern Med 89:*519–527, 1978
Reuler JB, Parker RA: Peritoneal dialysis in the management of hypothermia. *JAMA 240:*2289–2290, 1978
Southwick FS, Dalglish PH: Recovery after prolonged asystolic cardiac arrest in profound hypothermia: A case report

and review of the literature. *JAMA 243:*1250–1253, 1980
Stine RJ: Accidental hypothermia. *JACEP 6:*413–416, 1977
Trevino A, Razi B, Beller BM: The characteristic electrocardiogram of accidental hypothermia. *Arch Intern Med 127:*470–473, 1971
Weyman AE, Greenbaum DM, Grace WJ: Accidental hypothermia in an alcoholic population. *Am J Med 56:*13–21, 1974

Drowning and near drowning
Calderwood HW: The ineffectiveness of steroid therapy for treatment of fresh water near-drowning. *Anesthesiology 43:*642, 1975
Conn AW: Cerebral resuscitation in near-drowning. *Pediatr Clin North Am 24:*691–701, 1979
Fandel I, Bancalari E: Near-drowning in children: clinical aspects. *Pediatrics 58:*573–579, 1976
Hoff BH: Multisystem failure: a review with special reference to drowning. *Crit Care Med 7:*310–320, 1979
Knopp R: Near-drowning. *JACEP 7:*249–254, 1978
Levin DL: Near-drowning. *Crit Care Med 8:*590–595, 1980
Modell JH: Biology of drowning. *Ann Rev Med 29:*1, 1978
Ports TA, Deuel TF: Intravascular coagulation in fresh water submersion. *Ann Intern Med 87:*60–61, 1977
Orlowski JP: Prognostic factors in pediatric cases of drowning and near-drowning. *JACEP 8:*176–179, 1979
Young RSK, Zalneacitis EL, Dooling EC: Neurological outcome in cold water drowning. *JAMA 244:*1233–1235, 1980

Barotrauma and Decompression Sickness
Strauss RH (Ed): *Diving Medicine.* Grune and Stratton, New York, 1976
Strauss RH: Diving medicine. *Am Rev Respir Dis 119:*1001–1023, 1979
U.S. Navy Diving Manual, 1973

Smoke Inhalation
Agee RN, Long JM III, Hunt JL, et al: Use of Xenon[133] in early diagnosis of inhalation injury. *J Trauma 16:*218–224, 1976
Bartlett RH, Dressler DP, Horovitz JH, et al: Consensus report on smoke inhalation. *J Trauma 19:*913–922, 1979
Dyer RF, Esch VH: Polyvinyl chloride toxicity in fires. *JAMA 235:*393–397, 1976
Hunt JL, Agee RN, Pruitt BA: Fiberoptic bronchoscopy in acute inhalation injury. *J Trauma 15:*641–649, 1975
Luce EA, Chi Tsi SU, Hoopes JE: Alveolar-arterial oxygen gradient in the burn patient. *J Trauma 16:*212–217, 1976
Moylan JA, Chan C-K: Inhalation injury, an increasing problem. *Ann Surg 188:*34–37, 1978
Petroff PA, Hander EW, Clayton WH, et al: Pulmonary function studies after smoke inhalation. *Am J Surg 132:*346–351, 1976
Pruitt BA, Erickson DR, Morris A: Progessive pulmonary insufficiency and other pulmonary complications of thermal injury. *J Trauma 15:*369–379, 1975
Zawacki BE, Jung RC, Joyce J, et al: Smoke, burns, and the natural history of inhalation injury in fire victims. *Ann Surg 185:*100–110, 1977

Carbon Monoxide Poisoning
Finley J, Van Beek A, Glover JL: Myonecrosis complicating carbon monoxide poisoning. *J Trauma 17:*536–540, 1977
Goldbaum LR, Orellano T, Dergal E: Mechanism of the toxic action of carbon monoxide. *Ann Clin Lab Sci 6:*372–376, 1976
Kindwall E: Carbon monoxide poisoning. In Dairs JC, Hunt TK (Eds): *Hyperbaric Oxygen Therapy.* Undersea Medical Society, Inc, pp. 177–190, 1977

Larkin JM, Bcahos GJ, Moylan JA: Treatment of carbon monoxide poisoning: prognostic factors. *J Trauma* 16:111–114, 1976

Myers RA, Linberg RAM, Cowley RA: Carbon monoxide poisoning: the injury and its treatment. *JACEP* 8:479–484, 1979

Smith JS: Morbidity from acute carbon monoxide poisoning at three year follow-up. *Br Med J* 1:318–321, 1973

Winter PM, Miller JN: Carbon monoxide poisoning. *JAMA* 236:1502–1504, 1976

Radiation Accidents

Beeson PN, McDermott W (Eds): *Radiation Injury*. Textbook of Medicine, 14th Edition, Vol. 1, 1975. W. B. Saunders, Philadelphia, pp. 66–72

Bond VP, Fliedner TM, Cronkite EP: Evaluation and management of the heavily irradiated individual. *J Nuc Med* 1:221–238, 1960

Casarett GW: *Radiation Histopathology*, Vols. I and II, CTC Press, Boca Raton, Florida, 1980

Catsch A, Kawin B: *Radioactive Metal Mobilization in Medicine*. Charles C Thomas, Springfield, IL, 1964

Cember H: *Introduction to Health Physics*. Pergamon Press, NY, 2nd Edition, 1976

Dalrymple GV, Goulden ME, Kollmorgen GM, et al: *Medical Radiation Biology*. W.B. Saunders, Philadelphia, 1973

Hounam RF: The removal of particles from the nasopharyngeal (NP) compartment of the respiratory tract by nose blowing and swabbing. *Health Phys* 28:743–750, 1975

Hübner KF, Fry SA (Eds): *The Medical Basis for Radiation Accident Preparedness*. Elsevier North-Holland, New York, NY, 1980

International Atomic Energy Agency, 1969. *Handling of Radiation Accidents*, Proceedings of IAEA/WHO Symposium, Vienna, May 19–23, 1969, STI/PUB/229, International Atomic Energy Agency, Vienna.

International Atomic Energy Agency, 1971. *Manual on Radiation Haematology*, Technical Reports Series No. 123, International Atomic Energy Agency, Vienna.

International Atomic Energy Agency, 1978. *Manual on Early Medical Treatment of Possible Radiation Injury with an Appendix on Sodium Burns*. Vienna (IAEA Safety Series, No. 47)

Joint Commission on Accreditation of Hospitals. *Accreditation Manual for Hospital*—1980 Edition, JCAH, Chicago, IL, 1980

Lincoln TA: Importance of initial management of persons internally contaminated with radionuclides. *Am Indust Hygiene Assoc J* 37:16–21, 1976

Love RA: Planning for radiation accidents. *Hospitals* 38:7–14, 1964

National Council on Radiation Protection and Measurements. *Radiological Factors Affecting Decision Making in a Nuclear Attack*. Report No. 42, Nov. 15, 1974. *Protection of the Thyroid Gland in the Event of Releases of Radioiodine*. Report No. 55, 1977. C/P NCRP Publications PO Box 3107, Washington, DC 20014

National Council on Radiation Protection and Measurements, 1978. *Instrumentation and Monitoring Methods for Radiation Protection*. Washington, DC (NCRP Report No. 57)

National Research Council, Committee on the Biological Effects of Ionizing Radiations. 1980. *The Effects on Populations of Exposure to Low Levels of Ionizing Radiation: 1980*. National Academy Press, Washington, DC (BIER III)

NCRP Report 39, Basic Radiation Protection Criteria. Issued January 15, 1971.

NCRP Report 65, Management of Persons Accidentally Contaminated with Radionuclides. Issued April 15, 1981.

Sanders, SM Jr: Excretion of Am^{241} and Cm^{244} following two cases of accidental inhalation. *Health Phys* 27:359–365, 1974

Saenger EL: Hospital planning to combat radioactive contamination. *JAMA* 112–113, 1963

Saenger EL: Medical aspects of radiation accidents. United States Atomic Energy Commission, 1963.

United Nations 1977. Report of the United Nations Scientific Committee on the Effects of Atomic Radiation (UNSCEAR), *Sources and Effects of Ionizing Radiation*, 1977 Report to the General Assembly, Publication Sales No. UN E. 77. IX. 1

U.S. Nuclear Regulatory Commission, Regulatory Guide 8.29, "Instruction Concerning Risks from Occupational Radiation Exposure", July 1981

U. S. Nuclear Regulatory Commission, Rules and Regulations, Title 10, Chapter 1, Code of Federal Regulations, Part 19, "Notices, Instructions and Reports to Workers: Inspections"

U. S. Nuclear Regulatory Commission, Rules and Regulations, Title 10, Chapter 1, Code of Federal Regulations, Part 20, "Standards For Protection Against Radiation"

Waldron RL, Danielson RA, Schultz HE, et al: Radiation decontamination unit for the community hospital. *Am J Roentgen* 136:977–981, 1981

Weidner WA, Miller KL, Latshaw RF, et al: The impact of a nuclear crisis on a radiology department. *Radiology* 135:717–723, 1980

World Health Organization, 1960. *Diagnosis and Treatment of Acute Radiation Injury*, Proceedings of a Scientific meeting jointly sponsored by the IAEA and WHO, October 17–21, 1960. World Health Organization, Geneva

Animal Bites

General

Berzon DR: Animal bites in a large city—A report on Baltimore, Maryland. *Am J Publ Health* 62:422–426, 1972

Hubbert WT, McCullough WF, Schurrenberger PR: *Diseases Transmitted from Animal to Man*, Charles C Thomas, Springfield, IL, 1975

Kahrs RF, Holmes DN, Poppensiek GC: Diseases transmitted from pets to man: An evolving concern for veterinarians. *Cornell Veterinarian* 68:442–459, 1978

Steele JH: A bookshelf on veterinary public health. *Am J Publ Health* 63:291–311, 1973

Strassburg MA, Greenland MA, Marron JA: Animal bites: Patterns of treatment. *Ann Emerg Med* 10:193–197, 1981

Dog Bites

Callaham M: Prophylactic antibiotics in common dog bite wounds: A controlled study. *Ann Emerg Med* 9:410–414, 1980

Klein D: Friendly dog syndrome. *NY State J Med* 66:2306–2309, 1966

Parris HM, et al: Epidemiology of dog bites. Public Health Reports, United States Public Health Service 74:891–903, 1959

Human Bites

Mann RJ, Hoffeld TA, Farmer CB: Human bites of the hand: Twenty years of experience. *J Hand Surg* 2:97–104, 1977

Peeples E, Boswick JA, Scott FA: Wounds of the hand contaminated by human or animal saliva. *J Trauma* 20:383–389, 1980

Pasteurella Multocida

Francis DP, Holmes MA, Brandon G: *Pasteurella multocida.* Infections after domestic animal bites and scratches. *JAMA 233:*42–46, 1975

Gump GW, Holden RA: Endocarditis caused by a new species of Pasteurella. *Ann Intern Med 76:*275–278, 1972

Hawkins LG: Local *Pasteurella multocida* infections. *J Bone Joint Surg 51A:*363–366, 1969

Hubbert WT, Rosen MN: *Pasteurella multocida* infection due to animal bite. *Am J Publ Health 60:*1103–1108, 1970

Jarvis WR, Banko S, Snyder E, et al: *Pasteurella multocida* osteomyelitis following dog bites. *Am J Dis Child 135:* 625–627, 1981

Lucas GL, Bartlett DH: *Pasteurella* infection in the hand. *Plast Reconstr Surg 67:*49–53, 1981

Patton F: *Pasteurella multocida* septicemia and peritonitis in a cirrhotic cocktrainer with a pet pig. *N Engl J Med 303:*1126–1127, 1980 (Letter to Editor)

Stevens DL: Antibiotic susceptibilities of human isolates of Pasteurella multocida. *Antimicr Ag Chem 16:*322, 1979

Swartz MN, Kunz LF: Pasteurella multocida infections in man. *N Engl J Med 261:*889–893, 1959

Tindall JP, Harrison CM: Pasteurella multocida infections following animal injuries, especially cat bites. *Arch Dermatol 105:*412–416, 1972

Plague

Butler T, Levin J, Linh NN, et al: Yersinia pestis infection in Vietnam. *J Infect Dis 133:*493–499, 1976

Finegold KJ: Pathogenesis of plague. *Am J Med 45:*549–554, 1968

Kaufmann AF, Boyce JM, Martone WJ: Trends in human plague in the U.S. *J Infect Dis 141:*522–524, 1980

Reed WP, Palmer DC, Willams RC, Jr, et al: Bubonic plague in southwestern United States. *Medicine 49:*465–486, 1970

Von Reyn CF, Weber NS, Tempest B, et al: Epidemiologic and clinical features of an outbreak of bubonic plague in New Mexico. *J Infect Dis 136:*489–494, 1977

Tularemia

Guerrant RL, Humphries MK, Butler JE, et al: Tick borne oculo-glandular tularemia. *Arch Intern Med 136:*811–813, 1976

Kloch CE, Olsen PF, Fukushima T: Tularemia epidemic associated with the deerfly. *JAMA 266:*149–152, 1973

Roueché B: Annals of Medicine: The New Yorker: August 4, pp. 49–57, 1980

Tularemia acquired from a bear. *MMWR,* February 1980

Young LS, Bicknell DS, Archer BG, et al: Tularemia epidemic: Vermont 1968. Forty-seven cases limited to contact with muskrats. *N Engl J Med 280:*1253–1260, 1969

Rocky Mountain Spotted Fever

Hazard GW, Ganz RN, Nevin RW, et al: Rocky Mountain spotted fever in the eastern United States. *N Engl J Med 280:*57–62, 1969

Hechemy KE: Laboratory diagnosis of Rocky Mountain spotted fever. *N Engl J Med 300:*859–860, 1979

Babesiosis

Deforges JF, Quinby F: Babesiosis abroad. *N Engl J Med* Editorial *295:*103–104, 1976

Jacoby GA, Hunt JU, Kosinski KS: Treatment of transfusion-transmitted babesiosis by exchange transfusion. *N Engl J Med 303:*1098–1100, 1980

Ruebush TK, Cassaday PB, Marsh HJ, et al: Human babesiosis on Nantucket Island. *Ann Int Med 86:*6–9, 1976

Western KA, Benson KA, Gleason NN, et al: Babesiosis in a Massachusetts resident. *N Engl J Med 183:*854–856, 1970

Rat-Bite Fever

Cole JS, Stoll RW, Bulger RJ: Rat-bite fever. *Ann Int Med 71:*979–981, 1969

Rogosa M: Streptobacillus and Spirillum minus, the causative agents of two distinct rat-bite fevers. Chapter 26 in Blair JE, Lennette E and Truant J (Eds), *Manual of Microbiology,* 1970

Roughgarden JW: Antimicrobial therapy of rat-bite fever: A review. *Arch Intern Med 116:*39–54, 1965

Cat-Scratch Disease

Carithers HA, Carthers CM, Edwards RO, Jr: Cat scratch disease. Its natural history. *JAMA 207:*312–316, 1969

Margileth AM: Cat scratch disease: Non-bacterial regional lymphadenitis. The study of 145 patients and a review of the literature. *Pediatrics 42:*803–818, 1968

Warwick WJ: The cat scratch syndrome, many diseases or one disease? *Prog Med Virol 9:*256–601, 1967

Rabies

Anderson LJ, Sikes RK, Langkos CW: Post exposure trial of human diploid cell strain. *J Infect Dis 142:*133–138, 1980

Corey L, Hattwick MA: Treatment of persons exposed to rabies. *JAMA 232:*272–275, 1975

Houff SA, Burton RC, Wilson RW, et al: Human to human transmission of rabies virus by a corneal transplant. *N Engl J Med 300:*603–604, 1979

Meyer, HW: Rabies vaccine. *J Infect Dis 2:*287–289, 1980

Plotkin SA: Rabies vaccination in the 1980's. *Hosp Pract* (November):65–72, 1980

Porras C, Barboza JJ, Fuenzalida E, et al: Recovery from rabies in man. *Ann Intern Med 85:*44–48, 1976

Rabies Prevention: Recommendation of Immunization Practices Advisory Committee (ACIP) *MMWR* 29, #23, June 13, 1980

Simian Herpes B Virus

Davidson WL, Hummeler R: Herpes B virus infection in man. *Ann NY Acad Sci 85:*970–979, 1968

Hull: The Simian viruses: Chapter 3 in Kaplan (Ed): *The Herpes Viruses.* Academic Press, New York, pp. 389–425, 1979

Snake Bites

Garfin SR, Castilonia RR, Mubarek SJ, et al: Role of surgical decompression in treatment of rattlesnake bites. *Surg Forum 30:*502–504, 1979

Glass TG: Early debridement in pit viper bites, *JAMA 235:*2513–2516, 1976

Goldstein EJC, Citron DM, Gonzalez H, et al: Bacteriology of rattlesnake venom and implications for therapy. *J Infect Dis 140:*818–821, 1979

Grace TG, Omer GE: The management of upper extremity pit viper wounds. *J Hand Surg 2:*168–177, 1980

Parrish HM, Badgley RF, Carr CA: Poisonous snake bites in New England. *N Engl J Med 263:*788–793, 1960

Russell F: Jaws that bite. *Emerg Med 10:*25–40, 1978

Russell F, Carlson RW, Wainschel J, et al: Snake venom poisoning in the United States. *JAMA 233:*341–344, 1975

Sutherland SK, Coulter AR, Harris RD: Early management of bites by the eastern diamond back rattlesnake. *Am J Trop Med Hyg* (March 30):497–500, 1981

Spider Bites

Editorial: Spider bites. *Lancet* 2:509, 1969

Gorham JR: The brown recluse spider, Loxosceles reclusa and necrotic spider bite—a new public health problem in the U.S. *J Envir Health 31:*138, 1968

Hunt GP: Bites and stings of uncommon arthropods. 1. Spiders. *Postgrad Med 70:*91–102, 1981

Scorpion Stings

Horen WP: Insect and scorpion sting. *JAMA 221:*894–898, 1972

Hunt GR: Bites and stings of uncommon arthropods. *Postgrad Med 70:*107–114, 1981.

Stahnke HL: Arizona's lethal scorpion. *Arizona Med 29:*490, 1972

Hymenoptera Stings

Barclay WR: Emergency treatment of insect sting allergy. *JAMA 240:*2735, 1978

Golden DB, Valentine MD, Sobotka AK, et al: Regimens of hymenoptera venom immunotherapy. *Ann Intern Med 92:*620–624, 1980

Hunt KJ, Valentine MD, Sobotka AK, et al: Diagnosis of allergy to stinging insects by skin testing with hymenoptera venoms. *Ann Intern Med 85:*56–59, 1976

Lichtenstein LM, Valentine MD, Sobotka AK: A case for venom treatment in anaphylactic sensitivity to hymenoptera sting. *N Engl J Med 290:*1223–1227, 1974

Marine Diseases (General)

Halstead BW: Poisonous and venomous marine animals of the world. Volumes 1 and 2. (Government Printing Office), 1965 and 1967

Erysipeloid

Case 16, 1978: Erysipelothrix rhusiopathiae septicemia. *N Engl J Med 298:*957–962, 1978

Grieco MH, Sheldon C: Erysipelothrix rhusiopathiae. *Ann NY Acad Sci 174:*523–532, 1970

Klarder J: Erysipeloid as an occupational disease. *JAMA 111:*1345–1348, 1938

Nelson E: Five hundred cases of erysipeloid. *Rocky Mountain Med J 52:*40–42, 1955

Price J, Bennett W: The erysipeloid of Rosenbach. *Br Med J 2:*1060–1062, 1951

Seal Bite

Beck B, Smith TG: Seal finger: An unsolved medical problem in Canada. Technical Report of the Fisheries Research Board of Canada, No. 625. Arctic Biological Station, Fisheries and Marine Service. (Quebec: Ste. Anne de Bellevue), 1976

Hillenbrand FKM: Whale finger and seal finger. *Lancet 2:*680–681, 1953

Markham RB, Polk F: Seal finger. *J Infect Dis 1:*567–569, 1979

Coelenterata

Drury JK, Noonan JD, Pollack JG, et al: Jelly fish sting with serious hand complications. *Injury 12:*66–68, 1980

Hartwick R, Callanan U, Williamson J, et al: Disarming the box-jelly fish: Nematocyst inhibition in Chironex fleckeri. *Med J Australia 1:*15–20, 1980

CHAPTER 11

Infectious Diseases in the Emergency Ward

HARVEY B. SIMON, M.D.

Infectious diseases are among the most important problems for which patients seek medical care in the emergency ward; their spectrum ranges from acute medical emergencies such as bacterial meningitis and septic shock to subtle diagnostic puzzles such as fever of unknown origin. The etiologic agents span a diverse range of bacteria, viruses, fungi, and parasites, which may involve any organ system. Modern antimicrobial chemotherapy provides the means to eradicate many of these infections, but these drugs must be administered with care. The initial evaluation of the patient in the emergency ward is often crucial; in the case of life-threatening sepsis, diagnosis and therapy must proceed without delay, and even in less dramatic situations, the emergency ward work-up may provide the only opportunity to collect diagnostic specimens before therapeutic intervention alters the microbial flora. Because of their frequency, seriousness, and treatability, this chapter will concentrate on the emergency management of acute bacterial infections.

GENERAL APPROACH TO THE PATIENT WITH SUSPECTED INFECTION

Evaluation of the patient with suspected infection is directed toward answering two basic questions: (1) What organ system is involved? Does the patient have a localized infection such as pneumonia or pyelonephritis or a generalized infection such as bacteremia? (2) What is the etiologic agent? Is the pneumonia, for example, caused by the pneumococcus or by a gram-negative bacterium? The answers to these questions depend on a detailed history, a meticulous physical examination, and approriate laboratory procedures, particularly Gram stains and cultures.

History

Many items should be stressed when taking the history of a patient with suspected infectious disease:

(1) Host factors. Is the patient normally healthy, or does he have an underlying disease that may make him unusually susceptible to infection? For example, patients with malignant conditions (especially lymphoma, leukemia, and myeloma), diabetes, neutropenia, or sickle cell anemia and patients receiving corticosteroids or other immunosuppressive drugs may become infected with unusual, opportunistic pathogens or may be unable to respond normally even to the common pathogens. For such patients, a vigorous approach to diagnosis and therapy is required. Patients with foreign bodies in place, such as a prosthetic heart valve, are also particularly vulnerable to infection.

(2) Epidemiology. Has the patient traveled to areas where he may have been exposed to "exotic" infections such as typhoid fever or malaria? Has the patient been exposed to animals or birds that may transmit infection? Even common pets may be implicated, such as the cat (cat-scratch fever and *Pasteurella multocida* cellulitis from scratches or bites, toxoplasmosis from fecal contamination), parakeet (psittacosis), and turtle (salmonellosis). Bites of stray dogs, skunks, and bats are potentialy serious because of the possibility of rabies. Has the patient been exposed to other persons with communicable diseases such as influenza or tuberculosis? Have other persons in the community been ill recently? Does the patient's occupation provide clues to unusual infections, such as brucellosis or Q fever in slaughterhouse workers?

(3) Antibiotics. Has the patient been receiving antibiotics that may alter susceptibility to infection by favoring growth of drug-resistant organisms?

Does the patient have any drug allergies that may alter the physician's choice of therapeutic agents? Are there underlying medical problems, such as renal failure, that may influence therapy?

(4) Symptoms and clinical course. An important element in the history is to evaluate the course of the illness. Was the onset sudden or gradual? Is the illness rapidly progressing or smoldering? Symptoms such as headache, altered consciousness, cough, dyspnea, flank pain, and dysuria are especially helpful in localizing the infection. If the patient is unable to answer clearly, a friend or relative can often provide important information.

Physical Examination

A detailed physical examination is necessary. Vital signs must be measured carefully; hypotension, severe respiratory distress, or extreme hyperpyrexia may require immediate treatment. Although fever is an important clue to infection, the emergency physician must remember that many patients with infections are afebrile, and in other patients, fever may develop from noninfectious causes. The skin and mucous membranes may provide crucial information. For example, petechial eruptions may suggest meningococcemia or Rocky Mountain spotted fever, pustular lesions may indicate gonococcemia or staphylococcal endocarditis, an erythroderm with desquamation may suggest toxic shock syndrome, splinter hemorrhages and conjunctival petechiae may be clues to endocarditis, and macular or vesicular eruptions may reflect many viral infections. Similarly, the ocular fundi should be examined; Roth's spots suggest endocarditis, and choroidal tubercles may be the only physical finding in patients with miliary tuberculosis. Enlarged lymph nodes should be sought. Examination of the chest may disclose pneumonia or empyema, and cardiac examination may reveal evidence of endocarditis or pericarditis. Abdominal findings may disclose hepatomegaly or splenomegaly, or may indicate an abscess or peritonitis, as may rectal and pelvic examinations. Evaluation of the musculoskeletal system may reveal septic arthritis or osteomyelitis, and neurologic evaluation may raise the possibility of meningitis or encephalitis.

Laboratory Evaluation

While a history should be taken and a physical examination performed in every patient with suspected infection, the clinical laboratory must be utilized more selectively. Once the infectious process can be localized to an organ system, that area should be studied intensively; in many patients,

however, the history and physical examination fail to define the source of fever. In these patients and in patients with multiple problems or a systemic toxic reaction, certain laboratory studies are essential:

(1) Complete blood cell count and differential. Polymorphonuclear leukocytosis with immature forms (a "shift to the left") suggests, but does not prove, bacterial infection. Toxic granulations, vacuoles, and Döhle's inclusion bodies in polymorphonuclear leukocytes strongly indicate bacterial infection, and these should be sought in all blood smears.

(2) Urinalysis. Pyuria and leukocyte casts strongly suggest a urinary tract infection.

(3) Posteroanterior and lateral chest x-ray films. Such films may disclose pneumonitis even in the absence of abnormalities on physical examination.

(4) Blood chemistries. Determination of the blood glucose level may reveal unsuspected diabetes, and is important in evaluating the significance of the glucose concentrations in other body fluids. Liver function tests are often helpful in defining obscure fevers.

(5) Examination of other body fluids. This is not always indicated, but may be lifesaving. If there is any possibility of meningitis, a lumbar puncture must be performed. Taps of pleural effusion, ascitic fluid, or joint effusion may be extremely informative; whenever possible, these procedures should be performed in the emergency ward before beginning antimicrobial therapy. Fluids should be examined directly by cell counts and differentials, and the concentrations of glucose and protein should be determined. Gram stains and cultures are mandatory.

(6) Cultures and Gram stains. These are critically important. The emergency ward evaluation of a patient with fever of undefined origin should include cultures of blood (at least two cultures, each from a separate venipuncture), urine (a clean voided specimen), and sputum (together with a Gram stain). If any other body fluids are obtained, they too should be examined by culture and a Gram stain.

Bacteriologic Procedures in the Emergency Ward

The cornerstone of management of an infectious disease is isolation and identification of the responsible pathogen. This requires the services of a professional bacteriology laboratory that is able to evaluate a specimen fully, which usually requires several days. However, because the physician is responsible not only for ordering the appropriate tests but also for interpreting the results, he must be familiar with bacteriologic principles. In addition, specimens should be collected and prepared for analysis before antimicrobial therapy is begun, and in many institutions, bacteriology technologists are not available during the evening and weekend hours when so many patients seek emergency care. The purpose of this section, therefore, is to discuss the bacteriologic procedures that the physician may have to perform. A few hours in the bacteriology laboratory will provide excellent practice.

Obtaining the Specimen

It is extremely important to obtain appropriate specimens before antibiotic therapy; in fact, antibiotic selection often depends on preliminary analysis of the specimen in the emergency ward. Techniques for obtaining specimens of sputum, urine, and other body fluids are discussed in later sections.

Blood cultures are necessary for almost all patients with serious infections. Since the blood must not be contaminated with normal skin bacteria, meticulous preparation is required:

1. With tourniquet in place, select vein.
2. Prepare skin twice with iodine solution.
3. Prepare skin with alcohol.
4. Obtain 10 ml of blood. If venipuncture is difficult and requires excessive manipulation, the likelihood of contamination has increased, and an alternative site should be sought.
5. Place 5 ml of blood into each of two blood culture flasks. Ordinarily, one flask contains dextrose-phosphate broth, and the other, thioglycollate broth. The flasks should be prepared either by flaming (screw cap) or with alcohol swabs (rubber-stopped top). Incubate at 37°C.
6. Repeat blood culture, using a different site, preferably after waiting at least 30 minutes.

Examining the Specimen

The specimen can be examined in the emergency ward within minutes. The macroscopic appearance may be very informative. Turbidity in cerebrospinal fluid, ascitic fluid, or urine often results from infection. A good sputum specimen from a patient with bacterial pneumonitis or bronchitis is usually thick, viscous, green, gray, or yellow. A foul odor from sputum or other body fluids often is an important clue to the presence of anaerobic organisms that require specialized diagnostic techniques and chemotherapeutic agents.

Microscopic evaluation is critical. Ideally, all specimens of sputum, cerebrospinal fluid, and other body fluids should be examined using the Gram-stain technique; this is helpful but not mandatory for unspun specimens of urine, since urinalysis and quantitative cultures can frequently provide equivalent data.

GRAM STAIN

1. Prepare smear by swabbing specimen on a clean glass slide. Air dry.
2. Heat fix by passing slide over Bunsen burner flame 2 or 3 times. Allow to cool.
3. Flood slide with gentain violet for 15 seconds. Rinse with water.
4. Flood slide with Gram's iodine for 15 seconds. Rinse with water.
5. Decolorize with 95% alcohol. This is the only step that requires experience. In the case of thin body fluids such as the cerebrospinal fluid, decolorization should render the specimen colorless; for this the alcohol should remain on the slide about 10 seconds. In the case of sputum or pus, the alcohol should be dropped onto the slide until the thinnest parts of the smear are colorless but the thickest parts retain a blue hue. After decolorization, rinse with water.
6. Flood slide with safranin for 15 seconds. Rinse with water.
7. Blot dry with filter paper and examine under oil immersion lens.

Interpretation of the Gram stain requires practice. The polymorphonuclear leukocytes should be examined first; in a properly stained smear, they appear pink. Next, the numbers and types of inflammatory cells should be evaluated; abundant polymorphonuclear leukocytes often reflect bacterial inflammation. Finally, the bacterial flora should be examined. Are the organisms gram-positive (blue) or gram-negative (red)? Are they cocci (round), bacilli (rod-shaped), or do they have an intermediate shape (coccobacillary)? Is more than one type of organism present? It is important to remember that help in interpreting results is available; slides can be saved and reviewed with a bacteriologist or pathologist.

Although the Gram stain is central to the evaluation of most bacterial infections, other procedures are required for the identification of certain organisms:

1. *Mycobacterium tuberculosis* and other mycobacteria—acid-fast stain.
2. *Cryptococcus meningitidis*—India ink preparation.
3. Fungi—fungal wet mount.
4. Nocardia and *Actinomyces israelii*—modified acid-fast stain.

5. *Corynebacterium diphtheriae*—methylene blue preparation.

6. Intestinal parasites—stool examination.

Because they are used less frequently, these techniques are not discussed here, but can be reviewed in standard texts.

Culturing the Specimen

Since many pathogenic bacteria are fastidious, it is important to culture specimens promptly. Many types of media are available (Table 11.1). In general, solid media are useful in providing quantitative estimates of the organisms present and in allowing study of individual bacteria, while liquid media enable just a few organisms to grow readily. Some media are *enriched* to enhance growth of the more fastidious organisms, while other media are *selective*, that is, designed to inhibit growth of the "normal flora," thus allowing the pathogens to grow.

When a specimen is inoculated on a solid medium, it should first be streaked across one quadrant of the culture plate with a sterile swab or loop (Fig. 11.1). Then, with a loop that has been flamed and allowed to cool, the specimen should be streaked across a second quadrant. This procedure should be performed twice more, flaming and cooling the loop each time. This will dilute the bacteria, enabling the technician later to select individual colonies for study.

When a liquid medium is used, the loop swab should be immersed in it and rotated several times. The mouth of the medium tube should be flamed before and after the specimen is introduced.

Anaerobic cultures require special mention. Numerous species of anaerobic bacteria reside in the upper part of the respiratory tract, in the gastrointestinal tract, and in the female genitourinary tract. It has become increasingly clear that these bacteria can be important pathogens. Infections that are particularly likely to be caused at least partly by anaerobes include abscesses, infections with foul-smelling pus, gas-forming infections, infections involving necrotic tissue, and other infections arising from respiratory, gastrointestinal, or genitourinary foci. Anaerobic bacteria will not grow in the presence of oxygen; hence, when they are suspected, specimens should be streaked on blood agar plates and cultured in anaerobic jars. Many devices can be used to remove oxygen from such jars either chemically or nonchemically; in addition, numerous media are becoming available to preserve anaerobic conditions even while the specimen is en route to the laboratory.

Bacterial cultures must grow at least 24 hours before they can provide diagnostic information, and to obtain complete data usually takes 2–3 days. What data can the laboratory provide? Identification of the bacteria in the specimen is of utmost importance, as is antibiotic sensitivity testing of possible pathogens to ensure optimal antimicrobial therapy. However, interpretation of results is the responsibility not only of those in the laboratory but also of the physician. The presence of a microorganism does *not* automatically implicate it in the patient's disease. Four considerations may assist in interpreting results:

(1) Contamination. Small numbers of organisms, unusual bacteria, or results inconsistent with clinical findings should raise the possibility of contamination.

(2) Normal flora. Although the cerebrospinal fluid and urine are normally sterile, some areas of the body such as the skin, the gastrointestinal tract, the female genital tract, and the upper part of the respiratory tract teem with bacteria that are ordinarily harmless in those locations. The laboratory personnel must select possible pathogens from all these bacteria; the physician must differentiate pathogens from harmless saprophytes.

(3) Tissue tropism. Certain bacteria are highly pathogenic in some areas of the body, but harmless in others. For example, the pneumococcus is a leading cause of otitis, sinusitis, and pneumonia, but although it frequently inhabits the nasopharynx, it never causes pharyngitis. When the laboratory reports growth of pneumococci from a throat swab, the clinician's reaction should be different from his reaction to the same organism from a sputum culture.

(4) Carrier state. Pathogens may be present without causing disease. For example, meningococci may be cultured from the throat or salmonellae from the stool of a healthy individual. Such findings may have greater significance for the epidemiologist than for the patient.

Thus far, only bacterial infections have been considered; the same laboratory principles apply to mycobacterial and fungal infections. Viruses, mycoplasmas, rickettsiae, and chlamydiae, however, are all important pathogens that require special culture techniques. The emergency physician can often suspect diseases caused by such organisms based on epidemiologic and clinical findings, and he can assist in the establishment of a definitive diagnosis by obtaining an "acute phase" serum sample and freezing it for later serologic study when a "convalescent phase" sample is also available.

SPECIFIC INFECTIOUS DISEASES

Before some of the infectious diseases seen in the emergency ward are considered, some caution-

Table 11.1.
Guide to cultures.

Specimen	Method of Procurement	Medium[a]	Other Studies
Blood	Sterile venipuncture	Dextrose phosphate broth, 5 ml THIO, 5 ml	
Pharynx	Throat swab	BAP CAP if patient <6 years (*Hemophilus influenzae*) TM in 5% CO_2 or Transgrow if gonococcus suspected Loeffler if *Corynebacterium diphtheriae* suspected	Methylene blue smear (if indicated)
Middle ear	Myringotomy	BAP CAP	Gram stain
Sinus	Surgical drainage or drainage from ostium	BAP CAP Anaerobic BAP	Gram stain
Sputum	Expectoration Nasotracheal suction Transtracheal aspiration	BAP MacC or EMB CAP if patient < 6 years or if *H. influenzae* suspected LJ if *Mycobacterium tuberculosis* suspected[b] SAB if fungus suspected	Gram stain Acid-fast smear (if indicated) Fungal wet mount (if indicated)
Lung aspirate	Needle aspiration	As for sputum plus anaerobic BAP	Cytology Pathology
Pleural fluid	Thoracentesis	As for sputum plus anaerobic BAP	Cell count and differential Glucose, protein, lactate dehydrogenase Cytology
Peritoneal fluid	Paracentesis	BAP MacC or EMB THIO Anaerobic BAP LJ if *M. tuberculosis* suspected[b]	Cell count and differential Glucose, protein, lactate dehydrogenase Cytology Acid-fast smear (if indicated)
Joint fluid	Arthrocentesis	BAP CAP in 5% CO_2 THIO LJ if *M. tuberculosis* suspected[b]	Gram stain Cell count and differential Glucose, protein, crystals, mucin Acid-fast smear (if indicated)
Urine	Midstream clean voided specimen Bladder tap (especially in children) Urethral catheterization	BAP MacC or EMB	Urinalysis Gram stain of unspun urine

Table 11.1. *continued*

Specimen	Method of Procurement	Medium[a]	Other studies
Cerebrospinal fluid	Lumbar puncture	BAP CAS in 5% CO_2 THIO LJ if *M. tuberculosis* suspected[b] SAB if fungus suspected	Gram stain Cell count and differential Glucose, protein Pressure (manometrics) India ink preparation (if indicated) Acid-fast smear (if indicated) Cytology (if indicated)
Wound Abscess	Swab or aspiration	BAP MacC or EMB CAS THIO Anaerobic BAP	Gram stain
Urethra Cervix	Swab	TM in 5% CO_2 or Transgrow	Gram stain
Skin	Aspiration	BAP MacC or EMB THIO	Gram stain
Stool	Stool sample or rectal swab	SS Selenite BAP Campy	Direct examination for ova and parasites (if indicated) Gram stain (if staphylococcal enterocolitis suspected) Methylene blue smear for leukocytes

THIO = thioglycollate broth; BAP = blood agar plate; CAP = chocolate agar plate; TM = Thayer-Martin agar; MacC = MacConkey agar; EMB = eosin-methylene blue agar; LJ = Löwenstein–Jensen slant; SAB = Sabouraud agar; CAS = chocolate agar slant; SS = Salmonella-Shigella agar; Campy = campylobacter (incubated at 42°C)

[a] All specimens should be incubated at 37°C.
[b] Or other media for *M. tuberculosis* such as Middlebrook 7H10.

ary words are in the order. First, patients are rarely seen with conditions as neatly defined as in this section; most patients pose problems of differential diagnosis. Second, spatial limitations make it necessary to emphasize problems that are common, serious, and treatable. Even so, generalizations are necessary, and the reader is invited to expand his understanding through the suggested readings. Third, neither diagnosis nor therapy stops in the emergency ward. Both the patient who is sent home and the patient who is admitted to the hospital require follow-up study to re-evaluate the validity of the emergency ward diagnosis and the efficacy of initial therapy. This is particularly true of infectious diseases, since the cultures and sensitivity tests that are so crucial to therapy require at least 24–48 hours.

Infections of the Respiratory Tract

Infections of the respiratory tract are among the most common infectious diseases seen in the emergency ward. Although they range in location and severity from simple upper respiratory infection to overwhelming bacterial pneumonia, the approach to diagnosis and therapy remains similar.

Sinusitis and Otitis

Often, sinusitis and otitis are caused by the same viruses that cause the common cold. However, bacterial pathogens can produce more serious infections in the sinuses or ears; bacterial infection, in fact, often occurs after a milder viral process. The signs and symptoms of sinusitis and otitis, as well as the value of local therapy to ensure ade-

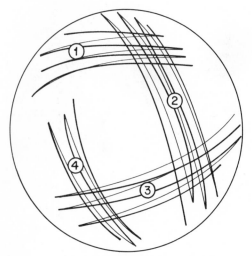

Figure 11.1.   Technique of streaking specimen on agar plate.

quate drainage of these potentially closed spaces, are discussed in Chapter 33. Identification of the bacterial pathogens responsible for such infections is complicated by two problems: (1) As previously mentioned, the upper part of the respiratory tract teems with microorganisms that constitute its normal flora. (2) The involved anatomic parts are inaccessible for direct culture except during operation. Cultures of the nasopharynx do not accurately reflect the disease process. Hence, therapy often is educated guesswork based on knowledge of the usual pathogens. Fortunately, the range of possibilities is limited. In adults, most cases of bacterial sinusitis and otitis are caused by the gram-positive cocci, including the pneumococcus, group A streptococci, and in occasional cases of sinusitis, *Staphylococcus aureus*. In children, the same organisms are frequently implicated, as well as *Hemophilus influenzae*. Recently, anaerobic bacteria have also been implicated in sinusitis. In adults, cloxacillin or other penicillinase-resistant penicillins are the preferred antibiotics (Table 11.2). Ampicillin is preferred for children. In the penicillin-allergic patient, cephalosporins, erythromycin, and clindamycin are acceptable alternatives; trimethoprim-sulfamethoxazole or erythromycin plus a sulfonamide may be useful in children. Table 11.3 lists appropriate dosages for mild infections. Most patients respond to oral administration of antibiotics without hospitalization.

Complications resulting from extension of infection to surrounding tissues include osteomyelitis, brain abscess, subdural empyema, and orbital cellulitis. These much more serious infections require immediate hospitalization, parenteral administra-

tion of large doses of antibiotics, and in the case of intracranial septic collections, surgical drainage.

Pharyngitis

In most patients, pharyngitis is mild; fever, sore throat, and occasionally dysphagia are the presenting symptoms. The major differential diagnosis is between viral infection and group A streptococcal pharyngitis. Even though high fever, cervical lymphadenopathy, pharyngeal exudate, and polymorphonuclear leukocytosis suggest streptococcal pharyngitis, throat culture is the only definitive means of diagnosis. If "strep throat" seems likely, antibiotic therapy can be started in the emergency ward. If the culture is positive, the patient should receive penicillin for 10 days to prevent rheumatic fever; if it is negative, antibiotics should be discontinued. In the penicillin-allergic patient, erythromycin is the drug of choice.

Both viral and streptococcal pharyngitis can sometimes become true medical emergencies. In patients with infectious mononucleosis, for example, the viral infection occasionally can cause sufficient edema to occlude the airway. These patients must be hospitalized and observed carefully, with tracheostomy immediately available. Fortunately, corticosteroids usually produce prompt improvement, obviating operation. Airway occlusion is also a threat if the streptococcus spreads from the pharynx to the soft tissues of the neck. Patients with this complication, called Ludwig's angina, are febrile and acutely ill, with a bullnecked appearance. Hospitalization and careful monitoring are mandatory; tracheostomy may be lifesaving, but penicillin alone is often sufficient. Streptococcal pharyngitis may lead to other serious local complications such as peritonsillar and retropharyngeal abscesses, but these infections have become rare since the introduction of penicillin.

Although many other bacteria can be cultured from the pharynx, only a few aside from the group A streptococci and *H. influenzae* in children cause pharyngitis. For example, pneumococci and *S. aureus* do not cause pharyngitis although they may be present in large numbers. Two bacteria that can cause pharyngitis are *Neisseria gonorrhoeae* and *C. diphtheriae*. Gonococcal infection is suggested by a history of orogenital exposure, and should be confirmed by culture on Thayer-Martin or Transgrow media. Diphtheria, which is suggested in a nonimmunized patient by membranous pharyngitis sometimes accompanied by bull neck, should be confirmed with a methylene blue preparation and culture of Loeffler medium.

Table 11.2.
Characteristics of some common bacterial pathogens.

Organism	Description	Medium	Usual Location	Common Infections	Antibiotic of Choice[a]	Alternative Antibiotics[a]
Gram-positive cocci Pneumococcus	Lancet-shaped in pairs or short chains	BAP	Nasopharynx	Pneumonia, bronchitis, otitis, sinusitis, bacteremia, meningitis	Penicillin	Cephalosporins[b] Erythromycin Clindamycin Chloramphenicol (for meningitis)
Staphylococcus aureus	Pairs, clusters, and clumps	BAP	Nasopharynx Skin Rectum	Skin infection, pneumonia, sinusitis, septic arthritis, bacteremia, endocarditis, osteomyelitis	Oxacillin[c]	Cephalosporins[b] Erythromycin Clindamycin Vancomycin (for endocarditis)
Group A streptococci	Pairs and chains	BAP	Nasopharynx	Pharyngitis, otitis, sinusitis, skin infection, osteomyelitis, septic arthritis, bacteremia, pneumonia	Penicillin	Cephalosporins[b] Erythromycin Clindamycin
Streptococcus viridans	Pairs and chains	BAP	Oral cavity	Endocarditis	Penicillin	Cephalosporins[b] Erythromycin Clindamycin Vancomycin (for endocarditis)
Enterococcus (group D streptococci)	Pairs and chains	BAP	Gastrointestinal tract Female genital tract	Urinary tract infection	Ampicillin	Variable
				Wound abscess, bacteremia, endocarditis, peritonitis	Penicillin and gentamicin for serious sepsis	Vancomycin alone or in combination with gentamicin for serious sepsis
Anaerobic streptococcus	Pairs and chains	Anaerobic BAP	Oral cavity Gastrointestinal tract Female genital tract	Pulmonary, brain, and abdominal abscesses; empyema	Penicillin	Clindamycin Erythromycin Cephalosporins[b]

Organism	Morphology	Culture media	Source	Disease	Drug of choice	Alternative drugs
Gram-positive bacilli						
Clostridium perfringens	Large rods	Anaerobic BAP	Gastrointestinal tract	Muscle, uterus, wound, bacteremia	Penicillin	Chloramphenicol, Clindamycin
Gram-negative cocci						
Neisseria gonorrhoeae	Bean-shaped diplococci	CAP or TM in 5% CO_2	Genitourinary tract	Urethritis, cervicitis, pharyngitis, septic arthritis, bacteremia	Penicillin	Tetracycline, Spectinomycin, Erythromycin, Cefoxitin, Chloramphenicol
Neisseria meningitidis	Bean-shaped diplococci	CAP or TM in 5% CO_2	Nasopharynx	Meningitis, bacteremia; Carrier state	Penicillin; Rifampin	Chloramphenicol; Minocycline
Gram-negative bacilli						
Escherichia coli	Rods	BAP, MacC	Gastrointestinal tract, Female genital tract	Intra-abdominal infection, urinary tract infection, bacteremia, neonatal meningitis, nosocomial pneumonia	Ampicillin	Cephalosporins[b], Chloramphenicol, Gentamicin, Tobramycin, Tetracycline, sulfisoxazole, or trimethoprim-sulfamethoxazole for urinary tract infection
Klebsiella pneumoniae	Rods with thick capsules	BAP, MacC	Gastrointestinal tract	Urinary tract infection, pneumonia, intra-abdominal infection, bacteremia	Gentamicin, tobramycin or cephalosporins[b]	Kanamycin, Amikacin
Proteus mirabilis	Rods	BAP, MacC	Gastrointestinal tract	Urinary tract infection, intra-abdominal infection, bacteremia	Ampicillin	Cephalosporins[b], Gentamicin or tobramycin
Indole-positive *Proteus* species	Rods	BAP, MacC	Gastrointestinal tract	Urinary tract infection, intra-abdominal infection, bacteremia	Gentamicin, tobramycin	Kanamycin, Carbenicillin[d], Cefoxitin or cefamandole[b]

Table 11.2. continued

Organism	Description	Medium	Usual Location	Common Infections	Antibiotic of Choice[a]	Alternative Antibiotics[a]
Pseudomonas aeruginosa	Rods	BAP MacC	Skin	Urinary tract infection, bacteremia, nosocomial infection	Gentamicin or tobramycin	Amikacin Carbenicillin
Bacteroides Oral	Thin filamentous rods	Anaerobic BAP	Oral cavity	Aspiration pneumonia, pulmonary and brain abscesses	Penicillin	Clindamycin Chloramphenicol Metronidazole
Gastrointestinal	Thin filamentous rods	Anaerobic BAP	Gastrointestinal tract Female genital tract	Intra-abdominal infection, wound abcess, bacteremia	Clindamycin or chloramphenicol	Carbenicillin[d] Cefoxitin[b] Metronidazole
Hemophilus influenzae	Small, coccobacillary	CAP	Nasopharynx	Adults—bronchitis, epiglottitis	Ampicillin[e] Chloramphenicol[e]	Tetracycline Cefamandole[b] Trimethoprim-sulfamethoxazole
				Children—otitis, sinusitis, pneumonia, meningitis, bacteremia, pharyngitis, bronchitis, epiglottitis		

BAP = blood agar plate; CAP = chocolate agar plate; TM = Thayer-Martin agar; MacC = MacConkey agar.

[a] Antibiotic of choice depends on sensitivity testing. Antibiotics listed are mostly likely to be effective at present, but sensitivities should be confirmed.

[b] Cephalosporins *must be used with caution in penicillin-allergic patients*. The standard cephalosporins are ineffective in meningitis but "third generation" drugs such as moxalactam have shown promise in limited experience with gram-negative meningitis.

[c] Nafcillin is an equally effective parenteral antistaphylococcal agent. Cloxacillin or dicloxacillin is preferred for oral administration in mild infections. If organisms are penicillin sensitive, penicillin is drug of choice.

[d] Ticarcillin, mezlocillin and piperacillin are similar to carbenicillin.

[e] Some strains of *H. influenzae* are ampicillin resistant. In life-threatening *H. influenzae* infections, chloramphenicol should be administered until sensitivities are known. Parenteral cefamandole is another excellent alternative (except for meningitis). In mild *H. influenzae* infections in penicillin-allergic patients, tetracycline or trimethoprim-sulfamethoxazole are preferred.

Epiglottitis

Another bacterial infection of the upper respiratory tract that is a true medical emergency is epiglottitis. This infection is much more common in children; when it occurs in adults, it is often fatal because of misdiagnosis. Presenting symptoms include fever, severe pharyngeal pain, dysphagia, and respiratory distress that can progress to asphyxia with alarming rapidity. The epiglottis is edematous, inflamed, and characteristically cherry red; attempts to visualize the epiglottis directly can lead to severe spasm and airway obstruction. Before a mirror, tongue blade, or culture swab is used, a lateral x-ray film of the neck should be taken. If the epiglottis is edematous, instrumentation is contraindicated. If no edema is apparent and if respiratory distress is only mild, indirect laryngoscopic examination may be undertaken with caution. Tracheostomy or endotracheal intubation by an experienced person should be performed if any sign of respiratory decompensation occurs. Most epiglottitis is caused by *H. influenzae*, with gram-positive cocci reported in a few cases. Ampicillin has traditionally been the drug of choice; however, ampicillin-resistant strains of *H. influenzae* are being recognized with increasing frequency, so chloramphenicol should also be administered until the sensitivity of the organism is known. Blood specimens should be cultured before therapy.

Bronchitis

Bronchitis is an infection of the lower part of the respiratory tract whose typical presenting symptoms are cough, sputum production, and low-grade fever. Auscultation of the lungs may be normal or reveal diffuse rhonchi from large-airway secretions. The chest x-ray film is normal. Viruses frequently cause bronchitis; in such cases, the sputum is clear and antibiotics have no role in therapy. Bacterial infections of the tracheobronchial tree frequently are accompanied by production of purulent sputum and a higher fever. Examination of the sputum levels reveals the causative organism. In otherwise healthy adults, the pneumococcus is the leading bacterial cause of bronchitis; in patients with chronic pulmonary disease and in children, *H. influenzae* is also common. Examination of sputum and therapy are discussed later with the types of pneumonia. Most patients with bronchitis respond well to oral administration of antibiotics without hospitalization. In patients with chronic pulmonary disease, however, even mild infections can cause respiratory failure requiring intensive therapy. In addition, in children with bronchitis, bronchospasm may develop that is severe enough to require bronchodilators and hospitalization.

Bacterial Pneumonia

Bacterial pneumonia often follows a viral infection of the upper part of the respiratory tract. The cardinal features suggesting bacterial pneumonia are fever, cough, and sputum production. Shaking chills, dyspnea, and pleuritic chest pain are often present as well. Physical examination frequently reveals signs of pulmonary consolidation in addition to tachypnea and tachycardia. Hypoxemia may be present if infection is severe, and it may lead to delirium or stupor. The white blood cell count and differential typically reveal polymorphonuclear leukocytosis. The chest x-ray film usually demonstrates infiltration that may range from dense consolidation of one or more lobes to a patchy bronchopneumonic pattern; the film may also provide evidence of two of the local complications of pneumonia, pulmonary abscess and empyema. Systemic complications of pneumonia include bacteremia and blood-borne infections such as septic arthritis and meningitis.

The differential diagnosis must take into consideration the types of nonbacterial pneumonia, such as those caused by viruses, mycoplasmas, and much less commonly, fungi. Tuberculosis occasionally may mimic acute bacterial pneumonia. Chronic pulmonary disease, including emphysema and bronchiectasis, may be misleading if previous chest x-ray films are unavailable. Noninfectious processes such as atelectasis, pulmonary infarction, pulmonary edema, and tumor also are confused sometimes with bacterial pneumonia.

In an emergency, the first concern is adequate oxygenation. Vital signs should be monitored, and arterial blood-gas levels should be determined if the patient is in respiratory distress, if he has a depressed level of consciousness, or if there is underlying pulmonary disease. Techniques for respiratory support are given elsewhere in this text. General supportive measures such as suppression of fever, chest physical therapy, and administration of expectorants should be employed promptly when needed. Virtually all patients with bacterial pneumonia require hospitalization and parenteral antibiotic therapy; occasionally, otherwise healthy young adults with mild pneumococcal pneumonia may be treated at home if follow-up care is close by.

The key to diagnosis is examination of sputum. In patients with bacterial pneumonia, it is typically thick and green to brownish, and it may be tinged

Dosage ranges for selected antibiotics.

Drug[b]	Route	Adult Dosage	Pediatric Dosage	Comments and Typical Indications
Penicillins[b]				
Penicillin V	PO	250 mg every 4–6 hours	30–60 mg/kg/day divided into 4 doses	Bronchitis, otitis, pharyngitis
Penicillin G procaine	IM	600,000–1.2 million units every 12 hours	25,000–50,000 units/kg/day divided into 2 doses	Bronchitis, otitis, pharyngitis, pneumococcal pneumonia
Penicillin G aqueous crystalline	IM	600,000 units every 6 hours	25,000–50,000 units/kg/day divided into 4 doses	Bronchitis, otitis, pharyngitis, pneumococcal pneumonia
	IV	1–4 million units every 4 hours	100,000–400,000 units/kg/day divided into 6 doses	Lower doses for streptococcal pneumonia, pulmonary abscess; highest doses for endocarditis, meningitis
Ampicillin	PO	250–500 mg every 4–6 hours	50–100 mg/kg/day divided into 4 doses	Otitis (pediatric), bronchitis, urinary tract infection
	IV	1–2 gm every 4–6 hours	100–400 mg/kg/day divided into 6 doses	Lower doses for pneumonia, pyelonephritis; highest doses for meningitis
Cloxacillin	PO	250—500 mg every 4–6 hours	50–100 mg/kg/day divided into 4 doses	Skin and soft-tissue infections, sinusitis
Oxacillin or nafcillin	IV	1–2 gm every 4 hours	50–200 mg/kg/day divided into 6 doses	Highest doses for endocarditis, meningitis, osteomyelitis
Carbenicillin	PO	1–2 tablets (382 mg/tablet) every 6 hours	50–65 mg/kg/day divided into 4 doses	Urinary tract infection only
	IV	4–6 gm every 4 hours	100–600 mg/kg/day divided into 4 or 6 doses	Lower doses for urinary tract infection; higher doses for bacteremia, pneumonia High sodium content
Cephalosporins[c]				
Cephalexin	PO	250–500 mg every 6 hours	25–50 mg/kg/day divided into 4 doses	Urinary tract infection, pharyngitis, skin and soft-tissue infections
Cephalothin Cefamandole Cefoxitin Cefotoxime	IV	0.75–2 gm every 4 hours	50–150 mg/kg/day divided into 4 or 6 doses	Lower doses for pyelonephritis; higher doses for pneumonia, bacteremia, endocarditis, osteomyelitis
Cefazolin	IV IM	0.5–1.5 gm every 6–8 hours	25–50 mg/kg/day divided into 3 or 4 doses	Same as for cephalothin; cefazolin less painful
Moxalactam	IV	0.5–2 gm every 8 hours	100–200 mg/kg/day divided into 3 or 4 doses	Same as for cephalothin; has shown promise in gram-negative meningitis (highest doses)
Erythromycin	PO	250–500mg every 6 hours	20–50 mg/kg/day divided into 4 doses	Pharyngitis, otitis in penicillin-allergic patients Toxicity: hypersensitivity
	IV	0.25–1 gm every 6 hours	30–50 mg/kg/day divided into 4 doses	Pneumonia, cellulitis in penicillin-allergic patients Toxicity: hypersensitivity, phlebitis

Drug	Route	Adult dosage	Pediatric dosage	Comments
Clindamycin	PO	150–300 mg every 6 hours	10–25 mg/kg/day divided into 4 doses	Infection with gram-positive cocci in penicillin-allergic patients (except meningitis), anaerobic infection Toxicity: hypersensitivity, colitis
Vancomycin	IV IM	300–600 mg every 6 hours	10–40 mg/kg/day divided into 4 doses	Life-threatening staphylococcal or enterococcal infection when penicillins and cephalosporins contraindicated Nephrotoxic—dosage must be reduced if patient has renal failure
	IV	250–500 mg every 6 hours	40 mg/kg/day divided into 4 doses	
Tetracycline	PO	250–500 mg every 6 hours	20–40 mg/kg/day divided into 4 doses	Much overused, rarely drug of choice; may stain teeth in children
Chloramphenicol	IV	250–500 mg every 6 hours	10–20 mg/kg/day divided into 4 doses	Potential marrow toxicity, use in serious infection only; use cautiously in newborns
	IV	0.25–1 gm every 6 hours	50–100 mg/kg/day divided into 4 doses	Oral form available, but rarely indicated
Aminoglycosides				
Kanamycin Amikacin	IM IV	7.5 mg/kg every 12 hours (maximal daily dose 1.5 gm)	Same as adult dosage	Toxicity: renal and VIII nerve
Gentamicin Tobramycin	IM IV	1.0–1.5 mg/kg every 8 hours	Same as adult dosage	Toxicity: renal and VIII nerve
Sulfisoxazole	PO	1 gm every 6 hours	150 mg/kg/day divided into 4 doses	Urinary tract infection Toxicity: hypersensitivity
Trimethoprim-sulfamethoxazole	PO	2 tablets every 12 hours	8 mg/kg/day (based on trimethoprim component) divided into 2 doses	Urinary tract infection Toxicity: hypersensitivity
	IV	3 mg/kg (based on trimethoprim component) every 8 hours	Same as adult dosage	Urinary tract infections and shigellosis (higher dose for *pneumocystis carinii*)

[a] Dosage ranges are for average-size adults and for pediatric patients beyond neonatal period with normal renal and hepatic functions. Adult dosages are expressed per individual dose while pediatric dosages are expressed in amount per day. Pediatric doses are given in accordance with kilograms of body weight; in older children, care must be taken not to exceed normal adult doses. In all patients, dosage must be individualized; see manufacturer's literature for more details. In most cases, intravenous antibiotics should be diluted in at least 100 ml of fluid and administered over approximately 60 minutes. Avoid mixing more than one medication in each infusion bottle. Only major toxicities are listed; consult manufacturer's literature for details. In addition, all antibiotics predispose the patient to superinfection.

[b] Hypersensitivity is a major toxic reaction; all cross-react—a patient allergic to one penicillin is allergic to all.

[c] Cephalosporins *must be used with caution in penicillin-allergic patients.* The standard cephalosporins are ineffective in meningitis but "third generation" drugs such as moxalactam have shown promise in very limited experience with gram-negative meningitis.

with blood. A good sputum specimen for microscopic examination and culture is crucial. If the patient cannot expectorate spontaneously, chest physical therapy, intermittent positive-pressure breathing with humidified air, or nasotracheal suction may be employed to obtain the specimen. If these fail, transtracheal aspiration may be performed. The Gram stain usually reveals abundant polymorphonuclear leukocytes, and often discloses the primary pathogen. The sputum should be cultured promptly, and blood cultures should also be obtained before administration of antibiotics (Table 11.1).

Pneumococcal Pneumonia. The pneumococcus is still the most common cause of bacterial pneumonia, accounting for from 30–60% of all cases. It affects all age groups, and is especially likely to be the agent infecting otherwise healthy ambulatory patients. Classic clinical features include abrupt onset of fever with a single rigor, cough with rusty sputum, and pleurisy. Radiologic evidence of lobar consolidation is typical, but infiltrates can be patchy, especially in patients with chronic pulmonary disease. Penicillin is the drug of choice (Tables 11.2 and 11.3). Tetracycline should *not* be administered because many pneumococci are now resistant to it. Therapy should be continued until the patient has been afebrile for 3–5 days; oral penicillin may be substituted in the last few days of treatment in uncomplicated cases. Bacteremia is a complication of pneumococcal pneumonia in about 30% of patients; fortunately, conditions resulting from blood-borne sepsis (septic arthritis, peritonitis, meningitis, and the like) are much less common. Sterile pleural effusions occur often, empyema is less frequent, and pulmonary abscess is rare.

Streptococcal Pneumonia. Although pneumonia caused by group A streptococci is uncommon, it has occurred in epidemics. It usually begins abruptly with fever, cough, chest pain, and severe debility. The distinctive clinical and radiologic feature is rapid spread in the lung, resulting in early development of empyema. Penicillin is the drug of choice. Therapy should be continued until clinical manifestations of infection are resolved, which usually requires at least 2 weeks. Pulmonary abscess, bacteremia, and metastatic infection are uncommon complications, as is postinfectious acute glomerulonephritis.

Staphylococcal Pneumonia. *S. aureus* causes up to 10% of all cases of bacterial pneumonia. Except in infancy when it can be a primary infection, staphylococcal pneumonia most commonly follows a viral infection of the respiratory tract, particularly influenza. It may also occur as a noso-

comial infection or as a result of bacteremic seeding of the lungs. These patients are usually extremely ill. *S. aureus* causes tissue necrosis, and the distinctive feature of staphylococcal pneumonia is the tendency to produce multiple small pulmonary abscesses. Healing usually leaves residual fibrosis. A semisynthetic penicillin such as oxacillin is the drug of choice (Tables 11.2 and 11.3). Therapy should be continued until both clinical and x-ray findings indicate healing; this usually requires at least 2–4 weeks. Empyema and pneumothorax are relatively common complications, and bacteremia with metastatic seeding of distant sites, including the endocardium, bones, joints, liver, and meninges, may also occur.

Hemophilus Pneumonia. *H. influenzae* commonly causes pneumonia in children less than 6 years old, often producing segmental or lobar consolidation or patchy bronchopneumonia; in older children, hemophilus pneumonia is rare. It is also uncommon in adults, exept in the elderly with underlying chronic pulmonary disease; in these patients a bronchopneumonic pattern is typical. Ampicillin is the antibiotic of choice (Tables 11.2 and 11.3). Now that ampicillin-resistant strains of *H. influenzae* are appearing, however, sensitivity testing is important; chloramphenicol is the drug of choice for these strains, but cefamandole has also proven useful. For *H. Influenzae* bronchitis, tetracycline and trimethoprim-sulfamethoxazole are useful alternatives to ampicillin for oral therapy. Therapy should be continued for 10–14 days. In children, bacteremia may develop, with metastatic infection (especially in the joints and meninges) or intrathoracic suppuration (pulmonary abscess or empyema). These complications are less common in adults, but hypoxia and respiratory failure may develop in elderly patients with chronic pulmonary disease.

Klebsiella Pneumonia. *Klebsiella pneumoniae* typically causes pulmonary infection in debilitated patients, especially alcoholics. Illness is usually acute, but chronic pneumonitis may occasionally occur. *K. pneumoniae* has a propensity to produce tissue necrosis, resulting in hemoptysis, dense lobar consolidation, and a high incidence of abscess. Gentamicin or tobramycin or a cephalosporin is the antibiotic of choice (Tables 11.2 and 11.3). Therapy should be continued until clinical and radiologic findings indicate resolution; this usually requires 3–4 weeks. Pulmonary abscess is part of the natural evolution of the disease, and empyema may also occur.

Other Gram-negative Bacillary Pneumonia. These serious infections, once rare, have increased over the past 15 years, accounting for up to 20% of cases of bacterial pneumonia in recent series. They occur typically as hospital-acquired infections in debilitated patients who frequently have received antibiotic therapy that has altered the respiratory flora. This type of pneumonia may result from aspiration of organisms from the upper part of the respiratory tract (often related to inhalation therapy) or from bacteremic seeding of the lungs. Bacteremic pneumonia is characterized by multiple small areas of infection in both lungs. Specific treatment depends on the etiologic agent. Gentamicin or tobramycin is the drug of choice before the results of cultures and sensitivity testing are available. Most patients with pneumonia due to gram-negative bacilli require at least 14–28 days of treatment. Complications include pulmonary abscess, empyema, and bacteremia with metastatic infection.

Aspiration Pneumonia. This type of pneumonia results from aspiration of bacteria from the mouth into the lower part of the respiratory tract. Infection is usually mixed, caused by the aerobic and anaerobic streptococci, Bacteroides, fusobacteria, and the like, that are harmless, normal flora in the upper airway but that are pathogenic in the parenchyma of the lung. Predisposing factors include alterations of consciousness resulting from drugs, anesthesia, alcohol, or trauma to the head, and diminution of the gag reflex. Patients usually are mildly to moderately ill, but can be severely ill, especially if pulmonary abscess or empyema occurs. In the usual aspiration pneumonia, the Gram stain of sputum reveals abundant polymorphonuclear leukocytes and mixed flora including grampositive cocci in pairs and chains and pleomorphic gram-negative bacilli. Penicillin is the drug of choice, and a 7-day course of therapy is usually sufficient. It must be stressed that both hospitalized and ambulatory patients receiving antibiotics may have altered respiratory flora, and aspiration of oral organisms in such individuals may result in staphylococcal or gram-negative bacillary pneumonia. Hence, aspiration in this setting requires broader antimicrobial coverage. Complications of aspiration pneumonia include pulmonary abscess and empyema, which are fairly common if therapy is delayed.

Legionnaire's Disease. Although Legionnaire's disease is often thought of in the context of epidemics which occur during the warmer months, it is also an important cause of sporadic cases of pneumonia throughout the entire year in all parts of the country. In fact, as many as 1% of all pneumonias may be caused by *Legionella pneumophila*. All age groups can be affected, but attack rates appear higher in older patients and in those with underlying diseases such as chronic obstructive pulmonary disease, neoplasia, and azotemia.

The typical patient with Legionnaire's disease becomes abruptly ill with high fever and rigors after a brief prodrome of myalgias, headache, and malaise. Cough is prominent but there is little, if any, sputum production; other pulmonary symptoms are tachypnea, dyspnea, and sometimes pleurisy. Diarrhea may be an important clue, and other extrapulmonary features may include encephalopathy and renal dysfunction.

The physical exam is usually nonspecific but may disclose confusion, rales, abdominal tenderness, and sometimes, relative bradycardia in addition to fever and "toxicity." Chest x-ray findings are variable, ranging from interstitial or patchy infiltrates to nodular consolidation; involvement may be confined to one lobe or may be diffuse. The white blood cell count is normal or mildly elevated. Other laboratory findings may include hypoxia, elevated liver enzymes, and abnormalities of the urinalysis and renal function tests.

In most cases, the emergency ward diagnosis of Legionnaire's disease depends on these clinical features. Laboratory confirmation is difficult. The sputum exam fails to disclose a pathogen. Cultures may be helpful but require specialized media (charcoal-yeast extract) and techniques. An indirect fluorescent antibody stain can make a rapid diagnosis but this test is not widely available. Serologic tests can confirm the diagnosis but require acute and convalescent serum.

The differential diagnosis of Legionnaire's disease includes the other causes of pneumonia without sputum production (see Nonbacterial Pneumonias, page 230). If Legionnaire's disease is suspected in the emergency ward, cultures and serologies should be obtained but treatment should not be delayed. Erythromycin is the drug of choice and is usually administered intravenously in doses of 500 mg–1 gram every 6 hours. Rifampin and tetracycline are active against most strains of *L. pneumophilia* in vitro, but clinical experience is limited.

Other Bacterial Pneumonia. Many other organisms, from *Bacillus anthracis* to the meningococcus, occasionally may cause bacterial pneumonia; patients require individualized therapy.

Other Intrathoracic Infections

Pulmonary Abscess. Patients with a pyogenic abscess of the lung are usually seen in the emergency ward with fever, cough, and if the abscess communicates with the bronchial tree, copious production of sputum. Pleurisy, hemoptysis, and dyspnea also may occur. In this respect, these patients resemble patients with pneumonia. Diagnosis depends on the chest x-ray film, which reveals abscess formation, often with air-fluid levels. As with pneumonia, the etiologic diagnosis depends on the Gram stain and culture of the sputum. The three basic causes of pulmonary abscess are:

(1) Aspiration of bacteria from the oropharynx into the lower part of the respiratory tract. This is the most common cause. Patients with the highest risk are those with depressed consciousness or an impaired gag reflex, such as alcoholics, patients who are heavily sedated or who are anesthetized, and patients with neurologic impairment. The α-hemolytic streptococci, together with the gram-positive and gram-negative oral anaerobes, are the causative organisms. The Gram stain of sputum reveals abundant polymorphonuclear leukocytes and mixed flora. Penicillin is the drug of choice, and clindamycin is the preferred alternative in penicillin-allergic patients. Some authorities advocate oral therapy on an outpatient basis, but we recommend hospitalization and parenteral treatment with moderate dosages (Table 11.3). Patients should have chest physical therapy, and should undergo postural drainage; many also require bronchoscopic examination to exclude an obstructing lesion.

(2) Necrotizing bacterial pneumonia. Staphylococci, Klebsiella, and other gram-negative bacilli are particularly likely to be the causative organisms of such abscesses, which are often small and multiple. Diagnosis and therapy are the same as for the underlying pneumonia, except that antibiotics dosage should usually be higher, with a longer duration of therapy.

(3) Bronchial obstruction. Foreign bodies and neoplasms frequently obstruct the bronchi, and bronchoscopic examination is essential. If obstruction is complete, it may be impossible initially to obtain a specimen of sputum. Cefoxitin is an excellent antibiotic with which to begin therapy in this situation, but it is important to relieve the obstruction subsequently, and to obtain specimens for a Gram stain and culture.

Empyema. Patients with empyema typically are seen in the emergency ward with fever and pleurisy. Dyspnea and respiratory insufficiency may occur, especially if the patient has underlying pulmonary disease. Although cough may be a prominent symptom, unless pneumonia is present such patients do not produce copious sputum.

Empyema may occur in several ways: it may be secondary to necrotizing pneumonia or a pulmonary abscess, in which case staphylococci, gram-negative bacilli, or mixed oral organisms are the most common agents; it may be caused by diaphragmatic penetration of an intra-abdominal septic process, such as a subphrenic abscess, in which case the intestinal flora are most common; or it may result from bacteremic seeding. The key to diagnosis and therapy is adequate drainage with thoracentesis performed in the emergency ward. The fluid is typically thick, and is foul smelling if anaerobes are present. Polymorphonuclear leukocytes are numerous, the glucose level is depressed, and protein and lactate dehydrogenase levels are elevated. Specimens should be cultured both aerobically and anaerobically (Table 11.1), and a Gram stain should be performed. If the source of infection is intestinal, antibiotic therapy should be directed at the gastrointestinal flora. Complete drainage is essential; if repeated thoracentesis is inadequate, drainage with a tube should be employed.

Nonbacterial Pneumonia. Patients with "atypical" or nonbacterial pneumonia are usually less acutely ill than those with bacterial pneumonia. This type of infection is most common in young adults, but can occur in any age group. Typically, patients are seen in the emergency ward with fever and a cough that is often nonproductive. Dyspnea, pleurisy, rigors, and frank pulmonary consolidation are uncommon; rales do occur. Chest x-ray examination may reveal infiltrates that are more extensive than suggested by physical findings; such infiltrates are often patchy and may be bilateral. The white blood cell count and differential are usually within normal limits.

The major causes of nonbacterial pneumonia are respiratory tract viruses and *Mycoplasma pneumoniae*. Epidemiologic findings are the key to diagnosis of the less common causes of nonbacterial pneumonia, such as Q fever in animal handlers and psittacosis after exposure to an infected bird. In mycoplasmal pneumonia, an elevated cold agglutinin titer is a useful clue to diagnosis, but is absent in at least one-third of cases. Absolute diagnosis depends on either specific serologic tests available through most state laboratories or culture with special media and techniques. Mycoplasmal pneumonia should be treated with either erythromycin or tetracycline, and most patients can be treated at home with oral antibiotics. Tetracycline is the drug of choice for Q fever and psittacosis.

Tuberculosis. Patients with tuberculosis also may be seen in the emergency ward with fever, cough, and pulmonary infiltrates. Primary tuberculosis, which is most common in children and young adults, may mimic atypical pneumonia clinically. Tuberculous pleuritis may occur. Postprimary or reactivation tuberculosis is a more frequent clinical problem, and usually involves the upper lobes, with formation of cavities in advanced cases. Diagnosis depends on skin tests and acid-fast smears and cultures of sputum. The smears should be made and studied in the emergency ward; however, cultures of these slow-growing organisms take 4–6 weeks. Patients with suspected pulmonary tuberculosis should be hospitalized for diagnosis and therapy. Respiratory precautions with well-ventilated single rooms and high-quality masks should be employed, and if the diagnosis is confirmed, epidemiologic investigation must be undertaken.

Infections of the Central Nervous System

Bacterial Meningitis

A true medical emergency, bacterial meningitis is fatal in virtually all patients who do not receive prompt, expert therapy; however, most of those who do receive appropriate treatment recover. Most patients have sytemic symptoms including fever and an acutely ill appearance. If the patient also has signs and symptoms of meningeal irritation including headache, stiff neck, and altered mentation, the diagnosis should be clear. Meningitis can be occult, however. Infants and very young children, for example, rarely have nuchal rigidity, and they may even be afebrile; elderly or debilitated patients may have only fever and altered consciousness. Because of the seriousness of this infection and the need for immediate therapy, any patient in whom bacterial meningitis is suspected should be vigorously evaluated.

Cardiovascular and pulmonary function must first be assessed. Many patients with meningitis have bacteremia, and septic shock may ensue (see pages 244–245 and Chapter 3). A brief history should be obtained, usually from a friend or relative. The physician immediately should ascertain whether the patient has any antecedent infection (particularly in the ears, sinuses, or lungs) and any drug allergies. Other details in the history will be important later, but because of the need for immediate action, the physician should next perform a physical examination. The skin should be examined for petechial or hemorrhagic lesions suggesting meningococcemia, and the ears and sinuses should be examined for a primary suppurative focus possibly extending to the meninges. Examination of the chest and sometimes even the abdomen also may reveal a septic focus responsible for bacteremia and resultant meningitis. The neurologic examination is of utmost importance. Patients with bacterial meningitis usually display altered mentation ranging from confusion or delirium to stupor or coma. Seizures may occur. Signs of meningeal irritation may be demonstrated by the patient's resistance to passive flexion of the neck (Brudzinski's sign) or by pain on extension of the leg with the hip flexed (Kernig's sign). Localizing signs should be sought; these are absent in most patients with bacterial meningitis, and their presence should raise the possibility of a focal lesion such as a brain abscess.

If the abbreviated examination suggests meningitis, the physician should proceed with the crucial diagnostic procedure, the lumbar puncture. The pressure of the cerebrospinal fluid is typically elevated in these patients, but tentorial herniation is uncommon after lumbar puncture. Nevertheless, if the pressure exceeds 400 mm H_2O, mannitol should be given intravenously before the cerebrospinal fluid is collected (see Chapter 15, pages 340–341).

The cerebrospinal fluid should be collected in at least four tubes. The fluid in the first tube should be used for a white blood cell count and differential, and if red blood cells are present, raising the possibility of a traumatic tap, the counts should be repeated with a sample from the fourth tube. The fluid in the second tube should be used for determination of glucose and protein levels, and a portion of the fluid in the third tube should be cultured using a blood agar plate, a chocolate agar slant, and thioglycollate broth (table 11.1). The remaining fluid in the third tube should be used for a Gram stain. Typical findings include an elevated white blood cell count usually between 500 and 20,000/mm.[3] Most of these cells are polymorphonuclear leukocytes. In addition, the protein level is usually somewhat elevated, ranging from 70–150 mg/100 ml. An important finding is a glucose level depressed to less than 50 mg/100 ml or to less than 50% of a simultaneously determined blood glucose level (Table 11.4).

In the patient with meningitis, other laboratory studies should include a complete blood cell count, differential, and urinalysis, as well as determination of the levels of serum electrolytes, blood urea nitrogen, creatinine, and blood glucose. A platelet count, prothrombin time, and partial thromboplastin time are important if the patient has hypotension or hemorrhagic cutaneous lesions (see Chapter 13, pages 285–286, for discussion of disseminated intravascular coagulation). Throat and blood cultures should be obtained, and sputum should be studied by a Gram stain and culture if possible. X-ray films of the chest, skull, and sinuses should be taken to look for a primary septic focus.

Definitive identification of the responsible bacterial pathogen requires 24–48 hours for culture results, but antibiotic therapy cannot wait. Fortunately, the Gram stain of the cerebrospinal fluid and the clinical findings provide sufficient information for the physician to choose an antibiotic in the emergency ward. Three major organisms account for most cases of bacterial meningitis:

(1) Pneumococcus. These gram-positive cocci occurring in pairs or short chains can cause meningitis in any age group, but particularly in adults; meningitis results from direct extension of the pathogens from an infected ear or sinus or from bacteremic spread from a pulmonary focus. The antibiotic of choice is penicillin, administered intravenously in high doses. In the penicillin-allergic patient, chloramphenicol or erythromycin should be administered, 4 gm/day in four doses for adults. Remember that first and second generation cephalosporins are ineffective therapy for meningitis, and even the third generation cephalosporins are not recommended for pneumococcal meningitis.

(2) Meningococcus. On the Gram stain, these organisms appear as bean-shaped, gram-negative diplococci. Meningococcal meningitis can occur at any age, but is particularly common in children and young adults. This potentially fulminating infection spreads from the pharynx to the meninges via the bloodstream; even if meningitis does not develop, meningococcemia can be fatal within hours. Petechial lesions on the skin may indicate disseminated intravascular coagulation; if this is confirmed by clotting studies, heparin may be of benefit. In hypotensive patients, corticosteroids may be helpful because of the possibility of associated adrenal hemorrhage. Neither heparin nor corticosteroids, however, are innocuous, and they should both be administered with caution. Cardiac function should be monitored in all patients; meningococcemia can cause myocarditis resulting in arrhythmias and congestive heart failure, as well as purulent pericarditis with tamponade. Meticulous circulatory and respiratory support is vital. Penicillin is the drug of choice. In the penicillin-allergic patient, chloramphenicol should be administered (Table 11.3).

Meningococcal meningitis is the only form of bacterial meningitis that is contagious, and in these patients, mask and gown precautions should be taken for the first 24 hours of therapy. Prophylactic treatment of contacts is difficult. Penicillin is ineffective when administered to persons in the carrier state, and most meningococci are now resistant to the sulfonamide compounds. The only effective antibiotics in this situation are minocycline and rifampin, but because of fewer side effects rifampin is generally preferred, 600 mg twice a day for a total of four doses in adults, 10 mg/kg twice a day for a total of four doses in children from 1–12 years, and 5 mg/kg twice a day for a total of four doses in children less than 1 year. Because of cost, side effects, and emerging drug resistance, therapy should be reserved for close contacts.

(3) *Hemophilus influenzae.* These small, gram-negative, coccobacillary organisms vary in size and shape. Bacterial meningitis caused by *H. influenzae* is common in children between 6 months and 6 years of age, but is uncommon in other age groups. The infection may originate in either the upper or lower part of the respiratory tract. Until recently, ampicillin was the drug of choice. In the last few years, however, ampicillin-resistant strains of *H. influenzae* have been isolated with increasing frequency. Because there is no room for error in the management of bacterial meningitis, it is best to begin treatment with chloramphenicol in the same doses as for meningococcal meningitis; if the causative organism is then proved sensitive to ampicillin, this drug can be administered instead, 12 gm/day intravenously in six doses for adults and 400 mg/kg/day in six doses for children.

While the three organisms discussed account for most cases of bacterial meningitis, in special circumstances other bacteria may be implicated:

(1) In the newborn, bacterial meningitis may be caused by a wide range of pathogens, including group B streptococci, *Escherichia coli*, and other enteric gram-negative bacilli, and it may be manifested by nothing more specific than failure to feed, often with hypothermia. Meningitis must be suspected in all newborns with sepsis, and a lumbar puncture must be performed. Until the results of cultures and sensitivity testing are available, patients with streptococcal infection should be treated with penicillin, and those with gram-negative bacillary infection should receive ampicillin and gentamicin. Penicillin and ampicillin dosages have been given; 1.5 mg/kg of gentamicin should be administered intramuscularly or intravenously every 8 hours. Since little gentamicin crosses the blood-brain barrier, this drug should probably also be administered intrathecally, 1 mg every 24 hours. If no organisms are seen on the Gram stain of the cerebrospinal fluid, the newborn with suspected bacterial meningitis should be treated with ampicillin and gentamicin until culture results are available.

(2) Staphylococcal meningitis is uncommon. Except in newborns, gram-negative bacillary meningitis is also rare. These both occur almost exclusively in the immunosuppressed, debilitated patient or as a complication of a neurosurgical pro-

cedure or penetrating head trauma. Until results of sensitivity testing are available, patients whose cerebrospinal fluid reveals gram-negative bacilli should be treated with ampicillin and gentamicin in the aforementioned dosages. Adults should probably also receive intrathecal gentamicin, 5 mg every 24 hours. As experience with moxalactam and cefotoxime increases, these third generation cephalosporins may become the agents of choice for meningitis caused by susceptible strains of gram-negative bacilli. Patients with staphylococcal meningitis should receive a semisynthetic penicillinase-resistant penicillin such as oxacillin.

(3) Other bacteria can also cause meningitis under special circumstances; examples include *Listeria monocytogenes* and various streptococci.

In some patients with bacterial meningitis, the initial Gram stain of the cerebrospinal fluid does not reveal the causative organism. As stated previously, most cases of bacterial meningitis beyond the neonatal period are caused by *H. influenzae*, pneumococci, or meningococci. In adults in whom the pathogen is unidentified, ampicillin is usually sufficient, but in children less than 6 years old, initial therapy with both ampicillin and chloramphenicol is best because of the existence of ampicillin-resistant strains of *H. influenzae*. If the patient is allergic to penicillin, therapy with chloramphenicol and erythromycin is recommended. If cultures of the cerebrospinal fluid become positive, therapy should then be directed toward the organism isolated.

Partly treated bacterial meningitis is a difficult problem for the emergency physician. Often, these patients have received oral antibiotics before being seen in the emergency ward. As a result, Gram stains and cultures of the cerebrospinal fluid may be negative, and the cerebrospinal fluid may even show a predominance of lymphocytes and a nearly normal glucose level. If blood and cerebrospinal fluid cultures remain negative, these patients should be treated in the manner discussed above for bacterial meningitis of uncertain cause.

Viral Meningitis

The course of viral meningitis is usually much milder than that of bacterial meningitis. Patients are commonly seen with fever and headache with or without photophobia and vomiting. Nuchal rigidity may be severe, but these patients are mentally alert and free of focal neurologic signs. Identical clinical findings can be produced by many viruses, including enteroviruses, some of the herpesviruses, and mumps virus. The specific diagnosis is usually difficult, but examination of the cerebrospinal fluid should suggest that a viral agent is responsible (Table 11.4). Typical findings include normal pressure, a normal glucose level, and a normal to slightly elevated protein level. The white blood cell count is usually less than $1000/mm^3$; early in the course of viral meningitis, polymorphonuclear leukocytes may predominate, but within 24 hours, almost all cells should be lymphocytes. Gram stains and bacterial cultures are negative. In general, patients with viral meningitis should be hospitalized for observation.

If polymorphonuclear leukocytes predominate in the cerebrospinal fluid from the initial lumbar puncture and if the patient appears ill, it is best to start administration of antibiotics before culture results are available. However, if polymorphonuclear leukocytes predominate in the cerebrospinal fluid but other findings are typical of viral meningitis, antibiotics may be withheld, with the patient closely observed and a lumbar puncture repeated in 12–24 huors.

Tuberculous and Fungal Meningitis

These are much less common than bacterial and viral meningitis. Patients typically are seen with a history of several days or weeks of fever, headache, confusion, and personality changes. Physical examination may reveal nuchal rigidity and cranial nerve palsies. Examination of the cerebrospinal fluid suggests the diagnosis. Typical findings include elevated pressure, an elevated protein level, a decreased glucose level, and fewer than 500 white blood cells/mm³ with a predominance of lymphocytes. In the most common type of fungal meningitis, cryptococcal meningitis, the Gram stain may reveal yeast forms; however, the India ink preparation is more specific. Cryptococcal polysaccharide may also be detected in the cerebrospinal fluid by immunologic tests. Specimens should be inoculated on Sabouraud agar if fungal meningitis is suspected and on Löwenstein-Jensen slants if tuberculosis is a possibility. Acid-fast smears should always be made when tuberculous meningitis is suspected, and chest x-ray films and skin tests can provide additional useful data. Amphotericin B is the drug of choice for most types of fungal meningitis; 5-fluorocytosine is a new agent that is proving useful in combination with amphotericin B. Combination therapy with isoniazid, rifampin and ethambutol is recommended for tuberculosis of the central nervous system.

The differential diagnosis of nonbacterial (aseptic) meningitis includes many conditions. Carcinomatous meningitis, sarcoidosis, and leptospirosis can all cause lymphocytic meningitis with a low glucose level in the cerebrospinal fluid; viral encephalitis, vasculitis, brain abscess, subdural

Table 11.4.
Typical cerebrospinal fluid findings in meningitis.

Type	Pressure	White Blood Cells/mm^3	Differential	Glucose	Protein	Other
Bacterial	Normal-elevated	500–20,000	Mostly polymorphs	Low, usually <50 mg/100 ml	Elevated	Gram stain positive in 80%
Partly treated	Normal-elevated	Usually <1000	Variable	Normal	Elevated	
Viral	Usually normal	Usually <1000	Polymorphs early, mostly mononuclear cells later	Normal	Normal-elevated	Viral cultures may be positive; blood serologies required for specific diagnosis
Tuberculous	Elevated	Usually <500	Mostly mononuclear cells	Low	Elevated	Acid-fast smears, culture on tuberculosis medium
Fungal	Elevated	Usually <500	Mostly mononuclear cells	Low	Elevated	India ink preparation, cryptococcal serologies on blood and cerebrospinal fluid

empyema, and osteomyelitis of the cranial bones can cause lymphocytic meningitis with a normal glucose level. Diagnosis and therapy of these conditions occur in the emergency ward rarely, and they will not be discussed further.

Gastrointestinal and Intra-abdominal Infections

The normal gastrointestinal tract has abundant bacterial flora; colonization is most dense in the colon, where fecal material contains approximately 1×10^{11} bacteria/gm. Infectious diseases involving the abdomen may be divided into very different categories: (1) serious acute infectious processes, such as peritonitis, cholecystitis, and intra-abdominal abscess, that result from entry of intestinal bacteria into normally sterile areas and that usually require surgical treatment; and (2) gastroenteritis caused by ingestion of toxins or pathogenic organisms that are not part of the normal flora. The diarrhea and vomiting that result from such ingestion may require rehydration in the emergency ward and occasionally hospitalization.

Surgical Abdominal Infections

Included in this category are many processes in which the integrity of the gastrointestinal tract is disrupted by an anatomic defect such as a perforated viscus or impaired drainage of the biliary tract that leads to bacterial overgrowth and infection. The clinical features of these illnesses, including appendicitis, diverticulitis, cholecystitis, peritonitis, and intra-abdominal abscess, are considered elsewhere in this text (Chapter 23). Prompt surgical therapy is required to correct the underlying anatomic defect in almost all of these situations; however, antibiotics also have an important role in treatment.

The proper choice of antibiotics in intra-abdominal infections depends on knowledge of the fecal bacteria. In all cases, blood cultures should be obtained in the emergency ward and cultures and Gram stains at operation. Even before a specific pathogen is isolated, antibiotics can be chosen directed at the "usual suspects." The most well-known constituents of the intestinal flora are the enteric gram-negative bacilli. E. coli is the most important of these aerobic organisms; others include Klebsiella, Proteus, and Enterobacter. Antibiotic sensitivities vary, but most strains of E. coli are sensitive to ampicillin, chloramphenicol, tobramycin, and gentamicin. A second group even more common in feces are the anaerobic gram-negative organisms, particularly *Bacteroides fragilis*. Because these slender bacilli are often involved in intra-abdominal infections, abscesses must specifically be cultured for anaerobes. The Bacteroides species present in the intestine are *not* sensitive to ampicillin or aminoglycosides, and a high percentage are now resistant to tetracycline. The antibiotics effective against most strains of *B. fragilis* are clindamycin, chloramphenicol, carbenicillin, ticarcillin, cefoxitin and metronidazole. A third group of organisms present in the intestine are the gram-positive bacteria. Anaerobes are also found in this category, including the clostridia and streptococci. Most organisms in this group are sensitive to ampicillin or penicillin and clindamycin. Finally, an aerobic streptococcus, the enterococcus, represents a special problem. Enterococci may be adequately treated with ampicillin alone in uncomplicated urinary tract infections, but in serious tissue infections or bacteremia, a combination of a penicillin (such as ampicillin) and an aminoglycoside (such as gentamicin) is required.

With this information, guidelines can be established for the initial choice of antibiotics in intra-abdominal infections. In the mildly to moderately ill patient with a localized condition such as appendicitis, cholecystitis, or diverticulitis, ampicillin alone may suffice, 1 gm intravenously every 3–4 hours for adults. In the more seriously ill patient with generalized peritonitis and possible bacteremia, a combination of antibiotics should be administered. Several combinations have proved effective, and at present, no one method is favored. Traditional combinations include: (1) clindamycin, 600 mg intravenously every 6 hours, with gentamicin, 1.5 mg/kg intramuscularly or intravenously every 8 hours in patients with normal renal function, and (2) ampicillin, 1 gm intravenously every 3–4 hours, with chloramphenicol, 2–3 gm/day intravenously in divided doses; all dosages are for adults. Another approach would be to administer cefoxitin alone in a dose at 1–2 grams intravenously every 4–6 hrs. None of these approaches, however, is effective against the enterococcus, so in the extremely ill patient, it may be necessary to start therapy with three antibiotics simultaneously—ampicillin and gentamicin plus either clindamycin or chloramphenicol. Because of problems concerning toxic reactions, hypersensitivity, superinfection, and cost, simultaneous administration of three drugs should be restricted to special circumstances, such as critical abdominal sepsis in the immunosuppressed patient. A two-drug regimen of carbenicillin or ticarcillin plus gentamicin should also cover the enterococcus, *B. fragilis*, and enteric gram-negative bacilli.

Gastroenteritis

Diarrhea and vomiting cause many patients to seek emergency care, and gastroenteritis is an important part of the differential diagnosis in these patients (see Chapter 12, pages 248–250). Many can be treated adequately at home, but children and elderly or debilitated persons may require hospitalization and intravenous rehydration. Measurement of vital signs, an abdominal examination, a hemogram, and determination of serum electrolyte levels serve to indicate whether a patient should be hospitalized. An epidemiologic history is important, and examination and culture of stool specimens may establish the etiologic diagnosis. Several important categories of gastroenteritis are caused by infectious agents.

Intoxication ("Food Poisoning"). Food products may be contaminated with bacteria that produce toxins. Since ingestion of the toxin rather than actual bacterial infection is responsible for the illness, these patients are afebrile, have normal white blood cell counts, do not have blood or leukocytes in the stool specimen, and do not require antibiotic therapy. Most cases of food poisoning are due to either *Clostridium perfringens*, with a 12- to 24-hour incubation period and diarrhea predominating, or *S. aureus*, with a 4- to 16-hour incubation period and vomiting predominating. *C. botulinum* may cause mild diarrhea, but this uncommon intoxication usually is seen as a neurologic emergency in which the patient has ocular and respiratory symptoms. Stool cultures are not helpful in the diagnosis of food poisoning; an epidemiologic history must be taken, food samples must be cultured, and assays for toxins must be performed.

Toxicogenic Bacterial Gastroenteritis. In some infections of the gastrointestinal tract, disease results from local production of bacterial toxins. Cholera is the best known example, but certain strains of *E. coli* and *Vibrio parahemolyticus* can also cause diarrhea by toxin production. Such patients are afebrile and have no blood or white blood cells in the stool specimen. Cholera is not endemic in the United States, but should be considered in patients who have been in endemic areas if symptoms include copious diarrhea, dehydration, and electrolyte imbalance.

Invasive Bacterial Gastroenteritis. Some bacterial pathogens cause diarrhea by invading the intestinal mucosa. In this manner, *S. aureus* sometimes causes enterocolitis in patients receiving broad-spectrum antibiotics. These patients are febrile, and stool specimens often reveal blood and polymorphonuclear leukocytes. Stool cultures yield abundant staphylococci. These patients require intravenous rehydration plus parenteral administration of antistaphylococcal antibiotics such as oxacillin or cephalothin.

Patients receiving antibiotics may also develop antibiotic-induced enterocolitis, which is caused by *Clostridium difficile*. The stool may contain blood and leukocytes but no enteric pathogens can be cultured. The diagnosis can be made by assaying the stool for *C. difficile* toxin. Oral vancomycin is the treatment of choice.

Certain strains of *E. coli* can also cause diarrhea by invading the mucosa. In these patients, clinical features resemble those of Salmonella gastroenteritis; diagnosis requires special techniques. Patients with nontyphoidal Salmonella gastroenteritis are seen with fever and diarrhea 1–3 days after ingesting contaminated food. Diarrhea may be bloody, and the stool specimen contains leukocytes. Such patients may require intravenous rehydration and antidiarrheal treatment, but antibiotics prolong the carrier state and should be reserved only for very sick persons. *Campylobacter fetus* causes gastroenteritis which is clinically very similar to salmonellosis, and is among the most common causes of bacterial enteritis. The diagnosis requires culturing the stool on special media at 42°C (see Table 11.1). Many patients recover spontaneously; but erythromycin is recommended for severe or protracted cases. Shigellosis has similar clinical features, although bloody diarrhea may be more severe. Most of these patients recover without antibiotics, but if the patient is seriously ill, ampicillin is an acceptable initial choice. The symptoms of typhoid fever are usually systemic rather than gastrointestinal; hospitalization and antibiotics therapy are mandatory. Parenteral therapy with chloramphenicol or ampicillin is recommended, but in special circumstances, oral trimethoprim-sulfamethoxazole may suffice.

Parasitic Gastroenteritis. Giardiasis and amebiasis are examples of such conditions. Diagnosis depends on epidemiologic findings and microscopic examination of a fresh stool specimen for ova and parasites. For further discussion, please see the section on protozoal gastroenteritis in medical gastrointestinal emergencies, Chapter 12.

Genitourinary Infections

Urinary Tract Infections

Infections of the urinary tract are much more common in females, except in infancy when anatomic anomalies increase the incidence in males, and in the elderly when prostatism and bladder outlet obstruction predispose to infections in men. In all age groups, instrumentation of the urinary tract is a major cause of infection.

Although urinary tract infections may be asymptomatic, patients are likely to seek medical attention in the emergency ward because of local or constitutional symptoms or both. Suprapubic pain, dysuria, frequency of urination, and urgency usually reflect infection of the lower part of the urinary tract (cystitis); flank pain, fever, chills, nausea, and vomiting suggest infection of the upper part (pyelonephritis). In patients with cystitis, physical findings are absent or confined to suprapubic tenderness. Patients with prostatitis may have prostatic tenderness and sponginess on rectal examination, and patients with acute pyelonephritis may have high fever, prostration, and flank tenderness. Hypotension may occur, and suggests bacteremia. Although absolute differentiation of cystitis and pyelonephritis may be difficult based on clinical findings, the distinction is important because of differences in management.

In all patients, the key to diagnosis is the urinary specimen. Urinalysis may reveal white blood cells or red blood cells or both. White blood cell casts suggest pyelonephritis. Hematuria may occur even with cystitis and prostatitis. If the pH of the urine is alkaline, infection with a urea-splitting organism such as Proteus is likely. Normal results of urinalysis in a patient with signs and symptoms of pyelonephritis may indicate infection above a completely obstructed ureter.

Although urinalysis may strongly suggest a urinary tract infection, urine must be cultured to confirm the diagnosis and to identify the responsible pathogen. Because the perineum and distal part of the urethra are colonized by numerous bacteria, a clean voided "midstream" specimen is essential. In infants and children, percutaneous suprapubic aspiration of urine from the bladder may be the best way to obtain an uncontaminated specimen. In adults, urethral catheterization is occasionally necessary, but because this procedure carries a significant risk of introducing pathogens, it should be avoided when possible. Urine should be cultured on both blood agar and on MacConkey or eosin-methylene blue agar. If specimens cannot be inoculated promptly, the urine should be refrigerated. In addition to urinalysis and culture, a Gram stain of *unsedimented* fresh urine can be extremely valuable in making a rapid diagnosis. The presence of organisms on such a stain suggests significant bacteriuria, with more than 100,000 organisms/ml.

Urinary cultures reveal gram-negative bacilli in most patients with infection of the urinary tract.

E. coli is the most common pathogen, especially in women with uncomplicated infections. Among the gram-positive organisms, the enterococcus (a group D streptococcus) is most likely to be the etiologic agent. *S. aureus* is an uncommon pathogen in the urinary tract, and its presence may indicate either bacteremic seeding of the kidney with or without abscesses or a prostatic abscess. Although other pathogens can also cause urinary tract infection, unusual organisms should raise the possibility of contaminated specimens, and cultures should be repeated. Negative cultures in patients with pyuria or other urinary tract symptoms are sometimes caused by prostatitis, urethritis, vaginitis, cervicitis, or urinary tract tuberculosis. Rarely, infection with fastidious bacteria such as *H. influenzae* or Brucella species can result in sterile pyuria. Adenovirus infection can cause hemorrhagic cystitis.

Although urinary cultures and sensitivity testing determine the optimal choice of antibiotics, administration of antibacterial agents should be started as soon as the specimen is cultured, and the choice should be re-evaluated when results become available. Patients with cystitis respond well to oral antibacterial therapy. First infections in ambulatory patients are almost always caused by E. coli with broad antibiotic sensitivities; in such circumstances, sulfonamide compounds such as sulfisoxazole are excellent (Table 11.3). Patients with uncomplicated cystitis respond well to either conventional 10–14 day treatment regimens or to single-dose therapy with amoxacillin, trimethoprim-sulfamethoxazole, or sulfisoxazole.

In patients who have recurrent infections, who have recently been receiving antibiotics, or who have been hospitalized and catheterized, infection may be due to sulfa-resistant organisms. Single dose treatment is not appropriate. Antibiotic sensitivity testing is mandatory for these patients; before results are available, ampicillin, cephalexin, tetracycline, and trimethoprim-sulfamethoxazole are all acceptable agents. Some physicians prefer nitrofurantoin; we have found this drug useful for chronic and recurrent infections. Intravenous pyelograms should be obtained in patients with recurrent cystitis. High fluid intake should be encouraged in all patients, and all should be instructed to return for follow-up urinalysis and culture after completing therapy.

Although persons with acute pyelonephritis respond to a similar range of antibiotics, most patients should initially be treated in the hospital with parenteral antibacterial agents. These patients may be severely ill, with high fever and leukocytosis. Since gram-negative bacteremia may occur, blood cultures should be obtained before antibiotic therapy. Septic shock may develop, and vital signs must be closely monitored. In the severely ill patient and when Proteus, Pseudomonas, or Enterobacter is suspected, gentamicin or tobramycin is generally the drug of choice for initial therapy; results of sensitivity testing may then allow a change to a potentially less toxic drug. In less critically ill patients, intravenous ampicillin or a parenteral cephalosporin may be administered initially. Other useful drugs include tetracycline, chloramphenicol, kanamycin, amikacin and trimethoprim-sulfamethoxazole. Maintenance of adequate hydration is important, and often requires administration of intravenous fluids in the first few days of treatment. Renal function must be evaluated, and intravenous pyelograms are indicated in most patients. Because pyelonephritis tends to recur, follow-up urinalysis and culture are important.

In addition to requiring medical therapy, some patients with urinary tract infections require emergency surgical evaluation. This occurs most often when urinary flow is obstructed by a calculus, stricture, or tumor, or by prostatic hypertrophy, as discussed in Chapter 25.

Genital Infections

Infections of the genital organs are common. Many are minor conditions that can be managed with topical agents on an outpatient basis, such as vaginitis due to *Candida albicans* or *Trichomonas vaginalis*. Others, such as prostatitis and epididymitis, usually are caused by the same organisms that cause urinary tract infections, and may be managed with the same oral antibiotics. However, epididymitis can progress to extreme local swelling with intense inflammation and pain as well as fever and leukocytosis; these patients require hospitalization, parenteral antibiotics, immobilization, analgesics, and sometimes operation. Nongonococcal urethritis is a common venereal infection whose chief symptom in men is a watery to purulent urethral discharge. The cause is uncertain, but chlamydiae have recently been implicated and tetracycline is the drug of choice. Certain uncommon infections of the genitalia such as chancroid, lymphogranuloma venereum, and granuloma inguinale also respond to antibiotics or sulfonamides.

Infection caused by herpes simplex virus may result in genital lesions (herpes progenitalis) in both sexes; although this condition can be painful, it rarely leads to serious complications. Because neonatal herpes can be devastating, genital herpes in pregnant women presents a special problem.

Although there is no curative treatment at present, topical acyclovir ointment provides symptomatic benefit for primary genital herpes.

Syphilis. Caused by *Treponema pallidum*, syphilis is an increasingly common venereal disease. Asymptomatic patients may be seen because of recent sexual exposure to a person with known or suspected syphilis; serologic testing should be performed, and these patients should also be examined to exclude gonorrhea. If exposure is certain, patients can be treated on epidemiologic grounds. In primary syphilis, patients are seen with a highly infectious, painless, ulcerated chancre, usually on the genitalia. In secondary syphilis, patients have systemic illness that includes fever, malaise, lymphadenopathy, and cutaneous lesions characteristically involving the palms and soles. Secondary syphilis is also infectious. All patients with syphilis should be reported to local public health authorities, and contacts should be identified and treated. The treatment for incubating primary and secondary syphilis is the same, consisting of benzathine penicillin G, 2.4 million units total by intramuscular injection at a single session, or procaine penicillin G, 600,000 units/day intramuscularly for 8 days. Penicillin-allergic patients should receive tetracycline or erythromycin, 500 mg four times a day for 15 days. Follow-up evaluation with repeated serologic testing is necessary to ensure adequacy of treatment.

Gonorrhea. This is the most common venereal disease seen in the emergency ward; caused by *N. gonorrhoeae*, it may display a broad spectrum of clinical features. Both men and women may be asymptomatic; diagnosis of the carrier state depends on urethral and cervical cultures and epidemiologic history. Urethritis in men and cervicitis in women often are indicated by pain, discharge, and dysuria. In men, a Gram stain of the urethral discharge is highly diagnostic, revealing gram-negative intracellular diplococci; in women, the Gram stain is less reliable. Specimens from all patients should be inoculated promptly on Thayer-Martin or Transgrow media; cultures from the urethra in men and from the cervix and anus in women are best. A serologic test for syphilis should also be performed. Patients with uncomplicated gonorrhea respond well to several antibiotic regimens: (1) procaine penicillin G, 4.8 million units intramuscularly, plus probenecid, 1 gm orally; (2) ampicillin, 3.5 gm orally, or amoxacillin, 3.0 gm orally plus probenecid, 1 gm orally; (3) spectinomycin, 2 gm intramuscularly; and (4) tetracycline, 0.5 gm orally four times a day for 5 days (a total of 20 doses). Cultures should be repeated after therapy. As with other venereal infections, gonorrhea should be reported to public health authorities and contacts should be identified and treated.

Other Gonococcal Infections. Pharyngitis or proctitis may be caused by *N. gonorrhoeae*. Diagnosis depends on a detailed sexual history and appropriate cultures. These infections may be more difficult to manage; the procaine penicillin regimen in the preceding paragraph is acceptable for initial therapy, but cultures after treatment are essential, and further therapy with higher doses may be required. In women, gonococci may also cause acute pelvic inflammatory disease, with fever, leukocytosis, and lower abdominal pain and tenderness. In milder cases of salpingitis, therapy may be started with penicillin or ampicillin in the previously stated dosages, followed by ampicillin, 500 mg orally four times a day for 10 days. Tetracyline, 500 mg orally four times a day for 10 days, is also acceptable for outpatient management of mild pelvic inflammatory disease. However, patients with more severe illnesses, including frank pelvic peritonitis and suspected pelvic abscess, should be hospitalized and treated with intravenous penicillin, approximately 10 million units/day. Oral ampicillin may be substituted when clinical improvement becomes apparent. Gonococcal infection can also become disseminated, with fever, leukocytosis, pustular or petechial rash, and arthritis. These patients should be hospitalized, cultures obtained, and intravenous penicillin administered approximately 10 million units/day. Oral ampicillin may be substituted after 3 days if clinical improvement occurs. Tetracycline is an acceptable substitute in the penicillin-allergic patient.

Nongonococcal Pelvic Inflammatory Disease. Not all pelvic inflammatory disease is caused by the gonococcus. Women with clinical features of pelvic inflammatory disease and with a negative history of exposure to gonorrhea should be hospitalized, and cultures should be obtained. Nongonococcal pelvic inflammatory disease may be caused by any of the intestinal flora discussed previously, including the enteric gram-negative bacilli and Bacteroides. Often, no specific organism can be implicated. Antibiotic therapy is similar to that for other intra-abdominal infections. Intravenous ampicillin is acceptable initial therapy, but if the patient fails to respond or is acutely ill, regimens such as cefoxitin, or clindamycin and gentamicin, or penicillin and chloramphenicol should be considered.

Infections of Bones and Joints

Bacterial infections of bones and joints are among the most important infections seen in the emergency ward. Although these infections are rarely life threatening, a vigorous approach to diagnosis and treatment is required to preserve joint function and to avoid chronic osteomyelitis.

Acute pyogenic infections of the skeletal system usually produce constitutional symptoms, including fever, chills, and anorexia. Pain, swelling, and inflammation, together with impaired function of the infected bone or joint, often pinpoint the site of infection. In such patients the diagnosis is not difficult, although the differential diagnosis must include crystalline arthritis (gout and pseudogout), rheumatic disease, and other hypersensitivity states, as well as trauma, viral infection (especially rubella and mumps), and tuberculosis. Occasionally the diagnosis may be occult; this is especially true in children and when the axial skeleton is involved.

Laboratory evaluation reveals leukocytosis and an elevated erythrocyte sedimentation rate in most patients. Work-up should also include blood cultures, studies directed at the noninfectious diseases just mentioned, and a search for other sites of infection that may have led to bacteremic seeding.

Septic Arthritis

The cause of septic arthritis may be bacteremic seeding, direct spread of infection from contiguous bone or muscle, a penetrating injury, or postoperative infection. This disease can occur in all age groups, and may involve any joint, although infections of the knees, hips, elbows, and shoulders are most common. X-ray examination usually reveals only soft-tissue swelling. Pyogenic arthritis is most often monoarticular, but multiple joints may be involved, especially in patients with gonococcal arthritis.

The gonococcus is the most common cause of septic arthritis in sexually active persons. The meningococcus can also cause septic arthritis, but does so much less commonly. In all age groups, gram-positive cocci are important causes of this disease; *S. aureus* is more common than the pneumococcus or streptococcus. *H. influenzae* may cause septic arthritis in children. Enteric gram-negative bacilli may be responsible in debilitated patients and in drug addicts, as well as after trauma and in infections of the vertebral disc spaces.

The key to diagnosis is examination of the joint fluid. Arthrocentesis should be performed as soon as possible (see Illustrative Techniques 10). In the patient with typical septic arthritis, the joint fluid is viscous and purulent with a high number of white blood cells (usually 20,000–200,000/mm^3), most of which are polymorphonuclear leukocytes. The glucose level is depressed (less than 50 mg/ 100 ml or less than 50% of the blood glucose level), and the mucin clot is poor. A Gram stain of the joint fluid is essential, and fluid should promptly be inoculated on blood agar and chocolate agar and in thioglycollate broth (Table 11.1).

The choice of antibiotics depends on the organism isolated. If analysis of the joint fluid and the clinical findings suggest septic arthritis, antibiotic therapy should not be delayed until culture results are available. If the gonococcus or meningococcus is suspected, penicillin is the drug of choice. For gram-positive cocci, oxacillin or nafcillin should be administered initially, with a change to penicillin if pneumococci or sensitive streptococci are cultured. In the presence of *H. influenzae*, ampicillin or chloramphenicol should be administered, depending on the results of sensitivity testing. These results also determine the choice of drug for gram-negative bacilli, but gentamicin or tobramycin is acceptable until these data are available. Antibiotics should be administered parenterally in high doses. Intra-articular administration is unnecessary, and may be harmful.

Pyogenic arthritis is a closed-space infection, and drainage is required to avert permanent damage. In peripheral joints, immobilization and repeated arthrocentesis are usually sufficient, but if an effusion cannot be completely tapped, operation is necessary. Because of its delicate blood supply, early surgical drainage of the hip joint is advisable.

Acute Osteomyelitis

Hematogenous seeding or direct extension from a contiguous focus may result in acute osteomyelitis. *S. aureus* is the most common cause of this disease, but other organisms may be involved, such as Salmonella in patients with sickle cell anemia, Pseudomonas in drug users, gram-negative bacilli in persons with vertebral osteomyelitis, and even rare organisms such as *P. multocida* after a cat bite. Because of this range of organisms, direct examination of the infected tissue is necessary unless other studies such as blood cultures or Salmonella agglutination titers are diagnostic; this involves either needle biopsy or open surgical biopsy. Histologic examination is important to exclude other processes such as tumor and tuberculosis. Roentgenograms do not show bony changes for several weeks, although soft-tissue swelling may be apparent. Bone scans may indicate osteomyelitis earlier, and the serum alkaline phosphatase level may be elevated. Again, the Gram stain and cultures are diagnostic. Pus or bone specimens or both should be inoculated on blood agar and chocolate agar, in thioglycollate broth, and also on a blood agar plate to be incubated anaerobically. If *M. tuberculosis* or fungi are suspected, special media must be used. The choice of antibiotics follows the principles discussed in relation to septic arthritis. High-dose parenteral therapy is required, usually for 4–6 weeks. Such vigorous and prolonged treatment is necessary to avoid chronic osteomyelitis, which responds poorly to antibiotics and which may require multiple surgical procedures.

Infections of Skin and Soft Tissue, Including Wounds

The skin is unique among the organ systems in that many of its pathologic conditions are visible on direct inspection. Since rash is a symptom that many patients find alarming, cutaneous lesions often cause patients to go to the emergency ward for care.

Table 11.5 lists the possible causes of rash and fever in the acutely ill patient. Many of these diseases are viral infections or drug-induced hypersensitivity states (see Chapter 20, pages 443–444 and 448–449).

Cutaneous infections may result from direct inoculation of bacteria or from hematogenous seeding. The cutaneous stigmata of meningococcemia and gonococcemia were mentioned earlier; it is important to remember that in either of these infections, fever and petechial, purpuric, or pustular lesions may be the presenting symptoms. Blood cultures are essential, as is a full workup that includes careful examination for primary sites of infection. In addition, fluid should be aspirated from pustular lesions, since a Gram stain may disclose gram-negative diplococci and culture may reveal Neisseria.

Similar cutaneous lesions may result from other types of bacteremia. Staphylococcal sepsis may cause pustules, and endocarditis due to any organism can lead to hemorrhagic, pustular, or infarcted lesions resembling those in some patients with vasculitis. Sepsis due to Pseudomonas may lead to ecthyma gangrenosum, with large necrotic lesions. Any bacteremia, but especially those due to gram-negative bacilli, can cause purpuric lesions that often indicate disseminated intravascular coagulation.

Certain bacterial infections which are localized to areas of the body remote from the skin can produce fever and a systemic illness with prominent rash by the mechanism of toxin production. Well known examples include scarlet fever (usually caused by group A streptococcal pharyngitis) and the scalded skin syndrome (*S. aureus* of phage

Table 11.5.
Rash and fever in the acutely ill patient: diagnosis according to type of lesion.

Macules or Papules	Vesicles, Bullae, or Pustules	Purpuric Macules, Papules, or Vesicles
Drug hypersensitivities	Drug hypersensitivities	Drug hypersensitivities
Scarlet fever	Dermatitis from plants	Bacteremia[b]
Erythema infectiosum (fifth disease)	Rickettsial pox	Meningococcemia (acute or chronic)
Measles (rubeola)	Varicella (chicken pox)[a]	Gonococcemia
German measles (rubella)	Generalized herpes zoster[a]	Staphylococcemia
Enterovirus infections (ECHO and Coxsackie)	Disseminated herpes simplex[a]	Pseudomonas bacteremia
Adenovirus infections	Eczema herpeticum[a]	Subacute bacterial endocarditis
Typhoid fever	Disseminated vaccinia[a]	Enterovirus infections (ECHO and Coxsackie)
Secondary syphilis	Eczema vaccinatum[a]	Rickettsial diseases
Typhus, murine (endemic)	Variola[a]	Rocky Mountain spotted fever
Rocky Mountain spotted fever (early lesions)	Enterovirus infections (ECHO and Coxsackie), including hand-foot-mouth disease	Typhus, louse-borne (epidemic)
Pityriasis rosea	Toxic epidermal necrolysis	Allergic cutaneous vasculitis
Erythema multiforme	Erythema multiforme bullosum	
Erythema marginatum		
Systemic lupus erythematosus		
Dermatomyositis		
"Serum sickness" (manifested only as wheals)		

[a] Characteristic lesion is an umbilicated papule or vesicle on an erythematous base.

[b] Often present as infarcts.

(Reproduced by permission, from Fitzpatrick TB, et al (eds): *Dermatology in General Medicine.* © 1971, McGraw-Hill Book Company.)

group II). A newly recognized disorder which belongs in this category is the toxic shock syndrome (TSS). TSS occurs primarily in menstruating women using tampons but has occurred in occasional nonmenstruating women and men with localized staphylococcal infections. Clinical features include high fever, hypotension, and a diffuse scarlatiniform eruption with hyperemia of mucous membranes, involvement of palms and soles, and late desquamation. Diarrhea, myalgias, headaches, encephalopathy, abnormal liver function tests, azotemia and pulmonary infiltrates often are present and reflect the characteristic involvement of multiple organ systems. Blood cultures almost always are negative since the disease is caused by a circulating toxin rather than bacteremic spread of infection. However, staphylococci often can be isolated from the vagina of menstruating females or from localized infections in others. Therapy should include antistaphylococcal antibiotics and vigorous cardiovascular support.

Among the other illnesses that can cause fever and petechial lesions of the skin, Rocky Mountain spotted fever deserves special mention. Despite its name, this disease is found nationwide, with most cases coming from the Atlantic seaboard, especially Virginia and North Carolina. Rocky Mountain spotted fever is caused by a rickettsia transmitted to human beings by the bite of infected ticks, usually between the months of April and August. Patients are seen with fever, chills, severe headache, photophobia, myalgia, and rash that often involves the palms and soles. Mental changes are common, and approximately 50% of patients have splenomegaly. Characteristic laboratory findings include thrombocytopenia and normal white blood cell counts, although polymorphonuclear leukocytes and band forms can predominate. Meningococcemia and atypical measles are the most common misdiagnoses in these patients. Because rickettsiae cannot be cultured under ordinary conditions, serologic tests are needed to confirm the diagnosis. However, mortality is high and therapy must be immediate; if the diagnosis seems probable according to clinical and epidemiologic findings, tetracycline or chloramphenicol should be administered, 2 gm/day for adults.

Direct inoculation of organisms into the skin may produce several other disease syndromes. The most common organisms involved are *S. aureus* and group A streptococci. Either of these may cause impetigo, with crusting, superficial lesions. Deep, localized abscesses such as furuncles, carbuncles, and paronychial lesions are caused by staphylococci. Patients with these infections are usually free of systemic findings, and respond well to soaks and oral antistaphylococcal antibiotics, although surgical drainage may hasten recovery. These same organisms can also cause much more serious infections of the skin, including erysipelas lymphangitis, and cellulitis. Such patients require hospitalization, parenteral administration of antibiotics, and a full workup including blood cultures. Antistreptolysin O titers may sometimes be helpful in diagnosing streptococcal infections. Aspiration of infected skin for a Gram stain and culture should be attempted, although these studies are often negative; if no material can be obtained by direct aspiration, a small amount of sterile saline *without* antibacterial preservatives can be injected and then aspirated. The bacteria causing these infections are so characteristic that administration of antistaphylococcal antibiotics may be started before culture results are available; patients should receive high-dose parenteral therapy until the infection is considerably resolved.

Although streptococci and staphylococci are responsible for most primary cutaneous infections, many other bacteria may also cause cellulitis. In children, cellulitis due to *H. influenzae* has a characteristic blue to purple appearance. In immunosuppressed patients, gram-negative bacilli can occasionally cause devastating cutaneous infections. Perirectal and perineal infections may be caused by these and other intestinal flora. *C. diphtheriae* is a rare cause of skin infection in nonimmunized patients. Finally, animal contact may be responsible for many uncommon infections, including cellulitis from *P. multocida* (cats), lesions due to Erysipelothrix (fish), anthrax (cattle and sheep), and tularemia (many wild species). An epidemiologic history provides the essential clue in these cases.

Thus far, the focus has been on normal skin, but when the integrity of the skin is altered by trauma, burns, or operation, virtually any organism can cause infection; often, multiple species produce synergistic infection. Accurate etiologic diagnosis requires a Gram stain and aerobic and anaerobic cultures of any exudate, blood cultures, and x-ray examination for gas and foreign bodies. Early surgical drainage and débridement of infected wounds and abscesses are important. A few organisms cause relatively characteristic infections in these circumstances. For example, group A streptococci typically cause early infection (sometimes within 12–24 hours of injury) associated with high fever and a watery, nonpurulent exudate. Therefore, low doses of penicillin or other antistreptococcal antibiotics are recommended during the first few days after a contaminated wound or burn is sustained. *Pseudomonas aeruginosa* is one of the most common pathogens of burned skin. The resultant infection may produce a characteristic musty, sweet odor, and illumination of the infected area with Wood's light may reveal green fluorescence due to bacterial pigment. Cultures are necessary to confirm the diagnosis, and gentamicin or tobramycin, alone or with carbenicillin, is the drug of choice. Anaerobic infections may produce foul-smelling pus. A variety of organisms, including group A streptococci, anaerobic streptococci, and gram-negative bacilli, either singly or in combination can cause many serious necrotizing infections of the skin, subcutaneous tissue, and muscle, including cutaneous gangrene, necrotizing fasciitis, and necrotizing myositis. Patients with these conditions have pronounced systemic toxic reactions and rapidly advancing infections. In addition to administration of high doses of parenteral antibiotics (usually a penicillinase-resistant penicillin and an aminoglycoside until culture results are available), these patients require immediate aggressive surgical débridement of all devitalized tissues.

Clostridial species can cause many types of wound infection. Wound botulism caused by C. botulinum is rare. Tetanus, which can result from contamination with either the vegetative cells or spores of C. tetani, may occur even in patients with minor lesions, but is more common after contamination of deep wounds that have devitalized tissues. The key to management of this disease is prevention. The wound must first be cleaned and debrided. The need for active immunization with tetanus toxoid or passive immunization with tetanus immune globulin (human) is determined by the patient's immunization history and the nature of the wound (Table 11.6). C. perfringens (C. welchii) and other species may be present in wounds

Table 11.6.
Tetanus prophylaxis in wound management.

History of Tetanus Immunization, doses	Clean, Minor Wounds		All Other Wounds	
	Td	TIG	Td	TIG
Uncertain	Yes	No	Yes	Yes
0–1	Yes	No	Yes	Yes
2	Yes	No	Yes	No[a]
3 or more	No[b]	No	No[c]	No

Td = tetanus and diphtheria toxoids, adult type; TIG = tetanus immune globulin (human), 250–500 units intramuscularly.

[a] Yes, if wound is more than 24 hours old.

[b] Yes, if more than 10 years since last dose.

[c] Yes, if more than 5 years since last dose.

(Modified with permission, from *Morbidity and Mortality* 30 (no. 33:420, 1981.)

merely as surface contaminants without causing significant disease. However, these same organisms can cause localized infection or spreading anaerobic cellulitis. Such patients are febrile, but do not have systemic toxic reactions. Gas is produced in the involved areas, but pain is minimal and the skin is not discolored. High doses of penicillin with local drainage produce excellent results. Much more serious is clostridial myonecrosis or gas gangrene, in which patients are febrile, delirious, and often hypotensive. The infected tissues are edematous, with discoloration of skin and often bleb formation. Gas is produced deep in the tissue planes, and infection advances rapidly. Pain is intense. Large gram-positive bacilli are evident in Gram stains of the exudate, but spore formation is rare and polymorphonuclear leukocytes are characteristically scant. Specimens must be cultured anaerobically when clostridial infection is suspected. Therapy requires high doses of penicillin, 20–30 million units/day for adults, and immediate, aggressive surgical débridement with complete excision of all infected tissues. Hyperbaric oxygen should be considered if available. Horse antiserum directed against clostridial toxins is available, but is not of proved benefit and should probably be reserved for rare instances of high-grade clostridial bacteremia with intravascular hemolysis; this occurs most commonly in patients with uterine myonecrosis after septic abortion.

Not all gas-forming infections are caused by clostridia. Many aerobic and anaerobic bacteria, especially the gram-negative bacilli, can produce gas in tissues. Patients with diabetes are particularly susceptible to gas-forming infections. The choice of antibiotics is dictated by the results of Gram stains and cultures, but broad coverage such as administration of oxacillin and chloramphenicol or clindamycin and gentamicin is usually advisable until results are available. Surgical drainage and débridement are also important.

A final problem concerning wound management is the possibility of rabies in the patient with an animal bite. Human rabies is rare in the United States today, with only one or two cases reported each year, and rabies in domestic animals has also become uncommon. However, rabies among wild animals appears to be increasing. Because this disease is almost invariably lethal, the main concern is prevention. Any wound should immediately be washed thoroughly with copious amounts of soap and water. If bacterial infection is present or seems likely, antibiotics should be administered; penicillin is the recommended antibiotic for many animal and human bites. The need for prophylactic immunization against rabies depends on the species of animal involved. Table 10.21 lists the current recommendations of the United States Public Health Service. Fortunately, human rabies immune globulin is now available, and should be administered when antiserum is required. Similarly, the new human diploid cell rabies vaccine (HDCV) is a major advance in active immunization against rabies.

Cardiac Infections

Bacterial Endocarditis

Patients with bacterial endocarditis constitute only a small minority of individuals receiving medical care in the emergency ward; however, the emergency physician must be fully knowledgeable in the management of these life-threatening infections. Endocarditis is classically divided into two types. First is subacute bacterial endocarditis, which usually occurs in patients with congenital or acquired (rheumatic or calcific) valvular heart disease. The most common causative organism is *S. viridans*. These streptococci, whose virulence is ordinarily low, are part of the normal oral flora; however, they commonly cause transient bacteremia, especially after dental manipulations, and they then may establish foci of infection on the previously damaged valve. Many other organisms can also cause subacute bacterial endocarditis. Symptoms include fever, anorexia, and weight loss, often of weeks' or even months' duration; congestive heart failure may also develop or may worsen as a result of infection. Neurologic manifestations may be striking, and subacute bacterial endocarditis should be considered in any patient with a cerebrovascular accident and fever. Physical examination usually reveals a murmur, but this may seem insignificant or may even be absent. Classic features include petechiae, Roth's spots, splinter hemorrhages in the nails, painful lesions of the fingertips (Osler's nodes), and splenomegaly. These findings require weeks to evolve, however, and are often absent when the patient is first examined. The same is true of abnormalities revealed by laboratory testing. Anemia is common, and the white blood cell count may be elevated or normal. Urinary sediments are often abnormal, and subacute bacterial endocarditis should be considered in patients with fever and renal failure of uncertain cause, especially in the elderly. The erythrocyte sedimentation rate is elevated, and the rheumatoid factor, reflecting chronic inflammation, is positive in about half the patients.

The second type of endocarditis is acute bacterial endocarditis. The pace of this condition is greatly accelerated because the disease classically results from more virulent organisms that produce destructive lesions even on previously normal valves. Many organisms have been implicated in acute bacterial endocarditis. *S. aureus* is most common; endocarditis due to this pathogen may follow bacteremia from even a minor infection such as a furuncle, or it may arise from an inapparent primary site. This is an extremely serious infection, and most patients with high-grade bacteremia due to *S. aureus* should be treated for it even if murmurs and other traditional indications of endocarditis are absent. Enterococci also cause acute bacterial endocarditis, often after a primary gastrointestinal or genitourinary disorder. Pneumococci are now uncommon causative agents. Among drug addicts a broad variety of organisms, including gram-negative bacilli, have been implicated. Although the clinical and laboratory features of acute bacterial endocarditis may include all the findings of the subacute type, in typical cases the peripheral manifestations are less pronounced and fever and acute systemic illness are more prominent. Congestive heart failure can fulminate if valve damage is severe.

The role of the emergency physician is to suspect the diagnosis of endocarditis and to order the crucial diagnostic procedure, the blood culture. In patients with indolent illness consistent with subacute bacterial endocarditis, six specimens for culture can be drawn in a 24- to 48-hour period before instituting antibiotic therapy. However, in acute disease the patient's condition may rapidly deteriorate, and therapy should not be so delayed. If acute bacterial endocarditis appears likely, four to six specimens for culture can be obtained with separate venipunctures in the course of 2 to 3 hours, and administration of antibiotics can be started. Most patients with endocarditis have high-grade bacteremia, and blood cultures are often all positive. In all patients, high doses of antibiotics should be administered parenterally for 4–6 weeks, with patients carefully observed for complications, including congestive heart failure, emboli, and mycotic aneurysms. Antibiotic therapy should be guided by sensitivity testing, and whenever possible, serum bactericidal levels should be determined. Until these data are available, penicillin, 20 million units/day, is the ideal first choice for adults with subacute bacterial endocarditis. Oxacillin, 12 gm/day, with gentamicin, 1.0–1.5 mg/kg every 8 hours if renal function is normal, is acceptable for initial treatment of patients with suspected acute bacterial endocarditis.

Pericarditis

Another cardiac condition that may require emergency treatment is pericarditis (see Chapter 6, pages 102–103). Many of the causes of pericarditis are noninfectious, including myocardial infarction, tumor, trauma, uremia, myxedema, and vasculitis. Among the infectious causes, viruses are most common. Patients with viral pericarditis usually have pericardial pain and may be febrile, but they usually do not have leukocytosis or severe systemic reactions. Pericardial tamponade is uncommon. Diagnosis is usually based on clinical criteria, but can sometimes be confirmed by serologic testing or, if specialized facilities are available, viral isolation. Therapy depends on symptoms, with anti-inflammatory agents such as indomethacin being particularly useful. Prognosis is generally excellent, although pain may recur in some patients, and rarely, early tamponade or late constrictive pericarditis may develop. Tuberculous pericarditis, which is much less common, may be indicated by fever and hemodynamic compromise. Pain is often less severe and the course is usually subacute, with the possibility of late calcific pericarditis. The tuberculin skin test is positive in most patients, but pulmonary tuberculosis may or may not be coexistent. Pericardiocentesis (see Section 5, "Illustrated Techniques") or biopsy or both provide the definitive diagnosis. A final form of pericarditis, which is also rare but which constitutes a true emergency, is purulent pericarditis. This can develop after a thoracic operation, from direct extension of bacterial pneumonia, or by bacteremic seeding. Patients are usually febrile and acutely ill; the condition rapidly progresses to tamponade and death if untreated. Pericardiocentesis is necessary for diagnosis in most cases. The fluid contains a high number of white blood cells with a predominance of polymorphonuclear leukocytes, a low glucose level, and a high protein level. A Gram stain and aerobic and anaerobic cultures are mandatory (Table 11.1). Studies for tuberculosis and fungal processes should be performed if there is any doubt as to diagnosis. Surgical drainage of the pericardium is required in almost all patients. Although *S. aureus* and pneumococci were previously the most common causes of purulent pericarditis, many organisms have been implicated recently; antibiotic therapy must therefore be individualized, based on the Gram stain, presence or absence of another septic focus, and clinical features.

Bacteremia and Septic Shock

Many of the acute infections that have been discussed may be accompanied by bacteremia, the clinical expression of which may be obvious or occult. Often, patients have a serious underlying disease such as diabetes, cirrhosis, or leukemia, or they may have had recent medical or surgical therapy involving Foley catheters or intravenous lines. The signs and symptoms of a primary infectious process such as pyelonephritis, cholecystitis, or pneumonia may predominate. High fever is common, and shaking chills are suggestive of bacteremia. Neither finding is invariable, however; patients with uremia and those receiving corticosteroids may even be afebrile. As mentioned earlier, patients with bacteremia may have purpuric, pustular, or necrotic cutaneous lesions. Even in the absence of pulmonary infection, tachypnea may be striking, and often may lead to respiratory alkalosis. Confusion and disorientation may be pronounced, especially in the elderly; although these signs should always raise the possibility of infection of the central nervous system, the metabolic and circulatory effects of bacteremia alone can produce toxic encephalopathy. Tachycardia is characteristic, and in patients with underlying heart disease, angina or congestive heart failure may develop.

A dread complication of bacteremia, septic shock constitutes a true medical emergency. All the clinical considerations just discussed apply to the bacteremic patient in whom septic shock develops. In the earliest stages, clinical findings may be those of "warm shock"; the patient is alert, with warm, dry skin. However, without treatment the classic syndrome of "cold shock" ensues; the skin becomes clammy and cold, with mottled cyanosis, and the patient becomes obtunded. Hypotension is a cardinal feature of septic shock, although some patients may have normal blood pressure early in the process. Even more common is the patient who has hypotension without true septic shock; however, management of hypotension in the presence of fever and possible bacteremia should always be approached vigorously.

True septic shock involves inadequate tissue perfusion, the clinical manifestations of which vary. Inadequate renal perfusion results in oliguria and a low concentration of sodium in the urine, poor perfusion of the coronary arteries can lead to myocardial ischemia or arrhythmias or both, and compromised cerebral perfusion may cause confusion or coma. Impaired peripheral blood flow results in vasoconstricted cutaneous vessels and diminished pulses.

The laboratory manifestations of septic shock are also variable. Polymorphonuclear leukocytosis with band forms often occurs. Thrombocytopenia may develop with or without coagulation disorders suggesting disseminated intravascular coagulation. Hypoxia may be present, and blood-gas levels may indicate respiratory alkalosis or metabolic acidosis or both. The level of lactate in the blood is often elevated in acidotic patients. Azotemia develops if renal perfusion remains poor.

The patient with septic shock requires immediate attention. Vital functions should be supported (see Section 1, Life Support), first securing an adequate airway. Arterial blood-gas levels should be determined and oxygen should be administered if indicated. A central venous pressure line is indispensable, and an intra-arterial line to monitor blood gases and pressure is helpful. A Foley catheter should be inserted to monitor urinary output. A rapid history and physical examination are essential, as is a complete laboratory evaluation to determine a primary site of infection. The importance of complete cultures, especially of the blood and urine, cannot be overemphasized. It is also important to screen for noninfectious causes of shock, including myocardial failure, pulmonary emboli, pericardial tamponade, and hemorrhage, and other causes of volume depletion such as pancreatitis.

Therapy for septic shock is multifaceted. Volume replacement is of primary importance. Crystalloids such as normal saline and Ringer's lactated solutions can be administered on a trial basis, but colloids such as albumin and blood are usually more effective. Volume expanders should be administered rapidly until the central venous pressure reaches 10–12 cm H_2O; some patients with chronic pulmonary disease may require even higher filling pressures, but further volume expansion must be approached with caution. Acidosis and other metabolic abnormalities should be corrected. If shock persists after fluid and electrolyte therapy, vasoactive drugs must be administered. There is no consensus as to which agents are best, and therapy must be individualized. Dopamine, a catecholamine that appears extremely promising, is presently suggested initially. Isoproterenol has long been a mainstay of therapy. Occasionally, epinephrine or norepinephrine is necessary when other drugs fail to provide satisfactory perfusion. Detailed information about these drugs is presented in Chapter 3, pages 48–51. Even more controversy surrounds the use of corticosteroids in patients with septic shock. Some physicians advocate large doses of glucocorticoids, but these are not of proved clinical benefit. If the patient has disseminated intravascular coagulation, heparin may be useful. Although vasodilating drugs are sometimes administered, their usefulness is unproved.

In patients with septic shock, although survival often depends on metabolic, respiratory, and circulatory support, vigorous antimicrobial therapy is also necessary. The initial choice of antibiotics should be based on the primary site of infection. For example, gentamicin may be indicated for gram-negative sepsis arising from the urinary tract, and combinations such as clindamycin and gentamicin or a penicillin and chloramphenicol may be preferred for sepsis originating from an intestinal or pelvic focus. The choice of antibiotics for specific infectious processes has been detailed earlier in this chapter. But what of the patient whose condition appears septic and in whom no focus can be identified in the emergency ward? Although cultures and other tests may provide an etiologic diagnosis within a few days, antibiotic therapy must be administered much sooner. Even though most cases of septic shock are caused by gram-negative organisms, gram-positive bacteria can cause clinically identical syndromes, so initial antibiotic coverage must be broad. High doses of oxacillin and gentamicin or tobramycin are recommended in these circumstances. In the penicillin-allergic patient, cephalothin or clindamycin can be substituted for oxacillin (Table 11.3). Because muscle perfusion is inadequate for reliable drug absorption in patients with septic shock, drugs should be administered intravenously. If gentamicin or tobramycin is administered, the dosage must be adjusted to the patient's renal function. The first dose should be 1.5 mg/kg, but the time between doses should be prolonged according to the severity of renal failure; in many patients it may be better to substitute another drug.

Hyperpyrexia

Thus far, fever has been discussed only as a sign of an underlying disease process. While infectious diseases are the most common causes of fever, it can also be caused by many other processes. In fact, extremely high body temperatures are often due to noninfectious causes such as heat stroke, thyroid storm, malignant hyperthermia of anesthesia, and disorders of the hypothalamus.

In otherwise healthy patients, temperatures of 103°F (39.4°C) or 104°F (40°C) may be well tolerated and may not require treatment. However, fever often causes deleterious effects that do indicate a need for antipyretic therapy. Uncomfortable symptoms such as anorexia, myalgia, confusion, lethargy, and chills respond to lowering of the body temperature. In young children, febrile convulsions can result from temperatures higher than 104°F even without underlying neurologic problems; therefore, antipyretic therapy should be employed routinely in this age group. Hyperpyrexia has profound metabolic consequences, including elevation in oxygen consumption and accelerated tissue catabolism. As a result, the cardiovascular system is faced with increased demands, and fever can precipitate myocardial ischemia or congestive heart failure or both in patients with heart disease. Extreme hyperpyrexia with a temperature of 105°F (40.6°C) or higher may directly cause tissue damage, including changes in the vascular endothelium. In patients with extreme hyperpyrexia, disseminated intravascular coagulation, acidosis, and cardiovascular collapse can develop.

In the emergency ward, the patient's respiratory, metabolic, and circulatory status must first be stabilized. Since extremely high fever can cause shock, these patients should be treated like patients with septic shock. A work-up to diagnose the underlying disorder should be undertaken without delay, and specific therapy should be directed by the findings. Any complications, such as seizures, congestive heart failure, or disseminated intravascular coagulation, should be treated, as well as the fever itself. Antipyretic therapy may include both chemical agents and physical cooling. Among the drugs available, both aspirin and acetaminophen act directly on the hypothalamus to lower its thermal set point. Doses up to 1.2 gm can be given to adults orally or rectally and repeated every 4 hours. Caution must be exercised, since elderly patients and those with certain conditions such as Hodgkin's disease and typhoid fever may react adversely to antipyretic agents. Phenothiazine compounds are sometimes useful, but their effectiveness has not been completely elucidated and their use in extreme pyrexia is still experimental. The technique of physical cooling depends on the seriousness of condition. If the fever is being well tolerated, a hypothermic mattress or sponging with alcohol or ice water may suffice. Since these are uncomfortable procedures, they should be reserved for patients in whom rapid reduction of temperature is mandatory. Under more serious circumstances such as heat stroke, more extreme cooling may be required, in which case immersion in an ice water bath is recommended. Other measures such as iced gastric lavage, ice water enemas, and iced peritoneal dialysis are both less effective and more cumbersome. Once body temperature has been reduced to a safe level, physical cooling should be discontinued to avoid hypothermia.

GUIDELINES FOR ANTIBIOTIC THERAPY IN THE EMERGENCY WARD

The number of antimicrobial agents available to the physician is great, and new drugs are rapidly being marketed. This section is not intended to provide a comprehensive review of antibiotics but rather to present some guidelines likely to be useful in the emergency ward:

(1) Antibiotics treat bacterial infection, not fever. It is important to evaluate the condition of each patient following the general approach on pages 215–216 to arrive at a tentative diagnosis before starting administration of antibiotics.

(2) In general, antibiotics do not *prevent* infection. "Prophylactic antibiotics" are beneficial only in few special circumstances.

(3) Antibiotics have disadvantages, including possible toxic effects, potential sensitization of the patient, and selection of resistant organisms that can superinfect the patient. Capricious use of antibiotics can result in resistant organisms throughout the hospital and community. In addition, many antibiotics are expensive.

(4) New antibiotics should be compared critically with established agents. Many "new" drugs are minor modifications of standard drugs and are often more expensive. Toxic reactions may become apparent long after introduction of the new agent.

(5) Appropriate cultures and Gram stains should be obtained *before* starting antibiotic therapy.

(6) The patient must be treated specifically. Although the acutely ill patient may initially require broad antibiotic therapy, the goal should always be to select as specific a program of treatment as possible. Results of cultures and sensitivity testing and any other data that may become available should always be used to re-evaluate therapy.

(a) Administer as few drugs as possible. Direct therapy at the specific pathogen or pathogens isolated from the patient.

(b) Administer drugs that will penetrate the infected tissues.

(c) Administer the least toxic drugs available. If the patient also has renal or hepatic disease, this should be considered in choosing the drug and its dosage.

(d) Administer bactericidal rather than bacteriostatic drugs when possible.

(e) Choose the route of administration, dosage, and duration of therapy appropriate for the specific infection being treated.

(f) Monitor the patient's condition for effectiveness of treatment, toxic reactions, hypersensitivity, and superinfection.

(g) Administer the least expensive drugs available when possible.

(h) Beware of drug incompatibilities.

Table 11.3 summarizes some properties of selected antibiotics. This material is not exhaustive; alternative drugs of similar efficacy may be available, and new drugs are being introduced frequently. The current literature should be consulted for details.

Suggested Readings

American Academy of Pediatrics: *Report of the Committee on Infectious Disease*, ed 17. Evanston IL, American Academy of Pediatrics, 1974

Beeson PB, McDermott W, Wyngaarden JB (Eds): *Textbook of Medicine*, ed 15 Part 9, Microbial Diseases. Philadelphia, WB Saunders, 1979, pp 227–564

Gardner P, Provine HT: *Manual of Acute Bacterial Infections: Early Diagnosis and Treatment*. Boston, Little, Brown, 1975

Garrod LP, Lambert HP, O'Grady F: *Antibiotic and Chemotherapy*, ed 5, Edinburgh, Churchill Livingstone, 1981

Hoeprich PD (Ed): *Infectious Diseases: A Modern Treatise of Infectious Processes*, ed 2. Hagerstown, MD, Harper & Row, 1977

Isselbacher KJ, Adams RD, Brownwald E, et al (Eds): *Harrison's Principles of Internal Medicine*, ed 9 Part 4, Disorders Caused by Biologic and Environmental Agents. New York, McGraw-Hill, 1980, pp 539–918

Krugman S: *Infectious Diseases of Children*, ed 7. St. Louis, CV Mosby, 1980

Mandell GL, Douglas RG, Bennet JE (Eds): *Principles and Practice of Infectious Diseases*, New York, John Wiley & Sons, 1979

Medical Letter on Drugs and Therapeutics, Choice of antimicrobial drugs. 24:21–28, March 1982

Rubenstein E, Federman DD (Eds): *Scientific American Medicine*, Section 7, Infectious Diseases, New York, Scientific American, 1982

CHAPTER 12

Medical Gastrointestinal Disorders

JAMES M. RICHTER, M.D.
JOSEPH L. PERROTTO, M.D.

Editor's note: This medical chapter on gastrointestinal disease includes the broad subjects of diarrhea, hemorrhage, hepatic and proctologic disorders. The separation of gastrointestinal diseases into medical and surgical components is arbitrary. Additional coverage is provided, therefore, in Chapter 23 (Abdominal Emergencies).

The emergency physician has to cope with an increasing variety of medical disorders, many of which are related to the digestive tract. This chapter reviews some common gastrointestinal problems seen in the emergency ward for which the physician must initiate diagnostic and therapeutic procedures.

DIARRHEA

One of the most common problems seen in the emergency ward is diarrhea. Since therapy for diarrhea varies with the clinical findings, it is important to take a pertinent history, perform an appropriate physical examination, and obtain certain diagnostic studies.

The history should include information about the foods eaten during the previous 72 hours, recent travel, contacts with other persons with diarrhea, current medical problems (for example, diabetes mellitus), and medications. In addition, the patient should be questioned about the onset of the diarrhea (acute or gradual), the amount and duration, the character of stool (including presence of blood), and any concomitant fever, nausea, vomiting, or abdominal pain.

Physical examination in the emergency ward initially is directed toward assessing the state of hydration and clinical toxicity of the patient. The seriously ill patient requires careful observation and fluid replacement regardless of the cause of the diarrhea. A complete examination is desirable, but special attention should be directed toward the abdomen and rectum. The stool specimen should be examined for gross and occult blood with the Hemocult test; in addition, a methylene blue stain for polymorphonuclear leukocytes is helpful in the diagnosis of inflammatory and infectious diarrheas (Table 12.1 and 12.2).

The following sections discuss common causes of diarrhea with regard to their clinical features and treatment.

Viral Gastroenteritis

The most common causes of acute sporadic diarrhea are viruses such as enteroviruses, reoviruses, and adenoviruses. Typically the patient has fever, headache, and malaise, and may have nausea, vomiting, or upper respiratory tract symptoms. The stools are watery, and there is no blood or pus. Diarrhea usually resolves in 5–7 days. Since these illnesses are self-limited and since viral isolation techniques are expensive, a specific etiologic diagnosis is neither indicated nor obtained. Therapy is principally directed at symptoms, with fluid replacement being of primary importance, especially in children. Aspirin or acetaminophen is taken for fever and myalgias. Bismuth subsalicylate (Pepto-Bismol), 30 ml every 4 hours, or diphenoxylate hydrochloride with atropine sulfate (Lomotil), 2.5–5.0 mg every 6 hours, may be taken for control of symptoms.

Bacterial Gastroenteritis

Bacteria may cause acute diarrhea by producing a toxin in contaminated food, by invading the gastrointestinal mucosa, or by producing a toxin after they are ingested. Foods contaminated by staphylococcal toxin, often custard-filled pastries or processed meats, produce nausea, vomiting, abdominal cramps, and diarrhea within a few hours of ingestion. Symptoms usually last less than 12 hours. Similarly, foods contaminated by *Clos-*

Table 12.1.
Causes of acute infectious diarrhea.

Virus
    Parvovirus-like agent
    Reovirus-like agent
    Enterovirus
Bacterial toxins
    Staphylococcal toxin
    Clostridial toxin
Bacteria
    Salmonella
    Shigella
    Escherichia coli
    Campylobacter fetus
    Yersinia enterocolitica
    Vibrio cholerae
Protozoa
    Amoeba
    Giardia lamblia

Table 12.2.
Fecal leukocytes in acute diarrhea.

Present	Absent
Salmonella	Viruses
Shigella	Staphylococcal toxin
Escherichia coli, invasive	*Clostridium perfringens*
Campylobacter fetus	toxin
Amebiasis	*E. coli,* toxinogenic
Pseudomembranous colitis	Cholera
Ulcerative colitis	Giardiasis
Crohn's disease	Amebiasis
	Most drug-associated
	diarrhea

tridium perfringens toxin, which have often been warmed on steam tables, induce diarrhea and abdominal cramps, beginning 8–24 hours after ingestion and lasting about 24 hours. Both conditions are distinguished by common-source outbreaks and the lack of fever.

In the United States, acute diarrheal illness often is caused by ingestion of Shigella, Salmonella, *Escherichia coli,* or *Campylobacter fetus.* These diseases are most common among children, but may occur at any age. Typically, shigellosis begins 24–72 hours after ingestion of the bacteria, with fever, toxicity, bloody diarrhea, nausea, vomiting, and cramps. Frequently, the disease is more subtle and may be difficult to distinguish clinically from other diarrheal illnesses. It usually resolves in less than 7 days. Symptoms of salmonellosis develop 12–36 hours after ingestion of the bacteria, with watery diarrhea, cramps, nausea, vomiting, and fever. Salmonellosis is often nonspecific, and there is usually no visible blood in the stool. It usually resolves in less than 5 days, but may persist for up to 2 weeks. A wide spectrum of diarrheal

illness may be caused by *E. coli,* which causes diarrhea by mucosal invasion or toxin production. Toxinogenic strains cause a profuse watery diarrheal syndrome with cramps and low-grade fever. This is commonly experienced as traveler's diarrhea. Invasive strains produce a disease characterized by fever, severe cramps, and bloody diarrhea. Recently, *Campylobacter fetus* has been recognized as a major cause of acute diarrhea in the United States. The clinical illness is similar to shigellosis, often with prominent rectal bleeding. The illness resolves spontaneously over 7–14 days, but may recur for 6–8 weeks.

Sigmoidoscopic examination of patients with invasive bacterial diseases reveals diffuse erythema, edema, and friability, but no discrete ulcers. This is often not distinguishable from acute ulcerative colitis.

Most acute diarrheal illnesses should be managed by hydration and by waiting for spontaneous resolution. Hydration often can be maintained by oral administration of fluids, even in patients with profuse diarrhea. Solutions containing electrolytes and sugars are best, but milk products should be avoided since acquired lactase deficiency is common, particularly in children. Patients in whom dehydration or electrolyte abnormalities develop should be admitted for parenteral therapy.

Antibiotics should not be used routinely for acute bacterial diarrhea. They have little effect on the course of the disease, and they may prolong an asymptomatic bacterial carrier state. Ampicillin is the first choice for the treatment of salmonellosis, but patients who are very ill or allergic to penicillin may require chloramphenicol. Elderly, debilitated patients and those who may not tolerate bacteremia, such as patients with sickle cell anemia or prosthetic heart valves, may benefit from antibiotic therapy by its ability to limit distant complications. Trimethoprim-sulfamethoxazole, ampicillin, or a single dose of tetracycline may be given for shigellosis. Erythromycin is presently recommended for campylobacterosis. Its role in the treatment of this disease is not clearly defined, but it probably should be given to toxic patients or individuals who are at risk for transmitting the disease. Traveler's diarrhea may be prevented by taking doxycycline, 100 mg daily prophylactically. Please see Chapter 11, for further discussion of antibiotic choices in bacterial diarrheas.

Absorbent preparations commonly are used to treat the symptoms of uncomplicated acute diarrhea. Solutions of kaolin and pectin have no proved benefit, but seem to be harmless; they should not be relied on, however, in the treatment of severe diarrhea. Bismuth subsalicylate has recently been shown to be effective therapy for the symptoms of traveler's diarrhea, and may be helpful in other forms of simple diarrhea. Diphenoxylate hydrochloride and loperamide hydrochloride effectively treat diarrhea by directly inhibiting the motility of the gastrointestinal smooth muscle. Diphenoxylate and loperamide are derived from meperidine, but have fewer central nervous system effects. They should be used cautiously, if at all, in conditions in which toxic megacolon is possible. Use also should be restricted in bacterial diarrheas because they may prolong the course of shigellosis. The usual dose of diphenoxylate is 2.5–5.0 mg every 4 hours up to 20 mg/day. Loperamide is given in a dose of 2 or 4 mg every 4 hours up to 16 mg daily. Dosage often can be decreased for maintenance after initial control of the diarrhea. Opiates are potent antidiarrheal agents, but carry a higher risk of abuse. They are particularly useful when their coincident analgesic activity is needed. Tincture of opium, 0.5–1.0 ml, paregoric, 4 ml, or codeine, 30–60 mg, is given orally every 4 hours.

Protozoal Gastroenteritis

Amebiasis can cause an intermittent, chronic diarrheal syndrome or a severe fulminating condition with a presentation similar to that of acute, fulminating ulcerative colitis. A history of travel is significant because active disease occurs primarily in persons who have been in tropical areas. Recently, amebiasis has become common among active male homosexuals in the United States without a history of travel. Findings on physical examination are usually nonspecific, and in many patients, sigmoidoscopic examination may not be helpful because the cecum is the primary site of infection. In some patients, however, shallow ulcers may be seen, with normal mucosa between them. Other patients may have diffuse ulceration similar to that seen in ulcerative colitis or bacillary dysentery. Microscopic examination of fresh stool specimens by an experienced observer is the primary diagnostic test. Examination of at least three specimens usually is necessary to exclude the diagnosis of amebiasis. Examination of a wet saline stool preparation or of a scraping from the base of a rectal ulcer is most likely to show typical trophozoites with ingested red blood cells. Recently, serologic tests for amebiasis have proved helpful, especially in patients with coincident hepatic disease. A plain x-ray film of the abdomen should be obtained in seriously ill patients to exclude the possibility of toxic megacolon or intestinal perfo-

ration. Once the diagnosis of amebic disease is established, the patient should be treated with metronidazole (Flagyl), 750 mg three times a day for 10 days. Alternative therapy is diiodohydroxyquin (Diodoquin), 650 mg three times a day for 21 days, tetracycline, 250 mg every 6 hours for 10 days, and chloroquine, 500 mg twice a day for 2 days followed by 250 mg twice a day for 19 days. Severe intestinal infection may be treated with dehydroemetine, 1.0–1.5 mg/kg to a total of 1 gm, tetracycline, 1 gm/day in four divided doses, and diiodohydroxyquin, 650 mg four times a day for 21 days, followed by chloroquine, 500 mg twice a day for 2 days and then 250 mg twice a day for 19 days.

Giardia lamblia is a frequent cause of acute or chronic diarrhea in the United States. A history of travel in certain countries (for example, Russia) or known endemic areas should alert the physician to the possibility of giardiasis. Giardiasis is often asymptomatic, and diarrhea may be intermittent. Stools are loose, greasy, or watery. Mucus often is present, but blood is rare. Mild steatorrhea and malabsorption occasionally may develop. Although some stool specimens contain cysts or trophozoites, diagnosis often depends on microscopic examination of biopsy specimens from the small intestine or duodenal aspirates. Metronidazole, 250 mg three times a day for 7–10 days, or quinacrine hydrochloride (Atabrine), 100 mg three times a day for 7 days, is effective therapy.

Drug-Associated Diarrhea

Because drugs are frequently associated with acute diarrhea (Table 12.3), a careful medication history should be obtained by the emergency physician. Ingestion of large amounts of caffeinated beverages or alcohol may cause diarrhea. Patients frequently experience diarrhea in the course of taking medications such as magnesium-containing antacids or quinidine. Some patients who take laxatives are seen with diarrhea because of misunderstanding or because of the psychological need to be ill and to receive attention.

Antibiotics are now recognized as an important cause of acute diarrhea. Almost all antibiotics have been associated with diarrhea, but most cases are associated with clindamycin or ampicillin. Many patients have an uncomplicated course of frequent loose stools, whereas others have a toxic reaction and acute pseudomembranous colitis. In most cases, examination of the stool specimen reveals a cytotoxin produced by *Clostridium difficile*, which seems to cause the colitis. The diagnosis is based on clinical findings, the presence of pseudomem-

Table 12.3.
Drugs associated with acute diarrhea.

Magnesium-containing antacids
Caffeine
Antibiotics, especially clindamycin and ampicillin
Quinidine
Alcohol
Colchicine
Guanethidine
Laxatives

branes on sigmoidoscopic examination, and *C. difficile* cytotoxin in the stool specimen. Withdrawal of the antibiotic is the mainstay of therapy, but vancomycin, 125–500 mg orally every 6 hours, or cholestyramine (Questran) 2–4 gm orally every 6 hours, is often helpful.

Inflammatory Bowel Disease

Diarrhea is a cardinal symptom in several chronic inflammatory diseases of the intestine. Patients with ulcerative colitis or Crohn's disease may be seen in the emergency ward, and require prompt and thorough evaluation.

Ulcerative Colitis and Toxic Megacolon

Patients with ulcerative colitis usually have mild to severe bloody diarrhea, crampy abdominal pain, and tenesmus. A history of diarrhea, rectal bleeding, or pain is often present. Symptoms persisting more than 2 weeks help exclude infectious causes other than amebiasis. Extracolonic manifestations may include fever, uveitis, dermatitis, and arthritis. Sigmoidoscopic examination is important in establishing the diagnosis because virtually all patients with ulcerative colitis have rectal involvement. The examiner will see a fiery red, friable mucosa that easily bleeds with the touch of a cotton swab. Methylene blue stain of the mucosal exudate demonstrates polymorphonuclear leukocytes, but culture of the stool specimen or exudate is negative for enteropathogenic bacteria. Stool specimens should be examined to exclude amebiasis. Leukocytosis and anemia are present in more severe cases. Serum electrolyte levels should be measured and corrected if needed. In patients with clinical toxicity, a plain x-ray film of the abdomen should be examined for toxic dilatation of the colon of more than 5.5 cm. Barium enemas, anticholinergic drugs, and opiates should not be administered to seriously ill patients because of the possibility of precipitating this condition. Seriously ill patients should be hospitalized and fluids and electrolytes replaced intravenously; blood replacement may also be necessary. High

doses of corticosteroids (prednisone or prednisolone, 50–60 mg/day) should be administered orally or parenterally. Patients with toxic megacolon are difficult to treat, but available data favor colectomy soon after fluid and electrolyte imbalances have been corrected. Less severely ill patients can be treated with lower doses of corticosteroids or sulfasalazine, depending on their clinical status. In patients in whom the diagnosis is not firmly established, corticosteroid therapy should be withheld until infectious diseases can be excluded.

Crohn's Disease

Patients with Crohn's disease often are seen with mild to severe diarrhea with or without blood, and with abdominal pain that may be indistinguishable from ulcerative colitis. Intestinal obstruction and acute ileitis are other common emergency presentations of Crohn's disease. Frequent clinical features include perirectal fistulas and tenderness in the lower right periumbilical area. A mass of thickened, tender small intestine sometimes may be palpated. Sigmoidoscopic examination is helpful if the rectum is involved, but this is much less frequent than in ulcerative colitis. Inflammation secondary to Crohn's disease characteristically shows linear ulcerations and a cobblestone appearance in the mucosa. A biopsy specimen can be obtained from the rectum for pathologic examination. A complete blood cell count may show leukocytosis, and the hematocrit may be decreased secondary to blood loss.

Therapy includes parenteral fluid and electrolyte replacement in the acute phase and administration of corticosteroids in doses similar to those given for acute ulcerative colitis to reduce intestinal inflammation. Sulfasalazine is helpful in milder cases with principally colonic inflammation. Patients with intestinal obstruction are treated with nasogastric suction, intravenous fluid and electrolyte replacement, and parenteral administration of prednisone or prednisolone, 40–60 mg initially. If these measures fail, surgical resection of the involved area is indicated.

Neoplastic Disease

Patients with colonic carcinoma or adenomatous polyps may seek treatment in the emergency ward with diarrhea due to partial obstruction of the intestinal lumen. These patients often have a history of rectal bleeding, anorexia, weight loss, constipation, or pain. Physical examination may reveal an abdominal mass or tenderness with an enlarged, hard liver and a friction rub. On rectal examination, the physician may palpate the tumor or a rectal shelf. A stool guaiac test is usually positive. When cancer or polyps are suspected, sigmoidoscopic examination followed by a barium enema or colonoscopy usually demonstrates the lesion.

Malabsorptive Disease

A common reason for diarrhea and intestinal gas in many patients is lactose intolerance. It may be difficult to obtain an exact historical correlation between milk or milk-product ingestion and diarrhea, but if the physician suspects this problem, the patient can be treated empirically or a lactose tolerance test can be performed. If test results are positive, a clinical response can be expected to a lactose-free diet.

Patients with steatorrhea usually complain of chronic diarrhea and weight loss. The stools are often large, foul-smelling, pasty, and floating. The patient should be questioned about problems in childhood thay may suggest nontropical sprue (celiac disease). A history of living in Puerto Rico or India suggests tropical sprue. A history of alcohol abuse or chronic pancreatitis points toward pancreatic insufficiency. In patients in whom malabsorption is suspected, a thorough physical examination is necessary, as well as complete blood cell counts, serum chemistries, and qualitative or quantitative examination of stool specimens for fat. After fat malabsorption is documented, studies are directed toward distinguishing small bowel disease from pancreatic insufficiency. The usual initial test is the D-xylose test, which is abnormal in small bowel disease. Pancreatic function tests are abnormal in pancreatic insufficiency, but are not widely available. A therapeutic trial of pancreatic enzymes usually is sufficient. Small bowel biopsy and radiographs are indicated when results of the D-xylose test are abnormal, and they usually provide the diagnosis. Pancreatic calcifications on a plain x-ray film suggest chronic pancreatitis, but more extensive study with ultrasound and pancreatography may be needed to exclude pancreatic cancer.

Celiac disease is treated with gluten restriction, and tropical sprue responds to administration of vitamin B_{12}, folic acid, and broad-spectrum antibiotics. In endemic areas, broad-spectrum antibiotics may have to be given for more than 6 months. Treatment of pancreatic insufficiency includes a low-fat, high-calorie diet and pancreatic enzyme replacement.

Functional Bowel Disease

When patients who usually are constipated have diarrhea, rectal examination may indicate the problem to be fecal impaction. In such a case, diarrhea is resolved soon after disimpaction. A high-fiber diet or bulk laxative should help prevent recurrence.

Many patients have crampy abdominal pain with a history of alternating diarrhea and constipation, and no change in weight. These patients have been given diagnoses of spastic colon, mucous colitis, and irritable bowel syndrome. After appropriate clinical, laboratory, and x-ray examinations, they should be treated with reassurance and a high-fiber diet. Patients should take bran or a bulk laxative such as psyllium hydrophilic mucilloid (Metamucil), the dosage of which must be adjusted relative to bowel movements. Anticholinergic medications alone or in combination with sedatives may help patients with cramps.

Certain patients who have been thought to have irritable bowel syndrome may have decreased absorption of bile salts in the ileum, and this may cause a detergent effect in the colon, resulting in diarrhea. This most often occurs after cholecystectomy. Cholestyramine, 4–16 gm/day, is helpful.

Psychiatric problems commonly are seen in the emergency ward, and a gastrointestinal complaint such as diarrhea may be the presenting symptom. The history and physical examination usually indicate the need for referral to an internist or gastroenterologist, who may suggest psychiatric consultation.

GASTROINTESTINAL HEMORRHAGE

Upper Gastrointestinal Hemorrhage

Patients with upper gastrointestinal hemorrhage usually present with hematemesis, melena, hematochezia, or shock. The earliest possible estimate of quantity and rate of blood loss is the key to initial management of acute hemorrhage. Initial management includes placement of large intravenous catheters, rapid infusion of fluids, crossmatching of blood, and monitoring of vital signs. Every patient with gastrointestinal bleeding should be treated as if hypovolemic shock were about to develop. Once sufficient data have accumulated to justify a less urgent approach, such emergency measures can be modified or discontinued. Unfortunately, it is too common to treat the patient casually until hypotension unexpectedly signals massive hemorrhage.

After volume therapy is underway, the specific diagnosis may be addressed. A history of dyspepsia or previous peptic ulcer disease often is obtained in patients bleeding from ulcers. Patients with hematemesis usually have lesions above the ligament of Treitz. Recent violent vomiting followed by hematemesis suggests a gastroesophageal mucosal tear (Mallory-Weiss syndrome). A history of alcohol abuse may predispose the patient to esophageal varices, gastritis, or gastroduodenal ulceration. Therapy with aspirin, nonsteroidal anti-inflammatory agents, or high-dose corticosteroids may cause erosions or ulcerations of the stomach or duodenum. Previous gastric surgery raises the possibility of an anastomotic ulceration or recurrent carcinoma.

Physical examination may reveal orthostatic hypotension and an increased pulse rate, indicating significant blood volume loss (decrease in systolic blood pressure more than 10 mm Hg, and pulse rate increase more than 20 beats/min). The presence of jaundice, hepatosplenomegaly, ascites, or spider angiomas indicates chronic hepatic disease and suggests the possibility of variceal bleeding. Enlarged lymph nodes, liver, or spleen may suggest a malignant disease. Black tarry stool in the rectum is characteristic, but a normal guaiac-negative stool may be found early in acute hemorrhage. Hematochezia is seen in rapid upper gastrointestinal bleeding and in many episodes of lower intestinal bleeding, especially from the right colon. If there is no history of hematemesis, a nasogastric tube must be passed to determine whether the blood is coming from the upper gastrointestinal tract and to ascertain whether bleeding is active. A nasogastric aspirate is considered negative when guaiac-negative bilious material is obtained or if only guaiac-negative material is found after 2 hours.

A complete blood cell count, platelet count, and prothrombin time, and partial thromboplastin time should be obtained, as well as crossmatching for up to 8 units of blood.

When a specific diagnosis is needed immediately to guide surgical or medical management, esophagogastroduodenoscopy should be performed. This is best done after fluid resuscitation is underway and the patient is hemodynamically stable. Although routine endoscopic examination has not been shown to prolong short-term survival, gastrointestinal hemorrhage is a sign of a serious pathologic process, and a specific diagnosis allows more intelligent management. This is especially true in the patient with hepatic disease. If endoscopy fails to provide a diagnosis or if a lesion is found that is amenable to vasopressin infusion, angiographic examination may be helpful. Bleeding usually must be greater than 0.5 ml/min to be localized angiographically. With this information, a specific operation can be performed if medical measures fail. Barium contrast studies are not helpful in the emergent situation because, although they may demonstrate a lesion, they provide no evidence that the lesion is the bleeding source.

Major Causes

Although initial therapy for all upper gastrointestinal bleeding is fluid replacement and supportive care, subsequent therapy is aimed at the cause of the bleeding. Gastroesophageal mucosal bleeding secondary to a Mallory-Weiss tear is treated conservatively with adequate fluid and blood replacement, because 80% of these patients stop bleeding spontaneously. If bleeding continues, it may be arrested by angiography with selective infusion of vasopressin. If this fails, an operation should be performed with oversewing of the tear.

The most common cause of copious upper gastrointestinal bleeding is peptic ulcer disease. An ulcer may erode into the large gastroduodenal or pancreaticoduodenal arteries causing massive blood loss. Many patients with bleeding from a peptic ulcer have no previous history of ulcers. If there is a large amount of bleeding into the proximal portion of the duodenum, blood usually refluxes into the stomach and is vomited or recovered on aspiration of the gastric contents. Occasionally, however, the blood is lost entirely into the distal portion of the gastrointestinal tract, and is manifested by black or maroon stools. If bleeding is ongoing, endoscopic or angiographic examination will either establish the diagnosis or will provide sufficient information that the physician may infer the presence of a bleeding ulcer. Lavage of the stomach is useful in clearing blood clots and in judging the rate of blood loss, but recovery of only small amounts of blood from the stomach does not exclude extensive ongoing loss into the distal portion of the gastrointestinal tract. Signs of hypovolemia and increased vigor of peristaltic activity provide additional evidence of continuing blood loss.

When bleeding appears to be due to peptic ulcer disease, medical therapy usually is begun although it probably has little effect on the bleeding itself. Cimetidine, an inhibitor of acid secretion, is given, 300 mg orally or intravenously every 6 hr. Alternatively, antacid can be given hourly by nasogastric tube, the amount depending on the pH of the gastric fluid. The gastric contents are aspirated before every hourly instillation and the pH is checked with pH paper so that sufficient antacid can be instilled to keep the pH above 4. If bleeding continues in patients with a gastric ulcer, gastritis, or a Mallory-Weiss tear, angiography may be employed to infuse vasopressin via the left gastric artery (see Chapter 35, pages 806–810). The decision whether to operate or to continue medical management must be made quickly when hemorrhage is massive. New techniques are being developed that use electrocautery or laser coagulation of bleeding ulcers at endoscopic examination. These techniques, however, are not generally available and their usefulness has not been fully assessed.

Hemorrhage from esophageal varices often is severe and requires prompt and effective therapy. Because bleeding occurs directly into the esophagus, copious hematemesis is common. The patient often describes blood welling up in the mouth, rather than forceful vomiting. Many patients have a history of previous upper gastrointestinal bleeding and of chronic liver disease, alcohol-abuse hepatitis, or jaundice. All patients with hepatic disease and hemorrhage should have special attention directed to the blood clotting function, and correction with vitamin K, fresh frozen plasma, and platelets as necessary. If hemorrhage is substantial or continuing, early endoscopic examination usually is wise in order to document the presence of varices and to exclude a bleeding peptic ulcer or gastritis, which frequently coexist.

Vasopressin then is infused intravenously through a peripheral line at the rate of 0.1–0.4 unit/min. If this does not control the bleeding quickly, a Sengstaken-Blakemore tube with Boyce modification of the esophageal component should be passed for tamponade of the bleeding varices. The tubing should be well lubricated and passed via the nose into the stomach. The gastric balloon should then be inflated with 200–300 cc of air and pulled back into the gastroesophageal junction under 1–2 lb of traction. After the position of the tube is checked by x-ray study, the esophageal balloon is inflated to 40 mm Hg, and after bleeding stops, it is deflated to the minimum pressure necessary for control of any further bleeding. The use of intermittent suction helps monitor the rate of bleeding. If bleeding is controlled for 24 hours, the esophageal balloon is decompressed, but suction is maintained. If no bleeding occurs for 24 additional hours, the gastric balloon is decompressed. An alternative method of balloon tamponade is use of the Linton balloon tube. This is a single gastric balloon tube, the effectiveness of which is based on compression of the collateral veins supplying the esophageal varices by distention of the balloon in the gastric fundus coupled with traction on the tube; 200–300 cc of air is placed in the balloon and 1–2 lb of traction are applied to the tube. Variceal hemorrhage and the use of balloon tubes pose a substantial threat of aspiration. Most patients require endotracheal intubation to protect the airway. Caution must be exercised in the use of any tube that involves balloon distention of the lower part of the esophagus. A balloon that is overdistended in the distal esophagus or a gastric balloon that is drawn back into the esophagus may result in esophageal necrosis or rupture. When medical therapy does not stop the bleeding, either the portal circulation should be decompressed via a portosystemic shunt or varices should be obliterated by ligation or endoscopic sclerosis, depending on the status of the patient and the experience of the attending personnel.

Aortoenteric fistulas are almost always a complication of an implanted graft after aortic resection. The diagnosis should be considered in any patient with gastrointestinal bleeding and previous operation on the aorta or iliac vessels. Surprisingly, bleeding from such fistulas is not always profuse. Aortic aneurysms can give rise spontaneously to fistulas into the duodenum, but these are exceedingly rare. The therapy is surgical.

Lower Gastrointestinal Hemorrhage

Intestinal bleeding below the ligament of Treitz usually is evidenced by the passing of bright red blood or maroon stools. As with acute upper gastrointestinal hemorrhage, the initial assessment must quickly focus on determination of the hemodynamic status of the patient and the rate of the bleeding. Initial therapy and further evaluation then may proceed simultaneously. An accurate history is important to determine the onset, duration, and character of the bleeding, as well as associated symptoms, such as abdominal pain or diarrhea.

Physical examination may reveal telangiectasias (hereditary hemorrhagic telangiectasia), osteomas or lipomas (Gardner's syndrome), rectal polyps, or cancer. Laboratory tests include a complete blood cell count, prothrombin time, partial thromboplastin time, platelet count, and blood typing and crossmatching. A nasogastric tube should be passed and gastric contents aspirated for an hour or until blood or bile is recovered in order to rule out hemorrhage from the upper gastrointestinal tract. Sigmoidoscopic examination then should be performed to ascertain the presence of cancer, polyps, inflammatory disease, or hemorrhoids in the rectosigmoid colon. In patients with bloody diarrhea, infectious causes should be investigated. If the bleeding site is not determined by sigmoidoscopy, angiographic examination should identify the location of the lesion in the patient who is actively bleeding. Angiography also may reveal evidence of arteriovenous malformations, which may be seen in the small intestine but which are more commonly observed in the cecum or ascending colon (angiodysplasia). Colonoscopy is being used increasingly in patients with lower gastrointestinal bleeding in whom the rate of bleeding is not fast enough for it to be seen by angiography. This technique also has been helpful in patients who bleed from ischemia, because the site can be observed and a biopsy specimen can be taken. In young patients, the possibility of Meckel's diverticulum should be considered. This lesion should be demonstrated by angiographic examination in the actively bleeding phase. At other times, it may be detected by technetium scanning.

If the site of intestinal bleeding is found by angiography, vasopressin can be infused to control blood loss. In patients with angiodysplasia, the physician may be able to cauterize the arteriovenous malformation at colonoscopic examination. If these measures do not stop the bleeding, the involved area should be surgically excised. The barium enema in patients with lower gastrointestinal bleeding is the least effective method of determining the cause or site of hemorrhage, and if it is used initially, it may preclude angiography or colonoscopy for an extended period while the patient has cleansing enemas.

The small intestine may be the source of massive bleeding from an ulcerated Meckel's diverticulum, Crohn's disease, hamartomatous tumors in patients with Peutz-Jeghers syndrome, and jejunal diverticula similar to that seen in patients with bleeding colonic diverticula. Angiographic examination is the most accurate method and is often the only method other than laparotomy by which the site of bleeding can be established.

Any major bleeding in the colon usually leads to the passage of maroon and red stools, although slow bleeding from the right colon and right portion of the transverse colon may be manifested by melena only. Massive colonic bleeding may originate from diverticula. Many diverticula arise at sites where major blood vessels penetrate the muscle wall, and bleeding is usually the result of erosion into one of these vessels. The typical history of bleeding diverticula is the passage of huge, bloody stools without preceding symptoms, followed by faintness. Angiographic examination provides the only specific means of diagnosis; if it cannot be employed, barium studies may be performed to assist the surgeon in planning a possible emergency operation.

Recently, the increased use of angiographic examination in the diagnosis of acute lower gastrointestinal hemorrhage has demonstrated angiodysplasia of the colon to be an important cause of bleeding. Patients are typically elderly and may have aortic valvular disease. There is often a history of previous bleeding with an inconclusive evaluation. Presently, diagnosis depends on angiography that demonstrates the arteriovenous malformations even in the absence of active bleeding. Lesions are usually present in the right colon, but may be found in the remainder of the colon or small intestine. Often, multiple lesions are found. Standard therapy is right colectomy, but some physicians report success with electrocoagulation of lesions via colonoscopy.

Inflammatory bowel disease may present as acute lower gastrointestinal bleeding. The patient usually has a history of diarrhea, abdominal pain, or previous colitis. Diagnosis usually is established by sigmoidoscopy.

Hemorrhoidal bleeding occasionally may be profuse enough to be frightening. In this instance, sigmoidoscopic examination is of primary importance. Portal hypertension or some form of bleeding disorder should be suspected in the patient whose bleeding is voluminous enough to constitute an acute, serious hemorrhage. Tumors of the colon, including polyps, may bleed, but seldom enough to provoke hypovolemia.

HEPATIC DISEASE

Patients with hepatic disease are seen in the emergency ward with jaundice, upper abdominal pain, abdominal swelling, encephalopathy, or malaise. The first two symptoms also may be due to primary biliary disease, which is discussed in more detail in Chapter 23.

The nature of the course of the illness should be determined. The onset of fever, anorexia, malaise, dark urine, abdominal discomfort, and perhaps jaundice over a few days is characteristic of viral hepatitis. A long history of intermittent abdominal pain or indigestion might suggest cholelithiasis, which coupled with jaundice would point to choledocholithiasis. Sudden onset of high fever, jaundice, and clinical toxicity, especially with the history of gallstones, is characteristic of cholangitis. Previous hepatobiliary disease may suggest a recurrence or exacerbation of a more chronic disease.

Careful questioning regarding alcohol consumption is always important. Drug use, especially use of antituberculous chemotherapeutic agents, methyldopa, phenothiazines, and estrogens (including oral contraceptives) may provide important insights (Table 12.4). An occupational history should be taken, particularly regarding work in institutions where hepatitis is endemic or where

Table 12.4.
Drugs reported to cause hepatic injury.

Drug	Incidence	Mechanism	Pattern of Injury	Comment
Anesthetic agents				
Chloroform	High, dose-related	Direct toxicity	Hepatocellular	May cause massive hepatic necrosis
Halothane	Low	Hypersensitivity	Hepatocellular	
Antibiotics				
Erythromycin estolate	Low	Hypersensitivity	Cholestatic	
Tetracycline, oral	Low	Indirect toxicity	Hepatocellular	
Tetracycline, intravenous	High, dose-related (>2 gm/24 hr)	Indirect toxicity	Hepatocellular	Particularly in pregnancy, characterized by small fat droplets in hepatocytes
Sulfonamides	Low	Hypersensitivity	Mixed	
Penicillin	Very low	Hypersensitivity	Hepatocellular	
Anti-inflammatory agents				
Acetaminophen	High, dose-related	Direct toxicity	Hepatocellular	Only seen with overdose, when fulminant hepatic failure may occur
Salicylates	High	Direct toxicity (?)	Mixed	Clinical disease rare, transaminase elevations with levels >25 mg/100 ml
Antimetabolites and immunosuppressive agents				
Azathioprine	Low	Indirect toxicity	Mixed	Irreversible hepatic failure reported
Chlorambucil	Low	Indirect toxicity	Cholestatic	
6-Mercaptopurine	10–35%	Indirect toxicity	Mixed	
Methotrexate	Low, dose-related	Indirect toxicity	Mixed	Progression to cirrhosis suggested but not proved
Antituberculous agents				
Isoniazid	Low	Metabolic idiosyncrasy (related to acetylation rate)	Hepatocellular or mixed	
Rifampin	Low		Hepatocellular	
Para-aminosalycylic acid	1%	Hypersensitivity	Mixed	
Ethionamide	3–5%	Metabolic idiosyncrasy	Hepatocellular	

Hormones				
Methyltestosterone	Jaundice: low	Metabolic idiosyncrasy	Bland cholestasis	No evidence for hepatic inflammation, but jaundice may be severe
	High, dose-related interference with hepatic excretory function	Indirect toxicity	Peliosis	
Synthetic estrogens (e.g., mestranol)	Jaundice: very low	Metabolic idiosyncrasy	Bland cholestasis	
	High, dose-related interference with hepatic excretory function	Indirect toxicity		
Synthetic progestational agents ("19-Nor" compounds)	Jaundice: low	Metabolic idiosyncrasy	Cholestatic	May be potentiated by estrogens
	High, dose-related interference with hepatic excretory function	Indirect toxicity		
Psychotropic drugs				
Phenothiazines	Low (exception: 1–3% with chlorpromazine)	Hypersensitivity	Cholestatic	
Miscellaneous				
α-Methyldopa	Low	Hypersensitivity	Mixed	
Phenytoin	Low	Hypersensitivity	Mixed	
Oxyphenisatin	Low	Metabolic idiosyncrasy	Mixed	Reversible chronic active hepatitis reported
Propylthiouracil	Low	Hypersensitivity	Hepatocellular	
Methimazole	Low	Hypersensitivity	Cholestatic	
Thiazide diuretics	Very low	Hypersensitivity	Cholestatic	

(Modified by permission from Zimmerman HJ: Drug-induced hepatic injury. In Samter M, Parker C (Eds): *Hypersensitivity to Drugs*, Vol. 1. Elmsford, NY, Pergamon Press, 1974.)

potential hepatotoxins such as carbon tetrachloride or vinyl chloride are used. Needle exposure to drugs, blood products, or persons with known hepatitis may point to viral hepatitis. A recent operation on the biliary tract may suggest a surgical complication, or a history of a malignant condition may suggest metastatic disease.

Physical examination is important to assess the patient's general health and to determine the presence of fever and manifestations of chronic hepatic disease, such as spider angiomas. For jaundice to be clinically apparent, the serum bilirubin level must be more than 2.0–2.5 mg/100 ml. An offensive, sweet smell of the breath (fetor hepaticus) also may indicate chronic hepatic disease. Lymphadenopathy suggests mononucleosis, viral hepatitis, or malignant disease, and arthritis and dermatitis may indicate acute or chronic viral hepatitis. The abdomen should be examined for signs of ascites, such as shifting dullness and distention. Shifting dullness may be determined by percussing the abdomen with the patient supine and then with the patient on his side. Next, the liver should be measured by percussing it over the right side of the chest onto the right side of the abdomen; normal breadth is 8–10 cm. The liver should be palpated to determine whether it is tender, and the firmness, smoothness, or nodularity of its edge should be established. The presence of a palpable gallbladder and splenomegaly should be determined. A positive stool guaiac test may indicate a gastrointestinal tumor metastatic to the liver or obstructing the bile ducts. Neurologic examination always should be performed to determine neuropathy, ophthalmoplegia, the level of consciousness, and the presence of asterixis.

Patients with jaundice should have a complete blood cell count, including reticulocytes. Blood urea nitrogen and serum electrolyte levels are helpful in determining the severity of hepatic dysfunction and of fluid and electrolyte disturbances that often occur. Prothrombin time and platelet count are frequently abnormal, and reflect the severity of hepatic injury and the bleeding potential. Liver function tests should be performed, depending on the historical and physical findings and the questions that the clinician needs answered. The adolescent with a few days of malaise and dark urine may require only a serum glutamic oxaloacetic transaminase determination to confirm the diagnosis of acute hepatitis and a prothrombin time to assess the severity of the hepatic damage. The older adult with abdominal pain and jaundice needs fractionated bilirubin and alkaline phosphatase determinations, as well as a transaminase measurement. If the alkaline phosphatase and direct bilirubin levels are elevated, suggesting biliary tract disease, an ultrasound study may be indicated as well. Patients with chronic hepatic disease require assessment of hepatic synthetic function such as albumin and prothrombin time.

Hepatitis

Viral Hepatitis

Several viruses may produce acute hepatitis. Hepatitis virus A is a frequent cause of acute hepatitis, especially in children and young adults. Formerly known as infectious hepatitis or short incubation hepatitis, viral hepatitis type A is passed by fecal-oral transmission. The illness is usually not severe, and has an excellent prognosis. There is no known carrier state, and illness never progresses to chronic hepatitis. Hepatitis virus B causes serum hepatitis or long incubation hepatitis in persons of all ages. The virus often is passed by parenteral contact with blood products, but nonparenteral transmission has frequently been reported, particularly between sexual contacts. Hepatitis B surface antigen is often detectable early in the disease, and usually disappears as hepatitis B surface antibody is produced. In about 5% of patients, the antigen persists. Hepatitis B surface antibody provides immunity to subsequent infection. Usually the precise virologic diagnosis is not needed initially, except for prognosis and prophylactic treatment of contacts.

As serologic techniques for identifying cases of hepatitis due to virus A and virus B have improved, it is now clear that there is a third principal hepatitis virus. Sufficient studies have been performed to demonstrate that it is not another widely recognized virus. Therefore, until it is identified and characterized, it has been designated "non-A, non-B." This agent (or these agents) is responsible for 90% of viral hepatitis occurring after blood transfusion and probably 20% of sporadic hepatitis in the community. The disease tends to be indolent, with a significant number of anicteric cases and a substantial frequency of subsequent chronic hepatitis, especially in post-transfusion cases. Infectious mononucleosis (Epstein-Barr virus) can also produce hepatitis. In this type of infection, pharyngitis and adenopathy are evident.

The diagnosis of acute viral hepatitis is based on the clinical features and a serum transaminase level that is characteristically very high. The alkaline phosphatase level usually is elevated modestly, but is less strikingly abnormal than the transaminase level. The bilirubin level is often high and is composed of both direct and indirect reacting fractions.

Most patients with viral hepatitis can be cared for at home. Pregnant or elderly patients may do better in the hospital with bed rest. Patients with abnormal clotting ability or encephalopathy should be admitted for observation and specific therapy. Patients who cannot maintain hydration by themselves also should be hospitalized for parenteral fluid administration. The principal therapy for all patients is supportive and includes rest, fluids, good nutrition, and abstinence from alcohol.

The complications of acute viral hepatitis usually arise from infection with hepatitis virus B. A prothrombin time greater than 2 seconds more than control and a bilirubin level greater than 20 μg/dl are the most reliable predictors of poor prognosis. In the early period, acute or subacute hepatic necrosis can develop, which is indicated by symptomatically severe hepatitis complicated by signs of hepatic failure such as ascites, encephalopathy, or coagulopathy. Recent data suggest that corticosteroids are not beneficial in this circumstance and that they actually may be detrimental; supportive care is probably the only treatment available.

Patients with viral hepatitis should maintain good personal hygiene to limit transmission of the virus. When blood is drawn from patients with viral hepatitis type B, needles and syringes should be disposed of carefully and the tubes of blood should be labeled as potentially infectious. Household contacts of patients with viral hepatitis type A should be treated with immune serum globulin, which is approximately 90% effective in inhibiting the clinical manifestations of acute hepatitis (Table 12.5). The recommended dose is 0.5 ml for patients weighing less than 50 lb, 1 ml for patients weighing from 50–100 lb, and 2 ml for patients weighing more than 100 lb; this will protect contacts for 4–8 weeks. Larger doses protect longer, and are appropriate for persons traveling to or residing in en-

demic areas. Close contacts, especially sexual partners of patients with viral hepatitis type B, should receive immune serum globulin, 0.07 ml/kg, if their test results are negative for hepatitis B surface antigen and antibody. Persons exposed to viral hepatitis type B via needle should be given hyperimmune serum globulin when available. A hepatitis B vaccine is now available for pre-exposure prophylaxis and is probably also helpful for postexposure prophylaxis. Hopefully, more detailed information will be forthcoming soon.

Alcoholic Hepatitis

Some persons who drink substantial quantities of alcohol over prolonged periods have hepatic disease. The liver may acquire fatty change, hepatitis cirrhosis, or frequently, combinations of these. In the emergency ward, alcoholic hepatitis or complications of cirrhosis are frequent problems. Patients with alcoholic hepatitis are seen with jaundice, dull pain in the right upper abdominal quadrant, vomiting, and fever. The transaminase level invariably is elevated, but is not as high as often is observed in viral hepatitis. In addition, the alkaline phosphatase level is significantly elevated and is often three to five times the upper limit of the normal range. Because of the coincidence of chronic liver disease, evidence of hepatic insufficiency, such as a prolonged prothrombin time and hypoalbuminemia, frequently is present. Therapy is abstinence from alcohol, supportive care, and specific therapy for complications, such as encephalopathy, bleeding, and ascites. Hospitalization is often required.

Toxin-Induced Hepatitis

Patients may be seen in the emergency ward with hepatitis induced by toxins such as acetaminophen, carbon tetrachloride, and the toxin

Table 12.5.
Recommendations for acute viral hepatitis immunoprophylaxis.

Exposure	Type	Immune Serum Globulin, Dosage
Household or intimate contacts	Hepatitis A	0.02 ml/kg intramuscularly up to 2 ml
	Hepatitis B	0.07 ml/kg intramuscularly up to 5 ml; repeat in 1 month for sexual contacts
	Unknown or non-A, non-B	0.07 ml/kg intramuscularly up to 5 ml
Percutaneous (needle-stick)	Hepatitis B (exposed person hepatitis B surface antigen and antibody negative)	Hyperimmune globulin 5 ml intramuscularly; repeat in 1 month
	Unknown or non-A, non-B	0.07 ml/kg intramuscularly up to 5 ml
	No evidence of hepatitis B or clinical hepatitis	No prophylaxis

produced by the *Amanita phalloides* mushroom. Many drugs also cause hepatitis either because of hypersensitivity or because of variable metabolism of the drug. Table 12.4 lists certain medications and their hepatotoxic effects. The major therapy for this type of problem is withdrawal of the offending agent. Corticosteroids occasionally are given for hypersensitivity reactions, but the efficacy of this therapy is unclear.

Acetaminophen is emerging as an important cause of toxic liver injury, because of its increasing use. It is safe in normal doses, but in massive overdose—more than 25 gm and sometimes as little as 10 gm in adults—serious toxic injury of the liver regularly occurs. This may be substantially prevented if treatment with N-acetyl-L-cysteine is begun from 12–24 hours. The presently recommended regimen is 140 mg/kg orally followed by 70 mg/kg every 4 hours for 3 days. Current information is available at the Rocky Mountain Poison Center (800–525–6115).

Cirrhosis

In the United States, cirrhosis usually is caused by alcohol or chronic hepatitis. The major related problems in the emergency ward are the associated complications—bleeding, encephalopathy, and ascites. Bleeding already has been discussed; encephalopathy and ascites are considered in the following sections.

Hepatic Encephalopathy

Hepatic encephalopathy is a complex metabolic disturbance in neurologic function characterized by alterations of consciousness, neurologic signs, and asterixis. It occurs in patients with severe acute or chronic hepatocellular disease, often with extensive portosystemic shunts. Disturbances in mentation with forgetfulness and elation are the earliest signs. This state is followed by confusion, drowsiness, and asterixis. The stages of hepatic encephalopathy are listed in Table 12.6. The emergency physician must be careful to exclude other causes of altered consciousness such as meningitis in a febrile patient or intracranial hemorrhage in a trauma victim.

After hepatic encephalopathy is recognized, the nature of the underlying hepatic disease and the precipitants of the encephalopathy need to be defined. Hepatic failure may occur acutely in patients with fulminant hepatitis due to viruses or hepatotoxins such as alcohol or carbon tetrachloride. In pediatric patients, Reye's syndrome is a possibility, in which prodromes of upper respiratory tract illness typically precede coma and hypoglycemia. In patients with chronic hepatic disease with portosystemic shunting, hepatic coma may develop as a result of intestinal bleeding, increased protein ingestion, hypokalemia secondary to diarrhea or diuretics, hypovolemia, viral or bacterial infection, drug ingestion (for example, narcotics or sedatives), or abdominal disease (for example, acute pancreatitis or a perforated viscus).

Family or friends should be questioned about previous medical history, exposure to toxins, diet, use of intravenous and other drug usage, exposure to others with hepatitis, and use of alcohol. Physical examination is helpful in determining signs of chronic hepatic disease, such as spider angiomas, jaundice, hepatosplenomegaly, and ascites. Moreover, evidence of trauma is critical because of the possibility of cerebral hemorrhage. Fever indicates the possibility of infection, such as peritonitis or pneumonia. The physician should assess the degree of dehydration utilizing the clinical findings and often a central venous pressure measurement. A stool specimen should be studied for occult blood, and a nasogastric aspirate obtained to determine the presence of active or previous bleeding (coffee-ground material) or recently ingested drugs.

Table 12.6.
Stages of hepatic encephalopathy.

Stage	Mental State	Tremor (Asterixis)	Electroencephalogram[a]
Prodrome	Euphoria, mild confusion, slow mentation	Often present, but slight	Changes usually absent
Impending coma	Confusion, drowsiness	Present	Changes usually present
Stupor	Marked confusion; sleepy but arousable	Present if patient can cooperate	Changes almost always present
Coma	Unconsciousness; may respond to pain	Absent (no muscle tone)	Changes often present

[a] The electroencephalogram abnormalities are characterized by paroxysms of bilaterally synchronous high-voltage slow waves in the Δ range (1.5–3/sec), alternating with normal α waves.
(Adapted by permission from Schiff L: *Diseases of the Liver*, ed. 3. Philadelphia, JB Lippincott Co., 1969, p. 378.)

Patients with encephalopathy may be seen in the emergency ward in markedly varying conditions ranging from mild confusion to coma (Table 12.6). In the patient with impending coma, the physician may be able to elicit asterixis, but this is difficult in the stuporous or comatose patient, who cannot maintain a sustained posture. The blood ammonia level frequently is elevated in patients with hepatic encephalopathy and is useful when the cause of the encephalopathy is not clearly hepatic. The electroencephalogram is also abnormal in patients with either impending coma, stupor, or coma, but this tool is not usually available to the emergency physician.

X-ray films of the chest and abdomen should be taken to exclude the possibility of pneumonia or a perforated viscus. Lumbar puncture should reveal normal cerebrospinal fluid in patients with hepatic coma.

All patients with hepatic coma should be admitted to an area of the hospital where they will receive constant attention from nurses and physicians. Therapy consists of withdrawal of the offending drug, reduction of dietary protein, and correction of electrolyte and fluid imbalance. Hypokalemia may require administration of large amounts of potassium chloride, 100–300 mEq orally or intravenously during the first 2–3 days. The patient with hyponatremia, peripheral edema, and ascites may require fluid restriction to less than 1500 ml/day and dietary sodium restriction to less than 500 mEq/day. Bacterial infections should be treated with the appropriate antibiotics. Gastrointestinal bleeding should be managed as discussed previously. In addition, cathartics and enemas should be administered on the first day of hospitalization to decrease the intestinal absorption of nitrogenous substances. Lactulose, 30 ml every 4 hours, is given until diarrhea begins and then is decreased to a dose that produces two soft bowel movements daily. Alternatively, neomycin, 500–1000 mg, with sorbitol may be given every 6 hours.

Ascites

Patients with acute alcoholic hepatitis, fulminant viral hepatitis, or chronic hepatic disease may be seen in the emergency ward with ascites or peripheral edema or both. These patients are typically hypoalbuminemic, and have an increased portal pressure. They behave as if they are dehydrated with an active secondary aldosterone mechanism, resulting in peritoneal and interstitial fluid retention. In addition to a full clinical and serum chemical evaluation, it is important to perform paracentesis to exclude the diagnosis of bacterial, mycobacterial, or carcinomatous peritonitis.

Treatment of ascites secondary to cirrhosis includes restriction of sodium, usually to 500 mg/day, and often restriction of fluid to 1200–1500 ml/day to prevent hyponatremia. Diuretic therapy is begun with spironolactone and is increased until sodium diuresis begins and urinary potassium loss decreases below 20 mEq/liter. Later, thiazides or loop diuretics may be given to raise the fluid loss to 400 ml daily. Diuretics must be used carefully since they can cause hypokalemia and depletion of extracellular fluid with resultant encephalopathy. Therapeutic paracentesis should be reserved for patients with significant respiratory embarassment due to pressure under the diaphragm. When used, it should be limited to 1 liter because a rapid shift of fluid from the plasma into the peritoneal cavity can lead to circulatory embarassment.

PROCTOLOGIC CONDITIONS

A variety of anorectal problems commonly are seen in the emergency ward. A thorough history and an appropriate physical examination are always helpful in determining the nature and cause of the symptoms. Inspection of the perianal area and anoproctoscopic examination are necessary diagnostic procedures, and familiarity with these techniques is essential.

Hemorrhoids

Patients with hemorrhoids usually are seen with bleeding, perianal pain, or pruritus ani. Most pain and bleeding arise when the vascular anal cushions prolapse through the anal canal and are congested by the internal sphincter on forceful defecation. Stool softeners and bulk laxatives are the mainstay of treatment. A thrombosed external hemorrhoid that is quite painful can be treated by injecting 1% lidocaine hydrochloride (Xylocaine) with epinephrine into the hemorrhoid and incising it, evacuating the clot, coagulating the bleeding areas, and using Gelfoam or Oxycel to control hemorrhage. Bleeding internal hemorrhoids are treated with stool softeners, bulk laxatives, hot tub baths, lubricants, and hydrocortisone suppositories. The emergency physician must resist the temptation to attribute all anorectal bleeding to hemorrhoids unless the bleeding hemorrhoid can be visualized. Patients with rectal carcinoma or polyps too often are diagnosed initially as having hemorrhoidal bleeding.

Fissure-in-ano

Patients with acute anal fissures usually are seen in the emergency ward because of rectal pain (especially with defecation) or mild bleeding or both. In men, acute fissures tend to occur in the posterior midline; in women, anterior fissures tend to be more common. Fissures secondary to Crohn's disease are typically multiple, and are less likely to be acute. Acute fissures are diagnosed visually; with the patient in the prone position, the buttocks are gently drawn apart. Proctoscopic examination is recommended, but may not be possible because of the pain. The treatment of acute fissures is to soften stools and to decrease pain and spasm. This is accomplished by having the patient use a bulk laxative and stool softener, a topical anesthetic, and sitz baths.

Chronic fissures extend to the internal sphincter and are associated with an edematous skin tag ("sentinel pile"). This type of fissure may be related to Crohn's disease, and these patients need to be examined thoroughly because of this possibility. Other possibilities include adenocarcinoma and tuberculous or syphilitic ulcers. Patients with chronic fissures should be referred for further evaluation.

Anorectal Fistula

Anorectal fistulas are inflammatory tracts that originate in an abscess in the longitudinal muscle layer which have an internal opening in the mucosa of the anal canal or rectum and an external opening in the perianal skin. Diagnosis often is made by a history of recurrent rectal discharge and recurrent perianal abscesses. The examiner should note the position of the fistulas in relation to the anal opening to determine the expected position of the internal opening. Next, by palpating the skin between the fistula and the anal canal, the physician may feel an indurated area that indicates the direction of the fistula. If digital examination of the anal canal is performed then, the extension of the fistula may be felt. Afterward, a blunt probe may be used to determine the internal opening; this is best done by someone experienced in the technique. If Crohn's disease is suspected as a result of examination, a thorough evaluation is indicated, including sigmoidoscopy, barium enema, and small-bowel x-ray films. Definitive therapy is surgical.

Pruritus Ani

Perianal itching can be caused by several conditions, and it is necessary to take a broad history and to examine the patient with particular attention to dermatologic lesions in other parts of the body. Many patients may have pruritus ani because of improper cleansing after defecation, he-

morrhoids, fissures, fistulas, or rectal prolapse. Several dermatologic disorders may cause perianal eruptions and itching, and it is important to inspect the skin over the entire body as well as in the perianal area.

Candida albicans can cause perianal irritation and pruritus, especially in patients with poorly controlled diabetes mellitus, patients receiving broad-spectrum antibiotics, and patients receiving corticosteroid therapy. Diagnosis is confirmed by microscopic examination of a scraping of the lesion.

Infectious anogenital warts of viral origin that cause perianal itching are frequent in homosexuals. Patients with this condition should undergo anoscopic examination because the warts can extend to the dentate line. Treatment consists of weekly applications of 25% podophyllin in benzoin until the warts have disappeared. Herpes simplex also can occur in the perianal area, and is manifested by erythematous macules and vesicles. This infection can be treated by keeping the lesions clean and dry.

Pinworms can cause pruritus ani and can be diagnosed by placing a piece of transparent tape against the anus in the early morning for several hours and then examining it with a microscope. Scabies is another problem that causes pruritus, as does infestation with crab lice, which must be searched for carefully. Both conditions can be treated with gamma benzene hexachloride (Kwell) lotion or shampoo.

Psoriasis may be seen in the perianal area without the scales seen in other parts of the body, but examination of the remainder of the skin may suggest the diagnosis. Topical corticosteroids and coal tar preparations are standard treatment for this condition. Lichen planus occurs in the perianal area, and almost always is manifested in other areas of the skin as well. It must be differentiated from secondary syphilis.

Venereal Disease

Many bacterial infections can occur in the anorectal area. Common among these is the primary chancre of syphilis in the anal canal of homosexuals. This may appear to be only a superficial erosion in the anorectal area. On further examination, these patients are noted to have enlarged inguinal nodes. Specific diagnosis is made by demonstrating *Treponema pallidum* by means of darkfield microscopy of serum from the area of the chancre. Results of serologic testing may not be positive until weeks after the occurrence of the primary chancre. Secondary syphilis is manifested by anal macules and condyloma latum in the perianal area, macules on the hands and soles of the feet, and generalized lymphadenopathy. The diagnosis of secondary syphilis is made by means of positive serologic testing.

Therapy is directed at treating not only the patient but also the patient's contacts for the previous 3 months in the case of primary syphilis and for the previous year in the case of secondary syphilis. Antibiotic therapy consists of procaine penicillin G, 600,000 units/day intramuscularly for 10 days, or erythromycin, 500 mg orally four times a day for 2 weeks. The patient definitely should receive follow-up care.

Gonorrheal infection of the rectal mucosa also is seen in the emergency ward. This disease causes mild symptoms of pain on defecation, tenesmus, and rectal discharge. On examination, the sphincter is lax, and proctoscopic examination reveals mild inflammation, friability of the rectal mucosa, and mucus. Specific diagnosis is made by means of a Gram stain of the pus, which shows the intracellular gram-negative diplococci, and culture of *Neisseria gonorrhoeae* on Thayer-Martin agar.

The treatment of gonorrheal proctitis is 2.4 million units of procaine penicillin G intramuscularly with 1 gm of probenecid orally. Patients allergic to penicillin can be treated with 2 gm of specti-nomycin. These patients and their sexual contacts should receive follow-up care, including repeated cultures.

A common problem in homosexual men is nonspecific proctitis, which may have a clinical presentation similar to that of gonococcal proctitis. These patients should be evaluated thoroughly for parasitic and less common venereal diseases. If no cause is found, tetracycline, 1 gm/day for 10 days may be tried. The sexual partner also should be evaluated for venereal disease.

Suggested Readings

Black M: Acetaminophen hepatotoxicity. *Gastroenterology* 78:382–392, 1980

Blaser MJ, Berkowitz ID, LaForce FM et al: Campylobacter enteritis: Clinical and epidemiological features. *Ann Intern Med 91:*179–185, 1979

Boley SJ, DiBlase A, Brandt LJ, et al: Lower intestinal bleeding in the elderly. *Am J Surg 137:*57–64, 1979

Eastwood GL: Does early endoscopy benefit the patient with active upper gastrointestinal bleeding? *Gastroenterology 72:*737–739, 1977

Seeff LB, Hoofnagle JH: Immunoprophylaxis of viral hepatitis. *Gastroenterology 77:*161–182, 1979

Sleisenger RH, Fordtran JS (Eds): *Gastrointestinal Disease: Pathophysiology, Diagnosis, and Management.* 2nd ed, Philadelphia, WB Saunders, 1978

Wright R, Alberti KGMM (Eds): *Liver and Biliary Disease.* London, WB Saunders, 1979

CHAPTER 13

Hematologic Emergencies

LEONARD ELLMAN, M.D.

This chapter will focus on hematologic conditions that require immediate diagnostic or therapeutic intervention and that are likely to be seen in the emergency ward. An effort will be made to present the basic laboratory tests necessary for effective diagnosis.

HEMOLYTIC ANEMIA

Signs of Hemolysis

Hemolysis refers to premature destruction of red blood cells. The hallmark of hemolysis is a decreasing hematocrit without signs of blood loss. If erythroid production in the bone marrow increases sufficiently to compensate for the hemolysis, the hematocrit will remain stable, but the reticulocyte count will be persistently elevated and will suggest the presence of hemolysis. An elevated reticulocyte count immediately suggests hemolysis. However, the absence of reticulocytosis does not exclude hemolytic anemia since the bone marrow may be suppressed for a variety of reasons and may be unable to respond appropriately to the decreasing red blood cell count. Most cases of hemolysis are due to *extravascular* destruction of red blood cells by phagocytic cells in the liver and spleen, in which case hemoglobin is largely converted to bilirubin. Less commonly, hemolysis is *intravascular* and is characterized by the unique finding of free hemoglobin in the plasma and urine; if hemoglobinemia and hemoglobinuria persist, hemosiderinuria may develop. This is detected by performing the Prussian blue stain on the urinary sediment. Signs common to both intravascular and extravascular hemolysis include depressed or absent serum haptoglobin, indirect hyperbilirubinemia, the presence of serum methemalbumin, and elevated concentrations of serum lactate dehydrogenase (particularly in intravascular hemolysis) and urinary urobilinogen. The routine blood smear may also strongly suggest hemolytic anemia if spherocytes or fragmented red blood cells are present (Fig. 13.1). Intracellular organisms that cause hemolysis may also be seen on occasion (Fig. 13.2). On physical examination, jaundice, scleral icterus, and splenomegaly suggest a hemolytic process.

If hemolytic anemia develops suddenly (for example, after a transfusion reaction), presenting features may include back and abdominal pain, vomiting, headache, chills and fever, and occasionally shock. In the presence of hemoglobinuria, oliguria and renal failure may develop. More commonly, acquired hemolytic anemia develops insidiously and is characterized by pallor, jaundice, and the usual signs and symptoms of anemia such as fatigue, dyspnea, and palpitation.

Conditions That May Mimic Hemolysis

Certain conditions occasionally can be confused with hemolytic anemia. Occult hemorrhage with a brisk bone marrow response may be difficult to distinguish from hemolysis, particularly if the hemorrhage has occurred internally so that hyperbilirubinemia results from the reabsorption of hemoglobin breakdown products. Brisk recovery from iron, folate, or vitamin B_{12} deficiency may also mimic hemolysis because of the combination of anemia and a high reticulocyte count. Myoglobinuria resulting from severe muscle injury may suggest hemolysis because the red urine may be mistaken for a sign of hemoglobinuria. Myoglobin, however, is a protein of small molecular weight, and it is rapidly cleared from the plasma. In contrast, when hemoglobinuria is present, the plasma usually remains pink for several hours since the larger size of the hemoglobin molecule leads to a slower clearance by the kidney. Definitive identification of the urinary pigment can be made by means of electrophoresis or spectrophotometry.

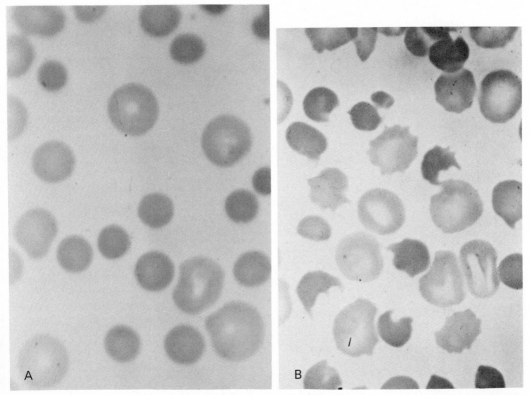

Figure 13.1. Hemolytic anemia. **(A)** Spherocytes, which are generally smaller than normal red blood cells, perfectly round, and lacking in central pallor. They are the hallmark of immune hemolytic anemia and hereditary spherocytosis. **(B)** Fragmented red blood cells, which result from shearing trauma to red cell membrane and which indicate microangiopathic hemolytic anemia.

Classification of Hemolytic Anemia

Discussion of all of the causes of hemolytic anemia is beyond the scope of this chapter. Distinctions can be made, however, that will assist the physician in making a differential diagnosis. *Intravascular hemolysis* vs. *extravascular hemolysis* is one such distinction. Hemoglobinemia, hemoglobinuria, and hemosiderinuria in patients with intravascular hemolysis immediately call attention to the disorders listed in Table 13.1, many of which require immediate therapy. Hemolytic anemia may also be classified as *inherited* or *acquired*. The inherited disorders are frequently characterized by a family history of the disease, and are usually due to a fundamental defect in synthesis of the red blood cell membrane, an enzyme, or globin. Patients with congenital hemolytic anemia frequently have a history of recurrent anemia and icterus, often first noted in childhood. Congenital hemolytic anemia may be first suspected because of gallstones at a young age.

Major categories of inherited hemolytic disorders include:

(1) Defects in the red blood cell membrane, as in hereditary spherocytosis, elliptocytosis, and stomatocytosis. These disorders are readily diagnosed by examination of the blood smear.

(2) Defects in the Embden-Meyerhof pathway of glycolysis, as in pyruvate kinase deficiency. These disorders are rare, and special enzyme tests are required to confirm the diagnosis.

(3) Defects in the hexose monophosphate shunt pathway, the most common of which is glucose-6-phosphate dehydrogenase deficiency.

(4) Defects in globin structure, as in unstable hemoglobin disease. These disorders are also rare and require specialized tests.

Glucose-6-Phosphate Dehydrogenase Deficiency

Among the inherited disorders, the most likely to be encountered in an emergency setting is a deficiency of glucose-6-phosphate dehydrogenase (G-6-PD), a key enzyme in the hexose monophos-

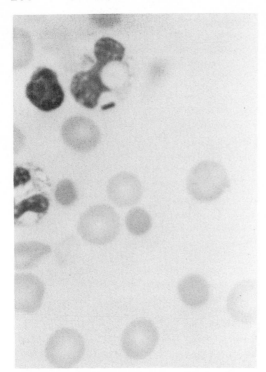

Figure 13.2. Hemolysis may result from *Clostridium perfringens* septicemia. Ingested bacteria may be present in polymorphonuclear leukocytes. Also note presence of spherocytes.

Table 13.1.
Conditions in which hemolytic anemia is predominantly intravascular.

Immunohemolytic anemia
  Acute or delayed transfusion reaction
  Paroxysmal cold hemoglobinuria
  Some cases of Coombs'-positive, warm autoimmune hemolytic anemia
  Some cases of cold agglutinin disease
Disorders associated with red blood cell fragmentation, eg, malfunctioning prosthetic heart valve
Infection
  Falciparum malaria
  Clostridial sepsis
Complications due to chemical agents
  Acute drug reaction in patient with glucose-6-phosphate dehydrogenase deficiency
  Arsine poisoning
  Snake and spider venoms
  Intravenous infusion of distilled water
Thermal injury
Physical injury, eg, march hemoglobinuria
Paroxysmal nocturnal hemoglobinuria

phate shunt. Normal function of this pathway is required for the red blood cell to withstand oxidative stress that otherwise leads to denaturation of hemoglobin and intravascular hemolysis.

Disorders due to G-6-PD deficiency are common in the black population and to a much lesser extent in persons from the Mediterranean basin, the Middle East, and Thailand. Since the gene for G-6-PD activity is carried on the X chromosome, inheritance is sex-linked. In the United States, 10–12% of black males and 1–2% of black females have G-6-PD deficiency.

The mechanism of hemolysis in the common variety of G-6-PD deficiency occurring in blacks is due to premature loss of G-6-PD activity as the red blood cell ages. As the bone marrow responds with the production of reticulocytes, G-6-PD activity increases because of the younger population of red blood cells. As a result, episodes of G-6-PD hemolysis in the black population are usually mild and self-limited. No specific therapy is required except omission of drugs that induce hemolysis; blood transfusion is rarely required. In contrast, in many of the forms of G-6-PD deficiency in the white population, there is severe lack of G-6-PD

activity; these forms are characterized by chronic hemolytic anemia with severe exacerbations after exposure to oxidative stress.

In the absence of oxidative stress, the peripheral blood of blacks with G-6-PD deficiency appears normal. During a hemolytic crisis, cells containing Heinz bodies (globules of denatured hemoglobin) may be transiently present when blood smears are made with supravital stains such as brilliant cresyl blue. Heinz bodies may be noted while performing a reticulocyte count since the stain used is a supravital stain. Many screening tests for G-6-PD deficiency are widely available; results may be falsely negative during the acute phase of hemolysis as a result of the elevated reticulocyte count.

Table 13.2 lists the principal agents causing G-6-PD hemolysis. If these agents are taken in sufficient amounts by normal persons, a similar hemolysis may develop. It is important to note that stressful physical situations in general, such as bacterial infections and diabetic ketoacidosis, can induce hemolysis in G-6-PD deficient individuals in the absence of the ingestion of oxidative medications.

Acquired Hemolytic Anemia

Although acquired hemolytic anemia may have an insidious onset, it is not associated with the features that suggest a congenital hemolytic anemia, such as episodes of anemia and jaundice in

Table 13.2.
Drugs associated with hemolysis in persons with glucose-6-phosphate dehydrogenase deficiency.

Antimalarial agents
  Primaquine phosphate
  Pamaquine
  Chloroquine
  Quinacrine hydrochloride (Atabrine)
Sulfonamide compounds
  Sulfanilamide
  Sulfisoxazole (Gantrisin)
  Salicylazosulfapyridine (Azulfidine)
  Sulfacetamide (Sulamyd)
  Sulfamethoxypyridazine
Antibiotics
  Nitrofurantoin (Furadantin)
  Chloramphenicol[a]
  Para-aminosalicylic acid
Analgesics
  Aspirin
  Phenacetin
Miscellaneous
  Quinine[a]
  Quinidine[a]
  Procainamide hydrochloride (Pronestyl)
  Probenecid
  Vitamin K (water-soluble analogues)

[a] Not hemolytic in blacks.

Table 13.3.
Immune hemolytic anemia.

Acute or delayed transfusion reaction due to incompatible blood
Autoimmune hemolytic anemia due to warm-reactive antibodies
  Idiopathic
  Secondary
    Lymphoproliferative disease
    Other malignant disease
    Systemic lupus erythematosus and other autoimmune disorders
  Drug induced (penicillin, quinidine, quinine, chlorpropamide, α-methyldopa (Aldomet), L-dopa, etc.)
Autoimmune hemolytic anemia due to cold-reactive antibodies
  Cold agglutinin disease
    Idiopathic
    Secondary
      Lymphoproliferative disease
      Mycoplasmal infection
      Infectious mononucleosis
  Paroxysmal cold hemoglobinuria

childhood, a family history of anemia, and gallstones. The acquired hemolytic anemias that have clinical importance may be classified in two main groups: immune disorders in which antibodies and complement play a major role in red blood cell destruction, and secondary conditions in which red blood cell destruction results from physical trauma to the cell from chemicals and toxins, infectious agents, or microangiopathic processes. Tables 13.3 and 13.4 list the types of acquired hemolytic anemia and their causes.

Autoimmune Hemolytic Anemia

The hallmark of autoimmune hemolytic anemia (AIHA) is a positive *direct Coombs' test*, which reveals the presence of antibody and complement on the red blood cell surface. If such antibody is also present in the serum, it can be detected by means of the *indirect Coombs' test*.

In terms of clinical presentation and laboratory findings, it is convenient to divide AIHA into warm AIHA, in which the antibody combines with the red blood cell optimally at 37°C, and cold AIHA, in which the antibody combines optimally at 0–4°C and shows progressively decreased affinity for the red blood cell antigens at higher temperatures. In addition to a positive direct Coombs'

test, cold AIHA is characterized by a high titer of cold agglutinins (more than 1:200). In this test the highest dilution of the patient's serum is determined that will cause agglutination of type O red blood cells in the cold. In contrast with warm AIHA, in which the antibody is of the IgG class, cold agglutinin disease is due to an IgM antibody.

AIHA can be acute and fulminating, but more commonly it is chronic and insidious. In patients with cold agglutinin disease, acute exacerbations with hemoglobinemia and hemoglobinuria may occur after exposure to the cold. In such patients, Raynaud's phenomenon or passing dark urine after cold exposure may be the first recognized abnormality. Slight to moderate splenomegaly is the most common physical finding in both warm and cold types. Examination of the blood smear is of considerable value. In warm AIHA, the characteristic findings are large numbers of spherocytes and often many polychromatophilic cells representing reticulocytes. In cold AIHA, spherocytosis is less common, and the blood smear more frequently shows large clumps of red blood cells. Both warm and cold AIHA may be secondary to underlying disorders (Table 13.3), and the precipitating factor should be sought in any patient with this diagnosis.

In the management of AIHA, transfusions should be avoided if possible, since the transfused cells will be hemolyzed just as rapidly as the patient's red blood cells. In fact, crossmatching

Table 13.4.
Additional types of acquired hemolytic anemia.

Microangiopathic hemolytic anemia
   Prosthetic valves and cardiac abnormalities
   Hemolytic-uremic syndrome
   Disseminated intravascular coagulation
   Thrombotic thrombocytopenic purpura
   Hemangioma
   Disseminated carcinoma
   Malignant hypertension
Infectious disease
   Clostridial sepsis
   Bartonellosis
   Malaria
   Toxoplasmosis
   Leishmaniasis
Anemia due to chemicals, drugs, or venoms
   Chemicals and toxins
     Naphthalene
     Nitrofurantoin (Furadantin)
     Sulfonamides
     Sulfones
     Phenacetin
     Phenylhydrazine
     Para-aminosalicylic acid
     Phenol derivatives
     Arsine
     Water
     Copper
Anemia due to physical agents
   Thermal injury
   March hemoglobinuria
Miscellaneous
   Hypophosphatemia
   Paroxysmal nocturnal hemoglobinuria
   Spur-cell anemia in severe hepatic disease

may be very difficult since the autoantibody, which frequently is present in the patient's serum, may react with virtually all units of blood in the blood bank. In this case, the unit of blood showing the weakest reaction pattern in vitro can be administered, with careful monitoring and cessation of the transfusion if signs of increased hemolysis develop.

Three-fourths of patients with warm AIHA respond initially to prednisone, 1 mg/kg/day. Unfortunately, most patients relapse as the corticosteroid is tapered, and splenectomy often becomes necessary. Most patients with cold AIHA related to infection require no treatment aside from warmth and rest, since the illness is transient. Management of chronic cold agglutinin disease is not very satisfactory, however, since corticosteroids and splenectomy are usually of little value. Keeping the patient warm and transfusing packed red blood cells when necessary is often the prin-

cipal form of therapy. Red blood cells should be washed in saline before transfusion to remove complement, which may exacerbate the hemolysis in cold AIHA. In all chronic hemolytic states, the folic acid requirement increases, and folic acid should be administered prophylactically.

SICKLE CELL ANEMIA

Pathophysiologic Principles

Sickle cell anemia (homozygous sickle cell disease) is the most common genetic disease seen in clinical practice. As a result of many years of research, much is now known about the cause of this condition. Normal adult human hemoglobin (hemoglobin A) consists of two α and two β chains. In sickle cell anemia, a single amino acid substitution of glutamic acid for valine occurs on the β chains, resulting in substantial alterations in the physicochemical properties of the hemoglobin molecule (hemoglobin S). In addition to a change in the electrophoretic mobility of the hemoglobin, erythrocytes from patients with homozygous sickle cell disease assume the sickle shape when they are deprived of oxygen. Sickling also is fostered by a decrease in pH. When enough cells have assumed the sickle shape, blood viscosity increases considerably and reduced blood flow results. Local impairment of circulation leads to further hypoxia and acidosis, and this engenders further sickling. A cycle occurs in which more and more cells become sickled, causing local blockage of the circulation and ischemic infarction. This sequence can occur in virtually any organ of the body, leading clinically to the painful "sickle crisis."

Sickle Cell Trait

Sickle cell anemia is inherited as a recessive gene according to Mendelian law. In the heterozygous state, sickle cell trait, only one β locus is affected and the red blood cell contains approximately equal amounts of hemoglobin A and hemoglobin S. The structure of the red blood cell is normal, and no anemia is present. Sickle cell trait is found in 8–11% of the black population in the United States and to a much smaller extent in persons of Greek, Italian, and Middle Eastern ancestry. Since the red blood cells in a person with sickle cell trait contain both hemoglobin A and hemoglobin S, they require much greater deoxygenation before sickling develops. As a result, sickle crises occur only during extreme conditions of deoxygenation such as flying in an unpressurized aircraft.

There are few established complications of

sickle cell trait. The structure of Henle's loop facilitates sickling in this area, leading to dysfunction of the loop and hyposthenuria. Painless hematuria, more commonly from the left kidney, is the most frequent complication of medical significance. Hematuria occasionally may be prolonged and recurrent, and may respond to treatment with diuretics or intravenous alkali. Priapism, occlusion of the central retinal artery, and splenic infarction are rarely reported. The longevity of persons with sickle cell trait appears to be normal.

Homozygous Sickle Cell Disease

In homozygous sickle cell disease, both β loci are affected, and the patient has only hemoglobin S, except for residual amounts of fetal hemoglobin (hemoglobin F). The clinical problems of sickle cell anemia can be divided into three major categories:

(1) Repeated episodes of vascular occlusion with pain, fever, and end-organ damage (sickle crisis). The pain, which usually is described as gnawing, gradually increases in the course of several hours; it commonly involves the extremities, the joints, the abdomen, and the chest, although it may affect virtually any organ. There are generally no specific clinical or laboratory findings that identify the episode as sickle crisis. Diagnosis may be aided by the prior experience of the patient, since many have a consistent pattern of pain. At times, however, it may be extremely difficult to differentiate sickle crisis from other conditions such as pulmonary embolism, appendicitis, or cholecystitis.

(2) Chronic hemolytic anemia due to the short survival time of the rigid sickle cells. The hematocrit value is usually from 20–30%.

(3) Frequent, severe infections, including Salmonella osteomyelitis, pneumococcal pneumonia, pneumococal meningitis, and mycoplasma pneumonia. Many factors appear to contribute to the high incidence of severe infection; the factors include functional asplenia, lack of bacterial opsonins, impairment of activity of the complement pathway, and defective phagocytic activity. Local factors such as stasis and tissue necrosis also may be important in bacterial growth. Persons with sickle cell anemia respond to infection poorly, and prompt antibiotic therapy should be started for presumed infection, especially if the pneumococcus is suspected.

Special mention should be made of pulmonary complications. In persons with sickle cell anemia, occlusive phenomena may develop in the pulmonary arteries. In addition, marrow and fat emboli from infarcted bone marrow, as well as emboli from peripheral veins, occur with considerable frequency. Pulmonary infection is also extremely common. Hence, elucidation of the cause of chest pain and lung infiltrates may be extremely difficult. The value of lung scanning and pulmonary angiographic examination in this setting has not yet been clearly established. Transtracheal aspiration and bronchial brushing may be helpful in recognizing bacterial infection, and possible sepsis should be treated vigorously.

Laboratory Tests

Sickle cells (Fig. 13.3) are not seen on a routine blood smear of the peripheral blood from a patient with sickle cell trait. Thus, the presence of sickle cells indicates sickle cell anemia or a major variant such as sickle cell-hemoglobin C disease.

The sickling phenomenon can be induced by several maneuvers that depend on the deoxygenation of hemoglobin. Sodium metabisulfite is the classic agent used to induce sickling in sickle cell anemia or sickle cell trait. This screening test largely has been replaced by commercially prepared tests, such as the Sickledex test, that allow rapid detection of hemoglobin S on the basis of its

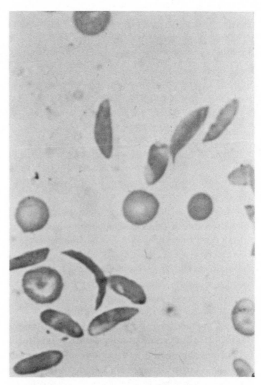

Figure 13.3. Sickle cell anemia. Peripheral blood smear with sickle cells characterized by pointed configuration at both ends of cell.

decreased solubility in high phosphate buffer solutions. Electrophoresis of hemoglobin on various media such as paper or cellulose acetate remains the definitive method for identification of hemoglobin S. It also readily allows differentiation between sickle cell trait and homozygous sickle cell anemia.

Therapy

Since painful episodes are often precipitated by infection, fever, and perhaps excessive cold, measures that prevent or remedy these conditions are important. Vigorous hydration and analgesics have remained the mainstay of therapy for the painful crisis. Patients with sickle cell anemia are likely to become dehydrated because of chronic hyposthenuria. Dehydration is a particular danger because it increases the concentration of hemoglobin S in the red blood cells, and therefore increases the tendency for sickling. Since acidosis enhances sickling, some physicians recommend administration of sodium bicarbonate and sodium lactate for alkalization. However, use of these agents remains controversial.

Transfusion with several units of normal blood or exchange transfusion to dilute the percentage of sickled cells is probably beneficial in patients with life-threatening complications such as impending cerebral infarction. Transfusion therapy before a surgical procedure is useful in decreasing sickle crises during and after operation, and may also be useful in patients with almost constantly recurring crises. Limited exchange transfusion may also decrease the duration of painful crises. Transfusion therapy, however, has the associated complications of hepatic and iron overload, and may lead to development of minor blood group incompatibilities that make future transfusions more difficult.

Administration of oxygen to patients with painful crises offers little benefit, and if it is continued, it may lead to suppression of red blood cell production and exacerbation of anemia. Oxygen, however, should be given liberally to patients with cardiopulmonary disease or pneumonia. Hyperbaric oxygen therapy has been utilized with uncertain results in intracerebral sickling.

Many agents have been employed in attempts to abort painful crises, usually without significant benefit. Enthusiasm for urea, one of the newer agents, has largely disappeared. Potassium cyanate prevents sickling in vitro as a result of "carbamylation" of the terminal nitrogen atom on the hemoglobin molecule. Carbamylation inhibits the sickling process, and also increases the oxygen affinity of hemoglobin S, which indirectly decreases the tendency for sickling. Unfortunately, clinical trial with potassium cyanate has failed to show a decrease in the incidence of painful crises, and has been associated with the development of cataracts and peripheral neuropathy.

Related Syndromes

Other types of hemoglobin present in the red blood cell along with hemoglobin S can significantly influence the extent of sickling. For example, hemoglobin S-thalassemia tends to be milder than sickle cell anemia because the presence of hemoglobin F, hemoglobin A, and hemoglobin A_2 tends to solubilize the hemoglobin S. Similarly, sickle cell-hemoglobin C disease is usually milder than sickle cell anemia because hemoglobin C has less of a tendency for sickling than hemoglobin S. Homozygous hemoglobin C disease is also milder than sickle cell anemia, but vascular occlusive crises do occur. Hemoglobin C trait is asymptomatic.

METHEMOGLOBINEMIA

Methemoglobin is hemoglobin with its iron atom in the oxidized, ferric state rather than the usual ferrous state. Methemoglobin is not capable of carrying oxygen reversibly as is hemoglobin. When the concentration of methemoglobin rises, the result is tissue hypoxia, which is clinically evident as cyanosis. Methemoglobinemia should be suspected whenever cyanosis occurs in a patient with normal arterial blood-gas oxygen saturation. An easy screening test is to draw a small amount of blood from a cyanotic patient and shake it with air. If the blood fails to become red, the cyanosis is not due to hypoxia and methemoglobinemia is strongly suggested. Definitive diagnosis involves spectrophotometric determination in the laboratory. The normal amount of methemoglobin is less then 1% of total hemoglobin. Patients with methemoglobin levels of 10–20% are asymptomatic, but higher levels are associated with headache, dizzyness, dyspnea, tachycardia, and stupor. When the level rises to 70%, death occurs rapidly.

Methemoglobinemia can be inherited, or acquired by normal individuals as a result of toxic exposures. The two hereditary varieties are very rare and include M hemoglobins, abnormal hemoglobins which promote oxidation of the iron in hemoglobin, and deficiencies of the nicotinamide adenine dinucleotide (NADH) methemoglobin reductase enzyme system, which normally reduces the small amounts of naturally occurring methemoglobin. Patients with the congenital varieties are generally asymptomatic despite being cyanotic. The extremely rare individual with homozygous deficiency may have mental retardation. Acquired methemoglobinemia in normal individuals results from exposure to a variety of oxidant agents. Nitrites and nitrates are the most common causes of acquired methemoglobinemia. Sodium nitrite, which is used as a preservative, has caused many cases due to accidental poisoning. Infants and young children are particularly vulnerable to high concentration of nitrates in the water supply, which most commonly occurs from water run-off containing fertilizers used in agriculture. Certain medications which have oxidant properties, such as antimalarials (see Table 13.2) are another cause of acquired methemoglobinemia in normal individuals when taken in excess. Methemoglobinemia also can be acquired as a result of excessive skin absorption of oxidant dyes such as aniline compounds.

For the asymptomatic patient with acquired methemoglobinemia, no treatment is necessary aside from omitting the toxic drug. If the patient has a methemoglobin level greater than 20–30% and is symptomatic, oxygen administration may be helpful. Efforts should also be made to eliminate the toxic agent through catharsis or gastric lavage. Methylene blue can also be used to reduce the methemoglobin to hemoglobin. The dose is 3–5 mg/kg orally, or 1–2 mg/kg by slow intravenous infusion; repeated doses may be needed.

MEGALOBLASTIC ANEMIA

Diagnosis

Clinical Features

Anemia due to vitamin B_{12} or folic acid deficiency is a common cause of severe anemia encountered in the emergency ward. Because megaloblastic anemia develops gradually, there is sufficient time for hemodynamic compensation to occur, and patients may look well despite profound anemia. Moderate neutropenia and thrombocytopenia are also frequently present, although complications due to infection and bleeding are uncommon. In addition to the general features of anemia such as weakness and shortness of breath, patients with megaloblastic anemia often have glossitis and mild jaundice. Patients with vitamin B_{12} deficiency often suffer from peripheral neuropathy or degeneration of the posterior and pyramidal tracts of the spinal cord (combined systems disease), resulting in paresthesia, loss of vibration and position sense, muscular weakness, difficulty in walking, and occasionally, psychotic behavior.

Folic acid deficiency may cause mental slowness and, rarely, mild dementia, but does not cause significant organic nervous system disease.

Laboratory Tests

The diagnosis of megaloblastic anemia is usually easy to make from the blood smear and from the bone marrow aspirate (sternal or iliac crest). The peripheral smear is characterized by giant macrocytes and hypersegmentation of the neutrophils, that is, neutrophils with six or seven nuclear lobes or more than 5% with five nuclear lobes (Fig. 13.4). As a result of the macrocytes, the mean corpuscular volume is elevated, often with values as high as 120–130. The bone marrow is also characteristic, with a hypercellular appearance and dissociation between nuclear and cytoplasmic development of the erythroblasts, the nucleus maintaining a primitive appearance with fine, lacy chromatin despite normal maturation of the cytoplasm. The myeloid series is characterized by large, abnormally shaped bands and metamyelocytes. The reticulocyte count is very low, particularly when the degree of anemia is considered. The serum lactate dehydrogenase concentration is frequently substantially elevated, and the indirect bilirubin level is mildly elevated.

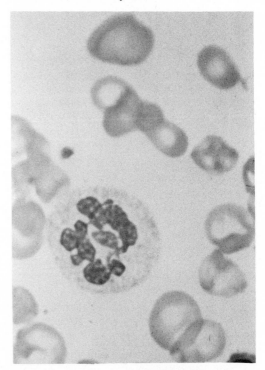

Figure 13.4. Megaloblastic anemia. Blood smear is noteworthy because of hypersegmented polymorphonuclear leukocytes and macrocytes.

It is often possible to determine whether vitamin B_{12} or folic acid deficiency is present from the patient's history (Table 13.5). However, confirmation depends on measurement of the serum levels of the two vitamins, and it is essential to obtain results of these tests before starting therapy. The presence of achlorhydria and the absence of gastric intrinsic factor as demonstrated in the Schilling test help confirm the diagnosis of pernicious anemia.

Therapy

It is usually possible to establish which of the two deficiencies is the cause of megaloblastic anemia and to treat the patient with the appropriate vitamin. Vitamin B_{12}, 100–1000 µg/day intramuscularly for 7–10 days, or folic acid, 2–5 mg/day orally, is adequate initial therapy. If the cause of megaloblastic anemia is unclear, treatment can be started with both vitamins until the results of

Table 13.5.
Causes of megaloblastic anemia.

Vitamin B_{12} deficiency
    Pernicious anemia
    Gastrectomy
    Intestinal absorptive defects
        Ileal resection
        Regional enteritis
        Celiac disease
        Malabsorption syndrome
    Competitive parasites
        Fish tapeworm
    Diverticula and blind loop syndrome
    Vegetarian diet very deficient in vitamin B_{12}
Folic acid deficiency
    Poor diet
        Alcoholism
        Food faddism
        Gastrectomy
        Other
    Impaired absorption
        Intrinsic intestinal disease
        Malabsorption syndrome
    Increased requirement
        Pregnancy
        Tumor
        Hemolytic anemia
    Drugs
        Folate antagonists
            Methotrexate
            Trimethoprim
            Pyrimethamine
        Phenytoin
        Oral contraceptives
        Triamterene
        Barbiturates
        Tetracycline

serum folate and B_{12} determinations are available. Transfusion is usually unnecessary because of the rapid response to the hematinics. If symptoms such as angina or congestive heart failure are due to severe anemia, packed red blood cells should be administered slowly.

Potassium supplements are also recommended in patients with normal renal function along with vitamin replacement because of the danger of hypokalemia that may develop during the initial hematologic response. Sudden death during this period may result from arrhythmias induced by hypokalemia.

ERYTHROCYTOSIS AND POLYCYTHEMIA

Classification

The upper limit of the hematocrit value in healthy men is 54%, and in healthy women it is 49%. *Relative erythrocytosis* refers to the situation in which the hematocrit is elevated because of a decrease in plasma volume. Relative erythrocytosis usually has a brief course, and is due to such causes as excessive diuresis, severe diarrhea or vomiting, and profuse sweating. Therapy consists of fluid replacement and correction of the underlying cause of volume depletion.

A few persons, who are usually young men, have a chronic form of pseudoerythrocytosis that has been referred to as *Gaisböck's syndrome* or *stress erythrocytosis*. Although the hematocrit level may be as high as 60%, the red blood cell mass is not increased. Complaints include headache, dizziness, and paresthesia, but symptoms are usually not alleviated by phlebotomy. It is doubtful that stress erythrocytosis is a true clinical entity, and no specific therapy is indicated.

True increases in the red blood cell mass occur in *secondary erythrocytosis* and *polycythemia vera*. Secondary erythrocytosis refers to an absolute increase in the red blood cell mass unassociated with a myeloproliferative disorder. The white blood cell count and the platelet count are normal. Causes of secondary erythrocytosis can be divided into two major categories (Table 13.6). The first category includes conditions associated with appropriate increases in the erythropoietin concentration resulting from tissue hypoxia. Severe pulmonary disease, in which oxygen saturation is less than 90%, and cyanotic congenital heart disease are the most common examples. The second category includes lesions resulting in inappropriate erythropoietin elaboration, such as tumors, cysts, and various renal conditions.

The absolute erythrocytosis of polycythemia

Table 13.6.
Causes of secondary erythrocytosis.

Appropriate erythropoietin production due to decreased oxygen transport
  High altitude
  Inadequate functioning hemoglobin
    Hemoglobin Chesapeake, etc.
    Congenital methemoglobinemia
  Pulmonary disease with oxygen saturation < 90%
  Cyanotic congenital cardiac disease with right-to-left shunt
  Cigarette smoking with elevated carbon monoxide level in blood
Inappropriate erythropoietin production unrelated to oxygen transport
  Malignant lesion in kidney, liver, adrenal gland, lung
  Benign disease
    Uterine myoma
    Renal cyst
    Hydronephrosis
    Cerebellar hemangioma
    Pheochromocytoma
    Cushing's syndrome
  Exogenous agents
    Cobalt
    Testosterone

vera is part of a panmyelopathy characterized by leukocytosis, thrombocytosis, basophilia, splenomegaly, hepatomegaly, and pruritus, especially after bathing.

Therapy

The relation between blood viscosity and hematocrit is characterized by a steep curve; small increases in the hematocrit level above 60% lead to substantial increases in the blood viscosity. The symptoms and signs of polycythemia vera can be attributed primarily to the expanded blood volume and to the slowing of the blood flow that results from the increased viscosity. The main form of emergency therapy for polycythemia vera is phlebotomy. Morbidity and mortality are decreased considerably by lowering the hematocrit to the normal range, and this fact is particularly important for patients with polycythemia vera who are to undergo a surgical procedure. In these patients, phlebotomy should be performed on an emergency basis, if necessary, before operation. Blood obtained by phlebotomy may be stored and then used for replacement during operation if it is needed. Long-term treatment of polycythemia vera may involve use of radioactive phosphorus or alkylating agents to suppress the bone marrow in addition to phlebotomy.

The decision to perform phlebotomy for secondary erythrocytosis resulting from appropriate elaboration of erythropoietin, as in chronic pulmonary disease or cyanotic congenital heart disease, is less clear-cut. Erythrocytosis in these situations usually is regarded as a compensatory response to tissue hypoxia. Nonetheless, phlebotomy should be performed if the increased blood volume and viscosity appear to be related to symptoms such as congestive heart failure or impending vascular thrombosis. Return of the red blood cell mass to normal improves pulmonary vascular resistance in patients with cor pulmonale and erythrocytosis. If phlebotomy is performed, time must be allowed for equilibration of vascular volume.

HYPERVISCOSITY SYNDROME

Blood viscosity increases substantially in both polycythemia and sickle cell anemia. However, the term "hyperviscosity syndrome" usually is applied only to situations in which serum viscosity increases as a result of greatly increased concentrations of abnormal plasma proteins. The hyperviscosity syndrome is a prominent feature of Waldenström's macroglobulinemia, and is less commonly seen in patients with multiple myeloma and Sjögren's syndrome. The hyperviscosity syndrome has certain characteristic features, including bleeding from mucous membranes; visual disturbance and retinopathy consisting of venous engorgement, hemorrhages, and occasionally papilledema; neurologic disorders such as headaches, seizures, and coma; congestive heart failure; and severe lethargy. It is unusual for a patient to become symptomatic until the serum becomes four times as viscous as water (normal viscosity of serum is less than 1.5 that of water). In an emergency, the viscosity of water and serum can be estimated with a white blood cell pipette and a stopwatch by measuring the time it takes the meniscus to fall from above the bulb to below the bulb of the pipette.

A patient with symptomatic hyperviscosity syndrome should undergo plasmapheresis. Two to four units of plasma daily can be removed, allowing time for equilibration of the plasma volume; if necessary, saline solution or colloid can be infused to maintain vascular volume. Plasmaphresis is greatly facilitated on the centrifugal type of cell separator (Celltrifuge, American Instrument Company). This device was developed to allow selective isolation and removal of granulocytes or platelets, but it also allows efficient plasma exchange. Plasmapheresis tends to be less effective for hyperviscosity due to multiple myeloma or Sjögren's syndrome, since the abnormal protein is less restricted to the intravascular compartment. Long-term therapy for the hyperviscosity syndrome involves chemotherapy, usually with an alkylating agent.

GRANULOCYTOPENIA

Leukopenia refers to depression of the total white blood cell count to fewer than 3500 cells/mm^3; *neutropenia* and *granulocytopenia* refer to a total neutrophil (or granulocyte) count of fewer than 1500 cells/mm^3. Susceptibility to infection becomes a serious problem when the neutrophil count decreases to fewer than 1000 cells/mm^3, and is extremely hazardous when the count is fewer than 500 cells/mm^3. *Agranulocytosis* describes almost complete disappearance of granulocytes from the blood.

The major causes of neutropenia are listed in Table 13.7. Biopsy of the bone marrow often is valuable in the evaluation of leukopenia, particularly in determining whether a primary disorder of the marrow is present. Neutropenia may be due to severe sepsis, and is associated with a high mortality in this setting. A careful drug history is a necessity since drugs are the principal cause of acute neutropenia is clinical practice. Table 13.8 lists the most important drugs causing neutropenia.

Agranulocytosis

The form of neutropenia with the most striking presentation is acute drug-induced agranulocyto-

Table 13.7.
Causes of neutropenia.

Infection
  Typhoid fever
  Rickettsial infection
  Malaria
  Kala-azar
  Viral infection
  Overwhelming infection
    Miliary tuberculosis
    Septicemia, especially in debilitated patients
Aplastic anemia
Myelophthisis
  Myelofibrosis
  Leukemia
  Carcinoma or granuloma involving bone marrow
Hypersplenism
Megaloblastic anemia
Felty's syndrome
Systemic lupus erythematosus
Drugs
Miscellaneous
  Cyclic neutropenia
  Hypothyroidism
  Anaphylactoid shock
  Other

Table 13.8.
Drugs and physical agents causing neutropenia and agranulocytosis.

Agents that produce marrow hypoplasia in all persons if given in sufficient doses
  Ionizing radiation
  Benzene
  Chemotherapeutic agents
    Nitrogen mustard
    Chlorambucil
    Cyclophosphamide
    Phenylalanine mustard
    Methotrexate
    6-mercaptopurine
    5-fluorouracil
    Cytosine arabinoside
    Daunomycin
    Adriamycin
    Other
Drugs that occasionally cause neutropenia as result of individual sensitivity
  Analgesics
    Aminopyrine
    Phenylbutazone
    Indomethacin
  Sulfonamide compounds
  Thiazide diuretics
  Oral hypoglycemic agents
  Phenothiazines
  Antithyroid drugs
    Propylthiouracil
    Methimazole
  Antimicrobial agents
    Chloramphenicol
    Isoniazid
    Cephalothin
    Semisynthetic penicillins
  Antihistamines

sis. This usually is due to myeloid suppression in the bone marrow after many days to weeks of drug therapy. Less commonly, acute agranulocytosis develops almost immediately after use of a drug as a result of an immune form of peripheral granulocyte destruction mediated by an antibody.

The onset of agranulocytosis is indicated by high fever, shaking chills, sore throat, and oral ulceration. The appearance of the bone marrow is variable; there may be a substantial decrease in myeloid elements or there may be adequate numbers of promyelocytes and myelocytes but markedly decreased numbers of more mature forms (so-called maturation arrest). Occasionally, the bone marrow appears entirely normal. Other diseases that may be confused with acute agranulocytosis include aleukemic leukemia, aplastic anemia, and overwhelming bacterial infection with secondary severe granulocytopenia due to bone marrow suppression.

Initial therapy for agranulocytosis is omission of the offending agent or drug. Table 13.8 lists the more common drugs causing agranulocytosis, but since virtually any drug can induce this condition, it is usually necessary to omit all of the drugs that the patient is taking. Intensive broad-spectrum antibiotic coverage with bactericidal agents such as oxacillin and gentamicin should be instituted after bacteriologic cultures have been obtained. Lack of granulocytes may make the site of infection difficult to detect. For example, minimal infiltrates on a chest film and anal ulcers may be significant and should be monitored. High-grade septicemia is common in this group of patients, and is the usual cause of death. The general care of the patient is important, and careful attention should be given to oral and anal hygiene to prevent the occurrence of serious ulceration. Corticosteroids have not been proved effective in the treatment of agranulocytosis, and their use should be discouraged. With prompt omission of the offending agent, good supportive care, and antibiotic therapy, the condition of most patients can be kept stable until the granulocyte count becomes normal. For the patient whose infection is advancing and becomes life-threatening, consideration should be given to the daily administration of granulocyte transfusions harvested on a cell separator from a healthy ABO compatible donor.

LEUKOSTASIS CRISIS IN ACUTE MYELOID LEUKEMIAS

Patients with acute myeloid leukemia and acute monocytic leukemia who present with blast cell counts greater than $100,000/mm^3$ are at high risk of developing intravascular leukostasis. This leukostasis occurs in the small arteries of the lung or brain, but also may occur in other organs. The leukemic aggregates are associated with hemorrhage and infarction in the white matter of the brain and, to a lesser extent, in the lung. The leukostasis syndrome must be considered a medical emergency and physicians should be aware of the need for prompt treatment. A single, daily, oral dose of hydroxyurea, 50–100 mg/kg with a maximum dose of 6 gm/day, is effective in rapidly reducing the blast count and can be instituted in the interval before consultation or referral. Conventional chemotherapy for acute leukemia can be initiated simultaneously, but its peak effect does not occur for several days. If central nervous system symptoms have already become evident, emergency cranial irradiation is indicated; leukapheresis of the patient on a cell separator machine

should also be considered since it is highly effective at rapidly reducing the white count on a temporary basis.

The risks of cerebral and pulmonary leukostasis are much less in patients with acute lymphoblastic (lymphocytic) leukemia, probably because myeloblasts and monoblasts are larger than lymphoblasts and the mass of circulating leukocytes is much greater. The leukostasis syndrome does not appear to occur despite the height of the white count when the cells are mature as in chronic lymphocytic or chronic myelogenous leukemia.

COMPLICATIONS OF CHEMOTHERAPY

The armamentarium of chemotherapeutic agents is rapidly expanding and the potential toxicity of these agents is very large. The majority of chemotherapeutic agents are cytotoxic and affect all rapidly dividing cells. Hence, bone marrow depression with thrombocytopenia and granulocytopenia is very common and is the most frequently encountered serious complication of chemotherapy. Patients may require intensive supportive care including platelet and granulocyte transfusions for periods of intense or prolonged bone marrow depression associated with bleeding or infection.

Mucositis involving the mouth, alimentary tract and vagina manifested as oral and vaginal sores, and nausea and diarrhea are also frequently encountered. Treatment is supportive. Certain chemotherapeutic agents have unique toxicities unrelated to mucositis and bone marrow depression and these problems are summarized in Table 13.9.

BLEEDING DISORDERS

The rapid arrest of hemorrhage after injury is an extremely important defense mechanism. Although it is customary to consider platelets and the coagulation factors separately, the distinction is largely one of convenience since there is an integral relation between platelets and the coagulation cascade.

Platelets are essential for sealing tiny leaks that continuously develop in the walls of small blood vessels. In addition, they are the first defense in the presence of tissue injury. When tissue injury occurs and endothelial tissue is exposed, platelets adhere at the injured site. After adhesion, other platelets aggregate, adding to the adherent platelets. Aggregation is mediated both by adenosine diphosphate released by adherent platelets and possibly by collagen from the exposed vascular wall. Thus, platelets are essential for the formation of a primary hemostatic plug. Platelet aggregation may also induce constriction of the injured vessel

Table 13.9.
Non-hematologic complications of commonly used chemotherapeutic agents.

Agents	Complications
Vincristine (Oncovin)	Peripheral neuropathy Constipation, ileus Syndrome of inappropriate antidiuretic hormone secretion
Doxorubicin (Adriamycin)	Cardiac arrhythmia
Daunorubicin	Congestive heart failure
Bleomycin (Blenoxane)	Pulmonary infiltrates Pulmonary fibrosis Erythroderma Fever Hypotension
Busulfan (Myleran)	Pulmonary fibrosis
Cyclophosphamide (Cytoxan)	Sterile hemorrhagic cystitis Syndrome of inappropriate secretion of antidiuretic hormone Pulmonary fibrosis
Mithramycin (Mutamycin)	Renal toxicity
Nitrosoureas (BCNU, CCNU, methyl CCNU)	Renal toxicity Hepatic toxicity Pulmonary fibrosis
Methotrexate	Hepatic toxicity
Streptozitocin	Renal toxicity
Cis-Platinum	Renal toxicity Hemolytic anemia Ototoxicity
Procarbazine (Matulane)	Dermatitis Myalgias Arthralgias
Dimethyl-triozeno-imidazole-carboxamide (DTIC)	Influenza-like syndrome

wall through release of serotonin, a powerful vasoconstricting agent. Vasoconstriction assists hemostasis by reducing blood flow in the injured vessel.

While the primary hemostatic plug is forming, the exposed vascular endothelium and thromboplastins released by the injured tissue activate the coagulation cascade, which leads to deposition of fibrin in and around the platelet plug. The fibrin strengthens the plug and helps anchor it to the wall of the blood vessel. The clot then begins to contract, and a permanent hemostatic plug is formed.

The coagulation cascade (Fig. 13.5) involves the sequential interaction of the coagulation factors, each factor being activated by the one preceding it. The end point of the process is generation of large amounts of fibrin clot. The coagulation cascade has traditionally been divided into two overlapping pathways, the intrinsic and the extrinsic. All of the factors required for the intrinsic system are present in the circulating blood, and the system is assayed by the partial thromboplastin time (PTT). Injury to the vessel wall exposes collagen, which initiates the intrinsic system by activating Factor XII (Hageman factor). Lipid from platelets and calcium are required at several points in the pathway.

The extrinsic coagulation system, which is monitored by the prothrombin time (PT), depends on release of tissue thromboplastin from damaged cells or vascular endothelium. The tissue thromboplastin together with Factor VII activates Factor X. The remainder of the sequence is identical to that of the intrinsic system, with generation of fibrin clot. Although called the extrinsic system, this pathway is also intravascular, and contributes to fibrin formation along with the intrinsic system.

COAGULATION CASCADE

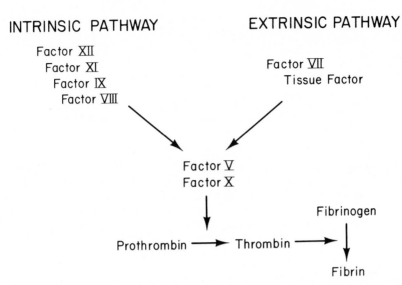

INTRINSIC PATHWAY　　　　EXTRINSIC PATHWAY

Factor XII
Factor XI
Factor IX
Factor VIII

Factor VII
Tissue Factor

Factor V
Factor X

Fibrinogen

Prothrombin ⟶ Thrombin ⟶

Fibrin

Figure 13.5. Coagulation cascade, which involves sequential interaction of coagulation factors with generation of fibrin. Both the intrinsic pathway, monitored by partial thromboplastin time, and the extrinsic pathway, monitored by prothrombin time, operate in vivo.

Evaluation of the Bleeding Patient

The clinical evaluation of a bleeding patient must include a careful history. It is important to determine whether the patient has a newly acquired bleeding disorder or a life-long disorder associated with bleeding at the time of circumcision, dental extraction, or menstruation, or after trauma. A family history of bleeding also may be informative in determining the presence of a congenital coagulation disorder. Hemophilia and Christmas disease occur almost exclusively in males since these are inherited, sex-linked conditions. In contrast, von Willebrand's disease is inherited as a dominant disorder, and occurs equally in males and females. A history of drug use should be obtained to determine whether the patient is receiving anticoagulants or drugs that impair platelet function. It is also important to seek information by means of the history and physical examination relating to possible underlying disease such as leukemia, uremia, and hepatic disease, since they affect the hemostatic process in well-defined ways.

Further information may be obtained from the type of bleeding. Most petechiae are due to thrombocytopenia. Widespread ecchymosis with hematuria and melena are common in patients with acquired coagulation defects such as defects resulting from sodium warfarin (Coumadin) or heparin excess and disseminated intravascular coagulation. In contrast, hemarthrosis and soft-tissue bleeding are characteristic of congenital coagulation defects such as hemophilia.

Laboratory Tests

The platelet count, bleeding time, PT, and PTT are an excellent set of screening tests for the bleeding patient. If results are normal, it is extremely unlikely that bleeding can be attributed to a coagulation defect.

Platelet Count. In most hospitals, platelet determinations are performed by direct count with a phase-contrast microscope or on an electronic counter. The normal count is 150,000–350,000 platelets/mm^3. Bleeding due to thrombocytopenia is unusual if the value is more than 70,000–90,000 platelets/mm^3. If a platelet count is not immediately available, a good estimate can be obtained from the blood smear; the oil immersion field normally contains 10–30 platelets, and significant thrombocytopenia can easily be detected.

Bleeding time. It is necessary to have not only adequate numbers of platelets but also platelets that function normally. Platelet function can be determined by measuring the bleeding time with Ivy's method: 40 mm Hg of pressure is maintained on the arm with a blood pressure cuff, and an incision 1 cm long and 1 mm deep is made on the volar surface of the forearm. The edge of the incision is gently blotted with filter paper at 30-second intervals. Bleeding for longer than 8–9 minutes suggests a disorder of platelet number or function. The bleeding time can be made more reproducible and accurate through use of a template and scalpel blade holder to ensure an incision of standard dimensions (Fig. 13.6). A spring-activated device (Simplate, General Diagnostics Co., Raritan, NJ) has become available and is recommended because of its ready availability and reproducibility of results. The bleeding time is not influenced by anticoagulation with sodium warfarin or by coagulation factor deficiencies. The bleeding time may be transiently elevated after large dose (10,000 U) bolus intravenous heparin injections.

Prothrombin Time. Tissue thromboplastin (whole brain extract) is added to plasma, and the time required for clotting is measured; the normal range is 11–13 seconds. The PT tests the integrity of the extrinsic system, and is routinely used to monitor oral anticoagulant therapy with coumarin derivatives.

Partial Thromboplastin Time. This test monitors the intrinsic system, and is performed in a similar manner to the PT except that an "incomplete" thromboplastin such as cephalin is substituted for whole brain extract. A surface-active agent such as kaolin is added to ensure complete activation of the contact factors (XII and XI). The normal PTT ranges from 25–40 seconds, depending on the technique employed. The PTT becomes prolonged when a factor in the intrinsic or common portion of the pathway is less than 25%.

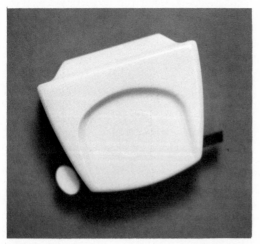

Figure 13.6. Bleeding-time kits that make the test more accurate and reproducible are now commercially available (Simplate, General Diagnostics Co.).

Specific Factor Assay. A sample of the patient's plasma is mixed with plasma from a congenitally deficient individual with zero factor activity. The clotting time of the mixture allows determination of the amount of the coagulation factor in the patient's plasma. Pooled plasma from a large number of healthy persons is used to define 100% activity. However, there is considerable variation of factor levels in healthy individuals, and the normal range for each factor is approximately 50–150%.

Normal Plasma Mix. This test determines whether abnormal results of a coagulation test are due to deficiency of a coagulation factor or are due to a circulating anticoagulant such as heparin or an antibody to a coagulation factor. A 1:1 mixture of the patient's plasma and normal plasma is made, and a PT, PTT, or specific factor assay is then performed. The 50% concentration of normal plasma in the mixture is adequate to correct for any factor deficiencies in the patient's plasma. Alternatively, if a circulating anticoagulant is present, the coagulation test will remain prolonged despite the addition of normal plasma.

Thrombin Time. A standardized amount of commercial thrombin is added to the patient's plasma. This test examines only the terminal portion of the coagulation cascade. The clotting time is usually about 20 seconds, depending on the technique. Prolonged thrombin times occur in severe hypofibrinogenemia, in the presence of heparin, and in the presence of large amounts of fibrin degradation products. The rare disorders in which fibrinogen fails to function normally (dysfibrinogenemia) are also characterized by a prolonged thrombin time. The thrombin time is not influenced by coumarin anticoagulants.

Fibrin Degradation Products. Increased amounts of fibrin degradation products (also called fibrin split products) occur in conditions in which there is excessive activation of the fibrinolytic system with digestion of fibrin. Increased concentrations of these substances are the hallmark of disseminated intravascular coagulation and primary fibrinolysis. Several methods are available for determination of the fibrin degradation products, including a rapid, accurate slide agglutination technique (Thrombo-Wellco-test).

Fibrinogen Level. Fibrinogen can be determined quantitatively by several techniques that measure the fibrin clot directly, or it can be estimated less accurately by tests such as the thrombin time.

Fibrin Stabilizing Factor (Factor XIII). Factor XIII deficiency, a rare disorder associated with delayed bleeding, is detected by determining the stability of the clot in either a 1% solution of monochloroacetic acid or a 5 M solution of urea for 2 hours. Premature dissolution of the clot indicates Factor XIII deficiency.

Vascular Purpura

If results of coagulation tests are normal, the bleeding patient may have a vascular defect. These are usually associated with underlying systemic illnesses (Table 13.10). Careful examination of the skin is necessary to note the pathognomonic findings of telangiectases in Osler-Weber-Rendu disease, palpable petechiae in Henoch-Schönlein purpura, and corkscrew hairs in scurvy, as examples of the more common types of vascular purpura.

Thrombocytopenia

The risk of bleeding increases in patients with fewer than 70,000–80,000 platelets/mm^3, and spontaneous hemorrhage is common with fewer than 30,000 platelets/mm^3. In patients with fewer than 10,000 platelets/mm^3, life-threatening hemorrhage occurs frequently.

Classification

In evaluating thrombocytopenia, the physician must distinguish between impaired production of platelets by the bone marrow and accelerated peripheral sequestration or destruction of platelets. A classification of the causes of thrombocytopenia according to this distinction is provided in Table 13.11.

Bone marrow examination is important in the

Table 13.10.
Classification of vascular purpura according to defect.

Vascular defects
  Henoch-Schönlein purpura
  Infection
    Bacterial endocarditis
    Rocky Mountain spotted fever
  Nonthrombocytopenic drug purpura
  Hereditary hemorrhagic telangiectasia (Osler-Weber-Rendu disease)
Extravascular defects
  "Senile" purpura
  Ehlers-Danlos syndrome
  Marfan's syndrome
  Cushing's syndrome
  Scurvy
Unclassified
  Dysglobulinemic purpura
  Purpura simplex
  "Autoerythrocyte sensitization"

Table 13.11.
Causes of thrombocytopenia.

Decreased platelet production
  Bone marrow replacement
    Neoplastic disease
    Leukemia
  Megaloblastic anemia
  Marrow injury from drugs, radiation, or chemicals
  Aplastic anemia
  Advanced uremia
  Acute alcohol ingestion
  Severe sepsis
  Drug toxicity
Abnormal distribution
  Splenomegaly
Dilution
  Transfusion with large amounts of thrombocytopenic blood and colloid
Increased platelet destruction
  Purpura after viral infection
  Drug-induced purpura
  Idiopathic thrombocytopenic purpura
  Secondary immunologic purpura, eg, lymphoma
  Purpura after transfusion
Nonimmune platelet consumption
  Disseminated intravascular coagulation
  Thrombotic thrombocytopenic purpura

evaluation of thrombocytopenia. When thrombocytopenia is due to decreased marrow production of platelets, the bone marrow usually shows hypoplasia, infiltration with malignant cells or granuloma, fibrosis, or megaloblastic changes. In cases of excessive peripheral destruction of platelets, the bone marrow usually appears normal and contains normal or increased numbers of megakaryocytes. The megakaryocytes characteristically appear young—nonbudding and with few nuclear segments. In such cases, the blood smear usually shows the platelets to be large, often as large as red blood cells, reflecting the increased production rate of young platelets, which are larger than platelets that have circulated for a few days.

The response to transfusion with 8–10 units of platelets may be helpful in distinguishing the two mechanisms of thrombocytopenia. In patients with thrombocytopenia due to excessive peripheral destruction of platelets, little or no increase in the platelet count is evident 2–3 hours after transfusion. In patients with impaired marrow production of platelets, however, an increase of approximately 10,000 platelets/mm^3 for each transfused unit may be expected in the absence of brisk bleeding, high fever, or prior sensitization to platelet antigens by multiple transfusions or pregnancy.

Increased peripheral destruction of platelets can be divided into two categories: immune and nonimmune. The most frequent cause of nonimmune peripheral thrombocytopenia is hypersplenism. The spleen normally acts as a reservoir for approximately one-third of the peripheral platelet pool, but with splenomegaly this proportion may increase to 75 or 80%. Abrupt thrombocytopenia due to traumatic injury to platelets occurs after extracorporeal circulation in cardiac operations. Thrombocytopenia also is encountered frequently as a result of severe bleeding followed by massive blood transfusion with products that are relatively platelet poor. This cause of thrombocytopenia can be corrected by platelet transfusion. Thrombocytopenia is also characteristic of disseminated intravascular coagulation and of thrombotic thrombocytopenic purpura, a rare illness in which the patient has microangiopathic hemolytic anemia, fever, renal failure, and neurologic symptoms.

If thrombocytopenia appears to be immune, a careful search should be made for an underlying cause such as a drug, systemic lupus erythematosus, or a lymphoproliferative disease. Thrombocytopenia after a viral illness is common in children, and is usually self-limited. If no underlying cause is apparent, the illness is considered idiopathic.

Among the causes of immune thrombocytopenia, it is important to consider that drug-induced thrombocytopenia can occur even after years of symptom-free use of a drug. Although certain drugs such as quinine, quinidine, and sulfonamide derivatives are the most common offending agents, any drug may be implicated. In a patient with thrombocytopenia without a clear-cut cause, all current medications should be omitted. If the thrombocytopenia is drug induced, it should disappear within 2 weeks after withdrawal of the drug. However, the patient may maintain a lifelong susceptibility to recurrence of thrombocytopenia with use of the same drug.

Post-transfusion purpura is extremely rare, and occurs almost exclusively in women. Thrombocytopenia develops about 1 week after blood transfusion. This entity may be confused easily with idiopathic thrombocytopenic purpura, and the diagnosis depends on the temporal relation to transfusion and demonstration of a unique antibody to platelet antigen. Exchange transfusion has been proposed as a means of treating the thrombocytopenia.

Prolonged heparin administration has been associated with thrombocytopenia through both immunologic and nonimmunologic mechanisms. Patients receiving heparin should have periodic platelet counts determined, and the heparin may need to be discontinued in the presence of a falling count.

Therapy

General Measures. Avoidance of trauma, especially to the head, is important. Intramuscular injections and medications that interfere with platelet function such as salicylates should be avoided. Straining at bowel movements should be prevented by liberal use of stool softeners and laxatives. Platelet transfusions may be of great value in patients with thrombocytopenia due to decreased marrow production of platelets; they are unlikely to be of more than transient value when the cause is hypersplenism, disseminated intravascular coagulation, or immune peripheral destruction. However, in the patient with significant bleeding, large numbers of platelet transfusions may be of some benefit despite the short survival time of the transfused platelets. If chronic thrombocytopenia is likely, as in aplastic anemia, persons matched for HL-A antigen are the most suitable platelet donors, and platelet transfusion may be feasible for a long period without development of sensitization to the transfused platelets.

Immune Thrombocytopenia. High dose corticosteroid therapy—usually prednisone, 1 mg/kg—is generally effective in raising the platelet count in patients with immune thrombocytopenic purpura within 7–10 days. Unfortunately, many patients relapse as the dosage is tapered, and splenectomy then becomes necessary.

If life-threatening bleeding develops before corticosteroids have become effective, emergency splenectomy is indicated. Approximately three-fourths of patients respond well to splenectomy, and the platelet count improves substantially within 24 hours of operation in most of these patients. Once the splenic pedicle has been clamped, transfused platelets can be expected to have a relatively normal survival time and can be administered to support the patient during operation. Platelet transfusion also may be of benefit before splenectomy for the patient with severe bleeding despite the very short survival of the infused platelets in immune thrombocytopenia.

Platelet Dysfunction

Despite adequate numbers of platelets, a bleeding diathesis may develop if the platelets fail to function properly. In recent years, several congenital platelet disorders have been delineated that usually cause mild to moderate bleeding syndromes characterized by easy bruising, menorrhagia, and excessive bleeding after operation. Many drugs impair platelet aggregation (Table 13.12), and with some, such as aspirin, the defect is present for the life of the platelet. Significant bleeding due to the antiplatelet effect of drugs is unusual, but cannot be ignored if the bleeding time is prolonged and results of other coagulation tests are normal. In this situation, more sophisticated tests of platelet function such as use of platelet aggregometry may confirm the defect. Transfusion with 8–10 units of normal platelets corrects the prolonged bleeding time. Advanced uremia and dysproteinemia also cause acquired platelet dysfunction. Uremic patients require dialysis to correct the platelet functional defect.

Thrombocytosis

Considerable increase in the platelet count is associated with both thrombosis and hemorrhage. The risk of complications becomes great when the count exceeds 2–3 million platelets/mm^3. Thrombocytosis may be due to a primary myeloproliferative disease, or it may result from several other disorders, including hemorrhage, iron deficiency, a malignant process, arthritis, and infection. Complications due to thrombocytosis are more commonly associated with the myeloproliferative disorders. Treatment is not well established. If the increased platelet count is directly associated with a hemorrhagic or thrombotic complication, it may be decreased rapidly by thrombocytopheresis. After thrombocytopheresis, nitrogen mustard, 10 mg/m^2, should be administered intravenously. If the need for reducing the platelet count is less urgent, nitrogen mustard or an oral alkylating agent such as busulfan (Myleran), 6–8 mg/day, may be administered without thrombocytopheresis. Heparin, aspirin, and dipyridamole have been used as prophylactic agents against thrombosis, but may aggravate hemorrhage. Splenectomy may severely accentuate thrombocytosis, and should be performed only after careful consideration in a patient with significant thrombocytosis.

Congenital Coagulation Factor Deficiencies

Table 13.13 lists the features of the congenital coagulation factor disorders. With the exception of hemophilia and Christmas disease, which are sex linked, and von Willebrand's disease, which is

Table 13.12
Drugs that inhibit platelet function and potentially prolong bleeding time.

Aspirin and other anti-inflammatory agents[a]	Dextran
Motrin	Anticoagulants
Indomethacin	Heparin (high concentrations inhibit collagen-induced aggregation)
Phenylbutazone	
Sulfinpyrazone	Androgens
Phenothiazines[a]	Phenformin hydrochloride (DBI)
Chlorpromazine	Clofibrate (Atromid-S)
Promethazine hydrochloride	Sympathetic blocking agents
Tricyclic antidepressants[a]	Phentolamine
Imipramine hydrochloride (Tofranil)	Dihydroergotamine
Amitriptyline hydrochloride (Elavil)	Dibenzylchlorethamine (Dibenamine)
Desipramine hydrochloride (Norpramin)	Phenoxybenzamine hydrochloride (Dibenzyline)
Nortriptyline hydrochloride (Aventyl)	Propranolol
Antihistamines[a]	Colchicine
Diphenhydramine hydrochloride (Benadryl)	Vinca alkaloids
Chlordiazepoxide hydrochloride (Librium)	Vinblastine sulfate (Velban)
Diazepam (Valium)	Vincristine
Flurazepam hydrochloride (Dalmane)	Glyceryl guaiacolate
Dipyridamole (Persantine)	Monoamine oxidase inhibitors
Methylxanthines	Nialamide
Caffeine	Diuretics
Theobromine	Ethacrynic acid
Aminophylline (high doses)	Nitrofurantoin (Furadantin)
Local anesthetics	Carbenicillin
Cocaine	
Procaine	
Lidocaine (Xylocaine)	
Dibucaine (Nupercaine)	

[a] Major offenders that commonly prolong the bleeding time test.

Table 13.13.
Congenital disorders of blood coagulation factors.

Factor	Inheritance	Sex Distribution	Frequency	Comments
XII (Hageman)	Recessive	Male Female	$1/10^6$	No bleeding disorder
XI	Recessive	Male Female	$1/10^6$	Often mild and not discovered until adulthood
IX Christmas disease Hemophilia B	Sex-linked	Male	$10/10^6$	Frequently severe
VIII Hemophilia A	Sex-linked	Male	$60–80/10^6$	Frequently severe
von Willebrand's disease	Dominant	Male Female	$60–80/10^6$	Also has a platelet defect manifested by prolonged bleeding time, decreased platelet adhesiveness, and abnormal aggregation to ristocetin
X	Recessive	Male Female	$1/10^6$	Usually mild Acquired variety with amyloidosis
V	Recessive	Male Female	$1/10^5$	Usually mild to moderately severe
VII	Recessive	Male Female	$1/10^6$	Usually mild to moderately severe
II (prothrombin)	Recessive	Male Female	Rare	Moderately severe
I (fibrinogen)	Recessive	Male Female	Rare	Usually severe

inherited as a dominant trait, the congenital coagulation deficiency states are inherited as autosomal recessive traits and are extremely uncommon. Since the coagulation factors are required for generation of the fibrin that supports the primary platelet plug, deficiencies in any of the coagulation factors may be expected to lead to development of a fragile clot. Delayed bleeding after trauma is characteristic of coagulation factor deficiencies. The severity of the disorder depends on the amount of the coagulation factor present. The normal range for each coagulation factor is approximately 50–150%. Levels of 0–2% are associated with severe disease, and are characterized by spontaneous bleeding into joints and soft-tissue spaces and severe hemorrhage after trauma. Persons with levels from 3–5% have moderate disease with less frequent episodes of spontaneous bleeding, and persons with levels more than 5% often have mild disease that may not be detected until operation.

Therapy

Local measures such as immobilization and application of cold compresses to a joint with hemarthrosis are important. Persons with congenital coagulation factor deficiencies should avoid drugs that impair platelet function, since they may exacerbate the tendency to bleed. The major form of therapy, however, is replacement of adequate amounts of the deficient factor.

Concentrates of plasma coagulation factors are available for the major congenital coagulation deficiencies, allowing replacement therapy without the risk of volume overload. The intensity of replacement therapy depends on the severity of the deficiency and the site of bleeding. For example, spontaneous bleeding into a joint in a hemophiliac patient can usually be managed on an outpatient basis with a single large infusion of Factor VIII concentrate, which corrects the factor deficiency for several hours. Bleeding into vital organs or into soft-tissue spaces that threatens to cause nerve compression or other serious damage, trauma to the head, and major surgical procedures require vigorous replacement therapy to maintain the factor level at more than 30% (the level at which the PTT is normalized) for 7–10 days.

Calculation of Replacement Therapy. Replacement therapy is calculated in terms of the "unit," which represents the amount of coagulation factor in 1 ml of normal plasma. The number of units

Table 13.14.
Replacement therapy.

Deficiency	Replacement	Initial Dosage/ kg Body Weight	Maintenance Dosage/ kg/day	Metabolic Half-life
				hr
Factor II (prothrombin)	Plasma	20 units twice a day	15–20 units	50–80
	Prothrombin concentrate	40 units	15–20 units	
Factor V	Fresh-frozen plasma	15–25 units	15–20 units	24
Factor VII	Plasma	5–10 units	5 units, 4 times a day	5
	Prothrombin concentrate	5–10 units	5 units, 4 times a day	
Factor VIII				
Hemophilia A	Cryoprecipitate	1 bag/2–4 kg	1 bag/4–8 kg twice a day	12
	Glycine precipitate	40 units	20 units twice a day	
von Willebrand's disease	Plasma	10 units	10 units	24
	Cryoprecipitate	1 bag/10 kg	1 bag/10 kg	
Factor IX				
Christmas disease	Plasma	30–60 units	5–10 units twice a day	20–30
	Prothrombin concentrate	30–60 units	5–10 units twice a day	
Factor X	Plasma	10–15 units	10 units	20–60
	Prothrombin concentrate	10–15 units	10 units	
Factor XI	Plasma	10–20 units	5 units	40–80
	Prothrombin concentrate	20 units	10 units	

administered depends on the patient's size, the half-life of the infused factor in the circulation, and the distribution between intravascular and extravascular compartments. Pertinent data on replacement therapy for major bleeding episodes are given in Table 13.14. In each case, it is imperative to test the adequacy of replacement therapy by ascertaining that the specific factor assay increases to the appropriate level or that the screening test— such as PTT in hemophilia A, von Willebrand's disease, Christmas disease, and Factor XI deficiency—remains corrected at all times.

Hemophilia. Two forms of Factor VIII concentrate are available. When frozen plasma is thawed at 4°C, the fibrinogen precipitates as a sludge containing much of Factor VIII. When this cryoprecipitate is removed, the Factor VIII of a unit of plasma can be concentrated into a volume of 10–15 ml. The major disadvantage of the cryoprecipitate is that the amount of Factor VIII may vary greatly, leading to difficulty in accurate replacement therapy. In addition, cryoprecipitate must be preserved at −40°C. The second source of Factor VIII for replacement therapy, glycine precipitate, is assayed by the manufacturer, and

the number of units of Factor VIII is printed on the container. This preparation is usually more expensive.

Different clinical situations require different levels of circulating Factor VIII:

(1) Minor episodes such as spontaneous hemarthrosis usually respond to a single large infusion, which maintains the level of Factor VIII above 30% for 12 hours and above 5% for 36–48 hours.

(2) Moderate bleeding or bleeding after minor trauma requires Factor VIII replacement until it is clear that bleeding has stopped.

(3) Major surgical procedures and significant trauma require full, therapeutic doses for 7–10 days.

A new approach to the treatment of bleeding in patients with mild hemophilia and von Willebrand's disease is the use of the vasopressin analogue deamino-8-D-arginine vasopressin (DDAVP), which stimulates both factor VIII activity and fibrinolytic activity when given intravenously before minor surgical procedures. The mechanism of action is not entirely clear. When used in conjunction with the fibrinolytic inhibitor, ε-aminocaproic acid (EACA), plasma replacement products may be avoided for the coverage of minor surgical procedures such as dental extraction. The use of DDAVP has not been associated with significant rises in blood pressure and it has been well tolerated. It is anticipated that this drug will be available in the United States in the near future.

Inhibitors of Factor VIII. In a small percentage of patients with severe hemophilia and occasionally in patients with mild disease, specific antibodies against Factor VIII develop, leading to resistance to Factor VIII infusions. This is detected either by failure of the PTT or Factor VIII assay to return to normal after replacement therapy or by development of a progressively larger requirement for Factor VIII. Specific assays to quantitate the level of inhibitor are available.

Development of an inhibitor severely complicates management. The traditional approach has been to try to overwhelm the inhibitor by administering enough Factor VIII to saturate all inhibitor molecules. This massive amount of Factor VIII is usually administered along with immunosuppressive agents such as cyclophosphamide and corticosteroids to prevent a further anamnestic increase in the amount of inhibitor. The higher the titer of the inhibitor, the less likely it is that this form of therapy will be successful. A new approach involves the administration of commercially prepared prothrombin concentrate (Factors II, VII, IX, and X), which contains activated coagulation factors able to "bypass" the inhibitor. Several promising reports have appeared regarding this approach in patients with high titers of inhibitor whose bleeding fails to improve after the administration of large amounts of Factor VIII concentrate. The usual dose is 70–100 Factor IX units/kg repeated at intervals of 8–12 hours. Complications such as thrombosis, disseminated intravascular coagulation, and a high incidence of hepatitis have also been reported. The risk of thrombosis or disseminated intravascular coagulation appears particularly high in patients with hepatic disease, and prothrombin concentrate should be used in this condition only when the patient has life-threatening bleeding. Since prothrombin concentrate contains prothrombin, thrombin can appear spontaneously during transit or storage. It is therefore important to perform the preinfusion stability check as outlined in the package insert. To decrease the risk of thrombotic complications further, 5 units of heparin should be added for each milliliter of reconstituted material. This amount of heparin does not prolong the clotting time after infusion. The patient's condition should be monitored during infusion to detect intravascular clotting, and infusion should be stopped promptly if any signs of this occur.

von Willebrand's Disease. A mild to moderately severe bleeding disorder, von Willebrand's disease is characterized by deficiency of Factor VIII and a prolonged bleeding time. The severity of the condition often fluctuates. Platelet aggregation is normal with the standard aggregating reagents such as adenosine diphosphate and epinephrine, but is decreased with ristocetin; platelet adhesiveness is also decreased. In contrast with hemophilia A, von Willebrand's disease is inherited as an autosomal dominant trait, and is thus found in both females and males. Recent investigations have demonstrated that Factor VIII antigenic material is present in normal amounts in hemophilia A, but is functionally inactive. In contrast, in von Willebrand's disease, the amount of Factor VIII antigenic material is decreased in proportion with the decline in Factor VIII functional activity. Patients with von Willebrand's disease appear to lack an early intermediary compound in Factor VIII synthesis that can be supplied to them in cryoprecipitate or plasma, including plasma from a patient with hemophilia A. As a result, these patients have an increase in Factor VIII after transfusion that is larger than would be predicted from the amount of Factor VIII infused. Plasma and cryoprecipitate lead to correction of both the Factor VIII deficiency and the bleeding time, but glycine precipitate does not lead to correction of the latter. Because of this, plasma or cryoprecipitate is recommended (Table 13.14). As previously mentioned in the section on hemophilia, intravenous DDAVP may correct the hemostatic defect in von Willebrand's disease without the need to resort to cryoprecipitate infusion.

Christmas Disease (Hemophilia B). Deficiency of Factor IX shows striking similarities to hemophilia A in terms of clinical manifestations and replacement therapy. Factor IX equilibrates with the extravascular compartment to a greater extent than Factor VIII, necessitating a larger initial infusion. This is counterbalanced by the longer metabolic half-life of Factor IX. Factor IX deficiency can be corrected by plasma infusion (often requiring simultaneous diuretic administration) or prothrombin concentrate (Table 13.14). Because of the potential complications associated with prothrombin concentrate, this material should be reserved for major bleeding episodes.

Factor XI Deficiency. This deficiency can usually be corrected with infusion of plasma (Table 13.14). Potential volume overload can be managed with diuretics. Prothrombin concentrate is frequently contaminated with Factor XI, and may be useful for the patient with large plasma requirements. Before administration, the prothrombin concentrate should be assayed to determine its Factor XI content.

Disseminated Intravascular Coagulation

This is a paradoxical disorder involving both abnormal clotting and bleeding. Disseminated intravascular coagulation results from aberrant activation of the coagulation cascade, leading to depletion of coagulation factors and platelets. The fibrinolytic system is activated secondarily, and as a consequence, hemostasis is compromised further because of lysis of fibrin, fibrinogen, and Factors V and VIII, as well as elaboration of fibrin degradation products that impair fibrin polymerization and platelet aggregation. Table 13.15 lists the major clinical situations in which disseminated intravascular coagulation is encountered, and Table 13.16 lists criteria for diagnosis.

Disseminated intravascular coagulation may

Table 13.15.
Conditions associated with disseminated intravascular coagulation.

Sepsis, especially gram-negative bacteremia
Malignant disease, especially prostatic carcinoma and acute promyelocytic leukemia
Obstetric complication
Brain injury
Burns
Hemolytic transfusion reaction
Fat embolism
Severe hepatic disease
Extensive operation involving prolonged hypotension
Purpura fulminans
Microangiopathic hemolytic anemia
Thrombotic thrombocytopenic purpura

range in severity from an asymptomatic state to fulminant hemorrhage. Treatment emphasizing cure or palliation of the underlying disorder may be sufficient. Replacement therapy with platelets, fresh-frozen plasma, and a source of fibrinogen such as cryoprecipitate may improve hemostasis, although it may exacerbate thrombotic complications. Use of heparin remains controversial. Although heparin frequently may improve coagulation, its effect on survival appears to be negligible since patients tend to die from the underlying disorder. Heparin should probably be reserved for patients who have significant hemorrhage as a result of well-documented disseminated intravascular coagulation. In this instance, continuous intravenous infusion of heparin, 10,000–24,000 units/day, with monitoring of coagulation and adjustment of dosage is indicated. Signs of improvement include increase in fibrinogen and platelet levels, decrease in fibrin degradation products, and improvement in hemostasis. Fresh-frozen plasma should be administered along with the heparin to replace depleted coagulation factors. If bleeding appears to increase as a result of heparin, protamine sulfate should promptly be administered.

Primary Fibrinolysis

This is a rare disorder that may be difficult to distinguish from disseminated intravascular coagulation. However, patients with primary fibrinolysis do not have thrombocytopenia or fragmented red blood cells on blood smears, and they have somewhat higher levels of Factors V and VIII. Primary fibrinolysis is much less common than disseminated intravascular coagulation, and should only be considered in the setting of prostatic carcinoma or operation, severe hepatic disease, or a thoracic operation. In patients with well-established primary fibrinolysis, antifibrinolytic therapy may be started with EACA, 4 gm initially

Table 13.16.
Criteria for diagnosis of disseminated intravascular coagulation and primary fibrinolysis.

Finding	Disseminated Intravascular Coagulation	Primary Fibrinolysis
Thrombocytopenia	+	−
Prolonged prothrombin time	+	+
Prolonged partial thromboplastin time	+	+
Prolonged thrombin time	+	+
Hypofibrinogenemia	+	+
Elevation of level of fibrin degradation products	+	+ +
Depression of Factors V and VIII	Usually substantial	Usually moderate
Microangiopathic blood smear	±	−

followed by 1 gm/hr either intravenously or orally. EACA therapy on rare occasions has been associated with thrombotic complications, especially in patients with disseminated intravascular coagulation who have not received prior heparin therapy.

Circulating Anticoagulants

In addition to their occurrence in congenital coagulation disorders, circulating anticoagulants against Factors V, VIII, IX, and XI may occur spontaneously or associated with a collagen vascular disease. They are detected by finding that prolonged coagulation times and factor assays fail to be corrected when the plasma is mixed with an equal volume of normal plasma. Rarely, severe hemorrhage will require the type of measure discussed under "Inhibitors of Factor VIII," page 284.

ANTICOAGULATION

The decision to use anticoagulants involves consideration of the risks of hemorrhage vs. the risks of thrombosis and embolism. In general, anticoagulants should not be administered to patients with active bleeding from the gastrointestinal, genitourinary, or pulmonary tracts; severe hypertension; a hemorrhagic diathesis; cerebrovascular hemorrhage; or pericarditis complicating acute myocardial infarction. Hemorrhage in a patient receiving anticoagulants should raise the suspicion that an occult pathologic process may have been uncovered as a result of anticoagulation, especially if the results of coagulation tests used to monitor the anticoagulation are in the therapeutic range.

Heparin

Heparin is the drug of choice for anticoagulation in the acute situation. A naturally occurring mucopolysaccharide derived principally from beef lung and hog intestine, heparin interferes with coagulation at several points in the coagulation cascade; among its effects are inhibition of the action of thrombin and inhibition of activated Factors XI, IX, and X. Sodium heparin is available in solutions containing 1,000, 5,000, 10,000, 20,000, and 40,000 USP units/ml. In most solutions, 1 mg of heparin contains approximately 150 units. Dosage should be prescribed in units rather than in milligrams.

Administration

Intravenous injection is the preferred route of administration. The initial dose is usually a bolus of 5,000–10,000 units, followed by either a contin-

uous infusion of 500–2,000 units/hr by a pump or repeated injections of 5,000–10,000 units every 4–6 hours. Although the intermittent method is more convenient, recent studies have suggested that continuous infusion is associated with fewer hemorrhagic complications. Anticoagulation with heparin should be monitored by means of coagulation tests. The most commonly employed are the PTT, with a therapeutic range from 1.5–2.5 times the control value, and the Lee-White method for determination of clotting time, with a therapeutic range from 2–3 times the control value. If heparin is administered by continuous infusion, the coagulation test may be performed at any time; if administration is intermittent, blood should be drawn just before the next dose of heparin.

Toxicity

Hemorrhage is the major side effect, occurring in approximately 3–7% of patients in large series. Allergic reactions such as urticaria, conjunctivitis, bronchospasm, and hypotension are uncommon. Thrombocytopenia has recently been reported as a frequent complication of prolonged heparin infusion, and the platelet count should be monitored. Osteoporosis may occur after prolonged use.

Antidote

Heparin is rapidly metabolized in the liver and kidney. A heparin antagonist is necessary, therefore, only when anticoagulation must be reversed within 4 hours after a dose. Protamine sulfate is the agent of choice, completely reversing the effect of heparin within minutes. It is administered slowly in the course of 3–5 minutes in a solution of 2 mg/ml. Immediately after a dose of heparin is administered, the number of milligrams of protamine sulfate necessary to neutralize the heparin is equal to the heparin dose in milligrams, which is calculated by dividing the number of USP units in the heparin dose by 150. Protamine sulfate neutralizes more heparin units derived from hog intestine than from beef lung. Hence, knowledge of the source of the heparin is helpful for accurate neutralization. One hour after the dose of heparin has been administered, the amount of protamine sulfate should be decreased by half. The maximal amount safely administered is 100 mg. As a result of its highly basic charge, large amounts of protamine sulfate interfere with coagulation and may lead to a hemorrhagic diathesis.

Coumarin Derivatives

The coumarin derivatives, such as sodium warfarin (Coumadin) and bishydroxycoumarin (Dicumarol), antagonize vitamin K, resulting in depression of hepatic synthesis of prothrombin (Factor II) and Factors VII, IX, and X. After coumarin therapy is started, the individual factor activities decrease at varying rates; Factor VII is the first to decrease in activity because of the short half-life. As a result of the longer half-life of Factors X and II, it may take from 40–90 hours for amounts to decrease to therapeutic levels. Although coumarin therapy is monitored by the PT, it also leads to prolongation of the PTT.

Administration

Dosage is regulated by the PT. The therapeutic range of the PT should be established by each laboratory, but is usually 1.5–2.5 times the control value, which corresponds to 10–25% of control activity. Initiation of anticoagulation can be efficiently undertaken by administering 10 mg of sodium warfarin daily for 3 days, with further adjustment of anticoagulation by means of daily PT determinations and sodium warfarin doses until a stable maintenance dose is established.

Toxicity

The major toxic reaction is hemorrhage. The principal drugs that interact with coumarin compounds are listed in Table 13.17. Coumarin crosses the placental barrier, and its use during pregnancy must be monitored carefully to prevent neonatal hemorrhage. Coumarin compounds are also teratogenic during the first trimester of pregnancy. Necrosis of subcutaneous fatty tissue (coumarin

Table 13.17.
Drugs that interact with coumarin compounds.

Potentiation of action
  Indomethacin
  Cimetidine
  Sulfinpyrazone
  Clofibrate
  Quinidine, quinine
  Salicylates
  Sulfisoxazole
  Tolbutamide, chlorpropamide
  Phenytoin
  Chloramphenicol
  Cholestyramine
  Dextrothyroxine
Retardation of action
  Barbiturates
  Ethanol
  Oral contraceptives
  Griseofulvin
  Glutethimide
  Rifampin

necrosis) is a rare complication occurring on the 3rd to 10th day of therapy. It is not related to excessive anticoagulation, and its cause is unclear. Other unusual reactions include rash, nausea, diarrhea, fever, jaundice, leukopenia or thrombocytopenia, and vasculitis.

Antidote

The effect of a coumarin derivative can be neutralized by administration of vitamin K. For moderate or severe bleeding, 10–25 mg may be given slowly intravenously. The PT may begin to be corrected within 1 hour, and is often within normal limits by 8 hours. A somewhat slower response occurs after intramuscular injection. For mild bleeding, 5–10 mg can be administered orally with correction expected within 12–24 hours.

Immediate correction of a prolonged PT due to a coumarin derivative can be achieved by infusion of 2–6 units of plasma along with vitamin K administration; this is often indicated for major hemorrhagic complications. Plasma infusion alone is also useful for partial correction of an excessively prolonged PT without interrupting anticoagulation with administration of vitamin K.

Elective Operation

The anticoagulant should be discontinued. After the PT decreases to less than 1.5 times the control value, operation can be performed. Therapy can be resumed after the procedure has been completed.

THROMBOLYTIC THERAPY FOR ACUTE PULMONARY EMBOLISM AND DEEP VENOUS THROMBOPHLEBITIS

A National Institute of Health Consensus Conference in 1980 recommended thrombolytic therapy rather than heparin anticoagulation as the primary treatment for certain patients with deep venous thrombophlebitis and pulmonary embolism. Although heparin is effective in reducing the formation of venous clot and decreasing the likelihood of recurrent embolism, it is unable to dissolve the thrombus. In contrast, thrombolytic agents are able to lyse clot and potentially are able to alleviate the hemodynamic and vascular complications of thrombosis. Streptokinase (SK) and urokinase (UK) are two commercially available agents that induce thrombolytic activity by activating plasminogen with generation of the proteolytic enzyme plasmin. Both agents are expensive; since UK is several times more expensive than SK, it is recommended that the use of UK be restricted to individuals who have become sensitized to SK as a result of streptococcal infections or prior use of SK.

A major prospective, controlled study has investigated the use of SK in pulmonary embolism. Although a 24-hour infusion of SK was shown to result in more rapid lysis of embolic clot than heparin, ventilation perfusion scans were no different after 7 days and the mortality was no different between the heparin and SK treated groups. Hence, the use of SK in pulmonary embolism probably should be limited to those patients with massive pulmonary embolism showing hemodynamic instability who would normally be candidates for pulmonary embolectomy.

In patients with deep vein thrombophlebitis, SK reduces the risk of pulmonary embolism to the same degree as heparin, but also helps to preserve venous valves and prevent the postphlebitic syndrome, particularly in the more serious cases involving the femoral or iliac veins. SK, therefore, can be recommended in any patient with deep thrombophlebitis involving the femoral or iliac veins which is less than 7 days old.

To limit the bleeding complications of SK, the drug should be administered only in an area where close monitoring and supervision are available. All invasive procedures should be avoided except carefully performed venipuncture. No anticoagulants or drugs which impair platelet function should be given concurrently with SK. Major contraindications to the use of SK include surgery less than 10 days ago, signs of recent trauma, ongoing menses, recent gastrointestinal bleeding, and intra-arterial diagnostic procedure within the past 10 days (excluding uncomplicated arterial blood-gas studies), cerebrovascular accident within the past 2 months and severe hypertension. Some of these contraindications may be outweighed in patients with massive pulmonary emboli and hemodynamic instability.

A fixed dosage schedule of SK has been found to result in sufficient activation of plasminogen in 95% of patients. The initial loading dose of 250,000 U in normal saline is administered over 30 minutes followed by a constant infusion of 100,000 U/hr via an infusion pump. It is recommended that 4 hours after initiation of SK, and every 12 hours thereafter, a thrombin time and hematocrit be checked. A thrombin time test 2–6 times normal indicates an appropriate fibrinolytic state. If the thrombin time remains normal, or if it is greater than 6 times normal, one should seek consultation for dosage adjustment. The SK is continued for 24 hours for pulmonary embolism and 72 hours for phlebitis. Thrombolytic therapy should not be considered a substitute for anticoagulant therapy and following completion of SK, anticoagulation is mandatory. Heparin, without a loading dose, is begun once the thrombin time is less than twice control, which is usually 2–4 hours after stopping the SK. This is followed by conventional coumadin therapy.

Mild allergic reactions occur in up to 15% of patients treated with SK, usually in the form of urticaria, pruritus, flushing, nausea, and headache. Mild fever occurs in up to one-third of patients given SK. The most feared complication is bleeding which most often occurs at the sites of skin incisions and blood vessel punctures. Serious bleeding may be controlled by stopping the SK infusion, and the administration of fresh-frozen plasma and/or the antifibrinolytic agent, EACA (Amicar), 4 grams over 1 hour followed by 1 gm/hr by continuous infusion.

Suggested Readings

Allgood JW, Chaplin H, Jr: Idiopathic acquired autoimmune hemolytic anemia: A review of forty-seven cases treated from 1955 through 1965. *Am J Med 43*:254–273, 1967

Bell WR, Meek AG: Guidelines for the use of thrombolytic agents. *New Engl J Med 301*:1266–1270, 1979

Beutler E: Glucose-6-phosphate dehydrogenase deficiency. *Br J Haematol 18*:117–121, 1970

Blatt PM, Lundblad RL, Kingdon HS, et al: Thrombogenic materials in prothrombin complex concentrates. *Ann Intern Med 81*:766–770, 1974

Brody JI, Goldsmith MH, Park SK, et al: Symptomatic crises of sickle cell anemia treated by limited exchange transfusion. *Ann Intern Med 72*:327–330, 1970

Colman RW, Robboy SJ, Minna JD: Disseminated intravascular coagulation (DIC): An approach. *Am J Med 52*:679–689, 1972

Corrigan JJ, Jr, Jordan CM: Heparin therapy in septicemia with disseminated intravascular coagulation: Effect on mortality and on correction of hemostatic defects. *N Engl J Med 283*:778–782, 1970

Fairbanks VF, Fernandez MN: The identification of metabolic errors associated with anemia. *JAMA 208*:316–320, 1969

Fillmore SJ, McDevitt E: Effects of coumarin compounds on the fetus. *Ann Intern Med 73*:731–735, 1970

Grund FM, Armitage JO, Burns CP: Hydroxyurea in the prevention of the effects of leukostasis in acute leukemia. *Arch Intern Med 137*:1246–1247, 1977

Harris JW, Kellermeyer RW: *The Red Cell; Production, Metabolism, Destruction: Normal and Abnormal*, revised ed. Cambridge, Harvard University Press, 1970

Jacobson LB, Longstreth GF, Edgington TS: Clinical and immunologic features of transient cold agglutinin hemolytic anemia. *Am J Med 54*:514–521, 1973

Kabins SA, Lerner C: Fulminant pneumococcemia and sickle cell anemia. *JAMA 211*:467–471, 197

Koch-Weser J: Editorial: Coumarin necrosis. *Ann Intern Med 68*:1365–1367, 1968

Koch-Weser J, Sellers EM: Drug interactions with coumarin anticoagulants. *N Engl J Med 285*:487–498, 547–558, 1971

Ratnoff OD: Editorial: Prothrombin complex preparations: A cautionary note. *Ann Intern Med 81*:852–853, 1974

Sherman LA: Therapeutic problems of disseminated intravascular coagulation. *Arch Intern Med 132*:446–453, 1973

Solomon A, Fahey JL: Plasmapheresis therapy in macroglobulinemia. *Ann Intern Med 58*:789–800, 1963

Sullivan LW: Differential diagnosis and management of the patient with megaloblastic anemia. *Am J Med 48*:609–617, 1970

Wasserman LR: The management of polycythaemia vera. *Br J Haematol 21*:371–376, 1971

Wessler S: Anticoagulant therapy—1974. *JAMA 228*:757–761, 1974

Yankee RA, Grumet FC, Rogentine GN: Platelet transfusion therapy: The selection of compatible platelet donors for refractory patients by lymphocyte HL-A typing. *N Engl J Med 281*:1208–1212, 1969

CHAPTER **14**

Metabolic and Endocrine Emergencies

GILBERT H. DANIELS, M.D.

Consideration of the metabolic problems encountered in an emergency ward encompasses a broad spectrum of biophysiologic abnormalities. Any presentation of the subject is based on an arbitrary classification of the disease processes and endocrine organs involved. This discussion is divided into five components: (1) metabolic emergencies involving carbohydrate metabolism and ketoacidosis, (2) adrenal emergencies, (3) thyroid emergencies, (4) emergencies of hypercalcemia and hypocalcemia, and (5) a consideration of hyponatremia and hyperkalemia.

METABOLIC EMERGENCIES

Diabetic Ketoacidosis

Diabetic ketoacidosis was almost always fatal 50 years ago, but today, knowledge of the relevant pathophysiologic processes, combined with the availability of insulin, permits remarkably successful therapy. In most medical centers, the overall mortality due to diabetic ketoacidosis is less than 10%, and in uncomplicated series, mortality should be less than 2%.

Pathophysiologic Principles

The central role of insulin in normal intermediary metabolism is depicted in Figure 14.1, which schematically shows the three major target and storage tissues to be considered—the liver, muscle, and adipose tissue. Insulin serves as the "storage" (anabolic) hormone for glucose, amino acids, and free fatty acids, which are stored as glycogen, protein, and triglycerides, respectively:

A steady supply of *glucose* is mandatory for normal function of the central nervous system. The so-called counter-regulatory hormones (for example, epinephrine, glucagon, growth hormone, and cortisol) maintain or elevate the blood glucose level to help ensure the supply. Insulin is the only major hormone that lowers the blood glucose level. This is accomplished in part by promoting storage of glucose as glycogen in the liver and inhibiting the de novo formation (gluconeogenesis) and release of glucose by this organ. Insulin also facilitates glucose transport into muscle and subsequent glycogen synthesis, and stimulates passage of glucose into fat cells, where it is converted to glycerol phosphate and free fatty acids and then stored as triglycerides.

Transport of *amino acids* into muscle, their subsequent conversion into protein, and inhibition of degradation of these proteins also result from the action of insulin.

Free fatty acids, the major energy source of the body, are stored as triglycerides in the fat cells. Insulin facilitates transfer of these triglycerides from the plasma into the fat cells, and prevents their breakdown (lipolysis) to free fatty acids and glycerol by inhibiting the enzyme responsible for such degradation. This enzyme is called the "hormone-sensitive lipase" because it is stimulated by many of the counter-regulatory hormones.

Given these considerations, it is easy to perceive the ultimate consequence of insulin deficiency to be diabetic ketoacidosis. Diabetic ketoacidosis results from an absolute lack of insulin or from a relative lack associated with "stress" and increased concentrations of the counter-regulatory hormones. The inhibition of lipolysis and glycogenolysis by insulin occurs at much lower insulin concentrations than stimulation of glucose transport and storage. Gluconeogenesis seems to have intermediate sensitivity to insulin. Although the effects of insulin deficiency on carbohydrate and lipid metabolism are complex and intertwined, for the purposes of discussion, they may be dissociated and considered separately (Fig. 14.2); clinically, these effects may be dissociated as well.

Carbohydrate Metabolism. Insulin deficiency

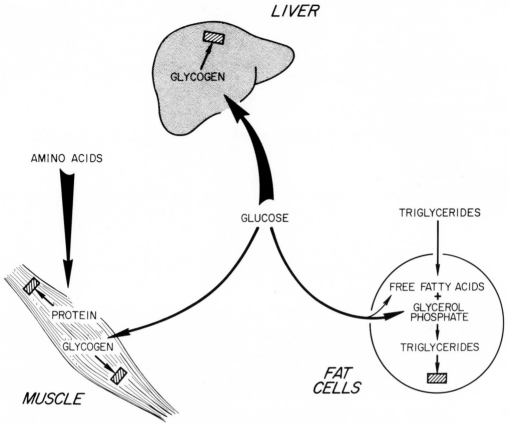

Figure 14.1.   Effects of insulin.

leads to marked hyperglycemia. Although the overall utilization of glucose by insulin-sensitive tissues is diminished, the brain continues to utilize large quantities even in the absence of insulin. Hence, underutilization alone should not result in severe hyperglycemia. In the presence of insulin deficiency, however, conversion of hepatic glycogen to glucose increases substantially. In addition, glycogen in muscle breaks down to yield lactic acid that is also converted to glucose by the liver. Insulin deficiency increases glucose production by two mechanisms: (1) activity of the appropriate hepatic enzymes increases significantly, and (2) the supply and uptake of substrates for gluconeogenesis also increases because of accelerated protein degradation in muscle (yielding amino acids—especially alanine and glutamine) and lipolysis in adipose tissue (yielding glycerol).

Lipid Metabolism. With severe insulin deficiency, insulin restraint on lipolysis is lost and triglycerides in the fat cells are hydrolyzed to glycerol and free fatty acids. The free fatty acids are transported to the liver, where they are oxidized to acetyl Coenzyme A and preferentially utilized for ketone body production; acetoacetic acid and β-hydroxybutyric acid are the "ketone bodies" produced by the liver, acetone being generated from acetoacetic acid by nonenzymatic decarboxylation. The preferential shunting of free fatty acids to ketone body production is facilitated by glucagon excess. Released from the liver, the ketone bodies apparently overwhelm their usual disposal mechanism, namely, oxidation by muscle. It is likely that insulin is necessary for the normal peripheral utilization of ketone bodies.

Clinical Correlations. As the blood glucose level increases, so does the serum osmolality. Water moves out of the cells, and cellular dehydration may occur. As the capacity of the kidney for glucose reabsorption is exceeded, glycosuria develops. Osmotic diuresis results in the loss of water and electrolytes, more water being lost than sodium or potassium. Acetoacetic acid and β-hydroxybutyric acid are strong acids whose increased production results in metabolic acidosis. Excreted in the urine as sodium and potassium salts, these ketone bodies further exacerbate the electrolyte losses. The intravascular volume contraction leads to secondary hyperaldosteronism which exacerbates the potassium loss.

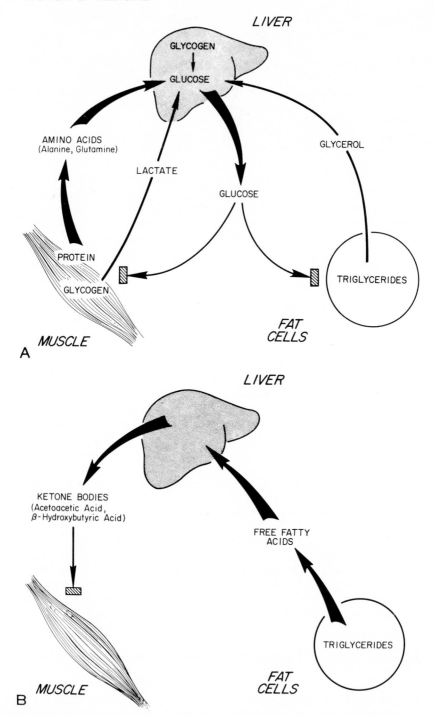

Figure 14.2. Effects of insulin deficiency on (**A**) carbohydrate metabolism and (**B**) lipid metabolism.

Diagnosis

Clinical Features. Diabetic ketoacidosis may develop during the course of known diabetes or may be the initial indication of disease. A history of the "three P's" may be obtained from the patient or the patient's relatives or friends. An episode of *p*olyuria and *p*olydipsia of several days' duration consequent to loss of a large amount of glucose in the urine, as well as *p*olyphagia, may precede ketoacidosis. Unexplained recent weight loss is common in younger patients, reflecting both muscle and adipose tissue breakdown. A history of visual disturbances may be a clue to new onset diabetes or worsening control. Muscle cramps may occur, perhaps related to fluid and electrolyte losses.

Anorexia follows the development of ketosis; nausea and vomiting may occur, thereby exacerbating the dehydration. If the patient is ketotic and unable to maintain oral intake, he or she should be hospitalized for intravenous fluid replacement even if frank acidosis has not yet developed. Although abdominal pain may occur related to ketoacidosis and abdominal tenderness is common, especially in children, in adults such symptoms should suggest an underlying precipitating event, such as pancreatitis or cholecystitis.

Whenever an acute abdominal emergency is suspected in a patient with diabetic ketoacidosis, the ketoacidosis should be vigorously treated for 3–4 hours. If the abdominal signs disappear, the metabolic derangement is the important clinical situation. If the abdominal findings persist, the patient will be better able to tolerate surgery after treating the ketoacidosis.

The patient's appearance is often dominated by signs of dehydration. The combination of dehydration and good urinary output should always suggest diabetic ketoacidosis. Dehydration may be mild, manifested by decrease in skin turgor or orbital resistance or absence of axillary sweat; moderate, with postural tachycardia or hypotension; or severe, resulting in frank shock. Despite hypotension, the skin often remains warm, flushed, and dry because of metabolic acidosis and considerable volume depletion.

If the patient is febrile, infection must be assumed. However, hypothermia may be present in diabetic ketoacidosis even in the presence of serious infection. Deep, labored respiration (Kussmaul's respiration) is a consequence of metabolic acidosis that is usually evident when the pH of the arterial blood is between 7.0 and 7.24. With more profound degrees of acidosis, respirations may become shallow. The patient's breath may have a fruity ketone (acetone) odor, and the patient may be alert, lethargic, or less commonly, comatose. Hypertonic dehydration leading to brain cell dehydration and ketosis itself are probably both contributory. It is important to remember that in all cases of coma, hypoglycemia should be considered and prophylactically treated (see pages 301–304).

Clinical Studies: A rigorous definition of diabetic ketoacidosis would include a blood glucose concentration over 250 mg/dl, serum ketones strongly positive in an undiluted serum specimen with an arterial pH less than 7.25 or a serum bicarbonate concentration less than 10 mEq/l. However, the attending physician can diagnose diabetic ketoacidosis within minutes with the aid of glucose reagent strips (e.g., Dextrostix) and nitroprusside reagent for serum ketones (e.g., Acetest tablets or Acetone test). Therapy, thus, can commence before definitive laboratory confirmation has been made.

Several caveats are worth noting. Dextrostrips are sensitive to heat, light, and moisture and should be kept fresh in a tightly closed container. Fluoride-containing tubes should not be used to collect blood for this test. The accuracy of the strips is enhanced with the aid of a reflectometer. The Acetest tablets should be crushed prior to use. Undiluted serum may interfere with the reagent and a dilution of serum should be used before concluding that serum ketones are negative. The nitroprusside reagents react to acetoacetate and less so to acetone (a nonacidic neutral compound.). However, the dominant ketone body in the circulation is β-hydroxybutyrate, and is not measured by this reagent. Reagent strips for ketones (e.g., Ketostix) should not be employed.

Although the initial blood glucose level may be less than 250 mg/dl and rarely less than 100 mg/dl in diabetic ketoacidosis, this situation almost always occurs in patients with known diabetes who have continued on a regimen of insulin. It has recently been recognized in patients on the ambulatory insulin pump as well. Thus, a blood glucose level less than 250 mg/dl does not exclude the possibility of diabetic ketoacidosis, but indicates that intravenous administration of glucose should be started immediately to permit administration of additional insulin without the hazard of hypoglycemia.

A strongly positive test for serum ketones may occur in alcoholic ketoacidosis as well. However, the blood glucose is usually less than 250 mg/dl in such patients. In alcoholic ketoacidosis, intravenous glucose is usually sufficient without concomitant insulin. However, whenever the distinction between alcoholic ketoacidosis and diabetic ketoacidosis is in doubt, with only slight elevation of the blood glucose, it is safer to administer both glucose and insulin.

The magnitude of serum ketone elevation is one important indication of the severity of the ketoacidosis. For determination of the serum ketone level, five crushed Acetest tablets should be placed separately on a sheet of filter paper. Serum from a centrifuged, clotted blood sample is then diluted serially with 2, 4, 8, and 16 parts of water or saline solution, and one or two drops of each dilution and of the undiluted serum are placed on the respective tablets. After 3 minutes, the color is determined. Deep purple represents a strong reaction and the highest dilution at which a strong reaction is noted is the value recorded—a serum ketone test strongly positive at 1:8 dilution, for example. β-hydroxybutyrate is not detected by this test.

Other immediate studies should include measurement of blood glucose, sodium, potassium, chloride, bicarbonate, blood urea nitrogen, amylase, and arterial blood-gas levels; a complete blood cell count; urinalysis; and an electrocardiogram. Appropriate specimens for culture, including blood, should be taken.

Therapy

The hallmarks of comprehensive therapy include an intensive care setting, individualization of treatment, and monitoring of the clinical and chemical progress of the patient so that appropriate adjustments can be made. A flow sheet recording the patient's status, laboratory data, and therapy is indispensable.

Initial Adjunctive Therapy. At the outset of therapy, several simple measures should be considered. Administration of oxygen may increase tissue oxygenation, thereby improving mental status. In obtunded patients, an endotracheal tube must be inserted. Gastric atony is a regular finding that often results in aspiration; a nasogastric tube should be passed and the stomach emptied. If the patient is alert, the nasogastric tube can then be removed, but in the obtunded patient, it should be left for further suctioning. The gastric contents often may be black and viscous, and guaiac tests may be positive. A Foley catheter should not be placed initially; however, if the patient does not urinate after intravenous administration of 500 ml of fluid, a catheter should be placed. In the obtunded, severely hypotensive patient, a Foley catheter may be necessary. Elderly patients and children with long-standing diabetes may require a central venous pressure line during fluid administration to avoid circulatory overload. Rarely, a pulmonary artery catheter will be necessary in patients with severe cardiac or pulmonary disease.

Specific Therapy. In the specific therapy for diabetic ketoacidosis (Table 14.1), administration of insulin alone is insufficient, even though insulin deficiency precipitated the metabolic and clinical abnormalities. In sequence, the patient must receive volume replacement, insulin, possibly bicarbonate, potassium, and glucose. In practice, both insulin and volume replacement must be started simultaneously as soon as the diagnosis is established.

Volume Replacement. The volume deficits are surprisingly large, averaging 10% of body weight or 6–8 liters of water, and from 300–500 mEq or more of sodium. Initial therapy is determined by the severity of the dehydration. For patients with frank shock or a minimal urine flow, plasma expanders are necessary. With moderate dehydration, normal saline is sufficient, the first liter being given over 30 minutes. The subsequent choice of fluids remains controversial. However, preservation of intravascular volume seems to be of paramount importance. A second liter of normal saline can be given over 1 hour. Subsequent infusions should be either normal saline or half-normal saline (0.45%) at a rate of 500 ml/hour, until the central venous pressure reaches 5–7 cm of water or the clinical signs of dehydration begin to disappear. When the patient is nearly adequately rehydrated, half-normal saline at 250 ml/hour can be administered. If the initial sodium concentration is greater than 150 mEq/l or rises to 155 mEq/l during therapy, half-normal saline should be substituted at that time. Extremes of hypo- and hypernatremia are to be avoided. In fully alert patients who are no longer nauseated, oral fluids can supplement intravenous infusion.

Insulin. Insulin therapy is critical in reversing the spiraling sequence of metabolic decompensation. However, much of the initial fall in blood glucose concentration is due to dilution of intravenous fluids. Only insulin will inhibit lipolysis and help correct ketosis. Insulin too is necessary to inhibit the ongoing gluconeogenesis. There is no "correct" amount of insulin and the optimal route of administration is still controversial. Only rapidly acting insulin (e.g., crystalline zinc insulin CZI, Actrapid, or others) should be used. Although fears of "insulin resistance" in diabetic ketoacidosis led to the use of heroic doses of insulin in the past, it appears that "low" or "modest" dose intravenous insulin by infusion provides a simple, reliable means of controlling diabetic ketoacidosis. Although doses as low as 4 units/hour can control the situation there is no merit to picking the lowest possible dose and no harm in using somewhat higher doses.

An intravenous bolus of 10 units can be given, followed by an infusion of 0.15 units/kg/hour or 10 units/hour. Although a variable quantity of insulin adheres to glass and plastic tubing, if a sufficiently concentrated solution is employed

Table 14.1.
Diabetic ketoacidosis: treatment.

Therapy	Dosage	Comments
Volume replacement	Moderate: 1 liter of normal saline intravenously over 30–60 min; 500 ml/hr subsequently until central venous pressure increases or dehydration disappears Severe: Add plasma, albumin (Albumisol) to above	Usual fluid deficit: 5–7 liters Usual sodium deficit: 300–500 mEq Monitor central venous pressure if indicated Subsequent fluids should be hypotonic (0.45% saline)
Insulin (alternatives)[a]		
Constant intravenous infusion	10 units intravenous bolus; then 50 units in 500 ml of normal saline, 100 ml/hr (10 units/hr)	Discard first 25 ml If blood glucose does not respond in 1–2 hrs, double the insulin dosage
Intramuscular insulin	15–20 units initially; 10 units/hr subsequently	Do not use in hypotensive patients If blood glucose does not respond in 1–2 hrs, double the insulin dosage
Hourly intravenous insulin	10 units intravenous bolus each hour	If no response in 1–2 hrs, double the insulin dosage or change to constant infusion
Bicarbonate	44–88 mEq intravenously over 1 hour; repeat as necessary	Indications: shock, pH <7.1, serum bicarbonate <5 mEq/liter
Potassium	Potassium chloride, 40 mEq/liter of intravenous solution	Administer when serum potassium enters normal range if urinary output satisfactory Usual potassium deficit: 200–500 mEq
Glucose	5% or 10% dextrose intravenously in water or saline, depending on blood glucose level and volume status 50 ml of 50% dextrose for hypoglycemia	Indication: persistent ketosis when blood glucose concentration decreases to 250–300 mg/dl

[a] Use only regular insulin (e.g. crystalline zinc insulin, CZI).

(e.g., 50 units in 500 ml), this is not a practical problem. Additional safety can be achieved by running the initial 25 ml out through the tube to "saturate" insulin binding sites. A pediatric infusion set is quite effective in delivering the insulin. If an infusion pump is available, 100 units of insulin can be added to 100 ml normal saline. Although albumin has been recommended to prevent insulin binding, a small amount of the patient's blood drawn into the infusion apparatus will suffice. Insulin can then be infused at a similar rate as above.

This regimen provides for a controlled fall in the blood glucose. Independent of dilution effects, the blood sugar can be expected to fall at the rate of 75–100 mg/dl/hour. The use of intravenous insulin by constant infusion provides great flexibility in the management of uncontrolled diabetes, whether it be diabetic ketoacidosis, or early decompensation in a hospitalized or ambulatory diabetic.

It is important to realize that if the intravenous line stops, or becomes disconnected, the patient will receive no insulin. If the blood glucose does not begin to fall in 1 hour, the concentration or the rate of the infusion should be doubled, and so on each hour. The intravenous infusion systems are superior to traditional methods of intravenous plus subcutaneous insulin in that hypoglycemia and hypokalemia appear to be minimized.

The half-life of insulin is short (4–6 minutes), hence the effect of an intravenous bolus of insulin is only 20–30 minutes. Despite this theoretical reservation, hourly intravenous insulin boluses (e.g., 10 units/hour) appear to be as effective as insulin infusions. Another alternative is hourly intramuscular (deltoid) injections. After an initial dose of 15–20 units, approximately 10 units/hour can be administered. Intramuscular insulin should not be employed in patients with severe hypotension.

The more traditional methods of insulin administration (e.g., intravenous plus subcutaneous insulin) are also effective; however, the variable rate of delivery of insulin from the subcutaneous sites makes these regimens somewhat less desirable.

Although these schedules simplify the initial decision regarding insulin administration, they do not alter the need for intensive monitoring of the patient's condition, and subsequent decisions regarding insulin administration must be determined by assessing the patient's response. If no change in blood glucose level is noted in the course of 1–2 hours, the dosage must be increased.

Bicarbonate. Acidosis in diabetic patients results from ketone body production (ketoacidosis) and, to a lesser degree, from poor tissue perfusion (lactic acidosis). In most cases, the acidosis is easily corrected with insulin and volume replacement alone. However, if peripheral vascular collapse is present, bicarbonate should be administered, 44–88 mEq intravenously in the course of 10–15 minutes. Also, if the pH of the arterial blood is less than 7.1 or if the serum bicarbonate concentration is less than 5 mEq/liter, bicarbonate should be administered at the rate of 44–88 mEq/hour until those values are exceeded. The bicarbonate should be added only to hypotonic fluids (e.g., 0.5 N [0.45%] Saline) to prevent severe hypernatremia. Profound acidosis antagonizes the action of catecholamines, such as norepinephrine, that are required for normal peripheral vasoconstriction and maintenance of blood pressure, and in patients with profound shock, bicarbonate may be lifesaving.

Most patients do not require bicarbonate therapy. Furthermore, excessive administration of bicarbonate may result in metabolic alkalosis and arrhythmias. In addition, hypokalemia may develop precipitously after bicarbonate therapy, increasing early potassium requirements substantially. Theoretical dangers of bicarbonate therapy include development of paradoxical cerebrospinal fluid acidosis and unfavorable shifts in the oxygen-hemoglobin dissociation curve.

Potassium. Striking potassium deficits are almost invariably present in patients with diabetic ketoacidosis. Deficits average about 5 mEq/kg of body weight (350 mEq in a person weighing 70 kg), but may range up to 10 mEq/kg. Although large quantities of potassium are lost in the urine, the serum potassium concentration is usually normal or elevated. This paradox is a consequence of the acidosis, which causes a shift of potassium ions from cells to plasma, as well as a consequence of insulin deficiency *per se* which prevents the entry of potassium into cells. Although peaked T waves on the electrocardiogram indicate an elevated serum potassium concentration, they may also occur with acidosis alone. Less than 5% of patients have initial hypokalemia; those who do should receive vigorous potassium replacement therapy immediately.

Once therapy with insulin and fluid replacement has been started, the serum potassium concentration may plummet. This is partly due to dilution by fluids that do not contain potassium and partly due to entry of potassium into the cells. As acidosis is corrected and insulin administered, potassium enters cells. As stated previously, bicarbonate therapy may accelerate the development of hypokalemia.

As soon as the serum potassium concentration enters the normal range (3.5–5.0 mEq/liter)—provided that good urinary output has been established—potassium chloride, 30–40 mEq/liter of intravenous solution, should be administered. Oral potassium salts may be given as well. The serum potassium level should be monitored at least every 2 hours to avoid a fatal arrhythmia, especially if the patient is receiving digitalis.

Glucose. If insulin therapy is adequate a decrease in the blood glucose level should be noted within a few hours. When the blood glucose concentration decreases to between 250–300 mg/dl (usually between 4–8 hours), special care must be taken. If the acidosis and ketosis have disappeared, insulin therapy can be diminished but must not be stopped. If ketosis persists, intravenous glucose should be administered to allow insulin to be given to speed the clearance of ketone bodies and yet avoid hypoglycemia. When glucose is required it should be given at a rate of 250 ml/hour of D5 solutions or 125 ml/hour of D10 solutions (12.5 gm/hour of glucose) depending upon the volume status of the patient at the time.

Although the serum ketones are an important indicator of the severity of the diabetic ketoacidosis, they are somewhat less useful in following the course of the disease. The disappearance of ketones in the blood and urine is, of course, a favorable clinical sign. However, the ketones may be slow to clear due to the shift in equilibrium between acetoacetate and β-hydroxybutyrate. As the acidosis is corrected, the ratio of acetoacetate to β-hydroxybutyrate rises as the concentration of β-hydroxybutyrate falls. Only the acetoacetate is measured by the nitroprusside reagent and its concentration may not change while the total ketone bodies decline. This improved state should be reflected by a decline in the anion gap, which does measure the hidden anion (β-hydroxybutyrate).

Phosphate. Severe phosphate deficits may occur in diabetic ketoacidosis. Although serum phosphate concentrations are often normal or elevated, intracellular organophosphates are depleted, including 2,3 diphosphoglycerate (2,3 DPG), the red cell organophosphate which facilitates oxygen unloading from hemoglobin. During the course of therapy for diabetic ketoacidosis, serum phosphate concentrations often fall dramatically. There has been a recent trend to supplement phosphate with intravenous therapy in nonoliguric patients (e.g., 5 mmoles/hour of intravenous phosphate as the potassium salt). Although theoretically attractive, such therapy does not appear to be necessary, and has not been shown to influence morbidity or mortality. Furthermore, symptomatic hypocalcemia may occur if the phosphate infusion rate is too vigorous.

Subsequent Management. The nasogastric tube, Foley catheter, and central venous pressure line should be removed as soon as possible, if it has been necessary to use them. The nasogastric tube can be removed when the patient becomes alert, and the central venous pressure line need not be left in place once normal volume status has been re-established.

Increased cerebrospinal fluid pressure occurs commonly during the course of therapy of diabetic ketoacidosis. Fortunately, coma or death due to documented cerebral edema is rare. If the mental state begins to deteriorate after a period of improvement, the fundi should be examined for papilledema. Although their efficacy has not yet been demonstrated, therapy for cerebral edema with mannitol and high-dose glucocorticoids should be considered in the appropriate clinical setting. Hyponatremia may predispose to this dreaded complication and should be avoided.

Arterial blood gases should be monitored. As in all cases of metabolic acidosis, a rising Pco_2 and a falling pH constitute a poor prognostic sign; they suggest that the patient is tiring and mandate assisted ventilation.

A vigilant watch for hypoglycemia must continue, although this is less likely if insulin has not been administered subcutaneously. It is worth reemphasizing the need for continuous glucose infusion once the blood glucose enters the range of

250–300 mg/dl. Once acidosis has been corrected, insulin should be administered subcutaneously at 4-hour intervals, based on the blood glucose, until the serum ketone test is no longer strongly positive and urinary ketones are no longer present in large amounts. Administration of intermediate acting insulin (e.g., NPH or lente insulin) should be started the following morning. Common errors in the management of diabetic ketoacidosis are summarized in Table 14.2.

Vascular thrombosis is a common concomitant of diabetic ketoacidosis, either as a precipitating event or a consequence of the dehydration. Low-dose subcutaneous heparin therapy can be considered in appropriate situations. Renal failure can develop during the course of therapy and dialysis may need to be instituted in certain cases.

Precipitating Factors

Once therapy has been started, the cause of the decompensation must be sought (see Table 14.3). Newly diagnosed diabetes, insulin omission, and infection are the most common offenders. The

Table 14.2.

Diabetic ketoacidosis: common errors in management.

Failure to individualize therapy
Insulin infusions becoming disconnected
Failure to increase rate of insulin infusion if patient not responding
Insufficient salt and volume replacement
Failure to begin potassium therapy when (K^+) enters normal range
Excessive bicarbonate
Failure to administer glucose when blood glucose levels enter 250–300 mg/dl range
Premature cessation of insulin therapy
Inadequate surveillance for delayed hypoglycemia
Failure to begin intermediate-acting insulins (NPH or lente) when ketosis has cleared
Inadequate search for precipitating cause
Failure to follow laboratory abnormalities in serial fashion and to maintain flow sheet of progress

Table 14.3.

Diabetic ketoacidosis: precipitating factors.

Newly diagnosed diabetes
Insulin omission
Infection
Myocardial infarction (may be silent) or cerebrovascular accident
Intra-abdominal emergencies including pancreatitis
Trauma
Pregnancy
Surgery

temperature may not be elevated despite infection, and the white blood count may be elevated in the absence of infection. Prophylactic antibiotics should not be used, but a careful search for infection, particularly of the urinary and respiratory tracts, should be initiated. The serum amylase is commonly elevated in diabetic ketoacidosis, although pancreatitis is rare. Salivary rather than pancreatic amylase may account for the confusing amylase elevation. Virtually any major stress can lead to diabetic ketoacidosis in a predisposed individual. It is equally important to remember that other conditions may cause coma, for example, subdural hematoma, drugs including ethanol, and meningitis. These must be considered even if frank ketoacidosis is evident. Although no precipitating cause is found in 10–20% of patients with diabetic ketoacidosis, a vigilant search must be made in every case.

Diabetic ketoacidosis is easier to prevent than to treat. Patients must be instructed not to omit insulin therapy when they become ill; rather, insulin dosage often needs to be increased. Oral intake must be sustained and perhaps augmented if additional insulin is administered. If the patient is nauseated, fruit juices, soft drinks, and bouillon can provide palatable sources of fluid, glucose, and sodium.

Hyperglycemic Hyperosmolar Nonketotic Coma (HHNC)

Severe hyperglycemia without ketosis is being recognized with increasing frequency, although unfortunately often in its late stages. In contrast, with diabetic ketoacidosis, hyperglycemic, hyperosmolar nonketotic coma has a mortality that still approaches 50%. It is unproven, but seems likely that the long delay in recognition, advanced age of the patients, and severity of underlying medical conditions are all important in this unacceptably high mortality. This syndrome often occurs in "mild" diabetics or in those with previously unrecognized diabetes, leads to initially subtle and then progressive deterioration in mental status and is most commonly misdiagnosed as "stroke" in the emergency ward.

Pathophysiologic Principles

Although relative insulin deficiency is present, only the carbohydrate side of the insulin deficiency schema is apparently affected (Fig. 14.2A). The explanation for the absence of ketosis remains elusive. It is possible that sufficient insulin is present to prevent lipolysis, but insufficient to prevent gluconeogenesis and stimulate glucose uptake. Additional effects of increased osmolality on intermediary metabolism are being explored.

As the blood glucose begins to rise, glycosuria develops. If renal perfusion is adequate, the kidney serves as a "drain" for the excess glucose, but if urinary output begins to decrease or if renal failure is present, the blood glucose increases substantially. The increased thirst often results in drinking of fruit juices or other high sugar beverages, further raising the blood glucose. Although intrinsic renal disease may account for a reduced urinary output, such a decrease more commonly represents decreasing glomerular filtration as a consequence of these fluid losses. Progressive lethargy, dehydration, and obtundation result and oral intake diminishes. The consequence is a striking elevation of the blood glucose and often the serum osmolality, resulting in profound cellular dehydration. The impaired mental state is best correlated with the magnitude of the serum osmolality elevation.

Diagnosis

The diagnosis may be unsuspected until an elevated blood glucose level is revealed by a "routine" laboratory test. Kussmaul's respiration and an acetone odor to the breath are absent. Patients tend to be middle-aged or older, and may have a history of Type II ("maturity-onset") diabetes. Signs of dehydration may provide the only clinical clue. Coma is common, and focal neurologic abnormalities, including seizures, may dominate the clinical findings. The common misdiagnosis is stroke.

To meet accepted criteria for hyperosmolar nonketotic coma, the blood glucose concentration must be more than 600 mg/dl, the serum osmolality more than 350 mEq/l, and the serum ketone reaction less than strong in undiluted serum. Lesser degrees of hyperglycemia and hyperosmolality may of course be present, and should be treated with similar care. At the other end of the scale, a severe hyperosmolar state may be part of diabetic ketoacidosis. Since the advent of intravenous insulin infusions, the arbitrary distinction between these syndromes is of somewhat less importance.

The osmolality may be measured precisely in the clinical laboratory, but a quick estimation is often helpful in establishing a diagnosis:

serum osmolality =

$$2\,[Na^+] + \frac{BUN}{2.8} + \frac{blood\ glucose}{18}$$

The osmolality and the serum sodium concentration [Na$^+$] are both expressed as mEq/liter, and the blood urea nitrogen (BUN) and blood glucose concentrations are expressed as mg/dl.

Therapy

Although mild to moderate degrees of acidosis may be present in patients with hyperosmolar nonketotic coma, profound acidosis is usually absent. With this exception, the therapeutic considerations are similar to those pertaining to diabetic ketoacidosis.

Volume Replacement. Volume deficits often exceed those of diabetic ketoacidosis, perhaps reflecting a longer prodromal period before clinical recognition. Deficits in excess of 10 liters are not unusual. Half of the volume lost should be replaced within the first 8–12 hours if possible. If profound dehydration with hypotension is present, the initial solutions should include plasma expanders. Although 0.9% (normal) saline is a hypertonic fluid (308 milliosm/liter), it is relatively hypotonic for these patients and is the initial therapy of choice to maintain adequate intravascular volume. Guidelines are similar to those for initial fluid management in diabetic ketoacidosis. In this older age group, close attention to volume status is of even greater importance, to prevent extremes of intravascular volume depletion and circulatory overload.

Insulin. The initial fall in blood glucose concentration in these patients reflects dilution by intravenous fluids and increased urinary losses secondary to improved renal perfusion. Insulin should be administered as in diabetic ketoacidosis, with constant intravenous infusions providing a controlled method of decreasing the blood glucose. When the blood glucose reaches 300 mg/dl however, constant infusions of insulin can be discontinued. Regular insulin (CZI) can be given subcutaneously at 4-hour intervals based on the blood glucose, until the next morning when intermediate acting insulins (e.g., NPH or lente) should be started.

Bicarbonate. The mild to moderate degrees of acidosis that have been noted are not adequately explained by decreased tissue perfusion (lactic acidosis) or renal insufficiency (uremic acidosis). Unless shock is present, bicarbonate therapy is rarely indicated.

Potassium. Severe potassium deficits are the rule. The initial serum potassium concentration is often closer to normal than those in diabetic ketoacidosis, reflecting the lack of severe acidosis. Potassium chloride, 30–40 mEq/liter, should be added to intravenous infusions once a good urinary output has been established.

Glucose. Intravenous administration of glucose should be started when the blood glucose concentration has decreased to between 250–300 mg/dl.

Phosphate. Profound phosphate depletion is much less common than in diabetic ketoacidosis with normal red cell 2,3 DPG levels usually being present. Although controversy continues about the utility of phosphate in patients with diabetic ketoacidosis, there is even less indication for this therapy in patients with hyperglycemic hyperosmolar coma.

Precipitating Factors

Some of the initiating events are similar to those that may precipitate diabetic ketoacidosis. Infection is important, and a rather high prevalence of gram-negative bacterial infection has been noted, especially pneumonia and urinary tract infections. Drugs play a more important role here, including thiazide diuretics or furosemide, phenytoin, glucocorticoids and occasionally propranolol and diazoxide. In addition, peritoneal dialysis, burn patients, demented or obtunded individuals, particularly those receiving intravenous glucose (e.g., hyperalimentation) are all well represented in series of patients with this diagnosis. The increased intake of solutions containing carbohydrates early in the course of dehydration may be important in ambulatory patients. Myocardial infarctions, cerebrovascular disease, and renal failure are particularly prevalent in these patients. Of the surviving patients, many require no diabetic therapy after the episode of hyperglycemic hyperosmolar coma has resolved.

Alcoholic Ketoacidosis

Alcoholic ketoacidosis is not a manifestation of diabetes, but may be confused with diabetic ketoacidosis. In this situation, persons with chronic alcoholism who have been drinking continually become nauseated and increasingly anorexic. Food intake ceases, and alcohol intake often ceases as well. Nausea increases and vomiting develops, occasionally with abdominal pain. Other presenting features include hyperpnea and possibly pancreatitis.

It appears that the lipid or ketone body pathway (Fig. 14.2B) is activated without necessarily activating the carbohydrate pathway. Acidosis is often severe. Although this is a ketoacidosis, the serum ketone concentration may be only mildly increased as assessed by testing with Acetest tablets;

for example, there may be less than a 4+ reaction for undiluted serum. This is due to a predominance of β-hydroxybutyrate (not measured by Acetest tablets) over acetoacetate, as well as concomitant lactic acidosis. The blood glucose concentration ranges from hypoglycemic to moderately hyperglycemic levels.

The pathophysiologic mechanisms are unclear. During starvation, insulin deficiency is present and this permits lipolysis and ketogenesis to occur. However, ketoacidosis is not a concomitant of the "normal" starved state and the role of ethanol and stress on the release of free fatty acids, inhibition of insulin release and hepatic ketogenesis remains unresolved. In most patients, the glucose tolerance test is normal after recovery.

The nondiabetic patient with such a typical history should receive intravenous or intramuscular thiamine (25 mg), intravenous fluid and electrolytes, large quantities of intravenous glucose, and bicarbonate if the arterial blood pH is less than 7.1. If the blood glucose level is greater than 250 mg/dl it appears judicious to administer insulin (CZI, 10 units/hour by intravenous infusion) along with intravenous glucose (12.5 gm/hour).

Lactic Acidosis

Lactic acidosis is a syndrome, not a disease. Severe metabolic acidosis due to accumulation of lactate may occur in many diseases.

Pathophysiologic Principles

Lactic acid is the end product of anaerobic glycolysis. All lactic acid is derived from pyruvic acid, a reaction catalyzed by lactate dehydrogenase (LDH):

$$NADH + pyruvate + H^+ \overset{LDH}{\rightleftharpoons} NAD^+ + lactate$$

where NADH = nicotinamide adenine dinucleotide. Under aerobic conditions, glucose in muscle and other tissues is partly oxidized to pyruvate. Under anaerobic conditions, the pyruvate is preferentially converted to lactate and released into the bloodstream. The liver has a great capacity for lactate metabolism, lactate being converted back to pyruvate. Several alternative pathways are available for pyruvate, including further oxidation to carbon dioxide and water with the storage of energy in the form of ATP, free fatty acid synthesis, and resynthesis into glucose (followed by release from the liver, completing the Cori cycle).

Under normal circumstances, skeletal muscle, red blood cells, and skin are the major contributors to the blood lactate pool. The liver and kidney are instrumental in lactate removal. In pathologic states, cellular oxidation of glucose may be impaired by poor tissue perfusion, poor tissue oxygenation, or metabolic poisons. Under these circumstances, virtually any tissue may produce a large amount of lactic acid. Impaired lactate removal is usually present in pathologic states, as the removal capacity for lactate is quite high under normal circumstances.

Lactic acidosis is now commonly separated into type A, in which circulatory collapse or hypoxia are primary, and type B, where the lactic acidosis has other causes. The clinical situation may be confusing, in that profound lactic acidosis can secondarily result in vascular collapse.

Diagnosis

The recognition of lactic acidosis depends on the recognition of metabolic acidosis. Vascular collapse or unexplained air hunger require assessment of acid-base status by means of arterial blood-gas determination. The presence of vasodilation and "warm shock" should suggest the presence of severe acidemia or overwhelming sepsis. Arterial blood with a pH less than 7.4, with a decreased P_{CO_2} or serum bicarbonate level, establishes the diagnosis of metabolic acidosis. Even if the pH is close to normal (e.g., 7.35–7.39), a decreased P_{CO_2} or serum bicarbonate concentration is still a valuable indication of ongoing metabolic acidemia (with respiratory compensation).

When a strong acid (such as lactic acid, represented by HA) is added to a solution of bicarbonate (such as plasma), carbon dioxide is produced:

$$HA + NaHCO_3 \rightleftharpoons$$
$$Na^+ A^- + H_2CO_3 \rightarrow H_2O + CO_2 \uparrow$$

Neutralization of the acid results in the formation of anions (A^-); these are the anions that contribute to the anion gap. In the presence of metabolic acidosis, the anion gap should be determined. The anion gap is equal to the serum sodium concentration minus the sum of the serum bicarbonate and serum chloride concentrations, normal being less than 12 mEq/liter. (If the serum potassium concentration is also considered, normal is less than 15 mEq/liter.) If the anion gap is more than 12 mEq/liter, one of the causes listed in Table 14.4 must be considered. It is usually fairly easy to exclude uremia, ketoacidosis, and drug ingestion, leaving lactic acidosis as the diagnosis.

Lactate can be measured directly as well, and in most clinical laboratories, the result can be known within several hours. A lactate concentration greater than 5 mEq/liter in a sick patient with metabolic acidosis indicates that lactic acidosis is at least contributory. Determination of the pyru-

Table 14.4.
Metabolic acidosis with anion gap.

Type	Anion in Excess
Lactic acidosis	Lactate
Ketoacidosis (diabetic or alcoholic)	β-hydroxybutyrate
	Acetoacetate
Uremic acidosis	Phosphate
	Sulfate
Drug-induced acidosis	
Ethylene glycol	Glycolate, oxalate
Methyl alcohol	Formate[a]
Paraldehyde	[a]
Salicylates	[a]
Chloral hydrate	[a]

[a] Uncertain.

vate level is more time-consuming, adds little information, and is unnecessary for diagnosis. The white blood count is often elevated in acute metabolic acidosis. The uric acid level is often markedly elevated, due to inhibition of renal excretion of urate by the elevation of blood lactate.

Precipitating Factors

Increased lactate production is a regular finding in the shock state and frequently occurs with regional underperfusion as well. Frank lactic acidosis is less common. When the shock or underperfusion is corrected, this type A lactic acidosis can be expected to disappear as well. Profound hypoxia, whether local or systemic, stimulates increased lactate production and depresses lactate clearance by the liver.

Type B lactic acidosis is much less common and can be further subdivided. In Type B1, a number of common disorders are found, including diabetes mellitus, renal failure, infections, liver disease, and leukemia. Type B2 includes drug-induced lactic acidosis and is less prevalent now that phenformin is no longer prescribed. Ethyl alcohol (ethanol) inhibits the hepatic disposal of lactic acid presumably by increasing the levels of NADH in the liver. Lactic acidosis may be precipitated or exacerbated by ethanol. Sorbitol and fructose infusions fall within this category as well. Type B3 includes a disparate group of hereditary enzyme defects.

Therapy

Therapy must be directed at the underlying disorder. In Type A lactic acidosis, tissue perfusion should be improved with volume replacement or cardiotonic agents when indicated. Hypoxia should be corrected, with assisted ventilation if necessary. Bicarbonate should be administered intravenously to maintain the arterial pH above 7.2.

The quantities of bicarbonate necessary will be quite variable (see below). Arterial blood-gas determinations must be serially repeated to monitor the effects of therapy.

There may be considerable clinical overlap in patients with type B lactic acidosis, in that vascular collapse may be present if the arterial pH is less than 7.1. Offending drugs should be omitted and any treatable underlying disease identified and treated as well. With vascular collapse, volume replacement will be necessary. Bicarbonate is required, often in heroic amounts, with thousands of milliequivalents administered in some cases. If the acidemia is severe and ongoing, 5% (600 mmole) $NaHCO_3$ may be required.

Loop diuretics such as furosemide or ethacrynic acid are often necessary to prevent volume overload. If sodium overload occurs in the face of such therapy, peritoneal dialysis may be necessary to remove excess sodium. The use of vasodilator therapy to allow adequate bicarbonate therapy has been successful and has the theoretic advantage of opening unidentified areas of regional underperfusion. Nitroprusside has been used but other vasodilators may be tried. Methylene blue (1–5 mg/kg intravenously) can decrease hepatic levels of NADH and may help correct the lactate accumulation but is rarely lifesaving. The experimental drug dichloracetate holds promise as a stimulator of pyruvate dehydrogenase, providing an alternative route for pyruvate other than to lactate production. It is effective in correcting lactic overproduction in experimental situations and its role in clinical lactic acidosis is being explored. Thiamine administation (several hundred mg intravenously) seems reasonable, particularly in alcoholic patients. The role of insulin with glucose therapy is being explored as well.

Hypoglycemia

The challenge of hypoglycemia lies in its recognition rather than its management. The type of hypoglycemia requiring treatment in the emergency ward is usually that which occurs after a variable period of fasting. Reactive hypoglycemia occurring within 4–5 hours after a meal is a benign condition and rarely requires immediate therapy; it may occasionally accompany fasting hypoglycemia. By far, the most common cause of hypoglycemia is insulin administration.

The immediate treatment is administration of glucose. Once treatment has been started, the amount of glucose and the duration of therapy can safely be determined. The physician must then also seek the underlying cause. Although the manifestations of hypoglycemia may vary considerably, one specific rule must be followed: any obtunded or comatose patient seen in the emergency ward should be treated immediately with 50 ml of a 50% glucose solution after blood has been drawn for determination of the glucose content.

Pathophysiologic Principles

During the normal fasting state (4 or more hours after the last meal), the blood glucose level begins to decrease and insulin release is inhibited. The liver provides glucose to maintain the amount in the blood, preventing hypoglycemia. Glycogen breakdown, and synthesis and release of glucose are both contributory. The substrates for glucose synthesis (lactate, the amino acids alanine and glutamine, and glycerol) are derived from muscle and fat breakdown. Cortisol, glucagon, growth hormone, and epinephrine—the counter-regulatory hormones—may provide substrates for glucose production. This process is similar to that occurring in insulin deficiency described in Figure 14.2A, and the net result is provision of an adequate glucose supply for the brain. Most instances of hypoglycemia are caused, in part, by inability of the liver to provide the necessary glucose. Rarely, increased peripheral utilization alone is at fault.

Insulin. Inappropriate elevation of insulin can cause substrate flow to the liver to halt and increased peripheral utilization of glucose, as well as termination of glucose production by the liver. The net result is severe hypoglycemia. This situation is most commonly due to insulin injections, oral hypoglycemic therapy with sulfonylurea compounds, and insulinomas. Drug interactions (for example, between sulfonamides and sulfonylureas) and hepatic or renal insufficiency may precipitate hypoglycemia in patients receiving long-term oral hypoglycemic therapy. Liver glycogen is adequate or increased in insulin-induced hypoglycemia, and alternative substrates such as free fatty acids or ketones are diminished by the action of insulin on fat cells.

Inhibition of Glucose Synthesis. Alcohol is the most common drug known to inhibit glucose synthesis; inhibition occurs because the increased NADH generated by ethanol oxidation depletes hepatic pyruvate by converting it to lactate. As long as the alcoholic continues to eat, hypoglycemia will not develop. However, when hepatic glycogen reserves are depleted, after a variable period of starvation, alcohol-induced inhibition of glucose synthesis can result in profound hypoglycemia. It is easy to confuse the clinical findings with those of alcoholic stupor, and this lethal error has

often been made. Severe starvation may result in decreased gluconeogenic substrates and hence hypoglycemia.

Salicylates in massive quantities can produce hypoglycemia, perhaps by inhibition of glucose synthesis. The glycogen storage diseases of infancy are rare causes of hypoglycemia. In these conditions, hereditary defects are present in the enzymes necessary for glucose production by the liver.

Intrinsic Hepatic Disease. Hypoglycemia is rare in patients with cirrhosis unless terminal hepatic failure develops. However, acute yellow atrophy, toxic hepatic damage, and Reye's syndrome can produce severe hypoglycemia.

Lack of Counter-regulatory Hormones. Cortisol deficiency alone, as in Addison's disease, or in association with growth hormone deficiency, as in hypopituitarism, may result in fasting hypoglycemia, especially in children.

Other. Fasting hypoglycemia may develop during pregnancy since the fetus has an obligatory glucose requirement. In infants with ketotic hypoglycemia, the liver is apparently insufficiently provided with substrates. Rarely, hypoglycemia is a consequence of nonpancreatic neoplasms, but the mechanism remains elusive. Prolonged exertion such as marathon running may result in hypoglycemia. Hypoglycemia may be a manifestation of sepsis or severe renal failure. Drugs such as propranolol and disopyramide (Norpace) have rarely been implicated.

Clinical Features

For convenience, the symptoms of hypoglycemia may be considered as "catechol-like" and "neuroglucopenic." A rapid fall in the blood glucose level results in release of the catecholamines epinephrine and norepinephrine, which tend to increase the amount of blood glucose. The symptoms and signs of catecholamine excess include anxiety, palpitations, tremor, diaphoresis, weakness, hunger, cool moist skin, pallor, and tachycardia. Increased systolic and decreased diastolic blood pressure may be present. Catechol-mediated symptoms occur when the blood glucose level falls rapidly, being absent with gradual decrease in the blood glucose level or with sustained or chronic hypoglycemia. Autonomic neuropathy in the diabetic patient or β-adrenergic blockade with propranolol will prevent signs and symptoms of catechol excess. Propranolol should be avoided or used with great caution in insulin-requiring diabetics; other drugs such as metoprolal may be safer. Alcohol-induced hypoglycemia often lacks signs of catechol excess, for unclear reasons.

When the central nervous system is deprived of

its principal source of energy, glucose, a variety of neuroglucopenic signs and symptoms may develop. Mental changes are common, and may range from lethargy, mild confusion, or difficulty in concentrating to personality changes or profound coma. Grand mal seizures may occur, and unilateral signs identical with those of a cerebrovascular accident may be present. These are all reversible if therapy is not delayed too long. However, it is important to recognize that, whereas response to glucose infusion is diagnostic, lack of response to a single bolus does not exclude the diagnosis of hypoglycemia.

Additional signs and symptoms may also be helpful. Nocturnal hypoglycemia may be characterized by nightmares, night sweats, early morning headaches, or occasionally, angina during sleep. Hypoglycemia causes hypothermia probably due to increased peripheral vasodilatation and sweating, which may be appreciated by studying the patient's temperature chart for inappropriate dips or failure of the temperature to rise from early morning to late evening. Chronic hypoglycemia, as in patients with insulinoma, may lead to increased caloric intake and weight gain, and may occasionally be associated with chronic sensory-motor neuropathy. Trismus may occur in patients with alcoholic hypoglycemia.

Specific Diagnosis and Therapy

If hypoglycemia is suspected, or in the presence of an acute neurologic condition (such as seizures, cerebrovascular accidents, or coma), blood should be drawn for a glucose determination by the laboratory and by Dextrostix and 50 ml of a 50% glucose solution should be administered intravenously. If it is certain that insulin-induced hypoglycemia is present, an alternative therapy is glucagon 1 mg by intramuscular injection, a rapidly acting therapy which may spare veins in diabetics with recurrent hypoglycemia. In suspected alcoholics, 25–50 mg of thiamine should also be administered to prevent an acute episode of Wernicke-Korsakoff syndrome. Even in the absence of obvious response to intravenous glucose, the blood glucose concentration should be estimated quickly with Dextrostix reagent strips. A laboratory determination revealing a blood glucose level less than 40 mg/dl or a plasma glucose level less than 45 mg/dl is diagnostic.

Coma which is apparently due to hypoglycemia, but does not reverse after glucose administration can be quite difficult to manage. Continued intravenous glucose to maintain the blood glucose level around 150–180 mg/dl is advisable, often requiring D10 solutions with concomitant insulin. Therapy for cerebral edema should be instituted with dexamethasone and/or mannitol. A search for other causes of coma, including drugs, trauma and continued seizure activity should be performed. A computed tomogram of the brain should be performed.

When blood is drawn, a specimen should be set aside in a green top (heparinized) tube for possible insulin assay. The combination of fasting hypoglycemia and inappropriately elevated insulin levels indicates insulin-induced hypoglycemia, which may be due to insulin therapy, oral hypoglycemic agents, or insulinoma. Much time can be saved and expense avoided if this simple expedient is followed. Surreptitious insulin injections (factitious hypoglycemia) in a nondiabetic patient can be detected if anti-insulin antibodies are present in serum. A blood specimen should also be set aside for cortisol assay if the cause of hypoglycemia is not obvious. In hypoglycemia, cortisol secretion and therefore the plasma cortisol level normally increase; if this does not occur in the presence of hypoglycemic symptoms, adrenal insufficiency or hypopituitarism is likely especially in children. The possibility of willful insulin overadministration in a suicide attempt should be kept in mind.

If insulin therapy is the cause of the hypoglycemia, intramuscular glucagon (1 mg) or intravenous glucose (25 gm) will suffice for the acute management. Dietary instructions and a careful review of the insulin regimen should be undertaken as well. If an oral hypoglycemic drug is responsible, the patient must be hospitalized. The hypoglycemia may last for days or weeks, particularly if chlorpropamide is the etiologic agent and it may recur several times after initial seemingly successful therapy. This may, in part, be related to increased insulin release by the sensitized pancreatic β cell in response to bolus glucose therapy. In these patients, continuous intravenous infusion of glucose, adequate oral food intake, and frequent monitoring of the blood glucose level are mandatory. Since a liter of 5% dextrose in water contains only 50 gm of glucose, a 10% or 20% solution should be administered with intravenous boluses of 50% dextrose as necessary. If hyperglycemia (blood glucose level more than 100 mg/dl) cannot be established in 4–6 hours with this therapy, hydrocortisone hemisuccinate (100 mg) should be added to each liter of solution. In particularly refractory situations, diazoxide, a drug which inhibits insulin release from the pancreas, should be administered.

Alcohol-induced hypoglycemia is particularly treacherous, because the diagnosis is often missed.

The alcoholic who is stuporous from hypoglycemia may be thought to be drunk, and grand mal seizures may be interpreted as withdrawal seizures ("rum fits"). Alcoholics should not be permitted to "sleep it off" unsupervised. Glucose and thiamine should be administered intravenously, and patients should be observed for increasing obtundation. After correction of alcoholic hypoglycemia, hospitalization is not required. The brain utilizes 5–6 gm/hour of glucose. In this situation, in contrast to the insulin-induced hypoglycemia, increased peripheral utilization is not playing a role and 10 gm/hour of glucose should suffice for maintenance therapy until the patient is eating. It is important to realize that alcoholic ketoacidosis can coexist with alcoholic hypoglycemia.

Profound hepatic failure is usually obvious, and must be managed with adequate caloric intake, at least 100 gm of carbohydrates each day, either orally or parenterally to spare muscle protein. With persistent hypoglycemia, larger quantities of glucose may be required.

Hypoglycemia is preventable in many patients. Otherwise healthy persons with diabetes should not decrease oral intake or increase exercise without decreasing the dosage of insulin. Diabetics with intermittent symptoms at home should be taught to test their blood by finger-stick analysis to exclude hypoglycemia. Chlorpropamide should not be administered to any patient with renal failure, and tolbutamide should not be given to patients with abnormal hepatic function. Drugs known to potentiate the action of the sulfonylurea compounds must be avoided.

ADRENAL INSUFFICIENCY AND HYPOPITUITARISM

Adrenal Physiology

The adrenal cortex produces three major classes of hormones: glucocorticoids or "sugar" hormones, mineralocorticoids or "salt" hormones, and androgens or "sex" hormones. Deficiency of either glucocorticoids or mineralocorticoids may be life-threatening. Adrenal androgen deficiency is of less consequence, and is not considered in this chapter.

Cortisol is the major glucocorticoid in human beings. Adrenocorticotropic hormone (ACTH), a pituitary hormone, controls the synthesis and release of cortisol from the adrenal gland. Normally, decrease in cortisol production leads to increased release of ACTH, and cortisol administration leads to decreased release of ACTH.

ACTH deficiency, as in hypopituitarism, leads to cortisol deficiency.

As the principal glucocorticoid, cortisol has many functions: It is required to sustain a normal blood glucose level, and is also necessary for maintenance of blood pressure, permitting normal sympathetic control of arterial tone. In addition, it contributes to normal appetite, sense of well-being, energy, mental acuity, and the ability of the kidneys to excrete extra water. In the absence of cortisol, the percentage of eosinophils and lymphocytes in the peripheral circulation increases.

Most importantly, cortisol enables the body to respond adequately during stress. The unstressed adrenal glands secrete 15–20 mg of cortisol daily, but they are capable of at least ten times that output. In the presence of major stress, such as an operation, sepsis, or trauma, 200–300 mg of cortisol must be produced to sustain life. With lesser degrees of stress, smaller amounts of cortisol are required. It is this ability to respond to stress that makes the adrenal cortex so critical. Lesions of the adrenal cortex may be difficult to diagnose since destruction of 90% of the tissue may result in few or no everyday symptoms, although profound debility will occur in times of stress.

Aldosterone is the most potent of the mineralocorticoids. Volume depletion is the major stimulus for aldosterone production, mediated by angiotensin II. Decrease in either intravascular volume or renal perfusion causes renin production by the kidney and subsequent generation of angiotensin II in the blood. Since ACTH does not contribute substantially to aldosterone control, aldosterone production tends to be unaffected by pituitary disease.

The role of the mineralocorticoids aldosterone and desoxycorticosterone is more limited than that of cortisol, but is equally important, since these hormones defend against loss of intravascular volume by promoting sodium reabsorption in the distal renal tubules. Sodium is conserved, and in its place, potassium and hydrogen ions are excreted. It is logical, therefore, that hyperkalemia is another important stimulus for release of aldosterone, and aldosterone is important in defending against hyperkalemia.

Addison's Disease

Destruction of the adrenal cortex (Addison's disease) may occur relatively slowly, as in patients with tuberculosis or autoimmune disease, or it may occur more rapidly, for example, as a result of bilateral adrenalectomy or adrenal hemorrhage.

With destruction of this tissue, both mineralocorticoid and glucocorticoid functions are lost.

Diagnosis

Clinical Features. The history may include weight loss with poor appetite, fatigue, lethargy, postural dizziness, and impaired ability to concentrate. Delayed recovery from either a minor illness, such as influenza or gastroenteritis, or a major stress, such as an operation, is important historically. Salt craving develops as a consequence of salt loss via the kidneys. Severe symptoms may develop in the summer months as additional salt is lost through the skin or during hospitalization, when access to salty snacks or oral intake may be limited. The patient may have gastrointestinal symptoms, such as nausea, vomiting, and severe abdominal pain; the mechanism of such symptoms is uncertain. Acute symptoms may develop in a patient with known Addison's disease when concurrent illness develops, and the patient neglects to increase his/her dose of glucocorticoids.

Hyperpigmentation is the most valuable clue to Addison's disease, although with rapid adrenal destruction there may not be sufficient time for hyperpigmentation to develop before the patient becomes critically ill. As cortisol deficiency develops, ACTH is secreted, causing the skin to darken. Pigmentation may be generalized, with the appearance of a suntan that is often sustained, and brownish, almost dirt-like pigmentation may also appear over the extensor surfaces, such as knuckles, elbows, and knees. Pigmentation of the lips and buccal mucosa is characteristic. Scars formed since the onset of Addison's disease become hyperpigmented, but older scars do not. Vitiligo, a patchy depigmentation of the skin, may also be present, suggesting the autoimmune nature of adrenal destruction.

High fever may be present with severe illness, even in the absence of infection. Hypotension is common, ranging from mild postural hypotension to frank shock, and is due to loss of arterial tone (cortisol deficiency) and diminished intravascular volume (mineralocorticoid deficiency). The combination of low blood pressure with fever and abdominal pain may mimic a surgical emergency.

Hyponatremia occurs frequently, and results from renal salt loss and impaired renal excretion of water. Hyperkalemia is a consequence of the decreased exchange of sodium, potassium, and hydrogen ions. Metabolic acidosis may result for similar reasons. Hypoglycemia is more likely to develop in infants with Addison's disease than in adults. Lymphocytosis and eosinophilia may be present. Suprarenal calcifications on plain x-ray films of the abdomen may be a valuable indication of tuberculous Addison's disease.

The manifestations of Addison's disease are summarized in Table 14.5, and the pathogenesis

Table 14.5.
Addison's disease: manifestations.

Site	History	Physical Examination	Laboratory Finding
General	Anorexia Lethargy Weight loss Salt craving[a] Delayed recovery from illness or operation Impaired ability to concentrate	Fever	Hyponatremia Hyperkalemia[a] Acidosis[a] Hypoglycemia Lymphocytosis Eosinophilia
Cardiovascular	Postural dizziness	Postural hypotension or shock Volume depletion[a]	
Skin	Prolonged suntan[a]	Hyperpigmentation[a] Vitiligo[a]	
Gastrointestinal	Nausea Vomiting Abdominal pain		
Genitourinary		Absent axillary and pubic hair in women	

[a] Absent in ACTH deficiency (hypopituitarism or ACTH suppression).

of addisonian crisis is given in Table 14.6. In the absence of a classic presentation, the diagnosis should be considered in every patient with unexplained hypotension, hyperpigmentation, "failure to thrive" after a major or minor stress (especially a surgical procedure), unexplained weight loss, tuberculosis, hyponatremia, hyperkalemia, hypoglycemia, or eosinophilia.

Clinical Studies. Since Addison's disease requires lifelong therapy, establishment of a definitive diagnosis is mandatory after the crisis has passed. A plasma cortisol level within normal limits (approximately 10–15 μg/dl) during major stress is inappropriately low, and a value below normal at such a time is almost diagnostic of Addison's disease. In unstressed patients, a normal plasma cortisol level or 24-hour excretion of 17-hydroxysteroids is compatible with decreased adrenal reserve, and does *not* exclude the diagnosis of adrenal insufficiency.

Initial therapy (see below) should not be discontinued during diagnostic testing, but dexamethasone, 2–4 mg/day in four divided doses, should be administered rather than cortisol; 1 mg of dexamethasone is equivalent to 20–30 mg of cortisol. Such small amounts of this potent glucocorticoid do not interfere with plasma or urinary corticosteroid measurements.

An attempt to stimulate the adrenal gland with ACTH is the diagnostic test of choice. ACTH should be administered according to a standard protocol such as synthetic (1–24) ACTH, 25 units intravenously in 500 ml of 5% dextrose in saline solution in the course of 8 hours on 3 consecutive days. In persons without adrenal insufficiency, the plasma cortisol level will increase to more than 30 μg/dl and the 17-hydroxysteroids will at least double to a value of 15 mg/day by the end of the third day's infusion.

In ambulatory patients in whom Addison's disease appears unlikely, a rapid test can be performed to exclude it conclusively. Synthetic ACTH, 25 units, is administered by intravenous

bolus or intramuscular injection and the plasma cortisol level is measured before and 1 hour after injection. Only synthetic ACTH should be given. An increase to more than 17 μg/dl excludes the diagnosis of Addison's disease. If these results are not achieved, however, more prolonged ACTH stimulation should be carried out.

Once the diagnosis is established, patient education is extremely important. In addition to wearing a Medic Alert bracelet or necklace, the patient should have an identification card providing the diagnosis and current therapy.

Therapy

Although the definitive diagnosis of Addison's disease depends on measurement of corticosteroid levels in plasma or urine, therapy must be started immediately in sick patients with the suspected diagnosis. Blood should be drawn for a cortisol determination, and cortisol should be administered intravenously. Dextrose and saline solutions are required as well.

Glucocorticoids. Intravenous administration of cortisol in the form of hydrocortisone sodium succinate may be lifesaving (Table 14.7). The dose should approximate the normal adrenal output during maximal stress, namely, 300 mg/day. Since the half-life of cortisol is at most a few hours, injections should be repeated, 75 mg intravenously or intramuscularly every 6 hours after an initial 100-mg intravenous bolus or cortisone hemisuccinate. A similar regimen of cortisol administration is required in patients with known Addison's disease who are about to undergo a major surgical procedure or who have another major illness. In the presence of persistent hypotension a continuous intravenous infusion of cortisone hemisuccinate should be employed.

The emergency situation often subsides within a few days; as this happens, the dosage of cortisol should be tapered by 50% each day until maintenance therapy is reached.

Volume Replacement. Cortisol alone is insufficient in the presence of volume depletion. More than 20% of the extracellular fluid volume may be lost. Deficits of 3 liters or more are common in hypotensive patients. The choice of fluid is 5% dextrose in saline to restore sodium and to prevent hypoglycemia. The rate of administration depends on the age and clinical status of the patient; central venous pressure monitoring is desirable in elderly patients and in those with known cardiac disease. Hospitalized patients with Addison's disease should receive saline solution intravenously if oral intake is limited for any reason.

Table 14.6.
Addisonian crisis: pathogenesis.

Condition	Cause
Hypotension	↓ Cortisol
	↓ Mineralocorticoid
Hyperpyrexia	↓ Cortisol (?)
Hyperpigmentation	↑ ACTH
Hyponatremia	↓ Cortisol
	↓ Mineralocorticoid
Hyperkalemia	↓ Mineralocorticoid
Hypoglycemia	↓ Cortisol

ACTH = adrenocorticotropic hormone.

Table 14.7.
Addison's disease: therapy.

Type	Dosage	Comments
Emergency[a]		
Volume and glucose replacement	5% dextrose in normal saline to replenish volume	
Glucocorticoid	Hydrocortisone hemisuccinate, 100 mg intravenously, and hydrocortisone hemisuccinate 75 mg intramuscularly or intravenously every 6 hours	
Mineralocorticoid	Desoxycorticosterone acetate (DOCA), 5 mg intramuscularly 2 times a day, or fludrocortisone acetate (Florinef), 0.05–0.2 mg/day orally	For persistent hypotension or hyperkalemia
Long-term		
Glucocorticoid	Hydrocortisone or cortisone acetate, 20–35 mg/day orally (2/3 dose at 8 a.m., 1/3 dose at 3 p.m.), or prednisone, 5–10 mg/day orally (2/3 dose at 8 a.m., 1/3 dose at 3 p.m.)	For minor stress, double dosage; for major stress, see above
Mineralocorticoid	Fludrocortisone acetate, 0.05–0.2 mg/day orally	

[a] Only glucocorticoid therapy is required in patients with hypopituitarism or ACTH suppression.

The response to saline administration may be dramatic. In fact, in hypotensive patients, Addison's disease is often unrecognized because of the favorable response to saline administration. The cycle of alleviation of hypotension with saline solution followed by recurrence when administration is discontinued may occur several times before adrenal insufficiency is recognized.

Mineralocorticoids. Administration of mineralocorticoids may help prevent further loss of sodium. In large dosages, 200–300 mg/day, cortisol does have significant mineralocorticoid effects, particularly when saline solution is administered concomitantly. However, mineralocorticoids should be administered: (1) if the blood pressure remains low despite saline; (2) if hyperkalemia persists; and (3) if a synthetic glucocorticoid such as prednisolone is used instead of cortisol (1 mg of prednisolone is the equivalent of 4 mg of cortisol). Mineralocorticoid is often required as the dosage of cortisone is diminished. Desoxycorticosterone acetate, 5 mg intramuscularly twice a day, or fludrocortisone acetate (Florinef), 0.05–0.2 mg/day orally, is recommended.

Long-term therapy is considered in Table 14.7. Patients with adrenal insufficiency must be instructed to increase corticosteroid dosage during illness or stress, however minor. Any patient who has a decreased oral intake or a severe fluid loss such as might result from vomiting or diarrhea should be hospitalized. Patients should be instructed in injection technique and provided with injectable drugs so that corticosteroids can be administered intramuscularly before arriving at the hospital. In such a situation, 100 mg of hydrocortisone sodium succinate is recommended.

ACTH Suppression and Hypopituitarism

ACTH deficiency results in cortisol deficiency, mineralocorticoid function being spared. The most common cause of ACTH lack is pituitary suppression after long-term corticosteroid (glucocorticoid) therapy. After weeks to months of therapy with supraphysiologic doses of corticosteroids, the ability of the pituitary gland to release ACTH during stress is lessened for as long as 6–9 months, and adrenal cortisol response is similarly impaired. The therapeutic implications are clear:

(1) All patients being treated with pharmacologic doses of corticosteroids (for example, more than 25 mg of cortisone or 5 mg of prednisone daily) need additional therapy during stress. If the stress is major, such as an operation or sepsis, 300 mg of cortisol or an equivalent corticosteroid are required—hydrocortisone sodium succinate 75 mg intramuscularly every 6 hours, or methylprednisolone sodium succinate, 20 mg intramuscularly or intravenously every 6 hours. Patients with known adrenal insufficiency or hypopituitarism require similar therapy.

(2) Any patient who has received pharmacologic doses of corticosteroids for more than 4 weeks during the past year may need similar therapy during stress and should be prophylactically

treated with corticosteroids during any surgical procedure.

Diagnosis

In adults, pituitary surgery and pituitary tumors are the most common causes of panhypopituitarism. Single or multiple hormone deficiencies may develop slowly or rapidly. Although growth hormone production ceases first, the consequences of this deficiency are usually unrecognized in adults. Gonadotropin (follicle-stimulating hormone and luteinizing hormone) deficiency usually occurs next, resulting in amenorrhea or oligomenorrhea in women and loss of libido in men. Thyroid-stimulating hormone and ACTH deficiencies usually develop last, and the consequences may be life-threatening. The presence of multiple hormone deficiencies should always suggest the possibility of hypopituitarism. Visual field abnormalities, especially bitemporal hemianopsia, may be a valuable clue to a pituitary tumor. Patients with pituitary tumors causing acromegaly, Cushing's disease, or galactorrhea may have pituitary insufficiency as well. Pituitary apoplexy (sudden hemorrhage into a pituitary tumor), which is rare, may be manifested by severe headache, visual field defects, depression of consciousness, meningismus, and occasionally other cranial nerve palsies. Sudden loss of adrenal cortical function may occur, whereas other pituitary deficits even when present, are slow to develop clinically.

Sheehan's syndrome, postpartum pituitary insufficiency, is easily recognized by the failure of menses to resume, inability to breast-feed, and generalized debility from thyroid and adrenal insufficiency that may follow postpartum hemorrhage. Pituitary insufficiency during pregnancy is particularly likely to develop in diabetic patients.

The life-threatening consequences of hypopituitarism are those of cortisol and thyroid hormone deficiency. Hypothyroidism is discussed on pages 313–317. Cortisol deficiency from hypopituitarism or ACTH suppression may be extraordinarily difficult to diagnose if it occurs alone. Many of the most valuable clinical indications leading to the recognition of Addison's disease are lacking, including hyperpigmentation and hyperkalemia. Although hypotension is present, volume depletion is not, unless the patient has had recurrent vomiting or diarrhea. Hypopigmentation may be present. Hyponatremia is often noted, and may be profound. The explanation for these findings is the lack of ACTH with preservation of aldosterone function. A history of weight loss, poor response to stress, gastrointestinal symptoms, and

"collapse" all may be recorded. The presence of concomitant hormone deficiencies (for example, thyroid or gonadal) may be a valuable finding. Patients in whom corticosteroids have recently been discontinued may experience arthralgia.

The presence of clinical Cushing's syndrome in a severely ill patient should suggest the possibility of exogenous glucocorticoid therapy with possible cortisol deficiency syndrome due to glucocorticoid withdrawal.

The definitive diagnosis of hypopituitarism or ACTH suppression requires pituitary stimulation by means of an insulin tolerance test or a metyrapone test or by inference, short or prolonged ACTH stimulation tests, details of which can be found in standard endocrinology texts.

Therapy

The immediate therapy is intravenous glucocorticoid replacement, as in Table 14.7. Mineralocorticoid therapy is unnecessary. Patients usually do not require volume replacement, and indeed, water restriction may be necessary because of hyponatremia. If concomitant adrenal and thyroid deficiencies are present, corticosteroid replacement must be started first. Thyroid hormone replacement can precipitate adrenal crisis in such a situation unless glucocorticoids are administered at the same time.

THYROID EMERGENCIES

Thyroid Storm or Decompensated Thyrotoxicosis

The drama and crisis of thyroid storm are implicit in its name. This exaggerated state of hyperthyroidism is, fortunately, now rare. Modern advances in the diagnosis and therapy of conventional hyperthyroidism, as well as intensive care for the decompensated thyrotoxic patient, have had a significant impact.

Early recognition and prompt therapy of hyperthyroidism are of utmost importance. When hyperthyroidism is complicated by concomitant illness, symptoms are likely to be exacerbated, and early hospitalization is recommended. Longstanding untreated hyperthyroidism is likely to result in failure of specific organ systems. Although the decompensated thyrotoxic patient is critically ill, an excellent response to an orderly sequence of therapeutic maneuvers may be expected.

Pathophysiologic Principles

The thyroid gland produces both thyroxine and triiodothyronine. In addition, thyroxine released from the gland is converted to triiodothyronine. Approximately 99.98% of thyroxine, as well as 99.8% of triiodothyronine, is bound to protein. It is the free, nonprotein-bound hormone that is metabolically active. The manifestations of severe hyperthyroidism are related to overproduction of thyroxine and triiodothyronine and apparent over-activity of the sympathetic nervous system. The distinction between severe hyperthyroidism and thyroid storm is qualitative: the blood levels of thyroid hormones do not differ in these conditions. The failure of various thyroid hormone target organs may be due to either untreated thyrotoxi-cosis itself or concomitant illness, and indicates the need for intensive medical care.

Diagnosis

Clinical Features. The diagnosis of hyperthy-roidism may be obvious in the younger patient with classic signs and symptoms (Table 14.8). However, in the elderly, only minor indications may be present, many of which are cardiovascular. Exacerbation of underlying heart disease, atrial

fibrillation refractory to digitalis, insidious onset of congestive heart failure, unexplained sinus tachycardia, atrial tachyarrhythmias, or progres-sive angina pectoris may be the only sign in con-junction with a slightly enlarged thyroid gland. Elderly patients may seem apathetic, with weak-ness, weight loss, and debility often mimicking neoplastic disease. When an additional illness or insult is present, the manifestations may become more severe (Table 14.9).

Although fever may be present in uncompli-cated hyperthyroidism, an elevated temperature should be considered as a sign of a potentially serious process. Even minor infections may pro-duce a dramatic febrile response, and a careful search for sepsis is mandatory. The pulse rate is usually elevated disproportionately in relation to the temperature.

The cardiac, gastrointestinal, and sympathetic nervous system are most likely to become decom-pensated. Overwhelming congestive heart failure—particularly right-sided—may develop, as well as the other cardiac symptoms mentioned. Vomiting may occur, and diarrhea may be debi-

Table 14.8.
Hyperthyroidism: manifestations.

	History	Physical Examination
General	Weight loss with good appetite Heat intolerance	
Skin		Warm, moist, smooth Onycholysis Pretibial myxedema (Graves' disease)
Eyes	Burning Tearing Diplopia	Lid lag, stare Exophthalmos, soft-tissue swelling, extraocu-lar muscle paresis, corneal involvement (Graves' disease)

Neck	Enlargement	Goiter
		  Diffuse
		  Nodular

Respiratory	Dyspnea	
Cardiovascular	Palpitations Angina pectoris	Sinus tachycardia Atrial fibrillation Increased systolic blood pressure Decreased diastolic blood pressure Scratchy systolic ejection murmur Congestive heart failure, right-sided more se-vere than left-sided
Gastrointestinal	Diarrhea	
Genitourinary	Nocturia Hypomenorrhea	Gynecomastia
Neuromuscular	Tremor Weakness	Peripheral and bulbar myopathy Brisk deep tendon reflexes
Psychiatric	Emotional instability Hyperkinesia Insomnia Anxiety	

Table 14.9.
Decompensated thyrotoxicosis; manifestations.

High fever
Cardiac decompensation
  Failure
  Arrhythmias
Gastrointestinal decompensation
  Diarrhea
  Vomiting
Neurologic deterioration
  Agitation
    Restlessness
    Delirium
  Apathy
    Myopathy
    Torpor
    Stupor
    Coma

litating. Although the blood flow to most organs increases in patients with hyperthyroidism, flow to the liver remains relatively constant despite increased metabolic demands, and hepatic decompensation may result. Central nervous system activation may be indicated by restlessness, severe agitation, or delirium. On the other hand, myopathy both of the peripheral and bulbar musculature may be so profound that patients become lethargic, stuporous, or comatose; this is often complicated by repeated aspiration.

Iodine excess may precipitate hyperthyroidism in patients with nodular goiters. This situation may be particularly treacherous in patients with coronary disease undergoing angiographic procedures or patients with arrhythmias treated with iodine containing drugs such as amiodarone.

Clinical Studies. Laboratory tests can confirm the diagnosis of hyperthyroidism, but are usually not a good index of its severity. In patients with hyperthyroidism, the total serum thyroxine level is usually elevated. To separate hyperthyroidism from other conditions that falsely elevate the total serum thyroxine level (namely, an elevated level of binding protein, which is commonly due to estrogens), either the triiodothyronine resin (T_3 resin) or the free thyroxine level is determined, both of which are usually elevated in hyperthyroidism. With an elevated level of binding protein, the patient is not hyperthyroid, the T_3 resin is decreased, and the free thyroxine is normal. Patients occasionally have so-called T_3-toxicosis, in which the concentrations of total and free thyroxine in the blood are normal, but the total triiodothyronine level is elevated. These tests take one to several days to complete. However, in an emer-

gency, therapy must be started before laboratory confirmation.

Therapy

The prognosis for the patient with severe decompensated thyrotoxicosis has improved substantially as specific therapeutic measures have become available (Table 14.10).

General Measures. The hyperpyrexic patient may require acetaminophen or cooling blankets while the search for infection proceeds. Attention to hydration is of utmost importance. Copious amounts of hypotonic fluid may be lost through the skin, and occasionally, large amounts of sodium and potassium may be lost if the patient has diarrhea. Glucose and soluble B vitamins should also be administered.

Blockade of Thyroid Hormone Synthesis. Both propylthiouracil (PTU) and methimazole (Tapazole) block the synthesis of thyroid hormone. Methimazole is ten times as potent and has a longer half-life, but propylthiouracil prevents some of the peripheral conversion of thyroxine to triiodothyronine. When large doses are used at frequent intervals, as in thyroid storm, propylthiouracil is the drug of choice. These agents are not commercially available for parenteral administration, although hospital pharmacies may be able to formulate such a preparation in an emergency. Patients with decompensated thyrotoxicosis should receive propylthiouracil, 200–250 mg, or methimazole, 20–25 mg, every 4 hours either orally or by nasogastric tube if necessary. In contrast, patients with uncomplicated hyperthyroidism receive propylthiouracil, 100 mg, or methimazole, 10 mg, every 6 or 8 hours.

Although complete blockade of thyroid hormone synthesis can be achieved within hours, clinical response may not be apparent for weeks or months because the large stores of thyroid hormone within the thyroid gland must be dissipated before euthyroidism is achieved, and neither propylthiouracil nor methimazole blocks release of these hormones.

Blockade of Thyroid Hormone Release. Although iodide is the substrate for thyroid hormone synthesis, in pharmacologic doses it blocks the release of hormone from the thyroid gland, especially from the diffuse toxic goiter. To prevent the administered iodide from being directed into new hormone stores, synthesis must be adequately blocked. For this reason, iodides should be given approximately 1 hour after therapy with propylthiouracil or methimazole. Sodium iodide, 1–2

Table 14.10.
Decompensated thyrotoxicosis: therapy.

Measure	Agent
General	
Reduction of fever	Acetaminophen, cooling blanket, sponge bath
Hydration	Intravenous fluids as necessary
Administration of vitamins	Soluble B vitamins
Administration of glucose	5% dextrose solution
Blockade of thyroid hormone synthesis	Propylthiouracil, 200–250 mg every 4 hours orally or by nasogastric tube
	or
	Methimazole, 20–25 mg every 4 hours orally or by nasogastric tube
Blockade of thyroid hormone release	Iodides
	Sodium iodide, 1–2 gm/day intravenously
	or
	Supersaturated solution of potassium iodide, 5 drops orally every 4 hours
Blockade of peripheral effects	Sympatholytics
	Propranolol, 1–5 mg intravenously or 20–40 mg orally every 4 hours
	or
	Reserpine, 0.25–2.5 mg intramuscularly every 4–6 hours
	or
	Guanethidine, 1–2 mg/kg/day orally
Inhibition of thyroxine to triiodothyronine conversion	Propylthiouracil (see above)
	Propranolol (see above)
	Glucocorticoids
	(e.g., Dexamethasone 2 mg intravenously or intramuscularly every 6 hours)
Therapy for cardiac disease	
Atrial fibrillation	Digoxin (increased requirements)
	Propranolol or other β-adrenergic blockers as required
Congestive heart failure	Digoxin plus diuretics
	Sympatholytics subsequently, if necessary

gm/day intravenously, or a supersaturated solution of potassium iodide, 5 drops orally every 4 hours, is effective. In general, the use of iodides is reserved for emergency situations.

Lithium shares with iodide the ability to block release of thyroid hormone. Although still considered an experimental agent for thyrotoxicosis, it has the potential advantage over iodides of not serving as a hormone substrate.

The half-life of thyroxine in plasma is approximately 7 days; that of triiodothyronine is 1 day. Although these periods are somewhat shortened in hyperthyroidism, it is obvious that the effects of blockade of hormone release are relatively slow to appear.

Blockade of Peripheral Effects. There is no known specific antagonist to the actions of thyroid hormone. Many of the manifestations of thyroid hormone excess mimic those of an overactive sympathetic nervous system, for example, tachycardia, tremor, diaphoresis, and weight loss. Although there is no direct evidence for sympathetic overactivity, several sympatholytic agents have been introduced into the therapeutic regimen for severe thyrotoxicosis. Used in conjunction with the previously mentioned modes of therapy and less commonly by themselves, these agents have proved remarkably successful.

The most effective agent appears to be propranolol, a β-adrenergic antagonist. Propranolol has the additional advantage, not shared by other β-adrenergic blockers, of partially inhibiting conversion of thyroxine (T_4) to triiodothyronine (T_3). Intravenous doses of 1–5 mg or oral doses of 20–

40 mg every 4 hours may dramatically improve the patient's condition within minutes to hours. In some situations, 200 or more mg by mouth every 4–6 hours may be necessary. The lower doses should be tried first. In the presence of congestive heart failure, propranolol should be administered very cautiously, and it is possible that newer β-adrenergic antagonists will be safer. Propranolol is contraindicated in patients with asthma, and may not be of benefit in the hyperthyroid patient without tachycardia.

Reserpine, 2.0–2.5 mg intramuscularly every 4–6 hours, is an alternative. However, a lower dose, such as 0.25–1.0 mg, may be effective and should be tried first. Reserpine should not be administered when sedation is considered undesirable.

Guanethidine, 75–100 mg/day orally, is also effective. Although hypotension may develop, significantly low blood pressure has not been common.

Inhibition of T_4 to T_3 conversion. Under ordinary circumstances, 85% or more of circulating triiodothyronine (T_3) is derived from peripheral conversion of thyroxine (T_4). T_3 is a more active hormone with T_4 possibly serving as a prohormone or precursor hormone for T_3. In hyperthyroidism, relatively more T_3 is produced from the thyroid gland. However, peripheral tissue T_3 production contributes a significant amount to the circulating T_3 concentration. Glucocorticoids have been part of the regimen for thyroid storm for years. Thyroid hormone accelerates the degradation of cortisol. However, frank adrenal insufficiency has not been recognized in thyroid storm in the absence of established Addison's disease. Recently, glucocorticoids such as dexamethasone have been shown to partially impair T_4 to T_3 conversion, providing a reasonable excuse to continue this firmly entrenched modality of therapy. Propranolol but not other β-adrenergic agents contributes to this impaired conversion as well. Glucocorticoids are additive to propylthiouracil in terms of peripheral T_4 to T_3 conversion.

Therapy of Congestive Heart Failure. In addition to exacerbating underlying heart disease, thyrotoxicosis can precipitate congestive heart failure in a previously normal heart. The striking increase in cardiac output often results in predominantly right-sided failure, and treatment may be difficult. The initial therapy should be administration of digitalis and diuretics. Sympatholytic agents may be administered later if response to therapy is inadequate. Since propranolol has myocardial depressant effects that are independent of its β-adrenergic blocking effects and that may exacerbate congestive heart failure, guanethidine and reserpine may be safer in this situation. Administration of these agents should follow conventional therapy. Newer, pure β-blockers will surely receive additional trials in this situation.

Digitalis must be administered to patients with atrial fibrillation. Since the space of distribution for digoxin is increased in patients with hyperthyroidism, larger doses than usual may be required. The ventricular response may slow to between 100 and 120 beats/min, but further increases in dosage are more likely to result in digitalis toxicity than in ventricular slowing. β-adrenergic blocking agents such as propranolol may be helpful in reducing the rate further.

Removal of Thyroid Hormone. Large quantities of thyroid hormone can be removed by peritoneal dialysis or plasmapheresis. This is usually not necessary, and has not been shown to improve the prognosis in decompensated thyrotoxicosis.

Precipitating Factors

Untreated hyperthyroidism may range from mild to severe, and exacerbations are usually related to an identifiable precipitating factor. In patients with hyperthyroidism, the following may be particularly dangerous: operation, infection, trauma, delivery, diabetic ketoacidosis, and certain drugs such as parasympatholytic and sympathomimetic agents. Symptoms of hyperthyroidism may worsen for a few days after therapy with iodine 131, and radioactive therapy is best deferred in acutely ill patients.

Before the development of effective antithyroid drugs, thyroid storm usually occurred as a result of thyroidectomy in untreated or iodide-treated thyrotoxic patients. Even now, extrathyroidal operation on patients with unrecognized hyperthyroidism can precipitate a crisis, particularly if atropine is used as a preanesthetic agent. Sepsis represents the major decompensating event today, and thyrotoxic patients with infections require special care. As stated previously, hospitalization should be considered for any patient with thyrotoxicosis and a concurrent illness.

Preparation for Operation

Currently, every thyrotoxic patient who undergoes operation—whether thyroidectomy or other surgical procedure—must receive specific preoperative preparation. Patients should be treated with propylthiouracil or methimazole until a euthyroid state is achieved. In addition, a supersaturated solution of potassium iodide, 3 drops orally twice a day, should be administered to reduce the vascularity of the thyroid gland during the 10 days before thyroid operation. Recently, patients have successfully been treated with β-blockade alone before thyroidectomy. Sufficient drug must be given to decrease the pulse (after exercise if possible) to the 80–90/minute range. This may require 1000 mg or more of propanolol per day. The drug must be given up to and including the morning of surgery and continued for several postoperative days, even if a thyroidectomy has been performed. If tachycardia appears in the recovery room, intravenous propranolol should be administered. Failure to adhere to these rigid guidelines may allow thyroid storm to develop.

Emergency operation for an unrelated condition is occasionally necessary in thyrotoxic patients. Survival in such a situation may depend on the use of sympatholytic agents, especially the β-adrenergic blocking agents. Atropine and scopolamine should be avoided as preanesthetics. Haloperidol has recently been implicated as a precipitant of thyroid storm. In addition, prophylactic administration of propylthiouracil or methimazole, as well as iodides, is recommended.

Myxedema Crisis

Severe, complicated hypothyroidism (myxedema crisis) usually develops as a result of the body's inability to handle additional insults, either endogenous or exogenous. It may occur with or without coma, and is a highly lethal disorder, with reported mortalities between 50 and 75%. Death from severe hypothyroidism is particularly tragic in light of the ease with which uncomplicated hypothyroidism can be treated. The fact that myxedema crisis develops after admission to the hospital in about 50% of cases emphasizes the need for early recognition and treatment of hypothyroidism. Although myxedema may be easy to recognize, mild hypothyroidism is often an extremely subtle process. Symptoms may be nonspecific or absent, and clinical indications may be easily overlooked.

Pathophysiologic Principles

As soon as hypothyroidism is suspected, the question of primary vs. secondary disease must be raised. Primary hypothyroidism refers to failure of the thyroid gland itself. It is most commonly caused by Hashimoto's thyroiditis (autoimmune thyroiditis), radioactive iodine therapy, and thyroid operation, and it accounts for 95% of all cases of hypothyroidism. As the thyroid gland begins to fail, the pituitary gland attempts to compensate with increased production of thyroid-stimulating hormone (TSH). The earliest sign of a failing thyroid gland, therefore, is an increase in the serum TSH level. Secondary hypothyroidism results from disease of the pituitary gland or hypothalamus, with resultant failure of TSH release.

Goiter usually indicates primary disease; loss of axillary and pubic hair, diminished libido, or amenorrhea may indicate a pituitary origin. An elevated TSH level on radioimmunoassay confirms the diagnosis of primary hypothyroidism. If the TSH level is not elevated in a hypothyroid patient, secondary hypothyroidism is present.

The distinction betwen primary and secondary disease is important because of its influence on therapy. Thyroid hormone accelerates the metabolism of cortisol in the liver, and normally, this results in release of ACTH from the pituitary gland and compensatory cortisol secretion. When the pituitary gland fails, many trophic hormones in addition to TSH are not produced, ACTH being particularly notable. If ACTH release is deficient, the addition of thyroid hormone may precipitate adrenal failure by inactivating the small amounts of cortisol that are being produced. In this setting (hypopituitarism), cortisol must be administered before thyroid hormone.

Diagnosis

Clinical Features. The cardinal features of hypothyroidism are listed in Table 14.11. Apathy may dominate the clinical findings, and as a result, the patient may deny all symptoms. On the other hand, depression may be striking, and may be accompanied by many somatic complaints.

The pulse rate may be normal, and the diastolic blood pressure is often elevated. Hypothermia is frequently not diagnosed because of failure to shake the mercury in the thermometer to below 96°F (35.6°C). Exophthalmos may be the only residual manifestations of previously treated hyperthyroidism (Graves' disease). Cutaneous manifestations such as dryness, swelling, and carotenodermia are common, and periorbital edema is a regular finding. A thyroidectomy scar may be a valuable clue to early hypothyroidism; however, radioactive iodine therapy leaves no clues. Delay in the relaxation phase of the deep tendon reflexes (especially of the ankle and biceps) is helpful, but may occur in hypothermia from any cause. Proptosis (exopthalmos) may be a clue to previously treated Graves' disease. The absence of any of these findings does not exclude the diagnosis of hypothyroidism.

Clinical Studies. In general, in patients with severe hypothyroidism, values for the conventional thyroid function such as serum thyroxine, and serum free thyroxine are all low. These tests,

Table 14.11.
Hypothyroidism: manifestations.

	History	Physical Examination	Laboratory Findings
General	Intolerance to cold Weight gain with de- creased appetite Obesity (rare) Radioactive iodine therapy	Hypothermia	Decreased thyroxine, free thy- roxine, T₃ resin Increased thyroid-stimulating hormone (primary hypothy- roidism) Elevated cholesterol, triglycer- ides, sedimentation rate, cre- atinine phosphokinase, cere- brospinal fluid protein
Cardiovascular		Sinus bradycardia Increased diastolic blood pressure Cardiomegaly Distant heart sounds	
Skin		Dry, cool, coarse, thickened Carotenodermia Patchy alopecia Periorbital edema	
Mouth		Enlarged tongue	
Neck	Thyroidectomy scar	Goiter	
Gastrointestinal	Constipation	Ileus	
Genitourinary	Menorrhagia (primary hypothyroidism) Amenorrhea (second- ary hypothyroidism)		
Neurologic	Muscle cramps Paresthesias Unsteadiness	Ataxic gait Delay in relaxation of deep tendon reflexes Obtundation	
Psychiatric	Lethargy Depression Mental slowing	Apathy Psychosis Myxedema "wit"	

however, may fail to confirm the diagnosis of hypothyroidism even when clinical evidence is present. For example, the normal range of the serum thyroxine is 4–11 μg/dl. However, each individual maintains a serum thyroxine level within a narrower range, for example, 8–9 μg/dl. If the thyroid gland fails, this level will decrease, but will stay within the "normal" range. In addition, pregnant women and those using oral contraceptives normally have an elevated serum thyroxine level because of an elevated level of binding proteins, and such patients may have thyroid failure with a thyroxine level in the range of 8–9 μg/dl. Thus, since the serum TSH level increases concomitantly with decrease in serum thyroxine, the only way to diagnose early hypothyroidism may be to measure the serum TSH in every patient with suspected hypothyroidism. The clinical recognition of such patients is important if one is to diagnose hypothyroidism early. However, such mild hypothyroidism is unlikely to precipitate myxedema crisis.

Many patients with a low serum thyroxine measurement do not have hypothyroidism. Such patients may have a deficiency of thyroxine-binding globulin, in which case the T₃ resin will be elevated. In hypothyroid patients, low normal or frankly low T_3-resin values are the rule.

Radioactive iodine uptake studies are of almost no value in the diagnosis of hypothyroidism, and are not recommended.

Therapy

The factors precipitating myxedema crisis, the manifestations, and therapy (Table 14.12) are closely related and are discussed together in this section. Therapy must begin before laboratory confirmation of the diagnosis. Myxedema crisis or coma is a problem of general medical care, and the components can be treated even if the diagnosis of hypothyroidism is not initially considered.

Hypoventilation. Carbon dioxide retention and narcosis commonly cause coma in the patient with myxedema. Arterial blood-gas levels must be monitored in the hospitalized hypothyroid patient. Respiratory failure in this setting has several causes. Hypothyroid patients have a decreased respiratory response to conventional stimuli such as hypoxia and carbon dioxide elevation. An enlarged tongue may fall back into the oropharynx, causing obstruction of the upper part of the respiratory tract. Sedative drugs administered either routinely or because of bizarre behavior can easily depress respiration in these patients. Patients with borderline hypothyroidism may become profoundly hypothyroid when exposed to iodides. This is particularly devastating when the iodides are prescribed for underlying pulmonary disease (for example, expectorants with iodides or a supersaturated solution of potassium iodide) since

Table 14.12.
Myxedema crisis: manifestations, prevention, and therapy.

Manifestation	Prevention	Therapy
HYPOventilation	Monitor blood gases Avoid sedatives	Institute assisted ventilation Perform tracheostomy early if necessary
HYPOmetabolism of drugs	Avoid sedatives, narcotics, iodides, lithium, preanesthetic medications Delay elective operation Alert anesthesiologist if emergency operation required If digitalis required, use in decreased dosage	
HYPOthermia	Avoid cold exposure Suspect infection with "normal" temperature	
HYPOresponsiveness to infection	Suspect infection even with "normal" temperature and physical examination Monitor frequently: chest x-ray, white blood cell count, urinalysis	Administer antibiotics as infections are identified
HYPOnatremia	Avoid excess fluids	Restrict fluid
HYPOadrenalism		Administer hydrocortisone sodium hemisuccinate, 75 mg intramuscularly or intravenously every 6 hours after 100 mg intravenously ("sick" primary hypothyroidism and all secondary hypothyroidism)
HYPOglycemia	Monitor blood glucose	Administer dextrose solution intravenously
HYPOtension	Administer steroids to "sick" hypothyroid patients Avoid sedatives Search for infection	Avoid pressor agents Administer cortisol Administer colloid Treat infection as indicated
HYPOtonia	Suspect ileus with "surgical abdomen" Administer mild laxatives as prophylaxis Search for silent urinary tract infection	
HYPOthyroidism	Place patient in intensive care unit	Administer L-thyroxine, 100–200 μg intravenously, then 100 μg/day either orally or intravenously

the subsequent hypothyroidism exacerbates the preexistent respiratory problem.

Myxedema develops and reverses slowly. Several weeks may be required to reverse the clinical state. Patients with severe ventilatory failure require intubation. If oversedation is not a causative factor, tracheostomy may be necessary until the underlying hypothyroidism responds to therapy.

Hypometabolism of Drugs. Many drugs are metabolized or excreted more slowly in the hypothyroid patient. Routine administration of sedatives, narcotic analgesics, or preanesthetic drugs, as well as anesthesia itself, can precipitate coma in the borderline or frankly hypothyroid individual. Sedatives and narcotics are contraindicated in patients with suspected hypothyroidism, and elective operation should be avoided until the patient is almost euthyroid. If emergency operation is required, preanesthetic medications can be omitted, and the anesthesiologist should be notified of the diagnosis. It is surprising how well surgery is tolerated in patients with moderate and even severe hypothyroidism, particularly when the diagnosis is recognized preoperatively and adequate precautions are taken.

Certain drugs can precipitate hypothyroidism in susceptible persons or cause myxedema in patients with borderline hypothyroidism. The most notable agents are the iodides, which inhibit thyroid hormone synthesis and release, and lithium, which also inhibits thyroid hormone release.

The heart size is often enlarged in patients with hypothyroidism. In myxedematous patients this may be due to a benign pericardial effusion requiring no specific therapy (tamponade is extraordinarily rare). Congestive heart failure is unusual in hypothyroidism, but digitalis might mistakenly be administered because of cardiac enlargement. Digoxin metabolism is impaired because of a decreased space of distribution; if conventional doses are administered, higher blood levels of digoxin will result, and digitalis toxicity will develop. If digitalis is required in the hypothyroid patient, it should be used sparingly and with great caution.

Hypothermia. Myxedema should be considered in any hypothermic patient. Hypothermia is important for several reasons. The lower the temperature, the worse the prognosis. Fewer than 15% of patients survive temperatures less than 90°F (32.2°C) in the setting of myxedema crisis. Cold weather and exposure may precipitate coma. Also, infection may be undetected because of the absence of fever. A "normal" temperature in a profoundly hypothyroid patient should always prompt a careful search for infection.

Hyporesponsiveness to Infection. The placid demeanor, apparently stable temperature, and lack of complaints of the hypothyroid patient may be misleading. Pneumonia will be missed on the basis of physical examination alone, since shallow respirations make examination difficult and cough is often absent. Patients will not complain of dysuria.

Frequent chest x-ray films, white blood cell counts, and urinalyses are necessary if infections are to be recognized early and if fatal sepsis is to be avoided. Prophylactic administration of antibiotics is not indicated, however.

Hyponatremia. The glomerular filtration rate is diminished in patients with hypothyroidism, probably because of decrease in intravascular volume. This results in impaired ability to excrete water. Hyponatremia results if hypotonic fluids are administered in excess. Inappropriate secretion of antidiuretic hormone is an alternative explanation for the hyponatremia.

The therapy and prevention of hyponatremia involve avoidance of an excess of free water. In severe cases, fluids must be restricted to less than 800–1000 ml/day. Although the intravascular space is contracted in hypothyroidism, there is an excess of whole body sodium that is located in the myxedema fluid. Therefore, sodium should be avoided as well. If volume replacement is necessary, colloid is the therapy of choice.

Hypoadrenalism. Patients with secondary hypothyroidism due to failure of the pituitary gland commonly have adrenal insufficiency as well. It is less recognized, however, that patients with severe primary hypothyroidism have relative adrenal insufficiency. Although their basal production of cortisol is adequate, hypothyroid patients may have an inadequate cortisol response to stress. Cortisol therapy is recommended, therefore, not only in all patients with secondary hypothyroidism but also in acutely ill patients with primary hypothyroidism. The doses are similar to those for ACTH deficiency (see pages 307–308). If emergency operation is necessary, corticosteroids should be administered.

Hypotension. Drug sensitivity, relative or absolute adrenal insufficiency, or occasionally sepsis may induce hypotension. The intravascular volume tends to be decreased, making colloid the initial therapy of choice. The myxedematous patient is thought to be refractory to catecholamines unless thyroid hormone is administered first. In addition, arrhythmias may develop if pressor agents and thyroid hormone are administered simultaneously. Given these two considerations, pressor agents are probably best avoided.

Hypotonia. Intestinal hypotonia may lead to ileus and may mimic obstruction; prophylactic administration of a mild laxative is recommended. Distention of the intestine may result in seeding of the blood by gram-negative organisms and, occasionally, gastrointestinal bleeding. In patients with atony of the bladder, stasis and infection may develop. To treat these complications properly, the underlying cause must be recognized.

Hypoglycemia. Hypoglycemia is a rare complication of hypothyroidism. It is much more common in patients with secondary hypothyroidism, but may complicate primary hypothyroidism with devastating consequences. The therapy is intravenous glucose. Seizures are common in the presence of hypoglycemia.

Hypothyroidism. It is not an error to consider hypothyroidism last. Most patients with coma or hypothyroid crisis respond favorably if attention is paid to all the complications previously mentioned.

In patients with uncomplicated hypothyroidism, small doses of L-thyroxine orally are recommended, with increments at 2- to 4-week intervals. The severity of the hypothyroidism, the duration of symptoms, the extent of cardiac disease, and the increasing age of the patient all dictate a lower initial dose. Recommended doses of L-thyroxine are 25–50 µg/day for older or sicker patients and 100–150 µg/day for younger patients or those with milder disease. Full replacement therapy with L-thyroxine varies with the individual, but commonly ranges from 50–200 µg/day.

Higher doses of L-thyroxine have been recommended for myxedema crisis—up to 500 µg as initial intravenous therapy. This approximates the whole body deficit of thyroxine in patients with hypothyroidism. We, however, are not convinced that the dose of thyroid hormone is the critical variable, and recommend an intermediate dose, 100–200 µg intravenously followed by 100 µg/day intravenously or orally.

Others have advocated administration of triidothyronine. This agent is not commercially available for parenteral administration, although it can be prepared in hospital pharmacies. Although the rapid termination of action that occurs after stopping this drug is thought to be an advantage, the rapid onset of action may be a considerable disadvantage, leading to cardiac arrhythmias and death.

Careful studies on thyroxine to triiodothyronine conversion have not been reported in myxedema crisis. In the face of sepsis or shock, impaired conversion might play a clinically important role. Although triiodothyronine therapy might be considered in such circumstances, there are no data to suggest that it is helpful or necessary.

Some patients who show considerable improvement after a few days of therapy die within a few weeks. The reason for this is unclear. We recommend intensive care monitoring for at least 2 weeks in all such critically ill patients with hypothyroidism. Although the patient may not appear to be critically ill, the presence of severe hypothyroidism with the above complications warrants such precautions.

CALCIUM EMERGENCIES

Physiologic Principles

Calcium in the blood circulates in bound, complexed, and ionized forms. Although all three are measured when the serum calcium level is determined, only the ionized calcium exerts important biologic effects. In some laboratories, the ionized calcium can be measured directly; this may be helpful in certain situations.

Approximately 45% of circulating calcium is bound to serum proteins. Roughly 0.8 mg is bound to each gram of albumin and 0.2 mg to each gram of globulin. For simplicity, the following rule can be adopted: an increase or decrease of 1 gm/dl in the serum albumin concentration causes a corresponding increase or decrease of approximately 1 mg/dl in the serum calcium concentration.

The serum calcium level, together with the serum albumin level, becomes elevated with dehydration or with prolonged tourniquet application before blood letting, but the ionized calcium concentration remains normal. Similarly, hypoalbuminemic states result in decrease in the total serum calcium concentration. With a normal serum albumin level of approximately 4.5 gm/dl, the normal serum calcium concentration is 8.5–10.5 mg/dl. However, an albumin concentration of 2 gm/dl corresponds to a total calcium concentration of 6.5–8.4 mg/dl, the ionized calcium remaining within normal limits. To correct for this, a second rule must be invoked: the serum albumin concentration must be measured whenever the serum calcium concentration is determined.

The concentration of ionized calcium is maintained within narrow limits in the blood predominantly through the action of parathyroid hormone. Increase in the serum calcium concentration suppresses parathyroid hormone production; decrease stimulates production. Parathyroid hormone mobilizes calcium from bone with the aid of vitamin D. Bone resorption releases phosphate in addition to calcium, and since parathyroid hormone facilitates urinary excretion of phosphate, a low serum phosphate value may indicate excess parathyroid hormone. In addition, parathyroid hormone increases absorption of calcium from the urine and, indirectly, from the diet.

Calcium is absorbed from the duodenum and upper part of the small intestine predominantly under the influence of vitamin D. Absorbed from the diet or synthesized in the skin, vitamin D must be hydroxylated by the liver (25-hydroxylation) and subsequently by the kidneys (1-hydroxylation) to become fully active. Decreased serum phosphate and parathyroid hormone appear to contribute to 1-hydroxylase activation. The fully active compound, 1,25-dihydroxycholecalciferol, both increases bone resorption and is necessary for the action of parathyroid hormone on bone resorption.

Calcitonin, a peptide hormone synthesized by the thyroid gland, retards bone resorption. In pharmacologic doses, calcitonin can lower the serum calcium level. However, its role in normal physiology remains unclear.

Hypercalcemia

Recognition of severe hypercalcemia without laboratory testing is extremely difficult if not impossible. Therefore, the serum calcium level of every patient with a disordered state of consciousness must be determined. The physician should also remember that a normal serum calcium level in the presence of hypoalbuminemia may, in fact, represent early or important hypercalcemia. Awareness of the possibility of hypercalcemia often leads to early and successful therapy.

Hypercalcemia can often be prevented if appropriate precautions are observed. Patients with hyperparathyroidism, cancer, or accelerated bone resorption as in Paget's disease may be susceptible to lethal hypercalcemia if they are immobilized, dehydrated, or treated with thiazide diuretics, since immobilization increases resorption of calcium from bone, and dehydration and thiazide diuretics prevent excretion of calcium in the urine. Hypercalcemia is particularly likely to develop after therapy for certain neoplasms, for example, breast carcinoma treated with estrogens or androgens. A surprising number of patients who enter the hospital with a normal serum calcium level become hypercalcemic as a result of immobilization or fasting, and all patients at risk should be kept well hydrated and should be encouraged to walk. Thiazide diuretics should not be administered to such patients.

Diagnosis

To provide optimal therapy, the physician must estimate the probable cause of the hypercalcemia (Table 14.13). In our experience, more than 90% of hypercalcemic patients have either a malignant tumor or primary hyperparathyroidism, the former being more common.

Clinical Features. Prodromal symptoms may develop with slight to moderate elevation of the serum calcium level. These symptoms depend on the level of calcium itself and not on the cause. Gastrointestinal symptoms include constipation, anorexia, nausea, and vomiting. Nausea and vomiting may cause dehydration, reducing renal calcium excretion and exacerbating hypercalcemia. As a result, a cycle may develop, terminating in coma or death. Polyuria and polydipsia are apparently related to the impaired renal concentrating ability induced by hypercalcemia, and increased urinary losses may begin a similar dehydration cycle. Central nervous system changes range from subtle depression, impaired memory, or difficulty in concentrating to lethargy, stupor, or coma. A history of any of these symptoms in a comatose patient should raise the suspicion of hypercalcemia.

Physical examination is rarely informative. Hypertension may develop with acute hypercalcemia. Tachycardia and, less commonly, bradycardia or irregular rhythms may occur, but are also nonspecific. Chronic hypercalcemia may cause band keratopathy, that is, calcific deposits at the limbus of the eye. These deposits occur at the junction of the cornea and the sclera, in the parenthesis distribu-

Table 14.13.
Hypercalcemia: causes.[a]

Common
Spurious
Laboratory error
Tourniquet
Dehydration (eg, with Addison's disease)
Malignant condition (especially breast and lung carcinoma, multiple myeloma)
With bony metastases
Without bony metastases (?ectopic hormone production)
Primary hyperparathyroidism
Uncommon
Granulomatous disease (sarcoidosis, berylliosis, tuberculosis, histoplasmosis, blastomycosis)
Vitamin D or A intoxication
Thyrotoxicosis
Milk-alkali syndrome
Paget's disease with immobilization
Renal transplantation

[a] Any of these may be exacerbated by thiazide diuretic therapy.

tion ("3 o'clock and 9 o'clock"), and may occasionally be demonstrated by shining a penlight obliquely at these areas. The absence of deep tendon reflexes may be another clinical sign. A parathyroid adenoma is rarely palpable. A careful search for malignant neoplasms is imperative, with particular attention to breast nodules or mastectomy scars.

Clinical Studies. The electrocardiogram may provide the first clinical indication of hypercalcemia. A shortened Q-T interval suggests this condition, particularly when a prior normal electrocardiogram is available for comparison. It is important to remember that hypercalcemia sensitizes the myocardium to digitalis, and digitalis toxicity may develop in this setting.

In general, any feature indicating chronic hypercalcemia favors primary hyperparathyroidism as the diagnosis; examples include prior laboratory confirmation of hypercalcemia, renal calculi, and nephrocalcinosis. It is extremely unusual for a malignant tumor to cause sustained hypercalcemia of several years' duration. A decreased glomerular filtration rate is regularly observed with severe hypercalcemia itself; therefore, an elevated blood urea nitrogen level does not necessarily imply chronicity of hypercalcemia or irreversible renal failure. A low fasting serum phosphate value favors but does not establish the diagnosis of hyperparathyroidism. Oral or intravenous glucose also lowers the serum phosphate level, and values determined while the patient is receiving glucose or after meals should be ignored. Parathyroid hormone causes loss of bicarbonate through the kidneys, and an elevated serum chloride level with a decreased serum bicarbonate concentration suggests parathyroid hormone excess. Although ability to measure parathyroid hormone has aided differential diagnosis considerably, this test takes too long to be of benefit in a hypercalcemic emergency.

Rouleaux on a peripheral blood smear suggest multiple myeloma, which should be confirmed with protein electrophoresis or immunoelectrophoresis or both. Diffuse hyperglobulinemia is characteristic of sarcoidosis.

When the clinical condition permits, the following radiologic studies should be obtained: chest films (pulmonary malignant process, hilar adenopathy, or interstitial pattern of sarcoidosis); kidney-ureter-bladder films (renal stones or nephrocalcinosis); bone survey or scan (metastatic disease or Paget's disease); hand and clavicular films (subperiosteal resorption pathognomonic of hyperparathyroidism); intravenous pyelogram (hypernephroma); and breast xerograms (cancer). Nor-

mal radiologic results exclude neither hyperparathyroidism nor a malignant lesion.

Therapy

Hypercalcemia may result from excess calcium absorption, excess bone resorption, or decreased calcium excretion (Table 14.14). A combination of these factors is often at fault. Therapy should not be more toxic than the disease. The therapy of hypercalcemia due to a malignant process is usually based on hope for other therapeutic interventions in the future. Patients who were clearly dying before development of hypercalcemia should probably not be treated, but whenever the prognosis is in doubt, hypercalcemic patients should receive treatment (Tables 14.15 and 14.16).

Prevention of Calcium Absorption. To eliminate excess calcium from the diet, consumption of dairy products and calcium-containing antacids such as Tums should be discontinued. Except in patients with the milk-alkali syndrome, this unfortunately has little immediate effect on the serum calcium level. Vitamin D and newer analogues should be discontinued.

The effects of vitamin D on calcium absorption may last for months. In patients with vitamin D intoxication or hypersensitivity (for example, sarcoidosis), rapid reversal of hypercalcemia may be accomplished with administration of glucocorticoids, such as prednisone, 40–60 mg/day in divided doses. Drugs such as phenytoin or phenobarbital may accelerate the metabolism of vitamin D.

Increase in Urinary Calcium Excretion. Calcium appears in the urine in conjunction with sodium. Dehydration rids the urine of sodium and prevents calcium excretion. Rehydration with oral fluids

Table 14.14.
Hypercalcemia: physiologic mechanisms.

Increased calcium absorption
  Vitamin D intoxication
  Sarcoidosis
  Milk-alkali syndrome
Increased bone resorption
  Hyperparathyroidism
  Malignant disease
  Hyperthyroidism
  Paget's disease, especially with immobilization
  Vitamin D intoxication
  Sarcoidosis
Decreased calcium excretion
  Hyperparathyroidism
  Above conditions in combination with dehydration or administration of thiazide diuretic compounds

Table 14.15.
Hypercalcemia: drug therapy.

Agent	Dosage and Route	Indications	Contraindications	Comments	Toxic Reactions
Corticosteroids Prednisone or Hydrocortisone	15 mg 4 times a day orally or intravenously 75 mg 4 times a day orally or intravenously	Sarcoidosis, vitamin D intoxication, malignant disease, emergency	None in acute situation	Never sole form of emergency therapy PPD prior to chronic use if possible	Hyperadrenocorticism
Mithramycin	25 μg/kg intravenously as bolus or over 4 hours	Emergency only, ideally in hypercalcemia of malignancy	Thrombocytopenia, bleeding disorders	Wait 48–72 hours before repeating dose	Thrombocytopenia, renal and hepatic damage
Normal saline with Furosemide	200 ml/hr intravenously (minimum) 40–100 mg intravenously every 2 hours as needed	Emergency only	Cardiac disease, congestive heart failure, renal failure	Requires intensive care unit, replacement of urinary volume and electrolytes	Congestive heart failure, hypokalemia, hypomagnesemia
Salmon calcitonin	100 MRC units intramuscularly every 8 hours	Emergency only	None	Limited efficacy May be potentiated by glucocorticoids	Nausea, vomiting
Phosphorus Oral	1–4 gm/day elemental phosphate orally	Symptomatic moderate hypercalcemia		Avoid antacids Administer between meals	Diarrhea
Intravenous	50 millimoles elemental phosphate intravenously over 6–8 hours	Emergency only	Renal failure, hyperphosphatemia		Metastatic calcifications, renal failure, hypocalcemia

PPD = purified protein derivative; MRC = Medical Research Council.

Table 14.16.
Hypercalcemia: therapeutic protocol.

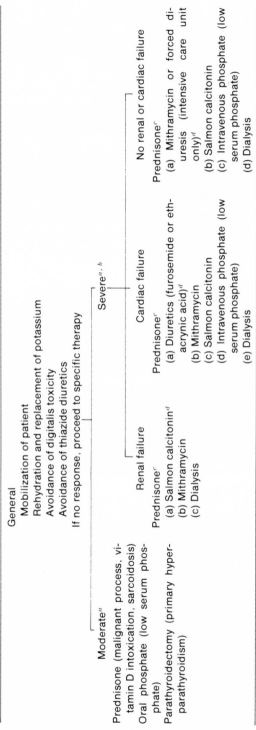

General
Mobilization of patient
Rehydration and replacement of potassium
Avoidance of digitalis toxicity
Avoidance of thiazide diuretics
If no response, proceed to specific therapy

Moderate[a]

Prednisone (malignant process, vitamin D intoxication, sarcoidosis)
Oral phosphate (low serum phosphate)
Parathyroidectomy (primary hyperparathyroidism)

Severe[a,b]

Renal failure
Prednisone[c]
(a) Salmon calcitonin[d]
(b) Mithramycin
(c) Dialysis

Cardiac failure
Prednisone[c]
(a) Diuretics (furosemide or ethacrynic acid)[d]
(b) Mithramycin
(c) Salmon calcitonin
(d) Intravenous phosphate (low serum phosphate)
(e) Dialysis

No renal or cardiac failure
Prednisone[c]
(a) Mithramycin or forced diuresis (intensive care unit only)[d]
(b) Salmon calcitonin
(c) Intravenous phosphate (low serum phosphate)
(d) Dialysis

[a] Moderate: serum calcium < 15 mg/100 ml, alert but symptomatic patient. Severe: serum calcium > 15 mg/100 ml or comatose patient.
[b] Emergency parathyroidectomy may be lifesaving in patients with primary hyperparathyroidism.
[c] Prednisone should never be the sole therapeutic agent in hypercalcemic emergencies, but should always be administered in conjunction with one or more of the measures listed below.
[d] If no response, proceed to (b), etc.

and salty foods may be adequate for prevention or treatment of mild hypercalcemia. Potassium should be replaced, and thiazide diuretics should not be prescribed.

With markedly symptomatic or severe hypercalcemia, large amounts of intravenous fluid containing sodium are often required. "Forced diuresis" with saline solution and potent diuretics, such as furosemide or ethacrynic acid, is effective, but is potentially dangerous and should never be performed outside of an intensive care setting. The central venous pressure should be monitored to prevent fluid overload. In severe cases, a minimum of 200 ml/hr of normal saline solution with intravenous furosemide in sufficient quantity (40–100 mg every 2 hours) is necessary to sustain the diuresis. Fluid administration must match urinary volume. In addition, urine should be analyzed for potassium and magnesium, and the amounts lost should be replaced, potassium replacement being mandatory.

Isotonic sodium sulfate solution has been suggested as an alternative to normal saline because it contains more sodium per liter and because sulfate complexes calcium in the urine. However, these advantages are outweighed by the disadvantages of sodium overload and hypernatremia. Ethylenediamine tetra-acetic acid (EDTA) complexes calcium, facilitating its urinary excretion, but nephrotoxicity limits its use.

If other measures fail, peritoneal dialysis or hemodialysis with calcium-free solutions should be considered.

Decrease in Bone Resorption or Increase in Bone Formation. Corticosteroids have an important but limited role in the treatment of hypercalcemia. Prednisone in vitamin D intoxication and sarcoidosis has already been discussed. Similar doses of corticosteroids are sometimes effective in hypercalcemia due to a malignant process, especially multiple myeloma, lymphoma, leukemia, or breast cancer; they have no effect on hypercalcemia due to hyperparathyroidism, however. Although they are part of the emergency therapy for hypercalcemia, corticosteroids should never be the only therapy in that setting, because of variable efficacy and delayed clinical response.

Mithramycin, an antineoplastic agent, is one of the most effective agents in the correction of hypercalcemia. The recommended dosage, 25 μg/kg as a single intravenous bolus, is much lower than the tumoricidal dose of this drug. Although we prefer to reserve this therapy for hypercalcemia due to a malignant condition, mithramycin may be the therapy of choice for emergency treatment of hypercalcemia refractory to rehydration. The effects of a single injection appear in the course of hours and last for 2–5 or more days. Therapy should not be repeated in less than 48 hours, and repeated therapy is reserved almost exclusively for patients with carcinoma. Toxic effects include thrombocytopenia, as well as renal and hepatic damage.

Salmon calcitonin is a safe, but only modestly effective means of lowering the serum calcium; a simple therapeutic regimen is 100 Medical Research Council (MRS) units intramuscularly every 8 hours. This will usually lower the serum calcium level acutely but rarely to within the normal range. The therapeutic effect often wears off after 48 hours. Recently, it has been suggested that prednisone (30–60 mg/day in three divided doses) may be synergistic with calcitonin and appears to prevent the loss of effectiveness of calcitonin or "escape" phenomenon. Calcitonin's safety makes it the initial drug of choice in patients with cardiac, renal, or hepatic disease.

Phosphate can be quite effective in the management of hypercalcemia. The mechanism of action is not completely known, but increased deposition of calcium in bone is one of the effects. Unfortunately, calcium tends to be deposited in other tissues as well. If the patient has hyperphosphatemia, this mode of therapy should be avoided.

With moderate, symptomatic hypercalcemia, 1–4 gm/day orally of elemental phosphate is preferred. Antacids bind phosphate and should not be given concurrently. Diarrhea may develop and limit the dosage. Intravenous phosphate has been employed in comatose patients, the magnitude of calcium decrease being directly proportional to the amount of phosphate infused. The dangers of intravenous phosphate are significant, and this therapy should be considered only in extreme emergencies. It is recommended that no more than 50 millimoles of phosphate be infused in the course of 6–8 hours. When larger amounts are administered, therapy is more effective, but renal failure and soft-tissue calcification become more frequent. The serum calcium level may continue to decrease for several hours after an infusion of intravenous phosphate is completed, and this must be kept in mind if additional phosphate is being considered.

In some cases of "ectopic hormone hypercalcemia", prostaglandins appear to mediate the hypercalcemia, in the absence of bony metastases. Prostaglandin inhibitors such as indomethacin are occasionally effective in decreasing the serum calcium in such patients and are worth a 24- to 48-hour trial.

The diphosphonates are pyrophosphate analogues which inhibit bone resorption. The currently licensed diphosphonates are effective in treating Paget's disease, but ineffective in hypercalcemia. The newer analogues (particularly dichloromethylene diphosphonate) are still experimental but appear to be very effective when administered intravenously in treating the hypercalcemia of malignancy. As oral agents, they hold great promise for the outpatient chronic treatment of hypercalcemia of malignancy when antitumor therapy has failed or is being tried.

The definitive therapy for parathyroid hormone-induced hypercalcemia is parathyroidectomy. Emergency operation is indicated if progressive renal failure appears or if the calcium level is refractory to the above modes of therapy. If possible, the patient's condition, including the calcium level, should be stabilized before surgery is performed. Additional medical adjuncts prior to the surgical therapy of hyperparathyroidism include estrogen administration (appears to inhibit action of parathyroid hormone), cimetidine therapy (appears to inhibit release of parathyroid hormone), and dichloromethylene diphosphonate (inhibits bone resorption).

Therapeutic Protocol. In the alert patient whose serum calcium level is less than 15 mg/dl (mild or moderate hypercalcemia), hydration and mobilization may be adequate therapy (Table 14.16). If there is no response and the patient is symptomatic, phosphorus should be administered orally, particularly if the serum phosphate value is low. Corticosteroids are an alternative in patients with a malignant process or a condition considered responsive to corticosteroids.

In the comatose patient or the patient whose serum calcium level is more than 15 mg/dl (severe hypercalcemia), intravenous hydration and corticosteroids are required initially. If no decrease in the serum calcium level is noted during the next several hours, the decision regarding further therapy may be difficult. For a malignant condition, mithramycin is clearly the therapy of choice. It may also be useful as onetime therapy in hypercalcemia of unknown cause. If an intensive care unit is available, forced diuresis is an acceptable alternative in young patients without heart disease. In the presence of renal failure, only calcitonin, mithramycin, or dialysis is effective. In patients with refractory hypercalcemia, intravenous phosphate can be administered. It should not be administered to patients with renal failure, and is most effective when the serum phosphate level is diminished. Emergency parathyroidectomy is oc-

casionally lifesaving if the diagnosis is firm and if the situation continues to deteriorate.

Hypocalcemia

Although the causes of hypocalcemia are many, the therapy, in general, is simple: administer calcium. In contrast with hypercalcemia, severe hypocalcemia is relatively easy to recognize because of signs of neuromuscular irritability; however, neuromuscular irritability alone does not necessarily imply hypocalcemia.

Diagnosis

Clinical Features. Numbness and tingling of the fingers and toes with perioral paresthesia are among the earliest symptoms of hypocalcemia, and are often accompanied by signs of tetany, such as carpal and pedal spasms. These findings, however, are nonspecific, the most common causes of such neuromuscular irritability being hyperventilation with metabolic alkalosis and, less often, hypomagnesemia. In patients with these signs and symptoms, the serum calcium should be measured immediately. Severe hypocalcemia may result in laryngeal spasm with stridor or in grand mal seizures, and should be treated as a genuine medical emergency.

Chronic hypocalcemia is associated with many nonspecific symptoms. Changes in mental status include general malaise, torpor, anxiety, neurosis, depression, delusions, and even psychosis. Spasms may occur in both smooth and voluntary muscles, and patients may complain of vague muscle cramps, diplopia, difficulty in swallowing, abdominal cramps, or bronchospasm.

Physical examination may be very informative. In the absence of obvious signs of neuromuscular irritability such as twitching, latent tetany can be unmasked with the Chvostek or Trousseau maneuver. The Chvostek test is performed by tapping the facial nerve anterior to the ear. Unilateral contraction of the facial muscle, such as twitching of the lip, is a positive sign; ipsilateral contraction of the eyelid is a more specific response. The Trousseau test renders nerves temporarily ischemic, bringing out latent tetany. The blood pressure cuff is inflated to a pressure above systolic and maintained at that level for 3 minutes. Carpal spasm with wrist flexion and finger adduction (main d'accoucheur) is a positive response. Chvostek and Trousseau tests can be negative in hypocalcemic patients, and positive tests need not indicate hypocalcemia. These tests may provide important information, however, when hypocalcemia is suspected.

An operative scar on the neck should suggest the possibility of hypocalcemia, whether it is the result of surgical treatment for thyroid disease, parathyroid disease, or an unrelated neoplasm. The deep tendon reflexes may be hyperactive in patients with mild to moderate hypocalcemia, but often disappear when hypocalcemia is profound.

Cutaneous changes indicating chronic hypocalcemia include dry scaly skin, eczema, brittle nails, thin or patchy scalp and eyebrow hair, absent axillary and pubic hair, and candidiasis. Dental hypoplasia suggests hypocalcemia dating from infancy. Cataracts regularly develop with sustained hypocalcemia. Pseudohypoparathyroidism, a rare syndrome of resistance to parathyroid hormone, is characterized by short stature, mental retardation, and short metacarpal bones. Although these symptoms may help establish the onset and duration of hypocalcemia, they are rarely useful in an emergency situation.

Clinical Studies. Lengthening of the Q-T interval on the electrocardiogram after correction for heart rate is a significant indication of hypocalcemia. In contrast with the Q-T lengthening seen with hypokalemia, no U waves are present. The serum albumin, creatinine, phosphate, magnesium, and blood urea nitrogen must be measured to determine the cause of the hypocalcemia.

Therapy

Emergency therapy for symptomatic hypocalcemia is intravenous administration of calcium. Vitamin D should *not* be administered in the emergency situation; with its long duration of action, it tends to complicate subsequent management by obscuring the cause of the hypocalcemia. In tetanic patients 200 mg of elemental calcium (20 ml of calcium gluconate or 22 ml of calcium glucoheptonate) should be administered over 5 minutes. In cases of severe hypocalcemia, this should be followed by 800–1000 mg of elemental calcium in 1000 ml of 5% dextrose solution to be infused over 12–24 hours. Calcium glucoheptonate and calcium gluconate contain 9 and 10%, respectively, calcium by weight, that is 100 ml of a 10% solution contains 9–10 gm of compound, but only 900–1000 mg of elemental calcium. Patients without parathyroid glands can be treated with 400 mg elemental calcium every 24 hours by constant intravenous infusion. However, in patients with bones avid for calcium, so called "hungry bones", up to 2000 mg or more per 24 hours will be required intravenously. It is important that the

serum calcium values be determined serially and the clinical response be monitored to ensure the desired therapeutic effect and to avoid overshoot. A serum calcium level of 7–8 mg/dl usually eliminates symptoms.

When hungry bones are not present, 400 mg of intravenous (elemental) calcium per 24 hours will usually suffice even in a parathyroidectomized patient. After parathyroid surgery with hungry bones, after parathyroid trauma or removal post thyroidectomy or after parathyroidectomy in renal failure patients, Vitamin D or its derivatives will usually be required. Vitamin D, 50,000 units/day will suffice, but the newer derivative, 1,25 dihydroxyVitamin D has the advantage of more rapid onset. Initial dosages of 1,25 dihydroxy-Vitamin D range from 0.5–2.0 μg/day. As soon as possible, calcium supplements should be changed from parenteral to oral. For chronic therapy, 1,25 dihydroxyVitamin D is still quite expensive and a switch to Vitamin D is reasonable.

A few warnings are necessary. Calcium chloride is sclerosing to veins, and should not be administered intravenously. Bicarbonate should never be added to a solution containing calcium, since calcium carbonate will precipitate. If the serum phosphate level is elevated when calcium therapy is begun, it must be lowered to avoid deposition of calcium in tissues. Oral antacids are recommended for this purpose. When calcium is being administered, the myocardium becomes sensitized to digitalis, and digitalis intoxication may develop. If neuromuscular irritability persists during calcium administration or if hypocalcemia develops rapidly after cessation of calcium therapy, magnesium deficiency may be at fault, requiring administration of magnesium sulfate, 40–60 mEq intravenously in the course of 4–6 hours if renal function is normal.

After the acute situation has been treated, the cause of the hypocalcemia must be determined.

Precipitating Factors

The differential diagnosis of hypocalcemia is listed in Table 14.17. The most common cause of a low serum calcium level is hypoalbuminemia. The ionized calcium value is normal in this situation, the patient is asymptomatic, and no therapy is indicated.

Hypocalcemia is a regular feature of renal failure, but emergency therapy is rarely required. The neuromuscular irritability of uremia is usually not due to the hypocalcemia. In patients with renal failure, lack of hypocalcemic symptoms is probably related to acidosis; hydrogen ions displace

Table 14.17.
Hypocalcemia: etiology.

Spurious
   Laboratory error
   Hypoalbuminemia
Decreased calcium absorption (increased parathyroid hormone production)
   Vitamin D deficiency
     Dietary lack
     Malabsorption (sprue, chronic pancreatitis)
   Vitamin D resistance
     Renal failure
     Phenytoin or phenobarbital administration
     Hereditary condition
Decreased bone release of calcium (decreased effect of parathyroid hormone)
   Severe vitamin D deficiency or resistance
   Parathyroid hormone absence
     Idiopathic
     Postoperative (parathyroidectomy)
       Permanent
       Transient (edema, ischemia, parathyroid gland suppression)
     Magnesium deficiency
   Parathyroid hormone resistance
     Pseudohypoparathyroidism
     Magnesium deficiency
Increased bone deposition
   "Hungry bones"
   Blastic tumors
Acute pancreatitis

---

calcium bound to albumin, increasing the ionized form. Conversely, rapid administration of alkali in such a setting can substantially decrease the ionized calcium, precipitating seizures or severe neuromuscular irritability.

Malabsorption of Vitamin D in conditions such as sprue or chronic pancreatitis is a common cause of hypocalcemia. Phenytoin (diphenylhydantoin) and phenobarbital have recently been shown to divert Vitamin D metabolism, preventing formation of active metabolites and causing functional Vitamin D deficiency. Inhibition of Vitamin D effect on bone is another possible mechanism of phenytoin-induced hypocalcemia and osteomalacia. In patients lacking Vitamin D, additional parathyroid hormone is secreted in response to hypocalcemia, and the serum phosphate level decreases because of the phosphaturic effect of parathyroid hormone.

In contrast, all forms of hypoparathyroidism are accompanied by hyperphosphatemia, the phosphaturic effect of parathyroid hormone being absent. Idiopathic parathyroid hormone deficiency is rare, and may be accompanied by mucocutaneous candidiasis and Addison's disease. Iatrogenic hypoparathyroidism is far more common, and most often occurs after parathyroid or thyroid operation. Parathyroid hormone resistance (pseudohypoparathyroidism) has already been mentioned.

Hypocalcemia after operation on the neck (especially parathyroid or thyroid operation) raises several important considerations. Permanent hypoparathyroidism may result from removal or destruction of the parathyroid glands. In patients who have undergone removal of a parathyroid adenoma, transient hypoparathyroidism may develop a few days after operation because of prior suppression of the parathyroid glands by the neoplasm, or it may develop days, weeks, or months later, resulting from ischemia of the residual parathyroid glands. Hyperphosphatemia is the indicator that one of these two situations exists. In patients with hyperparathyroidism or thyrotoxicosis, the serum calcium and phosphate levels may both decrease after operation, requiring temporary calcium therapy. This is due to hungry bones, that is, diversion of large amounts of calcium and phosphate into bone formation. The magnesium deficiency associated with hyperparathyroidism may result in hypocalcemia after operation, and postoperative hyperparathyroidism in rare cases is complicated by severe pancreatitis with attendant hypocalcemia. As in other instances of pancreatitis, the cause of hypocalcemia is unclear.

Severe hypomagnesemia may result from alcoholism, malabsorption, or diuretics, and has been shown to inhibit the release of parathyroid hormone or its action or both, resulting in hypocalcemia. Calcium administration transiently elevates the serum calcium level in this situation; however, hypocalcemia recurs rapidly unless magnesium is administered. Furthermore, neuromuscular irritability may not subside unless magnesium is administered as well as calcium.

SODIUM AND POTASSIUM EMERGENCIES

Hyponatremia

Renal Physiology

Hyponatremia is a consequence of impaired ability of the kidneys to excrete adequate amounts of dilute urine. In this setting, administration or ingestion of hypotonic fluids dilutes the serum sodium concentration and hyponatremia develops. To understand this fully, the manner in which kidneys excrete dilute urine must be considered.

The tonicity or osmolality of the blood is nor-

Table 14.18.
Hyponatremia: differential diagnosis and therapy.

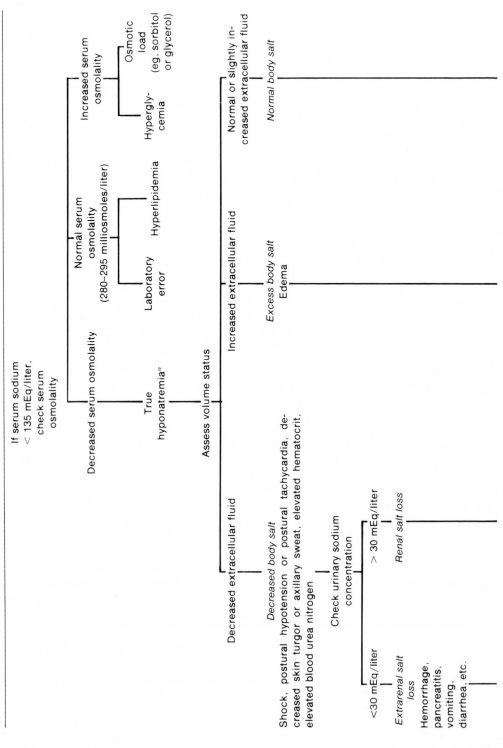

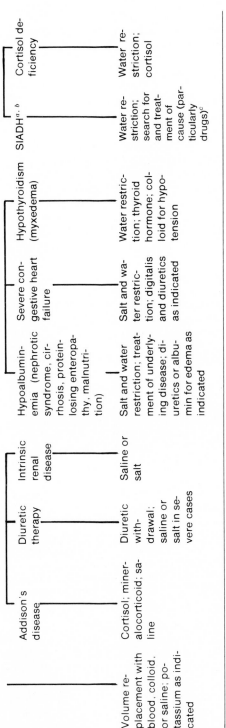

Addison's disease	Diuretic therapy	Intrinsic renal disease	Hypoalbuminemia (nephrotic syndrome, cirrhosis, protein-losing enteropathy, malnutrition)	Severe congestive heart failure	Hypothyroidism (myxedema)	SIADH[a,b]	Cortisol deficiency
Volume replacement with blood, colloid, or saline; potassium as indicated	Cortisol; mineralocorticoid; saline	Diuretic withdrawal; saline or salt in severe cases	Saline or salt	Salt and water restriction; treatment of underlying disease; diuretics or albumin for edema as indicated	Salt and water restriction; digitalis and diuretics as indicated	Water restriction; thyroid hormone; colloid for hypotension	Water restriction; search for and treatment of cause (particularly drugs)[c]	Water restriction; cortisol

[a] In an emergency, administer 3% saline solution, 500–1000 ml intravenously over 1–2 hours. In the presence of volume overload, diuretics should be administered as well.

[b] SIADH = syndrome of inappropriate antidiuretic hormone secretion; normal renal, adrenal, and thyroid function; blood urea nitrogen usually < 10 mg/dl, urinary sodium usually > 30 mEq/liter, urinary osmolality elevated inappropriately.

[c] Occasionally, demeclocycline or lithium are useful for chronic therapy.

mally maintained with narrow limits, 280–295 milliosmoles/liter (technically milliosmoles/kg); electrolytes constitute most of the osmotically active particles. The serum osmolality equals approximately twice the serum sodium concentration if the blood urea nitrogen and blood glucose concentrations are normal, these components also being osmotically active (see page 298).

Antidiuretic hormone (ADH) stimulates conservation of water by the kidneys. It is secreted from the posterior part of the pituitary gland, and is very sensitive to changes in the osmolality of the blood. Increased osmolality stimulates ADH release, resulting in concentration of the urine and correction of the the increased tonicity of the blood by the reabsorbed water. Severe volume depletion is a nonosmotic stimulus for ADH release by which intravascular volume is replaced.

Conversely, decreased serum osmolality inhibits release of ADH. If a healthy person drinks too much water, the excess is rapidly excreted by the kidneys in the form of dilute urine. This is because renal cells in the distal tubules and collecting ducts become relatively impermeable to water in the absence of ADH. In the absence of this hormone, when sodium is reabsorbed from the tubular fluids, water is left behind and dilute urine is excreted. The integrity of the barrier to water reabsorption requires the presence of cortisol as well as the absence of ADH; therefore, impaired ability to excrete dilute urine can result from the *presence of ADH* or the *absence of cortisol.*

Excretion of sufficient amounts of dilute urine also requires an adequate glomerular filtration rate, by which the filtrate is delivered to the diluting segments. In conditions in which renal perfusion is decreased, such as hypotension, increased sodium and water reabsorption occurs in the proximal renal tubules in an attempt to preserve or to expand the intravascular volume. As a result, flow to the distal segments is inadequate, and the ability to excrete normal quantities of dilute urine is impaired. Furthermore, the urine that *is* excreted may be less dilute than expected, and may even be hypertonic. There are two possible explanations for this. One is the imperfect barrier to water presented by the distal sites. If the urinary flow is sufficiently low, enough water will be reabsorbed that concentrated urine will result. Although the urine may be free of sodium, it will contain urea, the major solute in hypertonic urine. The other explanation is release of ADH by volume contraction; resultant water retention serves as a partial defense against hypotension. In such a situation, the attempt to preserve volume may override the usual osmotic stimulus to ADH release.

Thus, four requirements must be fulfilled for the excretion of sufficient amounts of dilute urine: the glomerular filtration rate must be adequate, ADH release must be inhibited, cortisol must be present, and the renal cells must remain impermeable to water.

Diagnosis and Therapy

The symptoms of hyponatremia are variable and rather nonspecific. Hyponatremia that develops rapidly is more likely to produce symptoms than that occurring more slowly. Symptoms include weakness, lethargy, anorexia, nausea, vomiting, headache, dizziness, and restlessness. Acute, severe hyponatremia may cause brain swelling with attendant delirium or convulsions, while chronic hyponatremia may be manifested by irritability or a personality change. When the serum sodium value decreases to less than 100 mEq/liter, objective motor weakness and loss of deep tendon reflexes may occur.

Decisions regarding therapy depend on clinical assessment of the state of sodium balance (Table 14.18). Excess and deficiency of whole body sodium can only be determined in this way, laboratory studies being of little help. The report of a low serum sodium value often results in routine administration of isotonic or hypertonic saline; this approach to therapy is irresponsible and may have dire consequences. The serum sodium concentration bears *no* relation to the amount of sodium in the body (Fig. 14.3). A low serum sodium level may be a consequence of water excess alone, in which case the sodium balance is normal and the only therapy required is water restriction. Hyponatremia may also occur with an excess of both water and sodium, the water excess predominating. Therapy in this instance consists primarily of water and sodium deprivation, but diuretics are often administered as well. Last, decrease in the serum sodium level may result from deficits of both salt and water, followed by hypotonic fluid ingestion or therapy. Saline or salt administration is then necessary.

Spurious Hyponatremia. When hyponatremia is reported, the serum sodium should immediately be measured again along with the serum osmolality. If the serum osmolality is not diminished, the hyponatremia is probably spurious (Table 14.18). Common causes of spurious hyponatremia include laboratory error and improper sampling—blood may have been drawn downstream from a rapidly flowing intravenous line, for example.

Severe hyperlipidemia may result in artifactual hyponatremia. The additional triglycerides separate the blood into a lipid compartment and an

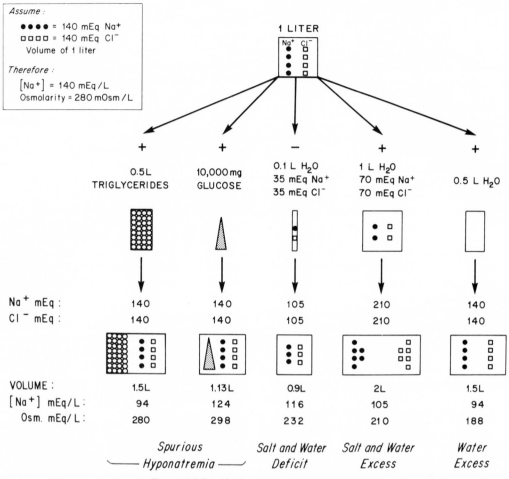

Figure 14.3. Mechanisms of hyponatremia.

aqueous compartment. The sodium concentration and osmolality of the aqueous phase are normal. Since the serum sodium concentration depends on the volume of the sample, the aqueous sodium content is diluted by the lipid compartment. The serum osmolality, however, is not influenced by the additional lipid, and is normal (Fig. 14.3). As a guide, an increase in the triglyceride concentration of 6000 mg/dl will result in a 5% decrease in the serum sodium concentration. The creamy appearance of the plasma will establish the diagnosis, and a search for the cause of the elevated triglyceride concentration can then be instituted.

When glucose is added to the intravascular compartment, it remains osmotically active and draws water to it. This movement of water out of the cells results in a decrease in the serum sodium concentration. An increase in the blood glucose level of 100 mg/dl will result in a serum sodium decrease of 1.6 mEq/liter. For example, a blood glucose level of 1000 mg/dl (900 mg/dl above

baseline) will decrease the serum sodium concentration from 144 to 130 mEq/liter independent of any sodium or water losses from the body. (Since 100 mg/dl of glucose represents 6 milliosmoles/liter, if enough water were attracted by the increase to maintain a constant blood osmolality, the electrolyte concentration would be expected to decrease by 6 milliosmoles/liter, half of which would be sodium. However, such a shift of water out of the cells would make the intracellular compartment hyperosmolar, and the osmolality must be constant throughout the body. Therefore, in actuality, a slight increase in the blood osmolality results from administration of glucose, and the sodium concentration decreases less than the theoretical 3 milliosmoles/liter.) Therapy in this situation must be directed toward the hyperglycemia rather than the hyponatremia.

Unmeasured osmotically active particles such as sorbitol or glycerol may cause similar changes.

Hyponatremia with Sodium Deficiency. Sodium

is primarily an extracellular cation, and sodium deficits result in a decrease in both intravascular and interstitial fluid volumes. Acute, severe depletion of intravascular volume, as in blood loss or pancreatitis, is easily recognized by a low central venous pressure in the presence of shock. Less severe volume loss may result only in postural hypotension or tachycardia.

Recognition of mild, chronic sodium depletion may be difficult. Such a deficit may be suggested by a history of vomiting, diarrhea, or diuretic intake; weight loss or persistently negative fluid balance in a hospitalized hyponatremic patient; and lack of axillary sweat. Decreased skin turgor in a well-nourished patient should also suggest sodium deficiency; the skin of the forehead should be pinched and then released, a slow relaxation rate indicating decreased turgor. The blood urea nitrogen value is commonly elevated, as is the hematocrit value if acute blood loss has not occurred.

Sodium loss may be extrarenal or renal. With extrarenal salt loss—as in sweating, vomiting, diarrhea, or pancreatitis—the glomerular filtration rate decreases, the blood urea nitrogen level may increase, and the urine is relatively free of sodium (less than 30 mEq/liter) because of salt conservation by the kidneys. Ability to dilute the urine is impaired, and hyponatremia will result *if* hypotonic fluids are ingested by the patient or administered by the physician.

Therapy for extrarenal salt loss is replacement of the underlying deficits. Severe loss of volume may require blood or plasma expanders. Lesser amounts of volume can be replaced with normal saline solution. Mild chronic sodium deficits can be managed with sodium-containing foods and fluids, salt tablets, or judicious administration of saline. Concomitant potassium deficits should be corrected as well. Hypotonic fluids should be excluded until volume is replaced, at which time the kidneys will be able to excrete dilute urine again. If the serum sodium level is less than 110 mEq/liter or if seizures are noted, 500–1000 ml of a 3% solution of hypertonic saline should be administered in addition to brisk volume expansion.

Hyponatremia in the presence of renal sodium loss can occur as a result of intrinsic renal disease, diuretic administration, or Addison's disease. Despite hyponatremia and clinical evidence of sodium deficiency, the urinary sodium concentration will be more than 30 mEq/liter. Diuretics and renal disease with salt-wasting result in excretion of isotonic urine. Even mild diuretics such as hydrochlorthiazide can lead to profound, often lethal, hyponatremia, particularly in older patients. If excess hypotonic fluids are provided, hyponatremia will result. In patients with Addison's disease, impaired ability to excrete dilute urine is a consequence of cortisol lack, resulting in "leaky" distal tubules as well as volume depletion itself. Saline administration may correct the volume depletion but not the hyponatremia, and renal salt-wasting in this setting may strongly indicate Addison's disease. Therapy with cortisol may be lifesaving for such patients.

Hyponatremia with Sodium Excess. Hyponatremia with total body sodium excess is characterized by edema. Severe hypoalbuminemia, as in patients with cirrhosis, nephrotic syndrome, protein-losing enteropathy, or severe malnutrition , leads to extravasation of fluid out of the intravascular compartment. Despite peripheral edema, the intravascular volume and glomerular filtration rate are diminished, resulting in impaired ability to excrete excess water. The hyponatremia is corrected with fluid restriction, and salt should be limited as well. Diuretic therapy or albumin administration is not necessary for the hyponatremia, but may be required for the edema.

In patients with severe congestive heart failure, the kidneys may be underperfused despite an increased intravascular volume, and hyponatremia may result. Therapy for heart failure includes digitalis, diuretics, vasodilators, and salt restriction; rigorous water restriction is required to treat the hyponatremia. Although not all patients with congestive heart failure have an impaired ability to excrete dilute urine, careful monitoring of the serum sodium levels is imperative if hyponatremia is to be prevented.

Hypothyroidism is another special example of this syndrome. The intravascular volume is often diminished, although excess sodium is present in the myxedema fluid. Impaired ability to excrete dilute urine is probably related to the diminished glomerular filtration rate, although inappropriate secretion of ADH has been postulated as well. Therapy requires fluid restriction and thyroid hormone administration. If hypotension is present, colloid may help replace volume and correct hyponatremia.

Hyponatremia with Normal Amounts of Body Sodium. This situation represents a state of water intoxication. There is no evidence for volume depletion, edema is absent, and renal function is normal. Such patients have a normal sodium balance, the urinary sodium excretion being equal to the sodium intake. This condition often results from inappropriate secretion of ADH; it may be mimicked by administration of certain drugs and by isolated cortisol deficiency. In the presence of adequate sodium intake, lack of urinary sodium (less than 30 mEq/liter) probably implies sodium depletion, and in this circumstance the diagnosis of water intoxication alone is suspect.

Inappropriate Section of ADH. The criteria for this syndrome include: (1) decreased serum sodium and serum osmolality; (2) normal renal function (glomerular filtration rate), with a blood urea nitrogen value usually less than 10 mg/dl; (3) normal adrenal and thyroid function; and (4) urinary osmolality inappropriately elevated in relation to the serum osmolality.

The last criterion requires amplification. A healthy person should be able to dilute urine to an osmolality of 50–75 milliosmoles/liter if large amounts of water are ingested. Blood hypotonicity should inhibit ADH release and result in similarly dilute urine. When the serum osmolality is decreased, a urinary osmolality more than 150 milliosmoles/liter is inappropriate, and indicates inability to dilute the urine maximally. Note that all forms of hyponatremia will be associated with inappropriately elevated urine osmolality, not just SIADH. Criteria 1–3 establish the diagnosis of SIADH.

Inappropriate secretion of ADH has many causes. It may occur after cerebral trauma or operation on the pituitary gland. Pulmonary lesions, including tuberculosis, abscess, and rarely pneumonia, may initiate this syndrome. Ectopic production of ADH by malignant neoplasms—especially oat cell carcinoma of the lung—is being recognized with increasing frequency. Narcotics and barbiturates may produce the syndrome rapidly through stimulations of ADH release. Vasopressin (ADH) infusion for gastrointestinal bleeding provides an exogenous source of the hormone. Chronic inappropriate secretion of ADH may develop with chlorpropamide therapy, and diuretic administration may mimic the syndrome if signs of volume depletion are subtle.

The therapy for hyponatremia due to inappropriate secretion of ADH is simple: restrict water while searching for a correctable cause, particularly drug intake. Total fluid intake may have to be decreased to 500–800 ml/day. Continued intravenous feeding is a notorious means of perpetuating hyponatremia. If normal saline solution is administered, hypertonic urine will be excreted, and hyponatremia may worsen.

If hyponatremia is life-threatening, in the presence of a serum sodium concentration less than 110 mEq/liter, coma, or seizures, for example, a 3% hypertonic saline solution should be administered, 500 ml intravenously in the course of 1–2 hours, followed by water restriction. If circulatory overload is feared, or develops, a loop diuretic such as furosemide should be administered before the hypertonic saline. Although furosemide will not allow for excretion of a dilute urine (the urine will be approximately isotonic—300 milliosmoles/liter), the excretion of isotonic urine with hypertonic fluid replacement will result in a rising serum sodium. The osmotic diuretic mannitol has the theoretical advantage of allowing water excretion out of proportion to solute and perhaps more rapid correction of the hyponatremia.

In chronic hyponatremia due to SIADH, water restriction will usually suffice but may be difficult to enforce. Both demeclocycline (but not other tetracyclines) and lithium cause a partial defect in water conservation by the kidney, which can be utilized to advantage in the SIADH situation. Demeclocycline is probably safer and can be administered in doses of 0.6–1.2 gm/day in divided dosages. There appears to be limited role for these agents in the acute situation as conventional therapy (above) usually suffices.

Cortisol Insufficiency. Cortisol deficiency alone due to hypopituitarism or pituitary suppression is a rare but important cause of water intoxication. In contrast with Addison's disease, lack of pigmentation and volume depletion may delay the diagnosis. The low serum sodium level responds to water restriction; however, cortisol must be administered to achieve a satisfactory clinical response.

Hyperkalemia

Physiologic Principles

Of the body potassium, 98% is intracellular; the low potassium concentration in the extracellular fluid is maintained within fairly narrow limits, 3.5–5.0 mEq/liter. Acidosis favors a shift of potassium from intracellular to extracellular sites, and alkalosis favors the reverse. Insulin deficiency is associated with decreased potassium tolerance (i.e., impaired ability to dispose of potassium loads).

Most urinary potassium results from the sodium/potassium-hydrogen ion exchange that occurs in the distal renal tubules and collecting ducts. This exchange requires the presence of aldosterone, the major mineralocorticoid. Hence, urinary potassium excretion is a consequence of tubular secretion, little being derived directly from glomerular filtration.

The requirements for normal potassium excretion include: (1) adequate glomerular filtration to deliver sodium to the distal tubules; (2) aldosterone or other mineralocorticoid hormones; and (3) renal tubules that respond to mineralocoroticoid hormones.

Precipitating Factors

If spurious causes are excluded, hyperkalemia can be considered to result from either excessive potassium input or impaired potassium excretion (Table 14.19). A combination of these two possibilities often exists.

Spurious Hyperkalemia. Minimal test-tube hemolysis may strikingly elevate the serum potassium concentration; this is a consequence of the extremely high intracellular potassium levels. Potassium release from platelets in vitro may lead to pseudohyperkalemia in patients with severe thrombocytosis. Heparin prevents such platelet lysis, and a normal plasma potassium level (heparinized tube) simultaneous with an elevated serum potassium level confirms the diagnosis of pseudohyperkalemia.

Excessive Potassium Input. Moderate to substantial increases in the serum potassium concentration may result from exogenous or endogenous

Table 14.19.
Hyperkalemia: mechanisms and diagnostic possibilities.

Spurious
    Laboratory error
    Hemolysis in vitro
    Platelet lysis associated with thrombocytosis (pseudohyperkalemia)

Excessive potassium input
    Exogenous
        Potassium salts
        Salt substitutes and low-salt milk
        Penicillin G therapy
        Transfusions with long-stored blood
    Endogenous
        Severe tissue injury (trauma, gangrene)
        Acidosis
        Insulin deficiency
        Intravascular hemolysis (clostridial sepsis)
        Hyperkalemic periodic paralysis

Decreased potassium excretion
    Decreased glomerular filtration rate
        Acute renal failure
        Chronic renal failure
        Sodium restriction
        Volume depletion producing poor renal perfusion
    Decreased sodium and potassium exchange
        Addison's disease
        Isolated aldosterone deficiency (renin deficiency, biosynthetic defect, heparin therapy)
        Drugs (spironolactone, triamterene or amiloride)

sources. Exogenous sources include oral and intravenous potassium salts, salt substitutes, low-sodium milk (potassium concentration of 60 mEq/liter) and penicillin G (potassium concentration of 1.7 mEq/million units). Although low-dose penicillin therapy represents little hazard, high-dose therapy, 20–40 million units/day, may lead to severe hyperkalemia unless the sodium salt is utilized. Banked blood is another important potassium source, the potassium leaking from the red blood cells with time. All these agents should be used with extreme caution in patients with an impaired ability to excrete potassium.

Endogenous sources of potassium are equally important. Acidosis may lead to profound hyperkalemia, as in diabetic ketoacidosis. Insulin deficiency in itself may prevent the translocation of potassium into cells. Tissue destruction, such as a crush injury or gangrene, may release massive amounts of potassium from damaged cells. Brisk intravascular hemolysis, as in clostridial sepsis, may result in death from hyperkalemia. The rare syndrome of hyperkalemic periodic paralysis is due to a potassium shift out of the cells, but the mechanism is unknown.

Impaired Excretion of Potassium. The simplest example of this is anuric renal failure, in which potassium excretion ceases and hyperkalemia develops. Acidosis soon follows and exacerbates the hyperkalemia. The physician should not only be aware of the possibility of hyperkalemia in patients with anuric renal failure but should also realize that with even minor decreases in the glomerular filtration rate, as in severe sodium restriction or minor volume depletion, sodium does not reach the distal tubules and potassium excretion is impaired.

When aldosterone is absent or its effect is blocked, potassium excretion diminishes. Aldosterone deficiency may occur with cortisol deficiency as part of Addison's disease, or it may be isolated, as in renin deficiency, biosynthetic defects, or heparin therapy. Aldosterone antagonism due to drug therapy with spironolactone is far more common, however. Both triamterene and amiloride are mild diuretics which appear to inhibit sodium-potassium exchange, independent of aldosterone. In general, potassium should *not* be administered with any of these drugs.

The urinary sodium concentration may help establish the cause of hyperkalemia. A urinary sodium concentration less than 30 mEq/liter implies decreased sodium delivery to distal sites, and sodium replacement is likely to help lower the serum potassium level by providing substrate for the sodium-potassium exchange. If the urinary sodium concentration is high, excessive administration of potassium or aldosterone deficiency or antagonism is likely.

Diagnosis and Therapy

The important manifestations of hyperkalemia are cardiac. Sudden death may occur without any previous clinical signs, although the electrocardiogram often contains important information regarding early potassium toxicity.

As the serum potassium level begins to increase, peaked T waves appear on the electrocardiogram (Fig. 14.4). In contrast with other causes of symmetrically peaked T waves, hyperkalemia is associated with a normal or decreased Q-T interval. With more profound hyperkalemia (serum potassium usually more than 8 mEq/liter), the P-R interval lengthens, P waves may disappear, and complete heart block may develop. The QRS complex widens, and may progress to sine waves. Ventricular arrhythmias are common. When ex-

posed to hyperkalemia, the heart is more sensitive to vagal influences, and such stimulation may lead to cardiac arrest. Hyponatremia, hypocalcemia, and acidosis all may exaggerate the cardiac effects of hyperkalemia.

If the serum potassium concentration is elevated, an electrocardiogram should be obtained immediately. Abnormalities compatible with the diagnosis of hyperkalemia dictate immediate therapy while the laboratory data are verified. A urinary sodium determination is helpful in planning therapy in this situation. If no electrocardiographic abnormalities are noted, the potassium in both serum and plasma (heparinized tube) should be measured again. Tubes should be carried to the laboratory immediately to minimize hemolysis.

In the hyperkalemic patient, administration of potassium and of drugs that impair potassium excretion must be discontinued, and large areas of necrotic tissue should be removed. However, these measures do not suffice in the emergency management of hyperkalemia (Table 14.20). If the serum

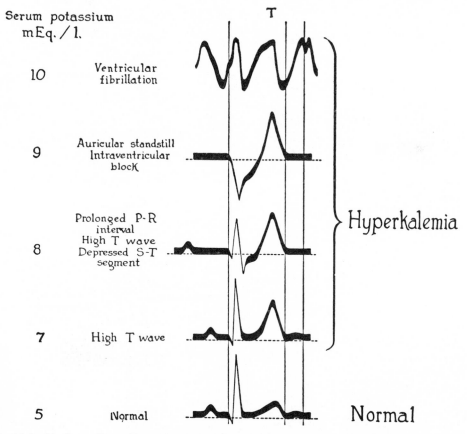

Figure 14.4. Electrocardiographic manifestations of hyperkalemia. (Modified with permission, from Burch GE, Winsor T: *A Primer of Electrocardiography*, 4th ed. Philadelphia, Lea & Febiger, 1960.)

Table 14.20.
Hyperkalemia: therapeutic protocol.

	Findings	Therapy	Agent and Dosage	Comments
General		Stop potassium administration Correct acidosis Stop drugs impairing potassium excretion Increase urinary sodium excretion by increasing sodium intake or by administering diuretics Remove necrotic tissue		Check for spurious hyperkalemia
Specific Mild	Serum potassium < 6.5 mEq/liter	Follow above steps		Consider diagnosis of Addison's disease if urinary sodium > 30 mEq/liter
Moderate	Serum potassium 6.5–8.0 mEq/liter or Peaked T waves on electrocardiogram	Follow above steps Administer ion-exchange resins	Sodium polystyrene sulfonate, 20 gm, plus sorbitol, 20 ml, 4 times a day orally, or sodium polystyrene sulfonate, 50 gm in 50 ml of 70% sorbitol solution, plus 100–150 ml water as retention enema	With circulatory overload or severe renal insufficiency, consider using calcium resin Retain enema at least half hour, repeat in 4 hours after a cleansing enema if necessary
Severe	Serum potassium > 8.0 mEq/liter or Widened QRS complex, heart block, or ventricular arrhythmia on electrocardiogram	Follow above steps Administer specified agents Employ peritoneal dialysis or hemodialysis if drug therapy is ineffective Administer ion-exchange resins as above when crisis passes	Sodium bicarbonate, 88 mEq/liter over 5 min intravenously and/or 50% glucose, 50–100 ml, plus insulin (CZI), 8–15 units as intravenous bolus[a] If above therapy ineffective, administer calcium gluconate, 1–2 gm over 5 min intravenously	Repeat in 15–20 min as needed Peak effect after 30 min Contraindicated in patients receiving digitalis, requires electrocardiographic monitoring

[a] In the absence of circulatory overload, an alternative to sodium bicarbonate and glucose in combination is 5% dextrose in 1 liter of normal saline, plus sodium bicarbonate, 88 mEq/liter over 30 min.

potassium level is more than 8 mEq/liter of if electrocardiographic changes *other than peaked T waves* are present, such as widening of the QRS complex or indications of heart block or a ventricular arrhythmia, administration of either sodium bicarbonate, insulin plus glucose, or intravenous calcium should be considered.

Sodium bicarbonate drives potassium into the cells even in the absence of acidosis, and may be lifesaving. Glucose with insulin is effective therapy because insulin transports potassium into cells, and the glucose prevents hypoglycemia. The peak effect of glucose plus insulin occurs after 30 minutes, however, and this may be too slow if the electrocardiogram shows signs of worsening hyperkalemia. Calcium directly antagonizes the effect of potassium on the heart, although it does not influence the serum potassium concentration. Calcium therapy is potentially hazardous, requires careful electrocardiographic monitoring, and should be avoided if the patient is receiving digitalis. Hypertonic saline solution antagonizes the effect of potassium on the heart to a lesser degree, and an alternative form of therapy is a "cocktail" containing dextrose, normal saline, and bicarbonate. If heart block is present and is not immediately reversed with medical therapy, a transvenous pacemaker should be inserted.

The effects of these agents are short-lived. Although with moderate hyperkalemia (serum potassium value from 6.5–8.0 mEq/liter and peaked T waves the only electrocardiographic indication) these slower forms of therapy may suffice, therapy directed toward a more sustained decrease in the serum potassium level should be instituted as well. Sodium intake should be increased if renal and cardiac functions are adequate. If the urinary sodium concentration is low, oral or parenteral salt administration will help return the potassium to normal levels. Ion-exchange resins such as sodium polystyrene sulfonate (Kayexalate) are effective, removing approximately 1 mEq of potassium for each gram of resin; the route of administration may be oral or rectal. Sorbitol is often administered in conjunction with resins to prevent constipation and to decrease absorption of the sodium leaving the resin. In patients with circulatory overload, the calcium form of the resin may be safer than the sodium form. If these measures do not suffice, hemodialysis or peritoneal dialysis against potassium-free solutions should be started.

It is important to avoid hypokalemia as a result of too vigorous therapy, particularly in patients receiving digitalis. The diagnosis of Addison's disease should be considered. Desoxycorticosterone acetate, 5 mg twice a day intramuscularly, or fludrocortisone acetate, 0.1–0.2 mg/day orally, in addition to cortisol is effective therapy.

Suggested Readings

Diabetic Ketoacidosis and Hyperosmolar Nonketotic Coma

Alberti KGMM: Low-dose insulin in the treatment of diabetic ketoacidosis. *Arch Intern Med* 137:1367–1376, 1977

Alberti KG, Hockaday TD, Turner RC: Small doses of intramuscular insulin in the treatment of diabetic "coma." *Lancet* 2:515–522, 1973

Arieff AI, Carroll HJ: Nonketotic hyperosmolar coma with hyperglycemia. *Medicine* 51:73–94, 1972

Beigelman PM: Potassium in severe diabetic ketoacidosis. *Am J Med* 54:419–420, 1973

Felig P: Diabetic ketoacidosis. *N Engl J Med* 290:1360–1363, 1974

Felts PW: *Current Concepts: Coma in the Diabetic.* Kalamazoo, MI, Upjohn Co., 1974

Fisher JN, Shahshahani MN, Kitabchi AE: Diabetic ketoacidosis: low-dose insulin therapy by various routes. *N Engl J Med* 297:238, 1977

Hare JW, Rossini AA: Diabetic comas: the overlap concept. *Hosp Prac* 14:95–108, May, 1979

Hockaday TD, Alberti KG: Diabetic coma. *Clin Endocrinol Metabol* 1:751–788, 1972

Johnston DG, Alberti KGMM: Diabetic Emergencies: Practical aspects of the management of diabetic ketoacidosis and diabetes during surgery. *Clin Endocrinol Metabol* 9:437–460, 1980

Keller U, Berger W: Prevention of hypophosphatemia by phosphate infusion during treatment of diabetic ketoacidosis and hyperosmolar coma. *Diabetes* 29:87–95, 1980

Kreisberg RA: Diabetic ketoacidosis: New concepts and trends in pathogenesis and treatment. *Ann Intern Med* 88:681–695, 1978

McCurdy D: Hyperosmolar hyperglycemic nonketotic diabetic coma. *Med Clin North Am* 54:683–699, 1970

McGarry JD: New perspectives in the regulation of ketogenesis. *Diabetes* 28:517–523, 1979

McGarry JD, Foster DW: Regulation of ketogenesis and clinical aspects of the ketotic state. *Metabolism* 21:471–489, 1972

Page MM, Alberti KG, Greenwood R, et al: Treatment of diabetic coma with continuous low-dose infusion of insulin. *Br Med J* 2:687–690, 1974

Soler NG, Fitzgerald MG, Bennett MA, et al: Intensive care in the management of diabetic ketoacidosis. *Lancet* 1:951–953, 1973

Alcoholic Ketoacidosis

Jenkins DW, Eckle RE, Craig JW: Alcoholic ketoacidosis. *JAMA* 217:177–183, 1971

Levy LJ, Duga J, Girgis M, et al: Ketoacidosis associated with alcoholism in nondiabetic subjects. *Ann Intern Med* 78:213–219, 1973

Miller PD, Heinig RE, Waterhouse C: Treatment of alcoholic acidosis. The role of dextrose and phosphorus. *Arch Intern Med* 138:67–72, 1978

Lactic Acidosis

Alberti KGMM, Nattrass M: Lactic acidosis. *Lancet* 2:25–29, 1977

Cohen RD, Iles RA: Lactic acidosis: diagnosis and therapy. *Clin Endocrinol Metabol* 9:513–527, 1980

Narins RG, Rudnick MR, Basti CP: Lactic acidosis and the elevated anion gap (I) and (II). *Hosp Prac* 15:125–125, May, 1980, 91–98, June, 1980

Oliva PB: Lactic acidosis. *Am J Med* 48:209–225, 1980

Taradash MR, Jacobson LB: Vasodilator therapy of idiopathic lactic acidosis. *N Engl J Med* 293:468–471, 1975

Hypoglycemia

Conn JW, Pek S: *Current Concepts: On Spontaneous Hypoglycemia.* Kalamazoo, MI, Upjohn Co., 1970

Fajans SS, Floyd JC, Jr: Fasting hypoglycemia in adults. *N Engl J Med* 294:766–772, 1976

Gale E: Hypoglycemia. *Clin Endocrinol Metabol* 9:461–475, 1980

Madison LL: Ethanol-induced hypoglycemia. *Adv Metab Disord* 3:85–109, 1968

Miller SI, Wallace RJ, Jr, Musher DM, et al: Hypoglycemia as a manifestation of sepsis. *Am J Med* 68:649–654, 1980

Seltzer HS: Drug-induced hypoglycemia: A review based on 473 cases. *Diabetes* 21:955–966, 1972

Adrenal Insufficiency

Amatruda TT, Jr, Hurst MM, D'Esopo ND: Certain endocrine and metabolic facets of the steroid withdrawal syndrome. *J Clin Endocrinol Metab* 25:1207–1217, 1965

Bayliss RIS: Adrenal cortex. *Clin Endocrinol Metabol* 9:477–486, 1980

Dixon RB, Christy NP: On the various forms of corticosteroid withdrawal syndrome. *Am J Med* 68:224–230, 1980

Graber AL, Ney RL, Nicholson WE, et al: Natural history of pituitary-adrenal recovery following long-term suppression with corticosteroids. *J Clin Endocrinol Metabol* 25:11–16, 1965

Mason AS, Meade TW, Lee JA, et al: Epidemiological and clinical picture of Addison's disease. *Lancet* 2:744–747, 1968

Melby JC: Drug spotlight program: Systemic corticosteroid therapy: Pharmacology and endocrinologic considerations. *Ann Intern Med* 81:505–512, 1974

Nerup J: Addison's disease—Clinical studies: A report of 108 cases. *Acta Endocrinol* 76:127–141, 1974

Thyroid Storm or Decompensated Thyrotoxicosis

Das G, Krieger M: Treatment of thyrotoxic storm with intravenous administration of propranolol. *Ann Intern Med* 70:985–988, 1969

Dillon PT, Babe J, Meloni CR, et al: Reserpine in thyrotoxic crisis. *N Engl J Med* 283:1020–1023, 1970

Ingbar SH: Management of emergencies. IX. Thyrotoxic storm. *N Engl J Med* 274:1252–1254, 1966

Mazzaferri EL, Skillman TG: Thyroid storm: A review of 22 episodes with special emphasis on the use of guanethidine. *Arch Intern Med* 124:684–690, 1969

McArthur JW, Rawson RW, Means JH, et al: Thyrotoxic crisis: Analysis of 36 cases seen at Massachusetts General Hospital during the past 25 years. *JAMA* 134:868–874, 1947

Menendez CE, Rivlin RS: Thyrotoxic crisis and myxedema coma. *Med Clin North Am* 57:1463–1470, 1973

Michie W, Hamer-Hodges DW, Pegg CA, et al: Beta-blockade and partial thyroidectomy for thyrotoxicosis. *Lancet* 1:1009–1011, 1974

Waldstein SS, Slodki SJ, Kaganiec GI, et al: A clinical study of thyroid storm. *Ann Intern Med* 52:626–642, 1960

Myxedema Crisis

Blum M: Myxedema coma. *Am J Med Sci* 264:432–443, 1972

Hausmann W: Myxoedema crisis. *Hormones* 1:110–128, 1970

Holvey DN, Goodner CJ, Nicoloff JT, et al: Treatment of myxedema coma with intravenous thyroxine. *Arch Intern Med* 113:89–96, 1964

Ridgway EC, McCammon JA, Benotti J, et al: Acute metabolic responses in myxedema to large doses of intravenous L-thyroxine. *Ann Intern Med* 77:549–555, 1972

Senior RM, Birge SJ, Wessler S, et al: The recognition and management of myxedema coma. *JAMA* 217:61–65, 1971

Calcium Emergencies

Binstock ML, Mundy GR: Effect of calcitonin and glucocorticoids in combination on the hypercalcemia of malignancy. *Ann Intern Med* 93:269–272, 1980

Elias EG, Evans JT: Hypercalcemic crisis in neoplastic diseases: Management with mithramycin. *Surgery* 71:631–635, 1972

Fulmer DH, Dimich AB, Rothschild EO, et al: Treatment of hypercalcemia: Comparison of intravenously administered phosphate, sulfate and hydrocortisone. *Arch Intern Med* 129:923–930, 1972

Goldsmith RS: Therapy of hypercalcemia. *Med Clin North Am* 56:951–960, 1972

Heath DP: The emergency management of disorders of calcium and magnesium. *Clin Endocrinol Metabol* 9:487–502, 1980

Jacobs TP, Siris ES, Bilezikian JP, et al: Hypercalcemia of malignancy: treatment with intravenous dichloromethylene diphosphonate. *Ann Intern Med* 94:312–316, 1981

Muggia FM, Heinemann HO: Hypercalcemia associated with neoplastic disease. *Ann Intern Med* 73:281–290, 1970

Schneider AB, Sherwood LM: Calcium homeostasis and the pathogenesis and management of hypercalcemic disorders. *Metabolism* 23:975–1007, 1974

Silva OL, Becker KL: Salmon calcitonin in the treatment of hypercalcemia. *Arch Intern Med* 132:337–339, 1973

Suki WN, Yium JJ, Von Minden M, et al: Acute treatment of hypercalcemia with furosemide. *N Engl J Med* 283:836–840, 1970

Hyponatremia

Ashraf N, Locksley R, Arieff AI: Thiazide-induced hyponatremia associated with death or neurologic damage in outpatients. *Am J Med* 70:1163–1168, 1981

Ayus JC, Olivero JJ, Frommer JP: Rapid correction of severe hyponatremia with intravenous hypertonic saline solution. *Am J Med* 72:43–48, 1982

Baylis PH: Hyponatremia and hypernatremia. *Clin Endocrinol Metabol* 9:625–637, 1980

Bartter FC, Schwartz WB: The syndrome of inappropriate secretion of antidiuretic hormone. *Am J Med* 42:790–806, 1967

Fichman MP, Vorherr H, Kleeman CR, et al: Diuretic-induced hyponatremia. *Ann Intern Med* 75:853–863, 1971

Fuisz RE: Hyponatremia. *Medicine* 42:149–170, 1963

Hantamn D, Rossier B, Zohlman R, et al: Rapid correction of hyponatremia in the syndrome of inappropriate secretion of antidiuretic hormone: An alternative treatment to hypertonic saline. *Ann Intern Med* 78:870–875, 1973

Katz MA: Hyperglycemia-induced hyponatremia—Calculation

of expected serum sodium depression. *N Engl J Med* *289*:843–844, 1973

Leaf A: The clinical and physiologic significance of the serum sodium concentration. *N Engl J Med 267*:25–30, 77–83, 1962

Michelis MF, Warms PC, Davis BB: An approach to the diagnosis and therapy of hyponatremic states. *Milit Med 140*:17–21, 1975

Moses AM, Miller M: Drug-induced dilutional hyponatremia. *N Engl J Med 291*:1234–1239, 1974

White MG, Fetner CD: Treatment of the syndrome of inappropriate secretion of antidiuretic hormone with lithium carbonate. *N Engl J Med 292*:390–392, 1975

Hyperkalemia

Levinsky N: Management of emergencies. VI. Hyperkalemia. *N Engl J Med 274*:1076–1077, 1966

CHAPTER 15

Neurologic Emergencies

EDWARD R. WOLPOW, M.D.

"Excuse me, but what is it like to have a blocked ear?"

" ... It's the only real sound in the universe, though it can be proved not to exist ... "

Halldór Laxness, *The Pigeon Banquet*

History-taking in neurology is often unsatisfactory. The damaged nervous system finds it difficult to give a good account of itself, and at times is totally unaware of flagrant deficits. Even when the complaint is fairly obvious, interpretation may be complex: the patient who states that his hand is numb may, in fact, have hypesthesia, paresthesia, spastic weakness, flaccid weakness, or ataxia. Still, careful conversation with the neurologic patient and his family is the most efficient way to gather data with which to make medical decisions, even in the emergency ward.

This chapter divides neurologic illness into major categories according to symptoms, and deals with differential diagnosis and therapy in each category. Sections concerned with general principles of lumbar puncture, electroencephalography, and intravenous therapy in neurologic patients are also included. The topics of poisoning and drug overdose, head injury, and a systematic discussion of stupor and coma are found in other chapters.

DIAGNOSTIC TECHNIQUES

Lumbar Puncture

Procurement of adequate quantities of uncontaminated cerebrospinal fluid (CSF) by puncture of the lumbar spinal subarachnoid space is essential to the diagnosis of many types of medical illness. Many guidelines have been established to achieve success, and careful planning before the lumbar puncture will allow the gathering of all relevant information from the sample. All too often, a second lumbar puncture is carried out soon after the first because care was not taken initially to secure the proper amount of CSF, resulting in inadequate workup.

In many neurologic conditions, lumbar puncture is not indicated, and in others it may be dangerous. Patients with brain tumors, particularly in the posterior fossa, should usually not be subjected to lumbar puncture, at least early in the workup, to avoid a lethal shift of cerebral tissue such as "herniation" of cerebellar tonsils, resulting in compression of the medulla oblongata. The presentation of brain tumor varies, however, and the diagnosis may not be evident when lumbar puncture is attempted. In general, evidence of increased intracranial pressure contraindicates lumbar puncture, yet there are several clinical settings in which it is essential, even if somewhat risky. A notable example would be when purulent meningitis is suspected.

Examination of the optic fundi provides information on the intracranial pressure. The earliest change at the optic discs reflecting increased pressure within the cranium is loss of the normal venous pulsations. Although absence of venous pulsations may not be very informative, their presence makes it likely that CSF pressure is not high. Tortuosity of retinal veins and erythema of the optic nerve head are next seen as CSF pressure rises, after which disc margins become blurred and hemorrhages may appear. Some patients with cerebral edema may have retinal edema as well, which can be seen with the ophthalmoscope. Chronically increased intracranial pressure produces characteristic changes in the radiologic appearance of the sella turcica (Fig. 15.1). Computed tomography of the brain is indicated before lumbar puncture if the question of tumor or the likelihood of raised pressure exists.

Another condition in which lumbar puncture is contraindicated is severe bleeding diathesis. In a patient with fewer than 40,000 platelets/mm^3, lumbar puncture presents the risk of spinal subarach-

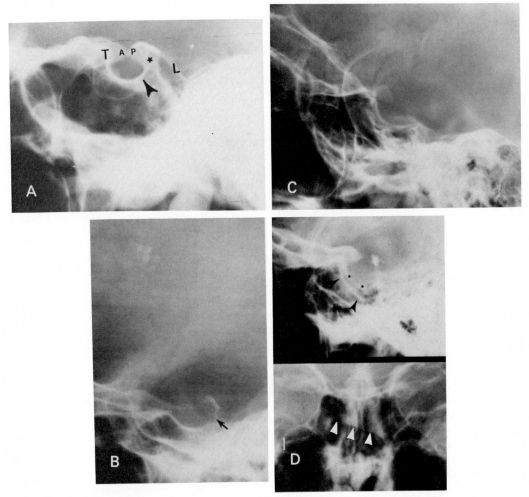

Figure 15.1. Sella turcica enlarged from standard skull x-ray films. In lateral views, anterior is to the left, posterior to the right. (**A**) Lateral view of normal sella turcica showing well-corticated floor. Note tuberculum (*T*) and prominent anterior (*A*) and posterior (*P*) clinoid processes, the latter overlying the dorsum sellae (***). The petroclinoid ligament (*L*) is densely calcified—a normal variant. Earliest change with increased intracranial pressure is erosion of floor where indicated by *arrow*. (**B**) Lateral view of sella turcica with increased intracranial pressure resulting from a glioma (note tumor calcification in upper part of figure). Posterior aspect of sella floor and base of dorsum sellae are eroded (*arrow*), whereas anterior part of floor appears normal. (**C**) Lateral view of sella turcica in patient with destruction of dorsum sellae as result of direct pressure from a suprasellar tumor. Sella is enlarged. (**D**) Top, lateral view of sella turcica in patient with a chromophobe adenoma of the pituitary gland with asymmetric enlargement. *Asterisks* mark location of normal side of floor, and *arrows* mark location of eroded side. Bottom, frontal view showing sloping floor (*arrows*) produced by asymmetric expansion of pituitary gland. (Courtesy of R. H. Ackerman, M.D.)

noid hemorrhage, which may develop slowly—even after the lumbar puncture is completed—and which may be severe.

Procedure

The patient should lie curled on his side, and the physician should be seated. If the physician is right-handed, it may be easier to manipulate the needle if the patient is in the left lateral decubitus position; the opposite is true for the left-handed

physician. Palpation of the lower part of the back will reveal dorsal spinous processes of the lumbar vertebrae. The preferred site for puncture is at the level of the superior iliac crest, which is usually between the third and fourth or fourth and fifth lumbar vertebrae.

After the superior iliac crest is located, the skin is cleansed. If iodine is used, a history of any related allergic reactions should be obtained, and the effect of topical iodine on subsequent thyroid studies should be considered, particularly in patients with dementia, confusion, or coma. The lumbar puncture needle should not be passed through iodine; whatever the primary cleansing agent, alcohol should be employed as the final wash.

Lidocaine (Xylocaine), 1 ml of a 2% solution, is infiltrated into the skin with a short 26-gauge needle. It is usually unnecessary to anesthetize more deeply. One minute or more may be required before the anesthetic agent takes effect.

Various gauges of lumbar puncture needle are available. A 20-gauge needle may be used in most instances. Although finer needles possess theoretic advantages, they may be difficult to use, especially in muscular patients, because the needle may be caught in muscle planes and veer off center. Needles without stylets should not be used; in children, such a needle may introduce a plug of skin into the lumbar theca that may later develop into an epidermoid tumor. The bevel of the needle should be oriented so that the fibers of the ligamentum flavum and dura mater are split rather than cut (Fig. 15.2A). The needle should puncture the anesthetic bleb a few millimeters from the entry point of the anesthetizing needle to avoid contamination by blood that might be at or beneath this site.

The patient is "curled up" by an assistant, with the bed horizontal. The needle is aimed roughly at the umbilicus. The "pop" that is said to be felt on entering the subarachnoid space is not, in fact, often distinctly experienced, and rather than risk too deep a penetration with possible violation of the intervertebral disc space, the stylet should be removed often as the needle is advanced. When the CSF flows freely, the needle may be turned 90 degrees so that the bevel faces the head of the patient.

CSF pressure should be measured before any fluid is removed. Normal values range from 80–180 mm CSF. The patient is allowed to uncurl to decrease intra-abdominal pressure. If ventilatory assistance is being employed, the respirator should be disconnected, if possible, since a positive-pressure apparatus will spuriously raise CSF pressure. Increased systemic venous pressure will also raise CSF pressure. Before the diagnosis of increased CSF pressure can be made, at least 10 minutes should pass before a high reading is officially recorded. If partial or total spinal block is suspected, bilateral compression of the neck with sufficient force to occlude the internal and external jugular veins will not result in the prompt rise in lumbar CSF pressure that would normally occur (Queckenstedt's test). If Queckenstedt's test is positive, an emergency myelogram is often indicated.

If the CSF pressure is less than 400 mm CSF, enough CSF should slowly be collected to ensure that all necessary laboratory tests can be performed; as much CSF should be taken as necessary, even if the quantity is 40 ml or more, since the total volume of human adult CSF is replaced several times each day. To determine the pH and partial pressures of oxygen (P_{O_2}) and carbon dioxide (P_{CO_2}), the CSF must be drawn in a closed system—usually a syringe attached to the stopcock.

The appearance of the CSF as it flows may partly determine how many test tubes of fluid are collected. If placement of the needle has caused local bleeding ("traumatic tap"), the CSF may initially be blood-streaked, and then may become clear. In such cases, it may be advisable to collect more CSF than originally planned, with the hope that the later samples will be free of blood cells on microscopic examination. On the other hand, traumatic tap can produce equal numbers of red blood cells in all tubes, even if five or more samples are collected. In patients with a partial CSF block at a spinal level, the first few milliliters may be yellow or orange because of large amounts of protein

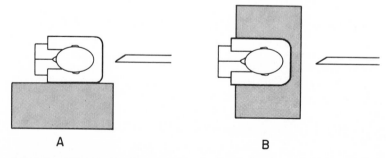

A   B

Figure 15.2.   Orientation of bevel of lumbar puncture needle. **(A)** Patient in decubitus position, viewed from top of head. **(B)** Seated patient, viewed from above.

(Froin's syndrome); later samples will contain decreasing quantities of protein as normal CSF flows past the partial block. In this situation, too, additional CSF may have to be collected. Measurement of pressure after the CSF is drawn is seldom indicated.

If CSF pressure is more than 400 mm CSF, no CSF should be collected until the pressure is lowered. With the needle in place and the pressure being recorded, intravenous mannitol should be administered, 1.5–2.0 gm/kg in a 30-minute period. If the patient is not fully awake, catheterization of the bladder is required since diuresis resulting from mannitol can be extremely rapid and voluminous. In virtually all patients with increased intracranial pressure, mannitol is successful in lowering lumbar pressure to safe levels (less than 300 mm CSF) so that CSF can be collected. An alternate method is to remove CSF very slowly (1–4 drops/min) until the manometer reading decreases to a safe level. This may require time that cannot be spared, as in patients with bacterial meningitis.

If lumbar puncture at the level of the superior iliac crest is unsuccessful, higher or lower puncture may be tried; cephalad, the procedure is safe only as far as the space between the second and third lumbar vertebrae. Another method is to have the patient sit at the edge of the bed, bent forward as much as possible. The lumbar puncture is then carried out as described in the preceding paragraphs, except that the bevel of the needle is turned 90 degrees (Fig. 15.2B) and the CSF pressure is measured in terms of estimated distance of the top of the manometer column above or below the foramen magnum.

After lumbar puncture, the patient should remain flat for at least 2 hours. The patient need not remain supine, but can be prone or on either side; in whichever position, the head should not be higher than the rest of the body. Headache and damage related to increased intracranial pressure or incipient pressure cones both result from leakage of CSF from the puncture site into the meninges after withdrawal of the needle. Although it is conventional to recommend that patients drink a lot of fluid after lumbar puncture, it is in fact, more reasonable to restrict fluid intake in order to reduce CSF pressure at the needle puncture site so that the puncture in the meninges can heal. Indeed, agents for lowering the CSF pressure, such as acetazolamide (Diamox), 250 mg orally three times a day, may be useful in the treatment of leakage or headache by virtue of retarding CSF production.

In some patients, lumbar puncture is not possible, for example, in the case of previous extensive lumbar bony fusions, "narrow lumbar canal syndrome," or burns or cutaneous infections of the lower part of the back. If collection of CSF is essential, puncture of the cisterna magna may be carried out, as well as lateral cervical puncture. These procedures should only be performed by physicians experienced in them, and they usually require radiographic monitoring.

Analysis of CSF

A description of the color and clarity of the CSF should be recorded. "Crystal clear water white" describes the normal specimen. Blood-tinged or frankly bloody CSF must be centrifuged as quickly as possible. Blood in the CSF begins to hemolyze rapidly; in general, the supernatant after a traumatic tap will appear normal, but the supernatant from a patient with a condition such as subarachnoid or intracranial hemorrhage, for example, will appear orange. An orange hue to spun CSF does not allow distinction between the presence of large amounts of protein and the products of hemolysis. In many cases, a blood sample for glucose determination should be drawn during lumbar puncture.

Laboratory studies of the CSF must be individualized. Although it is not possible to detail all of the variations, a few points should be highlighted. Bloody CSF should always be cultured, particularly if the clinical history is incomplete. The sequence of bacterial meningitis causing delirium, in turn leading to a fall with cerebral contusion and skull fracture, is not farfetched. Since the Gram stain is seldom informative when the CSF is bloody, culture may be the only clue to a life-threatening illness. After the bloody sample is centrifuged, the protein concentration of the supernatant should be determined. In a person with a peripheral count of 5 million red blood cells/mm^3 and a serum protein level of 5 gm/dl, blood in the CSF will increase the protein by 1 mg/1000 red blood cells; this amount may be subtracted in calculating the true concentration of CSF protein. Patients with subarachnoid hemorrhage alone tend to have CSF with no excess of protein, using this correction. In patients with intracerebral hemorrhage, however, the amount of protein is often much in excess of the corrected figure, suggesting parenchymal brain damage.

Staining of the CSF for microscopic study of cells or bacteria is often difficult. Before this is done, it may be useful to suspend the centrifuged button in a drop of the patient's serum to preserve cell structure.

Computed Tomography of the Brain

Within only a few years, computed tomography (CT) of the brain has become an indispensable adjunct to emergency care of patients with neurologic illness. With this noninvasive technique, the physician can rapidly collect information about the brain, meningeal spaces, and cranial bones and sinuses. Most importantly for emergency medicine, information is promptly provided on the presence of tumor (neoplasm, abscess, hematoma), cerebral edema, and resultant shifts of cerebral tissue. Blood is frequently visible in the subarachnoid space as a result of aneurysmal rupture. The only hazards are those due to use of intravenous iodinated contrast material, frequently employed to enhance various pathologic changes.

Since CT is a test of anatomy, it provides different information from tests of physiology, such as neurologic examination of the patient and electroencephalography (EEG). Most often, detailed data from both types of tests are necessary to resolve clinical problems effectively. In addition, fine anatomic detail in certain regions, such as the lower brainstem and sella turcica (Fig. 15.1), is beyond the resolution of current CT scanners. New nuclear magnetic resonance scanners (NMR), capable of defining these areas, are already on the "horizon", however.

Electroencephalography

Rhythmic impulses from the reticular formation of the brainstem normally excite the cerebral cortex, producing fluctuating levels of electrical excitation that are measurable from electrodes placed on the scalp; the recording that is produced is the EEG. As a *physiologic* test, this procedure differs qualitatively from most other special neurologic procedures, which are *anatomic*, for example, the plain x-ray film, isotopic scan, CT scan, angiographic examination, and pneumoencephalogram.

The EEG may be useful in a limited number of emergency situations. With a portable machine, a trained technician can begin to record in the emergency ward after only 5–10 minutes of setup time. Ten minutes of recording is usually adequate.

Seizures

EEG examination is seldom necessary to establish the diagnosis of seizures. It may, however, aid in distinguishing patients with true seizures from patients with hysterical attacks and from malingerers whose spells are designed to simulate epileptic attacks. Although EEGs recorded during either a generalized epileptic seizure or a hysterical or malingering attack are not likely to be interpretable because of the substantial artifact produced by movement, paroxysms (spikes or sharp waves) occur commonly in interictal records of patients with true cerebral seizures, but rarely in the records of neurotic or malingering patients. Also, grand mal seizures are usually followed by slowing of brain waves on the EEG, whereas hysterical or malingering attacks are not.

Acute Psychosis

Recording of brain waves may aid in the differential diagnosis of patients with acute psychosis. Tracings of patients with acute schizophrenia or manic-depressive illness are virtually always normal or nearly normal. Acute psychosis, though, may also be a presentation of metabolic derangements such as hypoglycemia, in which case generalized slowing on the EEG is evident. Encephalitis, particularly when caused by herpes simplex virus (acute inclusion-body encephalitis), is often manifested by psychotic behavior, even before fever or focal cerebral findings are evident. In this case, the EEG characteristically shows generalized, sharp slowing that is most prominent over one temporal lobe. Behavioral disorders also occur in children with subacute sclerosing panencephalitis and in adults with subacute spongiform encephalopathy (Creutzfeldt-Jakob syndrome). In both instances, characteristic paroxysmal EEG activity is likely to be present, and the history will reveal a subacute rather than acute onset of the behavioral disorder.

Coma

The differential diagnosis of patients with coma may also be aided by the EEG. Patients with severe, bilateral, lower brainstem disease may appear to be comatose, but they are actually wide-awake and paralyzed ("locked-in syndrome"). As long as upper brainstem and cerebral hemispheres are intact in these patients, the EEG will be normal. The presence of therapeutic or toxic amounts of several types of medication may be suggested by anterior fast (β) activity on the EEG. Most notable among these medications are barbiturates and benzodiazepine compounds such as diazepam hydrochloride (Valium), chlordiazepoxide hydrochloride (Librium), and flurazepam (Dalmane).

Irreversible Cerebral Cortical Damage

The EEG is one element in the diagnosis of "cerebral death" or, more accurately, irreversible cerebral cortical damage. Criteria for this include absence of the following: cerebral depressant drugs, hypothermia, any spontaneous movement (including breathing, twitching, shivering, and so on), and all reflexes (deep tendon reflexes, plantar reflexes, vestibulo-ocular reflexes, and pupillary reaction to light, loud noise, or stimulation of the skin of the neck). In addition, the EEG must show no cerebral activity more than 2 μv in amplitude for a half-hour. Furthermore, these signs must all be constant for 24 hours. The concept that irreversible cerebral cortical damage documented by these criteria or modifications of them may be the functional equivalent of death is new and controversial. As criteria evolve and life-sustaining technologic advances are developed, the decision whether a comatose patient has any potential for awakening may become the responsibility of emergency physicians. The role of the EEG in the diagnosis of irreversible coma should not be overestimated: although compared with the EEG a detailed neurologic examination is more difficult to perform and to interpret, it is more relevant to the issue.

INTRAVENOUS FLUID ADMINISTRATION

Few emergency ward activities are carried out with the aggressive zeal that characterizes the institution of intravenous fluid administration. With full appreciation of the legitimate need for central venous lines and other lines in distal arm veins, it should be stressed that the most common and serious error in the emergency treatment of patients with acute cerebral disease is infusion of intravenous fluid. In the course of several hours, 500 ml of 5% dextrose in water can be lethal to patients with brain tumor, acute stroke, acute head injury, or any other process in which cerebral edema is a factor, such as abscess or meningitis. While in the emergency ward, patients with acute cerebral disease should receive only as much intravenous fluid as cardiac and renal functions require (which is most often no fluid). Intravenous fluid is one of the first causes considered when a hospitalized patient shows signs of neurologic deterioration.

If it is necessary to start intravenous fluid administration either for measurement of central venous pressure or for infusion of medications, the least possible quantity should be given. A pediatric infusion system set at "keep open" will provide the smallest volume. Even better, however, is a heparin lock system in which there can be no flow at all much of the time. Patients with acute brain disease should virtually never receive salt-free intravenous fluid; either normal saline or 0.45% saline solution is indicated.

Two other considerations in intravenous fluid therapy are important. First, if a waking patient has hemiparesis or brachial monoparesis, it is desirable to insert the intravenous line in the paretic side so that the patient will be able to use the other arm. Second, the patient's extended arm should not be bound tightly for any length of time to an armboard with a sharp proximal edge halfway up the upper arm. The edge of such an armboard, which creases the triceps muscle, may injure the radial nerve, resulting in an incapacitating and painful wristdrop.

MENINGEAL IRRITATION

Pus and blood are the most common meningeal irritants, and bacterial meningitis, viral meningitis and encephalitis, and subarachnoid hemorrhage are the most common relevant illnesses. Resistance to passive flexion of the head is the hallmark of meningeal irritation. Such resistance is a *reflex* whose arc passes from meninges to spinal cord to paraspinal and limb musculature; when central nervous system activity is severely depressed, as in end-stage meningitis with coma, there is no "stiff neck," even in the presence of substantial meningeal irritation. In testing for resistance, the physician must distinguish between resistance to flexing the head and resistance to turning it. In meningeal irritative states, resistance to flexion is much greater than that to other neck movements, while in patients with severe cervical arthritis or parkinsonism, for example, there is approximately equal resistance to neck movement in any direction. Some patients with arthritis may have virtually no forward flexion because of a relatively fixed cervical spine, and this must be differentiated from the reflex resistance of meningeal irritation. Resistance to straight-leg raising, which provides comparable information about meningeal irritation, should be used to complement the results of testing for stiff neck.

Precipitating Factors

Meningitis

Headache, fever, and signs of meningeal irritation are the classic features of meningitis. Any or all of these features may be lacking, and the emergency physician must be aware of the possibility of early meningitis, especially in the patient with an altered mental state for no apparent reason. Physical examination must include careful inspection of the skin and tympanic membranes and a search for evidence of CSF leakage from the nose or ears. X-ray films of the chest and skull are essential, including adequate views of the paranasal sinuses and mastoid regions and CT scanning. When, however, the likelihood of purulent meningitis is very high (high fever, severe headache, marked meningismus), lumbar puncture should be performed before any radiologic test, including CT scanning. The CSF and antibiotic therapy in patients with meningitis are discussed in Chapter 11, pages 231–234.

Encephalitis

Encephalitis is most frequently viral. Headache is often prominent, and fever and meningeal irritation are commonly present. The most common nonepidemic etiologic agent is herpes simplex virus, which causes acute inclusion-body encephalitis. A small percentage of patients may exhibit typical "cold sores" on the mouth. Since the disease is necrotizing, cerebral edema can be severe and fatal, and the CSF may show both red and white blood cells. It is possible that the virus enters the brain via the nose, and the symptoms and distribution of the neuropathologic changes are in accordance with that postulation. The olfactory system is affected, and patients may complain of altered sense of smell or of olfactory hallucinations. When the sense of smell is tested, which is essential in all patients with suspected encephalitis, anosmia may be discovered. The medial temporal lobe is a common site of infection, which often occurs much more extensively in one hemisphere than in the other. Disordered behavior (acute psychosis) is common, and memory may be affected severely. The changes affecting the mental state may appear before other neurologic findings become evident, such as reflex asymmetry, hemiparesis, and so on. Small quick myoclonic jerks of the fingers may suggest the diagnosis. The EEG is always considerably abnormal, with diffuse, sharp slowing that is often more extreme in the affected hemisphere. The CT scan may show edema of one temporal lobe. The antiviral agent adenine arabinoside (Vidarabine) has been shown to be effective in the treatment of herpes simplex encephalitis, so prompt diagnosis, often including biopsy of brain tissues, is important.

The major immediate threat to the patient is cerebral edema, which is commonly massive and asymmetric. If the patient is comatose or deeply obtunded, especially if signs of herniation of the temporal lobe such as ipsilateral pupillary dilatation are evident, immediate lowering of intracranial pressure is essential and wide subtemporal surgical decompression may be indicated. Such

therapy is not now the sole alternative that it once was; this is because of the advent of rapidly acting antiedema agents, such as intravenous mannitol, 1.5–2.0 gm/kg in the course of 30 minutes, and glycerol, 1–2 gm/kg/day in divided doses via a nasogastric tube (glycerol will probably soon be widely available for intravenous use). High doses of corticosteroids should not be administered because of the possibility of enhancing spread of the virus to uninfected parts of the brain, and in addition, these agents do not cause antiedema effects until several hours after administration has begun. Minimization of fluid intake is essential. In severe cases, slow intravenous administration of phenytoin (Dilantin) is recommended to prevent seizures.

Encephalitis may accompany virtually all other common viral illnesses. Some etiologic agents, such as the virus that causes infectious mononucleosis, typically produce mild illness, while others, such as that responsible for eastern equine encephalomyelitis, cause devastating disease. Most often, the agent is not discovered, but samples of CSF, blood, throat washings, and stool should be collected in the emergency ward for viral studies in all patients with encephalitis. Treatment of increased intracranial pressure with fluid restriction and medication, together with close observation, is the therapeutic feature common to all these illnesses. Anticonvulsant therapy is not usually indicated.

Tumor

Meningeal irritation may occur with carcinoma or lymphoma of the meninges, and the clinical features strongly resemble those of infectious meningitis or encephalitis. Often, the CSF glucose level is extremely low, as it is in patients with bacterial meningitis. (Other noninfectious causes of a very low CSF glucose level are central nervous system sarcoidosis and blood in the CSF.) The correct diagnosis may be made by means of cytologic study of the CSF.

Tumor in the vicinity of the foramen magnum may reflexly produce a stiff neck. In this situation, neither blood nor pus is noted on lumbar puncture (which is particularly risky). If tumor in this region is suspected, the safest diagnostic approach is early CT scanning, followed, if necessary, by arteriographic examination to study the vertebral and basilar arteries and their branches.

Subarachnoid Hemorrhage

Blood in the CSF causes meningeal irritation, and primary subarachnoid hemorrhage from rupture of a saccular aneurysm is frequently the source. Typically, a sudden and excruciatingly severe headache develops, and in some patients, similar minor headaches may have occurred in the preceding days or weeks. Headache and stiff neck may be all that is noted on examination, but focal neurologic findings may indicate the site of the aneurysm. Aneurysms tend to occur where arteries of unequal diameter anastomose. The three most common locations are the junction of the anterior cerebral and anterior communicating arteries, the junction of the internal carotid artery and the posterior communicating artery, and the major sites of division of the middle cerebral artery above the temporal lobe. Lateralizing findings occur most commonly in patients with aneurysm of the middle cerebral artery. Since these aneurysms lie within the subarachnoid space, all bleeding may, in fact, be external to the brain. Bleeding into the brain is also possible, however, and rarely, bleeding is almost exclusively into the brain, with the result that no blood appears in the CSF on lumbar puncture. Examination of the optic fundi may reveal subhyaloid hemorrhages usually close to the optic disc and often comparable in size with the disc itself. This finding indicates that there is blood under high pressure in the CSF, and although it usually signifies primary subarachnoid hemorrhage, it may also accompany other types of intracranial hemorrhage.

In patients with a ruptured aneurysm, elevated blood pressure should be treated vigorously in the emergency ward. Slow intravenous administration of phenytoin is recommended for prophylaxis. Since the patient will die unless the aneurysmal bleeding stops, the emphasis should not be on swift lowering of intracranial pressure, even if the pressure at lumbar puncture is very high. (It may be argued that lowering of intracranial pressure will make further aneurysmal bleeding more likely.) If signs of herniation of the temporal lobe develop, however, or if neurologic function is rapidly declining, corticosteroid or mannitol therapy should be begun. The timing of arteriographic examination and surgical intervention is determined in consultation with the neurosurgeon. Usually, arteriography within the first 24 hours is recommended. CT scanning may reveal intracerebral hematoma or hydrocephalus, and often indicates the location of the aneurysm.

Several newer types of adjunctive therapy should be mentioned. The antifibrinolytic agent ϵ-aminocaproic acid (Amicar) has been recommended for patients with aneurysmal bleeding to help preserve the clot that eventually seals the bleeding point. The dosage is 1.5 gm/hr, orally or by slow intravenous invusion. The morbidity resulting from aneurysmal hemorrhage is often largely due to spasm of major cerebral arteries that is produced by nearby blood, which may last many days and which may lead to infarction distal to the aneurysm. Many pharmacologic agents are being studied either to prevent or to treat arterial spasm, but specific recommendations cannot as yet be made.

Other Nontraumatic Causes

Bloody CSF may also result from bleeding dyscrasias, which may produce intracranial hemorrhage; the most common factor is use of sodium warfarin (Coumadin) and heparin as anticoagulants. The prothrombin time, partial thromboplastin time, and platelet count should be determined in the emergency ward for all patients with bloody CSF. Anticoagulant hemorrhage may be intracerebral, subarachnoid, subdural, or epidural. Treatment is discussed in Chapter 13, pages 286–287. Vascular malformations may bleed within the brain tissue or external to the brain. If hypertension is present, it should be treated quickly. When primary intracerebral hemorrhage is not due to anticoagulant therapy or to a vascular malformation, the cause is virtually always hypertension. CT scanning reveals the hematoma and often the site of bleeding, and in most instances, the CSF is bloody. Therapy consists of lowering blood pressure to normal levels. In some conditions, such as hemorrhage into the cerebellum, surgical intervention should be considered; these syndromes are considered in more detail on pages 356–357. Intracranial hemorrhage in relation to head trauma is discussed in Chapter 27, pages 600–605.

SEIZURES

Grand Mal Status Epilepticus

General Considerations

The most dangerous and therapeutically demanding seizure disorder encountered clinically is grand mal status epilepticus. By this is meant either generalized, whole-body convulsions with loss of consciousness that are uninterrupted for more than 10 minutes or grand mal seizures leading to postictal coma followed by further grand mal seizures rather than by wakening. Although data are equivocal, it is reasonable to presume that grand mal status epilepticus may damage the brain, even if oxygen and glucose are adequate. Therapy to stop the seizures is therefore essential, and the sooner they are stopped, the less the chance for permanent brain damage.

Although a generalized convulsion may signify serious cerebral disease, it also indicates that much of the central and peripheral nervous system is intact. The classic tonic-clonic grand mal seizure requires that the cerebral cortex, the projection pathways to and from the thalamus, the cortico-bulbar and corticospinal efferent pathways, the bulbar and spinal motor neuron pool, the motor peripheral nerves, and the neuromuscular systems carry out a complex series of events. Structural or biochemical lesions that interfere with the functioning of the neuraxis at any of these levels may prevent or curtail the convulsion. There are several correlates to this. First is that the cessation of a series of seizures may indicate a worsening state of the neuraxis rather than improvement. If untreated hypoglycemia is present, for example, grand mal seizures may spontaneously end because the impulses can no longer be conducted by the brain. Irreversible coma and death may follow quickly if therapy is not begun. Since the postictal state after a series of grand mal seizures normally resembles deep coma, a period of anxious waiting follows the cessation of a long series of generalized seizures. A second correlate is that generalized seizures that are expressed as less than total body movements may indicate more profound nervous system damage than seizures in which all parts of the body participate. In patients with severe cerebral hypoxia, for example, generalized seizures may be expressed only by loss of consciousness with conjugate flickering movements of the eyes, since pathways through the brainstem to the spinal cord are too damaged to transmit the cerebral impulses for limb movement.

The most common serious threat to life during grand mal seizures is vomiting followed by aspiration of gastric contents, which frequently occurs before the patient has arrived in the emergency ward. The autonomic nervous system participates greatly in grand mal seizures—profuse salivation, for example, being a hallmark of the illness. Vomiting may occur as part of the seizure, during the alterations in autonomic activity that may take place. Another cause for vomiting in the seizing patient is the lay therapy directed toward the "myth of the swallowed tongue." The tongue is commonly bitten during grand mal seizures, and because of the gurgling and gasping that occurs, the well-meaning witness may place a finger into the patient's mouth, resulting not only in a bitten finger but also and more disastrously in gagging and vomiting. Teeth and parts of dentures may also be aspirated, either during the seizure itself or in attempts to liberate the patient's tongue. The

treatment of aspiration of a foreign body into the lungs is discussed in Chapter 22, page 487.

The autonomic changes are expressed by changes in blood pressure that may be dramatic, by alterations in pupillary size, and by many other physiologic responses, such as sweating and urination. Some patients die during grand mal status epilepticus, and as in patients with subarachnoid hemorrhage, death may occasionally be due to cardiac arrhythmia.

Therapeutic Protocol

When the patient is brought to the emergency ward, some clues regarding his history may be available, even if no witnesses, family, or friends accompany him. His belongings should be searched for medications and for cards identifying him as an epileptic or diabetic, for example. Needle puncture marks should be sought.

Particularly because of the likelihood of vomiting, the seizing or comatose patient should not be left supine, but should be turned on his side. If respiratory assistance is required, nasotracheal intubation may be the best and quickest method, particularly if the patient's jaws are clenched. If the seizure began before the patient was brought to the hospital, the possibility of head, back, and neck trauma deserves attention. Dislocation of one or both shoulders is common, and represents an orthopaedic emergency within the neurologic emergency. If the patient has fallen, the eyes may be injured, and the globes should be inspected for signs of trauma.

After respiratory and cardiovascular functions are assured, blood must be drawn for laboratory studies. In the patient with grand mal status epilepticus for whom no medical information is available, venous blood should be drawn for measurement of glucose, sodium, potassium, calcium, phosphorus, urea nitrogen, ammonia, phenytoin, and barbiturates, and for determination of toxic substances. As soon as possible after this, 50 ml of a 50% dextrose solution should be instilled rapidly as an intravenous bolus. Hypoglycemia as a possible cause of seizures will thus be treated even before the laboratory can provide a blood glucose value. If alcoholism is a factor, 50 mg of thiamine should be administered parenterally at the same time. A well-anchored intravenous line will be necessary, but in the seizing patient without a specific diagnosis, no fluid beyond what is required to provide medication should be delivered by any route. An arterial blood sample should be taken for determination of the pH, P_{O_2}, and P_{CO_2};

alkalosis lowers the threshold for seizures and hypoxia is not reliably determined by examination of skin color.

Anticonvulsant therapy is required next. Hypertrophied gums may indicate that the patient has ingested phenytoin for an extended period. Another indication that phenytoin may be present is absence of the tonic (stiffening) phase of grand mal, with only the clonic (shaking) movements observable. No peripheral signs reliably indicate the presence of therapeutic amounts of barbiturates. These facts are important because a combination of several classes of drugs (hydantoin compounds, barbiturates, and benzodiazepine derivatives) may lead to respiratory and cardiovascular depression. It is recommended that only two major anticonvulsants be administered to patients with ongoing seizures, and doses should be extended to therapeutic limits. The major anticonvulsants available in this setting include diazepam, phenytoin, and phenobarbital.

Intravenous diazepam is an effective anticonvulsant that frequently stops seizures in approximately one circulation time. The action may be short-term, and it may be necessary to administer boluses frequently. A bolus of 2–5 mg administered slowly into a small hand vein may stop seizures long enough to allow a well-anchored intravenous line to be placed and to intubate the patient if necessary. Additional 2–5 mg boluses should be administered as needed. An arbitrary limit of 60 mg in the course of 12 hours for an adult should not be exceeded. Diazepam should not be mixed in an intravenous bottle but only given in small, separate infusions. Intravenous diazepam does not supply the brain with a long-lasting anticonvulsant effect, and it is not sufficient by itself to protect the patient from further seizures, even if it succeeds in stopping ongoing seizures and allows the patient to waken. It is unlikely that oral diazepam has clinical usefulness as an anticonvulsant, and intramuscular absorption is incomplete, unpredictable, slow, and therefore of little or no use in therapy for ongoing seizures.

Phenytoin is the basic anticonvulsant for adults, whatever the type of seizure. Anticonvulsant action can be obtained within a few hours with intravenous infusion, which is the recommended route in patients with grand mal status epilepticus. Up to 1 gm as a slow, separate intravenous infusion delivered at a rate not faster than 100 mg in 5 minutes is the therapeutic dose for an adult. The medication is unstable when mixed with other intravenous solutions, and it should always be administered separately. Phenytoin should not be administered intramuscularly, since it is poorly and slowly absorbed and adequate levels in the blood are only reached many days after injection, if at all. Oral phenytoin is a standard anticonvulsant medication, but it also acts slowly; in patients who start receiving 100 mg orally three times a day, the level in the blood is often not in the therapeutic range in less than a week. Therefore, for emergency treatment of grand mal status epilepticus, the only acceptable route for this drug is intravenous. Treatment with 2–5 mg boluses of intravenous diazepam and up to 1 gm of intravenous phenytoin is adequate in most patients with seizures.

An alternative to diazepam is slow intravenous administration of phenobarbital, up to 1 gm in an adult. This medication acts rapidly, and is synergistic with phenytoin. It has a specific advantage over diazepam in the treatment of seizures due to barbiturate withdrawal, but it is more sedating and usually takes longer to act. It does, however, provide anticonvulsant effects for many hours after administration, which diazepam does not. It is not recommended that all three medications be used concurrently because of the danger of respiratory and cardiovascular depression. A combination of diazepam and phenytoin or phenobarbital and phenytoin should be chosen.

A less potent but useful adjunctive medication for seizures is paraldehyde. It is particularly recommended for patients with seizures in whom alcohol is a factor. It is not likely to replace the need for diazepam, phenytoin, or phenobarbital, but it may be used with them. Paraldehyde is an organic solvent, and plastic should be avoided in its use. Sterile abscesses can result if plastic syringes are used because of the plastic injected along with the drug. If care is taken to use glass syringes and metal needles with no plastic parts, 7 ml can safely be administered deep in each buttock. Common therapy in children is rectal administration of paraldehyde dissolved in oil. Intravenous paraldehyde has been recommended as a potent anticonvulsant, but use of plastic intravenous tubing contraindicates this route of administration.

A small number of patients in whom no correctable metabolic disorder is uncovered will fail to respond to full doses of medication as outlined. If, at this point, the duration of status epilepticus is more than 6–8 hours, general anesthesia should be induced because of the threat of brain damage due to continued generalized convulsions. General anesthesia guarantees cessation of seizures, but it may be many hours before it is possible to decrease the amount of anesthetic without seizure recurrence.

Paralytic agents such as curare stop the somatic expression of the seizure by neuromuscular blockade, but the real danger to the patient stems from excessive cerebral activity, which curare does not change and which still requires the types of therapy outlined. Curarization is not recommended since it does not solve the major difficulty, it makes neurologic monitoring much more difficult, and it may lead the physician to a false sense of accomplishment.

Known electrolyte disturbances should be corrected in preference to administration of high doses of anticonvulsants. Low sodium and calcium levels are particularly likely to cause intractable seizures. Hyponatremia in outpatients is most often due to salt-wasting diuretic medications, and in inpatients it is most often due to salt-poor intravenous fluids. Seizures in connection with drug withdrawals, notably alcohol (delirium tremens) and barbiturates, may be difficult to treat. Intravenous ethanol is not recommended in the therapy for alcoholic withdrawal, but fluid replacement, sedation, and anticonvulsants should be administered as needed. Lower doses of anticonvulsants should be administered in the presence of hepatic or renal failure.

Once the seizure stops, CT scanning should be carried out to look for tumor or blood. Chest and skull x-ray films may also be informative. If status epilepticus continues, however, and if meningitis or intracranial bleeding is a possibility, lumbar puncture should be performed, despite the associated risk. Subarachnoid hemorrhage and meningitis may both be manifested by intractable seizures, and much valuable time may be used in treating seizures before the serious underlying cerebral disease is diagnosed. Although fever may develop in the course of status epilepticus, its presence always necessitates lumbar puncture.

The typical single grand mal seizure lasts only 5–6 minutes, with wakening a few minutes later. Such patients are brought to the emergency ward after the seizure is over, and they may or may not have further seizures with or without treatment. A patient who has suffered his first grand mal seizure should undergo full medical and neurological examination; venous blood studies as previously outlined, CT scanning, EEG examination, radiologic examination of the skull, and a lumbar puncture should all be performed. The patient should also be hospitalized for a few days, particularly if the cause of the seizure is not obvious and he lives

alone. Oral administration of phenobarbital, 30 mg three times a day, will provide anticonvulsant action on the day it is begun; oral phenytoin, 100 mg three times a day, may require up to 1 week to achieve effective levels in the blood. In adults, phenytoin may be adequate alone, but the lag before it takes effect must not be overlooked. Because of the possibility of an allergic or other toxic reaction, phenytoin should not be administered intravenously unless it is essential; the patient who has recovered from his first grand mal seizure and whose neurologic status is normal does not usually require this route of therapy.

When phenytoin cannot be administered, primidone is an acceptable initial drug in adult epilepsy, especially the grand mal and temporal lobe types. Its effect is quick, but the dosage must be increased slowly to avoid drowsiness, which can be severe; 50–250 mg orally at bedtime may be increased to the usual dosage of 250 mg three times a day in about 3 weeks. One of the breakdown products of primidone is phenobarbital, and in fact, therapeutic doses of primidone usually result in higher blood levels of phenobarbital than do therapeutic doses of phenobarbital.

Carbamazepine is another first-line anticonvulsant drug for major seizures; it may be started at a dose of 200 mg/day and increased over 1–2 weeks to minimize drowsiness. Liver function, white blood cell count, differential, and platelet count must be carefully monitored in patients receiving this drug.

Other Types of Status Epilepticus

Aside from grand mal status epilepticus, two other types of status epilepticus may be encountered: partial continuous epilepsy and petit mal epilepsy.

Partial Continuous Epilepsy

Any focal seizure may recur for hours at a time. For example, a patient may come to the emergency ward complaining of uncontrolled rhythmic twitching for many hours of a thumb or great toe. If the focus is the temporal lobe, the seizure disorder may be behavioral, automatic (licking lips, rubbing hands, and so on), or emotional (fear, for example). All of the focal seizures are characterized by retention of consciousness and the tendency to stereotypy. This type of seizure is called partial continuous epilepsy (epilepsia partialis continua), and if the cerebral focus is small or deep, the EEG may appear normal or nonfocally abnormal, even while the seizure is occurring. The workup for seizures of this sort is the same as for grand mal seizures, but causes that imply focal cerebral disease are more likely. These include cerebral embolism, primary or metastatic brain tumor, scarring from old cerebral trauma, and cerebral vasculitis as in lupus erythematosus. Prevalence of partial continuous epilepsy in the hyperosmolar nonketotic state has been noted. The need to stop these seizures is not so strong as it is in patients with grand mal status epilepticus. In fact, to stop partial continuous epilepsy, it may be necessary to administer so much medication that the patient is put to sleep. It is not acceptable to trade an awake patient with focal seizures for a drugged-to-sleep patient without focal seizures. The most important therapeutic maneuver is to provide the patient with medication that will prevent the focal seizure from becoming generalized; intravenous phenytoin should be administered, up to 1 gm slowly. Although such therapy may not affect the focal seizure, it provides prophylaxis against grand mal seizures. Patients with partial continuous epilepsy should be hospitalized until the seizure ends.

Petit Mal Epilepsy

The syndrome of petit mal epilepsy consists of periods of loss of consciousness, which may be associated with loss of postural tone, and rhythmic myoclonic twitches of parts of the body (most characteristically, the eyelids), three per second, which correspond to a three-per-second spike-and-wave pattern on the EEG. Petit mal epilepsy occurs most often in children, who may have hundreds of attacks each day. Although it is a type of generalized epilepsy, there is usually no postictal somnolence nor paralysis. Attacks may blend together, producing hours of continuous seizures, and this is termed petit mal status epilepticus, which may be seen in adults as well as in children. Careful search for three-per-second myoclonic twitches should be made in any patient in a trance-like state, and the EEG may be useful in the differential diagnosis. Small quantities of intravenous diazepam, 2–5 mg boluses administered slowly, characteristically interrupt the seizures, allowing the patient to waken. The patient is often immediately able to converse and to act normally. Basic therapy for petit mal epilepsy usually includes ethosuximide (Zarontin), although acetazolamide, which has fewer potential side effects, may be tried first. As with partial continuous epilepsy, it is not essential to stop the seizures by all means available. Phenytoin is not usually help-ful in children with petit mal epilepsy, but it may be administered to adults with refractory seizures. A major neurologic workup for this condition is not indicated since it is virtually always idiopathic—known structural or biochemical lesions never produce this seizure pattern.

HEADACHE AND FACIAL PAIN

Tension headaches, particularly in the region of the occiput and cervical spine, afflict many persons, but few seek assistance in the emergency ward; patients with *headaches caused by depression* often seek emergency care, however. A dull ache "all over the head" is a frequent symptom of this common psychiatric illness, and although some features, such as the report of a headache that never goes away completely for a few weeks or months, may suggest the cause, the specific features of a mood disorder should be sought and the patient should be directed to the care of an internist or psychiatrist.

Although there are no laboratory tests to separate *migraine headache* from other types of headache, the clinical syndrome is usually sufficiently distinctive to allow correct diagnosis. Visual scintillations often precede the headache, which is typically confined to one side, hence the alternate designation, hemicrania. It is frequently experienced as originating behind one eye. The patient has usually had previous attacks, and there is often a family history of the illness. In women, the condition may worsen at or before menses, although various endocrine patterns may occur, for example, headaches only during pregnancy, headaches during menses but not during pregnancy, or headaches beginning at menopause. Nausea and vomiting, photophobia, and intolerance to loud noises complete the clinical presentation. In the variant known as cluster headache, there may be tearing of the ipsilateral eye and ipsilateral nasal discharge. The headache may be so severe that it mimics subarachnoid hemorrhage, and it may be necessary to perform CT scanning and lumbar puncture to exclude the possibility of intracranial bleeding. Analgesics, including parenteral narcotics, may be necessary to control the acute attack. Ergot preparations may be of little value during the most severe phase. In women, it is reasonable to discontinue any pills containing estrogens or progesterones permanently if possible, because of the risk of stroke.

Headache occurring with subarachnoid hemorrhage may or may not be associated with stiff neck, and a traumatic lumbar puncture in a patient with a severe attack of migraine may result in days of uncertainty regarding diagnosis. It is reasonable, however, to perform CT scanning and lumbar puncture on a patient with sudden onset of severe headache who has no history of migraine. This is particularly true if the patient has a neurologic deficit such as hemiparesis, even though such a deficit may result from migraine.

Headache that is prominent in the early morning may indicate high blood pressure. Headache from systemic hypertension may cause the patient to see a physician, who can then easily make that important diagnosis. Headache is also usually prominent in hypertensive encephalopathy, in association with fluctuating neurologic signs, seizures, and retinal arteriolar spasm.

Headache with fever requires lumbar puncture to exclude the diagnosis of meningitis or encephalitis. Two other important entities accompanied by both headache and fever are temporal arteritis (giant cell arteritis) and paranasal sinusitis. The former disease occurs in persons more than 40 years old, and typically produces unilateral temporal headache that is often associated with a focally tender and thickened superficial temporal artery. The erythrocyte sedimentation rate is nearly always elevated, and this test should be performed in the emergency ward if temporal arteritis is considered. Sudden, permanent ipsilateral blindness may occur in patients with acute temporal arteritis, and it is advisable to start corticosteroid therapy immediately if the clinical findings are sufficiently indicative. Temporal artery biopsy is a relatively simple procedure that should be performed in patients in whom this disease is suspected.

Most patients who complain of sinus headaches actually have migraine or tension headaches. The location of the paranasal sinuses, however, particularly the sphenoid sinus underlying the sella turcica, makes it crucial to consider the diagnosis of paranasal sinusitis in patients with fever and anterior headache or sinus tenderness. Skull and sinus x-ray films should be studied for evidence of fluid level, mucosal thickening, or erosive bony changes.

Increased intracranial pressure may produce headache, and it may be the only presenting symptom in patients with *brain tumor*, including neoplasms and abscesses. A brain tumor in any location, including the pituitary fossa, can produce severe headache or may become enormous without any headache at all. When a brain tumor produces headache, papilledema may also be present. Headache wakens some patients with brain tumor in the early morning, and then subsides as the day progresses. Ipsilateral headache is commonly present in patients with chronic subdural hematoma. In all these conditions, lumbar puncture is usually contraindicated. Patients admitted to the hospital with headache, papilledema, and increased intracranial pressure should be given as little fluid as possible orally and particularly intravenously. If the patient is obtunded or if the neurologic status is measurably deteriorating, the intracranial pressure should be lowered. This is achieved most rapidly with intravenous mannitol (bladder catheterization is obligatory) or with oral or intravenous glycerol. Corticosteroids are useful, but may take from several hours to 1–2 days to be maximally effective.

The clinical findings of increased intracranial pressure, headache, and papilledema may also be associated with no tumor (pseudotumor cerebri), a condition that is most often idiopathic but that may occur as either a toxic reaction to tetracycline or high doses of vitamin A, in association with tapering of exogenous corticosteroids, or in conjunction with cerebral venous sinus thrombosis. Diffuse cerebral edema occurs that can be treated in the same way as the increased intracranial pressure of true brain tumors.

Commonly occurring and potentially dangerous head and facial pains include several entities discussed elsewhere in this text, such as earache with otitis media, eye pain with acute glaucoma, and toothache. *Facial neuralgia* (trigeminal neuralgia or tic douloureux) is a neurologic condition in which pain occurs in one or more of the three divisions of the trigeminal nerve, often with a "trigger zone" that is extremely sensitive to touch. Attacks may produce what patients attest is the worst pain human beings can suffer. A patient with a severe attack should be hospitalized and given sedatives and analgesics. Patients with severe attacks and those who have had many unpredictable and disabling attacks in the course of months or years should be evaluated for suicidal tendencies. Long-term medical therapy, particularly with carbamazepine (Tegretol), may provide dramatic, permanent relief, and patients who do not respond or who cannot tolerate carbamazepine may benefit from the newer neurosurgical procedures, such as stereotactic radiofrequency lesions. It is important to understand that most patients with facial neuralgia can now be cured or substantially helped. This disease is virtually always idiopathic, although some patients experience trigeminal neuralgia as a symptom of another illness, such as multiple sclerosis. Less commonly, the region of the glossopharyngeal nerve is the site of an equally disabling neuralgia, and the patient suffers unpredictable attacks of pain in the posterior pharyngeal wall on one side. The need for sedatives and analgesics for the acute attack and the usefulness of carbamazepine for long-term therapy is the same as for trigeminal neuralgia.

DEMENTIA

Dementia is a special syndrome that may qualify as the worst of all possible acquired human afflictions. Although it seldom develops suddenly, it is remarkable how often it is the previously undiagnosed primary illness of persons brought to the emergency ward. Virtually all patients with this type of illness suffer temporary worsening in the presence of poorly controlled medical illness, notably infection but also congestive heart failure, anemia, and many other conditions. These maladies, rather than the underlying dementia, often cause the patient to be seen in the hospital. Although patients with curable forms of dementia are fewer than those who cannot be treated specifically, the possibility of surgically treatable disease such as normal-pressure hydrocephalus, chronic subdural hematoma, or benign operable tumor (for example, subfrontal meningioma) requires at least one hospitalization with intensive diagnostic testing. Hospitalization should also include workup for medically treatable causes, such as hypothyroidism, vitamin B_{12} deficiency, hypercalcemia, hyponatremia, hypoglycemia, brominism, barbiturate toxicity, and digitalis toxicity.

ACUTE FOCAL CEREBRAL DISEASE

Stroke is by far the most common acute, focal, nontraumatic cerebral disease. The three most important mechanisms of stroke are atherosclerotic thrombosis, embolism, and hemorrhage; ideally a reliable history will reflect one of the three. Other less common stroke mechanisms include low cerebral perfusion and arterial spasm.

Atherosclerotic Thrombosis

Thrombotic strokes tend to occur slowly and stutteringly, often in the course of many hours or even several days. Symptoms may fluctuate greatly—worsening and improving—in the hours of stroke development. At times, the stuttering evolution is obscured by sleep so that the patient wakens with a completed stroke. Cerebral thrombosis may occur either in the large cerebral arteries such as the internal carotid artery or the basilar artery or in the small penetrating end-arteries such

as the arteries branching from the basilar artery to feed small regions of the brainstem (Fig. 15.3).

Large Cerebral Arteries

In the absence of adequate collateral flow, thrombosis in the internal carotid artery (ICA) causes ischemic symptoms in the territories of the ipsilateral middle cerebral artery (MCA) and the anterior cerebral artery (ACA). The dominant hemisphere is virtually always the left, even for left-handed persons. When this hemisphere is affected, right hemiplegia, right hemianesthesia, right homonymous hemianopsia, aphasia, apraxia, and ocular deviation to the left may develop. Any part of this total presentation may occur as a major stroke evolves or as it is completed if there is good collateral circulation to the hemisphere. If only the territory of the cortical branches of the MCA is involved, the leg tends to be spared, the hand being more severely affected than the foot. In the nondominant (right) hemisphere, total infarction of the ACA and MCA territories causes left hemiplegia, left hemianesthesia, left homonymous hemianopsia, anosognosia (denial of illness), neglect of the left side of space, inability to deal with spatial problems (such as construction of a triangle of three sticks or a square of four), dysarthria, and deviation of the eyes to the right. If the territories of the ACA and MCA of one side have become completely infarcted, the patient is often obtunded, and higher cortical function testing may not be possible.

What most concerns the emergency physician are the individual symptoms of the full syndrome, indicating either a small stroke or ongoing, possibly reversible progression to a major deficit. It is important to emphasize that, in the territory of the ICA, thrombotic disease most often occurs in the neck arteries—the common carotid or internal carotid arteries—where the condition is potentially operable, and only rarely in the MCA or ACA.

If thrombosis in the region of the basilar artery is massive, death occurs rapidly because of major brainstem infarction. Symptoms of the complete syndrome, such as quadriparesis, ocular palsies, dysarthria, numbness of the face, or dizziness, may herald a major stroke.

Small Penetrating End-arteries

Cerebral thrombosis in the small penetrating end-arteries occurs virtually only in the presence of hypertension (blood pressure higher than 140/90 mm Hg) and produces small deep infarcts, termed lacunes. When many lacunes are present,

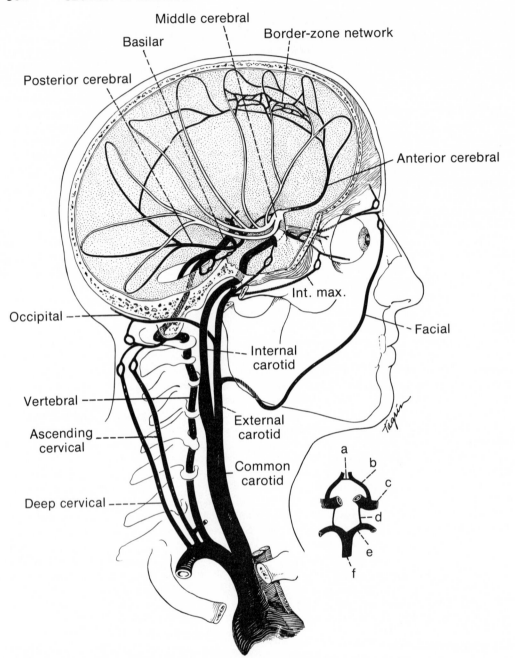

Figure 15.3. Arterial supply to the brain. Internal carotid artery gives rise to anterior cerebral and middle cerebral arteries, which supply most of the cerebral hemispheres. Internal carotid artery and all its branches are sometimes referred to as the "anterior circulation" of the brain. The "posterior circulation" consists of the intracranial branches of the two vertebral arteries, the midline basilar artery and its branches, and the posterior cerebral arteries arising from the "top" of the basilar. Anastomotic communications between major surface arterial territories occur via a "border-zone" network of vessels. In addition, the major cerebral arteries usually efficiently communicate, close to their origins, into a seven-sided polygon termed the circle of Willis (*inset: a* = anterior communicating artery; *b* = anterior cerebral artery; *c* = internal carotid artery; *d* = posterior communicating artery; *e* = posterior cerebral artery; *f* = basilar artery). (Courtesy of C. Miller Fisher, M.D.)

the neuropathologic terminology is lacunar state, and the clinical syndrome of dementia, shuffling spastic gait, dysphagia, dysarthria, and emotional lability known as pseudobulbar paralysis exists. The individual lacunes may be either symptomatic or asymptomatic. Certain stroke syndromes, such as pure hemiparesis without sensory loss or pure hemisensory loss without weakness, have been demonstrated to occur only as the result of such small deep lacunar infarcts. The EEG is normal, while strokes in regions of the MCA and ACA typically show focal slowing on the EEG. Long-term therapy for hypertension tends to prevent further lacunar strokes. *Acute* lowering of the blood pressure should not be attempted.

Transient Ischemic Attacks

Either type of thrombotic stroke, whether of a large artery or a small penetrating end-artery, may be heralded by a special neurologic event termed the transient ischemic attack (TIA). This is symptomatically a miniature stroke with neurologic findings lasting only up to 12 hours. The symptoms give a clue as to the territory of the artery involved; for example, numbness of the right hand and right side of the face lasting 1 hour suggests left ICA stenosis. If the patient arrives in the emergency ward earlier than 12 hours after the onset of symptoms, it may not be possible to decide if symptoms indicate a TIA or an evolving thrombotic stroke. TIAs are only rarely associated with major embolic or hemorrhagic strokes. Their mechanism is thought to be either intermittent local decrease of perfusion to a region of the brain ("hemodynamic crisis") or microembolization of platelet thrombi from the stenotic region of the artery. It is probable that both mechanisms are valid in different circumstances. The specific internal carotid territory syndrome of transient monocular blindess (amaurosis fugax) has been correlated, at times, with the ophthalmoscopic visualization of embolic material in the retinal arteries. The postulated mechanism of intermittent arterial spasm in TIAs is less likely to be proved valid.

Treatment

There are three options in the emergency ward for the management of a presumed thrombotic stroke or TIA. These are to watch (hospitalize and observe closely), to start heparin therapy, or to arrange for emergency angiographic examination with subsequent emergency endarterectomy in selected patients.

Basilar-Vertebral or Small Penetrating End-artery Disease. When symptoms indicate basilar-vertebral disease or disease in the territory of the small penetrating end-arteries, operation is not feasible. If symptoms fluctuate or progress, CT scanning or lumbar puncture should be carried out to exclude the possibility of hemorrhage or hemorrhagic infarction in the central nervous system, and heparin therapy should be started. If symptoms are stable, the decision to administer anticoagulants may be postponed, and if arteriographic examination is indicated, it may be performed electively, not as an emergency.

Carotid Artery Disease. The most controversial and challenging facet of emergency care for patients with cerebrovascular disease is that of carotid artery disease. The therapeutic plan for patients with carotid atherosclerosis depends on several premises. First, the ICA in the neck, where *endarterectomy* is feasible, is frequently the site of critical atherosclerosis (stenosis or ulcerated plaque) that threatens the cerebral territories of the MCA and ACA or the retina. Second, TIAs in this vascular territory can be identified clinically, and may herald the development of a major, permanently disabling stroke. Third, when patients have critical narrowing or ulcerated plaque of the ICA without having suffered a major stroke, endarterectomy is beneficial. Critical narrowing is defined as an internal diameter less than 2 mm on arteriographic examination.

At one end of the spectrum is the patient between 40 and 50 years old who has had several episodes within the previous 24 hours of tingling in the right hand, foot, and side of the face, associated with dysphasia and lasting 5 minutes. Neurologic examination is normal, but there is a bruit and decreased pulsation of the left carotid artery in the neck and decreased central retinal arterial pressure in the left eye. Emergency transfemoral arteriographic examination shows only a 1-mm lumen of the left ICA just above the bifurcation of the common carotid artery. There is adequate filling of the ipsilateral ACA and MCA branches but little evidence for good collateral circulation to these regions. The right ICA appears normal. In this case, emergency endarterectomy is recommended since it is reasonable to assume that there is an imminent risk of major infarction in the territory of the left ICA, should it become occluded. Even if total occlusion would not result in a stroke because of adequate collateral circulation, it is reasonable to attempt to open this major vessel to the brain since clot may form in the totally occluded ICA and embolize to vessels of the circle of Willis, producing fresh strokes. At the other end of the spectrum is the patient without neurologic complaints who has a bruit over one carotid artery and who may be seen to have, on arteriographic examination or at endarterectomy, a roughened wall resulting from atherosclerosis but neither significant narrowing nor an ulcerated plaque. Although complete statistics are not available for use in recommending whether one, both, or neither of these patients should be subjected to arteriographic examination followed by operation, recommendations must be made because all the presentations of ICA atherosclerosis are seen in the emergency ward.

The risk of arteriographic examination depends on many factors, but unquestionably the most important is patient selection. Arteriographic examination is usually transfemoral in patients with acute stroke. These patients tend to be elderly and hypertensive and to have extensive atherosclerosis. The procedure carries a risk of mortality or serious morbidity of approximately 2% even in the best of circumstances. This risk is scarcely less than that of endarterectomy itself. The decision to carry out emergency arteriographic examination in search of "surgical" carotid artery disease is one of the most difficult in emergency practice (Table 15.1).

There are many aspects to the *noninvasive examination* of cerebral hemodynamics, and it is necessary to establish what is implied by strong *vs.* weak noninvasive evidence. Unfortunately, no noninvasive technique or combination of techniques now available allows a high degree of certainty as to the status of the ICA, particularly

Table 15.1.
Indications for arteriography in carotid artery territory disease.

Emergency arteriography
  Transient ischemic attacks within preceding 48 hours
  Stuttering stroke in progress
  Small recent stroke with patient's condition stable or improving
Elective arteriography
  Transient ischemic attacks more than 48 hours previously
  Old stroke without new symptoms; strong noninvasive evidence
  Asymptomatic patient with strong noninvasive evidence
  Fresh massive stroke
Close follow-up study without arteriography
  Old stroke without strong noninvasive evidence
  Asymptomatic patient without strong noninvasive evidence

regarding the distinction between high-grade (pinpoint) stenosis and total occlusion. *Palpation* of the neck is the first diagnostic maneuver. In the presence of ICA stenosis, there is frequently a diminished pulse that can easily be felt. Failure to feel a decreased pulse, however, may reflect palpation of a patent external carotid artery or common carotid artery, even in the presence of a totally occluded ICA. Palpation of the ICA where there can be no confusion with other arteries is only possible in the tonsillar fossa, but reliable, accurate palpation in that location is not easily carried out, and lack of patient cooperation or tolerance may limit its usefulness. The palpable thrill or auscultated bruit indicates turbulent flow in the underlying vessel. Turbulent flow, however, does not necessarily correspond with hemodynamically significant stenosis, and a bruit is never heard if an artery is occluded or nearly occluded. The distinction between transmitted cardiac murmurs (especially in patients with aortic stenosis) and intrinsic carotid bruits is not always easily made, and of course, both may coexist. There are no branches of significant size from the ICA until it pierces the cavernous sinus; the ophthalmic artery is the first branch after this. The central retinal artery is a branch of the ophthalmic artery, and its pressure can be measured with an ophthalmodynamometer. *Measurement of central retinal pressures* can be mastered rapidly, but visualization of the fundus is necessary, and patients with cataract, nystagmus, or ocular deviation, as well as uncooperative patients, are poor candidates. Nevertheless, significant asymmetry of central retinal arterial pressures from both eyes is presumptive evidence that the pressure is low in the ICA on the side from which low ophthalmodynamometer readings have been obtained. Asymmetry of central retinal arterial pressures constitutes strong noninvasive evidence for ICA stenosis in a surgically accessible location, especially if the lower "diastolic" value is less than 30.

When the ICA is narrowed, the blood supply to the brain may pass via the branches of the external carotid artery through the orbit, reversing the normal direction of flow in the orbital vessels. It may be possible to determine the direction of flow with the use of a directional Doppler probe, and this, combined with other techniques such as thermographic examination of the face, provides further noninvasive data as to presumed surgical ICA disease. Techniques of noninvasive emergency study of the carotid system will evolve rapidly over the coming years, making easier the decision as to which patients to submit to arteriography.

If emergency arteriographic examination is not feasible, the rules for treatment of disease in the carotid territory are the same as those for treatment of basilar-vertebral or small penetrating end-artery disease, namely, if the symptoms are fluctuating or progressive, heparin therapy should be started if the CT scan or lumbar puncture reveals no blood in the CSF. Hypertension occurs more often in patients with stroke than in the general population, whatever the mechanism of the stroke. In the case of thrombotic disease, it is not recommended that blood pressure be lowered unless it is dangerously high. Usually, bed rest alone lowers blood pressure to a fairly safe level. Long-term therapy for stroke patients includes vigorous treatment of hypertension, but therapy should not be vigorous in the case of acute thrombotic disease of cerebral vessels.

Venous Thrombosis

Cerebral venous thrombosis may be encountered in many clinical settings. It may follow parturition, or it may be a sequel to infections of the middle ear or mastoids, especially in children. It may also accompany severe dehydration in infants or purulent meningitis at any age, and it tends to occur in the superior sagittal sinus or the large veins draining into it. The infarct is virtually always hemorrhagic, as opposed to the white infarct of arterial thrombosis, and it usually occurs on the cerebral cortical surface, producing a greatly epileptogenic region. Seizures are common in patients with cortical venous thrombosis, and uncommon in those with acute arterial thrombosis. Another syndrome that may be associated with cerebral venous thrombosis is pseudotumor cerebri, in which the patient has headache, generalized cerebral edema with increased intracranial pressure, and papilledema, but no evidence of a mass. Diagnosis of cerebral venous disease requires close attention to the venous phase of cerebral angiograms.

Embolism

Cerebral embolism is underdiagnosed. It occurs at least as frequently as cerebral thrombosis, and is the likely mechanism for the large number of strokes in which the onset is sudden and the deficit maximal from the start. Only rarely are there premonitory neurologic symptoms (TIAs). The origin of the embolic material may be the heart or a large vessel such as the aorta, innominate artery, or carotid artery, or it may be unknown.

Emboli of Cardiac Origin

Probably the first concern in the treatment of patients with acute embolic stroke is the possibility of acute myocardial infarction, which may cause emboli as a result of either endocardial damage or arrhythmias. This possibility must be considered in every patient with an embolic stroke, and serial electrocardiograms, serial serum enzyme determinations, and related studies must be obtained. The most common cardiac disease causing embolic stroke is atrial fibrillation, particularly when it is intermittent or associated with mitral valvular disease. Cardiac monitoring of patients with normal sinus rhythm and embolic stroke may reveal short episodes of atrial fibrillation or other arrhythmias; such monitoring should start in the emergency ward and continue for several days. Mitral valvular disease, particularly stenosis, also predisposes patients to embolic stroke. Much less common but potentially curable is left atrial myxoma, and it is reasonable to carry out additional noninvasive studies such as echocardiographic examination to look for this tumor in patients with embolic stroke of unknown source. Several types of endocarditis, including acute or subacute bacterial endocarditis, may produce cerebral emboli. Blood cultures and other tests for subacute bacterial endocarditis should be carried out in all patients. The CSF in patients with subacute bacterial endocarditis may contain small numbers of both red and white blood cells. Marantic endocarditis is a condition in which emboli are released from the heart in patients with carcinoma elsewhere; at times, stroke from this mechanism is the first indication of an occult malignant process. In all these situations, there may be concurrent embolization to other systemic arteries.

Emboli from Large Vessels

Emboli composed mainly of cholesterol may break free from atheromas in large vessels such as the aorta or common or internal carotid artery, causing symptoms in the brain or eye. Careful examination of the optic fundi may reveal these bright, shiny, sharp emboli. Platelets and fibrin from atheromatous ulcerated plaques may also embolize to the brain or eye. In this case, the optic fundi contain dull whitish or yellowish material. This type of embolus may originate in the common or internal carotid artery near its origin, and may constitute a stroke threat in a readily operable location without causing hemodynamically significant stenosis. In the case of an ulcerated plaque in the common or internal carotid artery in the neck without significant stenosis, results of the usual noninvasive tests such as palpation and measurement of central retinal arterial pressures are likely to be normal. It is mainly because of this type of remediable lesion that "small recent stroke with patient's condition stable or improving" is listed in Table 15.1, although a stroke of that description can, of course, also be thrombotic. A bruit may or may not be heard over such a lesion. Embolic strokes occur in the vertebrobasilar territory as well as in the carotid territory, and embolic material commonly passes through the vertebral and basilar arteries to enter one or both posterior cerebral arteries, causing varying degrees of unilateral or bilateral homonymous hemianopsia and memory loss.

Anticoagulation

As mentioned previously, arterial thrombosis produces nonhemorrhagic infarcts and venous thrombosis produces hemorrhagic infarcts. In embolic disease, the cerebral infarct may be of either type. Hemorrhagic infarction is always a possibility, and the lumbar puncture may not reveal red blood cells, especially in the case of a deep red infarct. It is, therefore, usually recommended that, when embolism rather than thrombosis is suspected, anticoagulation not be started on an emergency basis, but approximately 48 hours later. This is hazardous, especially since heparin may prevent a new embolus in the first 2 days after emergency treatment. Yet because of the risk of extending the zone of hemorrhage in a red infarct, emergency anticoagulation with heparin is not routinely recommended, although long-term anticoagulation is often indicated, for example, sodium warfarin in patients with cerebral embolization and atrial fibrillation.

Hemorrhage

Hypertensive intracerebral hemorrhage and primary subarachnoid hemorrhage from a ruptured saccular aneurysm (see pages 344–345) are the two most common types of nontraumatic intracranial hemorrhage. Only a small percentage of patients with intracranial hemorrhage survive without residual deficits.

The supratentorial region is the most common site for hypertensive intracerebral hemorrhage, particularly the region of the putamen and, less often, the thalamus. Patients with supratentorial cerebral hemorrhage usually experience slow onset of headache, which steadily increases over the next few hours or fractions of an hour with the evolution of neurologic signs depending on the location

of the hemorrhage. The presentation differs from that of cerebral embolism in that the neurologic deficit slowly worsens rather than being maximal at the start. It differs from cerebral thrombosis in that TIAs almost never occur, and the progression is that of smooth deterioration rather than the fluctuations characteristic of thrombosis. In the case of hemorrhage in the putamen, contralateral hemiplegia is common, and in thalamic hemorrhage there may also be downward deviation of the eyes with inability to elevate them above the horizontal plane. CT scanning reveals the hematoma and lumbar puncture virtually always reveals bloody CSF under elevated pressure. Medical therapy consists mainly of the emergency lowering of elevated blood pressure. Surgical approaches to emergency removal of intracerebral supratentorial hematoma must be considered, especially if a nondominant hemorrhage in the putamen bleeds forward, producing a large right frontal clot that by its size threatens to be lethal. Prognosis for patients with a large intracerebral hematoma is poor, however, with or without operation.

Approximately 20% of hypertensive intracerebral hemorrhages occur *below* the tentorium in the pons or cerebellum, and the disease profile in these cases is different from that of the supratentorial syndromes. *Acute pontine hemorrhage* most often produces coma very rapidly. The patient has bloody CSF, quadriparesis, small pupils that usually react to light, and evidence of destruction of the pathways for regulation of eye movement, such as paralysis of the conjugate lateral gaze to one or both sides or paralysis of abduction to one or both sides. There is no effective therapy.

In *acute cerebellar hemorrhage*, patients usually experience sudden devastating vertigo, often with ataxia so severe that the patient is unable to sit or stand from the onset of symptoms. The site of bleeding is usually deep within one cerebellar hemisphere, and the eyes may be deviated to the opposite side. Ipsilateral facial weakness, nystagmus, and dysarthria are common, and the CSF is almost always bloody. As the cerebellar hemisphere swells, the brainstem is in danger of compression, and the appearance of "long-tract signs"—hemiparesis, quadriparesis, or toes that turn up on plantar stimulation—indicates that death may be imminent even if the patient is fully conscious. Emergency radiographic confirmation of the cerebellar mass should be obtained. In patients with intracranial hemorrhage, particularly intracerebellar hemorrhage, CT scanning will quickly disclose the site of the hematoma. When long-tract signs develop or if the patient is breathing irregularly or is obtunded, the clinical features, along with the CT scan or presence of blood in the CSF, must suffice as the indication for emergency operation; removal of the hematoma from the cerebellum may be lifesaving. Once the decision to operate is made, some time may be gained by administering intravenous mannitol to lower the intracranial pressure rapidly.

Many bleeding disorders cause intracranial hemorrhage; the most common is iatrogenic and relates to the ingestion of sodium warfarin. Intracerebral hemorrhage resulting from sodium warfarin is often devastating, regardless of the site of hemorrhage. The importance of careful, frequent outpatient monitoring of persons receiving sodium warfarin cannot be stressed enough, nor is it possible to warn excessively against the use of this medication for any but the most rigid, clear-cut indications.

Hypertensive encephalopathy deserves attention since hemorrhages of various sizes may occur in the brain. This condition occurs in patients with longstanding, severe, untreated hypertension, and severe spasm of the retinal arterioles on examination of the optic fundi is a significant finding. Clinical features include headache, confusion, or obtundation associated with fluctuating major neurologic signs such as hemiparesis or aphasia, and seizures are often present as well. Blood pressure must be lowered quickly, and intravenous phenytoin should be administered.

Intracerebral hemorrhage in patients with normal blood pressure is usually due to arteriovenous malformation; such hemorrhage can occur with hypertension as well. These malformations may be of any size and in any location, and the symptoms may be trivial or catastrophic. In von Hippel-Lindau disease, retinal vascular malformations accompany those of the brain, which are usually in the posterior fossa, and examination of the optic fundi may be diagnostic.

Certain tumors metastatic to the brain, especially malignant melanoma, tend to bleed, and rarely, what appears to be primary intracranial hemorrhage is bleeding into a metastatic site.

Low Cerebral Perfusion

A special type of ischemic damage may occur during systemic hypotension. Sustained low blood pressure during massive blood loss, certain surgical procedures, or cardiovascular collapse and subsequent resuscitative efforts causes strokes limited to "watershed" or "border-zone" areas, by which is meant the most distal territories of the major arteries (Fig. 15.4). An agricultural irrigation system may be envisioned in which the water supply is deficient. Only fields close to the water source

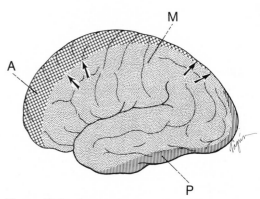

Figure 15.4. Lateral surface of left cerebral hemisphere showing arterial territories for anterior (*A*), middle (*M*), and posterior (*P*) cerebral arteries. In conditions of low blood flow, infarction occurs in the most distal fields of the territory of the middle cerebral artery (*arrows*). (Courtesy of C. Miller Fisher, M.D.)

receive sufficient fluid, and the distal fields suffer. The best-documented ischemic cerebral "distal field" is in the territory of the MCA; in patients with hypotensive stroke, nonhemorrhagic infarction is observed on the cerebral hemispheral convexities, mainly on the MCA side of the border zones between it and the ACA anteriorly and the posterior cerebral artery posteriorly. Because of the location of such an infarct on the surface of the brain, weakness of the upper extremities is the most common feature of anterior hemispheral border-zone infarcts. Ischemia is often bilateral, and when the posterior distal branches of the MCA are affected, aphasia and visual field cuts may also develop. This neurologic presentation may occur in the emergency ward in patients resuscitated from cardiac arrest. Prevention of further hypotension and administration of oxygen are the only therapies required, and in some cases, even patients with extremely severe clinical syndromes may eventually recover fully. There are other regions of the central nervous system both in the brain and in the spinal cord that are supplied by distal fields of feeding arteries, and a full description of all the permutations of low-flow syndromes is not yet available.

Arterial Spasm

The presumed mechanism for the neurologic deficits that accompany migraine is arterial spasm. It is not artificial to separate the two aspects of migraine—vasodilatory phenomena (see page 349) and ischemia—since not only may headache occur without any accompanying signs but also ischemic symptoms may occur without headache. Arterial spasm in patients with migraine may occur in any of the arteries serving the brain, and such spasm may even rarely be visualized in retinal arterioles during an attack. When both vasoconstrictive (ischemic) and vasodilatory (headache) symptoms occur in a single episode, the vasoconstrictive symptoms usually occur first. Although it is not entirely clear which arteries are responsible, it is evident that visual symptoms predominate over other types of ischemic symptoms in most cases. The flashing lights or zigzag lines of migrainous scintillations and the brightly lit shimmering polygonal figures (fortification spectra) are well known. Symptoms may be limited to one eye or to a homonymous half-field. Photophobia is often present as well. Rarely, a permanent visual deficit such as a homonymous quadrantic field cut may follow an attack. The vasospastic episodes may be in the territory of the MCA, with symptoms including hemiparesis, hemihypesthesia, or aphasia, or in the territory of the basilar artery, causing brainstem signs. Unusually persistent migrainous ischemic deficits should be managed like other cerebral thrombotic events, that is, with rapid heparin therapy after CT scanning or examination of the CSF for blood. Arteriographic examination is particularly hazardous in migrainous patients, especially during an attack. The likelihood of stroke with migraine is increased with administration of estrogens or progesterones, and such medication is contraindicated in women with a history of migraine.

Arterial spasm may also occur when irritative substances are present in the subarachnoid space, such as blood from subarachnoid hemorrhage or pus in patients with meningitis. Spasm of major arteries, such as the ICA as it enters the skull, may produce ischemia of large areas of the brain, giving rise to further neurologic deficits in patients with subarachnoid hemorrhage or meningitis. For these patients as well as for patients with vasospastic migraine, there is as yet no proved therapy for the spasm.

Nonvascular Conditions

Acute focal cerebral disease encompasses a few nonvascular conditions. Perhaps the most common is the acute attack of multiple sclerosis. A history of this illness is often obtained, simplifying the emergency diagnostic workup. Acute optic neuritis (loss of vision in one eye, often associated with some pain on eye movement, with or without erythema of the optic nerve head), sudden weakness of one limb, sudden diplopia, ataxia, and dizziness are among the neurologic presentations of this illness. Emergency therapy is not crucial.

Diagnostic studies may be required to exclude other conditions, for example, a myelogram to exclude a compressive spinal cord lesion in the patient with demyelinating myelitis. Exacerbations of multiple sclerosis may be precipitated by local or systemic infection. Urinary tract infection is particularly likely to occur in multiple sclerosis patients with myelopathy, and this possibility must be investigated scrupulously and vigorously treated. Elevation of body temperature worsens the neurologic state of most patients with multiple sclerosis, and hyperthermia of any cause should be treated with antipyretic agents.

Many metabolic abnormalities may cause asymmetric or focal cerebral symptoms; hypoglycemia and hyponatremia are often the etiologic agents. In patients with previous focal cerebral disease such as an old stroke with complete recovery, symptoms of the earlier focal cerebral lesion may reappear in the presence of a metabolic disorder such as uremia or hepatic failure.

NONACUTE PROGRESSIVE FOCAL CEREBRAL DISEASE

Intracranial *space-occupying lesions* cause most illnesses in this category. Excluded is the symptomatic acute hematoma (intracerebral hemorrhage, acute subdural hematoma, or acute epidural hematoma); included is the *chronic subdural hematoma*, as well as *cerebral abscess*. The most common lesion is *brain tumor* (neoplasm). Brain neoplasms and abscesses grow slowly, as do some chronic subdural hematomas. Regardless of cause, the syndrome that results is essentially the same: increased intracranial pressure from the mass produces headache that is often restricted to the same side as the mass; focal signs and symptoms relating to the location of the tumor develop; and finally, obtundation leading to coma ensues. If the mass is close to the cerebral cortex, focal or generalized seizures may occur. The patient may be seen in the emergency ward at any stage in the evolution of brain tumor. Some are seen with minor findings, and in these patients, results of a thorough workup may be negative, only to become positive at a later workup. Other patients arrive in the emergency ward with such extensive damage from increased intracranial pressure that the brain may be fatally injured. When the presentation is not that of headache alone or of seizures alone, the key to diagnosis is the slow progression of symptoms in the course of weeks or months—a pace never seen with cerebrovascular disease. Lumbar puncture should be avoided until other safer tests such as brain scanning can be carried out. Absence of retinal venous pulsations is a moderate contraindication and papilledema is a strong although not absolute contraindication to lumbar puncture. CT scanning, with and without contrast material, is the single best noninvasive test for diagnosis of brain tumor, although some conditions, such as chronic subdural hematoma and meningioma, are better diagnosed in some patients by radioisotope scanning than by CT scanning. Skull x-ray films may reveal demineralization of the dorsum sellae, which indicates chronically raised intracranial pressure. Exuberant growth of blood vessels to a meningioma may produce pronounced vascular grooves in the calvarium. Some brain tumors, such as oligodendroglioma and craniopharyngioma in children, are characteristically calcified, as may be the chronic subdural hematoma. Pituitary tumors may enlarge and distort the sella turcica. If the pineal gland is calcified, its position is a useful guide to whether midline cerebral structures are shifted. Echoencephalographic examination is a quick, safe, deceptively simple technique for assessment of cerebral midline shifts; it is reliable only when performed by experienced personnel.

Evidence for tumor elsewhere in the body must be sought, as well as evidence for pulmonary disease such as bronchiectasis, tuberculosis, or fungal disease, which may cause cerebral abscess. Brain abscess may also arise from infection of the middle ear, usually involving the temporal lobe, or from infection of the mastoids, usually involving the cerebellum.

When brain tumor is likely, it is reasonable to start anticonvulsant medication even in the absence of seizures, particularly if a supratentorial tumor is suspected; oral phenytoin is usually sufficient.

When a mass in the lateral hemisphere becomes sufficiently large, the danger of temporal lobe herniation develops. The medial edge of the temporal lobe squeezes into the tentorial notch, stretching the ipsilateral oculomotor nerve and producing ipsilateral pupillary dilatation; if herniation is severe, the mesencephalon will be damaged by compression, the posterior cerebral artery may be compressed (producing hemorrhagic occipital lobe infarction), secondary bleeding (Duret's hemorrhages) may occur in the brainstem, and the patient may become obtunded and die. This sequence can be hastened by lumbar puncture and can be slowed by therapy with agents such as intravenous mannitol that lower intracranial pressure.

The manifestations of several illnesses whose pattern is usually that of either acute attacks (for example, multiple sclerosis), rapid progression (for example, herpes encephalitis), or nonfocal cerebral disease (for example, subacute spongiform encephalopathy or Creutzfeldt-Jakob syndrome) may be subacute, progressive, and focal. Schilder's disease (encephalitis periaxialis diffusa), which is closely related to multiple sclerosis, typically produces a subacute progressive focal lesion in one cerebral hemisphere. This disease occurs in children, at times producing sufficient unilateral cerebral edema that it mimics brain tumor.

SYMMETRICAL WEAKNESS WITH OR WITHOUT SENSORY LOSS

In this category are many diverse illnesses. The correct diagnosis depends on knowing the anatomic distribution and time course of the illness, but that information is not always available.

Vascular Disease

In the field of vascular disease, only a few conditions are commonly seen with symmetrical findings. The junction of the anterior communicating and anterior cerebral arteries is one of the most common sites for intracranial aneurysm. Bleeding from an aneurysm in this location is frequently associated with spasm of both ACAs which lie close by. The result may be symmetrical leg weakness, since the area of the cerebral cortex controlling the leg lies in the territory of the ACA. If bleeding is substantial and cerebral edema develops, a bifrontal syndrome of ataxia, abulia (loss of spontaneous speech and action in the presence of full consciousness), and frontal reflexes (grasping, sucking, and the like) is also present. If bleeding is massive, the patient is comatose. However, weakness and hyperreflexia of the legs may be the only (or at least the earliest) features of aneurysmal hemorrhage of the anterior communicating artery, and a patient with bloody CSF and acute leg weakness should be treated as if he had an aneurysm in this location.

In the territory of the basilar artery, ischemia may produce either symmetrical or asymmetric symptoms. Hyperreflexic quadriparesis can occur alone at times, for example, in patients with ischemia of the ventral pons. Most brainstem strokes, however, are manifested by segmental features as well, such as ocular palsies and facial weakness, which indicate that the process is located in the brainstem. When spastic quadriplegia of a stuttering type occurs, especially with other brainstem signs such as paralysis of conjugate gaze and nystagmus, life-threatening ischemia of the brainstem may be present. CT scanning or lumbar puncture will quickly reveal the presence of certain hemorrhagic conditions of the posterior fossa, such as pontine hemorrhage or cerebellar hemorrhage, and if the CSF is not bloody, therapy with intravenous heparin may totally reverse the potentially fatal clinical state in a short time. Heparin therapy should be accompanied by placing the patient in a head-down position and by administering oxygen.

Rarely, the anterior spinal artery may be the site of thromboembolic disease. The ventral part of the spinal cord may become ischemic at any level, resulting in features of cord transection, such as spastic paralysis and sensory loss below the specific level, but with relative sparing of the sensory modalities of the dorsal part of the cord, such as sense of joint position and vibration. This is because the posterior part of the cord is nourished by the posterior spinal arteries. New techniques of transfemoral angiography are being perfected that allow visualization of the anterior spinal artery, but the diagnosis continues to be based on clinical findings. Anticoagulation with heparin is indicated.

Cord Transection

The spinal cord is long, soft, and narrow, and many disease processes, whether intrinsic to the spinal cord or pressing on the cord externally, may produce clinical indications of partial or complete cord transection. There are no reliable bedside rules to determine whether an acute or subacute segmental cord syndrome is due to a lesion that is intrinsic or extrinsic. Commonly, spastic or flaccid weakness and sensory diminution or loss are found below a particular dermatome level, and the distribution may be asymmetric. Physical examination should include percussion of each vertebral spinous process, since epidural abscess of the spinal cord at a particular level may be associated with vertebral osteomyelitis and tenderness at that level. Extramedullary compression may occur as a result of acute trauma with vertebral fracture, acute midline disc herniation, pus (especially when associated with vertebral osteomyelitis), and tumor (spread of metastatic tumor in the vertebrae, meningioma, or neurofibroma). In addition, compression of the spinal cord by hematoma may occur with a neck injury or as a complication of anticoagulation with heparin or sodium warfarin. The more acute the onset of the syndrome, the greater the urgency to carry out emergency myelographic examination and surgical decompression if compression of the spinal cord is revealed. Rarely, an intraspinal tumor such as glioma is manifested by sudden neurologic deterioration, perhaps because of bleeding into the tumor.

Many illnesses have the presentation of transverse myelopathy, multiple sclerosis and postinfectious myelitis being the most common. Some lymphocytes are usually observed in the CSF, and the protein level may be elevated. Seldom can the diagnosis of extrinsic spinal cord compression be excluded with such confidence in the emergency ward that myelographic examination is obviated. Acute, severe, necrotizing myelopathy may occur in heroin addicts, particularly if a single dose of heroin follows a period of abstinence. Although there is no specific therapy, myelographic examination should be performed, especially since addicts have a greater risk of infection than the general population and the diagnosis of vertebral osteomyelitis with epidural abscess must be excluded. More troublesome is the question of emergency myelographic examination in a patient with known multiple sclerosis who has an acute attack of transverse myelitis. Even in this setting, myelographic examination must be performed. The efficacy of corticosteroids or adrenocorticotropic hormone in the therapy of myelitis due to multiple sclerosis or occurring after infection is debatable, but this type of medication should probably be administered if myelographic examination demonstrates swelling of the spinal cord or if the syndrome worsens as the patient is followed. Catheterization of the bladder must be considered, since all acute spinal cord syndromes carry the risk of urinary retention, and in the presence of sensory impairment, the symptoms of bladder distention may not be obvious.

Paralytic Infectious Diseases

In this category are illnesses due to either bacterial toxins or invasion of the central nervous system by neurotropic viruses. In the diseases caused by toxins (tetanus, botulism, and diphtheria), full neurologic recovery is the rule if the patient can safely be brought through the acute phase of the illness. The CSF is normal in all three conditions. However, in the diseases caused by viral invasion of the central nervous system (rabies and poliomyelitis), the CSF contains cells and often raised protein levels, and when the acute illness is past, permanent neurologic deficits are likely because of the death of neurons.

Tetanus

Although tetanus is not strictly a "paralytic" disease, the patient with clinical manifestations of this illness may suffer such spasms of somatic musculature as to preclude normal muscular function. Death from respiratory failure may result, and over half of the more than 100 patients reported in the United States each year die of the illness. Since the portal of entry—the wound—may be inapparent and since only about one-third of patients with tetanus have cultures positive for *Clostridium tetani*, the diagnosis is made primarily on the basis of the clinical presentation. After an incubation period of from a few days to more than 2 weeks, neurologic signs and symptoms develop. Most often, spasms of cranial and cervical muscles are prominent early, with clenching of teeth (trismus, lockjaw) a characteristic feature. Painful spasms of limbs and trunk may be initiated by afferent stimuli such as touch, bright light, and noise, and respiration and swallowing may thereby be compromised. Involvement of the autonomic nervous system produces profuse sweating and potentially dangerous swings in blood pressure. Rarely, local muscle spasms occur only in the region of the portal of entry; much more commonly the disease is generalized. In the United States, noteworthy portals of entry for the bacteria are the venous puncture sites of drug addicts, the pelvis in the case of septic abortion, and wounds inflicted by lawnmowers.

Human tetanus immune globulin is the recommended therapy (see Chapter 11, page 242), although it does not counteract toxin already bound to nervous tissue. The painful spasms are best treated with small increments of intravenous diazepam, 2–5 mg, and it is important to minimize afferent stimuli to the patient. If complications such as secondary infection and hypoxia can be avoided, total recovery is the rule.

A syndrome of generalized muscular rigidity with severe trismus and sweating may occur as an idiosyncratic reaction to phenothiazine medications, and a history of the use of this class of drug should be sought. Parenteral administration of diphenhydramine hydrochloride, 25–50 mg, may quickly reverse this drug reaction, which in several ways can mimic tetanus.

Botulism

The extremely potent neurotoxin produced by *C. botulinum* causes botulism in about 25 persons a year in the United States, and approximately 6 persons die as a result. Home-canned food, especially vegetables canned at an alkaline pH, is often responsible, but in many cases the ingested food is never identified. Some cases of botulism in newborns have been traced to ingestion of honey. Rarely, botulism can follow introduction of the bacteria into a deep wound, where relatively anaerobic conditions essential to this organism's growth are met. Clinical symptoms usually begin within 24 hours of ingestion, and blurred vision, diplopia, dysphagia, and dysphonia are prominent. Generalized weakness is also often present, along with nausea, vomiting, and abdominal cramps. The pupils may be fixed and dilated, the sensorium is clear, and orthostatic hypotension may be prominent. Deep tendon reflexes are preserved in the presence of weakness, whereas in the Guillain-Barré syndrome they are most often depressed or lost.

Some of the patient's serum should be set aside for testing in animals for the presence of botulinus toxin, and in patients in whom a reasonably certain clinical diagnosis can be made, trivalent (ABE) antitoxin should quickly be administered. This can be obtained most rapidly by telephoning the Center for Disease Control in Atlanta, Georgia (404) 329–3311 during the day, or (404) 329–3644 at night and on weekends.

Diphtheria

Because of decreasing levels of immunity in the United States, especially among adults, almost 250 new cases of diphtheria occur each year, with approximately 10 deaths. Membranous pharyngitis or laryngitis is the key to diagnosis, but several types of neurologic involvement result from the toxin produced by *Corynebacterium diphtheriae*. In the first days of illness, the muscles of the pharynx underlying the membrane may become weak. Cranial motor polyneuropathy may develop in the next few weeks, and a peripheral neuritis virtually identical with Guillain-Barré syndrome may appear up to 3 months after the acute pharyngitis. Because of the specific effect of the toxin on myelin sheaths, nerve conduction velocities are greatly slowed, a characteristic shared with the Guillain-Barré syndrome. The neuropathic consequences of diphtheria are all totally reversible, although recovery may be slow.

Rabies

Rabies is a viral encephalitis that appears months after the virus enters the body at the site of the bite of a rabid animal. (Antirabies prophylaxis at the time of the bite is discussed in Chapter 11, pages 242–243 and Chapter 10, Table 10.21). Most domestic dogs in this country are immunized against rabies, and in recent years a greater threat to human beings has been posed by wild bats and skunks. Up to 1 year (usually 1–2 months) after the animal bite, the patient experiences paresthesias and pain at the site of the bite and exhibits a prodromal syndrome of fever and malaise. Within a few days of the premonitory symptoms, the encephalitic syndrome ensues, consisting of alternating agitation and depression and severe muscle spasms, especially reflex spasms of the larynx that make drinking impossible and extremely painful to attempt (hydrophobia). Other cranial nerves are affected in the brainstem, resulting in disorders of ocular and facial movement. The CSF usually contains lymphocytes and has an elevated protein content.

In recent years, it has become evident that some persons may recover if respiratory assistance, sedation, and treatment of other complications are vigorously carried out.

Poliomyelitis

Approximately 15 cases of this once epidemic disease now occur annually in the United States. Half or more develop as a complication of the ingestion of oral poliovirus vaccine (OPV), and a few instances of disease have occurred in persons in close contact with recent recipients of OPV. A minor upper respiratory tract illness or gastrointestinal upset with fever may precede the neurologic illness. In most patients with central nervous system involvement, the clinical presentation is simply one of aseptic meningitis, with stiff neck, fever, and inflammatory cells in the CSF; there is no feature of this type of poliomyelitis that allows it to be distinguished from any other viral meningitis. In a smaller number of patients, the central nervous system involvement takes the form of encephalomyelitis, resulting in rapid progression of paresis or paralysis of bulbar and limb musculature that is usually asymmetric. Before they are destroyed by the virus, motor neurons are first irritated, so in the earliest stages, coarse twitches and fasciculations appear, only to be superseded shortly thereafter by paralysis. Spasticity and a positive Babinski sign do not occur, and although paresthesias are common, no sensory loss can be documented. In the early stage of weakness, it is important to exercise the patient's muscles as little as possible—extensive, vigorous muscle testing should not be carried out if poliomyelitis is suspected. Serum should be set aside and pharyngeal washings and stool specimens should be cultured as soon as possible in an attempt to isolate the virus.

Diseases of the Peripheral Neuromuscular System

Rapid symmetrical paralysis may occur for many reasons, but the common element in therapy is respiratory maintenance. In emergency care, adequate respiratory support, often with endotracheal intubation, has priority over measures dealing with the specific disease. Those illnesses that cause rapid, profound weakness as part of a major systemic catastrophe, such as shock after massive blood loss, will not be considered here; what will be considered are the neurologic diseases mainly of the peripheral neuromuscular system. In this category, the two most common conditions are acute idiopathic polyneuritis and myasthenia gravis.

Acute Idiopathic Polyneuritis

Paralysis from acute idiopathic polyneuritis (Guillain-Barré syndrome) occurs frequently in all seasons and at all ages. Illness may be so severe that all somatic muscle is paralyzed for months, or it may be so mild that it is asymptomatic. Approximately half of the patients have had a recent viral illness. Association with infectious mononucleosis and infectious hepatitis occurs often enough that screening tests for these illnesses should be performed in all patients with the syndrome. Weakness and paresthesias usually begin distally in the lower extremities, and ascend in the course of days; paralysis may eventually be total. Muscles innervated by cranial nerves may be involved, with bifacial paralysis, extraocular muscle palsies, and weakness of phonation, chewing, swallowing, and breathing. On examination, the motor findings are always more prominent than the sensory findings; it is unusual to be able to map a hypesthetic zone in the feet, even in the presence of pedal paresthesia. An important diagnostic finding is depression or, more often, absence of all deep tendon reflexes, even in limbs with no other clinical signs. Although emergency studies of nerve conduction are usually unnecessary, the slowing of motor nerve conduction velocities in patients with acute idiopathic polyneuritis is usually profound, and may rapidly provide diagnostic evidence since few other illnesses and no other common illness produces such extreme slowing. The CSF contains high amounts of protein without cells ("albuminocytologic dissociation"), but early in the course of illness, the CSF protein level may be normal. Large alterations in blood pressure may occur spontaneously in severe or moderately severe cases. Progress of the disease may be unpredictable; for example, in patients with slight weakness of the ankles, the disease may quickly progress to respiratory embarrassment without the steady ascending pattern most patients demonstrate. It is necessary, therefore, to be wary whenever progression occurs, even if symptoms and signs appear trivial, such as weak toes with generalized hyporeflexia. All patients should be hospitalized until the symptoms of this monophasic illness begin to recede. Occasionally, attacks affect the respiratory and bulbar musculature almost exclusively, requiring rapid, effective respiratory support. In the absence of complications such as infection and pulmonary embolism, patients recover fully or almost fully. Second attacks are uncommon.

Corticosteroids are often administered, but there are no compelling data supporting such a practice. Indeed, in a paralyzed patient receiving corticosteroids, problems concerning osteoporosis, infection, and mental state are more difficult to manage, and routine use of these drugs is not recommended. Recent evidence indicates the benefit of prompt plasmapheresis in this disease.

Myasthenia Gravis

A chronic, recurrent disease, myasthenia gravis is characterized by attacks of gradual paralysis of somatic musculature, especially with exercise. Some degree of asymmetry may occur, especially in the eyelids, and the bulbar musculature, including extraocular muscles, may be severely involved. In this illness, an insufficient amount of acetylcholine is released by motor nerve endings; conventional therapy with neostigmine or pyridostigmine bromide inhibits cholinesterases that cleave acetylcholine, thereby allowing whatever is released to act longer. Either exacerbation of the disease (myasthenic crisis) or overdose of anticholinesterase medication (cholinergic crisis) may result in paralysis, and although some signs may indicate the cause (for example, fasciculations due to anticholinesterases), the distinction in practice may be difficult. A test injection of intravenous edrophonium chloride (Tensilon) has been recommended in dealing with this emergency dilemma: if the patient's condition improves, the crisis is myasthenic, and if it worsens, it is cholinergic. This diagnostic test is not always easy to interpret, however, and some patients with cholinergic crisis will not tolerate any worsening. In a severely weak myasthenic patient, it is better to stop all medications and to wait—intubating if necessary for respiratory embarrassment. The nasotracheal tube can be left in place for several days, during which time it will become clear which of the two crises was present.

The most common precipitant of decompensation in a myasthenic patient is respiratory tract infection. These patients may be extremely sensitive to the earliest features of a viral respiratory tract infection, and may appear in the emergency ward claiming that they feel as if they are getting weaker before pulmonary infection becomes evident on physical or radiographic examination. Generally, if a myasthenic patient claims he is rapidly getting weaker, *he should be hospitalized* and infection (particularly respiratory) should be suspected, even if weakness or evidence of infection cannot readily be confirmed by the physician. Several types of antibiotic may produce neuromuscular blockade similar to that of myasthenia gravis and should be avoided in myasthenic patients for fear of worsening the weakness. These include aminoglycosides such as kanamycin and neomycin, polypeptides such as colistin, and tetracyclines. Anesthetic agents in myasthenic patients must be chosen carefully. Recently, the efficacy of high doses of corticosteroids or adrenocorticotropic hormone has been demonstrated in therapy for myasthenia gravis. Although many patients improve with such treatment, myasthenic weakness characteristically worsens before improving when administration of these agents is begun, so hospitalization is mandatory for this mode of therapy. Plasmapheresis is often effective in short-term minimization of the severity of myasthenic weakness.

Myasthenic Syndrome (Eaton-Lambert Syndrome)

In myasthenia gravis, the patient is weak, and typically, exercise of an affected muscle quickly leads to diminished output (neuromuscular fatigue). Less commonly, muscular output increases with repetitive contractions of a tested muscle. This condition ("inverse myasthenia," "myasthenic syndrome," or Eaton-Lambert syndrome), which is much less common than myasthenia gravis, is associated with occult carcinoma, notably oat cell carcinoma of the lung. Therapy consists of administration of guanidine hydrochloride, not anticholinesterases. Distinction between myasthenia gravis and inverse myasthenia may be provided by electromyographic examination, since characteristic decrement of motor unit action potential occurs on repetitive stimulation of a motor nerve in patients with myasthenia gravis, and increment occurs in patients with inverse myasthenia. Further, the deep tendon reflexes are preserved and do not become fatigued in myasthenia gravis, while they are absent in myasthenic syndrome.

Periodic Paralysis

Patients with periodic paralysis have recurrent attacks of weakness of the four limbs, often sparing the musculature innervated by the cranial nerves. In some patients, the serum potassium level increases or decreases during an attack, and attacks may be precipitated in susceptible persons by pharmacologically increasing or lowering the serum potassium concentration. A family history of the disease is often obtained. Respiratory support, drawing of blood for appropriate electrolyte determinations, and hospitalization are all that is necessary in the emergency setting. If hypokalemia is present, potassium should be replaced slowly; it should not be infused quickly in the emergency ward. Relevant in the discussion of familial periodic paralysis is the fact that hypokalemia of any cause may produce profound weakness, and serum potassium determinations are required in all patients with generalized weakness of uncertain cause. Attacks of periodic paralysis in patients with a low serum potassium level tend to last longer (many hours) than those in hyperkalemic patients. Some patients with hypokalemia have coexisting and perhaps causative hyperthyroidism, and appropriate tests should be carried out to document thyroid function. Hyperkalemic periodic paralysis is often associated with clinical evidence of myotonia: sharp percussion of an affected muscle produces a slight depression that lasts for many seconds. Also, relaxation after an intense muscular effort, such as a strong grip, is extremely slow.

Acute Intermittent Porphyria

The only common type of porphyria that affects the nervous system is acute intermittent porphyria. Total paralysis may follow a severe attack. Many substances can precipitate an attack, the most common being barbiturates; these may inadvertently be administered during an attack of severe abdominal pain, which is typical of the illness. Diagnosis can rapidly be made by testing for porphobilinogen in the urine (Watson-Schwartz test), and this ought to be carried out in all patients with sudden unexplained paralysis. Respiratory support must be given, and barbiturates, sulfonamide derivatives, griseofulvin, and estrogens must be avoided.

Primary Disease of Muscle

Many types of inflammatory disease (polymyositis) and degenerative disease (muscular dystrophy) exist. Most are chronically or subacutely progressive, and are characterized by proximal symmetrical weakness. As with other slowly progressive neurologic illnesses, intercurrent infections, particularly of the urinary or respiratory tract, may cause deterioration of neurologic function. Infection must therefore be the first consideration in a patient with known dystrophy who becomes noticeably weaker within a short period. Despite the presence of inflammatory lesions in polymyositis, only a small number of patients have tender muscles. One exception is the patient with acute trichinosis, who may have extremely tender and weak muscles, fever, periorbital edema, and considerable peripheral eosinophilia. Therapy requires corticosteroids.

Paralytic Toxic Disease

Aside from the paralysis caused by bacterial toxins, as in patients with botulism or diphtheria, there are many other paralytic toxins, either occurring naturally or related to industrial technology. The bite of certain ticks may produce an ascending paralysis that closely resembles acute idiopathic polyneuritis in its temporal course and symptoms. The illness is abruptly terminated by removal of the tick. Antisera are available to treat the bites inflicted by some poisonous reptiles and insects. In certain industries, special toxicologic problems occur, such as chronic and acute cholinesterase inhibition in persons who work with organic insecticides. Accidental ingestion of tri-or-tho-cresyl phosphate has caused small but disastrous epidemics of irreversible paralysis in several settings around the world in the past century. Respiratory support and bladder catheterization if necessary are the emergency measures common to these types of paralysis.

Motor Neuron Disease

A common neurologic condition, motor neuron disease frequently results in death within 1–2 years of the onset of symptoms. When the upper motor neuron (corticobulbar and corticospinal tracts) is involved, spastic weakness and hyperreflexia with reflex dorsiflexion of the great toe (Babinski's reflex) are noted, but there is little muscle wasting. When the lower motor neuron is affected, atrophic weakness with visible fasciculations develops. Most often, the patient has both types of symptom. There are three major forms of motor neuron disease in adults. (Similar illnesses, such as Werdnig-Hoffmann paralysis, occur in children.) In *progressive bulbar palsy*, upper and lower motor neuron disease affects mainly the muscles innervated by cranial nerves, and life expectancy is the shortest of the three patterns because of respiratory failure compounded by aspiration and malnutrition. The most common form is *amyotrophic lateral sclerosis* (ALS), in which upper motor neuron symptoms predominate over lower motor neuron symptoms and the distribution is largely spinal, resulting in possibly severe involvement of the limbs. The least common form is *progressive muscular atrophy*, in which there is mainly lower motor neuron weakness that causes atrophy and fasciculations of four limbs with little spasticity. The final stages of all types of motor neuron disease may result in the patient's being seen in the emergency ward with acute respiratory failure. The history, the severe generalized wasting with fasciculations, and spasticity with hyperreflexia cannot be confused with other illnesses. In such patients, intubation followed by long-term respiratory life-support requires compassionate—and difficult—decision-making.

Weakness Associated with Psychiatric Syndromes

Although the term neurasthenia has lost some popularity, there is clearly a group of patients, most of whom are depressed, who complain of overwhelming weakness and easy fatigability. Testing of strength frequently shows what appears to be much more power than the symptoms suggest. Results of reflex testing and the remainder of the neurologic examination are normal. Recognition of the mood disorder is the key to diagnosis.

Many patterns of weakness and sensory loss may appear in the conversion symptoms of patients with hysterical neuroses and in the symptoms of malingerers. Paresthesia and weakness in the feet are common early indications of demyelinating myelopathy and of acute idiopathic polyneuropathy. When these signs occur in young women, the correct diagnosis is often delayed because of the tendency to consider the patient as hysterical. Differential diagnosis can be difficult, and the major caution in such a situation is to pay strict attention to the detailed neurologic examination.

DIZZINESS AND ATAXIA

Both the causes of an illness producing dizziness or ataxia and the anatomic site of the pathologic process (for example, cerebral hemispheres, brainstem, cerebellum, spinal cord, eighth nerve, labyrinth, or peripheral nerves) too often remain undetermined despite intensive investigation after hospitalization; the problems involved with diagnosis and decision-making in the emergency ward are still more difficult. In patients with light-headedness or an unsteady gait, nonembolic cardiac disease should first be considered, that is, low cardiac output with hypotension or low perfusion

resulting from congestive heart failure, myocardial infarction, or cardiac arrhythmia. Orthostatic hypotension should be sought specifically, since this is a common side effect of many medications, as well as a symptom of several diseases ranging from anemia to neuropathy, the most common being diabetes mellitus. Pulmonary and hematologic diseases such as anemia may result in hypoxemia, and may produce cerebral symptoms such as those of the cardiac disorders.

Dizziness is rarely a complaint in supratentorial structural cerebral disease, but may occur in certain patients with temporal lobe epilepsy. Therefore, when dizziness is associated with an altered psychic state (for example, dreaminess or fear), EEG examination and other appropriate diagnostic procedures for epilepsy should be performed. Patients with bilateral frontal lobe illness such as tumor or hydrocephalus walk badly, as if they had forgotten how. This has been called "gait apraxia," and its anatomic source is confirmed by observation of other evidence of bifrontal disease, such as grasping, snout and sucking reflexes, hypertonia of the legs, and abulia.

Regional blood flow to the brainstem may be compromised in patients with acute dizziness, and local hemodynamic events such as embolization, thrombosis, and steal need to be considered. Dizziness and ataxia occur in cerebrovascular disease, but almost always in the presence of other signs and symptoms. In addition to dizziness, thrombotic and embolic strokes involving the territory of the basilar artery or one of its penetrating paramedian or circumferential branches may be expected to produce one or more symptoms of dysarthria, numbness of the face or limbs, weakness or sensory loss in one or both sides of the body, hyperreflexia that includes jaw jerk, unilateral or bilateral facial paresis, ocular skew deviation, conjugate or nonconjugate gaze paresis, dysphagia, Horner's syndrome, and hiccups. When acute dizziness is accompanied by any of these features, brainstem localization is likely, and in the presence of a suggestive time course, stroke must be considered.

Certain mechanical maneuvers may precipitate transient brainstem ischemia, and relevant information should be sought in the history and physical examination. For example, some patients with narrowing of the vertebral artery, especially if it is associated with cervical spondylosis, may cause brainstem ischemia by turning the head strongly to one side, as in driving an automobile in reverse. In other patients, a combination of stenoses in thoracic, cervical, and cerebral vessels may lead to symptoms of brainstem ischemia after exercise involving one arm: blood that would usually flow to the brain may flow to the exercised arm (subclavian steal).

Ischemia or infarction involving the cerebellum alone is more difficult to differentiate from disease of the cochlea, but cerebellar-type ataxia of a limb or of the trunk may help reveal the process as intracerebral. Emboli that travel up the basilar artery may cause ataxia and dizziness, and may then move to the posterior cerebral arteries, causing ischemic symptoms such as homonymous visual field cuts and memory loss in those territories.

Vomiting and nystagmus, which often results in a complaint of blurred vision, may indicate lesions either in the brain or in the eighth nerve or inner ear. Episodes of dizziness along with tinnitus and hearing loss characterize Ménière's disease, and several other vertiginous diseases also have a labyrinthine origin. Diphenhydramine hydrochloride, 25–50 mg intramuscularly, may be useful for relief of symptoms. The only central nervous system illness with sudden catastrophic dizziness is acute intracerebellar hemorrhage, which is readily distinguished by hypertension, bloody CSF, and other neurologic findings.

Rarely, a cerebellar tumor may cause ataxia in the form of pure anteropulsion or retropulsion in the absence of other signs of cerebellar disease. The anatomic location is usually the vermis cerebelli, and since some potentially curable tumors such as hemangioblastoma occur in this location, vermian tumor must be suspected in the patient who consistently falls forward or backward. Anteropulsion or retropulsion in the absence of other physical findings may suggest the hysterical gait ataxia termed astasia-abasia, but in that condition, other indications of a hysterical neurosis are present and the patient tends to fall specifically in the direction of anyone nearby, rather than consistently forward or backward. A peculiar cerebellar ataxia that is often limited to the trunk and legs is seen in patients with chronic alcoholism, and is associated with degeneration of a characteristic region of the anterior part of the cerebellum; this condition is known as alcoholic cerebellar degeneration. In all patients with ataxia, blood and urine should be tested for toxins.

Detailed sensory testing in the limbs is essential to differentiate the cause of ataxia. Limb and trunk ataxia may be produced by many types of polyneuropathy. Reduction of joint position sense occurs in the ataxic neuropathies, and the Romberg test is positive. The most common types of ataxia-producing neuropathy are diabetic, nutritional (particularly alcoholic), carcinomatous, and uremic. Ataxia is also a feature of subacute combined degeneration with vitamin B$_{12}$ deficiency, in which the dorsal columns of the spinal cord are involved as well as the peripheral nervous system.

NERVE AND ROOT DISEASE

Types of acute and chronic nerve, root, and plexus disease occur often in medical practice, and patients with these syndromes commonly are seen in the emergency ward.

Cranial Nerves

Sudden cessation of function of the *oculomotor nerve* (III) with or without pain occurs often enough to deserve special mention. The total syndrome consists of severe ptosis of one eye, with the globe in a position of depression and abduction and the pupil large and fixed to light. In roughly one-third of patients, the cause is diabetes mellitus, and interruption of oculomotor nerve function is one of the most common types of diabetic mononeuropathy multiplex. There is a tendency for the pupil to appear normal when the cause is diabetes, but this is not reliably the case. Saccular aneurysm of the circle of Willis with or without rupture, particularly at the junction of the ICA and the posterior communicating artery, is the cause of sudden oculomotor nerve palsy in another third of patients. Many conditions affect the last third of patients with this syndrome, including migraine, periarteritis nodosa, and tumor deposit on the nerve. The patient should be treated as if he had an aneurysm, with hospitalization and sedation if necessary. Lumbar puncture may reveal blood in the case of aneurysmal rupture. A bruit may be heard over the eye in some patients with an aneurysm or arteriovenous malformation. Sudden loss of function of the *abducens nerve* (VI) resulting in failure of abduction of one eye, or of the *trochlear nerve* (IV), resulting in weakness of "down gaze" of the eye when it is adducted, is less common than sudden oculomotor nerve palsy, but diabetes mellitus and aneurysm remain likely possibilities in the differential diagnosis.

Rapidly progressing bilateral weakness of ocular abduction may be seen as one of the false localizing signs of increased intracranial pressure of any cause, while bilateral abducens nerve palsy in the setting of meningitis raises the possibility of tuberculosis as the etiologic factor. Virtually any combination of extraocular muscle palsy may occur in patients with myasthenia gravis, a disease that can be restricted entirely to the ocular muscles but that always spares the pupils.

Paralysis of extraocular muscles of one eye alone may be seen with sensory loss in the ophthalmic and maxillary divisions of the *trigeminal nerve* (V) (upper and middle portions of the face on one side) in patients with cavernous sinus disease, particularly thrombosis, a dreaded complication of paranasal sinusitis. Diagnosis is essential, since antibiotic therapy can be lifesaving. One totally paralyzed eye in a patient with diabetes mellitus or other debilitating disease such as uremia may be due to orbital phycomycosis (mucormycosis): crusted fungal lesions are virtually always visible in the nasopharynx, and prompt therapy with amphotericin B may result in total cure.

Sudden paralysis of the *facial nerve* (VII) is one of the most common human nervous disorders. It is first necessary to differentiate Bell's palsy from stroke; in fact, the patient is often convinced he has had a stroke. Although a small stroke in the pons might produce a syndrome indistinguishable from Bell's palsy, it is likely that a brainstem lesion would be associated with other symptoms, such as diminished sensation on the opposite half of the body, ataxia, and diminished extraocular movements. When facial weakness results from lesions rostral to the nucleus of the facial nerve in the pons ("supranuclear"), there is a tendency for the forehead muscles to be uninvolved, whereas lesions of the facial nerve itself, such as Bell's palsy, tend to affect both the upper and lower halves of the face equally. Further evidence that the facial weakness originates from the nerve rather than from the brain is loss of taste on the anterior two-thirds of the ipsilateral half of the tongue and hyperacusis (increased sensitivity to loud noises resulting from paralysis of the stapedius muscle) in the ipsilateral ear. The pinna or external ear canal may have a small region of decreased sense of pain and touch, and there is often an aching pain behind the ipsilateral ear. There is much controversy as to the optimal therapy for Bell's palsy, but the one undisputed therapeutic necessity is protection of the cornea. If the orbicular muscle of the eye is at all weak, a sterile dressing should be placed over the eye and the eye should be taped shut each night. The eye should the taped shut during waking hours as well if blinking on the affected side is faulty. A short course of oral corticosteroids has been recommended. Hospitalization is not normally necessary. Most cases of sudden unilateral facial palsy are idiopathic, and most patients recover completely. A small percentage of patients are seen with Bell's palsy due to involvement of the geniculate ganglion with herpes zoster. In these instances, characteristic vesicles may be seen on the tympanic membrane or in the external ear canal (Ramsay Hunt's syndrome).

Bilateral facial palsy of rapid onset should raise the possibility of widespread acute polyneuropathy (Guillain-Barré syndrome) or an infiltrating meningeal process such as sarcoidosis of the central nervous system.

Nerves and Roots of Limbs and Trunk

Many of the roots and nerves of the brachial plexus on one side can be involved in an acute, presumably inflammatory process whose suddenness of onset and frequently excruciating pain may mimic acute myocardial infarction. Most cases of *brachial plexus neuritis* are idiopathic, but some follow injection of a foreign substance, which is usually proteinaceous, such as a vaccine, but which may have other composition, such as heroin or penicillin. Brachial plexus neuropathy due to vaccine often develops in the setting of the signs and symptoms of serum sickness. There are often sensory and motor deficits, as well as pain in the limb, and the sympathetic chain in the thorax may be involved, producing the symptoms of Horner's syndrome—ptosis, small pupil, and decreased sweating—on that side of the face. Brachial plexus neuropathy may accompany many viral illnesses, such as infectious mononucleosis. It is necessary to exclude the diagnoses of traumatic cervical spinal disease and acute cervical radiculitis due to spondylosis or disc disease; in the case of spondylosis, usually only one or two roots are affected. If the illness is exceptionally painful, which happens frequently, or if cardiac or aortic disease cannot definitely be excluded, hospitalization with analgesics and sedation is necessary.

The painful radicular syndromes of herpes zoster (shingles) can result in diagnostic uncertainties before the characteristic rash erupts. The cutaneous distribution is usually one dermatome, but may occasionally be several adjacent dermatomes. The rash most commonly occurs on the thorax, and the pain is often burning, itching, and intense. Pain is the most salient feature, but diminished sensory modalities within the painful dermatome and motor weakness in the territories of the corresponding motor roots are not rare. A few white blood cells may be present in the CSF, and the protein level may be slightly elevated. Therapy for radicular herpes zoster infection with systemic corticosteroids may predispose the patient to spread of the infection within the central nervous system. Herpes zoster in the first or second division of the trigeminal nerve threatens the cornea. Herpes simplex virus may occasionally cause a painful radicular syndrome with the characteristic herpetic rash of grouped vesicles on an erythematous base. After recovery from radicular herpes zoster infection, some patients have long-term burning pain in the same region (postherpetic neuralgia). It is questionable whether the incidence of depressive psychiatric disease is more common in these patients. Therapy with analgesics and trials of phenytoin or carbamazepine should be undertaken. Ethyl chloride spray can be a useful adjunct in the therapy for postherpetic neuralgia.

Sudden loss of function, often with pain, in the territory of a major peripheral nerve is most often due to trauma. An exception is *diabetic mononeuropathy multiplex*. In the limbs, proximal nerves, particularly femoral or obturator nerves, are the most common sites. The patient with diabetic femoral neuropathy may suddenly experience intense pain in the anterior part of the thigh and paralysis of knee extension. On examination, there is sensory loss in the region of the knee, loss of the knee jerk, and weakness of the quadriceps muscle. Recovery is usually complete, but may take several months. Sudden mononeuropathy is also a feature of periarteritis nodosa.

Some nerves are particularly vulnerable to *trauma* because of their location. Even trivial injury at the lateral aspect of the knee can result in peroneal nerve palsy and footdrop. Intramuscular injections deep in the buttock may injure the sciatic nerve if there is not strict adherence to injecting only into the upper outer quadrant. Intradeltoid injections may injure the radial nerve (wristdrop) as it traverses the humerus. Overdose of many types of medication may cause a state of motionless sleep or light coma in which nerve and muscle may be injured by pressure or ischemia. In the case of widespread pressure injury to muscle, myoglobinemia may lead to renal damage.

Suggested Readings

Ackerman RH: Non-invasive carotid evaluation. *Stroke* 11:675–678, 1980

Argov Z, Mastaglia FL: Disorders of neuromuscular transmission caused by drugs. *N Engl J Med* 301:409–413, 1979

Brust JCM, Dickinson PCT, Healton EB: Failure of CT sharing in a large municipal hospital. *N Engl J Med* 304:1388–1393, 1981

Center for Disease Control (Atlanta, GA) Periodic (usually annual) USA surveillance, with updated commentary on: aseptic meningitis, botulism, diphtheria, encephalitis, Guillain-Barré syndrome, poliomyelitis, rabies, tetanus

Diamond S: Headache: Its diagnosis and management. *Headache* 19:113–192, 1979

Drachman DA, Hart CW: An approach to the dizzy patient. *Neurology* 22; 323–334, 1972.

Fisher CM: Vertigo in cerebrovascular disease. *Arch Otolaryngol* 85:529–534, 1967

Fisher CM: The anatomy and pathology of the cerebral vasculature. In: Meyer JS (Ed): *Modern Concepts in Cerebrovascular Disease.* New York, Spectrum Publications, 1975, pp. 1–41

Fröscher W: *Treatment of Status Epilepticus.* Baltimore, University Park Press, 1979

Guillain-Barré syndrome. (Proceedings of a conference sponsored by the Kroc Foundation.) *Ann Neurol 9 Suppl:* 1–148, 1981 Myasthenia gravis. (Festschrift to Professor J. A. Simpson). *J Neurol Neurosurg Psychiat* 43:561–659, 1980

Plum F, Posner JB: *The Diagnosis of Stupor and Coma*, ed 3. Philadelphia, FA Davis, 1980

Ruff RL, Dougherty JH Jr: Evaluation of acute cerebral ischemia for anticoagulant therapy: Computed tomography or lumbar puncture. *Neurology* 31:736–740, 1981

Sandok BA, Furlan AJ, Whisnant JP, et al: Guidelines for the management of transient ischemic attacks. *Mayo Clin Proc* 53:665–674, 1978

Siekert RG (Ed): *Cerebrovascular Survey Report for Joint Council Subcommittee on Cerebrovascular Disease.* NINCDS & NHLI, 1980

Vinken PJ, Bruyn GW (Eds): *Handbook of Clinical Neurology.* Amsterdam, North-Holland Publ. Co. 41 volumes, 1969–1979

Whitley RJ, Soong S-J, Hirsch MS, et al: Herpes simplex encephalitis. Vidarabine therapy and diagnostic problems. *N Engl J Med* 304:313–318, 1981

Wilder BJ, Ramsay RE, Willmore LJ, et al: Efficacy of intravenous phenytoin in the treatment of status epilepticus: Kinetics of central nervous system penetration. *Ann Neurol* 1:511–518, 1977

Wolpow ER, Schatzki SC, Buchwald LY: Electroencephalography and computed tomography of the brain. In: Stålberg E, Young RR (Eds): *Clinical Neurophysiology, Neurology 1.* London, Butterworths, 1981, pp. 296–324

CHAPTER 16

Approach to the Patient with Altered Consciousness

AMY A. PRUITT, M.D.

Editor's note: This chapter, new to the second edition, supplements the preceding chapter on neurologic emergencies by presenting a systematic approach to the patient with any alteration in state of consciousness. It is thus, with the possible exceptions of the cardiology chapters, an innovation to the format of this textbook in concentration on the symptomatic presentation of the patient.

Patients with acutely altered mental status present the physician with an array of medical, neurologic, and psychiatric diseases that challenge his emergency diagnostic and therapeutic skills. More than 10% of patients admitted for medical and surgical problems have a component of confusion superimposed on their illness, and conversely, 18% of patients seen in psychiatric outpatient settings have a medical illness that explains a significant part of their psychiatric problem. The accurate triage of such patients can mean the difference between successful reversal of the impairment and permanent neurologic damage. This chapter presents a general emergency ward approach to confused, agitated, stuporous, and comatose patients, and offers a multidisciplinary differential diagnosis of delirium and coma. Further discussion of specific causes of altered mental status can be found in other chapters.

DELIRIUM

Presentation

The confused patient is brought to the hospital because he is behaving inappropriately. Delirium is defined as a clouding of consciousness with reduced awareness of the environment. Prominent alterations in arousal and attention are the hall-marks: the patient may alternate between hyper-alert agitation and somnolence. Frequently worse at night, perceptual disturbances with hallucinations or misinterpretations are common. The patient may have increased or decreased psychomotor activity. These fluctuating features develop over minutes to a few days.

Certain patients are more susceptible to delirium, such as elderly patients, alcohol and other drug abusers, and patients with structural brain damage. Situations in which delirium is likely to develop include sleep deprivation, psychologic stress, sensory deprivations, drug changes, and seemingly trivial alterations in metabolic balance. The recognition of delirium should alert the examiner to begin a thorough medical evaluation, *since delirium is most often due to a primary problem outside the central nervous system.*

Differential Diagnosis

The differential diagnosis of delirium includes an extensive list of medical illnesses, a small group of psychiatric conditions, and a limited number of structural neurologic defects (Table 16.1).

"Medical" delirium has the largest number of causes. The apparent neurologic nature of the presentation should not fool the physician into neglecting basic cardiopulmonary and metabolic examination. Hypothermia or hyperthermia may be sufficient to greatly disorient an elderly patient, and may indicate sepsis. Similarly, hypoperfusion states with diminished cerebral blood flow due to a new myocardial infarction or cardiac arrhythmia may masquerade primarily as agitation rather than somnolence. Hypertensive encephalopathy with raised intracranial pressure may do the same.

A comprehensive list of metabolic abnormalities

Table 16.1.
Causes of delirium.

"Medical" delirium

  Altered temperature
  Hypoxia, hypercapnia
  Hypoperfusion—new myocardial infarct, slower
    heart rate
  Hypertensive encephalopathy
  Hypoglycemia
  Electrolyte imbalance
    Hypernatremia, hyperosmolar states
    Hyponatremia
    Hypercalcemia
  Endocrine imbalance
    Hyperthyroidism
    Hypothyroidism
    Addisonian crisis
    Cushing's syndrome
  Organ failure
    Liver
    Kidney
  Deficiency states
    Thiamin—Wernicke's encephalopathy
  Drugs
    Anticholinergics
    Barbiturates, opiates, sedative-hypnotics
    Alcohol
    Amphetamines, cocaine
    Carbidopa-levodopa (Sinemet)
    Zomax
    Cimetidine
    Lithium
    Withdrawal syndromes

"Psychiatric" delirium

  Acute manic states
  Acute schizophreniform psychoses
  Hysteria
  Homosexual panic
  Ganser's syndrome

"Neurologic" delirium

  Postictal states
  Psychomotor status epilepticus
  Postconcussive states
  Posthypoperfusion states
  Subarachnoid hemorrhage with acute hydroceph-
    alus
  Infection
    Encephalitis (herpes simplex)
    Meningitis (viral, bacterial, tuberculous)
  Vascular syndromes
    Nondominant parietal lobe infarct
    Mesial occipital or temporal cortex infarct
    Aphasia
      Wernicke's
      Transcortical motor and sensory
    Transient global amnesia
  Mass lesions
    Tumor
    Abscess
    Subdural hematoma

producing delirium would include every metabolic imbalance known, but the most common offending conditions are hypoglycemia, hyperglycemia, electrolyte imbalances, and organ failure with ammoniemia or hyperuricemia. In all these cases, rapid development of the metabolic abnormality results in a more florid presentation of central nervous system dysfunction, sometimes including seizures.

Although other vitamin deficiencies such as niacin and B_{12} deficiencies may produce delirious states, the most common deficiency that causes delirium is diminished thiamine reserve in alcoholic and malnourished patients. This critical syndrome is characterized by acute or subacute onset of confusion, nystagmus, oculomotor palsies (usually bilateral abducens palsies), and variable ataxia. Even if the syndrome is not seen on initial examination, it may be precipitated by a glucose load. Thus, in the emergency setting, any patient suspected to have thiamine deficiency should be given parenteral thiamine, 100 mg, before being given glucose. A smaller dose of thiamine may be sufficient to relieve the ocular symptoms, but the above dose with continued supplementation is advisable to prevent development of the irreversible memory deficit known as Korsakoff's syndrome.

The drugs causing delirium are listed in Table 16.1. Major offenders include drugs with central and peripheral anticholinergic properties, such as scopolamine, tricyclic antidepressants, antihistamines, phenothiazines, butyrophenones, and antidiarrheal compounds such as Donnagel and Lomotil. Peripheral signs of these drugs are mydriasis, tachycardia, urinary retention, fever, ileus, and dry mouth; central signs include hallucinations, ataxia, dysarthria, and myoclonus. Acute confusion and peripheral side effects may be reduced by administration of physostigmine, which should not be given in the presence of coronary artery disease, hyperthyroidism, bronchial asthma, or peptic ulcer. Administration of physostigmine results in lacrimation, salivation, and rhinorrhea. The acute dystonias seen with phenothiazines and butyrophenones such as haloperidol (Haldol) may be rapidly reversed by intravenous administration of benztropine mesylate (Congentin) or diphenhydramine hydrochloride (Benadryl).

Barbiturates, opiates, and sedative-hypnotic agents are less likely to cause a delirious state, but paradoxical reactions may occur. An excited, hyperalert state, often with headache, tachypnea, and dysesthesias, may be seen with cocaine ingestion, and a similar state is produced by amphetamines. Withdrawal syndromes from any of the above medications may produce confusion, mydriasis, tachycardia, or seizures. The examiner should carefully take an ingestion history, looking particularly for medications with a long half-life ("tranquilizers" such as diazepam [Valium] and chlordiazepoxide hydrochloride). Of particular importance is alcohol withdrawal, alcohol being the most commonly abused drug in most emergency ward presentations. Peaking at 12–24 hours after the last ingestion, withdrawal is marked by restlessness, tremors, and confusion with auditory and visual hallucinations. Actual seizures may occur in this same time interval and the patient may have a quiet, oriented period between the "rum fits" and full-blown delirium tremens.

A final reminder: the physician can never be too thorough in taking a medication history. Particularly in the organically impaired brain, very small changes in medication or very low doses of sedative-hypnotic agents may be sufficient to alter mental status.

"Psychiatric" delirium is a component of a smaller but equally difficult group of diagnoses. The hallmarks of psychiatric disease in this setting include inconsistencies in the mental status examination, with some high-level responses or consistently abnormal responses indicating that the patient has some understanding of the question. There may be highly variable performance, and the patient may have auditory rather than visual hallucinations. Ganser's syndrome is a denial of specific events, usually with the intent of avoiding prosecution. Several psychiatric medications, including lithium and tricyclic antidepressants, can be associated with tremors, agitation, and in some cases, seizures.

The group of neurologic disorders causing delirium is relatively small. Immediately after a seizure, patients may be confused, amnesic and extremely agitated. Progressive improvement should occur over several hours. Psychomotor status epilepticus has been confused with psychiatric disease; its hallmarks are a trance-like appearance, rhythmic movements of the tongue or lips, and repetitive, often complex stereotypical movements. Intravenous administration of diazepam may abruptly reverse the abnormality and clarify the situation. The classic temporal lobe features of disagreeable odor or lip smacking may be seen in patients without a history of seizures who have acute herpes simplex encephalitis.

Focal signs may be absent in many neurologic disorders. Post-traumatic confusion and confusion after an episode of hypoxic or ischemic injury should be suspected with the appropriate history. Steady improvement is expected, and deterioration should raise suspicion of epidural, subdural, or intracerebral hematoma. The sudden onset of hydrocephalus from a subarachnoid hemorrhage or third ventricular tumor may also be unaccompanied by headache or focal signs.

Neurologic syndromes with focal deficits indicating the underlying cause are predominantly vascular, although patients are occasionally seen who have a frontal or temporal lobe mass with an acutely altered mental state independent of seizure activity. Specific vascular syndromes are listed in Table 16.1. Right middle cerebral artery disease with nondominant parietal lobe infarction may result in agitation and concomitant left-sided weakness with inattention to the deficit. However, denial of illness occurs frequently in delirious patients. Similarly, although many delirious patients have word-finding difficulty, mesial occipital and temporal cortex infarction, particularly on the dominant side, may result in inability to form new memories and localizing symptoms of nominal aphasia and homonymous hemianopsia. Fluent aphasias may produce difficult diagnostic dilemmas, since schizophrenic speech must be distinguished from the "word salad" of Wernicke's aphasia or the echolalia of transcortical aphasia. A careful screen for primarily verbal problems (Table 16.2) should separate patients with a focal lesion from those without a focal deficit who may have some word-finding difficulty as part of the delirious state. Transient global amnesia is a syndrome of complete inability to form new memories that may last up to several hours. This may be a symptom of basilar artery insufficiency, or it may occur after head trauma or seizures.

A final word of caution concerning the differential diagnosis of delirium: there frequently may be more than one reason for the delirious state. Thus, a patient with Wernicke's encephalopathy may also be withdrawing from alcohol and may have ceased to eat and drink because of an infection or a subdural hematoma. A patient with seizures may fail to waken rapidly because of anoxic damage suffered during the seizure, and a patient with a markedly altered mental state with apparently trivial medication change or metabolic alteration may harbor an underlying dementia or other structural neurologic problem.

Evaluation

History

The confused patient frequently has little insight into his problem, and often a relevant history must be obtained from bystanders. Points of immediate significance include: (1) mode of onset, whether abrupt or insidious; (2) history of trauma; (3) history of cerebrovascular or cardiovascular disease; (4) history of underlying metabolic disease

Table 16.2.
Emergency "mini" mental status examination.

Procedure	Abnormalities and Significance
Describe the patient's condition	Establishes baseline
Include level of consciousness, coherence of speech, and types of movement (purposeful, asterixis, tremor, and so on)	
?Hallucinations	
Ask about orientation	Disorientation to person implies psychiatric disease
Test attention[a]	Normal = 7 digits forward, 5 backward
Digit span—recite numbers in monotone and have patient repeat immediately; recite random letters, asking patient to raise his hand every time you say certain letters	
Test short-term memory	Selective disturbance of new memory
Ask patient to memorize three to five objects and ask him 5–10 minutes later to repeat them	Postictal, postconcussive states, transient global amnesia, temporal infarction, herpes simplex encephalitis
Test long-term memory	Tests general level of intelligence/education, and
Ask about remote historical or biographic events	may indicate acute deterioration
Test object-naming ability	Specific nominal aphasia seen with left temporooccipital defects
Ask patient to identify several objects in room, including body parts	"Word salad" in Wernicke's aphasia to be distinguished from schizophrenic speech
	Echolalia to be distinguished from transcortical aphasia
	Look for associated visual field defects
Test ability to draw simple objects: square, star, cube, house	Tests right hemisphere function

[a] If patient is unable to perform these tests, it is unlikely he will be able to perform subsequent tests.

such as diabetes or renal failure; (5) history of seizures; (6) use of anticoagulants or presence of coagulopathy; (7) likelihood of intoxication or a suicide attempt (psychiatric history); and (8) knowledge of any complaint in the days or weeks preceding the illness, such as headache, loss of balance, depression, visual disturbance, or memory loss.

Examination

The delirious state can be assessed quickly with a "mini" mental status examination. Excellent expanded versions are available, but Table 16.2 allows quantitation of the degree of the disturbance, and aids in the triage of the medical, psychiatric, and neurologic causes of delirium, providing a hemispheric localization for the last.

The mental status examination can be performed only in patients whose level of attention permits it. A wide variety of focal neurologic findings should not be expected in metabolic delirium, and aphasia, apraxia, or memory disturbance should raise suspicion of a focal deficit. Isolated inability to form new memories in patients who do not appear agitated or confused may indicate Korsakoff's syndrome. Inconsistent performance should raise the suspicion of psychiatric delirium.

The general physical and neurologic examination of the delirious or comatose patient is directed toward distinguishing between medical and neurologic diseases (see page 370). Unlike in the comatose patient, some tests such as visual field testing can also be included.

Treatment

Emergency therapeutic maneuvers depend on assessment of the underlying cause for the altered mental state. General principles dictate a calm approach to the confused patient. A family member or other familiar person should be present with the patient in a well-lighted environment. Minimal restraint should be used, if possible, and the examination should be conducted at a pace that does not frustrate the patient. Sedation should be avoided until the underlying problem is evident. Electrolyte determinations and other metabolic studies should be performed early, and thiamin may be administered without harmful effects. If initial examination suggests a focal deficit, or if the patient has a history of trauma, computed tomography (CT) without contrast enhancement should be performed to look for hematoma or edema. Although sedation is undesirable, it may be necessary to obtain a high-quality scan. Lumbar puncture is required in all but a few settings. If there is a clear metabolic problem such as hypoglycemia and if the patient appears to be improving rapidly with correction of the abnormality, or if a patient with a known seizure disorder was witnessed to have a seizure and is improving rapidly, lumbar puncture may be omitted. Even if alcohol ingestion has been established, lumbar puncture should be considered to rule out infection. Repetitive seizures or psychomotor status epilepticus can be stopped with intravenous diazepam, 5 mg every 5–10 minutes with respiratory support on hand. Long-acting anticonvulsant agents should be started simultaneously (see Chapter 15, page 348). Acute psychiatric management is discussed in Chapter 18; antipsychotic agents with sedative properties such as chlorpromazine (Thorazine) may be useful in many agitated patients as soon as the type of disease underlying the altered mental state has been determined.

COMA

At the other end of the spectrum from the hyperalert, delirious patient is the person who over a period of minutes to days has become sleepy but rousable (stuporous) or unrousable (comatose). Perhaps even more than in the case of the delirious patient, rapid action is essential. The physician requires a systematic approach to focus his actions quickly and effectively.

Neuroanatomy

Whereas the list of diseases leading to coma is lengthy (Table 16.3), the neuroanatomic variations in altered consciousness are few. For any pathologic process to cause coma, it must produce bilateral dysfunction of the cerebral hemispheres either structurally or metabolically *or* it must damage the reticular activating system in the upper brainstem and diencephalon, again either structurally or metabolically. Thus, supratentorial lesions, infratentorial lesions, and metabolic processes may all lead to coma.

Table 16.4 summarizes the anatomic areas whose dysfunction leads to coma, and indicates the appropriate terminology. Finally, psychiatric unresponsiveness should be considered a fourth cause of "coma."

Differential Diagnosis

Initial diagnosis depends on the integration of available history and physical data to place the

Table 16.3.
Causes of coma.

Outside the central nervous system
  Metabolic causes
    Hypoxia
      Cardiopulmonary disease
      Carbon monoxide poisoning
    Ischemia
      Decreased cerebral blood flow due to myocardial infarction, congestive heart failure, pulmonary disease, hyperviscosity
    Hypoglycemia
    Hepatic failure
    Renal failure
    Hypothyroidism
    Adrenal insufficiency
    Acid-base or electrolyte imbalance
      Hyponatremia, hypernatremia
      Acidosis, alkalosis
      Hypercalcemia
      Hypophosphatemia
      Hypermagnesemia, hypomagnesemia
    Hypothermia, hyperthermia
  Exogenous poisons
    Barbiturates, opiates, alcohol, tranquilizers, bromides
    Psychotropic agents
      Tricyclic antidepressants
      Lithium
      LSD
    Heavy metals
    Organic phosphates
  Infection
    Meningitis
    Encephalitis

Within the central nervous system
  Supratentorial lesions
    Hemorrhage, traumatic and nontraumatic
      Subdural, epidural
      Intracerebral (lobar)
      Basal ganglia (putamen, thalamus)
      Intraventricular
      Subarachnoid
    Infarction
      Middle cerebral occlusion with edema or hemorrhage or both
    Tumor
    Abscess
  Infratentorial lesions
    Hemorrhage
      Cerebellar
      Pontine
      Posterior fossa (subdural, epidural)
    Infarction
      Basilar thrombosis
      Cerebellar infarction with edema
    Posterior fossa tumor
    Posterior fossa abscess
    Demyelinating disease
    Basilar migraine

Table 16.4.
Relationship of neuroanatomy to coma.

Damaged Site	Resulting State
Cortex	
Bilateral cerebral hemispheres	Coma (metabolic, structural)
Frontal lobes	Abulia, akinetic mutism
Unilateral hemispheric lesion plus edema or hemorrhage	Early local signs leading to coma
Brainstem/Diencephalon	
Hypothalamus	Hypersomnia
Brainstem reticular formation	Coma
Basis pontis	Locked-in or "de-efferented" state: patient awake but unable to respond

Table 16.5.
Physical examination of the comatose patient.

General examination: Is there an extracranial cause for the coma?

Observations	Abnormalities and Significance
Vital signs	Hypotension: shock, sepsis
	Hyperthermia: tricyclics, lithium, monoamine oxidase inhibitors, sepsis
	Hypothermia: phenothiazines, exposure, alcohol, myxedema
Head	Evidence of trauma, odor of alcohol, old burr holes
Eyes	Papilledema
Skin	Shock, needle tracks, hepatic disease, bleeding disorders, suicide attempts, endocarditis
Cardiopulmonary evaluation	Shock, arrhythmia, pneumothorax, pneumonia
Abdomen	Acute abdominal event precipitating shock

Neurologic examination: Is this a neurosurgical emergency? Is coma due to brainstem disease or to bilateral cerebral hemispheric disease?

	General description
Responsiveness:	Occasional appropriate verbal response
	Garbled speech
	No speech
Arousal:	Opens eyes to voice
	Opens eyes to gentle stimulation
	Opens eyes to noxious stimulation
	No response
	Brainstem assessment

Observations	Abnormalities and Significance
Pupillary reaction	
Equal and reactive	Likely metabolic cause for coma
Large, often fixed	Midbrain dysfunction or mydriatics
Pinpoint	Pontine dysfunction
Fixed, dilated	Medullary dysfunction or mydriatics
Spontaneous eye position and movements	Skew deviation: posterior fossa
Oculovestibular testing with warm and cool or ice water (check eardrums)	Dysconjugate response: infratentorial lesion
Corneas	Unilateral loss: infratentorial lesion
Respiratory pattern	Hyperventilation: acidosis, hypoxia, pontine disease, psychogenic origin
	Cheyne-Stokes: supratentorial or metabolic
Motor assessment	
Check tone, spontaneous movements—myoclonus, seizures, opisthotonos, swallowing, chewing	Lateralization: supratentorial origin, suggest metabolic low-level function
Blinking	Pons intact
Yawning, sneezing	Light coma
Deep tendon reflexes	Lateralization: supratentorial origin

cause of coma into one of the general categories just discussed. This will lead to effective initial emergency treatment. Using laboratory and radiologic data, the emergency physician can then make a more specific diagnosis.

Supratentorial lesions are usually accompanied by early signs and symptoms of focal cerebral dysfunction. Motor signs may be asymmetric, or the observer's history may suggest focal dysfunction at an early stage. Thus, the patient with an expanding right subdural hematoma will have early left hemiparesis followed by altered consciousness as both hemispheres are affected. As pointed out in Table 16.4, unilateral hemispheric disease alone is insufficient to cause coma. A patient with a large left middle cerebral infarct may be densely aphasic and hemiplegic, but is not comatose. Later deterioration in level of consciousness may be due to hemorrhage into the infarcted area or to edema caused by ischemic cell death.

Infratentorial lesions lead to more rapid onset of coma. The patient may briefly experience headache, vertigo, nausea, vomiting, diplopia, or other brainstem symptoms before losing consciousness. Localizing brainstem signs such as cranial nerve palsies and oculovestibular abnormalities may accompany coma. Unusual respiratory patterns such as hyperventilation or extremely irregular breathing are characteristic.

Metabolic causes of coma are heralded by more gradual progression from confusion or delirium through stupor to coma. Pupillary reactions may be preserved (unless a drug effect is present), and abnormal (symmetric) motor findings such as asterixis, myoclonus, and tremor may be seen. There may be increased ventilation (due to hypoxia or acidosis) or hypoventilation.

Psychogenic unresponsiveness is characterized by preserved pupillary reactions, active lid closure, nystagmus with caloric stimulation, normal motor tone, normal deep tendon reflexes, and either normal ventilation or hyperventilation.

Examination

The goal of physical examination is to determine which type of coma is present. The *general examination* seeks to establish a metabolic or infectious origin of the coma, and the *neurologic examination* attempts to characterize the type of intracranial abnormality leading to the comatose state.

Table 16.5 summarizes the sequence of the physical examination in the comatose patient. The patient is observed for signs of shock, metabolic derangement, or sepsis. The neurologic examination then attempts to sort out neurosurgical emergencies and to separate brainstem disease from

bilateral cerebral hemispheric disease. The patient is quickly observed for level of responsiveness and rousability. Assessment of eyes and pupils then localizes the lesion within the brainstem. A problem in diagnosis is failure of the pupils to react caused by mydriatic agents such as atropine, glutethimide, or other anticholinergics. Pinpoint, barely reactive pupils are seen both in pontine dysfunction and in opiate overdose.

Spontaneous eye movements and resting position offer many clues to localization. Skew deviation of the eyes can arise from an intra-axial brainstem lesion or from a compressive lesion in the posterior fossa. More specific clues to the level of brainstem dysfunction in the unresponsive patient are obtained by irrigating the external canals with ice water. In the comatose patient, intact brainstem function is indicated by conjugate deviation of the eyes toward the irrigated ear. Dysconjugate responses to caloric stimulation should suggest an infratentorial cause of coma. When eye movements and pupillary movements are disproportionately preserved compared with level of function, metabolic coma is likely. Observation of nystagmus with a cold water irrigation indicates either light stupor or an awake patient (who will be very nauseated).

Spontaneous movement indicates the patient's level of responsiveness, as well as laterality. Reflex movements to noxious stimuli may fall into recognizable patterns: extension of all limbs is consistent with decerebration, and flexion of arms with extension of legs indicates decortication. Asymmetries of tone should be recorded, and adventitial movements such as tremor or myoclonus suggest a metabolic origin. Deep tendon reflexes give further evidence of laterality.

The abbreviated neurologic examination outlined in Table 16.5 should provide the examiner with an idea of which part of the brain has malfunctioned. The physical examination should also give the physician a sense of the pace of the disease. The examiner should be aware of progressive signs warning of incipient herniation. The syndrome of uncal herniation results from intracranial lesions in the temporal lobe or lateral part of the cranium. Unilateral dilation of the pupil from oculomotor nerve compression occurs early in the patient's course. Impaired consciousness is not necessarily present at this stage, but motor signs will then appear, frequently with ipsilateral hemiparesis due to compression of the cerebral peduncle against the tentorium. Signs of brainstem compression then develop rapidly.

The central herniation syndrome results from more medial supratentorial lesions. Unlike in un-

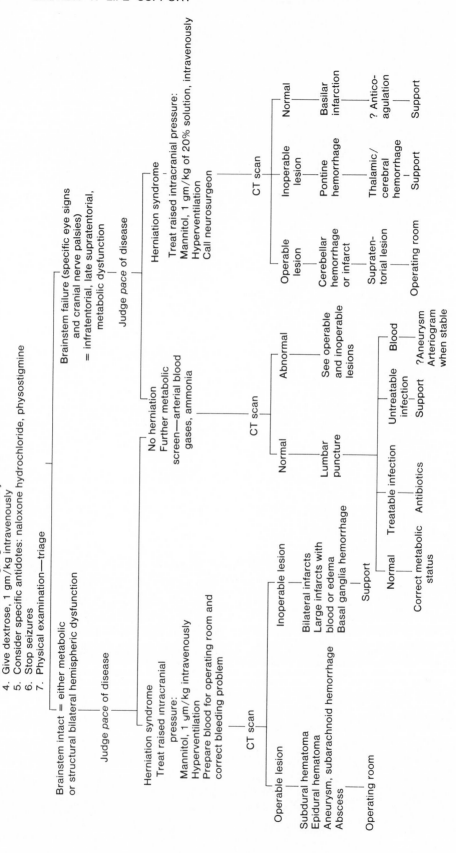

Figure 16.1. Schema (algorithm) of steps in triage/treatment of the comatose patient.

cal herniation, drowsiness occurs early as a result of direct pressure on the diencephalon from above. Respiration may be the Cheyne-Stokes pattern. Eye movements are full, pupils small, and reactive and motor signs possibly bilateral. With progression, level of consciousness decreases, respiration rate increases, pupils become midsized and unreactive, and decerebration may be observed, which then gives way to flaccidity with ataxic respirations in the medullary stage. *The early stage of the central herniation syndrome may be mistaken for metabolic coma with drowsiness, periodic respirations, and preserved eye movements.*

Treatment

The physician may have to perform several steps of the evaluation at once. While obtaining a history from family or friends (see pages 371–372), he must begin general supportive measures and carry out the examination that will lead to definitive therapy. Figure 16.1 summarizes the steps in initial emergency support and triage based on the physical examination.

Brainstem failure with incipient herniation is the most critical stiutaiton. The patient should be given mannitol, 1 gm/kg of 20% solution intravenously, followed by intubation and hyperventilation to decrease cerebral blood flow. Dexamethasone, 20 mg inravenously, may be given in addition, although its effects will not begin for several hours. A neurosurgeon may need to place a burr hole on the side of the dilating pupil in patients with uncal hernation before CT scanning. A CT scan without contrast enhancement should be obtained immediately. Potentially operable lesions include cerebellar hemorrhage and infarction. The former is usually seen in the setting of systemic hypertension or anticoagulation. Hallmarks are sudden occipital headache, nausea, vomiting, dizziness, and difficulty walking. Similar although usually less acute findings occur with ischemic infarction, which later can compress the contents of the posterior fossa and compromise brainstem function. Since it is virtually impossible to distinguish intra-axial brainstem lesions such as stroke from compressive lesions such as cerebellar hemorrhage or from late compressive effects of supratentorial lesions, the patient should be treated for a compressive lesion because these processes are potentially reversible. If the patient has a fluctuating ischemic deficit in the basilar territory, immediate anticoagulant therapy with heparin should be considered and blood pressure should be kept at adequate levels to assure perfusion.

If the brainstem is intact (eye movements, pupils, and oculovestibular movements preserved), the examiner should judge the pace of deterioration. A potential hazard at this point in the evaluation is that, in the early stages of central herniation, the patient may appear to be in metabolic coma. If there is no clear reason to suspect metabolic coma, the examiner should proceed as if treating raised intracranial pressure. If there is reason to suspect a coagulation disturbance, the patient should be given vitamin K, 10 mg intramuscularly, and fresh-frozen plasma and typed blood should be made available for use in the operating room. A CT scan should then be obtained. Operable lesions such as subdural hematoma or epidural hematoma should be treated immediately. Acute obstructive hydrocephalus can be relieved and abscesses drained. Inoperable lesions resulting in supratentorial coma include bilateral cerebral infarcts, large unilateral infarcts with edema or blood, and basal ganglia hemorrhages (see Chapter 27).

If herniation is not imminent, the examiner has more time to obtain further metabolic screening information. If data are unrevealing, a CT scan should be obtained. CT scanning will frequently reveal blood in subarachnoid hemorrhage and may give information about the location of an arteriovenous malformation or aneurysm. If findings are normal, a lumbar puncture should be performed to rule out treatable infection. Lumbar puncture should be a primary diagnostic procedure in coma only when infection is suspected. If CT scanning is unavailable in the emergency ward, arteriography or ultrasound studies should be performed if raised intracranial pressure is suspected.

At this point in the evaluation, all structural causes of coma should be excluded and any infection discovered, with laboratory studies in process that will reveal the metabolic abnormality in need of correction. In many cases, it is impossible to be sure of the diagnosis after examination alone. Late stages of any supratentorial or infratentorial lesion result in brainstem failure. Similarly, early stages of central herniation may mimic metabolic coma. In no patient in whom a structural lesion is suspected should a CT scan be omitted because of absence of focal signs, nor should any of the initial resuscitative and general support measures listed at the top of Figure 16.1 be omitted, no matter how focal the findings.

Some statistics may be useful for the emergency physician to remember as he begins examination and treatment of the comatose patient: of 500 consecutive patients with coma treated at New York Hospital, 326 had a metabolic cause, 101 had supratentorial lesions, 65 had infratentorial lesions, and 8 had psychogenic unresponsiveness.

Attention to examination and careful supportive therapy at each step should allow appropriate triage of each patient and should maximize the possibility of successful recovery from this life-threatening situation.

Suggested Readings

McEvoy JP: Organic brain syndromes in DSM-III (letter). *Am J Psychiatr 138:*124–125, 1981
Strub RL, Black FW: *The Mental Status Examination in Neurology.* Philadelphia, F. A. Davis Co., 1977

CHAPTER 17

Toxicologic Emergencies

PETER L. GROSS, M.D.
HOWARD S. SCHWARTZ, M.D.

Acute poisoning is a common medical emergency requiring rapid assessment and well-organized treatment. A successful outcome depends on (1) appropriate application of basic management principles and (2) recognition and treatment of specific complicating clinical problems. This chapter reviews the basic management principles and discusses the complicating clinical syndromes. Space does not allow a complete review of all poisons, drugs, and toxins, but selected agents are highlighted in an attempt to review both common and controversial management problems.

With more than 1 million poisonings each year, resulting in approximately 5000 deaths, emergency wards are frequently required to provide information as well as medical consultation concerning intentional and accidental overdose, poisoning, and toxic exposure. In some geographic areas, poison control centers also provide valuable assistance in answer to public and professional needs.

The emergency physician not only must have extensive knowledge of clinical toxicology but also must be prepared to assess and treat poisonings in all age groups. Approximately 70% of reported cases of poisoning in the United States involve children under the age of 5 years, the most common situation being accidental ingestion. Although unintentional poisoning also occurs in adults (as the result of factors such as confusion in dose and treatment schedules or the accidental ingestion or inhalation of toxins), deliberate toxic exposure is more likely in this age group. Suicide attempts or drug abuse problems require concurrent medical and psychiatric treatment and evaluation.

The patient with intentional poisoning may be difficult to evaluate because of depression or behavioral abnormalities. The underlying psychiatric state or the effect of the poison or toxin often makes history unreliable and compliance with treatment difficult. In addition, some patients are repeatedly seen with ingestions or complaints of drug abuse, perhaps diminishing the physician's suspicion of a true suicidal intent and making objective evaluation more difficult. Each patient must be approached calmly and dispassionately with a rational plan of assessment and treatment.

BASIC MANAGEMENT PRINCIPLES

Treatment of the poisoned patient may be divided into three parts: (1) general support, (2) removal of the drug by decreasing absorption or increasing elimination, and (3) specific treatment of complicating medical conditions, such as shock, seizure, cardiac arrhythmias, and respiratory failure.

General Support

The first priority for the emergency physician is general supportive care and resuscitative measures. Rapid attention must be given to the airway and adequacy of ventilation, as well as to blood pressure, cardiac rhythm, and level of consciousness. Once basic resuscitative or supportive measures have been instituted, attention can be given to specific management of the poisoning. Consideration of the pharmacokinetics and specific characteristics of the drug or toxic substance is secondary to the initial general support of the patient in almost all circumstances.

Estimation of Severity

The emergency physician must make an initial determination of the severity of a drug ingestion or poisoning, and must then continually reassess the patient's condition for signs of improvement or deterioration. Three factors contribute to the initial determination: (1) the patient's general status and level of consciousness on arrival, (2) the alleged drug and dose involved, and (3) any specific complicating clinical situations already present or possible with the particular agent.

Cardiorespiratory adequacy and level of consciousness should be noted and recorded. With regard to mental status, three conditions may be seen: awake, stuporous, or comatose. Table 17.1 provides a more detailed grading for depth of coma, but actual staging is less important than the recorded statement concerning reflexes, response to pain, and level of consciousness. Changes with time are extremely important indicators of improvement or deterioration.

The history from the patient may be unreliable, but it should be obtained and compared with available information from family, friends, or ambulance personnel in the attempt to determine the drug, dose, and time of ingestion or exposure. In the circumstance of illicit drug use, persons accompanying the patient tend to leave as soon as the patient is under a physician's care. The physician should obtain any information in a nonjudgmental manner, with attention to any home remedies already tried that might complicate the patient's clinical course.

A rough guideline to significant toxicity in adults with sedative, hypnotic, antipsychotic or antidepressant overdose is ingestion of 10–20 times the usual daily therapeutic dose. Standard toxicology texts or information resources should be readily available to the emergency physician to help with the patient's assessment, determination of the extent of toxicity, and estimation of severity.

Deep stupor, coma, or the presence of one or more of the conditions listed in Table 17.2 increases the gravity of the situation and may require admission of the patient for intensive care. Local institutional resources may vary, and some patients with mild ingestion or toxic exposure may be observed in the emergency ward and released after appropriate psychiatric assessment. Many pa-

Table 17.1.
Evaluation of level of consciousness.

Grade	Description
0	Fully conscious
1	Drowsy, but responds to verbal commands
2	Unconscious, but responds to minimal painful stimuli[a]
3	Unconscious, responds only to maximal painful stimuli
4	Unconscious, no response, loss of all reflexes

[a] Sternal rubbing with a knuckle is an adequate painful stimulus and is less dangerous than other methods.

Table 17.2.
Clinical situations complicating drug ingestion.

Hypotension or hypertension
Hypothermia or hyperthermia
Respiratory failure
Pulmonary edema
Aspiration pneumonia
Cardiac arrhythmia
Agitation, hyperactivity, or seizure
Anticholinergic syndromes
Oliguria or renal failure
Clinical relapse

tients who are still stuporous after several hours require brief hospital admission, and patients in whom the particular agent may cause ongoing or delayed complications require admission as well.

Diagnosis

When no history is available, drug overdose should always be considered in comatose patients with or without localizing neurologic findings, but rapid assessment to exclude other causes of this state is necessary. Possible diagnostic considerations include hypoglycemia, hyperglycemia, postictal state, head injury, hypothermia, intracranial bleeding, hepatic or uremic coma, meningoencephalitis, myxedema, and electrolyte imbalance. Some of these conditions may exist as complications of drug overdose when trauma, exposure, infection, or underlying disease is present.

In all patients with coma of unclear cause, 50–100 ml of 50% dextrose in water should be rapidly administered after blood is drawn for glucose determination, since it may be lifesaving should the diagnosis prove to be hypoglycemia. In debilitated or malnourished patients in whom Wernicke-Korsakoff syndrome may be a possibility, dextrose administration should be preceded by thiamine, 50–100 mg intravenously.

When respiratory insufficiency exists or when signs of narcotic abuse are present, such as pinpoint pupils or needle tracks, naloxone hydrochloride, 0.4 mg, should be given parenterally and repeated if necessary. Blood glucose, calcium, and electrolyte levels are often necessary in evaluation of the obtunded patient in whom the cause is unclear. Arterial blood-gas analysis is extremely useful both for assessment of ventilatory adequacy and for determination of acid-base disturbance that might lead to the suspicion of certain drugs with metabolic toxicity, such as methanol, ethylene glycol, and salicylates.

Creatine phosphokinase levels become elevated with rhabdomyolysis, and should be determined along with renal function when uncontrolled seizures occur or when ingested drugs have the potential to cause muscle injury, which may lead to renal failure. Pink or red urine may be an early clue to this possibility.

Drug Removal

Decreased Absorption

Induced emesis or gastric lavage may remove significant amounts of orally ingested drug if utilized properly. Data on the benefit of these techniques are limited to a small number of drugs, but the following guidelines are relevant to many common drug ingestions.

Depressed mental status contraindicates use of induced emesis or lavage because of the risk of aspiration. If the patient is stuporous or comatose, he should be intubated first with a cuffed endotracheal tube. Gastric lavage may then be performed safely. With most drugs, the efficacy of induced emesis or gastric lavage decreases with time, as gastric emptying and absorption take place. After approximately 4 hours, only an insignificant amount of drug may be returned unless the agent has significant anticholinergic properties that may slow gastric emptying and absorption.

Gastric lavage and induced emesis should never be utilized as punitive measures to discourage future ingestion. The inappropriate application of invasive procedures may lead to disastrous consequences. Patients who have ingested a minor amount often do well with supportive care only, with no attempt to remove drug from the gastrointestinal tract. A more serious ingestion, however, warrants consideration of induced emesis or lavage. Contraindications to these techniques include ingestions of strong alkali, corrosive agents such as lye or ammonia, and strong acids. Emptying the stomach after petroleum distillate ingestion remains controversial and is discussed on page 396.

Emesis. Ipecac is the first choice for inducing emesis in a serious overdose, if the patient is alert and relatively cooperative, and if fewer than 4 hours have elapsed since ingestion. It is a safe drug with little toxicity. The dose of syrup of ipecac is 15 ml orally in a 1-year-old to 5-year-old, 30 ml in older children, and 30–60 ml in adults. This must be followed by 6–8 ounces of water in children and four or five 8-ounce glasses of water in adults. Emesis will follow in approximately 20 minutes.

Apomorphine may be used alternatively. It is given parenterally in a dose of 0.1 mg/kg in adults and also requires that the stomach be filled with water. Emesis occurs in 3–5 minutes. Although its onset of action is faster than that of syrup of ipecac, it can produce hypotension and respiratory depression, and it requires time to prepare in fresh solution. In general, ipecac is preferred. Respiratory depression and hypotension secondary to apomorphine administration are reversible with naloxone hydrochloride.

Gastric Lavage. This technique may be utilized if there is no response to ipecac. This may occur with anticholinergic poisonings that are antiemetic. The patient must be alert and cooperative. If mental status is depressed even slightly, endotracheal intubation is necessary.

Data from animal experiments suggest that the spontaneous emesis is more effective in removing drugs, but serious ingestions may require lavage. Efficacy in humans demands proper technique. An Ewalds or similar large-bore tube (at least 28 French or larger) must be used to remove pill fragments. The patient should be in the left lateral decubitus position. With the stomach dependent and the pylorus uppermost, adequate mixing of lavage fluid and stomach contents occurs without excessive loss of fluid into the duodenum. The tube is passed through the mouth, preferably after topical anesthesia in the pharynx to diminish the likelihood of gagging and vomiting. Physiologic saline solution is preferred since water can induce a hypotonic intravascular state in children. In adults, a total of 5–10 liters of fluid is used, although many European centers advocate more than 20 liters. Lavage fluid should be brought to a temperature of approximately 37°C to avoid hypothermia.

Activated Charcoal. This agent may be used after the stomach has been emptied by either emesis or lavage. It should never be given simultaneously with ipecac since it will adsorb ipecac and prevent its action. After the stomach is emptied, 20–50 gm of charcoal is mixed in a slurry with 100–200 ml of water. The slurry can be given orally to a cooperative patient, or it can be instilled via the orogastric tube used for lavage. Activated charcoal binds many organic and inorganic chemicals with the exception of cyanide. It should be followed with a saline cathartic to decrease transit time of drug already in the intestine or bound to charcoal. Magnesium sulfate, 15 gm in adults and 250 mg/kg in children, is effective, as is sorbitol, 50–100 ml of a 70% solution.

Increased Elimination

Forced Diuresis. Some drugs may be removed by increasing urinary excretion. Forced diuresis refers to vigorous administration of intravenous fluids to rates of 200–400 ml/hr in adults, or 5 ml/ kg. This technique along with addition of potent loop diuretics is of benefit only with water-soluble, weakly protein-bound drugs that are excreted by the kidneys, such as phenobarbitol, meprobamate, amphetamines, and lithium salts. Forced diuresis is contraindicated in patients with congestive heart failure, shock, or renal failure. The procedure may be started in the emergency ward, but requires careful monitoring in an inpatient unit to assure electrolyte balance and prevention of volume overload.

Alkalization with sodium bicarbonate to produce a urinary pH of 8 further enhances removal of a drug whose pK is such that it remains ionized in the renal tubule at this pH. This is a useful adjunct to the treatment of overdoses with long-acting barbiturates, salicylates, and isoniazid. Excretion of certain other toxins is enhanced with systemic acidification. Phencyclidine hydrochloride and amphetamine excretion can be increased by acidifying the urine to a pH of less than 5 with ascorbic acid, 8 gm/day, or ammonium chloride, 2.75 mEq/kg every 6 hours orally or intravenously.

Dialysis. Although dialysis is not performed in the emergency ward, it is important for the emergency physician to recognize its place in the treatment of the poisoned patient. In general, peritoneal dialysis or hemodialysis is rarely necessary in most poisonings since supportive management usually suffices. Standard peritoneal dialysis or hemodialysis is only useful for removal of weakly protein-bound drugs and water-soluble substances. Phenobarbital, salicylates, lithium, and meprobamate, for example, can be removed by dialysis, but the technique has no advantage over forced diuresis and may result in increased morbidity. Standard dialysis is of no benefit with lipid-soluble drugs such as glutethimide or highly protein-bound drugs such as short-acting barbiturates, phenothiazine derivatives, tricyclic antidepressants, and benzodiazepines. Charcoal hemoperfusion (dialysis across a column of activated charcoal) is a specialized technique that may be of use with lipid-soluble or protein-bound drugs, but it requires systemic anticoagulant therapy and is associated with coagulation-factor consumption. It should be reserved for life-threatening overdoses with associated renal failure.

In the presence of renal failure, dialysis may be necessary both to support the patient and to remove a water-soluble, weakly protein-bound toxin. Dialysis is also indicated in methyl alcohol and ethylene glycol poisonings (see pages 395–396), and may be required in heavy-metal intoxications after administration of chelating agents. Table 17.3 summarizes the indications for dialysis and potential applications.

Complicating Medical Conditions

Many clinical situations can complicate the management of serious drug ingestions, and knowledge of the pathophysiology of these conditions can help the emergency physician administer proper therapy.

Blood Pressure

Hypotension is commonly seen in overdoses of sedatives, hypnotics, antipsychotics and antidepressants; it is principally caused by dilation of venous capacitance vessels. Unreplaced volume losses in the comatose patient can also contribute to hypotension. Phenothiazines produce venous pooling, but in high doses they can also cause decreased peripheral vascular resistance due to α-adrenergic blockade. In this setting, sympathomimetic amines with β-adrenergic actions, such as isoproterenol hydrochloride, epinephrine, and dopamine, may worsen the shock state by causing vasodilation. Volume replacement is often all that is necessary in drug-overdose-induced hypotension. If a pressor amine is required for a patient with phenothiazine ingestion, predominantly α-adrenergic agents such as phenylephrine hydrochloride or levarterenol bitartrate should be used.

Drug overdoses can also cause hypertension.

Table 17.3.
Dialysis indications and potential applications.

Indications
  Poisoning with water-soluble, poorly protein-bound drugs
  Extreme toxicity with hypotension or renal compromise
  Potentially lethal dose determined by history or blood levels

Dialyzable drugs with markedly increased clearance
  Acetaminophen
  Amphetamines
  Bromides
  Ethanol
  Ethchlorvynol
  Ethylene glycol
  Lithium
  Meprobamate
  Methanol
  Phenobarbital
  Salicylates

This may be a direct effect, as occurs with tricyclic antidepressants or monoamine oxidase inhibitors, or it may be a consequence of hypoxic brain injury. Drug-induced hypertension is often of short duration and requires treatment only if there is evidence of end-organ damage to the brain or heart. For drug-induced hypertension, rapid-acting agents such as nitroprusside should be used so that the effect may be quickly reversed.

Respiratory Failure

In the setting of poisoning or overdose, respiratory failure may have several causes, which may be independent or related. Most often, drug ingestion causes central nervous system depression with hypoventilation and carbon dioxide retention. Naloxone hydrochloride and assisted ventilation are the primary treatment.

Pulmonary edema may be responsible for respiratory failure in patients with drug overdose, most commonly when there has been parenteral narcotic abuse with heroin but also in instances of high-dose salicylate toxicity. The pathophysiology involves an alveolar-capillary leak syndrome, and in parenteral narcotic abuse, it may be a reaction to the adulterants of the drug mixture. The cause is unclear in salicylate poisoning, but in both circumstances, left ventricular function may be adequate and treatment consists of intubation and positive-pressure ventilation. High-dose corticosteroids have been advocated, but are not of proven benefit. Aspiration pneumonia can contribute to respiratory failure as a primary event or as an additional factor in ventilatory depression or pulmonary edema.

Temperature Variations

Hypothermia may complicate treatment of the poisoned patient, and is most commonly due to exposure of a comatose patient to ambient temperature below body temperature. Iatrogenic hypothermia may result from vigorous lavage with fluids at room temperature, and some drugs, such as phenothiazine derivatives, may have a direct effect on the hypothalamic temperature-regulating center. Hypothermia may contribute to the comatose state and to cardiorespiratory depression, and may be initially overlooked unless accurate rectal probe temperatures are obtained. In the absence of cardiorespiratory arrest, slow warming is preferred. Vigorous external rewarming should be avoided since it may cause peripheral vasodilation, vascular compromise, and further temperature drop.

Elevated temperature may be a direct effect of some drugs such as salicylates, tricyclic antidepressants, and other anticholinergic agents. Temperature elevation with salicylates is related to the associated hypermetabolic state; with tricyclic antidepressants and other anticholinergic drugs, peripheral heat loss is reduced and central nervous system thermoregulation may be affected.

Uncontrolled seizures or unrecognized infection may also contribute to hyperthermia. Fever always demands careful consideration of occult infection as a primary or secondary problem. Significant hyperpyrexia should be reduced with external cooling to minimize insensitive fluid losses and to reduce the impact of heat stress on already compromised organ systems.

Anticholinergic Syndromes

Atropine, antihistamines, phenothiazine derivatives, and tricyclic antidepressants may cause a spectrum of complications that are commonly referred to as anticholinergic syndromes. In addition, certain plants such as jimson weed, belladonna (deadly nightshade), bittersweet, and the *Amanita muscaria* mushroom may have anticholinergic properties (Table 17.4). Commonly available proprietary sleep-aids contain various antihistamines, usually methapyrilene or scopolamine (Table 17.5). These sleep-aids are widely advertised as safe, but their efficacy is doubtful and, in overdose quantities, they can cause serious poisoning.

Peripheral and central nervous system effects as well as cardiac arrhythmias are seen in patients with anticholinergic poisoning. Classical features include dry skin, flushing, mild fever, urinary retention, confusion, tachycardia, and mild hypertension. Hypotension may also occur in patients with a large overdose. Blurred vision with secondary mydriasis is common. Central nervous system effects include agitation, seizures, and confusion leading to stupor and coma in high doses. These drugs cause atrial and ventricular arrhythmias, as well as conduction disturbances, because of their quinidine-like effect on the heart. Cardiac and central nervous system features may be increased by coexistent fever, hypoxemia, or electrolyte imbalance.

Physostigmine, a cholinesterase inhibitor, may be administered to temporarily reverse peripheral, central, and cardiac effects of anticholinergic poisoning. Quarternary cholinesterase inhibitors such as neostigmine and edrophonium chloride are not effective in the reversal of central nervous system effects since they do not cross the blood-brain barrier. Anticholinergic drugs block parasympa-

Table 17.4.
Sources of anticholinergic poisoning.

Drugs and chemicals
  Atropine
  Belladonna
  Benactyzine hydrochloride
  Chlorpheniramine maleate
  Cyclopentolate hydrochloride
  Dicyclomine hydrochloride
  Diphenhydramine hydrochoride
  Homatropine
  Hyoscine (scopolamine)
  Hyoscyamus
  Isopropamide iodide
  Mepenzolate bromide
  Methantheline bromide
  Methapyrilene
  Phenothiazine derivatives
  Pipenzolate methylbromide
  Propantheline bromide
  Pyrilamine maleate
  Stramonium
  Tricyclic antidepressants
    Amitriptyline hydrochloride
    Desipramine hydrochloride
    Doxepin hydrochloride
    Imipramine hydrochloride
    Nortriptyline hydrochloride
    Protriptyline hydrochloride
Plants
  Amanita muscaria
  Belladonna (deadly nightshade)
  Bittersweet
  Black henbane
  Jerusalem cherry
  Jimson weed
  Lantana
  Potato tuber
  Wild tomato

thetic nerve endings and motor endplates and prevent the action of acetylcholine on muscle, glands, heart, and brain. Physostigmine reverses this effect by diminishing the cholinesterase-mediated metabolism, resulting in increases in acetylcholine (Fig. 17.1).

As an antidote for anticholinergic poisoning, physostigmine should be given with caution since cholinergic excess can result and too rapid infusion can cause seizures. Physostigmine may cause bronchospasm, as well as nausea, vomiting, and abdominal pain, and it is contraindicated in patients with asthma. It should only be given after initial stabilization of the airway and ventilation. In patients with peripheral or central manifestations of anticholinergic excess, it may be tried for the following conditions: malignant cardiac arrhythmias uncontrollable with standard drugs, hyper-

tension with end-organ compromise, and uncontrolled seizures. Patients in coma may respond to physostigmine given as a diagnostic test, but coma alone is not an indication for ongoing treatment, nor is a response totally diagnostic of anticholinergic poisoning. In adults, 2 mg intravenously can be given slowly over approximately 3–5 minutes. The half-life of the drug is 1–2 hours, and repeated doses may be necessary since the duration of action may be less than that of the anticholinergic compound.

Alternative therapeutic strategies for patients with anticholinergic poisoning involve use of lidocaine hydrochloride, propranolol hydrochloride, or phenytoin for serious cardiac arrhythmias and conduction disturbances, which may also benefit from sodium bicarbonate administration. Seizures may be treated with phenytoin, and severe hypertension with end-organ compromise will respond to rapid-acting agents such as nitroprusside, but appropriate monitoring should be available.

Seizures

Agitation, hyperactivity, and seizures may complicate drug overdose. Dystonic movements and extrapyramidal reactions may be seen with phenothiazine overdose and should be distinguished from seizures. Careful observation of the patient after assuring adequacy of the airway often provides the clue, since posturing is frequently characteristic. Dystonic reactions may be reversed by diphenhydramine hydrochloride (Benadryl), 25–50 mg intravenously. Restraints should be applied to any patient in danger of injuring himself, but sedation should be used with great care, lest it be additive to the central nervous system depressant effects of the drug overdose.

Overdoses of propoxyphene, tricyclic antidepressants, and phenothiazine derivatives may cause seizures directly, but central nervous system hypoxemia, coexistent trauma, electrolyte disturbances, and underlying seizure disorders may also be contributory. Uncontrolled seizures can lead to rhabdomyolysis and pigment-induced renal failure; hyperthermia may also result. Intravenous phenytoin is the treatment of choice for seizures in patients with drug overdose. Diazepam and barbiturates should be avoided because they may contribute to central nervous system depression.

Renal Failure

Commonly abused drugs are usually not nephrotoxic, and when oliguria and acute renal fail-

Table 17.5.
Commonly available sleep aids.

Product (Manufacturer)	Scopolamine	Antihistamine	Analgesic
Compoz Tablets (Jeffrey Martin)		Methapyrilene hydrochloride, 15 mg; Pyrilamine maleate, 10 mg	
Dormin Capsules (Dormin)		Methapyrilene hydrochloride, 25 mg	
Nervine Capsule-Shaped Tablets (Miles)		Methapyrilene hydrochloride, 25 mg	
Nervine Effervescent Tablets (Miles)		Methapyrilene fumarate, equivalent to 25 mg of hydrochloride	
Nervine Liquid (Miles)		Methapyrilene fumarate, equivalent to 5 mg of hydrochloride/ml	
Nite Rest Capsules (Amer. Pharm.)	Aminoxide hydrobromide 0.25 mg	Methapyrilene hydrochloride, 50 mg	
Nytol Capsules & Tablets (Block)		Methapyrilene hydrochloride, 50 mg/cap., 25 mg/tab.	
Quiet World Tablets (Whitehall)		Pyrilamine maleate, 25 mg	Aspirin, 227.5 mg; Acetaminophen, 162.5 mg
Relax-U-Caps (Columbia Medical)		Methapyrilene hydrochloride, 25 mg	
Sedacaps (Vitarine)		Methapyrilene hydrochloride, 25 mg	
Seedate Capsules (Amer. Pharm.)	Aminoxide hydrobromide, 0.125 mg	Methapyrilene hydrochloride, 25 mg	
Sleep-Eze Tablets (Whitehall)		Pyrilamine maleate, 25 mg	
Sleepinal Capsules (Thompson)		Methapyrilene hydrochloride, 50 mg	
Sominex Tablets & Capsules (J. B. Williams)	Aminoxide hydrobromide, 0.25 mg/tab., 0.5 mg/cap.	Methapyrilene hydrochloride, 25 mg/tab., 50 mg cap.	Salicylamide, 200 mg/tab. or capsule
Somnicaps (Amer. Pharm.)		Methapyrilene hydrochloride, 25 mg	
Tranqium Capsules (Thompson)		Methapyrilene hydrochloride, 50 mg	
Tranquil Capsules (North American)		Methapyrilene fumarate, 25 mg	Sodium salicylate, 25 mg; Acetaminophen, 25 mg
Twilight Capsules (Pfeiffer)		Methapyrilene hydrochloride, 25 mg	Salicylamide, 300 mg

From: *Handbook of Nonprescription Drugs.* American Pharmaceutical Association, Washington, DC, Sixth Edition, 1977.

PATHOPHYSIOLOGY OF ANTICHOLINERGIC SYNDROME

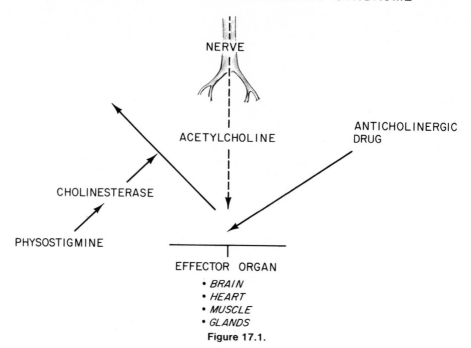

Figure 17.1.

ure occur, the condition is often a consequence of renal hypoperfusion and shock. Pigmented urine secondary to rhabdomyolysis may occur with phencyclidine hydrochloride and drugs associated with prolonged seizures, and it may contribute to renal failure. With anticholinergic drugs, urinary retention may occur. The bladder should be palpated; if it is distended, use of a Foley catheter will establish the diagnosis.

Clinical Relapse

Clinical relapse is a feature of many drug ingestions. A patient who awakens after several hours of care may still require observation. Anticholinergic drugs may have slowed gastrointestinal uptake because of drug-induced ileus or delayed gastric emptying, and the patient's condition may deteriorate after initial improvement. In a multiple drug overdose, the effect of one agent may wane before the effect of a second agent becomes maximal. In addition, drugs such as glutethimide and phencyclidine hydrochloride are highly lipid-soluble and have enterohepatic circulation resulting in a waxing and waning course.

Psychiatric Considerations

Treatment of the poisoned patient does not end with control of clinical complications. Psychiatric evaluation is essential to establish the intent or suicidal risk and to determine the social supports available to the patient. Many overdoses that are medically not serious are actually high risk because of the psychiatric implications.

After a patient's medical condition becomes satisfactory, a psychiatrist or trained psychiatric nurse or social worker should assist in the determination of suicidal intent. The patient must have a clear mental status for the psychiatrist or psychiatric worker to make a complete assessment. If an emergency ward does not provide space for supportive care in a holding unit, the patient will often have to be admitted until a complete psychiatric evaluation unencumbered by a drug-depressed mental state is possible. The environment in the emergency ward and hospital must offer protection from further self-induced injury as well. Restraints may be necessary, and equipment such as knife blades, needles, and drugs should not be in the immediate vicinity of the patient.

Each patient must be viewed as being at a high risk until all of the data are available to judge completely the potential for serious injury. It is far better to admit the patient for supportive short-term care than to run the risk of a repeated attempt with a fatal outcome.

Many patients do not have to be hospitalized if supportive help is available on an outpatient basis and if family supports are strong. The elderly, alcoholic, drug-dependent, or psychiatrically high-risk patient with a violent method or with an attempt involving little likelihood of rescue will usually require hospitalization, as will psychotic and severely depressed patients.

Whereas poisonings in children are most often accidental, such an event may be a manifestation of social disorder in the home, parental neglect, or frank child abuse by a parent or sibling. The emergency physician and psychiatric staff must be alert to this phenomenon and must involve appropriate community resources if further injury is to be prevented.

SPECIFIC POISONINGS

In this section, the treatment of selected poisonings is discussed. The selections represent an effort to address both common and controversial problems facing the emergency physician. A list of clinical papers relating to these and to less common poisonings is supplied at the end of this chapter.

Narcotics

Poisoning with narcotics is a common problem in the United States. When it is associated with parenteral drug abuse, there is often coexistent medical illness. When the patient's condition is stabilized, the physician must be alert to common infectious complications. Hepatitis is often seen, as well as local and systemic bacterial infections such as skin abscess, cellulitis, septicemia, endocarditis, septic thromboembolism, and occasionally, tetanus.

Overdose with opiates results in central nervous system and respiratory depression with hypotension. Pulmonary edema may occur, perhaps related to adulterants in the injected drug mixture, such as quinine, lactose, and fruit sugars. The pupils are commonly pinpoint, except in the case of meperidine hydrochloride where the pupils are normal to slightly dilated. Support of the airway and administration of the narcotic antagonist naloxone hydrochloride to reverse respiratory depression are first measures. Repeated doses of naloxone are often required, since the half-life of the drug is often longer than that of the antagonist.

Determination of the route of overdose administration is very important. Emesis or lavage has no efficacy if the drug has been parenterally injected, but should be utilized in oral ingestions if the patient is alert. In comatose patients with oral ingestions, the stomach should be emptied after the airway has been intubated. Concurrent aspirin or acetaminophen toxicity may complicate the patient's course when a narcotic has been ingested

in fixed combinations with these agents. Blood levels are necessary to determine coexistent toxicity and to guide therapy.

Corticosteroids have been advocated for pulmonary edema resulting from opiate overdose, but there are no good scientific data to support this. These patients require intubation, positive-pressure ventilation, and intensive care.

Barbiturates

Barbiturates are sedative drugs that are frequently abused in the United States and elsewhere. They are responsible for nearly 20% of the hospitalizations resulting from acute poisoning in the United States. Barbiturates are usually classified according to the duration of clinical action, which is determined by the rate of absorption, lipid solubility, serum binding, and mode of metabolism. Absorption from the intestine is limited by the rate of dissolution and dispersal in the gastrointestinal contents. Barbiturates are absorbed more rapidly if taken with ethanol or on an empty stomach.

Short-acting barbiturates such as amobarbital, sodium pentobarbital, and secobarbital have a duration of therapeutic action of 4–6 hours. They are primarily metabolized to inactive products by the liver. Toxic effects usually occur at blood levels of 3 mg/dl and higher; in most cases, this requires ingestion of 5 mg/kg of drug in children and 4 mg/kg in adults.

The long-acting barbiturates such as phenobarbital are excreted mainly unchanged by the kidneys, and have a therapeutic life of 12–24 hours. Serum levels above 8 mg/dl are toxic if the barbiturate is taken "acutely," but tolerance occurs and many patients on long-term therapy are asymptomatic with high blood levels. Ingestion of 8–10 mg/kg acutely produces a toxic level.

Respiratory depression is the major toxic effect assessed clinically and with arterial blood-gas analysis. Aspiration pneumonia is common, and necrotizing pneumonia is a frequent cause of death in these patients. Pulmonary edema is seen occasionally and is usually due to fluid overload and coexistent myocardial impairment. Hypothermia may occur as a result of depression of temperature regulation in the brainstem. Cutaneous bullae are seen frequently and are helpful in diagnosis, although they are not specific for barbiturate intoxication. They occur over pressure areas within a few hours after drug ingestion.

Treatment is primarily supportive, with attention to airway management. Positive-pressure ventilation is necessary if ventilatory failure is present; the patient should be observed for pneumothroax throughout the hospital course since many pulmonary infections are necrotizing and cause blebs that can rupture into the pleural space.

Shock should be treated by correction of hypoxemia and acidosis and by plasma expansion. Forced diuresis with systemic alkalization to produce a urinary pH of 8 enhances excretion of long-acting barbiturates. Urinary output should be advanced to 3–6 ml/kg/hr with careful attention to electrolyte and volume status. Hemodialysis can be used, but should be reserved for extreme toxic reactions and for the patient with renal failure. With short-acting barbiturates, forced diuresis or hemodialysis offers no benefit since these drugs are relatively more protein-bound and liver metabolized. Charcoal resin hemoperfusion can be considered for patients with severe intoxication from short-acting barbiturates.

Salicylates

Salicylate poisoning remains the most commonly reported poisoning in the United States, occurring frequently in children less than 6 years old. Intentional poisoning in adults is common, but accidental overdose occurs in the adult population as well. In such a situation, the patient is seen in the emergency ward with altered mental status, and the major indicator as to cause is an unexplained metabolic acidosis. A dose of 150 mg/kg is usually associated with toxicity (35 tablets or 10 gm in adults), although toxicity can vary, with fatalities in adults reported after ingestion of 10–30 gm but survival reported with a single dose in excess of 100 gm. The prevalence of salicylates in poisonings relates in part to the large number of salicylate products on the market. Among these is the highly toxic methyl salicylate found in wintergreen oil and linaments. One teaspoon of this preparation provides 3 gm of salicylate and is a source of considerable toxicity in children, who may be attracted to the bottle by its color or smell.

With either purposeful or accidental mild salicylate intoxication, salicylism occurs, characterized in the clinical setting by tinnitus, diminished hearing, and vertigo. With more moderate doses, nausea and vomiting occur along with hyperventilation and confusion. More severe toxicity is associated with tachycardia, hyperpyrexia, and mental torpor, with seizures, coma, cardiorespiratory compromise, and pulmonary edema at the extreme.

Salicylic acid salts are rapidly absorbed from the gastrointestinal tract, but absorption of commercial products varies in relation to tablet dissolution and gastric motility. Although the drug is usually well absorbed in the stomach and small intestine and bound in part (50–80%) to albumin, tablets occasionally combine to form a large bolus that may continue to be absorbed for several days. Free salicylate is conjugated in the liver and eventually excreted by the kidneys.

Saturation of hepatic metabolic pathways occurs rapidly in overdoses, but may also occur slowly with increased therapeutic doses or decreased intervals of administration. The half-life of the drug is therefore variable, increasing from 4 hours with a low dose to as much as 30 hours in patients with salicylate toxicity. Accidental self-poisoning in the adult is produced by this changing half-life that allows a progressive increase in the level of salicylate in the blood.

Salicylates stimulate the central respiratory drive center, causing hyperventilation, hypocapnia, and initially, respiratory alkalosis in adults. Renal loss of bicarbonate occurs in compensation. Children are more commonly acidemic on presentation, with buffering capacity overwhelmed. In mild cases, adults may have a relatively normal pH along with renal compensation. In extreme situations, however, respiratory center depression occurs, with carbon dioxide retention and respiratory acidosis adding to the metabolic acidosis caused by the lactate and keto acids produced by the effect of salicylate on the Krebs cycle.

Salicylate excess also interferes with carbohydrate metabolism. Depletion of tissue stores of glucose may result in hypoglycemia, but hyperglycemia may also occur because of the variability of metabolism, level of tissue stores, and rate of consumption. Hypoglycemia may be worsened by nausea, vomiting, and diminished oral intake.

Hyperpyrexia can occur, and is occasionally severe. Increased heat production by inefficient oxidative phosphorylation may not be eliminated rapidly enough to maintain homeostasis since the sweating mechanism may be impaired in a dehydrated, vomiting patient.

Microscopic gastrointestinal bleeding is common with therapeutic doses of salicylates, and increased bleeding has been assumed for larger toxic doses. The incidence of massive bleeding is low despite the multiple effects that salicylates produce on the hematologic system, including interference with prothrombin production and platelet function and an increase in capillary permeability. Acute renal failure occurs rarely and is usually a result of dehydration and hypotension.

Laboratory studies are helpful in the evaluation and treatment of salicylate poisoning. Arterial blood-gas levels should be used to determine the acid-base status of the patient. Substantial hypoglycemia and hypokalemia occasionally develop, and should be treated. Hypokalemia may be due to intracellular shifts owing to early alkalosis or to renal and gastrointestinal losses. If the patient is acidotic, the degree of hypokalemia may be underestimated.

Plasma salicylate levels more than 30 mg/dl can cause a toxic reaction, with moderate toxicity usually seen at levels of 30–70 mg/dl and severe toxicity at levels in excess of 70–100 mg/dl (Table 17.6). Because of the variability of absorption and tissue saturation, one blood-level determination may not reflect the peak, and reliance should be placed more on serial determinations and on other clinical and laboratory findings. A rising blood level may also suggest that tablets have agglomerated in the stomach. Even after 4–6 hours, gastric lavage or emesis may be of benefit. Forced diuresis should be employed with attention to cardiac status to avoid volume overload, particularly in patients with severe poisoning in whom pulmonary edema may develop as the result of an alveolocapillary leak syndrome and in whom it may be worsened by volume excess. Sodium bicarbonate, 2–3 mg/kg intravenously, to normalize or slightly alkalinize serum pH and increase urinary pH to 8 enhances urinary excretion in the acidemic patient. Hemodialysis is indicated in cases of severe toxicity with cardiac impairment and pulmonary edema, or when there is major compromise to renal function.

Acetaminophen

Increased use of acetaminophen as an antipyretic and analgesic has led to its appearance as a common overdose agent, either alone or in fixed combination with other analgesics such as propoxyphene, oxycodone, and codeine. In adults, 10–15 gm can produce serious toxicity and may be fatal. The blood level is the key to determination of potential toxicity; ideally, the blood level should be determined and then repeated after several hours to confirm the need for therapy (Fig. 17.2).

The liver is the major organ affected by acetaminophen toxicity, and the clinical features of the poisoning may be divided into three phases. In the early phase, up to 24 hours after ingestion, the patient may have mild anorexia, nausea, vomiting, and diaphoresis, but occasionally there may be little evidence of toxicity unless other drugs have been simultaneously ingested. This underscores the importance of the history, since the patient may be seen in the emergency ward with depression or suicidal ideation without the usual signs of drug overdose. Early recognition of this

Table 17.6.
Clinical features of salicylate intoxication.

Level of Toxicity	Manifestations
Mild (<30 mg/dl)	Salicylism with tinnitus, deafness, nausea
Moderate (30–70 mg/dl)	Salicylism, vomiting, confusion, fever, acid-base and electrolyte disturbances
Severe (>70 mg/dl)	Pulmonary edema, cardiorespiratory failure, coma

poisoning is important to the therapeutic outcome.

In the second phase of acetaminophen toxicity, from 24–48 hours, the patient may feel initially improved, but abnormal liver function will be detectable and pain in the right upper abdominal quadrant may develop as hepatic toxicity proceeds. In the third phase, from 2–5 days, the sequelae of hepatic necrosis occur, with jaundice, coagulopathy, and encephalopathy.

Acetaminophen is rapidly absorbed from the gastrointestinal tract, with peak levels occurring in 30–60 minutes at therapeutic doses. The drug is metabolized in the liver by the cytochrome P-450 mixed function oxidase system to an active intermediate metabolite that is normally detoxified by conjugation with glutathione. In overdose situations, glutathione is depleted, allowing increased intermediate metabolites that are toxic to liver cells. These intermediate metabolites bind to hepatic microsomes and cause cell death.

Treatment of acetaminophen poisoning requires administration of a sulfhydril-containing substitute for glutathione. If it is given early after ingestion, hepatic injury may be substantially reduced. Methionine and cysteamine have been shown to be effective, but acetylcysteine is currently the drug of choice. These agents provide sulfhydril groups that bind the toxic intermediate metabolites. The stomach should be emptied, but charcoal should not be used since it will adsorb acetylcysteine. Blood samples should be drawn for determination of acetaminophen level, but if the history suggests the potential for toxicity and less than 24 hours have passed since ingestion, therapy should be started and either continued or stopped when blood-level results are available. Table 17.7 summarizes the dosage schedule for acetylcysteine, which may be given orally or by nasogastric tube. If more than 24 hours have passed since ingestion, supportive measures should be used without acetylcysteine. Nausea and vomiting may occur as side effects, but in general, the drug is adequately tolerated.

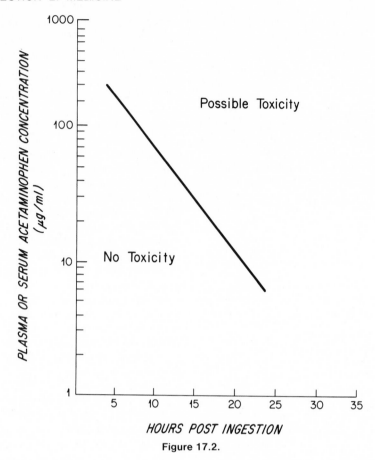

Figure 17.2.

Table 17.7.
Treatment of acetaminophen poisoning.

Empty stomach with induced emesis or lavage as appropriate.

Do not use activated charcoal.

If < 24 hours since ingestion, administer acetylcysteine in a 20% solution diluted 1:3 in cola, grapefruit juice, orange juice, or water:
140 mg/kg orally in loading dose
70 mg/kg orally every 4 hours for 68 hours (17 doses)

Start treatment pending confirmation by blood-level determination. If > 24 hours since ingestion, provide supportive measures.

Benzodiazepines

The benzodiazepine group of drugs (diazepam, chlordiazepoxide hydrochloride, oxazepam, and others) are among the most commonly prescribed pharmaceuticals in the United States. Used primarily as antianxiety agents or as muscle relaxants, they are also frequently prescribed indiscriminately and patients are commonly seen in emergency wards with minor and major overdoses. These drugs have a wide therapeutic range and are relatively safe. Mild to moderate overdoses are associated with initial excitement followed by drowsiness, dysarthria, and confusion; more severe overdoses result in coma with respiratory depression. Overdoses of 1–2 gm require supportive measures, but fatalities have not been reported resulting solely from these drugs.

However, these drugs are also commonly seen in overdoses involving multiple pharmaceuticals or street drugs plus alcohol. In this setting, major morbidity may occur, and death can ensue that is often due to ventilatory depression. Toxicologic assays may determine the presence of these agents, but should not be solely relied on in clinical decision-making both because of the difficulty in assaying for the agents and because of the inherent unreliability of commercial assays themselves.

Reports of response to physostigmine have recently been published, but sufficient data are not available to warrant this treatment, with its risks of cholinergic excess. Supportive measures usually suffice.

Glutethimide

Glutethimide causes serious poisoning because a very small amount of the drug yields significant toxicity, particularly in combination with alcohol or other sedative hypnotic agents. As few as 10–20 500-mg tablets may cause death in adults.

The drug is highly lipid soluble, with relatively rapid intestinal uptake and concentration in brain and adipose tissue. Although blood levels are easily determined, they do not always correlate with the clinical findings or with the severity of the poisoning.

Glutethimide overdose is similar to barbiturate intoxication in that stupor, coma, respiratory depression, and hypotension are key features. Glutethimide may be associated with a fluctuating mental status that is probably related to changing levels of the drug in the blood and brain. Hyperthermia is associated with coma and may develop slowly over 24 hours. The skin may be dry and flushed as in anticholinergic poisonings, and the pupils are often widely dilated.

The stomach should be emptied with emesis or lavage. Reports have advocated lavage with castor oil emulsion, which may theoretically absorb the drug in the stomach. Standard lavage followed by administration of activated charcoal is preferable, as the efficacy of castor oil lavage is unproven. The airway must be protected to prevent aspiration of lavage material, particularly if castor oil is used.

Since the drug is lipid soluble, forced diuresis is of no benefit, and vigorous volume expansion may overwhelm a hypokinetic cardiovascular system and result in pulmonary edema. Lipid hemodialysis has been attempted, but charcoal hemoperfusion is probably the preferred treatment in severe cases complicated by hypotension and shock.

Amphetamines

The amphetamines are noncatecholamine sympathomimetic drugs that stimulate both the α- and β-adrenergic nerve endings, producing central nervous system and cardiorespiratory stimulation. In therapeutic doses, these drugs may temporarily diminish fatigue and improve the patient's sense of well-being, but in overdoses of 15–25 mg/kg, a toxic delirium may give way to seizures, hyperpyrexia, and cardiovascular compromise.

Chronic amphetamine abuse may lead to amphetamine psychosis manifested by paranoia delusions, and hallucinosis, but with preservation of orientation and memory. Chronic abuse may also be associated with nausea, vomiting, diarrhea, and weight loss. In chronic intravenous use, necrotizing angiitis and intracerebral hemorrhage have been described.

The drug is rapidly absorbed over 1–2 hours. Metabolism of 30–40% of the parent drug takes place in the liver, followed by excretion of metabolites along with free drug via the kidneys. With a pK of 9.9, amphetamines have a pH-dependent urinary excretion pattern that is enhanced by acidification and delayed by alkalinization.

If the drug has been taken orally, the stomach should be emptied and charcoal administered. Patients who are extremely agitated or anxious can be calmed with haloperidol, 2–5 mg, or chlorpromazine, 1 mg/kg every 4–6 hours. Severe hypertension with end-organ compromise should be treated with either phentolamine or phenoxybenzamine hydrochloride, nitroprusside, or diazeoxide. Severe hyperthermia can mimic heat stroke, and may be associated with coagulopathy and acute renal failure. Temperature elevations will respond to vigorous external cooling, with chlorpromazine administration to prevent shivering and further temperature elevation.

Since some of the drug is excreted unchanged in the urine, forced diuresis with systemic acidification will enhance removal. Either ammonium chloride, 2.75 mEq/kg every 6 hours intravenously or by nasogastric tube, or ascorbic acid, 8 gm/day, can be given in both acute and chronic poisonings. Dialysis greatly enhances clearance, but is rarely needed if adequate supportive measures are instituted.

Tricyclic Antidepressants

Drugs of this group (amitriptyline hydrochloride, imipramine hydrochloride, nortriptyline hydrochloride, protriptyline hydrochloride, desipramine hydrochloride, doxepin hydrochloride, and others) are common causes of hospitalization for drug overdose in the adult population in certain areas of the United States. The large number of antidepressants should not be a source of confusion in management since their clinical presentation is similar. Poisoning with tricyclic antidepressants usually occurs as a suicide attempt by a depressed individual, and is not generally part of street drug abuse.

Doses of 1.5–3.0 gm of tricyclic drugs result in serious poisonings with potentially fatal outcomes. The clinical features are those of initial central nervous system excitation followed by depression with seizures and anticholinergic syndromes, hypertension followed by hypotension, and cardiac effects including atrial and ventricular arrhythmias and conduction disturbances. There may be mild temperature elevation, urinary retention, and a progressively deteriorating course despite good initial management.

Blood levels of more than 1000 ng/ml correlate with significant toxicity, but measurements are usually not rapidly available and may be unreliable. However, Biggs et al. (1977) has shown that this level, which is highly associated with the risk of serious cardiac arrhythmias, seizures, coma, and the need for ventilatory support, correlates with prolongation of the QRS interval on the electrocardiogram. In the absence of prior conduction disease, QRS-interval prolongation of .10 msec or more should be sought as an indicator of major toxicity.

Treatment of tricyclic ingestions involves standard initial supportive measures. These drugs are antiemetic, but administration of ipecac early after ingestion may still be of benefit. In more serious ingestions with central nervous system and respiratory depression, the airway should be intubated, the stomach lavaged, and activated charcoal instilled, followed by administration of a saline cathartic. The anticholinergic properties of the drug result in ileus with delayed gastric emptying and possibly delayed intestinal uptake; as a result, efforts to remove drug from the gastrointestinal tract may be beneficial even after 3–4 hours.

Cardiac arrhythmias are most often supraventricular, but serious ventricular arrhythmias (ectopy, tachycardia, and fibrillation) occur because of quinidine-like effect of these drugs. These arrhythmias are more likely in the setting of hypoxemia, acidosis, and underlying ischemic cardiac disease. The risk of developing late cardiac arrhythmias with tricyclic antidepressant poisoning is controversial, and decisions on the need to admit and monitor patients with less serious poisonings (without hypotension, respiratory depression, or seizures) must be made in the absence of good data to guide the emergency physician.

Suggested guidelines regarding this issue include the following:

(1) Patients with ventricular arrhythmias or conduction disturbances on admission to the emergency ward or developing within several hours of observation should be admitted and monitored until arrhythmias cease.

(2) Patients with no arrhythmias or anticholinergic findings who are mentally alert enough for psychiatric treatment probably have a low risk for late significant arrhythmias.

(3) Patients with anticholinergic findings and sinus tachycardia of more than 110 beats/min may require monitoring until the clinical course is defined more clearly.

Physostigmine can be administered to reverse the central and peripheral anticholinergic effects of tricyclic antidepressants, but many tricyclic poisonings can be treated conservatively without it. Rapid bolus administration may precipitate seizures in patients with tricyclic poisoning, and severe bradyarrhythmias or asystole may occur. In general, physostigmine should be utilized for diagnosis in patients with unexplained coma and associated anticholinergic findings, since better alternatives exist for treatment of cardiac arrhythmias, seizures, and hypertension. Hypotension resulting from anticholinergic and tricyclic agents is generally poorly responsive to physostigmine, unless it is strictly due to reversible tachyarrhythmia.

Serious ventricular arrhythmias in patients with tricyclic antidepressant poisoning should be treated with intravenous lidocaine hydrochloride, 50–75 mg intravenously, followed by a 1–4 mg/min infusion. Small doses of propranolol hydrochloride, 1 mg/min up to 5 mg total, may be of benefit in the absence of cardiac failure and volume overload, and bretylium tosylate, 5–10 mg/kg intravenously, may be used for refractory ventricular tachycardia or fibrillation. Systemic alkalinization with 1–2 ampules of sodium bicarbonate or by means of transient hyperventilation of the intubated patient has been reported to be successful adjunctive therapy for ventricular arrhythmias caused by tricyclic antidepressants, even in the absence of acidosis. The mechanism of this effect is not completely understood.

Physostigmine for ventricular arrhythmias has theoretical benefit, but should be used as a backup to other therapies, because of the risk of cholinergic excess. Phenytoin reverses tricyclic-induced atrioventricular block and conduction disturbances, and may also diminish ventricular ectopy. Its use, however, in patients with tricyclic-related QRS-interval prolongation and a stable hemodynamic pattern has not yet been fully evaluated.

Hypotension usually responds to intravenous volume expansion with crystalloid or colloid. In general, sympathomimetic agents should be avoided, but when necessary, levarterenol bitartrate is a good choice since it provides some α-adrenergic peripheral vasoconstriction without significant cardiac effects.

Seizures should be treated with intravenous phenytoin, a 50- to 100-mg bolus slowly over 5 minutes, repeated to a total dose of 800–1000 mg as necessary. Barbiturates and diazepam should be avoided because of their additive effect to central nervous system or respiratory depression. Physostigmine, 1–2 mg given slowly intravenously, may help abort seizures in tricyclic antidepressant overdose, but should be used cautiously since a more rapid bolus may precipitate or prolong seizures.

These drugs are highly protein-bound and poorly water soluble, so forced diuresis and standard hemodialysis are of no benefit. In severely poisoned patients with refractory hypotension, charcoal hemoperfusion should be considered.

Phenothiazines

Phenothiazine derivatives are commonly given for their antipsychotic effects and for the treatment of nausea and vomiting. These drugs may be divided into three classes, aliphatic, piperidine, and piperazine compounds. The pharmacologic effects of each group are slightly different, but in general, piperidine compounds (for example, thioridazine hydrochloride) and aliphatic compounds (for example, chlorpromazine) produce sedation and hypotension rather than central nervous system excitation in overdoses, whereas piperazine compounds (for example, perphenazine) tend to have an excitatory phase with agitation and extrapyramidal effects before central nervous system depression occurs.

In major overdoses of 2–4 gm, the clinical features include confusion, delirium, seizures, and coma with anticholinergic stimulation. Extrapyramidal reactions, including posturing, oculogyric crisis, and muscle spasm in the face and neck, may be confused with seizure activity. Hyperthermia may occur on an anticholinergic basis or secondary to hypothalamic effects, but hypothermia has also been reported with exposure. Cardiac effects are in part anticholinergic, with a quinidine-like toxicity producing conduction disturbances and atrial and ventricular arrhythmias. Hypotension is due to both phenothiazine-induced α-adrenergic blockade and splanchnic vasodilation with relative hypovolemia. Respiratory depression occurs when the doses are sufficient to cause coma.

Although as little as 2 gm of a phenothiazine derivative can cause death in adults, patients on chronic maintenance therapy may survive much higher single overdoses. In children, 350 mg of chlorpromazine has been reported to cause death.

Although these agents are antiemetic, ipecac may be of benefit soon after ingestion and before the development of sedation. If a major overdose is suspected and the patient is stuporous or comatose, the airway should be secured, lavage performed, and activated charcoal instilled. Extrapyramidal reactions often respond rapidly to diphenhydramine hydrochloride, 25–50 mg intravenously, which may be repeated if necessary. Seizures should be treated with phenytoin.

The emergency physician should treat phenothiazine-induced hypotension with volume expansion. Sympathomimetic agents are rarely needed. However, if a pressor agent is required, agents with β-adrenergic activity such as low doses of dopamine or isoproterenol hydrochloride should be avoided. These agents may worsen hypotension because of peripheral β-adrenergic vasodilation in the setting of phenothiazine-induced α-adrenergic blockade.

Patients with ventricular ectopy and conduction disturbances require cardiac monitoring. Supraventricular tachycardia is common, but rarely requires treatment. Quinidine and procainamide hydrochloride should be avoided in the treatment of ventricular ectopy since they may add to the cardiotoxic effects. Lidocaine hydrochloride, phenytoin, or propranolol hydrochloride may be given, with sodium bicarbonate as an adjunctive agent as in tricyclic antidepressant poisonings. Physostigmine may also be of benefit in patients with these arrhythmias.

Phenothiazine derivatives may be ingested in fixed combination with tricyclic antidepressants (Triavil) or as part of a multiple drug ingestion. Qualitative analysis for the presence of phenothiazines is not difficult for most toxicology laboratories, but quantitative analysis is unreliable since blood levels may not correlate with the patient's clinical course. Because these drugs are protein-bound, treatment with forced diuresis is of no benefit.

Cocaine

Increasing numbers of patients are being treated in emergency wards for toxic effects from cocaine, one of the most common recreational drugs of abuse. Although it is costly, it has been advocated as a relatively safe drug when used intranasally, but deaths have occurred by this route as well as by oral ingestion and intravenous injection.

Cocaine is an alkaloid extract of the leaves of *Erythroxylon coca.* A topical anesthetic, it blocks peripheral nerve conduction. Cocaine also has prominent central nervous system stimulation properties, and its illicit use depends on this phenomenon.

The drug is usually sold as a powder, adulterated with mannitol, sugars, or other drugs such as lidocaine hydrochloride, phencyclidine, or amphetamine. It is most often taken by intranasal insufflation, which is followed in 5–20 minutes by pharmacologic effects. Intravenous and pulmonary absorption is also rapid; oral administration results in absorption in the small intestine at a pK of 8.5, but gastric hydrolysis may diminish the effect.

Central nervous system stimulation begins rapidly, with a sense of euphoria and excitement associated with pupillary dilation and increased heart rate, blood pressure, and respiration rate. Occasionally, dysphoria occurs acutely, with confusion, apprehension, and hallucinosis. Chronic use may be associated with hallucinosis and a syndrome of schizophrenia with paranoia. In addition, the nasal septum may become perforated as a result of vasoconstriction and tissue loss.

Pharmacologic effects depend on dose and route of administration. In excessive doses, hyperthermia, seizures, coma, respiratory arrest, and ventricular arrhythmias may occur. Convulsions may follow relatively small doses 30–60 minutes after use. Cocaine-filled condoms ingested by drug dealers in smuggling activities have ruptured in the gastrointestinal tract, leading to sudden massive absorption and rapid cardiac arrest. Because of the risk of rupture with handling, operation rather than endoscopic examination is recommended for intact ingested condoms.

Treatment of cocaine ingestion involves protection of the airway, observation, and appropriate treatment of the cardiac rhythm. Residual drug on one nasal mucosa should be removed. Persistent seizures should be treated with phenytoin, body temperature should be lowered with external cooling, and severe hypertension with end-organ compromise should be treated with rapid-acting antihypertensive agents. Small doses of intravenous propranolol hydrochloride may antagonize the cardiopressor effects of cocaine, and some have advocated its use in patients with casual cocaine intoxication with hypertension, tachycardia, and behavioral changes. In animal experiments, pretreatment with chlorpromazine has been shown to block some of the cardiotoxic effects. Data to support clinical administration of these drugs are not yet available, and the emergency physician should proceed cautiously, with provision of supportive measures as the first priority.

Phencyclidine

Phencyclidine hydrochloride is an analgesic anesthetic agent similar to ketamine hydrochloride. Because of severe dysphoric reactions during its development, phencyclidine was discontinued for application in humans, although it is still used in veterinary medicine as Sernylan. The major current source in drug abuse and overdose is illicit manufacture. Phencyclidine is sold on the street in pill or powder form (usually misrepresented as tetrahydrocannabinol, mescaline, or LSD) or in marihuana mixtures ("supergrass"). Street vernacular referring to phencyclidine includes such terms as angel dust, crystal, goon, surfer, peace weed, and cyclones.

The clinical features of this intoxication depend on dose and route of administration, with smoking and inhalation in general causing a milder course than oral ingestion or the less common intravenous use. At low doses, agitation, excitement, and incoordination may be present, but a predominant feature is a blank stare with occasional catatonic mutism. The patient may appear inebriated. The pupils are usually in midposition and reactive with prominent nystagmus. Disorganized thoughts and a sense of altered body image may be present along with paranoid ideation.

At moderate to high doses, seizures, stupor, or coma with respiratory depression may occur. The eyes may remain open with reactive pupils, and nystagmus and vomiting may occur with risk of aspiration. Myoclonus and muscular rigidity can mimic seizure activity, and the anesthetic effect of the drug can cause diminished sensation. Considerable agitation may result, and the patient may be easily provoked into assaultive behavior, which can include homicide. Clinical findings may be marked by a relapsing course, and rhabdomyolysis may produce pigment-induced renal failure.

A dose of 5–10 mg of phencyclidine can produce moderate symptoms, with severe manifestations occurring after ingestions in excess of 10 mg. The drug produces sensory dissociation and blockade and is highly lipid-soluble with a pK of 8.6. Phencyclidine is metabolized in the liver, with urinary excretion of metabolites in low doses and excretion of free drug in high doses. The half-life varies with the dose, as hepatic metabolism becomes limiting. Enterohepatic circulation may prolong the half-life as well. As a weak base, the drug is readily ionized in an acidic environment and trapped within cells.

Low-dose intoxication should be treated in a quiet environment. Haloperidol may be used for sedation in cases of extreme agitation. The patient must be monitored carefully for central nervous system and respiratory depression at higher doses of phencyclidine. Intubation may be required and seizures should be controlled with phenytoin. If the drug has been taken orally, the stomach should be emptied.

Done and associates (Aronow and Done, 1978) have advocated continuous gastric suction and systemic acidification. Urinary concentration can be increased by acidification to 200 times the concentration in the blood to produce a urinary pH less than 5. Either ascorbic acid, 8 gm/day orally, or ammonium chloride, 2.75 mEq/kg by nasogastric tube or intravenously every 6 hours, can be given, and forced diuresis with the addition of a loop diuretic will maximize urinary excretion of the drug.

Methanol

Methyl alcohol or wood alcohol intoxication produces serious poisoning associated with severe metabolic acidosis. The degree of acidosis is disproportionate to the amount of acid produced by the toxin, and is due to interference with normal intermediary metabolism with consequent overproduction of metabolic acids (lactate and keto acids). The usual sources of methanol in poisonings are solvents, paint thinner, and Sterno. Methanol may be accidentally consumed as an ethanol substitute or taken in a purposeful suicide attempt.

Methanol is less inebriating than ethanol. It is oxidized to formaldehyde by alcohol dehydrogenase and then to formic acid. The toxicity of methanol is due to formaldehyde and formic acid, and becomes manifest slowly, usually appearing 12–24 hours after ingestion. Headache, nausea, vomiting, and dizziness are followed by central nervous system and respiratory depression. Visual impairment results from the toxic effects of formaldehyde and formic acid on the optic nerve and retina. The pupils may be dilated and optic disc hyperemia develops. Ingestions of 10–15 ml may result in significant visual impairment, and death has occurred after a 20-ml ingestion. The toxicity may vary, however, and survival has occurred after ingestions in excess of 100 ml.

Blood levels of 20–50 mg/dl suggest major toxicity, and treatment includes lavage or induced emesis in the first few hours after ingestion. Sodium bicarbonate must be administered intravenously to reverse acidosis.

Ethanol and methanol are both metabolized by alcohol dehydrogenase, but the metabolic rate of methanol is only 15% that of ethanol. Because of its affinity for alcohol dehydrogenase, ethanol competitively inhibits the metabolism of methanol and should be used in therapy when blood levels of methanol exceed 20 mg/dl. For intravenous treatment, a loading dose of absolute ethanol, 1 ml/kg, is given in 5% dextrose solution over 15 minutes, followed by 7–10 ml/hr to maintain a blood level of ethanol at 100 mg/dl. When methanol levels exceed 50 mg/dl or when acidosis is severe and resistant to bicarbonate therapy, hemodialysis is indicated in addition to ethanol therapy. On dialysis, intravenous administration of ethanol may have to be increased up to 50% to maintain the blood level of ethanol at 100 mg/dl.

Ethylene Glycol

Ethylene glycol, like methanol, produces severe anion gap acidosis due to the contribution of its metabolic products (aldehydes, glycolic acid, and oxalic acid) and its effect on intermediary metabolism, which causes the elaboration of lactic acid and keto acids. As in methanol ingestion, mild inebriation may occur without the odor of alcohol, but unlike methanol poisoning, ethylene glycol toxicity becomes manifest rapidly over several hours. Death in adults may occur with ingestions of approximately 75–100 gm of ethylene glycol.

Headache, nausea, vomiting, ataxia, and stupor may be followed by convulsions and coma in the first 6 hours. Cardiac failure, pulmonary edema, and respiratory failure often ensue by 24 hours, with oliguria leading to acute renal failure. Oxalate crystals may be present in the urine sediment and may be a clue to diagnosis. Diffuse oxalate crystal deposition occurs in other organs as well. Hypothermia and hypocalcemia may develop.

The treatment of ethylene glycol poisoning requires rapid diagnosis. In the absence of corroborative history, the diagnosis should be suspected in comatose patients with severe anion-gap metabolic acidosis. Toxicologic analysis will confirm the diagnosis and exclude salicylate, methanol, and paraldehyde ingestions. The clinical data and history will often help exclude causes of anion-gap acidosis unrelated to poisoning, such as diabetic ketoacidosis, lactic acidosis, and chronic renal failure.

The stomach should be emptied after the airway is protected, and vigorous sodium bicarbonate therapy may be required to control acidosis. The metabolic breakdown of ethylene glycol, like that of methanol, depends on alcohol dehydrogenase and may be blocked by the concurrent administration of ethanol. A blood level of 100 mg/dl of ethanol should be maintained with intravenous therapy; loading and maintenance doses are the same as for methanol. Intravenous administration of pyridoxine, 100 mg, and thiamin, 1 mg, have been advocated to direct metabolism of glycol to nontoxic metabolites, although this effect is not proven. Like methanol, ethylene glycol may be removed with dialysis, which should be undertaken promptly. Ethanol infusion rates must be increased on dialysis to maintain a blood level of 100 mg/dl.

In contrast to ethylene glycol and methanol, isopropyl alcohol (rubbing alcohol) does not pro-

duce metabolic acidosis. It is metabolized to acetone, and is inebriating like ethanol. Coma, gastritis, and aspiration pneumonitis may occur, but
death is uncommon. Treatment is supportive.

Petroleum Distillates

Petroleum distillate ingestion frequently occurs
in children. Approximately 100 deaths occur
yearly from this poisoning, 90% of which are in
children less than 5 years old. The most commonly
ingested products are kerosene, charcoal lighter
fluids, mineral seal oil preparations, turpentine,
and gasoline. As little as 0.5 ounce of ingested
petroleum distillate has occasionally caused death.

Death is produced by central nervous system
depression, cardiotoxic reactions, and complications of aspiration. The viscosity and surface tension of the fluid determine the aspiration hazard.
Distillates with lower viscosity and surface tension
tend to "creep" along the mucous membranes.
This is much more likely in patients who are
lethargic or convulsing.

The clinical findings are related to the respiratory, central nervous, and gastrointestinal systems.
Respiratory findings may be as mild as the frequent upper respiratory tract infections in this age
group, or they may be severe, with cyanosis, pulmonary edema, and hemorrhage. Breath holding
usually signals an attempt to protect the airway
from further aspiration of distillate and indicates
severe ingestion. Central nervous system depression and seizures are infrequently seen unless more
than 30 ml has been ingested. Local irritation of
the mucous membranes in the mouth and pharynx
occurs. Vomiting is frequent, and is usually accompanied by the characteristic odor of the hydrocar-
bon product. Diarrhea may also occur, and occasionally may be bloody. Furniture polish containing mineral seal oil products produces particularly
severe gastrointestinal symptoms.

Blood levels of hydrocarbons are extremely difficult to determine, but x-ray evaluation is helpful.
An x-ray film of the chest should be obtained in
all suspected cases, since there is often evidence of
pneumonitis in the absence of clinical signs and
symptoms. A double gastric fluid shadow on an
upright abdominal x-ray film can be seen after
giving the patient 4–8 ounces of water. This can
detect as little as 5 ml of petroleum distillate in the
stomach, thereby identifying cases of potential
toxicity.

Treatment of petroleum distillate ingestions has
been controversial, with gastric lavage, emesis, and
cathartics being both favored and opposed. The
controversy has been heightened by the product
labels on petroleum distillate packages. A typical

label states: "*In case of accidental ingestion, do not
induce vomiting. Call your physician immediately.*"
Cautious gastric lavage has been advocated, but
few physicians can perform this procedure in a
struggling, frightened child.

If the patient is coughing, wheezing, or dyspneic
with pulmonary findings on presentation, aspiration is likely to have already occurred, and further
gastric emptying is not necessary. If more than 1
ml/kg has been ingested, the current trend favors
gastric emptying with emesis induced by ipecac in
the alert patient. There is a risk of aspiration with
this method, but it is less than the risk of aspiration
after depression of consciousness. If the patient is
comatose, gastric lavage should be performed after
the airway is protected by a cuffed endotracheal
tube. Sympathomimetic drugs should be avoided
in these patients since life-threatening arrhythmias
may develop in a sensitized myocardium. Charcoal is of no benefit, but a saline cathartic may
help reduce gastrointestinal absorption. There is
no proven benefit to prophylactic antibiotics and
no data to support use of high-dose corticosteroids.

Data on decision-making for hospitalization
suggest that all patients with respiratory symptoms
and chest x-ray evidence of pneumonitis should be
admitted, whereas children who are asymptomatic
with normal physical findings and x-ray films and
who remain asymptomatic for 6–8 hours of observation may be safely discharged. Patients with x-
ray evidence of minor aspiration but without
symptoms may not require hospitalization, but the
emergency physician should base this decision on
the patient's availability for follow-up care and on
the family's reliability.

The toxicity of aromatic hydrocarbons (xylene,
toluene) and halogenated hydrocarbons (carbon
tetrachloride, trichloroethane) is distinct from that
of petroleum distillates. The aromatic hydrocarbons affect the gastrointestinal tract, the central
nervous system, and the bone marrow (marrow
suppression). Chronic use may also be associated
with renal tubular injury. The halogenated hydrocarbons cause severe hepatic and renal injury.
Aromatic and halogenated hydrocarbons should
be removed from the gastrointestinal tract as a
definite priority.

Mushrooms

Although there are more than 3000 species of
mushrooms, only about 50 are known to cause
toxic reactions, and more than 90% of lethal mushroom poisonings are attributed to the genus *Amanita*. Mushroom poisoning may vary from mild
gastrointestinal symptoms to severe hepatic, renal,
and neurologic toxicity. Table 17.8 summarizes

Table 17.8.
Classification of mushroom groups.

	Group						
	Cyclopeptide	Ibotenic	Muscarine	Psilocybin	Disulfiram-like	Gastrointestinal Irritant	Gyromitrin
Mushroom Genus species	*Amanita phalloides, verna, virosa Galerina autumnaus, marginata, venenata*	*Amanita muscaris, pantherine*	*Inocybe* many species *Clitocybe dealbata, virulosa*	*Psilocybe cubensis, eaerulescens, silvatic Panaeolus subbalteus*	*Coprinus atramentarius*	Many varied genera	*Gyromitra* many species
Toxin	Amanitine, phalloidine	Ibotenic acid, muscimol, pantherin	Muscarine	Psilocybin, psilocin, baeocystin	Monomethyl hydrazine	Unidentified	Gyromitrin
Onset of symptoms	10–20 hours	15–30 min	15–30 min	30–60 min	5–10 min	30–90 min	6–8 hours
Predominant signs and symptoms	Initial gastrointestinal toxicity, transient clinical improvement, terminal hepato- and nephrotoxicity	Anticholinergic and CNS disturbances	Cholinergic	CNS disturbances	Antabuse-like reaction, gastrointestinal toxicity	Gastrointestinal toxicity	Gastrointestinal toxicity
Treatment	Thioctic acid, supportive	Supportive, atropine contraindicated	Supportive, atropine	Supportive	Supportive, avoid alcohol	Supportive	Supportive
Prognosis	Poor; fatalities have been reported from one mushroom cap	Good; recovery is rapid and complete; deaths are rare	Good; death infrequently results from cardiac arrest and respiratory failure	Good; recovery is rapid and complete	Good; recovery is rapid and complete	Good; recovery is rapid and complete	Fair to poor; mortality may range from 2–4%

CNS = central nervous system.
Reproduced by permission from McCormick DJ, Avbel AJ, Gibbons RB: Nonlethal mushroom poisoning. *Ann Intern Med 90:* 332–335, 1979.

seven groups of toxic mushrooms according to their toxin.

The emergency physician can best judge the severity of these poisonings by combining clinical assessment with identification of the mushroom. Knowledge of local toxic species is of benefit, and often, poison control centers maintain a list of experts who are able to identify mushrooms from description or direct examination. Local mycologic societies are usually willing to provide such consultation, and the emergency ward should maintain a call list. Identification involves gross examination of the mushroom cap, stem, and bulb, and occasionally, microscopic examination of the spores.

Amanita phalloides (death cup), *Amanita verna*, and *Amanita virosa* (destroying angel) are among the most poisonous mushrooms. They produce toxins, phalloidine and amanitine, that interfere with RNA synthesis and cellular metabolism in the liver, kidneys, brain, and striated muscle. The clinical manifestations are divided into three phases. The first phase begins 10–20 hours after ingestion and is characterized by nausea, vomiting, abdominal pain, and profuse watery diarrhea. During the second phase, from 24–48 hours, the patient's condition improves as electrolytes and volume are replenished, but hepatic and renal damage takes place as evidenced both by liver function tests showing progressive hepatocellular dysfunction and by renal impairment. Within 3–4 days, marked liver failure ensues, with coagulopathy, acidosis, oliguric renal failure, and acute tubular necrosis. Cardiac arrhythmias and conduction disturbances may occur.

The use of emesis, gastric lavage, or charcoal is rarely of benefit in amanita poisonings since ingestion has often occurred 8–10 hours before the onset of symptoms. Supportive measures, volume and electrolyte replacement, and attention to the end-organ effects of coagulopathy, hepatic failure, and renal failure are necessary. Renal failure may require dialysis, but the toxins themselves are poorly dialyzable. Thioctic acid has been used in Europe and in the United States for amanita poisoning. The mechanism of action is not completely understood, nor is there complete agreement as to its efficacy. Early administration seems to correlate with the best results. The mortality rate among patients with amanita poisoning ranges from 50–80%.

Nonlethal mushroom poisonings tend to have an earlier onset of symptoms, and may be characterized by either gastrointestinal symptoms of nausea, vomiting, pain, and diarrhea or by neurologic dysfunction related to either cholinergic or anticholinergic manifestations. Hallucinosis, delirium, and coma may occur with bronchorrhea, lacrimation, and bronchospasm in cholinergic excess; tachycardia, fever, and seizures characterize the anticholinergic toxins.

Anticholinergic poisonings respond to supportive measures, and improvement has been reported after physostigmine administration in comatose and delirious patients. The toxin muscarine in the genus *Clitocybe* produces cholinergic excess that responds to supportive measures and atropine, 0.6–1.0 mg intravenously. The genus *Coprinus* produces an acute antabuse-type reaction with alcohol, resulting in moderately severe gastrointestinal symptoms but usually relatively rapid recovery over 24 hours.

ANTIDOTES FOR SPECIFIC POISONS

Several poisons require antidotes immediately to decrease morbidity and mortality. These include carbon monoxide, cyanide, nitrites and nitrates, and organophosphorus insecticide compounds.

Cyanide

Cyanide is one of the most rapidly acting of all poisons. It inhibits cytochrome B, one of the enzymes in cellular oxygen transport, by binding with the ferric (Fe^{3+}) component of cytochrome oxidase. Cyanides are present in rodent poisons and in the seeds of many fruits, including the peach, apple, plum, cherry, and apricot, and they are used industrially in electroplating and mining. They are absorbed through the skin and mucous membranes, and toxic amounts can be absorbed quickly via inhalation.

Symptoms appear soon after exposure; although most deaths are rapid, patients may survive for several hours and can be saved with prompt and proper treatment. An odor of bitter almonds is classic, but is not always present. Signs are due to the rapid development of tissue hypoxia.

Treatment is based on the principle of providing competitive ferric sites with which the cyanide can bind, thus freeing some of the ferric components of cytochrome oxidase. This is done by converting hemoglobin containing ferrous (Fe^{2+}) iron to methemoglobin with ferric sites, producing methemoglobinemia. Care must be taken to prevent a lethal level of methemoglobin. Methemoglobinemia can be produced by inhalation of amyl nitrite or intravenous infusion of sodium nitrite:

$$\text{hemoglobin} + \text{nitrite} \rightarrow \text{methemoglobin}$$
$$(Fe^{2+}) \qquad\qquad\qquad (Fe^{3+})$$

Some of the cyanide then binds to the methemoglobin:

methemoglobin + cytochrome oxidase-cyanide
→ methemoglobin-cyanide + cytochrome
oxidase

If thiosulfate is made available, thiocyanate is formed, which is nontoxic and can be excreted:

methemoglobin-cyanide + thiosulfate →
methemoglobin + thiocyanate + sulfite

The methemoglobin is reduced to hemoglobin by erythrocytic enzyme systems.

A prepackaged kit containing the necessary drugs is available (Eli Lilly & Company). The amyl nitrite should be replaced yearly. Amyl nitrite pearls should be broken and held under the nose while the sodium nitrite is being drawn into a syringe, and should be removed after the sodium nitrite is given. Oxygen should be administered during treatment. Sodium nitrite is infused intravenously, 10 ml of a 3% solution in a 2-minute period. Ideally, such treatment will produce a methemoglobin level of approximately 30% in adults. The adult dose produces fatal methemoglobinemia in children. The pediatric dose is 10 mg/kg or 0.33 ml/kg of the 3% solution. Immediately after administration of sodium nitrite, 50 ml of a 25% solution of sodium thiosulfate is given intravenously in the course of 1–2 minutes.

If the poisoning was the result of ingestion, gastric lavage should be performed with a 1:5000 solution of potassium permanganate. After lavage, 300 ml of the 25% solution of sodium thiosulfate should be instilled in the stomach. Symptoms may recur and can be treated in a manner similar to the initial treatment with one half the dose.

Contaminated skin and clothing can be cleansed with soap and water. Since cyanide can be absorbed through the skin, personnel must avoid becoming contaminated.

Nitrites and Nitrates

Nitrite and nitrate poisoning is unusual. Poisoning can result from nitrite-containing drugs used as coronary vasodilators. Nitrite is also used in meat processing for preservation and for prevention of discoloration. Nitrates are found in fertilizers and feedstock, and are converted to nitrites by intestinal bacteria. Beets, spinach, and carrots grown in soil containing large amounts of nitrite or nitrate have high concentrations of the toxin. Accidental poisoning also occurs in children whose milk formula has been contaminated with *Bacillus subtilis*.

The toxic state is produced by development of methemoglobinemia. Clinical findings include considerable cyanosis unresponsive to oxygen. Diagnosis can be confirmed by drying a drop of blood on filter paper and observing a brown color. A 1% solution of methylene blue can be infused intravenously, 0.2 ml/kg in the course of 5 minutes. Surface decontamination is important since the chemicals can be absorbed through the skin.

Organophosphorus Compounds and Carbamates

Organophosphorus compounds are used as insecticides, and the incidence of poisoning with them has increased since they have replaced recently banned DDT. These compounds are extremely toxic; one drop of undiluted parathion can be fatal. Most poisoning is due to occupational exposure in crop dusters, farmers, and florists, with absorption through the mucous membranes, skin, and lungs.

Organophosphates block the action of cholinesterase, so the action of acetylcholine released from nerve endings is unopposed. Cholinesterase activity in red blood cells can be measured, and is usually less than 30% of normal. Poisoning is manifested by the SLUD syndrome: *s*alivation, *l*acrimation, *u*rination, and *d*efecation. Pupils are usually small, but this sign can be unreliable. Other effects are fasciculations, muscular weakness, paralysis, ataxia, and coma. Death may be due to depression of central respiratory or circulatory centers, bronchoconstriction, excessive bronchial secretion, or paralysis of the respiratory muscles.

Treatment should not wait for confirmation from the laboratory. The initial treatment in a cyanotic patient is oxygen, after which intravenous or intramuscular atropine sulfate can be given, 2 mg initially (0.05 mg/kg in children). If atropine is given to a cyanotic patient, ventricular fibrillation is likely. Lack of a clinical response to small amounts of atropine is further evidence for poisoning of this type. The amount of atropine administered depends on the given patient, and salivation can be used as a clinical factor. When salivation decreases substantially, enough atropine has been given. Large amounts are often necessary, and a total dose more than 500 mg has been reported often. Usually, a total of 25–50 mg is necessary in a 24-hour period. Artificial ventilation with a respirator is usually indicated since the atropine often does not reverse the muscular paralysis. Frequent suction of the lower part of the respiratory tract is necessary to keep the patient from drowning in secretions.

After the diagnosis is confirmed and the symptoms are controlled with atropine sulfate, reactivation of cholinesterase can be accomplished by the use of oximes, which cleave the bond between the organophosphate and the cholinesterase. Pralidoxime chloride (Protopam), 1 gm intravenously in adults, can be given in a 2-minute period. This dose can be repeated after 1 hour if the exposure was severe. The dosage in children is 25–50 mg/kg. Pralidoxime chloride is effective if given within several hours of exposure.

Mild cases of poisoning can usually be treated with oral administration of pralidoxime chloride, and symptoms usually abate within 1 hour. The dose may be repeated as necessary. All patients, however mild the toxic state, should be closely supervised in the hospital for 24 hours. Seizures can be controlled with small doses of short-acting barbiturates since the anticholinesterase sensitizes the medullary depressant center. Morphine, aminophylline, succinylcholine, and phenothiazines are contraindicated.

Decontamination of skin and clothing is important. An alkaline solution should be used since this accelerates hydrolysis of the phosphate. Leather cannot be decontaminated and must be discarded properly.

Carbamates are used as insecticides, and poisoning produces signs and symptoms similar to those seen with organophosphorus compounds. The carbamates also combine with cholinesterase, but binding is reversible and the complex usually rapidly dissociates spontaneously. Treatment is similar to that for organophosphorus poisoning, with use of atropine sulfate as needed. However, oximes are not indicated and may be harmful.

Suggested Readings

Arena JM: Poisoning—treatment and prevention. *JAMA* 232:1271–1275, 233:358–363, 1975

Arieff A: Coma following non-narcotic overdose: management of 208 adult patients. *Am J Med Sci* 266:405, 1973

Davis JM, Bartlett E, Termini BS, et al: Overdosage of psychotropic drugs: a review. *Dis Nerv Syst* 29:157–164, 240–256, 1968

Greenblatt DJ, Shader RI: Acute poisoning with psychotropic drugs. In: Shader et al. (Eds): *Psychotropic Drug Side Effects: Clinical and Theoretical Perspectives.* Baltimore, Williams & Wilkins, pp. 214–234, 1970

Smith RP, Gosselin RE: Current concepts about the treatment of selected poisonings: nitrite, cyanide, barium and quinidine. *Ann Rev Pharmacol Toxicol* 16: 189–199, 1976

Winchester JF, Gelfand MC, Knepshield JH, et al: Dialysis and hemoperfusion of poisons and drugs—update. *Trans Am Soc Artif Intern Organs* 23:762–842, 1977

Specific Poisonings

Acetaminophen

Ameer B, Greenblatt DJ: Acetaminophen. *Ann Intern Med* 87:202–209, 1977

Medical Letter: Acetylcysteine for acetaminophen overdosage. *21*:98–100, 1979

Rumack BH, Peterson RG: Acetaminophen overdose: incidence, diagnosis and management in 416 patients. Pediatrics 62:898–903, 1978

Amphetamines

Angrist BM: Managing amphetamine toxicity. *Psychiat Ann* 8:443–446, 1978

Aspirin

Anderson RJ, Potts DE, Gabow PA, et al: Unrecognized adult salicylate intoxication. *Ann Intern Med* 85:745, 1976

Hill JB: Salicylate intoxication. *N Engl J Med* 288:1110–1113, 1973

Carbon Monoxide

Winter PM, Miller JN: Carbon monoxide poisoning. *JAMA* 236:1502–1504, 1976

Caustics

Campbell GS, Burnett HF, Ransom JM, et al: Treatment of caustic burns of the esophagus. *Arch Surg 112:* 495–500, 1977

Cocaine

Cohen S: Cocaine. *JAMA 231*:74–75, 1975

Haddad LM: Cocaine in perspective:1978 *JACEP 8*:374–376, 1978

Ethchlorvynol

Teehan BP, Maher JF, Carey JH, et al: Acute ethchlorvynol (Placidyl®) intoxication. *Ann Intern Med 72*:875–882, 1970

Ethylene Glycol

Levinsky NG: Severe metabolic acidosis in a young man—case records of MGH. *N Engl J Med 301*:650–657, 1979

Parry MF, Wallach R: Ethylene glycol poisoning. *Am J Med* 57:143–150, 1974

Peterson CD, Collins AJ, Himes JM, et al: Ethylene glycol poisoning: pharmacokinetics during therapy with ethanol and hemodialysis. *N Engl J Med 304*:21–24, 1981

Glutethimide

Chazan JA, Garella S: Glutethimide intoxication: A prospective study of 70 patients treated conservatively without hemodialysis. *Arch Intern Med 128*:215–219, 1971

Wright N, Roscoe P: Acute glutethimide poisoning: Conservative management of 31 patients. *JAMA 214*:1704–1706, 1970

Heavy Metals

Chisholm JJ: Poisoning due to heavy metals. *Pediatr Clin North Am* 17:591–597, 1970

Methanol

Bennett IL, Jr, Cary FH, Mitchell GL, Jr, et al: Acute methyl alcohol poisoning: A review based on experiences in an outbreak of 323 cases. *Medicine* 32:431–463, 1953

Keyvan-Larijarni H, Tannenberg AM: Methanol intoxication: Comparison of peritoneal dialysis and hemodialsis treatment. *Arch Intern Med 134*:293–296, 1974

Mushrooms

McCormick DJ, Avbel AJ, Gibbons RB: Non-lethal mushroom poisoning. *Ann Intern Med 90*:332–335, 1979

Paaso B, Harrison DC: A new look at an old problem: Mushroom poisoning. Clinical presentations and new therapeutic approaches. *Am J Med 58*:505–509, 1975

Narcotics

Thornton WE, Thornton BP: Narcotic poisoning: A review of the literature. *Am J Psychiatr 131:*867–869, 1974

Pesticides

Milby TH: Prevention and management of organophosphate poisonings. *JAMA 216:*2131–2133, 1971

Zavon M: Poisoning from pesticides: Diagnosis and treatment. *Pediatrics 54:*332–336, 1974

Petroleum Distillates

Brown J, Burke B, Dajani AS: Experimental kerosene pneumonia. *J Pediatr 84:*396–441, 1974

Shirkey H: Treatment of petroleum distillate ingestion. *Mod Treat 8:*580–592, 1971

Phencyclidine

Aronow R, Done AK: Phencyclidine overdose: An emerging concept of management. *JACEP 7:*56–59, 1978

McCarron MM, Schulze BW, Thompson GA, et al: Acute phencyclidine intoxication: Clinical patterns, complications and treatment. *Ann Emerg Med 10:*290–297, 1981

Stillman R, Peterson RC: The paradox of PCP abuse. *Ann Intern Med 90:*428–430, 1979

Phenothiazines

Barry D, et al: Phenothiazine poisoning. *Calif Med 118:*1–12, 1973

Benowitz NC, Rosenberg J, Becker DE, et al: Phenothiazine poisoning. *Med Clin North Am 63:*276–296, 1979

Tricyclic Antidepressants and Anticholinergic Poisonings

Biggs JT, Spiker DG, Petit JM, et al: Tricyclic antidepressant overdose: incidence of symptoms. *JAMA 238:*135–138, 1977

Brasheres ZA, Conley WR: Physostigmine in drug overdose. *JACEP 1:*42–48, 1975

Granacher RP, Baldessarini RJ: Physostigmine. *Arch Gen Psy 32:*375–380, 1975

Rumack BH: Physostigmine: Rational use. *JACEP 5:*541–542, 1976

Rumack BH: Anticholinergic poisoning: Treatment with physostigmine. *Pediatrics 52:*449–451, 1973

CHAPTER 18

Psychiatric Emergencies

WILLIAM H. ANDERSON, M.D.

Psychiatric emergencies refer to medical and psychologic disturbances manifested chiefly by acute alteration of behavior, thought, or feeling. Some of the conditions are life-threatening and, therefore, require immediate diagnosis and vigorous management. Others are less severe conditions that nevertheless are defined subjectively as emergencies by the patient or family, and so are likely to be seen by the emergency physician. The task of the emergency physician is to identify those conditions with risk of mortality or serious morbidity, to institute treatment, and to arrange adequate continued inpatient or outpatient care. In addition, the time and situation permitting, the physician may have the opportunity to intervene effectively in those less severe conditions that are defined as emergencies by the patient or his social environment. Among the first questions to address is "What acute disturbance has there been in this patient's medical, psychologic, or social condition that causes him to appear for emergency care *today*?" The problem of specific diagnosis usually presents little difficulty provided that general principles of patient management are observed. All too often the patient with an acute behavioral disturbance is evaluated inadequately because of the staff's assumption that the disturbance is willful or deliberate. Careful attention to standard examination procedures is essential. A complete history should be taken from the patient or persons accompanying him, the mental status should be evaluated, and an appropriate physical examination and relevant laboratory studies should be performed. The physician in charge must make every effort to resist the temptation to make a rapid and perhaps unsatisfactory disposition in an effort to rid the emergency ward of a disruptive patient. Numerous acute physiologic conditions can simulate the behavioral manifestations of schizophrenia, manic-depressive disease, or other "functional" psychiatric illnesses.

MAJOR LIFE-THREATENING CONDITIONS

This section will consider emergency situations that have the potential for fatality or serious morbidity. These include acute psychosis and suicidal and homicidal states.

Acute Psychosis

This condition constitutes a medical emergency. Victims of these disorders are in constant danger of acting on distorted perceptions or delusional ideas with the result that serious injury or death may occur inadvertently. In addition to this cardinal indication for early intervention, three other considerations demand that diagnosis and treatment proceed without delay. First, acute psychosis is generally a mental state of intense discomfort. Second, family and social relationships may be strained severely in the course of the episode. Third, psychotic symptoms may be the most visible indicators of subtle but serious acute medical conditions.

Acute psychosis refers to a spectrum of aberrant mental states characterized by rapid development of major disturbances of perception, cognition, affect, and reality testing. Schizophrenia, manic-depressive disease, and psychotic depression usually are classified as functional psychoses and are separated conceptually from organic psychoses that represent those disturbances of mental state that can be attributed to disorders of brain tissue function. The most critical problem for the emergency physician who evaluates the psychotic patient is differentiating between these two general classifications. Guidelines are summarized in Table 18.1.

Initial Examination

Exclusion of Organic Brain Disease. The first step is to take all of the necessary measures to

Table 18.1.
Differential diagnosis of acute psychosis.

Clinical Information	Organic	Functional
History		
Age	Most often > 40 years	Most often < 40 years
Onset	May be sudden	Usually over weeks
Physical examination		
Vital signs		
Temperature	Often elevated	Usually normal
Pulse, blood pressure	Often elevated	Usually normal
Head	Injury may be present	Injury absent
Autonomic signs (pathologic)	Present	May be present
Tympanic membranes	Bloody (with skull fracture)	Normal
Ocular fundi	May be papilledematous	Normal
Mental status		
Orientation	Impaired	Preserved
Recent memory	Impaired	Preserved
Hallucinations	Often visual, tactile, or olfactory	Usually auditory
Intellectual function	Impaired	Preserved
Insight	Often present	Usually absent
Neurologic examination		
Nystagmus	May be present	Absent
Pathologic reflexes	May be present	Absent
Tremor	May be present	Absent
Asterixis	May be present	Absent
Response to caloric test	May be impaired (coma)	Normal
Laboratory findings		
Complete blood cell count and sedimentation rate	May be abnormal	Normal
Urinalysis	May be abnormal	Normal
Chest and skull x-ray films	May be abnormal	Normal
Blood chemistries	May be abnormal	Normal
Electroencephalogram	Often abnormal	Normal

obtain a thorough history and to perform an adequate physical examination. Two problems must be overcome to accomplish this—the patient's agitation and discomfort, and on occasion, the resistance of the emergency ward staff. The patient's cooperation usually can be obtained by an attitude of gentle firmness on the part of the physician. He should explain procedures in a matter-of-fact, unambiguous manner without excessive discussion, exhortation, or argument. Occasionally, a patient may be so agitated that chemotherapy may be required before full examination. In such cases, the best choice of medication is a high-potency antipsychotic drug such as haloperidol (Haldol), 5–10 mg intramuscularly. Drugs of this class have relatively little sedative or hypotensive effect and, therefore, are less likely to complicate the clinical presentation than are barbiturates or other sedatives.

At times, the patient may resist an adequate medical evaluation, leaving the physician with the dilemma that to perform examination despite the patient's protest may constitute an assault, whereas to avoid examining him may be negligence. In general, a patient who comes to the emergency service with an acute psychosis may be presumed to have a potentially life-threatening condition. Good practice, therefore, requires that an evaluation at least adequate to exclude major illness be performed. While every effort must be made to be courteous, diplomatic, and gentle, the "assault" of performing an examination usually is more defensible than the negligence of refusing to assess an incapacitated patient.

The other problem that may make full evaluation difficult is the occasional negative attitude of the emergency ward staff. There is a tendency to regard the acute psychotic patient as having a "psychiatric" problem, by which some persons imply that the patient has no business in a medical emergency ward. Professional judgment may be impaired by anger or fear. The physician in charge may feel subtle pressure to make a quick disposition rather than a thorough evaluation. Under

Table 18.2.

Metabolic and structural disorders that may have psychotic features.

Space-occupying lesions in brain
    Primary tumor
    Metastatic carcinoma (lung, breast)
    Subdural hematoma[a]
    Brain abscess (bacterial or fungal infection, gumma, cysticercosis)
Cerebral hypoxia
    Pulmonary insufficiency[a]
    Severe anemia
    Diminished cardiac output[a]
    Toxicosis (e.g., carbon monoxide)
Metabolic and endocrine disorders
    Electrolyte imbalance[a]
    Hypocalcemia
    Thyroid disease (thyrotoxicosis and myxedema)
    Pituitary insufficiency
    Adrenal disease (Addison's disease and Cushing's syndrome)
    Hypoglycemia[a]
    Diabetes mellitus (ketoacidosis)[a]
    Uremia
    Hepatic failure
    Porphyria
Use of exogenous substances
    Alcohol (intoxication and withdrawal)
    Barbiturates and other sedatives (intoxication and withdrawal)
    Amphetamines
    LSD, PCP, and similar compounds
    Anticholinergic agents[a]
    Heavy metals
    Digitalis
    Corticosteroids
    L-dopa
    Reserpine
    Cocaine
    Bromide compounds
    Marihuana
    Carbon disulfide
    Isoniazid
    Cycloserine
    Disulfiram
Nutritional deficiencies
    Thiamine (Wernicke-Korsakoff syndrome)[a]
    Niacin (pellagra)
    Vitamin B_{12}
    Folate
Vascular abnormalities
    Intracranial hemorrhage[a]
    Lacunae due to hypertension
    Collagen disorders
    Aneurysm
    Hypertensive encephalopathy[a]
Infections
    Meningitis (bacterial, fungal, tuberculous)[a]
    Encephalitis (viral, e.g., herpetic)[a]
    Syphilis
    Subacute bacterial endocarditis[a]
    Typhoid fever
    Malaria
Miscellaneous conditions
    Normal-pressure hydrocephalus
    Temporal lobe epilepsy
    Huntington's chorea
    Alzheimer's disease
    Remote effects of carcinoma
    Wilson's disease
    Pancreatitis

[a] Indicates potentially severe acute illness that requires immediate diagnosis and treatment.

such circumstances, the physician may find that the ancillary help to which he is accustomed may not be forthcoming. Initial identifying data may not be collected by desk clerks, vital signs may not be evaluated, or the patient may not be assigned to an appropriate examining area. Such difficulties are understandable, and the specialist in emergency medicine ought to anticipate them. If he is not prepared to do all of the necessary procedures himself, continuing staff education may be required.

History. Every potential source of relevant present and past medical information must be explored. Most frequently, this information can be obtained from family or friends. Special inquiry should be directed to the possibility of head injuries, epilepsy, diabetes mellitus, endocrine disorders, ingestion of drugs or other foreign substances, cardiopulmonary disease, electrolyte imbalance, and hepatic and renal dysfunction (Table 18.2).

Even if the patient is mute or has a florid thought disorder, he may be able to provide some history. Such patients may be asked to show identification. Examination of the patient's wallet may provide medical information, phone numbers of relatives, or names of physicians. A severely depressed patient may be unable to give oral answers, but may be able to write "yes" and "no" or short sentences.

The patient's age is an important consideration. Acute functional psychosis is typically a disorder with onset after puberty and before age 40. The major exception to this is involutional melancholia, which may be suspected by the presence of profound depression, often with agitation, with onset after age 40. Excluding this entity, psychotic features appearing for the first time in the older age group should be presumed initially to have an organic cause.

Mode of onset is also a helpful feature in the

history. Acute psychosis that has developed in the course of minutes or hours suggests either a vascular, metabolic, toxic, infectious, or epileptic cause. Thus, intracranial hemorrhage, hypoglycemia, meningitis, temporal lobe epilepsy, or intoxications (for example, from amphetamines, LSD, or anticholinergic agents) should be suspected. Psychosis in a young person in whom florid symptoms develop over several weeks suggests the likelihood of a schizophrenic or manic-depressive condition. Insidious onset with barely perceptible personality change over months suggests a dementing illness. Since some of these are remediable, the cause always should be sought, although this is not usually the task of the emergency physician.

Physical Examination. A complete physical examination should be performed, although rectal and pelvic examinations are best deferred in the absence of specific indications. Even though vital signs frequently are neglected because of real or assumed lack of patient cooperation, they are of utmost importance and always should be recorded. The temperature is most critical. Mild elevations may exist (99–100°F; 37.2–37.8°C) in functional states such as acute catatonia, but fever usually implies an acute organic process and deserves full investigation. In such a case, meningitis and encephalitis, subacute bacterial endocarditis, collagen diseases, thyrotoxicosis, delirium tremens, and anticholinergic poisoning should receive special consideration.

The scalp should be examined carefully for evidence of laceration, contusion, or penetrating injury. Such injuries may not be noted in the history because of traumatic amnesia. Evidence of bleeding behind the tympanic membranes should be sought. Ecchymoses around the orbits or behind the ears may be suggestive. The optic fundi should be examined for signs of papilledema.

Signs of autonomic dysfunction may suggest a specific cause. The combination of fixed, dilated pupils, tachycardia, dry mucous membranes, urinary retention, and abdominal distention with absent bowel sounds is highly suggestive of anticholinergic poisoning. Profuse cold sweat, tachycardia, and peculiar brightness of the eyes suggest hypoglycemia. Acute amphetamine overdose may cause dilated pupils and tachycardia.

Mental Status. Careful systematic evaluation of the patient's mental status is often the most helpful procedure in making the differential diagnosis between organic and functional psychosis. Orientation, or the ability of the patient to recognize time and place, should be considered first. Disturbance of spatial and temporal orientation indicates acute organic disease. The patient with functional psychosis typically retains knowledge of the day of the week and of the place even in the presence of profound thought disorder. Severe temporal disorientation, such as incorrect identification of the year, suggests a more insidious organic disorder of brain function.

Recent memory should be evaluated next. The physician should ask the patient about recent actions and experiences, verifying the answers by consulting independent sources. Another method is to instruct the patient to name five objects and to request him to name them again after 5 minutes. Patients with functional psychosis usually have intact recent memory, but delirious and demented patients usually do not.

Hallucinations frequently accompany an acute psychotic process. The acute schizophrenic patient typically experiences auditory hallucinations. Visual, tactile, and olfactory phenomena are rare in acute functional psychosis, but often are present in acute organic brain syndromes, especially those secondary to a toxic or metabolic disturbance, infection, or epilepsy.

Preservation of intellectual function is typical of schizophrenia and manic-depressive disease. Measurements must be judged against standards of premorbid function, which often must be inferred from educational history. Simple arithmetic calculations are useful tests.

Evaluation of the patient's insight simply requires determining the degree of appreciation of illness. Patients with organic brain disease, even though possibly delusional or hallucinatory or both, often recognize that illness is present, but patients with schizophrenia or manic-depressive disease usually do not. However, this criterion is perhaps the least reliable in the evaluation of mental status.

Neurological Examination. A full neurologic examination always should be attempted. Certain aspects of this type of examination are more likely to yield positive findings in patients with an acute psychosis. Pathologic reflexes require little time to check and are highly suggestive when present. The plantar flexion, grasping, snout, sucking, and palmomental reflexes, as well as the glabellar response, should be investigated.

Myoclonus suggests diffuse brain disease, and nystagmus suggests sedative intoxication or Wernicke's encephalopathy. Tremor and asterixis indicate organic brain disease. In comatose patients in whom hysteria or catatonia cannot be excluded readily, the response to caloric stimulation of the external auditory canals may be helpful. Patients who generally are unresponsive because of hysteria or catatonia show a normal response. Irrigation with ice water normally causes nystagmus with the quick component away from the irrigated ear. In unconscious patients with intact brainstem function, conjugate tonic deviation toward the irrigated ear suggests a metabolic cause.

Before proceeding further, the physician should consider the possibility that the abnormal mental status may be early evidence of Wernicke-Korsakoff syndrome. This condition deserves special attention since it requires early aggressive treatment, and diagnosis in the emergency ward, therefore, is essential. Early in the course of the disease, patients may be confused without prominent evidence of alcohol intoxication or other signs such as nystagmus, ophthalmoplegia, or ataxia. This syndrome may occur in alcoholic patients and in those otherwise deprived of thiamine. When it is suspected, an initial dose of 100 mg of thiamine may be given intravenously.

Laboratory Evaluation. In some patients, diagnosis continues to be difficult despite the aforementioned methods of evaluation, and it usually is best to admit such patients for further evaluation. Laboratory studies that may be helpful include an electroencephalogram (including a sleep study when temporal lobe epilepsy is suspected) and a computed tomography (CT) scan. On admission, procedures routinely should include a complete blood cell count, sedimentation rate, urinalysis, chest film, electrocardiogram, serologic studies, and measurement of serum electrolytes, calcium, blood urea nitrogen, and blood glucose. Thyroid studies, Vitamin B_{12} and folate levels, liver function tests, and screening for toxic exogenous substances complete the workup.

Patients with signs and symptoms of organic brain disease should be admitted to establish an etiologic diagnosis. In other patients, the diagnosis of functional psychosis may be made, although the possibility of an organic cause must not be forgotten.

Suicidal and Homicidal Potential. The next problem that the emergency physician must evaluate is the risk of suicidal or homicidal activity. Any acute psychotic process significantly increases the possibility of such behavior. Patients with severe depressive symptoms as well may be presumed to have high suicidal potential. It is of cardinal importance to inquire directly about such ideas or intentions. Psychotic patients with persecutory delusions may have increased potential for homicide, since they may respond to the imagined threat with a preemptive defense. A more complete strategy for evaluation of these risks is described on pages 407–412. Patients with significant risk should be hospitalized in a setting that provides security appropriate to their condition. Those in whom the risk is less possibly may be treated on an outpatient basis; this requires an adequate system of social support during the acute phase of treatment.

Evaluation of Social Supports. Not every acutely psychotic patient requires hospitalization. Many can be treated effectively as outpatients with appropriate chemotherapy. For this to be a feasible option, however, a social support system of concerned and capable family members and friends is essential. Those patients who live alone or whose relatives and friends are of dubious helpfulness should be hospitalized. Family members often wish to deny the nature and severity of an acute psychotic illness and, therefore, are vulnerable to the patient's rationalizations that treatment is unnecessary. If, however, family or friends are able to provide ongoing supervision and protection and to ensure the patient's adherence to medication and appointment schedules, then outpatient management may be considered.

Initial Treatment

In patients with acute schizophrenic or manic psychosis, the cornerstone of initial treatment is the timely aggressive use of antipsychotic chemotherapy. With this type of regimen, the acute symptoms may subside substantially within 4–6 hours. Time and situation permitting, it is well worth such a trial in the hope that hospitalization may be avoided or that the illness may be brought toward remission more quickly.

Despite modern advances, hospitalization on a psychiatric ward carries with it certain disadvantages: social opprobrium is always present, undue pessimism concerning prognosis sometimes results, and finally, the cost of inpatient treatment is very high. To avoid these disadvantages, the physician must first establish that (1) the cause is not organic; (2) suicidal and homicidal danger is minimal; and (3) social supports for outpatient treatment are satisfactory. If these criteria are fulfilled, he may attempt to induce symptomatic remission with chemotherapy.

As a general rule, the high-potency antipsychotic medications such as haloperidol, trifluoperazine hydrochloride (Stelazine), and fluphenazine (Prolixin) are the drugs of choice in this situation. They are potent in their antipsychotic effect without the major side effects of sedation or hypotension that characterize the lower-potency antipsychotic agents such as chlorpromazine and thioridazine hydrochloride. Sedation is not an essential feature in the treatment of acute psychosis. In fact, it may be counterproductive since the patient may feel the increased discomfort of obtundation. While every antipsychotic drug has some sedative effect, in the high-potency preparations, it is minimal. A hypotensive effect occasionally limits the dosage of antipsychotic medication. The high-potency preparations also minimize this side effect when compared with the lower-potency drugs for equal therapeutic effectiveness.

A frequent side effect of the chemotherapy of psychosis is development of acute extrapyramidal reactions of the dystonic type. These usually occur within the first hours or days of antipsychotic drug use, and are uncommon after the first 2–4 weeks. They consist of involuntary contraction of the muscles of the face, neck, and throat. Swallowing may be difficult, and occasionally the airway is impaired. The incidence of this complication is markedly reduced by prophylactic treatment with benztropine mesylate (Cogentin), 2 mg orally twice a day beginning with the first dose of antipsychotic drug. Should the reaction occur despite this therapy, it may be treated with intravenous diphenhydramine hydrochloride (Benadryl), 50 mg.

Having chosen an appropriate antipsychotic drug, the physician should consider the dosage schedule and route of administration. The intramuscular route usually is preferred because of rapid onset of action and a high initial level in the blood. If this is not feasible, oral liquid medication may be satisfactory. Tablets are not always swallowed and may be hidden easily, with resulting confusion about the dose received.

An appropriate initial dose of haloperidol is 5 or 10 mg, depending on age, weight, and severity of illness. This dose may be repeated every 60 minutes until satisfactory improvement occurs, the patient sleeps, or a maximal dose of 100 mg has been administered. Optimal improvement usually occurs at doses between 15 and 40 mg, although higher doses occasionally are required. Under circumstances in which doses greater than 40 mg appear to be required, the diagnosis should be reassessed. Trifluoperazine hydrochloride is about half as potent as haloperidol, and fluphenazine is about 1½ times as potent. Doses may be adjusted accordingly. Careful observation during this period is necessary to note signs of excessive sedation, an extrapyramidal reaction, or hypotension.

The goal of initial treatment is to reduce psychotic symptoms sufficiently to make outpatient management feasible. Many patients respond favorably to the regimen described. Those in whom the psychosis is not abated must receive inpatient treatment.

Outpatient Follow-up Care

If the psychotic process has been brought to remission and if the other appropriate criteria are fulfilled (Fig. 18.1), outpatient follow-up care should be arranged. Outpatient treatment must include monitoring of chemotherapeutic requirements and psychotherapy directed at restoration of premorbid function and reparation of the social and family turmoil brought about by the psychotic process. A psychiatrist is usually best able to satisfy these requirements, and appropriate referral should be made. Pending transfer of the patient to the care of another physician, the emergency physician may find it necessary to continue chemotherapy for several days. Usually the total initial dose that was effective in bringing about remission should be continued on a daily basis by the oral route. The most frequent cause of relapse is premature reduction of medication. If sedation and extrapyramidal reactions are not excessive, this dose may be continued for days or weeks until reliable follow-up care is arranged. Occasionally, a larger dose is required. Recurrence of psychotic thinking or insomnia suggests the need for additional medication. A reduction of dosage is indicated when excessive sedation or extrapyramidal reactions occur.

If the patient is manic-depressive, maintenance chemotherapy might include lithium carbonate. This treatment is usually outside the scope of the emergency physician, and should properly be monitored by the psychiatrist to whom the patient is referred.

Suicide

Self-destruction is a common event frequently preceded by incomplete or "unsuccessful" attempts. Although it is listed as the tenth leading cause of death, the actual incidence is virtually impossible to determine since many apparent accidents may be suicides.

Since these considerations are well known and generally appreciated, it is curious that the patient who has attempted suicide receives remarkably little sympathy from medical personnel. Emergency ward staff often become angry when a patient with a self-inflicted injury arrives. The feeling that the patient should have "finished the job" and other such attitudes ought to be recognized since they may lead to inadvertent improper care. It is not difficult to appreciate the origin of such notions in the harassed emergency physician who may be busy with many accidents and injuries and who may, therefore, view the attempted-suicide patient as unnecessary extra work. Those whose

INITIAL EXAMINATION

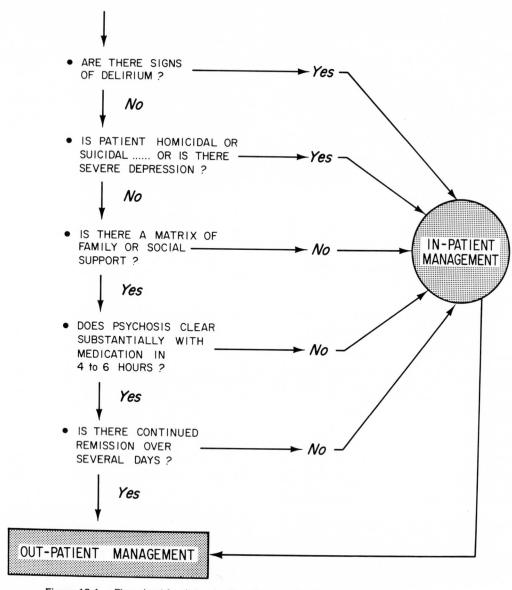

Figure 18.1.   Flow sheet for determination of appropriate inpatient/outpatient management.

lives are dedicated to the cure and amelioration of illness may find it difficult to have any empathic feeling for those whose actions so openly reject life as worthy of preservation. Although the emergency physician cannot always prevent the emergence of these feelings, he should make every effort to avoid compromise of patient care as a result.

Such subjective attitudes notwithstanding, evaluation and treatment would be relatively simple if all suicide attempts were equally serious. However,

the task is complicated by the fact that, like all other human illness, the degree of severity falls within a spectrum. At one end, the psychotic depressive who has swallowed a lethal dose of barbiturates before jumping in front of a subway train should obviously be hospitalized and intensively treated. At the other end, the adolescent who fails a minor examination and takes 6 aspirin before calling an ambulance may not require hospitalization. Seldom is the situation so clear-cut, however. Even attempts that appear minor may be an

Table 18.3.
Factors that increase degree of suicidal danger. [a]

Affirmation of suicidal intention

Psychosis (especially acute schizophrenic or manic-depressive)

Major depression (especially with insomnia or anorexia)

History of impaired impulse control

Contemplation or use of a violent method (e.g., subway train, shooting, hanging)

Alcohol or drug dependence

Social isolation (divorce, separation, friendlessness)

Previous suicide attempts

Family history of suicide or affect disorder

Recent major loss of self-esteem (e.g., loss of love or employment)

Subjective perception of helplessness and hopelessness

Presence of suicide note

Concurrent medical disease (serious, chronic, incurable)

Age (greater with advancing age, except for young psychotics)

Sex (men more than women)

[a] Factors are listed in descending order of seriousness.

early warning of a serious psychopathologic disturbance. In the emergency ward, it is best to assume that suicidal thoughts or actions are evidence of a serious morbid process. Ideally, every suicide attempt should be investigated by a psychiatric consultant called to the emergency ward. Since this is not always feasible, some guidelines are necessary to gauge the degree of imminent danger so that appropriate treatment plans can be made (Table 18.3). The following criteria should be considered before disposition of the patient.

Assessment of Suicidal Risk

Suicidal Intention. The simplest, most important means of evaluation is to ask the patient his intention; this is frequently neglected, however. By assessing the content and quality of the patient's answer, the physician obtains the single most valuable piece of information. Patients who state that they intend to take their lives should be believed, at least in the emergency ward evaluation. The physician is often reluctant to question the patient directly on this point, with the erroneous assumption that it may plant an idea in the patient's mind. Clinical experience shows that virtually every depressed person has entertained suicidal thoughts at some level and that the patient may be somewhat reassured by receiving implicit permission to discuss his thoughts or intentions. Questions such as "Have you been thinking of harming yourself

or taking your life?" tactfully stated can do no harm and may provide information not available by other means. Those who state their intention to attempt or to repeat suicidal behavior must have immediate psychiatric consultation.

Psychosis. As noted previously, the psychotic patient, especially when symptoms are acute, is in serious danger of inadvertent self-harm because of disordered perception and thought process. When suicidal ideation or attempt is added to an ongoing psychotic episode, the risk is extreme. Protective environment is mandatory at least until the major overt manifestations of psychosis are controlled. Psychoses with manic features are especially dangerous because of the intense and poorly directed energy available to these patients and because moods may be very labile. Even marked elevations of mood contain the seeds of profound depression. Patients with schizophrenic psychosis may have imperative auditory hallucinations ("Jump out the window!") or such intense persecutory delusions that death may seem a preferable alternative.

Major Depression. This criterion in the assessment of suicidal risk involves not only the subjective feeling of sadness or loss but also the symptoms suggestive of biologic involvement and termed endogenous. Insomnia is frequently profound, and the pattern is usually that of early morning wakening, although the patient may have difficulty in falling asleep as well. In addition, anorexia and weight loss may occur. Other suggestive symptoms are loss of libido, psychomotor retardation, and amenorrhea. When depression is substantial and accompanied by these symptoms, the risk of suicide is greatly increased. In a given patient, the risk can be greatest either as a depression is deepening or as it is getting better.

History of Impaired Impulse Control. Suicide or its attempt is often an impulsive act. Unlike most similar acts, it is irreversible—a notion which, curiously, may elude the patient. Those whose risk is greatest are those whose life-style is marked by the tendency to avoid realization of the implications of their actions. Prominent examples are reckless drivers, heavy drinkers, those with a poor employment history, and those with considerable family turmoil. Deficiencies of personality development that characterize the patient with poor impulse control not only make a specific suicidal act more probable but also suggest that other risk factors are likely to be increased.

Social Isolation. Those who can share distress are more fortunate than those who must bear it alone. The well-adjusted person with difficulties can nevertheless sustain himself by drawing on the psychic and material resources of friends and relatives. Those without families or friends have no such reserves on which to draw. While others may be rescued from the intention or consequences of a suicidal act, the isolated person enjoys no such likelihood.

Previous Suicide Attempts. Some physicians may believe that a history of previous suicide attempts suggests that future risk is less serious, presumably on the misconception that the first could not have been serious since the patient did not succeed. To the contrary notwithstanding, there is about a 10% chance of successful suicide within 10 years after a significant attempt.

Recent Major Loss of Self-esteem. Some persons depend on one or more extrinsic evidences of self-worth for their ego identity. These may include financial status, social position, or family harmony. Sudden and irrevocable loss of one of these supports may provide sufficient impetus for a major suicide attempt. Such an act may also be manipulative in the sense that it may be an attempt to restore the lost support. It is nevertheless perilous for the physician to assume that an attempt is manipulative and that it is therefore not serious.

Contemplation or Use of a Violent Method. Investigators in the area of the psychodynamics of suicide have repeatedly emphasized the importance of anger as a concomitant of self-destruction. Anger may provide the energy for the attempt to succeed. An index of the magnitude of the anger is the degree of violence it requires for its expression. Mutilation, shooting, hanging, or the use of painful corrosive poisons not only increases the likelihood of a successful suicide attempt but also suggests a high degree of anger.

Presence of a Suicide Note. Investigators have repeatedly noted an association between the use of a suicide note and the successfulness of the attempt. One suggestion is that the note represents an emotional testament to express the patient's intent after his death.

Concurrent Medical Disease. Maintenance of a well-integrated life with continued rewards requires acceptable physical health. When pain, weakness, and incapacity become constant companions, adaptive resources become depleted.

Sex. Although women are more likely to attempt suicide, men are more likely to carry the attempt to completion.

Age. In general, older patients are more vulnerable to completed suicide than are younger patients. However, suicide is the second leading cause of death in adolescents, exceeded only by accidents.

Alcohol or Drug Dependence. For several reasons, victims of alcohol or drug addiction have an increased risk for completed suicide. Impulse control is diminished during acute intoxications, social supports may be transitory or nonexistent, and there is a diminished capacity for adaptive restoration because of impaired sensorium.

Family History of Suicide or Affect Disorder. A family history of suicide has taught the individual, perhaps at an early age, that this method of ultimate escape is not without precedent and perhaps does not hold special personal, social, or religious opprobrium. Furthermore, suicide in first-degree relatives suggests the likelihood of an affect disorder, which has strong genetic components.

Treatment

An expressed suicide intention or overt attempt should ideally be managed by a psychiatrist in the emergency situation. Since this is not always possible, the emergency physician must make the best compromise available, given the resources of time and personnel. Those patients indicated by one or more of the previously discussed criteria to be at significant risk should be hospitalized and observed pending psychiatric consultation. Psychotic patients may be evaluated and aggressively treated on a medical ward. The physician may elect to transfer the patient to a psychiatric ward of a general hospital (ideally) or he may elect to send the patient to a psychiatric hospital. The physician is urged to become familiar with the available resources for management within the community.

The Homicidal and the Assaultive Patient

These patients can present the most disruptive and most difficult situations that the emergency physician must face. The usual means by which the emergency ward treats patients often become paralyzed in the presence of either threatened or overt violence.

General Considerations and Initial Management

Regardless of the cause of the episode, the most reasonable initial assumption is that overwhelming anger is the phenomenologic substrate. The physician must try to understand the anger before accurate diagnostic evaluation can proceed. Statements such as "Stop acting like a child" and "Control yourself" are often not helpful. Instead, the physician should try to assume that the anger may be partly justified, at least in principle if not in mode of expression or intensity. If possible, a relevant history should first be obtained from relatives or police officers. The patient should then be interviewed in surroundings of reasonable privacy and security. An initial statement such as "You appear very angry. Could you explain your feelings to me?" is often helpful. This allows the patient the opportunity to substitute verbal aggression for physical violence, and suggests the possibility that the physician may become an ally. After reasonable opportunity for expression of feelings, the patient is usually much more amenable to further history-taking and examination. Medication may then be offered with the suggestion that it will help the patient to be calm.

On rare occasions, violence may become overt in the emergency ward before peaceful methods of solution can be utilized. Since the safety of other patients and staff cannot be compromised, physical methods of control must be employed. Should this become necessary, the best strategy is use of overwhelming force. Several persons must work together to apply needed restraint. Ideally, these are security personnel with special training. Avoidance of unnecessary injury is sometimes facilitated by use of a mattress to immobilize the patient while restraint is applied.

Adjunctive chemotherapy is often indicated in the emergency ward. For patients in whom the diagnosis is unclear, the best choice is usually a parenteral high-potency antipsychotic drug such as haloperidol or thiothixine. The parenteral route is preferred because of greater speed of absorption. If the physician's judgment is to use oral medication, liquid preparations are preferred to tablets. One important exception to the use of antipsychotic agents is psychosis produced by large doses of anticholinergic drugs. Antipsychotic drugs make this condition worse. Fortunately, such a diagnosis is usually easy to make by history and physical findings. Barbiturates and other similar sedatives are inappropriate and may worsen assaultive behavior, unless it can be determined that the underlying cause is a withdrawal phenomenon such as barbiturate withdrawal or delirium tremens.

Oral medication should be liquid to ensure that the patient swallows it. It has the advantage that the patient begins to participate in his care but the disadvantage of somewhat slower absorption. Choices of drug and dosage must be individualized to the person and the situation. Chlorpromazine may be given in doses of 50 mg intramuscularly or 100 mg orally, repeated every half-hour if necessary. Haloperidol may be given in doses of 5–10 mg intramuscularly or orally every 30 to 60 minutes.

Specific Causes of Violent Behavior

Each of the following may represent the underlying difficulty in violent episodes:

(1) Catatonic excitement. A patient with a history of psychosis who has an unmanageable violent episode is likely to be experiencing the excited form of catatonia. He is usually oblivious to his surroundings and, if untreated, may die of exhaustion or injury. Treatment is the aggressive use of chemotherapy as discussed. On some occasions, electroconvulsive therapy may be necessary.

(2) "Delirious" mania. The patient has a history of manic-depressive disease. Treatment of the acute episode is the same as that for catatonic excitement.

(3) Paranoid delusions. The actively delusional patient is in constant danger of acting as if his delusions were true, planning and carrying out an aggressive defense against his imagined persecutors. In the emergency ward, he may appear brooding and quiet, but may still be capable of acting out homicidal plans. The danger is increased if symptoms are relatively acute and if delusions relate to a specific person or group. Imperative auditory hallucinations ("Kill your parents!") are likewise an ominous sign. Such patients require antipsychotic chemotherapy and a protective hospital environment until symptoms subside.

(4) Sedative intoxication and withdrawal. Sedatives can be responsible for acutely diminished impulse control. Such disability may occur with either a heavy intoxication or acute withdrawal from an addicting substance. Alcohol is the most notorious offending agent, but barbiturates and other sedatives must be considered as well. Some persons are susceptible to "pathologic" intoxication, which occurs with small amounts of alcohol.

Intoxicated states can usually be recognized by slurred speech, incoordination, ataxia, and vertical nystagmus. Treatment requires a quiet, protective environment with special nursing if possible to avoid such secondary emergencies as aspiration of vomitus. Physical restraint should be minimal and must not be used if the patient cannot be watched constantly. If chemical restraint cannot be avoided, the best choice is a high-potency antipsychotic agent such as haloperidol, which has relatively little hypotensive effect and sedative potentiation. The dose should be 5 mg intramuscularly.

Withdrawal states can be recognized by tremor, autonomic hyperactivity, diaphoresis, disorientation, visual hallucinosis, seizures, hyperreflexia, and mydriasis. Treatment requires controlled administration of a cross-tolerant sedative. Diazepam is a good choice. The initial dose may be 5 mg intravenously, administered slowly. Careful observation is required to avoid oversedation or respiratory depression. Oral diazepam may be used after initial control is obtained.

(5) Phencyclidine intoxication. This is a common cause of extreme or episodic violence. It may be suspected by a history of drug ingestion or inhalation. Physical findings include blank stare, labile mental status, nystagmus, ataxia, hypertension, and anesthesia (see Chapter 17, pages 394–395).

(6) Temporal lobe epilepsy. While frequently suspected as an underlying substrate to violence, seizure activity is an uncommon explanation. When it is suspected on historical grounds or because of the presence of aura, an electroencephalogram recorded during sleep may be confirmatory, but often is not. Anticonvulsant medication may be useful.

(7) Antisocial personality. Violent behavior occasionally may arise without any evidence of illness. This usually occurs in patients with a long history of criminal offenses or antisocial behavior. If no other evidence of medical or psychiatric illness is found, appropriate limit-setting should be employed, including consultation with law enforcement authorities.

Hospitalization

Hospitalization may be voluntary or involuntary. The latter is implemented only as a last resort when the physician has compelling evidence that the patient is in imminent danger of causing himself or another person serious harm because of the disordered mental state. The physician must become familiar with the law concerning involuntary hospitalization within his jurisdiction.

Psychosis by itself often does not justify involuntary hospitalization. If the possibility of serious harm is not imminent, the patient may refuse treatment as in any medical condition. However, a patient who is not formally homicidal or suicidal may require involuntary hospitalization if his judgment is so impaired that his safety is seriously compromised. For example, a manic patient may believe it is possible to walk 100 miles in subzero weather with inadequate clothing.

In most cases, voluntary hospitalization is accepted when the physician states his recommendation with conviction and firmness. Any ambiguity or uncertainty is likely to be magnified by the patient, who probably has a pathologic degree of ambivalence. It is essential to involve the family as much as possible in the decision to hospitalize.

This is not always easy, since the family's perceptions and concerns often vary considerably from those of the hospital staff. Some family members become excessively worried about minor symptoms, such as an acute extrapyramidal reaction, while others deny the significance of the most florid psychosis. All too often, family members resist acceptance of a psychiatric diagnosis with the outdated belief that such a diagnosis implies culpability for improper child-rearing or suggests the possibility of genetic taint.

Having accepted in principle the physician's recommendation for hospitalization, the patient or family may enter a phase of bargaining. The argument often consists of such statements as "I will stay in the hospital, but not tonight," "I must put my affairs in order first," or "I want to be on a medical ward but not a psychiatric ward." Such behavior may be symptomatic of the original illness, or it may be an attempt to deny the seriousness of the situation. Occasionally, it is a test of the physician's judgment and firmness. Once the decision to hospitalize is made, however, there must be no ambiguity in decisions to implement it. The patient must not be allowed to leave the hospital with the promise to return later.

Finally, those who resist all recommendations and who cannot be hospitalized involuntarily should be asked to indicate their intention by signing out "against advice." Since many patients are unwilling to do even this, a careful note should be made and witnessed in the hospital record.

After arrival on the ward, further management is facilitated by aggressive treatment. Patients may wish to sign themselves out soon after arrival unless treatment begins at once. When appropriate, antipsychotic medication should be prescribed and all necessary supervisory and nursing care ordered.

LESS SEVERE DISORDERS

Acute Anxiety Attacks and Hyperventilation

Anxiety is a symptom of many psychiatric conditions and some organic diseases. In addition, it may occur episodically in entirely healthy persons. Psychiatric conditions with manifest anxiety include incipient and acute schizophrenia, agitated depression, and transient situational disturbances. As always, the first concern of the emergency physician is to consider the possibility of an acute medical condition with psychiatric symptoms. The organic differential diagnosis includes effects of exogenous substances, metabolic disturbances, and cardiorespiratory conditions. Among exogenous substances, caffeine, amphetamines, corticosteroids, and withdrawal from alcohol or sedatives must be considered. Metabolic conditions of importance are hypoglycemia, electrolyte disturbances, hyperthyroidism, and pheochromocytoma. Cardiovascular and respiratory disturbances may include arrhythmia, mitral prolapse, asthma, congestive heart failure, and pulmonary embolism.

Commonly, however, none of these conditions is apparent. Typically, the patient appears at the emergency ward very frightened and agitated, with a history of shortness of breath of acute onset. The sensation may be described as the inability to take a deep-enough breath. Chest pain or pressure may be present, and muscular symptoms suggestive of hypocalcemia, such as carpopedal spasm, also occasionally may occur. The subjective sensation is one of impending doom. Sensory changes consist of paresthesias of the distal extremities and of the circumoral region. Most commonly, the acute anxiety attack is seen in young adults. It is unusual for a first attack to occur over the age of 35 years. When this constellation of findings appears without indication of other illness, the diagnosis of an acute anxiety attack is made.

Immediate treatment is directed at removal of physical symptoms. Since these are brought about by shift in the acid-base balance secondary to hyperventilation, restoring the balance brings quick relief. Among the most popular and inexpensive methods is use of a paper bag, which the patient holds over his mouth to rebreathe expired air and consequently to increase alveolar carbon dioxide. Rapid relief of symptoms is usual.

The next task is to demonstrate to the patient that his symptoms have resulted from simple hyperventilation. This is not always easy, and patients may cling for some time to the idea that they have had a "heart attack." One of the most dramatic and effective educational methods is to have the patient deliberately hyperventilate for several minutes or until symptoms are reproduced. This usually requires considerable encouragement by the physician, but is well worth the effort on those occasions when the patient is initially refractory to acceptance of a psychologic explanation.

By this time, the patient may be ready to accept the suggestion that "nerves" may have something to do with the symptoms. If approached diplomatically, most patients are able to relate some information concerning emotional turmoil that might have contributed to the emergent symptoms. The physician may now be tempted to prescribe one of the commonly used antianxiety agents such as chlordiazepoxide or diazepam. Generally, such prescription is premature at best. Often the attack is an isolated episode, and a few minutes of discussion will elucidate the psychodynamic or environmental cause. The physician does the patient much more service by sympathetic listening followed by firm reassurance than by mechanically prescribing a pill. Chemotherapy is seldom required.

Antianxiety agents do, however, occasionally have value in other situations. Chlordiazepoxide and diazepam are effective in the treatment of occasional anticipatory anxiety. Patients with phobias for air travel or public speaking, for example, may achieve satisfactory relief in a much more economical way than might be the case with psychotherapeutic treatment.

Chronic or frequent episodic anxiety is a different problem. If anxiety is severe and prolonged, psychiatric referral is appropriate for definitive diagnosis and management. Chronic use of sedatives and antianxiety agents is seldom effective, since tolerance grows and habituation is a possibility. Despite advertising claims, phenothiazines and similar compounds have little demonstrable action in anxiety relief. The unfortunate terms "major" and "minor" tranquilizers have increased confusion about this issue. It is well to remember that there are no "tranquilizers"—there are antipsychotic, antidepressant, and antianxiety agents. Each has its indications and likewise its limits of usefulness.

Insomnia

Difficulty with sleep is a frequent complaint late at night in the emergency ward, occasionally to the ironic amusement of a sleepy physician, who is often tempted to prescribe a single dose of sedative and hope that the matter will end there. A better strategy is to investigate the differential diagnosis of insomnia. Difficulty in sleeping can be a presenting symptom of virtually any psychiatric condition and numerous medical problems. Among the major psychiatric conditions frequently implicated are acute schizophrenia, manic-depressive disease, chronic abuse of amphetamines or cocaine, and incipient delirium tremens. Each of these usually presents no diagnostic difficulty after a brief history and examination.

Having excluded major disturbances, the emergency physician is often faced with treating a patient who gives a history of recent onset of inability to sleep with an absence of other symptoms. Occasionally a history of recent situational difficulty may be elicited—perhaps tension relating to an examination, a change in occupation, or family disharmony. Sometimes the cause of insomnia may be as simple as excessive use of caffeine or a restless new baby in the house. On careful history-taking and examination, most causes of insomnia may be elucidated without serious difficulty. There are, nevertheless, certain cases that remain refractory to investigation. The possibility must be considered that the patient may be a drug abuser hoping for a prescription for sedatives or even that he may be seeking sedatives with suicidal intention.

The general approach to treatment is to attempt specific therapy for the underlying condition if possible. Schizophrenic patients should receive antipsychotic medications on either an inpatient or outpatient basis. Manic patients can similarly benefit from such medications. Those with endogenous depression should receive tricyclic antidepressants. In general, however, it is not reasonable to begin treatment for these conditions in the emergency service.

Insomnia as a result of environmental events may respond to brief psychotherapy or to a short course of small amounts of sedatives at bedtime. Advice and reassurance, as well as courtesy and empathy, may have much more desirable long-term benefits than a casually written prescription for sedatives. After exclusion of specific clinical entities as causes of insomnia, the physician must decide what treatment, if any, is appropriate for so-called primary insomnia. Specific guidelines are as follows:

(1) Sedatives should not be prescribed if the cause of insomnia is inapparent. A transient situation occasionally may suggest the desirability of short-term bedtime sedation.

(2) Prescription of barbiturates should be avoided. They have a high abuse potential and relatively low index of safety, and they may agitate elderly patients.

(3) Prescription of sedatives for longer than a few days should be avoided. They lose effectiveness, and in addition, abuse potential may be increased.

(4) Flurazepam hydrochloride and related benzodiazepine compounds are among the safest and most effective short-term sedative-hypnotic agents.

(5) Although numerous hypnotic preparations have been marketed with considerable advertising fanfare, none shows special advantage over preparations mentioned previously, and some are much more dangerous and likely to lead to habituation.

(6) Sedatives should not be prescribed for patients with a history of alcohol abuse. Not only may alcohol and sedatives act synergistically with dangerous results but also alcoholism that is currently in remission may be reactivated by prescription of cross-tolerant drugs.

(7) When in doubt, medication should not be prescribed. For the physician to do otherwise is much more likely to complicate the situation than to be helpful.

Pain and Hypochondriasis

Occasionally, a patient will appear in the emergency ward with a complaint of severe pain for which no cause is immediately obvious or which seems disproportionate to the visible lesion or injury. If the patient is hostile or demanding or exhibits marked dramatic or histrionic behavior, the physician may be persuaded that the pain is psychogenic—a euphemism for saying that the patient is lying. Such patients represent extremely challenging diagnostic problems.

It must be remembered that pain is *always* "in the head" and that while personality factors may color its mode of expression or intensity, no reliable information as to cause necessarily need be implied. To assume otherwise sets the stage for the possibility of serious error.

The physician may be under the impression that the situation can be clarified by administration of a "pain-killing" placebo. This practice should be abandoned since it provides no useful information, and on discovery, which is frequent, it almost invariably leads to irreparable rupture of any rapport with the patient. This is not to say that placebo trials have no place. A significant number of patients respond to placebos, experiencing significant pain relief from inactive injections, regardless of the cause of pain. The properly executed trial requires informed consent, a well-controlled schedule of various analgesics as well as placebo, and an inpatient setting with the goal of determining the most effective schedule of medication for chronic pain. Such trials are inappropriate and impractical in the acute situation in the emergency ward.

Finally, it is wise to avoid the essentially pejorative labeling of a patient as hysterical or hypochondriacal. This not only interferes with clarity of diagnostic thinking but also may compromise future care if unsupported assumptions are made in the medical record. In a survey of 74 patients so labeled, Slater and Glithero found that three-fourths were seriously ill or had died in a 5- to 10-year follow-up period. Good medical practice demands suspension of such judgments before thorough diagnostic evaluation.

Family Turmoil

That couples and families come to the emergency ward for aid in solving domestic crises gives testimony to the frequent absence of other sources of counsel. On some occasions, one of the members first presents a nonspecific medical complaint, while on other occasions the physician is simply asked for emergency family therapy.

Most often, one member of the family is defined as the patient at the outset. The best strategy is usually to interview this person alone at first. Depending on the circumstances, the physician may then wish to interview other parties separately or together. This process is not always excessively time-consuming, although it can be. The most important task is to identify the possibility of such serious conditions as incipient psychosis, assault, and child-battering. Having excluded such possibilities, the physician may make appropriate referral to available family counseling. The main pitfall to avoid is coming to a premature conclusion and hence giving advice based on inadequate information. The emergency physician must not expect himself to be an accomplished single-visit family counselor, and should avoid accepting such a role if it is thrust on him. His obligations are to intercept nascent emergencies and to make impartial referrals when indicated.

Grief Reactions

Psychologic reaction to major personal loss is a commonly encountered difficulty in emergency practice. The reaction may be acute, as is the case when a relative is brought to the hospital dead on arrival, or symptoms may be delayed, causing a later visit to the emergency ward with symptoms either directly felt or displaced, perhaps as insomnia or as a gastrointestinal disturbance.

Often it is the unhappy task of the emergency physician to speak to relatives immediately after the death of a loved one. Occasionally, the physician may be under a mistaken impression that the relatives are already aware of the death. It is the physician's duty to inform them, which is best done in a gentle manner in a private setting. It usually is best to avoid unnecessary and unsolicited details, but all relevant questions should be answered. The well-integrated family may require little further assistance. Families without interpersonal resources may need the help of other professionals, such as a clergyman or lawyer. The physician should attempt to recognize this need and to arrange the appropriate referral. Occasionally, a sedative is helpful if especially severe reaction is noted.

Persons with protracted, delayed, or displaced grief reactions also may seek emergency assistance. The immediate task is to identify such grief as a probable cause for nonspecific symptoms such as insomnia, anorexia, anxiety, or depression. If the reaction appears unusually intense or if the patient does not show the expected gradual recovery in the course of several weeks, referral for short-term psychotherapy may be helpful.

SPECIAL PROBLEMS

Extrapyramidal Reactions

Reactions of the extrapyramidal system to phenothiazine compounds and related drugs frequently are encountered. Drugs most commonly implicated are the high-potency phenothiazines, such as trifluoperazine, prochlorperazine (Compazine), fluphenazine, and perphenazine (Trilafon), and haloperidol, a butyrophenone. The most common reaction seen in the emergency ward is dystonia that usually involves the facial muscles, the tongue, and the sternocleidomastoid muscles. Torticollis or an oculogyric crisis may occur. Also seen are akathisia, a syndrome of motor restlessness chiefly visible in the legs, and classic parkinsonian tremor.

Diagnosis is not difficult when a history of drug intake is known. Dystonia has been mistaken for a conversion reaction, possibly because the muscle spasm may respond transiently to suggestion or to treatment with a placebo. Occasionally, even tetanus may be suspected. The manifestations may provoke intense anxiety. Oculogyric crisis is especially troublesome in this regard.

Fortunately, the most severe symptoms of dystonia may be reversed readily by intramuscular injection of diphenhydramine hydrochloride, 50 mg, which brings about remission within 15 minutes. Intravenous administration is preferred if symptoms are very distressing or if there is any suggestion of respiratory difficulty. In such cases, the same dose should be given over 3–5 minutes. Complete remission of symptoms usually occurs within a few minutes.

The physician must then address the question of whether to maintain or to discontinue administration of the phenothiazine compound. It is helpful to contact the prescribing physician for guidance. If the drug has been given for a benign and self-limiting condition such as nausea or vomiting, it may be best to discontinue the offending agent. If, however, the medication has been prescribed for the treatment of psychosis, it is usually better to continue the phenothiazine, perhaps at a reduced dosage, allowing the prescribing physician to make further changes. The treatment of psychosis often requires use of phenothiazines in doses that may be expected to cause extrapyramidal reactions. These usually can be controlled satisfactorily with appropriate medication for drug-induced parkinsonism, such as benztropine mesylate, 1 or 2 mg twice a day.

After emergency treatment of the dystonia, remembering that phenothiazine compounds have a longer duration of action than diphenhydramine hydrochloride, the physician should prescribe benztropine mesylate or a similar agent for several days to avoid recurrence, even if the offending drug is to be discontinued.

Lithium Toxicity

Widespread use of lithium carbonate for the treatment and prophylaxis of manic-depressive disease raises the possibility that the emergency physician may see a patient with acute or subacute lithium toxicity. The therapeutic range is 0.6–1.2 mEq/liter. Levels more than 1.5 mEq/liter may be in the toxic range. Clinical expression of excess serum lithium concentration begins with tremor and proceeds to nausea, vomiting, slurred speech, ataxia, seizures, coma, and death.

Lithium concentration in excess of the therapeutic range may occur as a result of several situations. Acute suicidal overdose is the most serious and may result in very high serum concentrations. Chronic mild overdose due to the patient's misunderstanding of directions or the theory that "if a little is good, a lot is better" is also possible. Patients inadvertently placed on a low-salt diet as well as on lithium also may have a toxic reaction. Finally, diminished renal function that is primary, or that is secondary to decreased cardiac output, promotes a toxic state due to failure of excretion. In mild and moderate states of toxicity, treatment is directed at removal of the cause and administration of saline solution. In severe intoxications, lithium excretion may be enhanced by urea-induced diuresis, alkalization of urine, and administration of aminophylline.

Chronic Brain Syndromes

Patients with a chronic brain syndrome frequently are brought to the emergency ward by frustrated, desperate, or angry relatives with the demand that the hospital "do something." The precipitating event may be acute, such as an episode of assaultive behavior, or it may be a chronic accumulation of family frustrations. Frequently, the situation presents itself during night or weekend hours when the resources of the emergency ward are minimal for effective resolution.

This situation requires the services of a skilled and compassionate physician. On the one hand, he must avoid giving in to inappropriate family demands, while on the other, he must give due consideration to their problems within the context of optimal patient care.

The first consideration is to determine, if possible, whether the precipitating event might have been brought about by sudden deterioration of function from ongoing medical illness that might have a remedy. If this is the case, delicate negotiation with the family often can proceed to a conclusion satisfactory to all. Cardiopulmonary or renal failure and other metabolic derangements are common causes to be investigated.

In many cases, identification of a specific medical precipitant is not possible. The task then is to determine what balance of medical, psychologic, and social remedies best serves the patient within the context of his current situation. Paranoid ideation may be diminished or eliminated by relatively small amounts of antipsychotic medication. Often the best choice is a high-potency drug such as trifluoperazine or haloperidol, which may have little direct sedative or hypotensive effect. Night wandering or irritable agitation similarly may be diminished to an acceptable level.

Throughout the evaluation it must be remembered that nothing tends to upset the patient with chronic brain disease more than calling attention to his disabilities or asking him to perform mental status tasks that are beyond his ability. Extreme diplomacy is required during and after examination.

Optimal care of the patient may require a change in social environment. A family that is unable or unwilling to provide satisfactory care may make placement in a nursing home the most satisfactory alternative. Decisions of this nature with major long-term consequences often are best deferred for a few days until the situation can be clarified by further investigation of the social as well as medical status. If no immediate medical remedy can be found, a brief admission might be the most satisfactory alternative.

Drug Abuse

For the past 15 years, drug abuse, especially among the young, has come increasingly to the attention of physicians. The original cause is obscure, and patterns of incidence are constantly changing. Results of treatment are dubious. For the emergency physician, there are two problems. First, he must diagnose and treat the acute effects of drug overdose and the possible medical complications. Second, he must try to refer patients for ongoing treatment when this is appropriate.

Medical Complications

In addition to the specific pharmacologic hazards of each of the various drugs of abuse, there are some general complications that may occur secondary to septic parenteral injection. Hepatitis is the most widely recognized, but tetanus, septic pulmonary embolism, pulmonary granulomatosis, and malaria are also possibilities. Subacute bacterial endocarditis and septicemia may occur. Organisms most frequently seen are coagulase-positive *Staphylococcus aureus*, enterococcus, *S. albus*, and Candida species. Occasionally seen are *Escherichia coli*, Klebsiella, and Pseudomonas.

Heroin and Other Opiates

Overdose is the most serious acute complication to opiate abuse. Within the subculture of the abuser, a variety of myths concerning treatment have developed, with the result that arrival at the emergency ward may be delayed by attempts to resuscitate by means of home remedies such as bathing in ice and intravenous injection of saline solutions. Diagnosis is made by history taken from friends, sclerosis of veins, respiratory depression, and pinpoint pupils (except in the case of meperidine hydrochloride [Demerol] overdose, in which pupils may be normal or dilated.) Treatment requires a narcotic antagonist, preferably naloxone hydrochloride (Narcan), 0.4 mg initially. This may be repeated two or three times as necessary in the first few minutes after arrival. Naloxone hydrochloride does not have respiratory depressive properties and, therefore, is safer than other narcotic antagonists. Supportive cardiorespiratory care is also required.

Pulmonary edema secondary to opiate overdose is variable in its time of presentation. Because delayed onset is a possibility, patients with severe opiate intoxication should be observed carefully for 24 hours even if they respond quickly to narcotic antagonists.

During the withdrawal phase of opiate abuse, the patient may be seen in the emergency ward with profound subjective distress but without major evidence of physiologic compromise. The typical pattern of most opiate abusers is such that florid symptoms of withdrawal seldom occur. The presenting symptoms are usually agitation, nausea, and muscle cramps with concurrent signs of mydriasis, diaphoresis, and gooseflesh. The patient may insist on receiving narcotics. If he is to be admitted for other reasons or specifically for detoxification, it is appropriate to administer methadone hydrochloride, 5–10 mg intramuscularly, to diminish unnecessary suffering. Since this is a long-acting preparation and since habituation to large doses is unusual, these injections are seldom required more than two or three times in 24 hours. In some centers, outpatient withdrawal schedules using oral methadone hydrochloride have had some success when combined with a highly structured program of group therapy. Without such a program, outpatient withdrawal is hazardous and should not be attempted.

Amphetamines

Psychiatric emergencies after amphetamine abuse are of two types. First, as the result of a single acute overdose, a typical presentation of toxic delirium may be seen, with disorientation, visual and auditory hallucinosis, change in vital signs, tremor, and autonomic hyperactivity. The patient may have mydriasis, elevated blood pressure and pulse, and diaphoresis. Activity usually is frenetic. When these signs are prominent with a history of acute amphetamine abuse, the diagnosis is clear. Treatment requires supportive care and administration of antipsychotic medication. Unlike in the treatment of functional psychosis, small doses are effective. Haloperidol, 2–5 mg, or trifluoperazine, 5 mg administered intramuscularly, usually brings about rapid resolution.

Second, when amphetamines are taken in moderate doses for several weeks, another toxic syndrome may develop. Termed amphetamine psychosis, it is a chronic paranoid condition suggestive of schizophrenia with insidious onset and without the usual signs of organic psychosis. Orientation and recent memory are preserved. Auditory hallucinations, delusions, and ideas of reference are prominent. Physical signs are absent. Indeed, it is usually impossible to separate this condition from paranoid schizophrenia except by a history of chronic amphetamine use or by urinary screening for amphetamines. This syndrome usually disappears a few weeks after discontinuing the drug. Hospitalization generally is necessary to ensure this.

LSD and Similar Hallucinogens

Abuse of hallucinogens appears to be declining. Patients with dysphoric phenomena associated with their use may be seen in the emergency ward after friends have made unsuccessful attempts to "talk down" the patient. Typically, patients are manifestly anxious with signs of sympathetic hyperactivity. Visual hallucinosis is the chief finding. Some delusional activity also may be present. Insight is usually preserved at least partly, so the patient is able to give a history of drug ingestion. Treatment requires supportive care and reassurance from a sympathetic person in a quiet, private, moderately lighted room. Diazepam, 5–15 mg orally, is the medication currently favored by experienced clinicians. Phenothiazine compounds have been reported to exacerbate the psychotic reaction.

Phencyclidine

This pernicious analog of ketamine has sedative, anesthetic, hallucinatory, and seizure-generating effects. It is produced cheaply in small illicit laboratories. It cannot be detected reliably by the usual toxic screening procedures. Clinical findings include extreme lability of mental status, from catatonia to violence; a blank stare, nystagmus, and sympathetic overactivity may be seen. The patient must be protected by all available means, including rest in a moderately lighted room, with close supervision and possibly restraints. Medical management is discussed in Chapter 17, pages 394–395.

Marihuana

Adverse reaction to marihuana is uncommon despite widespread use of the drug. Like all intoxicants, it is capable of producing variations in mental status, not always with a pleasurable result. Panic attacks and paranoid reactions have been seen. Usual signs and symptoms of intoxication include euphoria, changes in perception of time and space, hunger, dry mucous membranes, tachycardia, and conjunctival injection. Use of potent preparations such as hashish can cause more profound effects, including hallucinosis. Treatment is supportive, with rest and reassurance, and recovery may be expected in a few hours. The occasional paranoid reaction, if persistent beyond that time, should be investigated further in an inpatient setting.

Barbiturates and Other Sedatives

Acute overdose with rapid progression to coma is a medical emergency, whereas chronic abuse may provoke a more psychiatric emergency. All of the sedatives, including alcohol, tend to bring about cortical release phenomena with consequent diminution of impulse control and deterioration of social behavior. Barbiturates and other drugs then may cause episodic violent outbursts.

An additional complication may be seen during withdrawal from barbiturates and other sedatives. The patient may become tremulous, hyperreflexic, and hallucinatory, and in severe cases may have clinical features similar to those seen with delirium tremens. Such patients require hospitalization,

carefully controlled reintoxication, and slow, controlled withdrawal. The schedule of withdrawal depends on the particular sedative involved. Frequent examination is necessary. It is wise to depend on physical signs for dosage decisions rather than on subjectively reported symptoms, since sedative abusers are not noted for truthfulness. Outpatient withdrawal attempts virtually always fail.

Anticholinergic Drugs

A wide variety of prescription drugs as well as over-the-counter medications contain anticholinergic substances that may be implicated in psychiatric emergencies. Overdoses may be accidental or deliberate, either with suicidal or recreational intention. Atropine, scopolamine (hyoscine), and stramonium are the active ingredients, and may be found in antisecretory preparations and sleep medications. Symptoms of overdose are dry skin and mucous membranes, mydriasis, tachycardia, gastrointestinal atony, tactile and visual hallucinations, and delusional activity. Physostigmine is a specific antidote, but should be used with caution as discussed in Chapter 17, pages 383–386. Because it has a shorter duration of action than some anticholinergic compounds, multiple injections may be necessary. Quaternary compounds such as neostigmine are ineffective in reversal of central nervous system effects since they do not cross the blood-brain barrier.

Follow-up Care

Having resolved medical psychiatric emergencies of drug abuse, the physician must address the question of further care. Unfortunately, the current state of treatment can point to few concrete results. The best strategy for the emergency physician is to become familiar with regional facilities that specialize in drug problems.

Suggested Readings

Anderson WH, Kuehnle JC: Diagnosis and early management of acute psychosis. *N Engl J Med 305:*1128–1130, 1981
Anderson WH: The physical examination in office practice. *Am J Psychiat 137:*1188–1192, 1980
Anderson WH, Kuehnle JC, Catanzano DM: Rapid treatment of acute psychosis. *Am J Psychiat 133:*1076–1078, 1976
Detre TP, Jarecki HC: *Modern Psychiatric Treatment*. Philadelphia, J.B. Lippincott, 1971
Hackett TP, Cassem EH (Eds): *Handbook of General Hospital Psychiatry*. St. Louis, C.V. Mosby Co, 1978
Louria DB, Hensle T, Rose J: The major medical complications of heroin addiction. *Ann Intern Med 67:*1–22, 1967
Plum F, Posner JB: *The Diagnosis of Stupor and Coma*, ed 2. Philadelphia, F.A. Davis, 1972
Shader RI (Ed): *Manual of Psychiatric Therapeutics*. Boston, Little, Brown and Co., Inc., 1975
Stern TA, Anderson WH: Benztropine prophylaxis of dystonic reactions. *Psychopharmacology 61:*261–262, 1979

CHAPTER 19

Neonatal and Pediatric Emergencies

JOHN T. HERRIN, M.B.B.S.
RONALD BENZ, M.D.
I. DAVID TODRES, M.D.
DEMETRIOS ZUKIN, M.D.
CARLA B. COHEN, M.D.
DOROTHY H. KELLY, M.D.

Editor's Note: This chapter is one of the more difficult to limit to appropriate size in a general textbook. Most subjects peculiar to neonatal and pediatric life are covered herein. When management does not differ significantly from that in adult practice, the topic may be treated in a specialty chapter—pneumonia is discussed in Chapter 11 (Infectious Diseases in the Emergency Ward), for example.

EMERGENCIES IN THE NEWBORN

Fifty percent of pediatric deaths occur in the neonatal period, and most of these occur in the first week of life. The physician dealing with an acute emergency in a newborn has an important role in decreasing mortality and particularly in preventing mental and physical handicaps in those infants who survive such an emergency.

Resuscitation at Birth

Asphyxiation in a newborn constitutes a medical emergency. The asphyxiated infant should be placed in a warm environment to prevent the complications of hypothermia, and the heart rate, respiration rate, and muscular tone should be assessed rapidly.

At birth, if the infant has respiratory depression but has good muscular tone and a heart rate greater than 100 beats/min, securing a clear airway may be the only measure required to re-establish normal respirations and heart rate. This may be done by means of pharyngeal suctioning and by briefly stimulating the infant on the soles of the feet. If normal respirations do not occur within 30–45 seconds, assisted ventilation with a bag and face mask and oxygen should be instituted until regular respirations are established.

If the heart rate is less than 100 beats/min and falling, and if the infant has absent respirations and markedly diminished muscular tone, respiratory support should be instituted immediately with a bag and face mask and oxygen, followed by endotracheal intubation with a 3.5-mm endotracheal tube for a full-term infant and a 3.0-mm endotracheal tube for a premature infant. The infant is ventilated at a rate of 25–30 breaths/min; the resuscitator must ensure that ventilatory efforts result in adequate bilateral chest excursion. An umbilical catheter is passed via the umbilical artery or vein (see Chapter 32, page 701), and sodium bicarbonate is administered, 2 mEq/kg over a period of 1 minute initially to correct metabolic acidosis. Repeated doses of sodium bicarbonate are given, depending on the results of arterial blood-gas analyses.

If the patient has asystole or severe bradycardia (less than 80 beats/min), cardiac massage (Fig. 19.1) should be carried out at the rate of 100 compressions/min while the patient is ventilated at 20 breaths/min, that is, at a ratio of 5 compressions to 1 breath. Infusion of a colloid solution such as a 5% serum albumin solution or of Ringer's lactated solution may be necessary to expand the intravascular volume when hypovolemia is suspected.

After these measures are performed, drug therapy may be necessary. Required agents include atropine, 0.03 mg/kg; sodium bicarbonate, 2 mEq/

419

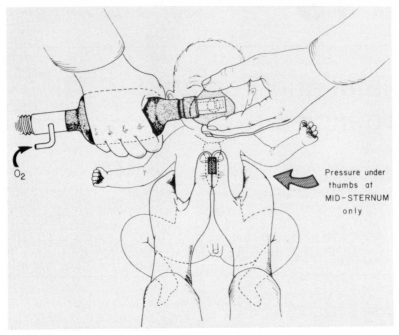

O2

Pressure under
thumbs at
MID-STERNUM
only

Figure 19.1.   Two-handed method of cardiac massage. Both hands encircle the chest and both thumbs are used for cardiac compression. (Reproduced by permission from Todres ID, Rogers MC: *J Pediatr 86:* 781–782, 1975.)

kg; elemental calcium, 10 mg/kg; epinephrine (1:10,000), 0.1 ml/kg; glucose (25% solution), 0.5 gm/kg; and isoproterenol, 0.1 μg/kg/min as a constant infusion. The drugs are administered preferably via an umbilical catheter; if this is not possible, they may be administered by intracardiac injection. Cardiac and pulmonary responses are monitored, and these agents are repeated as necessary.

The sick newborn is especially susceptible to cooling. Hypothermia leads to metabolic acidosis, cardiac depression, reduction in arterial partial pressure of oxygen (Pao$_2$), and respiratory depression—a series of events leading to an increase in morbidity and mortality. Measures to prevent hypothermia are paramount in the emergency care of any sick newborn. The temperature of the skin should be monitored and should be maintained at 96.8–97.7°F (36–36.5°C) by means of radiant heating devices during examination and treatment. The examining rooms must be heated generously at 75–80°F (23.9–26.6°C) to minimize radiant heat loss.

Although attention to the airway, respiration, circulation, and temperature is paramount in the asphyxiated infant, an attempt should be made to identify and to treat an underlying condition caus-

ing respiratory depression, such as heavy narcotic sedation of the mother. Once the infant's condition has been stabilized, arrangements should be made to transfer him to a neonatal intensive care unit for further definitive management of the underlying cause for the depression and of the possible sequelae of asphyxiation, including seizures and increased intracranial pressure.

Specific Conditions

Respiratory Distress

Respiratory distress in the newborn is an emergency. It is manifested by tachypnea, sternal and intercostal retractions, and grunting respirations; cyanosis indicates severe respiratory distress. The resultant hypoxemia is life-threatening and must be corrected immediately. Common causes of respiratory distress at birth are listed in Table 19.1.

Meconium Aspiration. Infants with meconium aspiration may have resultant severe chemical pneumonitis and severe hypoxemia, especially if the meconium is particulate. Meconium aspiration frequently is complicated by unilateral or bilateral pneumothorax. If the infant is in respiratory distress or if the meconium appears particulate, immediate endotracheal intubation and suctioning

Table 19.1.
Common causes of respiratory distress in newborns.

Respiratory depression and asphyxiation
Meconium aspiration
Effect of maternal drugs
  Narcotics
  Magnesium sulfate
  Anesthetic agents (general and local)
Hemorrhage and shock (abruptio placentae, placenta previa)
Hyaline membrane disease
Congenital heart disease
Pneumothorax
Congenital anomalies
  Choanal atresia
  Tracheoesophageal fistula
  Diaphragmatic hernia
  Hypoplastic lungs (Potter's syndrome)
  Lobar emphysema
  Laryngeal web
Traumatic delivery
  Cerebral trauma
  Spinal cord injury
  Recurrent laryngeal nerve palsy

are advised, followed by oxygenation with ventilatory support. Arterial blood-gas levels should then be monitored for assessment of the degree of respiratory failure to determine the necessary concentration of inspired oxygen and the amount of ventilatory support required. As soon as the infant's condition is stable, he should be transported to an intensive care unit.

Effect of Maternal Drugs. Opiates act on the infant as a depressant if they are given to the mother close to the time of delivery. Respiratory support should be given with a face mask and bag. If equipment is not immediately available, mouth-to-mouth or mouth-to-nose resuscitation may be necessary until the effects of the narcotics have worn off. The antidote naloxone hydrochloride may be administered, 0.01 mg/kg, to restore adequate respirations. Agents administered for general and local anesthesia have depressant effects, and if depressant concentrations have passed across the placenta to the fetus, assisted ventilation should be given until the effects of these drugs have worn off.

Hemorrhage and Shock. This condition should be suspected if the mother has a history of abruptio placentae or placenta previa, if twin-to-twin transfusion has occurred, or if the infant has suffered trauma involving the liver, spleen, or brain. The infant is pale, with tachycardia and a decreasing hematocrit. Hypotension is further evidence of shock, as is metabolic acidosis. A decreased urinary output is a valuable monitor of decreased intravascular volume; however, the newborn normally may not urinate for 16–20 hours after birth.

Therapy includes immediate restoration of an adequate circulating blood volume to correct metabolic acidosis due to poor peripheral circulation. Colloid solutions (5% serum albumin) or Ringer's lactated solution, 10–20 ml/kg over 10–15 minutes, may be given intravenously if blood is not available immediately. Further infusions are determined by the infant's condition and whether there is ongoing blood loss. The underlying cause of hypotension should be sought and definitive treatment undertaken. Once the infant's general condition is stable, he should be transported to a neonatal intensive care unit for further therapy.

Hyaline Membrane Disease. This condition is a leading cause of neonatal morbidity and mortality. It is often associated with prematurity, birth asphyxia, delivery by cesarean section, and maternal diabetes. In this condition, a lack of surfactant produces multiple areas of atelectasis and shunting with resultant hypoxemia. Shortly after birth (often within the first hour or two) hyaline membrane disease is manifested by grunting respirations, retractions, and cyanosis. A chest x-ray film will demonstrate the bilateral presence of reticulogranular densities. Arterial blood-gas levels will reflect hypoxemia and in more severe cases hypercapnia and acidosis.

Emergency therapy consists of keeping the infant warm and administering oxygen by means of a head box, for example, an Oxyhood. This allows a predetermined concentration of oxygen to be delivered and, thus, accurate assessment of the infant's progress by sequential arterial blood-gas monitoring. Efforts should be made to maintain the PaO_2 between 55 and 75 mm Hg to prevent hypoxemia on the one hand and the possible development of retrolental fibroplasia on the other. Metabolic acidosis should be corrected by administration of a colloid solution or Ringer's lactated solution when hypovolemia is suspected. If hypovolemia is not present, sodium bicarbonate solution should be administered intravenously, 2 mEq/kg over at least 30 minutes. Arterial pH should be rechecked and further doses of sodium bicarbonate should be administered if necessary.

Should prolonged apnea develop or should respiratory distress worsen as manifested by increased tachypnea and retractions with an increasing $PaCO_2$ (greater than 55–60 mm Hg), ventilation should be supported with a bag and face mask and oxygen at approximately 25 breaths/min. Endotracheal intubation may be necessary to secure optimal control of the airway and to provide more effective support of ventilation.

Infants with hyaline membrane disease may be hypovolemic, and intravascular volume should be expanded, if necessary, with 10–20 ml/kg of a colloid solution (5% serum albumin) or Ringer's lactated solution before the infant is transported. In addition, the level of glucose in the blood must be checked, since these infants are frequently hypoglycemic. Initial evaluation can be made by means of Dextrostix reagent strips, and the results can be confirmed by analysis of the blood glucose level. Hypoglycemia must be treated as an acute emergency.

Congenital Heart Disease. Newborns with symptoms including poor feeding, sweating, tachypnea, lethargy, cyanosis at rest, cyanosis with crying and feeding, or poor urinary output should be investigated for possible congenital heart disease.

On examination, the infant with congenital heart disease is often tachypneic and tachycardic and may be cyanotic. The femoral pulses should be evaluated for the possibility of coarctation of the aorta, and the liver should be palpated for evidence of cardiac failure. Rales in newborns suggest primary pulmonary disease rather than heart disease.

All newborns with persistent cyanosis must be evaluated urgently for an underlying cardiac lesion. Obstructive congenital cardiac lesions such as critical aortic stenosis, critical pulmonary stenosis, and coarctation of the aorta may cause rapid deterioration. In addition, the condition of a newborn with pulmonary atresia will worsen dramatically once the patent ductus arteriosus closes. The condition of an infant with total anomalous pulmonary drainage may deteriorate with increasing acidosis.

A chest x-ray film may reveal evidence of cardiac enlargement and increased or decreased pulmonary vascular markings. Electrocardiographic evaluation may provide additional information, especially with regard to either ventricular hypertrophy or hypoplasia. Arterial blood-gas analysis will indicate the degree of hypoxemia and metabolic acidosis. The degree of metabolic acidosis correlates with the severity of the cardiac lesion and indicates urgency for correction.

In stabilizing and transporting the sick newborn with a cardiac lesion, the physician must pay special attention to maintaining normothermia.

Hypothermia may result in hypoxemia and acidosis, and hyperthermia may aggravate an existent right-to-left shunt by producing peripheral systemic vasodilation in the presence of pulmonary vasoconstriction.

Pneumothorax. This condition should be suspected in every newborn with respiratory distress. It is particularly common in infants with hyaline membrane disease who receive positive-pressure ventilation and in infants with meconium aspiration. Small areas of pneumothorax may be well tolerated, but must be monitored closely in an intensive care setting. Larger areas of pneumothorax may produce a life-threatening emergency, and prompt action is essential.

In the nonacute situation, a chest x-ray film will clarify the diagnosis, since clinical signs such as unequal expansion of the chest and diminished breath sounds are more difficult to interpret in newborns than in older children or in adults. In the acute situation in which delay in diagnosis is life-threatening, a suspicion of pneumothorax warrants the introduction of a 20-gauge angiographic catheter into the third or fourth interspace at the anterior axillary line. This measure will relieve tension pneumothorax; a chest tube can be placed subsequently.

Convulsions

A convulsion in an infant may consist of a classic tonic-clonic seizure, but more often is manifested in more subtle ways such as eye rolling, slight twitching of the face or a limb, and apnea. The cause of most convulsions is obscure. Possible etiologic factors are listed in Table 19.2. Supportive therapy is critical. The infant must be given oxygen for asphyxia, and ventilatory support should be provided by a face mask and bag if the

Table 19.2.
Common causes of convulsions in newborns.

Hypoxia
Hypoglycemia
Hypocalcemia
Hyponatremia
Hypernatremia
Infection
Meningitis
Septicemia
Pneumonia
Drug withdrawal
Pyridoxine deficiency
Aminoacidemia

seizures interfere with ventilatory efforts. Initial drug therapy consists of phenobarbital, 5 mg/kg intravenously, repeated as necessary to control convulsions. The infant should be placed on its side to help maintain a clear airway and to prevent aspiration of gastric contents. If diagnostic workup for a metabolic disorder or infection is unrevealing, neurologic consultation should be sought for a definitive diagnosis and further management once the infant's condition is stable.

Hypoglycemia. This condition may be asymptomatic, or it may be manifested by apnea, convulsions, irritability or lethargy, and poor feeding. Hypoglycemia occurs commonly in infants of diabetic mothers and in infants who are premature or small for gestational age. If the Dextrostix reagent strip indicates a blood glucose level less than 35 mg/dl, the blood glucose level must be measured more accurately. However, treatment must begin before laboratory results are available; therapy consists of administration of 25% dextrose in water, 2 ml/kg intravenously, followed by continuous infusion of 10% dextrose in water, 100 ml/kg/day. Dextrose infusion must not be discontinued abruptly after correction of hypoglycemia because of the possibility of rebound hypoglycemia. The infant should be treated further in the neonatal intensive care unit.

Hypocalcemia. Infants with jitters, tremors, a high-pitched cry, or convulsions may be hypocalcemic. Shortly after birth, hypocalcemia may be found in premature infants, infants of diabetic mothers, or infants who have undergone exchange transfusion. Hypocalcemia also may occur 7–10 days after birth as a result of high-phosphate infant formulas, particularly soya formulas. The serum calcium level should be measured, the normal level being 8.5–11.0 mg/dl. Electrocardiographic demonstration of a prolonged QT interval provides further evidence of hypocalcemia.

The prognosis for recovery is excellent with prompt treatment consisting of elemental calcium administered initially in a dose of 10 mg/kg (0.5 mEq/kg) over 20–30 minutes, followed by a supplemental dose of 20–30 mg/kg/day. The amount of elemental calcium in three common calcium compounds is indicated in Table 19.3. Calcium salts are highly irritating to the tissues and must be infused through a free-flowing intravenous line. Rapid administration also may lead to bradycardia; therefore, the compound should be administered slowly and cardiac activity should be monitored carefully.

Hyponatremia. This condition is associated with excessive intake of water in the presence of impaired water excretion or excess sodium excretion. Symptoms include convulsions, lethargy, and coma; the serum sodium value is less than 120 mEq/liter. Treatment consists of immediate intravenous administration of 3% saline solution, 1 ml/kg (0.5 mEq/kg) over 15 minutes, followed by physiologic saline solution at maintenance levels while serum electrolytes and the clinical situation are assessed. Serial body weights provide the most reliable means of distinguishing water overload from salt depletion.

Hypernatremia. This condition is caused either by loss of free water in greater amounts than loss of sodium or by sodium overload; it is often associated with diarrhea following hyperosmolar feedings. It may also be associated with a renal concentrating defect or with a high temperature that aggravates water loss. Sodium overload can result from feeding with nonproprietary formulas or from administration of excess sodium bicarbonate in therapy for severe acidosis. Treatment is discussed on pages 428–430.

Infection. *Meningitis* at delivery may be associated with premature rupture of membranes. Symptoms in the newborn may include lethargy and poor feeding, apnea, hypothermia, hyperthermia, jaundice, irritability, and convulsions. The most common infecting organisms are group B β-hemolytic streptococci and *Escherichia coli*.

A lumbar puncture should be performed with a No. 22 needle (see Chapter 15, pages 343–344), and the cerebrospinal fluid should be analyzed. If results suggest meningitis, antibiotics should be administered immediately; a combination of ampicillin and gentamicin (Table 19.3) should be given intravenously. Meningitis is discussed further in Chapter 11, pages 231–234.

Septicemia at birth may be associated with prematurity and with early rupture of membranes. This condition should be suspected in any infant with convulsions, lethargy, poor feeding, hypotonia, jaundice, hypoglycemia, apnea, or respiratory distress. Specimens of blood, urine, and cerebrospinal fluid should be cultured, and cultures may also be taken from the mother's vagina. The organisms commonly associated with septicemia are group B β-hemolytic streptococci, *E. coli*, Proteus, and staphylococci.

Pneumonia in the newborn is manifested by tachypnea, retractions, lethargy, poor feeding, fever, hypothermia, and cyanosis in severe cases. A chest x-ray film will confirm the diagnosis. Specimens of tracheal aspirate and blood should be taken for culture and sensitivity testing. Blood culture is indicated because pneumonia in the

Table 19.3.
Neonatal dosages of common drugs and preparations.

Agent	Dosage	Route
Ampicillin	Age < 1 week:	
	100 mg/kg/day in two divided doses	IV
	Age > 1 week:	
	200 mg/kg/day in three divided doses	IV
Atropine	0.01–0.03 mg/kg	IV or IM
Calcium gluconate	10 mg/kg (9 mg/ml elemental calcium)	IV
Calcium gluceptate	10 mg/kg (18 mg/ml elemental calcium)	IV
Calcium chloride	0.3 gm/kg/day	PO
	10 mg/kg (27 mg/ml elemental calcium)	IV
Chloral hydrate	Sedative dose:	
	25 mg/kg/day	PO or PR
	Hypnotic dose:	
	50 mg/kg/day	PO or PR
Chlorpromazine (Thorazine)	0.5 mg/kg every 6–8 hours	IV, IM, or PO
Chlorthiazide (Diuril)	20–40 mg/kg/day in two divided doses	IV
d-Tubocurarine chloride	0.5 mg/kg initially followed by 0.15 mg/kg	IV
Dexamethasone sodium phosphate (Decadron)	0.1–1.0 mg/kg/day in four divided doses	IM
Dextrose (25% solution)	0.5–1.0 gm/kg	IV
Digoxin	Loading dose:	
	0.04–0.06 mg/kg/day in three divided doses	IV or IM
	Maintenance dose:	
	0.013–0.02 mg/kg/day	IV or IM
Diphenhydramine hydrochloride (Benadryl)	5 mg/kg/day in four to six divided doses	PO or IV
Epinephrine (1:1000, aqueous)	0.01 ml/kg	IV or SC
Furosemide (Lasix)	1 mg/kg as single dose	IV or IM
Gentamicin	Age < 1 week:	
	5 mg/kg/day in two divided doses	IV or IM
	Age > 1 week:	
	7.5 mg/kg/day in three divided doses	IV or IM
Heparin	1 mg/kg every 4 hours	IV
Hydrocortisone sodium succinate	2–5 mg/kg/day in four divided doses	IV
Insulin (crystalline zinc insulin)	0.5–1.0 unit/kg every 3 hours (titrate to desired effect according to serum glucose level)	IV
Iron (elemental)	6 mg/kg/day	PO
Isoproterenol (Isuprel)	0.1 μg/kg/min (titrate to desired effect)	IV constant infusion
Kanamycin	15 mg/kg/day in two divided doses	IV or IM
Magnesium sulfate (50% solution)	0.2 ml/kg every 4–8 hours	IM
Mercaptomerin (Thiomerin)	0.1–0.25 ml every 6 hours if necessary	IM
Morphine	0.1 mg/kg every 4 hours	IV or IM
Naloxone hydrochloride (Narcan)	0.02 mg repeated every 20 minutes as necessary	IV
Neostigmine bromide (Prostigmin)	0.06 mg/kg (after atropine, 0.03 mg/kg)	IV
Nystatin (Mycostatin)	100,000–200,000 units every 6 hours	PO
Oxacillin	Age < 1 week:	
	100 mg/kg/day in two divided doses	IV
	Age > 1 week:	
	200 mg/kg/day in three divided doses	IV
Pancuronium bromide (Pavulon)	0.1 mg/kg initially followed by 0.03 mg/kg as necessary	IV

Table 19.3.—*continued*

Agent	Dosage	Route
Penicillin (aqueous)	Age < 1 week:	
	150,000 units/kg/day in two divided doses	IV
	Age > 1 week:	
	250,000 units/kg/day in three divided doses	IV
Phenytoin	3–5 mg/kg/day in two divided doses	IV, IM, or PO
Pitressin (aqueous)	1–3 ml/day in three divided doses	SC
Prednisone	1–3 mg/kg/day in six divided doses	PO
Sodium bicarbonate	2–3 mEq/kg in single dose	IV
Theophylline	1.5 mg/kg every 3–4 hours (check blood levels)	PO
Vitamin A	Preventive:	
	600–1000 units/day	PO
Vitamin B_1 (thiamine)	Preventive:	
	0.5–1.0 mg/day	PO
	Therapeutic:	
	10 mg every 6–8 hours	IM
Vitamin B_6 (pyridoxine)	Anticonvulsant:	
	50 mg	IV
	Therapeutic:	
	2–5 mg/day	PO
Vitamin C	Preventive:	
	50–100 mg/day	PO
	Therapeutic:	
	600 mg every 4 hours	PO or IM
Vitamin D	400 units/day	PO
Vitamin E	25 international units/day	PO
Vitamin K_1	Preventive:	
	1 mg at birth	IM
	Therapeutic:	
	2.5–5.0 mg every 6–12 hours	IM

IV = intravenous; IM = intramuscular; PO = oral; PR = rectal; SC = subcutaneous.

newborn is considered a systemic illness and should be treated with systemic antibiotics.

Septicemia is treated with broad-spectrum antibiotics, pending results of cultures and sensitivity tests. In infants 1–3 days old, a combination of ampicillin and gentamicin (Table 19.3) should be administered initially. In older infants, initial treatment should include oxacillin as well to combat possible staphylococcal infection; ampicillin is administered for the possibility of β-hemolytic streptococcal infection. The infant with diagnosed or suspected sepsis is critically ill and must receive cardiopulmonary support and monitoring of metabolic status in an intensive care setting in addition to antibiotic therapy.

Drug Withdrawal. The infant of a mother addicted to heroin or methadone may have hyperirritability, yawning, sweating, diarrhea, and myoclonic jerks. If drug withdrawal is suspected, phenobarbital, 5–10 mg/kg, should be administered intramuscularly or intravenously. In addition, chlorpromazine hydrochloride, 2 mg/kg/day, and diazepam, 0.3 mg/kg/day, may be required.

Transportation

In all emergency situations, once the infant's condition has been stabilized, arrangements should be made to transfer him either to a neonatal intensive care unit within the hospital or to a regional neonatal intensive care center. The following guidelines are critical to the safe transport of the sick newborn:

(1) Equipment should include a special battery-charged transport isolation incubator with equipment for monitoring and for maintaining the infant's body temperature. Monitoring equipment should include a battery-charged cardiotachometer, a thermometer to measure incubator temperature, and a thermistor probe to measure cutaneous or rectal temperature. A constant infusion pump (Holter type) should be available for admin-

istration of fluid and drugs. In addition, respiratory therapy equipment including face masks, oxygen, endotracheal tubes (3.0 mm and 3.5 mm), oral airways, breathing bags, suction apparatus, catheters, and drugs should accompany the infant.

(2) A physician and a nurse qualified in emergency transport of infants must be present.

(3) Particular attention should be paid en route to maintaining normal body temperature, a clear airway, and adequate circulation and ventilation. The infant should be positioned on his side (facing the physician and nurse) if he is not intubated in order to maintain a clear airway and to reduce the risk of aspiration of gastric contents. This risk can be reduced further by emptying the stomach of the infant before he is transported.

(4) The transport ambulance must be kept warm to reduce radiant heat loss from the incubator to the environment.

(5) The referral intensive care unit should be notified as to the nature of the infant's illness and whether resuscitative equipment such as a ventilator should be available when the infant arrives.

The safe transport of a sick infant, however, primarily depends on the effectiveness of resuscitation in the emergency situation and the stabilization of the infant's condition before transport.

CPR

The common causes of cardiopulmonary arrest in the pediatric patient include sudden infant death syndrome, trauma, sepsis, airway obstruction from croup, epiglottitis and aspirated foreign bodies; and severe dehydration. Regardless of the cause, the basic ABCs of resuscitation outlined in Chapter 2 remain the same. Some special considerations for CPR in the child are listed below.

Table 19.4.
Endotracheal tube sizes.

Age	Tube size
	Internal Diameter mm (ID)
Premature infants < 1200 G	2.5
Premature infants > 1200 G	3.0
Newborn to 6 months	3.5
6 months to 18 months	4.0
Over 2 years-formula used:	
$\dfrac{\text{Age in Years}}{4} + 4.5$	

Note: These sizes are estimates and one should always have 3 tube sizes available—the estimated size, sizes below and above. Tubes should fit to allow adequate expansion of both lungs while allowing a leak around the tube at pressures of 25 cm of water.

Airway. A large number of the cardiopulmonary arrests occur secondary to upper airway obstructions. In the infant and young child, the tongue occupies a proportionally larger part of the mouth and pharynx than in the adult. Thus, such maneuvers as the jaw thrust, or placement of an oral airway may be required to provide a clear airway. The ideal airway is an endotracheal tube. Specific tube sizes for various ages is listed in Table 19.4.

Breathing. Patients should be given 100% oxygen. The tidal volume delivered should provide adequate inflation of the chest with each breath. On chest auscultation, the breath sounds should be equal on both sides. A common problem in the intubated child is inadvertent placement of the endotracheal tube in the right mainstem bronchus. In this situation, the breath sounds and chest excursion will be decreased in the left chest. Although the tidal volumes are proportionately lower in the child than the adult, the peak inspiratory pressures needed to provide adequate expansion of the chest may be the same for child and adult. The ratio of breaths to compressions is one to five in the infant and child, with a compression rate of 100/min in the first year of life, and 80/min thereafter. After 9–11 years of age, depending upon the maturity of the patient, adult compression rates should be employed—i.e., 60 compressions per minute.

Circulation. Since children undergoing frequent arrests have a preceeding history of fever and dehydration, a 10–20 ml/kg bolus of Ringer's lactate or isotonic saline may be necessary to correct hypovolemia. Compressions in the infant should be at midsternum, to a depth of ½–1 inch. The method of encircling the chest and compressing the sternum with two thumbs yields higher blood pressures than pressing on the sternum with the index and middle finger (Fig. 19.1). In the child 1–8 or 9 years of age, the heel of one hand over the lower half of the sternum and compression is used to a depth of 1–1½ inches. Patients over 9 years of age can receive compressions as in the adult, i.e., two finger breadths above the bottom of the sternum to a depth of 1½–2 inches, using two hands.

Drugs. All patients should receive a bolus of sodium bicarbonate and epinephrine regardless of the cause of the arrest. Sodium bicarbonate will buffer metabolic acidosis and epinephrine will increase α-adrenergic vascular tone and cardiac contractibility. Other selected drugs which may be useful in resuscitation are listed in Table 19.5. Neonatal drugs are listed in Table 19.3. Drugs should be administered via a large-bore venous

Table 19.5.
Pediatric resuscitation—emergency drugs and defibrillation.

Atropine	0.02 mg/kg maximum 0.5 mg/single dose
Sodium bicarbonate	2 mEq/kg
Calcium chloride	5 mg/kg elemental calcium = 0.15 ml/kg 10% solution
Epinephrine	0.1 ml/kg of 1:10,000 solution maximum 5 ml single dose
Xylocaine	1 mg/kg DRIP: 2 mg/kg/hr (120 mg/dl 5% dextrose water)
Isoproterenol	DRIP: 0.1 μg/kg/min (1 mg/dl 5% dextrose water) $\equiv$ 10 μg/ml
Dopamine	DRIP: 5–10 μg/kg/min (30 mg/dl 5% dextrose water) $\equiv$ 300 μg/ml
Defibrillation	2 watt-seconds/kg

catheter, e.g., external jugular vein, internal jugular vein, subclavian vein, femoral vein, or saphenous vein. If access to a major vein is not possible, intracardiac injection may be given. More recently, intratracheal instillation of epinephrine and atropine have been recommended.

Defibrillation. Patients with electrocardiographic demonstration of ventricular fibrillation should be shocked with an initial defibrillation setting of 2 joules/kg. This setting should be doubled if the initial attempt is not successful. Successful defibrillation often will depend upon appropriate correction of hypoxemia and acidosis.

Fluid, Electrolyte, and Metabolic Emergencies

Life-threatening metabolic emergencies (Table 19.6) may result from significant elevation or depletion of electrolytes and acid-base substrates or from an inability to utilize glucose and amino acids. Vital organ systems and cellular integrity are threatened, resulting in temporary or permanent damage or even in death. Despite biochemical differences, there are many similarities in the clinical findings. Common symptoms include failure to feed or to gain weight, vomiting, lethargy, weakness, alteration in consciousness or disorientation, and seizures. On the basis of these symptoms, a differential diagnosis must be made between sepsis or toxemia and a metabolic crisis.

The initial therapeutic approach utilizes the following scheme of priorities:

(1) Establish and maintain an adequate airway and respiration.

(2) Establish and maintain circulatory volume.

(3) Establish and sustain urinary flow.

(4) Take blood samples for diagnosis of the precipitating condition.

(5) Correct fluid, electrolyte, or acid-base abnormalities according to the results of tests.

(6) Admit the patient to the hospital for diagnosis of the underlying cause and for initiation of maintenance therapy.

A large-bore intravenous line should be estab-

Table 19.6.
Classification of pediatric metabolic emergencies.

Electrolyte abnormalities
  Hypernatremia
  Hyponatremia
  Hyperkalemia
  Hypercalcemia
  Hypocalcemia
Water-solute imbalance
  Water intoxication
  Hyperosmolar state
Acid-base abnormalities
  Acidosis
  Alkalosis (marked)
Disorders of carbohydrate metabolism
  Hyperglycemia
  Hypoglycemia
  Galactosemia
Inherited aminoacidopathy
Urea cycle abnormality
Iatrogenic emergency (usually resulting from inappropriate fluid therapy when excretory function is limited)
  Parenteral nutrition without adequate laboratory control
  Hypernatremia due to overadministration of sodium bicarbonate in neonatal emergency or in salicylate intoxication emergency

lished, preferably in a central vein, and blood samples should be taken for assessment of electrolytes, glucose, ketones, ammonia, blood urea nitrogen, creatinine, pH, Pa_{CO_2}, and bicarbonate. Circulatory volume is then replaced via this line with isotonic balanced saline solution such as Ringer's lactated solution or a 0.45% saline solution with added sodium bicarbonate (40 mEq/liter) at 20 ml/kg. Either solution is administered at a rate sufficient to maintain circulation. If no blood pressure can be recorded after this, a further rapid infusion of 20–30 ml/kg of solution is administered, followed over the next hour by another 20–30 ml/kg to establish urinary output. If the patient has not urinated, administration of the isotonic fluid to expand circulation should be continued;

volume expansion should be monitored by means of a central venous pressure line.

After initial resuscitation, diagnostic workup may continue with testing of the serum ketone level with Acetest tablets and the blood glucose level with Dextrostix reagent strips. Urine may be analyzed for glucose, electrolytes, and sediment. The patient should be hospitalized for further workup and therapy.

Dehydration

One of the most common causes of fluid and electrolyte imbalance in children is diarrheal dehydration (Table 19.7). Infants have a large insensible water loss and a large water turnover daily; either a decrease in intake or an increase in output produces major changes that do not occur in adults.

The parents should be asked about the frequency and amount of diarrhea and whether urinary flow has continued normally or has markedly decreased. Details of dietary intake including type of formula, solids, and details of preparation—"home made", or proprietory prepared—of any supplements given. In infants with marked fluid losses or poor fluid intake or both, oliguria is almost always present. Continuation of urinary output in the presence of severe diarrhea suggests polyuric states associated with renal abnormalities, obstruction, urinary tract infection, an electrolyte abnormality, or tubular dysfunction.

Clinical assessment of the degree of dehydration often is easier in infants since a record of frequent weights is available. A weight record is the best guide to fluid losses. In *hypotonic* and *isotonic dehydration*, clinical signs such as a change in skin turgor and eyeball tension are usually noticed by the parents when 3% of body weight has been lost. With loss of 5% of body weight, the skin over the thorax may "tent" on testing, and the eyes appear sunken because of decreased eyeball tension. Mucous membranes are moist rather than wet, and tend to dry out, particularly if the child breathes through the mouth or hyperventilates because of acidosis. Urinary output decreases, and the urine is more concentrated and has a low sodium level. With 8–10% weight loss, the child exhibits tachycardia, tachypnea, and a mild decrease in blood pressure, which often is preceded by an elevation because of catechol stimulation. If the process of dehydration is rapid, hypotension or even frank shock may occur at 8–10% of body weight loss. If it is more gradual in onset, changes are somewhat better tolerated, and a 12–15% weight loss may take place before shock ensues.

In small infants and in infants who are fed a high-salt formula such as boiled skim milk or salt-containing fluids and who have poor intake and diarrhea, *hypertonic dehydration* may occur. In hypertonic dehydration, the degree of dehydration is notoriously difficult to estimate clinically except by noting changes in eyeball tension and by reviewing the weight record. The skin may have decreased turgor with a peculiar "doughy" consistency. Most infants who have hypernatremia associated with diarrhea have some salt depletion, but the water loss has exceeded the salt loss. On the other hand, if the infant's weight has remained stable, indicating that water loss has not occurred, or if salt replacement has been excessive, salt intoxication may exist. Weight review is extremely important since treatment of salt intoxication requires removal of salt rather than replacement of water.

Critical Dehydration. Children in shock with hypotension and children with marked dehydration should initially be given an isotonic balanced saline solution such as those previously mentioned, 20 ml/kg. Once the child has passed urine for the second time in the hospital, potassium in the form of potassium chloride or potassium acetate, 20–30 mEq/liter, may be added to the fluid. Establishment of circulation is critical in patients with hypotonic or isotonic dehydration as well as in those with hypertonic dehydration and possible salt intoxication. After rehydration, a blood sample should be taken for an electrolyte profile.

In patients with a moderate degree of *isotonic* or *hypotonic* dehydration, rehydration after initial resuscitation is continued with a repair solution such as 5% dextrose in 0.25% saline with potassium added, 30–40 mEq/liter, or with a multielectrolyte solution such as Isolyte M or Ionosol T. All these solutions are administered intravenously, 2500–3000 ml/m^2/day (80–100 ml/kg/day). Reassessment should be made every 4–6 hours, and the dosage should be adjusted appropriately. If the degree of dehydration is marked, the solutions should be administered at a faster rate, 150–175 ml/m^2/hr (5–6 ml/kg/hr) over 6–8 hours followed by a slower rate of 2500 ml/m^2/day (80 ml/kg/day) for the next 16–18 hours. The patient should have no oral intake over this initial 24-hour period.

In cases of *hypertonic* dehydration, the circulatory volume is re-established, and the deficit gradually is replaced over 48 hours. The physician should search for damage due to hypernatremia and hyperosmolality, such as cortical vein thrombosis or lateral sinus thrombosis and subarachnoid hemorrhage. If the serum sodium level is ex-

Table 19.7.
Treatment scheme for dehydration.

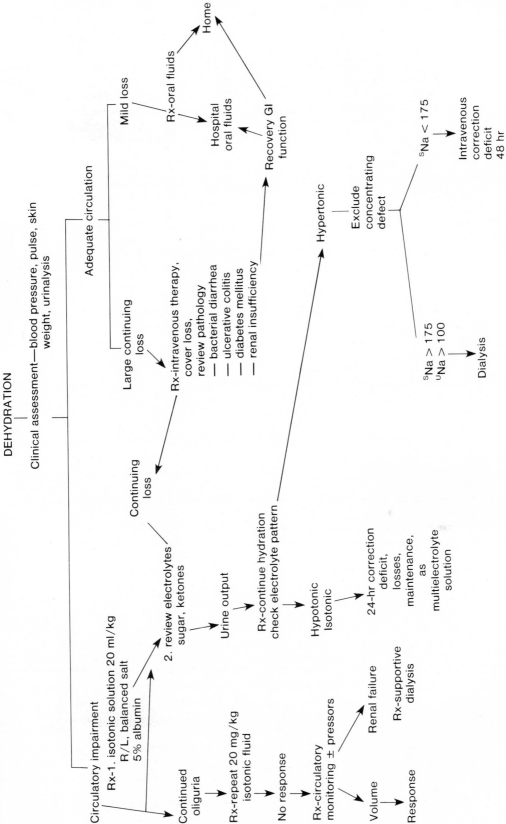

S = serum; U = urinary

429

tremely high (greater than 160 mEq/liter), the serum osmolality should be reduced slowly to prevent intracellular water intoxication, which may result in cerebral edema or pulmonary interstitial edema during rehydration. We recommend reduction of the serum osmolality by 2–3 milliosmoles/liter/hr while the serum sodium is decreased at a faster rate if possible, 2–4 mEq/liter/hr. This is accomplished by administration of a hyperosmolar solution to allow removal of sodium and its replacement with osmotically active particles of some other type. An ideal hyperosmolar solution is either a solution of 10% dextrose in 0.25% saline or a commercial multielectrolyte solution.

In patients with hypertonic dehydration, if the serum sodium level is greater than 175 mEq/liter after restoration of the circulation or if urinary output is difficult to re-establish, either peritoneal dialysis or hemodialysis may be necessary for removal of excess sodium and safe restoration of normal osmolality. Peritoneal dialysis should be instituted with modified dialysis fluid containing 2.5–4.25% glucose with a sodium concentration of 120 mEq/liter. The child should then be admitted to the intensive care unit for further therapy. It is important to monitor the patient's condition carefully in the early phase of dialysis, particularly if hypertonic dialysis solutions are used, to maintain circulation and a positive fluid balance.

Moderate and Mild Dehydration. This is more common than frank dehydration with circulatory collapse. In children with moderate dehydration, two conditions determine therapy—the ability of the child to maintain an oral intake and the degree of water loss through diarrhea. If diarrhea has remained the same or is decreasing and if the parents are competent to care for the patient at home, the child can be discharged after review and assessment in the emergency ward. If oral intake is inadequate and diarrheal losses excessive, oral intake should be discontinued and intravenous fluids should be administered. A repair solution such as Isolyte M or 5% dextrose in 0.25% saline with potassium is given to replace the deficit and to provide maintenance while continuing losses are assessed. If water losses do not seem excessive, the child should be given glucose fluids by mouth for the next 24 hours and then solid foods as tolerated. If oral fluid is tolerated and if water loss through diarrhea has not been extreme, the child may be discharged.

In milder cases, the child should be able to tolerate frequent small amounts of glucose fluids given orally in the emergency ward, with discharge to home after 4–6 hours on a regimen of frequent small clear fluid feedings and advancement to regular diet over 2–5 days as tolerated.

Dehydration Associated with Diabetic Ketoacidosis. A ketoacidotic state (see Chapter 14, pages 290–298) may be the first sign of juvenile diabetes mellitus, or it may occur in a patient with diagnosed diabetes, associated with infection or illness if insulin requirements have not been adjusted adequately. In addition, an adolescent with diagnosed diabetes may have ketoacidosis because his insulin requirement has changed or because he has neglected insulin therapy during an emotional crisis.

Children with ketoacidosis may have varying degrees of dehydration in addition to polyuria, polyphagia, and polydipsia. The diagnosis of diabetic ketoacidosis can be made by determining elevation of serum ketone and blood glucose levels with Acetest tablets and Dextrostix reagent strips, respectively. The diagnosis is established if the Acetest tablets indicate ketonemia and if the blood glucose level is greater than 200–250 mg/dl. After assessment of circulatory status, a large-bore intravenous line is placed for rehydration and insulin therapy. Blood samples should be sent for a complete blood cell count and for measurement of blood glucose, ketones, electrolytes, urea nitrogen, and arterial blood gases. The urine should be tested as soon as possible for glucose and ketones. Treatment is instituted after weighing the patient and clinically assessing the degree of hydration.

One method of treating diabetic ketoacidosis consists of volume replacement and intravenous infusion of insulin with frequent monitoring of plasma glucose concentration. Such a regimen provides insulin at a constant rate, thus maintaining serum insulin levels in the therapeutic range. With this therapy, the complications of hypokalemia and hypoglycemic rebound are uncommon. One unit of insulin is administered in each milliliter of a solution consisting of 1% albumin in physiologic saline. Such a solution is prepared by mixing 4 ml of 25% human serum albumin solution with 100 ml of physiologic saline solution and adding 100 units of crystalline zinc insulin. The solution is infused at a rate of 0.1 ml/kg/hr to produce a steady plasma insulin level between 100 and 200 microunits/ml. The blood glucose level is measured every 30 minutes during infusion; the level should decrease about 10% every hour. A daily insulin dosage schedule is initiated and insulin infusion is discontinued when the blood glucose level reaches 200–250 mg/dl, provided that acidosis has been corrected and the patient can tolerate a normal amount of glucose. Should the patient be unable to tolerate such an amount, intravenous insulin infusion may be continued at the rate of 0.1 ml/kg/hr and a separate infusion of 5% dextrose in water may be given, 1600–2500 ml/m^2/day (50–80 ml/kg/day), to maintain plasma glucose between 200 and 250 mg/dl.

Fluid and electrolyte replacement takes place concomitantly with insulin infusion. Sodium bicarbonate may be necessary in patients with severe acidosis, but is usually unnecessary after restoration of the circulatory volume. If the serum bicarbonate level is 10 mEq/liter or less, sodium bicarbonate should be administered in an isotonic solution prepared by adding 20 ml of 7% sodium bicarbonate solution (20 mEq of bicarbonate) to 100 ml of 5% dextrose in water. This solution should be infused until the serum bicarbonate level is 12–15 mEq/liter, whereupon sodium bicarbonate is discontinued unless continued monitoring demonstrates increasing acidosis. An excessive dose may be dangerous since a too rapid correction of metabolic acidosis may lead to respiratory alkalosis resulting from the lag in correction of cerebrospinal fluid acidosis.

Renal Failure

In renal failure, the kidneys lose their ability to excrete nitrogenous wastes and to maintain water and electrolyte balance. Three classifications of renal failure exist according to the producing mechanism: (1) prerenal—dehydration, sodium depletion, and protein loading; (2) parenchymal—glomerulonephritis and tubulointerstitial disease; and (3) postrenal—structural or intraluminal obstruction. Appropriate therapy requires the physician to determine which component or components are present.

Renal failure may be manifested as an acute episode or as acute decompensation in the presence of chronic renal failure; an emergency situation even may arise in the case of chronic progressive renal failure. Symptoms of renal failure include (1) change in conscious state, including somnolence, irritability, and seizures; (2) nausea, vomiting, and diarrhea; (3) generalized pruritus; (4) muscular twitching; and (5) tachypnea or Kussmaul's respiration. On auscultation, the physician may note cardiac arrhythmias or crackling rales signifying pulmonary edema. It must be remembered that oliguric renal failure is much more readily recognized than polyuric renal failure, yet approximately one-third of patients with renal failure have polyuria, particularly those with trauma, burns, crush injury with myoglobinuria, and obstructive uropathy with or without infection.

Life-threatening conditions associated with renal failure include circulatory collapse, severe metabolic acidosis, hypocalcemia, hyperkalemia, sepsis, water intoxication with or without pulmonary edema, and electrolyte imbalance manifested by neurologic symptoms.

Resuscitation. Therapy for renal failure is nonspecific; general guidelines are listed in Table 19.8. In the emergency ward, the first priority is treatment of life-threatening conditions. *Circulatory collapse* should be treated and circulatory volume should be maintained by administration of an isotonic balanced saline solution such as Ringer's lactated solution or 0.45% saline with sodium bicarbonate added, 20–40 mEq/liter. Once circulatory volume is re-established, infusion is continued at a slower rate.

Acidosis must be corrected concurrently with correction of hypocalcemia, since rapid correction of acidosis may lead to painful tetany or cardiac arrhythmias in a hypocalcemic patient. Acidosis is corrected by an initial infusion of 7% sodium bicarbonate solution administered over 5–10 minutes to provide 1–2 mEq/kg of bicarbonate. This is followed by a maintenance solution of 10% dextrose in water with sodium bicarbonate added to provide 1–2 mEq/kg/day of bicarbonate. This

Table 19.8.
Renal failure: general principles of therapy.

Treatment of correctable conditions
   Obstruction
   Infection
   Anemia or blood loss
   Dehydration
   Congestive heart failure
   Hypokalemia
   Hypercalcemia
Reduction of excretory load
   Dietary restriction of protein, potassium, sodium, phosphate
   Restriction of water intake to output plus insensible loss
   Adjustment of drug dosage to renal function (aminoglycosides, antibiotics, digitalis compounds)
Utilization of extrarenal routes of metabolism
   Binding of phosphate with aluminum hydroxide gel
Compensation for regulatory inadequacy
   Correction of acidosis with sodium bicarbonate
   Administration of vitamin D supplements
   Transfusion of packed cells for correction of anemia
Artificial replacement of renal function
   Dialysis on acute basis
   Transplantation on chronic basis

should be administered at 750 ml/m^2/day (25 ml/kg/day). *Hypocalcemia* is best treated by infusion of 10–20 mg/kg of elemental calcium (Table 19.3) over 20 minutes if the patient is symptomatic or over 6–12 hours if the patient has no symptoms.

In a patient with *hyperkalemia*, an electrocardiogram should be obtained. If no electrocardiographic changes are noted, acidosis should be corrected with a sodium bicarbonate solution as mentioned. An alternative initial infusion in children more than 2 years old or in those weighing more than 15 kg consists of one unit of crystalline zinc insulin in 8 ml of a 50% dextrose solution infused over 5–10 minutes to a total of 0.3 unit/kg of insulin. Initial infusion is followed by a maintenance infusion of sodium bicarbonate as mentioned until urinary output is established or dialysis is instituted.

If electrocardiographic changes are noted, treatment of hyperkalemia is urgent. First, elemental calcium, 10 mg/kg, should be administered in the form of 10% calcium gluconate over 5–10 minutes. This protective measure is followed by infusion of both the sodium bicarbonate solution and the insulin-glucose solution, followed by the maintenance solution of sodium bicarbonate.

In all hyperkalemic patients, if urinary flow greater than 0.5 ml/kg/hr has not occurred within 1–2 hours, ion-exchange resins such as sodium polystyrene sulfonate (Kayexalate) or dialysis or both may be required in addition to the maintenance solution. Sodium polystyrene sulfonate is administered orally or rectally, 1.0–1.5 gm/kg in 2–3 ml/kg of 10% sorbitol or 10% dextrose solution. Elemental calcium, 40 mg/kg/day in the form of 10% calcium gluconate or calcium gluceptate, should be added to the maintenance infusion, but the mode of administration should be changed to oral calcium supplements, 100–200 mg/kg/day of elemental calcium, as soon as it is practical. Oral administration of a phosphate-binding aluminum hydroxide gel providing 150–300 mg/kg/day of aluminum will assist in preventing hyperphosphatemia.

Generalized *sepsis* may be treated with an appropriate antibiotic, preferably one not requiring renal excretion. If a serious infection exists, administration of an aminoglycoside and a penicillin in a standard loading dose is advised. Maintenance levels of these agents are calculated on the basis of the results of cultures, measurement of renal function, and serum antibiotic levels.

Obstruction with pyuria and infection in an infant constitutes an emergency situation. Catheter or nephrostomy drainage is necessary, and may lead to rapid correction of azotemia. Postobstructive diuresis, defined as a urinary flow greater than 2 ml/kg/hr, may occur. The degree of diuresis can be forecast by preoperative measurement of the level of the blood urea nitrogen; the higher the level, the greater the diuresis. Since depletion of sodium and water may result from postobstructive diuresis, administration of intravenous fluid and monitoring of urinary electrolytes are necessary. A solution of 5% dextrose in 0.25% saline with sodium bicarbonate and potassium chloride added, 40 mEq/liter of sodium and 10–30 mEq/liter of potassium, approximately replaces the urinary electrolyte losses of postobstructive diuresis. This solution should be administered at 3500 ml/m^2/day (120 ml/kg/day). After 2 hours, a new hourly rate should be calculated by measuring the urinary output for the previous hour and adding 10 ml. In cases of oliguric renal failure, if there is difficulty in controlling levels of potassium or calcium, dialysis should be instituted early.

Pulmonary edema associated with renal failure and salt and water overload should be treated by dialysis. Respiratory support including positive-pressure ventilation may be necessary in addition to or preceding dialysis for removal of fluid.

Neurologic symptoms usually are associated with hyponatremia, water intoxication, or hypocalcemia. Altered consciousness, muscular twitching, or seizures require estimation of serum sodium, calcium, glucose, magnesium, urea nitrogen, and osmolality. Treatment consists of correction of the diagnosed abnormality. If hyponatremia exists in the presence of acute changes in consciousness or seizures, 3% saline solution should be administered intravenously, 1 ml/kg over 15 minutes. If neurologic symptoms are less acute and if urinary output continues or dialysis is contemplated, water should be restricted to 250 ml/m^2/day (80 ml/kg/day).

Transport. If the patient is to be transferred safely to an intensive care unit, circulatory status must be adequate, as measured by blood pressure and capillary refilling after blanching. Free water should be restricted to the minimal amount necessary to maintain an open intravenous line in case resuscitation is indicated. Before the patient is transported, hyperkalemia should be corrected by oral or rectal administration of sodium polystyrene sulfonate, 1 gm/kg in 2–3 ml/kg of a 10% sorbitol or 10% dextrose solution. Dialysis may be commenced before transfer by introducing the first fluid exchange and transporting the patient during the exchange period. If the time of transport will be longer than the exchange period, the patient's condition should be stabilized and 2–3 hours of peritoneal dialysis should be performed before transfer. Dialysis may then be resumed on arrival at the intensive care unit.

PEDIATRIC EMERGENCIES

Urinary Tract Infection

Urinary tract infection is a common condition in children, ranking second in incidence only to upper respiratory tract infection. Findings range from bacteriuria without symptoms to troublesome symptoms including frequency, dysuria, and a mild to moderate fever. Asymptomatic bacteriuria in children lacks the long history usually found in adults. Nonspecific symptoms that may herald a urinary tract infection, particularly in an infant less than 2 years old, include failure to thrive, vomiting, abdominal pain or distention, and constipation. Obvious toxemia and sepsis with pyuria also may be seen. If urinary tract infection is suspected, a specimen or urine should be taken for urinalysis and culture.

Obtaining a Urinary Specimen

Ideally the specimen should be obtained by a noninvasive technique, unless the child is too young to cooperate. In patients with signs of either toxemia or sepsis, urine should be obtained directly from the bladder either by suprapubic aspiration, which is preferable, or by urethral catheterization if adequate precautions are taken to minimize the risk of introducing pathogens during collection.

If it is possible, two clean-voided specimens of urine should be taken before treatment, especially in older children who have been toilet trained and who can void on command, and who will cooperate with adequate cleansing. In boys, the foreskin should be retracted and the glans and sulcus should be washed with sterile distilled water. Sterilizing soap may be an irritant; its use is unnecessary if sufficient water is employed. In girls, the labia are washed, separated, and washed again to ensure that the introitus has been adequately cleansed. The labia must be spread widely and preferably held apart during voiding. The urine is caught in a sterile container. A conical flask is ideal, since it is easier to hold and to manipulate than a bowl or basin. The specimen either should be cultured within a short time or should be refrigerated for up to 6 hours to prevent the growth of contaminant organisms before culture.

If suprapubic aspiration is to be performed, the child should not have voided recently. The bladder should be full on percussion before this maneuver is attempted. In newborns, the bladder is almost totally an abdominal organ. In older children, the bladder is in the pelvis, but the upper margin can be percussed if the bladder is full. The younger child is restrained by an assistant and the legs are placed in a frog-leg position with firm pressure on the middle to proximal femoral shafts to stabilize the pelvis. The skin of the abdominal wall is washed with iodine preparation solution. In girls, the assistant should compress the introital area to prevent voiding during the procedure; in boys, the urethra should be compressed. A No. 22 lumbar puncture needle, 1.5–3.0 inches long depending on the age of the child, is inserted over the bladder, the stylet is removed, and a 6- or 12-ml syringe is attached. The needle is advanced into the bladder; in newborns, it is held perpendicular to the skin and in older children it is held at an angle of 45 to 60 degrees. A "give" can be felt as the needle enters the bladder. Urine is aspirated, the needle is removed, and pressure is applied over the puncture site. After the needle is disconnected from the syringe, the urine for culture is placed in a sterile container.

At present, use of the antibody coating study of isolated urinary tract pathogens is becoming more prevalent, and after further evaluation it may become a standard diagnostic technique in pediatric medicine. If this test is contemplated, the urinary specimen is refrigerated. A specimen revealing pathogens on routine urinary culture then can be processed to demonstrate the fluorescent coating of bacteria found in the upper part of the urinary tract. In the future, such data may provide a better basis on which to plan the duration of antibiotic coverage.

Treatment

Patients with toxemia or sepsis should be treated differently from those with mild to moderate symptoms (Table 19.9). Fever (greater than 102°F) and a toxic appearance with pyuria signals an emergency situation, particularly in a newborn or a child less than 3 years old. In girls less than 3 years old and in all boys, an anatomic anomaly is probably the underlying cause of the infection. Therapy includes control of the infection and appropriate relief of a predisposing anomaly, which may consist of an obstruction at the urethral valves or ureteropelvic junction, megalocystis, megaloureter, or vesicoureteric reflux. In very young children, obstruction and acute infection may result in devastating damage to parenchymal tissue that interferes with subsequent development.

Control of infection initially requires antibiotic

Table 19.9.

Urinary tract infection: diagnostic and therapeutic protocol for pediatric patients.

Newborn and child of any age with toxic appearance and local tenderness
    Take blood specimen for culture and sensitivity testing
    Take urinary specimen for culture and sensitivity testing
    Institute drainage of urine
    Administer ampicillin and gentamicin intravenously
    Change to appropriate antibiotic on results of sensitivity testing
    Perform investigative studies early if symptoms persist or after 4–6 weeks if urinary sterility can be maintained
        Intravenous pyelogram
        Voiding cystourethrogram
        Cystoscopy
Child < 2 years without toxic appearance
    Take blood specimen for culture and sensitivity testing
    Take urinary specimen for culture and sensitivity testing
    Administer oral antibiotic
    Change to appropriate antibiotic on results of sensitivity testing
    Perform investigative studies early if symptoms persist or after 4–6 weeks if urinary sterility can be maintained
        Intravenous pyelogram
        Voiding cystourethrogram
        Cystoscopy
Child > 2 years without toxic appearance
    Take blood specimen for culture and sensitivity testing
    Administer oral antibiotic after results of sensitivity tests are available
    Perform investigative studies early if symptoms persist or after 4–6 weeks if urinary sterility can be maintained
        Intravenous pyelogram
        Voiding cystourethrogram
        Cystoscopy
Child > 4 years without toxic appearance
    Take urinary specimen for culture and sensitivity testing
    Administer oral antibiotic—single-dose ampicillin 1.5–3.0 gm depending on weight
    Repeat urinary culture in 48 hours and 2 weeks
    Treat for 6 weeks with conventional dosage if still positive at 48 hours
    No further treatment if urine sterile
or
    Administer conventional 2-week course of appropriate antibiotic determined from sensitivity testing

---

therapy and drainage of urine, with diagnostic evaluation as soon as possible. Pediatric dosages of commonly used antibiotics are given in Table 11.3 (see pages 225–226). After a specimen for culture has been obtained, ampicillin and gentamicin should be administered for 24–36 hours until definitive data from the cultures and the sensitivity tests are available. If the clinical situation has not improved by this time, a more appropriate antibiotic, as determined by sensitivity tests, should be administered. If the patient's condition has improved with initial antibiotic therapy, one of the initial antibiotics should be discontinued and treatment should be continued with an adequate dosage of the other. If the child continues to exhibit signs of toxemia or septicemia with fever after 48 hours of antibiotic therapy, an intravenous pyelogram should be obtained to determine whether high-grade obstruction exists; if it does, adequate urinary drainage must be carried out

before the infection can be controlled.

A child with mild or absent symptoms may be treated on an outpatient basis with sulfisoxazole or ampicillin for 10 days, at which time another urinary culture is obtained. Should the child remain febrile after 24–36 hours on this regimen, urinalysis and culture should be repeated. If infection is not controlled after 48 hours, intravenous pyelography should be performed to determine whether obstruction is present. If obstruction is suspected on the basis of roentgenographic studies, the child should be admitted for definitive therapy, including further investigation by means of cystoscopy or retrograde pyelography and perhaps surgical correction.

Recent studies have shown that single-dose therapy with ampicillin, gentamicin, or sulfamethoxazole-trimetheprim is as efficient as longer-term therapy for children with mild or absent symptoms.

Respiratory Conditions

Asthma

Asthma is defined as episodic and reversible bronchospasm that may be caused by allergic reaction or infection. Other causes of diffuse lower airway obstruction should be differentiated from asthma; these include bronchiolitis, pneumonia, aspiration of a foreign body, cystic fibrosis, and obstruction by a vascular ring.

Clinical findings in asthma include tachypnea, retractions, hyperinflation, a prolonged expiratory phase, and diffuse expiratory wheezing. In more severe cases, the patient may be cyanotic and agitated, and may purse his lips. In patients with poor tidal volume, expiratory wheezing may be absent. For further discussion of asthma, see Chapter 9, pages 158–166.

Treatment. The goals of treatment are correction of hypoxemia, identification and treatment of infection, correction of bronchospasm, and maintenance of adequate hydration.

If the patient is cyanotic or agitated, oxygen is administered by mask. A complete blood cell count and differential count should be obtained to confirm or exclude bacterial infection in the lungs, ears, or upper airway. A sample for arterial blood-gas analysis and a chest x-ray film should be obtained. Epinephrine (1:1000) should be administered for bronchospasm *after* a blood sample is drawn because this agent will falsely elevate the white blood cell count. It is administered subcutaneously, 0.01 ml/kg to a maximum of 0.35 ml; this dose may be repeated every 20 minutes for a total of three doses if wheezing does not subside. Adequate hydration should be instituted by intravenous infusion of physiologic saline solution or Ringer's lactated solution, 10 ml/kg over 30 minutes. Intravenous hydration is especially important if bronchospasm is severe. Initial administration may be followed by administration of a balanced electrolyte solution, 3000 ml/m^2/day (100 ml/kg/day). Oral hydration is acceptable in less severe cases. If bronchospasm resolves after initial epinephrine therapy, the child should be given long-acting epinephrine in aqueous suspension (1:200, Sus-Phrine), 0.005 ml/kg to a maximum of 0.2 ml subcutaneously, and should be discharged. An oral bronchodilating agent for 3–5 days at home usually is sufficient for children with this degree of asthma.

If initial specific therapy does not result in resolution of expiratory wheezing after three doses of epinephrine, the child should be admitted to the hospital. Aminophylline, 4–7 mg/kg, should be given intravenously over 20 minutes; this dosage should be repeated every 6 hours for 24 hours. Isoetharine hydrochloride with phenylephrine hydrochloride (Bronkosol), 0.5 ml diluted in 1.5 ml of physiologic saline solution, may be administered by nebulizer. Dexamethasone sodium phosphate (Decadron) or its equivalent, may be given intravenously, 0.3 mg/kg/day in four divided doses, for no more than 3–5 days. If bacterial infection is identified, the appropriate antibiotics should be administered; otherwise, antibiotics are generally unnecessary in the treatment of asthma.

Persistent severe distress with hypercapnia may require respiratory support by assisted ventilation. Any child who *may* require assisted ventilation by means of a respirator should be transferred to an intensive care unit.

Bronchiolitis

A clinical syndrome of wheezing and dyspnea, bronchiolitis usually occurs in children less than 18 months old. A significant number of children who have bronchiolitis at an early age have asthma later. The syndrome is clinically indistinguishable from asthma, and usually is caused by the respiratory syncytial virus. It often is preceded by symptoms of an upper respiratory tract infection. A chest x-ray film will demonstrate bilateral hyperinflation due to air trapping. Other possible causes of wheezing and dyspnea such as asthma, pneumonia, and tracheal or bronchial obstruction by a foreign body must be considered. Occasionally, laryngotracheitis and bronchiolitis coexist in the same patient. In bronchiolitis, wheezing does not respond to epinephrine injection.

Treatment. Treatment is aimed at improving oxygenation, maintaining hydration, relieving the excessive work of breathing, and allaying the patient's anxiety. All infants with bronchiolitis are hypoxemic, and may be hypercapneic in severe cases. In patients with severe bronchiolitis, arterial blood-gas levels should be monitored to assess the degree of hypoxemia in relation to the inspired concentration of oxygen. Very ill children may require endotracheal intubation and ventilatory assistance.

If intravenous hydration is required, a generous administration of physiologic saline or Ringer's lactated solution may be necessary, 3000 ml/m^2/day (100 ml/kg/day). However, children who need mechanical ventilation may benefit from restriction of fluid to minimize peribronchial edema and associated bronchiolar obstruction.

Children in minimal distress who live reasonably close to the hospital can be sent home; a cold mist vaporizer can be used until symptoms resolve. When there is evidence of severe hypoxemia and excessive work of breathing, close monitoring in an intensive care unit is necessary. Corticosteroids and antibiotics are not indicated. Most children with severe bronchiolitis receive bronchodilating agents because of the possibility that they might have asthma; in true bronchiolitis these agents do not appear to have any beneficial effect.

Ear and Throat Conditions

Epiglottitis and Croup

These conditions both may be manifested by respiratory stridor. Aspiration of a foreign body also should be considered in patients with this symptom.

Epiglottitis. This condition is life-threatening, since rapid swelling of the epiglottis and surrounding aryepiglottic folds can lead to total asphyxiation. The disease usually occurs in children between 2 and 7 years old. The patient is febrile, with signs of toxemia and severe air hunger. Because of inability to swallow, he may be drooling; aspiration of secretions may cause asphyxia. The disease usually is caused by *Hemophilus influenzae*.

The child who appears to have epiglottitis should not be disturbed. The hypopharynx should *not* be directly examined, since this may result in laryngospasm, increasing edema, asphyxiation, and death. Since anxiety will compound respiratory difficulty, a parent should be allowed within the sight of the child. Humidified oxygen should be administered by a face mask; a well supervised parent often can perform this function.

The diagnosis should be established by a lateral x-ray film of the neck; a physician who is prepared to intubate the trachea should be in attendance while the film is taken. Once the diagnosis of epiglottitis is confirmed, the child should immediately be taken to the operating room for nasotracheal intubation. Humidified oxygen is administered through the nasotracheal tube, and ampicillin, 300 mg/kg/day and chloramphenicol 100 mg/kg/day are administered intravenously. The child should be transferred to an intensive care unit.

Croup. Croup is manifested by a characteristic barking cough and inspiratory stridor. It usually is more gradual in onset and less severe than epiglottitis, and it is usually viral in origin. The child with croup is most often 6 months to 4 years old. Cough, stridor, and symptoms of an upper respiratory tract infection may have been present for days. The child should be kept as calm as

possible, usually by allowing the parent to remain with him. A lateral x-ray film of the neck should be obtained if there is any suspicion of epiglottitis. Treatment consists of administration of room air or oxygen with water vapor.

A child with mild disease and reliable parents may be discharged, and a cold mist vaporizer can be used at home. Moderate to severe croup requires admission to the hospital. A dramatic temporary improvement in symptoms can sometimes be achieved by aerosol application of 2.25% racemic epinephrine (Vaponefrin), 0.5 ml in 2.5 ml of normal saline by nebulizer with oxygen. This may be repeated every 2–3 hours; the heart rate should be monitored. Rebound increased stridor may occur 2–3 hours following racemic epinephrine. This therapy, thus, is inappropriate if the child is to be discharged home following treatment. The most severe cases of croup require tracheal intubation or tracheostomy. Uncomplicated cases of viral origin do not require antibiotic or corticosteroid therapy.

Streptococcal Pharyngitis

Group A β-hemolytic streptococcal infection of the pharynx is one of the most common diseases seen in children in the emergency ward. The physician should be aggressive in diagnosing this condition because of its serious sequelae, acute glomerulonephritis and rheumatic fever.

A diagnosis of "strep throat" cannot be made on clinical grounds alone, and is certain only when established by culture. The following manifestations, however, increase the probability of this diagnosis: (1) a history that includes either presentation during an epidemic of streptococcal infection or a close contact, especially a family member, who has infection proved by culture; (2) a fiery red pharynx with exudate; (3) petechiae on the soft palate; (4) swollen and tender anterior cervical nodes; (5) a high temperature; (6) a generalized scarlatiniform rash; and (7) diffuse abdominal pain.

Streptococcal pharyngitis can be mimicked by many viral infections; rarely, diphtheria has similar manifestations. The viral infection most commonly misdiagnosed as strep throat is infectious mononucleosis. Streptococcal pharyngitis is rarely seen in patients less than 1 year old and is most common during childhood.

Treatment. Treatment consists of a 10-day course of oral penicillin at home if the patient's parents are reliable. Because of the potential complications, we recommend treatment with antibiotics *on the first visit* if it seems likely that the patient will not return. In such patients, an alternative is one injection of benzathine penicillin G, 600,000 units in patients less than 6 years old and 1.2 million units in older patients. In the penicillin-allergic patient, erythromycin should be substituted for penicillin. Tetracycline may be administered to teenagers, but should be avoided in children because it may stain teeth. If streptococcal infection is proved by culture, the whole family should have cultures taken. The patient should remain out of close contact with other children (home from school) for the first 48 hours of antibiotic therapy to minimize the possibility of contagion.

Acute Otitis Media

Many febrile children seen in the emergency ward are diagnosed as having acute otitis media; although this disorder remains one of the most common in childhood, it is probably overdiagnosed. Care should be taken that fever due to a more serious disorder is not simply attributed to a "red ear."

Older children with this condition often complain of ear pain, but younger children may simply tug on the ear; infants may have such nonspecific signs and symptoms as irritability, poor feeding, and fever.

Examination of the ear always should include pneumatoscopy to assess movement of the tympanic membrane. For this procedure to be reliable, younger children must be adequately restrained by a parent if possible. The pneumatic otoscope is introduced into the external canal in such a way as to achieve a good air seal, and air is introduced into the ear canal. The movement of the pars flaccida and the rest of the tympanic membrane is observed. An erythematous, bulging, immobile eardrum with distorted landmarks and decreased light reflection confirms the diagnosis of acute otitis media. A red tympanic membrane with visible normal landmarks and mobility is not associated with acute suppurative otitis media. A retracted, immobile tympanic membrane with only slight redness may indicate serous otitis rather than acute otitis media.

The child should be examined thoroughly to exclude associated conditions such as mastoiditis and meningitis. Uncomplicated otitis requires no laboratory examination to confirm the diagnosis. Should the patient appear toxic, the physician may elect to perform a complete blood cell count with differential, blood cultures, and a lumbar puncture. Mastoiditis should be suspected if there is tenderness or redness over the mastoid tip, and all patients with chronic otitis media should be investigated for this condition. The diagnosis of mastoiditis is established by means of an x-ray film of the mastoid area.

Tympanocentesis to differentiate between viral and bacterial infection is unnecessary in the diagnosis and management of uncomplicated otitis, but can be performed if sepsis or meningitis is suspected since a Gram stain and cultures of middle-ear exudate may permit early identification of the infecting agent. Tympanocentesis is performed by introducing a fine needle into the most peripheral portion of the inferior anterior quadrant of the tympanic membrane. This technique also can be used to relieve pain due to an acutely tense eardrum. It is used rarely in emergency situations; an otolaryngologist should be consulted if it seems necessary. The emergency physician always must weigh the risk of damage to the middle ear against the benefit from the procedure.

At least 50% of all cases of otitis media are caused by viruses, but the physician should treat bacterial pathogens. The most common bacterial pathogen at all ages is *Streptococcus pneumoniae*. In patients less than 6 years old, *H. influenzae* accounts for 70–75% of cases. Other bacterial pathogens include *S. pyogenes*, *Staphylococcus aureus*, and anaerobic organisms.

Treatment. In children up to the age of 6 years, the drug of choice is oral amoxicillin, 40 mg/kg/day to a maximum of 750 mg/day, divided to 8-hourly doses for 10 days. Patients who do not respond to amoxicillin can be treated with sulfamethoxazole-trimethaprim, 10 mg/kg of trimethaprim divided as twice daily dosage. Penicillin-allergic children in this age group can be treated with a combination of erythromycin, 30–50 mg/kg/day, and sulfisoxazole, 100–150 mg/kg/day, orally for 10 days or sulfamethoxazole-trimethaprim. Older children are treated with penicillin, 250 mg orally four times a day for 10 days, and penicillin-allergic patients are given erythromycin, 250 mg orally, either three or four times a day or sulfamethoxazole-trimethaprim. Should vomiting or poor patient compliance preclude an extended course of oral medication, benzathine penicillin G may be given intramuscularly before discharge, 600,000 units for children less than 6 years old and 1.2 million units for older children. In the younger group, oral sulfisoxazole should be administered for the possibility of *H. influenzae* infection.

Acute otitis media with perforation is treated in an identical manner. Perforations associated with otitis media usually heal spontaneously. In all patients with otitis media, the ears should be re-examined in 10 days to assess the resolution of infection and the healing of perforations. A child with an unhealed perforation should be referred to an otolaryngologist.

Fever and pain should be treated with appropriate doses of aspirin or acetaminophen; codeine may be required for very severe pain. A topical anesthetic agent such as Auralgan otic solution can be instilled into the ear canal, and a cotton plug saturated with the same solution can be placed in the ear three to four times a day.

Fever

Children presenting to the emergency department with fever should be treated symptomatically with appropriate doses of aspirin or acetominophen, while search for the cause is undertaken. (Currently the American Academy of Pediatrics recommends *not* using aspirin in children who have, or might have, chicken pox or influenza, because of the possibility of Reye's syndrome.) If the fever persists, a tepid sponge bath will help in lowering the temperature. Infections, dehydration, or vigorous activity in hot environment provide major causes. In hot weather, vigorous activity can lead to fever which will fall once the child has rested in a cool environment.

History and Physical. During standard history and physical examination painful procedures such as otoscopy should be reserved for last. Physical signs which are not reliable in the child include: (1) *meningismus* in patients younger than 6–12 months of age with meningitis; (2) lack of wheeze, rales or rhonchi in the young child with pneumonia or chest x-ray. (Fever may be absent in infants despite a severe infection.)

Laboratory Tests. The choice of laboratory tests depends upon clinical status. In the child who appears severely compromised in any way, with lethargy, high fever, tachypnea, tachycardia or mottled skin, cultures of cerebrospinal fluid, blood, urine, stool, and sputum should be sent. Blood samples for complete blood count, platelet count (clotting parameters), electrolytes, glucose, blood urea nitrogen, creatinine, and liver function tests may be necessary. Chest x-ray should be performed even if the lungs sound clear.

A "nontoxic" child with fever and no obvious source should have a urine culture sent prior to discharge from the emergency department.The child with bacteriuria may have no pyuria. A urine culture should be performed even when the urinalysis is normal.

Nontoxic-appearing children under the age of 2 years with a rectal temperature greater than 102°F and a white blood count above 18,000 frequently have occult bacteremia. The bacteremia most commonly is due to the pneumococcus. Hence children in this special group should have a blood culture taken.

Therapy. Therapy should be directed toward the source of infection if present. Specific antibiotic regimes for specific infections are listed elsewhere in Chapter 11. Common pediatric infections including otitis media, urinary tract infections, croup and epiglottitis are discussed elsewhere in this chapter.

In the patient who appears "septic", but in whom no source of infection is found, broad-spectrum antibiotic therapy should be started as soon as all the cultures have been obtained. The most common pathogens for the child's age govern antibiotic choice, e.g., *E. coli*, Klebsiella, and the group B β-hemolytic streptococcus are common pathogens in the first 6–8 weeks of life. Streptococcal, pneumococcal, and meningococcal infections are common in patients 2–3 months of age and older. *H. influenzae* infections occur in infants and children younger than 6 years of age, and become increasingly rare thereafter. Staphylococcal infections occur in all age groups.

For the septic infant less than 2 months of age, the three-drug combination of ampicillin, oxacillin, and gentamicin is the most practical. For patients 2 months of age and over, the two-drug combination of chloramphenicol and oxacillin will cover the major pathogens. Community patterns of antibiotic resistance influence the choice of antibiotics.

Anaphylactic Reaction

An immediate and severe hypersensitivity to antigen, an anaphylactic reaction occurs within minutes to hours after contact. This rare reaction most often results from contact with the agents listed in Table 19.10.

Symptoms may include any combination of al-

Table 19.10.
Common agents causing anaphylactic reaction.

Penicillin (especially if given parenterally)
Foreign serum
Inhaled pollen
Insect stings (especially of bees, hornets, and wasps)
Diagnostic agents
    Bromsulphalein solution
    Iodinated materials
Local anesthetic agents
Antimetabolites

lergic phenomena, including itch, urticaria, wheezing, vomiting, and diarrhea. A severe episode of immediate hypersensitivity is life-threatening, and may involve laryngospasm, bronchospasm, and vascular collapse.

Treatment

Therapy for anaphylactic reaction is based on the following principles: (1) delay of absorption; (2) administration of sympathomimetic agents to stimulate the heart and to combat bronchospasm; (3) treatment of hypoxemia if present; (4) support of circulation by any necessary means; (5) counteraction of release of histamine by administration of antihistamines; and (6) management of the inflammatory response with corticosteroids. Patients with anaphylactic shock requiring cardiac support, intubation, and treatment with corticosteroids should be admitted to an intensive care unit.

To retard absorption, a tourniquet should be placed proximal to the injection site or sting, and a single dose of epinephrine (1:1000), 0.01 ml/kg to a maximum of 0.3 ml, should be injected subcutaneously at the site of antigen entry. In addition, epinephrine (1:1000) is given in a dose of 0.01 ml/kg to a maximum of 0.5 ml in a site distant from the affected extremity. In the presence of shock, this dose may be diluted in physiologic saline solution and administered intravenously; this dose may be repeated every 20 minutes while symptoms persist.

Volume replacement with physiologic saline or normal serum albumin in saline may be necessary to combat shock. All patients should have an intravenous line in place in case vascular collapse occurs. Severe shock is managed more easily and more accurately with an intravenous line in a central vein with close monitoring of the central venous pressure.

Bronchospasm that has not responded to epinephrine should be treated with aminophylline, 4–7 mg/kg administered intravenously over 20 minutes and repeated every 6 hours as necessary. Hypoxemia is treated with humidified oxygen administered by means of an endotracheal tube.

Diphenhydramine hydrochloride (Benadryl) is often used as an adjunct to therapy. An intravenous dose of 1 mg/kg may be given immediately. In severe anaphylaxis, corticosteroids should be administered. Dexamethasone sodium phosphate is given intravenously in a dose of 0.5 mg/kg.

Seizures

The details of seizure management are covered in Chapter 15, Neurologic Emergencies. Febrile seizures and the modifications of anticonvulsant dosages for the child provide special considerations in the pediatric patients.

Febrile Seizures. These are usually generalized, of short duration (lasting less than 15 minutes), and occur in children younger than 6 years. A family history of febrile seizures frequently is present. The seizure frequently has abated by the time the patient reaches the emergency department. As with other seizure patients, the basic principles of resuscitation are instituted as a rapid physical examination is performed. A check is made for meningismus. Laboratory studies for a *first* febrile seizure should include complete blood count, electrolytes, calcium, phosphorus, magnesium, blood urea nitrogen, creatinine, and glucose. A lumbar puncture is indicated to rule out meningitis in the first febrile seizure. The child with a first febrile seizure should be treated with fever control alone. Following a second febrile seizure, however, anticonvulsant therapy is instituted with phenobarbital, 5 mg/kg/day. This medication is usually continued on a daily basis until age 5.

In *status epilepticus* the basic ABCs of resuscitation are initiated. Oxygen is administered and a secure intravenous line established. Blood tests are sent, as for febrile seizures. Once a serum sample for glucose determination has been obtained, a bolus dose of D 25% W, 2–4 ml/kg should be administered without delay.

Further anticonvulsant therapy will vary depending upon the force of the convulsions. If the frequency and force of the seizures make it difficult to ensure adequate ventilation and reliable intravenous access, intravenous diazepam should be administered at a dose of 0.1–0.3 mg/kg, not to exceed 5–10 mg. Diazepam enters the cerebrospinal fluid rapidly, providing prompt seizure control. The effectiveness of diazepam is short-lived and seizures may recur if a second anticonvulsant is not given. Another problem with diazepam is that it can induce apnea; personnel capable of providing artificial ventilation must be on hand.

In the patient who is not compromised by the seizure, phenytoin, 10 mg/kg by slow intravenous infusion, is a useful first line drug. Electrocardiographic monitoring is wise during the administration of phenytoin. The intravenous line should be flushed with normal saline before and after administration. Phenytoin is absorbed poorly intramuscularly. A second bolus of Phenytoin 5–10 mg/kg should be given if seizure activity persists 15 minutes after the first bolus. (The total dose should not exceed 1 gm.) Phenytoin also is useful directly following diazepam administration to ensure that convulsion does not recur as the effect of diazepam decreases. After the second bolus of phenytoin, phenobarbital at a dose of 10 mg/kg can be given if the seizure persists. A second bolus of 5–10 mg/kg phenobarbital can be given if the first bolus fails to stop the seizure. Phenobarbital administration may induce hypoventilation making constant supervision necessary. If the seizure persists after phenobarbitol, a rectal dose 0.3 ml/kg of 10% paraldehyde, diluted with two parts Safflower oil may stop the seizure.

Near Drowning

A victim of a near drowning has damage to the lungs and vascular collapse, with hypoxemia, acidosis, and rarely, major electrolyte aberrations. Results of animal experiments indicating a predictable difference in blood volume and serum electrolytes between the victims of fresh and salt water immersion cannot be applied to humans, in whom the pathophysiology of both is identical.

Treatment. Therapy is aimed primarily at counteracting hypoxemia and acidosis. In addition, because the water often contains bacteria and other contaminants, potential infection should be treated with antibiotics, and the inflammatory reaction should be managed appropriately.

As soon as the patient arrives, the airway should be cleared of all foreign matter, and oxygen should be administered as soon as possible, by mask or endotracheal tube as the situation dictates. Tracheal intubation is the best way to prevent further aspiration. Since pulmonary edema may develop during the first 24 hours, the patient's respiratory status should be monitored closely both chemically and clinically, by means of arterial blood-gas and electrolyte determinations and frequent recordings of blood pressure, pulse, and urinary output. Pending results of serum electrolyte measurements, shock is treated most safely with plasma. In the absence of shock, an intravenous line should be established initially, and restricted fluid should be administered until electrolyte results are available. Only for severe acidosis should sodium bicarbonate be given intravenously, 1–2 mEq/kg. Mild acidosis is corrected by maintaining the circulation.

Aminophylline, 4–7 mg/kg, may be given intravenously to combat bronchospasm. Intravascular hemolysis, which may cause hemoglobinuria, should be treated by maintenance of the urinary output with mannitol and sodium bicarbonate. Aspiration of bacteria-laden water requires administration of an appropriate antibiotic to combat the known or presumed bacterial pathogens. Dexamethasone sodium phosphate, 1 mg/kg/day to a maximum of 20 mg, may help relieve the inflammatory response to aspiration as well as cerebral edema resulting from hypoxia but is of no proven benefit for the pulmonary complications of drowning. All victims of near drowning should be observed closely in the hospital for at least 48 hours.

Poisoning

More than 3000 deaths occur yearly in the United States from poisoning, many of which are in children less than 5 years old. A major reduction in morbidity and mortality will come primarily through more effective preventive measures, but a significant reduction also can result from urgent and appropriate therapy in the emergency ward. The possibility of poisoning must be considered in any sudden unexplained illness in a child. The aim of therapy is support of respiration, circulation, and renal and metabolic integrity until the toxin is identified or until the illness has been attributed to another cause. Even with definitive identification of the toxin and application of a specific antidote, general supportive care is required until the toxin is metabolized or excreted.

The pathophysiology of and emergency therapy for many specific poisonings in children and adults are discussed in Chapter 17. An additional poisoning common among children, which results in significant morbidity and mortality, is iron poisoning. The source is usually medicinal iron, which frequently is prescribed for pregnant women. The reported average lethal dose of elemental iron is 180 mg/kg; the minimal lethal dose, however, is as little as 600 mg (3 gm of ferrous sulfate). Symptoms usually occur within 30 minutes to 2 hours from the time of ingestion and include vomiting, bloody diarrhea, and drowsiness. The child's condition may appear to improve, but he may lapse into a profound coma within a few hours to 2 days. Hepatic injury is associated with the comatose phase, and a late complication of iron poisoning is stricture of the gastrointestinal tract, occurring 3–4 weeks after ingestion.

Treatment. Initial laboratory studies should include a complete blood cell count, determination of serum electrolyte and serum iron levels, and a plain x-ray film of the gastrointestinal tract to demonstrate the radiopaque tablets. Treatment consists of the following measures:

(1) Induction of emesis with ipecac syrup, 15 ml (1 tablespoon) orally, followed by 1 cup of milk or water. This is repeated in 20 minutes if necessary.

(2) If the amount ingested is estimated at 200 mg or more, and in all large ingestions unaccompanied by hematemesis, gastric lavage should be

performed with a 5% sodium bicarbonate solution. If the patient is comatose, the airway should be protected first with intubation.

(3) If shock or coma is present, fluids, blood, or plasma may be required.

(4) In severe cases associated with coma and shock, deferoxamine mesylate should be administered intravenously, 15 mg/kg/hr.

Battered Child

A child less than 16 years old who has been physically or emotionally abused or neglected is defined as a "battered child." A high index of suspicion is the key to diagnosing this syndrome. An inaccurate history or contradictory explanations for an injury, apparently trivial complaints requiring visits to many emergency facilities ("medical shopping"), and a history of multiple ingestions or frequent accidental injuries require fuller assessment and may lead to such a diagnosis.

During the physical examination, neglect is suggested if the child is poorly dressed and appears to be undernourished or unclean. Ecchymoses, lacerations, cigarette burns, fractures, and subdural hematomas, which may be unrelated to the present complaint, should arouse the examiner's suspicion. A fearful, passive, repressed child with inappropriate responses, poor interaction with his parents, and difficulty in establishing eye contact should alert the examiner to the possibility of neglect or battering or both.

Unusual parental interaction with the child, including accusatory or quarrelsome behavior and lack of concern, frequently can be noted during the examination. Parents are often aggressive and make hostile demands for the "best" in medical care, but may release information grudgingly, making evasive and contradictory statements, denying knowledge of the incident, or displaying irritation at being questioned. On occasion, the parents will belittle the injury and voice concern not for the child but for themselves. Such parents often lack empathy with the child and have inappropriately inflated expectations for his performance, perceiving him as an agent for meeting their needs rather than the opposite. A parent's frequent demands for medical care or admission or both for a minor problem may be a plea for help.

Treatment. All children at risk for battering or dangerous neglect should be admitted to the hospital to facilitate a multidisciplinary evaluation. Lengthy evaluation in the emergency ward is inappropriate, as is an accusatory or punitive approach toward the parents. An accurate and complete account of any pertinent verbal exchange should be recorded, as well as any objective observations regarding the interaction between parents and child. A radiologic skeletal survey should be obtained, including views of long bones, skull, and ribs. Hematologic studies to exclude a bleeding diathesis should be performed on children with ecchymoses. Photographs should be obtained as early as possible. If it is required, the emergency physician also should arrange consultation with an appropriate specialist such as an ophthalmologist, an orthopaedic surgeon, a neurologist, or a surgeon.

The emergency physician should familiarize himself with the statutes pertaining to child abuse and neglect in his state. In Massachusetts, if the parent or guardian refuses hospital admission, the physician must take the child into his custody with a court order. A report of inflicted injury is submitted by either the admitting physician or a social worker. Any mandated professional (physician, nurse, social worker, or teacher) is required by law to report suspected or definite abuse and neglect to the Division of Family and Children's Services of the Department of Public Welfare. Nonmandated individuals such as friends and neighbors may report directly to Children's Protective Services, a private statewide agency that will then make an appropriate referral.

Social Emergencies

Social emergencies such as teenage suicide, rape and complicated pregnancy require a social worker skilled in handling children and families in crisis as part of the emergency treatment team.

Medical aspects are outlined in appropriate chapters.

Suggested Readings

General

Barnett HL, Einhorn AH: *Pediatrics.* ed 15. New York, Appleton-Century-Crofts, 1972

Graef JW, Cone TE, Jr (Eds): *Manual of Pediatric Therapeutics.* Boston, Little, Brown and Co., Inc., 2nd ed., 1980

Pascoe DJ, Grossman M (Eds): *Quick Reference to Pediatric Emergencies.* Philadelphia, J.B. Lippincott, 1973

Reece RM, Chamberlain JW: *Manual of Emergency Pediatrics.* Philadelphia, W.B. Saunders, 1974

Roberts, KB: *Manual of Clinical Problems in Pediatrics.* Boston, Little, Brown and Co., Inc., 1979

Smith CA (Ed): *The Critically Ill Child: Diagnosis and Management.* ed 2. Philadelphia, W.B. Saunders, 1977

US Department of Health, Education, and Welfare, Public Health Service/Federal Drug Administration: *Handbook of Common Poisonings in Children.* HEW Pub. No. (FDA) 76-7004, 1976

Vaughan VC, III, McKay RJ (Eds): *Nelson Textbook of Pediatrics.* ed 10. Philadelphia, W.B. Saunders, 1975

Winters RW (Ed): *The Body Fluids in Pediatrics: Medical,*

Surgical, and Neonatal Disorders of Acid-Base Status, Hydration, and Oxygenation. Boston, Little, Brown and Co., Inc., 1973

CPR

Standards and Guidelines for Cardiopulmonary Resuscitation (CPR) and Emergency Cardiac Care (ECC). *JAMA 244:*453–512, 1980

Fever

Bratton L, Teele DW, Klein JO: Outcome of unsuspected pneumococcemia in children not initially admitted to the hospital. *J Pediatr 90:*703–706, 1977

McCarthy PL, Jekel JF, Dolan TF: Temperature greater than or equal to 40°C in children less than 24 months of age: A prospective study. *Pediatrics 59:*663–668 1977

McGowan JE, Bratton L, Klein JO, et al: Bacteremia in febrile children seen in a "walk-in" pediatric clinic. *N Engl J Med 288:*1309–1313, 1973

Roberts KB, Borzy MS: Fever in the first eight weeks of life. *Johns Hopkins Med J 141:*9–13, 1977

Otitis

Paradise JL: Otitis media in infants and children. *Pediatrics 65:*117–143, 1980

Urinary Tract Infection

Carvajal HF: Kidney and bladder infections. *Adv Pediatr 25:*383–413, 1978

CHAPTER 20

Emergency Management of Patients with Rash and Fever

THOMAS B. FITZPATRICK, M.D.
RICHARD A. JOHNSON, M.D.

The sudden appearance of rash and fever is frightening for the patient. Approximately 10% of patients seeking emergency medical care do so with a dermatologic complaint. Many of these acute disorders, such as contact dermatitis and sunburn, are managed more appropriately in an outpatient facility other than the emergency ward. Some dermatologic disorders, however, because of their life-threatening nature or because they are part of the syndrome of a life-threatening disorder, require prompt diagnosis and therapy. Cutaneous findings range from the subtle but diagnostic erythematous macules and pustules that occur with gonococcemia to toxic epidermal necrolysis in which the entire epidermis is necrotic.

Patients may complain of acute onset of both rash and fever. Many times, the cutaneous findings may be diagnostic in the emergency ward before confirmatory laboratory data are available. As in the problem of the acute abdomen, the results of laboratory tests such as microbiologic cultures, serologic titers, and skin biopsy may be available only after days to weeks. On the basis of a differential diagnosis, appropriate therapy—whether antibiotics, corticosteroids, or treatment of symptoms—may be started. One approach that has been effective in this differential diagnostic challenge has been to consider basic diseases according to the lesions: (1) macules and papules; (2) bullae or pustules or both; and (3) infarctive or purpuric lesions—macules, papules, and vesicles. The physician must scrutinize the types of primary lesion, their shape, and their distribution when the patient is first examined. The temporal evolution of the eruption may be key in supporting the definite diagnosis.

Finally, the physician should make use of the following laboratory tests immediately or within 8 hours.

(1) **Direct smear from the base of a vesicle.** This procedure, known as the *Tzanck* test, is performed by unroofing an intact vesicle, gently scraping the base with a curved scalpel blade, and smearing the contents on a slide. After air drying, the smear is stained with Wright's or Giemsa's stain and examined for multinucleated giant cells. These altered epidermal cells are present in the herpes simplex-herpes zoster varicella group but are not present in the vaccinia-variola group of viruses.

(2) **Gram stain of aspirates or scraping.** Organisms can be seen in the lesions of typhoid and in acute meningococcemia, and rarely in the skin lesions of gonococcemia.

(3) **Dark-field examination.** In the skin lesions of secondary syphilis, repeated examination of papules may show *Treponema pallidum*. This is not reliable in mucous membrane as nonpathogenic organisms are almost impossible to differentiate from *T. pallidum*.

(4) **Biopsy of the skin lesions.** A 3- to 4-mm trephine is used under local anesthesia. In many laboratories, this can be processed within 8 hours if necessary. A diagnosis can be made in instances of Rocky Mountain spotted fever, systemic lupus erythematosus, erythema multiforme bullosum, toxic epidermal necrolysis, herpes zoster, allergic vasculitis, and some bacteremias.

(5) **Blood and urine examinations.** Blood culture, rapid serologic test for syphilis, and lupus erythematosus preparation require 24 hours. Examination of urine sediment may reveal red cell casts in allergic vasculitis.

DISEASES MANIFESTED BY MACULES OR PAPULES (Table 20.1)

Drug Hypersensitivity

Eruptions due to drugs are common problems that may be accompanied by fever. Although

Table 20.1.
Differential diagnosis for the patient with acute onset of rash and fever: "spotted fevers" diseases manifested by macules or papules.

Disease	Clinical History	Physical Examination		Diagnostic Signs	Laboratory Data Available Within 8 Hours
		General	Dermatologic		
Drug hypersensitivity	More likely in atopy and in systemic lupus erythematosus Recent administration of new drug	Variable findings	Urticarial eruptions Exanthematous eruptions Eczematous eruptions Erythema multiforme Drug-induced systemic lupus erythematosus		White blood cell differential for eosinophilia
Erythema multiforme	Recent herpes simplex or mycoplasmal infection Drug exposure	Temperature to 104°F (40°C)	Target lesions characteristically on distal extremities, palms, and soles Lesions may become bullous Bullous and erosive lesions of conjunctival, oropharyngeal, nasal, and anogenital mucosa possible	Target lesions on extremities	Skin biopsy
Measles	Malaise, photophobia, barklike cough, upper respiratory tract catarrh	Conjunctivitis Temperature to 104°F (40°C)	Exanthem appears on 4th day of illness on forehead and behind ears; evolves *inferiorly and centrifugally during next 72 hr to involve face, trunk, and extremities* Initial pink discrete macules evolve into dull red confluent papules Exanthem fades during 6th–10th day of illness with residual brown staining and fine desquamation	Koplik's spots on buccal mucosa before rash—cluster of bluish-white spots with bright-red ring Eruption persists 6–10 days	

Disease	History	Physical Findings	Rash		Laboratory
Rubella	Older children, young adults May follow immunization in women Prodrome to rash may be absent or consist of mild headache, malaise, sore throat Arthralgia, especially in women	Suboccipital, postauricular, and posterior cervical lymph nodes enlarged Periarticular tenderness or arthritis with effusion	Red macules or petechiae on soft palate (Forchheimer's sign) Exanthem appears as pink macules that coalesce on face; *rash spreads during 24 hrs to involve trunk and extremities as face clears; by 4th day, trunk and extremities clear in contrast to measles*	Eruption spreads rapidly from face to trunk and legs; clears within 3 days	
Nonspecific viral syndromes	Malaise Nausea and vomiting Diarrhea Sore throat Headache	Fever Variable findings	Exanthematous or vesicular rash Possible enanthem		
Secondary syphilis	Sexually active individual Possible history of chancre occurring about 21 days after venereal exposure Sore throat, malaise, headache, fever, musculoskeletal pain appearing 6–12 weeks after chancre	Residual chancre possible Inguinal adenopathy associated with genital chancre Lymphadenopathy (suboccipital, postauricular, posterior cervical, epitrochlear)	Pink-tan macules to papules to scaling papules on trunk and extremities, especially palms and soles "Moth-eaten" alopecia Condylomata lata Mucous patches and split papules Annular lesions possible	Pink-tan macules to papules on palms or soles or both Herxheimer's reaction	Darkfield examination of lesion is diagnostic Rapid plasma reagent card test
Scarlet fever	Sore throat in patient in 1st decade of life Possible wound infection	Folliclar or membranous tonsillitis Painful regional lymph node enlargement	Punctate erythema on upper trunk, generalized within hours to days Face flushed, with perioral pallor Petechial lesions possible at body folds, especially antecubital fossae	Strawberry tongue, initially white with enlarged filiform papillae, then bright red	

Table 20.1.—continued

Disease	Clinical History	Physical Examination		Diagnostic Signs	Laboratory Data Available Within 8 Hours
		General	Dermatologic		
			Perifollicular hyperkeratosis resulting in sandpapery feel to skin. Desquamation of palms and soles		
Rocky Mountain spotted fever	Tick bite. Endemic area. Incubation period after tick bite of 7 days. Malaise, severe fever, chills, headache, myalgia, toxic reaction for 3–4 days	Temperature to 104°F (40°C). Muscle tenderness. Stiff neck. Splenomegaly	Erythematous macules on wrists and ankles in sick patient; in 6–18 hrs, rash spreads centrifugally to involve palms and soles and centripetally to extremities and trunk. During next few days, lesions may become papular and purpuric	Site of origin of rash (ankles and wrists are unique sites of origin among exanthems)	Skin biopsy shows *Rickettsia rickettsii* within vascular endothelial cells
Murine typhus	Excoriated rat flea bite. Endemic area (Southern USA)	Temperature to 102.2°F (39°C). Splenomegaly in 25% of patients	Rash appears on 5th day of illness. Centripetal erythematous macular and papular discrete eruption. Duration—evanescent to several days	Centripetal eruption in patient in endemic area	
Erythema infectiosum	Relatively asymptomatic	Temperature to 100.4°F (38°C). Unremarkable	Early "slapped-cheek" butterfly erythema of face. Later, pink macules and papules become confluent to form reticulate pattern on trunk and extremities. Rash may recur over several days	"Slapped-cheek" appearance in otherwise well child	

Disease	History	Physical Examination	Cutaneous Lesions	Distinctive Features	Laboratory
Exanthema subitum	Child 6 months to 4 years old who is febrile but asymptomatic for 3–5 days	Temperature from 100.4–104°F (38–40°C); Unremarkable	As defervescence occurs, exanthem appears; Discrete pink macules and papules mainly on trunk but also on proximal extremities; Exanthem disappears in 24 hr		
Salmonella infections	Fever, chills, headache, and constipation of 1 week's duration followed by diarrhea and abdominal pain	Temperature from 102.2–104°F (39–40°C); Bradycardia; Abdominal tenderness	Crops of 10–20 pink macules and papules 1–3 mm in diameter on lower chest, abdomen, midback; Lesions fade in 3–4 days and reappear 2nd week	Rose spots	
Infectious mononucleosis and viral hepatitis	Malaise, fatigue, jaundice, sore throat	Temperature to 102.2°F (39°C); Adenopathy; Splenomegaly; Pharyngitis	Urticarial, morbilliform, or erythema multiforme-like rash		Heterophil test; Hepatitis-associated antigen
Erythema marginatum	Fever, possible migratory arthritis, cardiac involvement, chorea; Usually a child	Temperature to 104°F (40°C); New murmurs, cardiomegaly, pericardial rub	Usually, flat or slightly raised erythema on trunk; Macules enlarge by 1 cm/day with central clearing, resulting in polycyclic or geographic pattern	Rapidly evolving circinate rash	
Systemic lupus erythematosus	Fatigue, rash, photosensitivity, Raynaud's phenomenon; Joint pains, chest pains, seizures	Arthritis; Pleural or pericardial rub	Butterfly rash; Scaling, erythematous, atrophic plaques (discoid lesions) on scalp, face, shoulders; Photosensitivity rash; Periungual erythema	Discoid lesions; Butterfly rash	Anemia; Leukopenia; Thrombocytopenia; Positive ANA; Skin biopsy specific
Serum sickness	Drug or serum exposure; Malaise, headache, myalgia, anorexia	Temperature from 102.2–104°F (39–40°C); Migratory polyarthritis; Generalized lymphadenopathy	Commonly, an urticarial-like eruption		

about 30 different patterns of drug eruption occur, only a few types are of sudden enough onset that the patient seeks emergency evaluation.

A period of sensitization is required with most drugs. Eruptions frequently appear 1–2 weeks after initiation of drug therapy. If the patient has been exposed to the drug previously, however, the eruption may begin within minutes to hours of reinstatement of the agent. In addition, eruptions may occur several weeks after drug administration has ceased. Patients who have an atopic disorder such as hay fever, asthma, or eczema or who have systemic lupus erythematosus appear to become sensitized to drugs much more frequently, especially the penicillins.

The most common type of drug eruption is urticaria, followed by the exanthematous eruptions, which resemble viral exanthems (measles-like or morbilliform) or scarlet fever (scarlatiniform). Seen less frequently are erythema multiforme, eczematous eruptions, toxic epidermal necrolysis (with potential bulla formation), and drug-induced systemic lupus erythematosus. Infectious mononucleosis also alters reactivity to ampicillin. In a series of patients with sore throats who have received ampicillin for presumed streptococcal pharyngitis or tonsillitis, 85–100% have been reported to have an exanthematous drug eruption. Although rashes do occur with infectious mononucleosis, the frequency without ampicillin is low (3%).

The exanthematous drug eruption in the febrile patient poses a diagnostic problem. Many viral infections are accompanied by exanthems. Both viral and drug eruptions appear relatively abruptly, that is, within 24 hours. Both types appear symmetrically and centripetally, which suggests a systemic cause rather than a topical or local cause. Drug eruptions are often a deeper red, that is, "drug red" compared with viral exanthems. Concomitant conditions such as coryza, an enanthem, pharyngitis, or gastroenteritis often are helpful in distinguishing between the two eruptions. However, often the patient with such a condition has taken a medication such as penicillin, which makes the distinction difficult. Peripheral eosinophilia occurs with drug eruptions and is useful evidence when detected in a differential white blood cell count.

The specific drug-induced eruptions, erythema multiforme and toxic epidermal necrolysis, are discussed separately (this page and pages 457–458).

Drugs that have been implicated in acute eruptions are listed in Table 20.2. In most situations, a suspected drug can be withdrawn, and if indicated, administration of an alternative agent can be started. Drug eruptions frequently begin to fade within a few days of discontinuance. In certain situations, for example, in cases of documented *Staphylococcus aureus* endocarditis and in cases of bacteremia being treated with nafcillin or oxacillin, the drug can be continued despite the appearance of an exanthematous eruption; the alternative agent in such a case would be the relatively toxic drug, vancomycin. In most such cases, the eruption fades. The physician must realize, however, that eczematous or exfoliative dermatitis may develop in some patients in whom drug administration is continued.

Therapy for drug eruptions is for the most part based on symptoms. Topical corticosteroids are beneficial for eczematous drug eruptions. Extensive eruptions with necrosis of skin or mucosa may resolve more quickly with oral prednisone, 60 mg in divided doses initially.

Erythema Multiforme

An acute reaction of the dermal vasculature, erythema multiforme is often related to drug administration (Table 20.2) or to infection (Table 20.3). Radiotherapy may also be causative. The triggering event is most commonly herpes simplex or drug administration. The clinical presentation varies from a mild eruption to one with fatal complications.

Prodromal symptoms of fever, malaise, myalgia, and arthralgia may occur. Many times, however, it is impossible to separate the symptoms of a precipitating infection from the prodrome of erythema multiforme. Also, a triggering drug may be given for early viral symptoms that cannot be distinguished from prodromal erythema multiforme.

Early lesions of erythema multiforme may appear to be urticarial wheals; however, unlike wheals, the lesions do not fade in 24–48 hours. Urticarial wheals are pruritic, whereas the lesions of erythema multiforme may be tender to painful. Individual lesions may evolve into hemorrhagic papules with central purpura encircled by a white edematous ring that is surrounded by a halo of erythema; this is the iris or target lesion. Frequently, bullous lesions occur that are erosive when located on a thin mucosal surface.

Lesions are more numerous on the distal extremities, especially the palms and soles. Mucosal involvement—conjunctival, nasal, oropharyngeal, and anogenital—is associated with higher morbidity and mortality. Bullae form at the junction of the epidermis and dermis. Involvement of keratin-

Table 20.2.
Common drug eruptions and causal agents.

Urticaria
  Adrenocorticotropic hormone
  Barbiturates
  Chloramphenicol
  Griseofulvin
  Insulin
  Opiates
  Penicillin

  Phenolphthalein
  Phenothiazines
  Salicylates
  Streptomycin
  Sulfonamides
  Tetracycline

Exanthematous eruptions (scarlatiniform, morbilliform)
  Aminosalicylic acid
  Antihistamines
  Barbiturates
  Gold salts
  Griseofulvin
  Hydantoins
  Meprobamate
  Penicillin

  Phenothiazines
  Phenylbutazone
  Quinacrine
  Streptomycin
  Sulfonamides
  Sulfones
  Thiazide diuretics
  Thiouracil

Erythema multiforme
  Barbiturates
  Chlorpropamide
  Hydantoins
  Hydroxychloroquine
  Penicillin

  Phenothiazines
  Phenylbutazone
  Phenolphthalein
  Sulfonamides
  Thiazide diuretics

Eczematous eruptions
  Chlorpromazine
  Meprobamate
  Penicillin

  Quinacrine
  Streptomycin
  Sulfonamides

Toxic epidermal necrolysis
  Chlorpropamide
  Barbiturates
  Hydantoins
  Phenolphthalein

  Phenylbutazone
  Sulfonamides
  Thiazide diuretics
  Tolbutamide

Table 20.3.
Infections precipitating erythema multiforme.

Herpes simplex
β-hemolytic streptococcal infection
Viral hepatitis
Infectious mononucleosis
Histoplasmosis
Influenza A
Mumps
Ornithosis
Mycoplasma pneumoniae infection
Salmonella infection
Vaccinia

ized skin usually does not result in significant morbidity; erosive mucosal lesions, however, may be followed by corneal scarring and aspiration pneumonitis.

In the differential diagnosis of erythema multiforme, hand-foot-and-mouth disease, herpetic gingivostomatitis, secondary syphilis, and Rocky Mountain spotted fever must be considered whenever mucocutaneous surfaces are involved.

Therapy for erythema multiforme should be based on the answers to three questions:

(1) Can a treatable precipitating event be identified? For example, if erythema multiforme occurs after a mycoplasmal infection, tetracycline or erythromycin should be given. If a drug is implicated, the drug should be withdrawn.

(2) Should the patient be hospitalized? The course and eventual extent of involvement cannot be predicted on initial examination. Patients with extensive cutaneous involvement with bullae and erosions and those with significant conjunctival or oropharyngeal erosion should be hospitalized for

topical therapy and observation. The major complication is corneal scarring after secondary infection. Death may occur following aspiration and pneumonitis.

(3) Should systemic corticosteroid therapy be started? In some cases, the vascular reaction may be halted by administration of 60–120 mg/day of prednisone or its equivalent; this effect has not been proved by controlled studies. All patients with conjunctival or oropharyngeal involvement or with extensive cutaneous involvement should receive corticosteroids as soon as the diagnosis is made. Once the disease process has been arrested, the corticosteroid dosage can be rapidly tapered. Erythema multiforme rarely flares after corticosteroids are discontinued.

Measles (Morbilli)

Many viral infections cause systemic illness accompanied by eruptions on both the skin and the mucosa. Measles has unique clinical symptoms and signs. The appearance of the exanthem is mimicked by other viral exanthems and drug eruptions, which thus are referred to as measles-like or morbilliform. Temporal evolution of an exanthem is often helpful in the identification of a specific viral syndrome in comparison with a single observation of the exanthem in the emergency ward.

Within 10–15 days after exposure to measles, symptoms of an upper respiratory tract infection with coryza and a hacking, bark-like cough may occur, accompanied by photophobia, malaise, and fever. If the patient is examined on or after the second day of febrile illness, Koplik's spots may be observed on the buccal mucosa opposite the premolar teeth. This pathognomonic exanthem is characterized by a cluster of tiny bluish-white papules with an erythematous areola. By the fourth day, the characteristic exanthem appears as erythematous macules and papules on the forehead and behind the ears. By the third to fifth day of rash, the eruption spreads centrifugally and inferiorly to involve the face, trunk, and extremities. The initial discrete lesions may become confluent. The exanthem fades gradually with residual yellow-tan stain due to mild extravasation and faint desquamation.

The incidence of measles has been greatly reduced as a result of childhood immunization. When infection does occur, treatment is based on symptoms in the uncomplicated case.

Rubella (German Measles)

Because of widespread childhood immunization, the incidence of rubella now is reduced considerably. Still at risk are those children who have not been immunized and young adults who have not had the illness or undergone immunization. A rubella-like illness in women frequently follows administration of the attenuated live rubella virus.

After an 18-day incubation period, a mild prodromal illness occurs. Adolescents and adults may complain of anorexia, malaise, conjunctivitis, headache, low-grade fever, and mild upper respiratory tract symptoms. These symptoms are absent to mild in young children. Lymphadenopathy frequently is present at this time. Postauricular, suboccipital, and posterior cervical lymph nodes are enlarged and tender. Mild generalized lymphadenopathy, as well as splenomegaly, may occur. Enlargement of lymph nodes usually persists for 1 week, but may last for months.

An enanthem of petechiae on the soft palate (Forchheimer's sign) may be seen during the prodromal illness. This finding is not pathognomonic for rubella, since petechiae may be seen in this location in infectious mononucleosis, which also is accompanied by prominent lymphadenopathy.

The exanthem begins as pink macules and papules at the hairline, which spread during the first 24 hours to involve the face, trunk, and extremities. By the second day, the facial exanthem may fade, whereas the discrete lesions on the trunk become confluent, creating a scarlatiniform eruption. The exanthem usually remains discrete on the extremities. Unlike in measles, by the end of the third day the eruption has faded without a residual yellow-tan color or fine scaling. Serologic studies indicate that the exanthem may not appear in 10–40% of known cases of rubella.

Involvement of the joints is uncommon in children and in men; it may be present, however, in 40% of women with naturally occurring rubella or with rubella after immunization with the attenuated virus. The small joints of the hands and feet, the knees, and the elbows may become painful and swollen. Arthralgia or arthritis occurs as the rash is fading and is confirmatory evidence of rubella in women.

Symptoms are mild and transient. Aspirin should be given to relieve the discomfort of headache, fever, lymphadenitis, and arthritis.

Nonspecific Viral Exanthems

Coxsackie viruses of both groups A and B, ECHO virus, reoviruses, and adenoviruses are associated with exanthems. In most cases, the symptoms and physical findings suggest a viral infection, which can only be confirmed by the costly methods of viral culture. Most of the exanthems are characterized by pink macules or papules or both on the trunk and extremities; vesicles and petechiae are rare. Enanthems have also been observed and are characteristic of viral exanthematous eruptive fevers. The cutaneous findings may be accompanied by fever, malaise, gastroenteritis, pharyngitis, or aseptic meningitis.

The diagnosis of a viral syndrome is made on clinical grounds, usually excluding treatable bacterial agents.

Secondary Syphilis

Asymptomatic dissemination of *T. pallidum* via the blood and lymphatics occurs from the inoculation site within the first few days after exposure. A chancre usually appears at the inoculation site within 21 days (range, 7–90 days), and heals spontaneously in 3–4 weeks.

Symptoms and lesions of secondary syphilis may develop 6–12 weeks after appearance of the chancre. Constitutional symptoms are present in fewer than one-half of patients with secondary syphilis. Early symptoms are sore throat (53%), malaise (42%), headache (24%), fever (14%), and musculoskeletal pain (9%). These symptoms alone are nonspecific. A physician trained during the past two decades might omit secondary syphilis from the differential diagnosis. The disease, however, has doubled in incidence during this time. A serologic test for syphilis should be considered for all patients with headache, sore throat, and lymph node enlargement.

Lymphatic involvement occurs in 70% of patients; in addition to the inguinal nodes, which may remain enlarged following a penile chancre, the suboccipital, postauricular, posterior cervical, and epitrochlear lymph nodes most frequently are enlarged, but are not tender. Generalized lymphadenopathy occurs less frequently. In the evaluation of a patient with generalized lymphadenopathy, qualitative and quantitative serologic tests for syphilis should be performed with initial noninvasive studies. It is better to make the diagnosis at this stage of the evaluation than after a lymph node biopsy. Rarely, the nodes may be tender. A tender mass in the inguinal region may be diagnosed as an incarcerated inguinal or femoral hernia, and emergency operation may be performed. Histologic study of the removed mass may show luetic lymphadenitis, which would then be confirmed by a serologic test for syphilis and a fluorescent treponemal antibody-absorption (FTA-ABS) test.

The earliest cutaneous lesions of secondary syphilis are symmetrical, discrete, pink-tan macules, which appear first on the chest and abdomen. The eruption is overlooked easily and is difficult to detect in blacks. The initial eruption may fade, may reappear, or may evolve into a papular eruption. The papules become rather firm and change from reddish brown to brown in older lesions. The surface initially is shiny, but later forms a thin scale. At this time, secondary syphilis may resemble pityriasis rosea. In time the lesions may become hyperkeratotic. In the papular stage, the lesions may be round, oval, or annular. On the palms and soles, early lesions become infiltrated and papular, covered with scale. Typical papules are seen on the penile shaft and glans.

Large, soft, moist papules (condylomata lata) occur on mucosal or macerated surfaces in the perianal and vulvar regions. These lesions have a high density of viable organisms. Darkfield examination can be performed within a few minutes to confirm the diagnosis. Hypertrophic papules occur on the oral mucosa as mucous patches and at the corners of the mouth as split papules. Perifollicular inflammation in the scalp results in patchy, "moth-eaten" alopecia.

Laboratory confirmation of syphilis can be made by identification of *T. pallidum* from a cutaneous lesion with a darkfield microscope. Qualitative and quantitative serologic tests for syphilis are always positive in secondary syphilis. Early in this stage the quantitative titer may be low and, therefore, may not be separable from a biologic false-positive test. The specific FTA-ABS test should be performed. The quantitative serologic test should be repeated at intervals for at least a year; in adequately treated cases of secondary syphilis the test usually becomes negative in 6–18 months.

Secondary syphilis can be treated with benzathine penicillin G, a total of 2.4 million units intramuscularly at a single session, or procaine penicillin G, 600,000 units/day for 8 days. Patients should be informed of Herxheimer's reaction, which may occur 12–24 hours after penicillin therapy. This reaction is characterized by a temperature up to 104°F (40°C) and a flu-like syndrome. In the penicillin-allergic patient, tetracycline or erythromycin, 500 mg orally four times a day for 15 days, should be given.

Scarlet Fever

Scarlet fever is an acute infection of the tonsils or skin by an erythrogenic exotoxin-producing strain of group A streptococcus. Erythrogenic toxin production depends on the presence of a temperate bacteriophage. Patients with prior exposure to the erythrogenic toxin have antitoxin immunity and neutralize the toxin; the scarlet fever syndrome therefore does not develop in these patients. Since several erythrogenic strains of β-hemolytic streptococcus cause infection, it is theoretically possible to have a second episode of scarlet fever. Strains of *S. aureus* can synthesize an erythrogenic exotoxin producing a scarlatiniform exanthem. Pharyngeal infection is manifested by acute follicular or membranous tonsillitis with anterior cervical lymphadenitis. Less frequently, the β-hemolytic streptococcus infects a surgical or other wound.

Vasodilation induced by erythrogenic toxin becomes clinically apparent within 2–3 days after the onset of infection. Finely punctate erythema is noted first on the upper part of the trunk. The face becomes diffusely flushed, contrasted with a perioral pallor. The eruption becomes confluent (scarlatiniform) on the chest as it spreads to the extremities. Erythema is most intense at pressure points and in the body folds. Linear petechiae (Pastia's sign) may be noted in the antecubital and axillary folds. The clinical intensity of the exanthem varies from mild erythema confined to the trunk to a more extensive purpuric eruption. Within 4–5 days the exanthem fades and is followed by brawny desquamation on the body and extremities and by sheet-like exfoliation on the palms and soles. In subclinical or mild infections the exanthem may pass unnoticed. In this case, the patient may seek medical advice only when exfoliation on the palms is noted.

Erythrogenic toxin also produces a characteristic enanthem. Early in the illness, the lingular mucosa becomes hyperkeratotic. Scattered red swollen papillae give the tongue the appearance of a white strawberry. By the fourth or fifth day, the hyperkeratotic membrane has been sloughed, and the lingular mucosa appears bright red, resembling a red strawberry. Punctate erythema and petechiae may occur in the palate. The diagnosis can be confirmed by throat or wound culture or by a rise in the antistreptolysin O titer.

Specific antibiotic therapy can be given with a single intramuscular injection of benzathine penicillin G, 600,000 units in infants and children up to 40 kg and 900,000 to 1.2 million units in heavier children and in adults, or with oral potassium penicillin V, 250 mg four times a day for 10 days. In the penicillin-allergic patient, a 10-day oral course of erythromycin, 40 mg/kg/day in children and 250 mg four times a day in adults, is effective. An alternative agent is cephalexin, 15 mg/kg/day for 10 days in children and 250 mg four times a day for 10 days in adults. The suppurative complications are eliminated in most cases and the nonsuppurative complications are greatly reduced.

Rocky Mountain Spotted Fever

Rocky Mountain spotted fever is caused by *Rickettsia rickettsii* and is transmitted to human beings by a tick bite. The disease is seasonal, and the incidence peaks in the summer, when man and the wood tick have the greatest mutual exposure. The patient should have a history of tick bite or of exposure in an endemic area.

After a mean incubation period of 7 days (range, 3–12 days) the patient experiences abrupt onset of fever, chills, malaise, headache, and musculoskeletal pain. The temperature may range from 103–104°F (39.5–40°C). The rash usually appears on the fourth day of the illness (range, 2–6 days). Pink macules that blanch with pressure are characteristically first noted on the wrists, forearms, and ankles. Within 6–18 hours, the rash spreads to involve the palms, soles, arms, thighs, trunk, and face. The lesions may become papular or purpuric or both. With extensive cutaneous vascular involvement, areas of necrotic skin may occur. The temporal evolution of the rash is quite helpful in the diagnosis. It must be kept in mind that a fatal form of the disease may occur without rash.

Cutaneous biopsy, with results available within 8 hours, may be helpful since rickettsiae can at times be demonstrated within the endothelial cells of the dermal vasculature. Specific complement fixation studies on acute and convalescent sera will confirm the diagnosis.

Treatment with tetracycline or chloramphenicol, 2 gm/day for adults, should be started early, especially if the patient has a history of tick bite in an endemic area, prodromal symptoms, and an exanthem on the wrists and ankles.

Murine (Endemic) Typhus

Murine typhus is a mild systemic disease caused by *R. mooseri*. This rickettsia is transferred from infected rats and mice to human beings by the bite of the rat flea. In the United States, reservoirs of infection occur along the southeast coast and along the Gulf of Mexico. In 1980, 81 cases of murine typhus were reported to the Center for Disease Control in Atlanta, Georgia, compared with 1163 cases of Rocky Mountain spotted fever, a more serious and more frequently detected rickettsial disease.

After an incubation period of 8–16 days, the

patient experiences a temperature to 102.2°F (39°C), chills, malaise, headache, nausea, and vomiting. The rash appears about the fifth day of illness and is characterized by a centripetal, truncal, macular to papular eruption. Involvement of the distal extremities is unusual. The rash may be evanescent or may last several days. Symptoms resolve in 9–14 days. The diagnosis is confirmed by detection of rising titers of specific complement-fixing antibodies.

The mortality from murine typhus is low. Administration of tetracycline or chloramphenicol, 2 gm/day, is followed by defervescence in 24–48 hours, together with abatement of the rash and symptoms.

Erythema Infectiosum

Erythema infectiosum is an acute mild illness with a characteristic exanthem. A viral cause is probable, but is not proved. The disease usually occurs in epidemics, and in that setting it is easier to identify. Sporadic cases may be difficult to diagnose with certainty.

Erythema infectiosum occurs most frequently in girls from 5 years old to puberty, but is also seen in boys and in adults. Prodromal symptoms are absent to mild. Malaise, headache, nausea and vomiting, coryza, sore throat, and musculoskeletal pain do occur. Adults tend to have more severe constitutional symptoms. The temperature is rarely higher than 100.4°F (38°C).

The exanthem begins with an erythematous plaque in a butterfly distribution on the face, creating a "slapped-cheek" appearance. The skin is hot and the eruption must be distinguished from erysipelas, scarlet fever, and lupus erythematosus. The plaque fades within a few days, leaving a dusky violet hue. As the facial eruption fades, an exanthem appears on the buttocks and extremities. Macular or urticarial lesions develop, which become confluent to form a characteristic annular, gyrate, or reticulate pattern. This latter eruption fades in 3–5 days, but may recur.

Usually a definitive diagnosis can be made by following the course of the illness over a week. Treatment of symptoms at times may be required.

Exanthema Subitum
(Roseola Infantum)

Exanthema subitum, as the name suggests, is characterized by the sudden appearance of a rash. Although thought to be viral, the agent has not been isolated. The disease is usually seen in children from 6 months to 4 years of age. Either the degree of contagiousness is low or the subclinical attack rate is high, since epidemics do not occur and the incidence of secondary cases within families is low. A temperature from 100.4–104°F (38–40°C) develops suddenly while the infant is otherwise asymptomatic. The fever is relatively constant for 3–5 days, after which defervescence occurs abruptly.

The exanthem develops coincidental with defervescence; it appears mainly on the trunk and to a lesser extent on the proximal extremities, neck, and face. Discrete pink macules and papules are seen. The exanthem is short-lived, usually lasting only 24 hours.

No confirmatory laboratory tests are available. Unless the patient has been examined during the febrile phase and subsequently with the exanthem, the diagnosis cannot be confirmed on clinical grounds.

Salmonella Infections
(Enteric Fever)

Salmonella typhi and other less virulent Salmonella species cause gastroenteritis followed by systemic illness. Symptoms begin days to several weeks after ingestion of contaminated food or water. Fever, headache, musculoskeletal aches, bronchitis, and constipation occur during the first week of illness. The temperature ranges from 102.2–104°F (39–40°C).

During the course of infection, the rose spots described by Osler develop in 75% of patients, and are accompanied by abdominal pain and diarrhea. In the second week of illness, successive crops of 10–20 pink papules 1–3 mm in diameter appear on the abdomen, lower part of the chest, and middle of the back. These lesions do not evolve further and fade in 3–4 days. New crops appear in the next 2–3 weeks. The lesions follow bacteremia, and salmonellae can be cultured and demonstrated on a Gram stain of a scraping from a lesion.

Today, most patients are treated early in the illness with the result that the classic lesions fail to appear. Administration of chloramphenicol or ampicillin is begun based on the presumptive diagnosis, and the diagnosis is confirmed by stool or blood cultures.

Infectious Mononucleosis and
Infectious Hepatitis

Both infectious mononucleosis and infectious hepatitis have been reported to occur with rashes during the early stage of the illness. In viral hepatitis the rash appears before jaundice develops.

Urticarial reactions are most common, but morbilliform and erythema multiforme eruptions also occur. Diagnosis is made either by means of the heterophil test or by detection of hepatitis-associated antigen.

Erythema Marginatum (Erythema Circinatum)

Erythema marginatum is part of the syndrome occurring in children with acute rheumatic fever, including fever, carditis, chorea, and possibly, migratory arthritis. The rash is noted in approximately 10% of patients. Macular or slightly raised erythema appears on the trunk and proximal extremities. While the borders of the erythema advance rapidly, the central area resolves. The evolving lesions result in annular, polycyclic, or geographic configurations. The rash may appear intermittently for months, but its presence does not correlate with the activity of the carditis.

Systemic Lupus Erythematosus

Systemic lupus erythematosus (SLE) is an intermittent, recurrent, systemic inflammatory disease in which 10% of patients may have fever or rash or both at any one period. Patients may have an acute presentation with arthritis, pleuritis, pleural effusion, pericarditis, myocarditis, psychosis, seizures, or thrombocytopenia. Cutaneous involvement may be of great diagnostic value before laboratory confirmation is available.

As seen in Table 20.4, patients with SLE may have many types of cutaneous involvement. The discoid lesion, a classic, scaly, erythematous plaque, is clinically distinct in many patients. Periungual erythema and telangiectasia are not diagnostic of SLE, but suggest a connective tissue disorder, that is, SLE, scleroderma, dermatomyositis, or rheumatoid arthritis. Urticaria is a nonspecific finding.

Serum Sickness

An infrequent systemic adverse drug reaction, serum sickness (Table 20.5) is a condition in which nearly all patients exhibit both fever and rash. In patients who are not sensitized, the reaction begins 8–12 days after exposure to the antigen. Fever is present from the onset of the reaction and persists throughout. Temperature elevation may be slight or high. Constitutional symptoms of headache, myalgia, malaise, and anorexia frequently occur. Physical examination shows migratory polyarthritis, mainly involving the distal large joints. Gen-

Table 20.4.

Cutaneous manifestations of systemic lupus erythematosus.

Manifestation	Dubois (520 patients)	Rothfield (240 patients)
	%	
Skin involvement	71.5	83.3
Rash	—	66.6
Erythematous butterfly blush	36.7	32.5
Discoid lesions	28.6	15.0
Maculopapular eruption	19.0	15.0
Purpura, ecchymoses, petechiae	19.8	6.2
Urticaria	6.9	9.1
Bullous lesions	0.4	4.5
Periungual erythema	1.1	10.0
Palmar erythema	—	8.7
Photosensitivity rash	9.1	22.9
Periorbital edema	4.8	5.8
Facial edema	4.6	18.3
Hyperpigmentation	8.4	5.8
Leg ulcers	5.6	9.1
Alopecia		
Diffuse	21.3	42.4
Patchy	3.6	9.5
Both diffuse and patchy	—	7.0
Mucosal ulcers	9.1	20.4
Raynaud's phenomenon	18.4	2.4
Digital gangrene	1.3	0.8

Table 20.5.

Drugs producing serum sickness.

Most frequently encountered
  Penicillin
  Serums
  Streptomycin
  Sulfonamides
  Thiouracil
Others
  Apresoline
  Barbiturates
  Hydantoins
  Iodides
  Phenylbutazone
  Quinidine
  Quinine
  Salicylates

eralized lymph node enlargement occurs and in severe cases is accompanied by splenomegaly.

A pruritic urticarial-like eruption, which may fade and recur over several weeks, occurs in 75% of patients. Morbilliform and scarlatiniform eruptions occur less frequently, and cutaneous vasculitis occurs rarely.

DISEASES MANIFESTED BY VESICLES, BULLAE, OR PUSTULES (Table 20.6)

Varicella (Chickenpox)

Herpesvirus varicellae is the cause of two distinct clinical infections: (1) varicella or chickenpox, a primary systemic infection; and (2) herpes zoster or shingles, which is usually an endogenous infection limited to cranial or peripheral sensory nerves and their corresponding dermatomes. Varicella is highly contagious, and most cases occur during childhood, when the constitutional symptoms and exanthem tend to be mild to moderate. In adults, however, systemic and cutaneous involvement may be more severe.

After an incubation period of 14–15 days, a prodromal illness of low-grade fever and mild constitutional symptoms occurs. In 1–2 days, the exanthem appears on the trunk with initial erythematous macules, or rarely, urticarial papules evolving into small vesicles in 24 hours; sometimes, large bullous lesions occur. The contents of the vesicles become turbid, and the vesicles become pustular with central umbilication. The lesions may rupture with crust formation. During the following 3–5 days, successive crops of vesiculopustules appear and further involve the trunk, the proximal extremities, and the face. Characteristically, lesions in all stages of evolution are present. With extensive involvement, lesions appear on the distal extremities, palms, and soles. Vesicles and erosions frequently occur on the oral mucosa. The ultimate number of vesiculopustules varies from few to profuse.

Crusted lesions usually heal in 1–3 weeks without scarring. Pruritus is common. Scratching the lesions increases the depth of cutaneous involvement and facilitates secondary impetiginization. If this occurs, scarring may result.

In adolescents and adults, asymptomatic pneumonitis may occur in one-half of the patients. Severe symptomatic varicella pneumonitis can develop. Varicella hepatitis frequently occurs in fatal cases.

The diagnosis of varicella can be confirmed in the emergency ward by demonstration of multinucleated giant epidermal cells within the vesicular fluid, the Tzanck test. Disseminated infection with herpes simplex virus is the only other cause of a generalized vesiculopustular eruption with multinucleated giant cells. Chest x-ray study is indicated in adults.

Treatment of uncomplicated varicella should be directed at alleviating pruritus and preventing secondary infection of erosions. An antihistamine should be given to make the patient drowsy to minimize excoriation. Shake lotions such as calamine lotions cool the skin by evaporation, but the residual powder tends to add to the bulk of the crusts. Impetiginization by a β-hemolytic streptococcus or *S. aureus* should be suspected in crusted lesions that increase in size or number. A Gram stain should be performed for gram-positive cocci within the polymorphonuclear leukocytes. If these are seen, the patient should be treated with erythromycin orally.

Herpes Zoster

Zoster or shingles is considered to be a reactivation of a latent *Herpesvirus varicellae* infection residing in the posterior root or cranial nerve ganglion after an episode of varicella. The virus replicates within the peripheral sensory nerve, and once the cutaneous nerve endings are reached, the characteristic dermatomal pattern of grouped vesicles on an erythematous base appears.

Associated with viral replication within the nerve, the patient experiences local pain, which may be dull, sharp, burning, or shooting. At this time, with no skin eruption, misdiagnosis may be made. The patient is afebrile. Crops of vesiculopustules on an erythematous base appear, at first posteriorly, that is, along the posterior branch of the intercostal nerve. A specific diagnosis usually can be made at this point with the history of pain and the demonstration of multinucleated giant epidermal cells in the vesicular fluid. During the next few days, crops of grouped vesicles continue to appear on the dermatome. The frequency of dermatomal involvement is as follows: thoracic (53–56%), trigeminal (10–15%), cervical (12–20%), lumbar (8–9%), and lumbosacral (2–4%). The extent of cutaneous involvement varies from scattered vesicles to confluent epidermal necrosis.

Mild hematogenous dissemination with a few vesicles outside the involved dermatome is common, occurring in approximately 15% of patients. Most cases of herpes zoster occur in otherwise healthy patients. Only if it is indicated by a complete history and physical examination should a workup for an underlying malignant condition be undertaken. Generalized herpes zoster involving skin and viscera usually develops in patients with an impaired immune response that is related to either lymphoma, leukemia, or immunosuppressive therapy. The prognosis for patients with gen-

Table 20.6.
Differential diagnosis for the patient with acute onset of rash and fever: "blistering fevers" diseases manifested by vesicles, bullae, or pustules.

Disease	Clinical History	Physical Examination		Diagnostic Signs	Laboratory Data Available Within 8 Hours
		General	Dermatologic		
Varicella	Exposure: chickenpox or shingles In children, mild constitutional symptoms In adolescents and adults, more severe constitutional symptoms; varying degrees of respiratory distress possible	Temperature 102.2°F (39°C)	Exanthem appears 1–2 days after onset of illness; vesiculopustules appear centripetally in crops over next 3–5 days Palms, soles, and oropharynx may be involved Crusted lesions heal in 1–3 weeks	Characteristic exanthem	Tzanck test shows multinucleated giant cells in vesicular fluid
Generalized zoster	Prodromal pain, which may be misdiagnosed as myocardial infarction, pleurisy, cholecystitis, appendicitis, pyelonephritis, renal colic, prolapsed disc, trigeminal neuralgia Lymphoma, leukemia, carcinoma Radiotherapy	Fever with dissemination outside dermatome	Grouped vesicles on erythematous base in dermatomal distribution Generalized vesicles	Characteristic eruption	Tzanck test shows multinucleated giant cells
Toxic epidermal necrolysis	Infant < 2 years old Adolescent or adult with drug exposure	Fever	In infant, erythema and tenderness of flexural epidermis, which shears off with trauma In adult, generalized erythema and shearing off of epidermis; mucosa may be involved	Nikolsky's sign	Skin biopsy Blood and skin cultures
Hand-foot-and-mouth disease	Exposure during epidemic summer months	Low-grade fever	Tender vesicles on hands and feet and in oropharynx	Tender oval vesicles on palms or soles	Negative Tzanck test

Eczema herpeticum	Inactive or active atopic dermatitis Exposure to "cold sore"	Regional lymphadenitis	Vesicles or well-demarcated erosions in eczematous skin; area of involvement varies	Vesicles in eczematous skin	Tzanck test shows multinucleated giant cells
Eczema vaccinatum	Inactive or active atopic dermatitis Recent vaccination or exposure to vaccination	Temperature to 102.2°F (39°C) Regional lymphadenitis	Umbilicated pustules in eczematous skin	Umbilicated pustules in eczematous skin	Gram stain reveals no bacteria Negative Tzanck test Skin biopsy
Rickettsial pox	Inoculation papule (eschar) present 3–7 days before onset of fever	Tender lymphadenitis in nodes draining inoculation papule Temperature to 104°F (40°C)	Generalized vesiculo-papular lesions	None	Negative Tzanck test

eralized herpes zoster depends on control of the underlying disease. Generalized herpes zoster usually can be diagnosed by noting a zosteriform eruption, a generalized vesiculopustular eruption, and multinucleated giant cells within the pustules. Rarely, there may be sensorineural involvement without a zosteriform eruption (zoster sine zoster) in patients with generalized varicella. In such a case, generalized infection with *Herpesvirus varicellae* can be distinguished from infection with herpes simplex virus only by viral tissue cultures of vesicular fluid, sputum, or blood.

Toxic Epidermal Necrolysis

Toxic epidermal necrolysis is characterized by epidermal necrosis of varying depth and extent. In newborns and infants, the disease, scalded skin syndrome, is caused by an exotoxin produced by *S. aureus*, phage type 71. The staphylococcus may colonize in the nose, conjunctivae, or umbilical stump without causing clinically apparent infection, but may elaborate an exotoxin that is carried hematogenously to the skin. In the newborn and infant, the toxin causes necrosis of the upper half of the viable epidermis.

Patients are brought for emergency evaluation because of the sudden occurrence of irritability, possibly mild fever, and tender skin. On examination in the early stage, erythema and tenderness are noted in the flexural areas of skin in the neck, axillae, antecubital fossae, and inguinal folds. The epidermis may shear off if a frictional force is applied to it (Nikolsky's sign). Within 1 or 2 days, all the skin may appear erythematous. Frank formation of bullae does not occur.

Staphylococcal scalded skin syndrome responds quickly to antibiotics. In the newborn, hospitalization and treatment with intravenous oxacillin, 200 mg/kg/day in divided doses every 4 hours, is preferable. Hospitalization also is indicated for infants when there is extensive sloughing of skin or if it is questionable whether the parents will provide adequate care. With reliable home care and mild involvement, dicloxacillin, 30–50 mg/kg/day, can be given orally. Baths or compresses to exfoliating or crusted areas, followed by application of a topical agent such as bacitracin ointment, will optimize the rate of epidermal regrowth.

In the adult, staphylococcal exotoxin is rarely a factor in toxic epidermal necrolysis. Drugs are common etiologic agents. In some cases, the cause is undetermined. The drugs most frequently implicated are the hydantoins, barbiturates, sulfonamides, thiazide diuretics, oral hypoglycemic agents, and phenylbutazone. The reaction may occur within a few days of initiation of a new drug or it may occur after the same drug has been taken for many years. Within 24–48 hours the entire epidermis, as well as the mucosa of the conjunctivae, nose, and oropharynx, may become necrotic. The epidermis shears off when the patient moves or is examined. Skin usually shows necrosis of the epidermis to the basal layer, which creates the clinical impression of a second-degree thermal burn. Extracellular fluid usually does not accumulate beneath the epidermis as bullae since there is little vascular damage. Initially the patient may be remarkably alert but in pain after stripping of the epidermis, or he may be obtunded.

Optimal care is given if the patient is hospitalized and treated as a burned patient. Epidermal necrosis usually stops within a few days; occasionally a patient may benefit from a short course of prednisone or its equivalent, 60–120 mg/day. Intravenous fluid replacement is not of the magnitude required in a burned patient since vessels are not damaged and there is little leakage of interstitial fluid. Because mucosal involvement occurs, secondary infection of the conjunctivae must be prevented with use of erythromycin ointment. Frequent suctioning must be performed to prevent aspiration pneumonitis when the oropharynx is denuded and the patient has difficulty in swallowing secretions. The mortality in older patients with drug-induced toxic epidermal necrolysis approaches 50%.

Enteroviral Infection

Hand-foot-and-mouth disease is a mild condition caused by Coxsackie A16 virus that produces characteristic mucocutaneous findings. As with other enteroviral infections, hand-foot-and-mouth disease occurs in epidemic outbreaks in late summer.

Systemic symptoms are mild to minimal and include low-grade fever, vague malaise, and tenderness of the lesions. In a few patients, these symptoms may be more intense and may be accompanied by myalgia, arthralgia, or diarrhea.

Within 24 hours after the prodromal symptoms, a vesicular eruption appears on the hands and feet and in the oropharynx. On the palmar and plantar surfaces, the vesicles are characteristically elongated or oval. The individual vesicles are tender and are surrounded by a red areola. There may be fewer than a dozen lesions confined to the hands and feet or there may be hundreds of lesions involving the extremities and buttocks. When an extensive exanthem occurs, varicella may be considered, but is ruled out by the centrifugal density of the lesions and a negative Tzanck test. The mucosal lesions may appear at any site in the oropharynx, and unlike in herpetic gingivostomatitis, they are not associated with submandibular lymphadenopathy. Oral vesicular lesions are fragile and quickly evolve into erosions. Although the three sites frequently demonstrate vesicles, some patients do not simultaneously have lesions on the hands and feet and in the mouth. Treatment is based on symptoms.

The Boston exanthem is a fairly characteristic clinical syndrome associated with ECHO 16 virus. Epidemics occur during the summer. The disease is more frequent in young children; adults, however, are more symptomatic. Children become mildly febrile with a temperature to 102.2°F (39°C) for 1–2 days. Youngsters may complain only of a mild sore throat associated with chills, headache, muscle aches and pains, prostration, and cramping abdominal pain. Associated with defervescence, a pink to salmon-colored macular and papular eruption appears on the face and upper part of of the chest. In some patients the exanthem becomes generalized, involving the palms and soles but clearing in 1–5 days. Treatment is based on symptoms.

Herpes Simplex Virus Infections

Herpes simplex virus causes several clinical syndromes that are characterized by both rash and fever. Only 10–15% of persons have symptomatic primary herpesvirus infection. The incidence of past infection as indicated by the presence of circulating antibodies varies according to conditions of overcrowding or poor hygiene. In more affluent groups, 25% have evidence of past infection, compared with 95% in some poorer socioeconomic groups.

The most frequent symptomatic manifestation of primary infection is acute gingivostomatitis. Patients have fever (temperature to 102.2°F [39°C]), malaise, and tender lesions in the mouth. There may be a history of recent exposure to someone with a cold sore. On examination, vesiculopustules can be seen at any site on the oropharyngeal mucosa, lips, and skin about the mouth. The submandibular lymph nodes are usually enlarged and tender. The diagnosis is confirmed by demonstration of multinucleated giant cells with a Tzanck test. Constitutional symptoms usually resolve within a week and oral erosion within 2 weeks. Subsequent to this, herpesvirus may remain latent in the patient for a lifetime. Treatment is based on symptoms, and includes aspirin, irrigations of the mouth with hydrogen peroxide solution, and application of a topical anesthetic such as viscous lidocaine (Xylocaine) or dyclonine hydrochloride (Dyclone).

In patients with altered skin, that is, atopic dermatitis or thermal burns, large areas of skin may become infected with herpesvirus. Patients with minimal or even inactive atopic dermatitis are subject to either endogenous or exogenous infection of extensive areas of skin (eczema herpeticum). Since patients with eczema may scratch and rupture herpetic vesicles, both intact vesicles and sharply demarcated erosions may be seen; the patient may have fever and lymph node enlargement. Diagnosis is made by means of the Tzanck test. Treatment is based on symptoms, and should include baths or moist compresses to debride crusted areas. Topical corticosteroids should not be applied to eczematous skin in patients with active eczema herpeticum.

Some patients have recurrent erythema multiforme with recurrent episodes of herpes labialis. Patients may be febrile and have two types of vesiculobullous disease simultaneously. Patients with frequent episodes of recurrent herpes labialis and symptomatic disabling erythema multiforme are candidates for short-term oral corticosteroid therapy to halt the natural evolution of each episode of erythema multiforme.

Generalized herpes simplex may follow a primary or recurrent herpetic infection or eczema herpeticum. A temperature to 104°F (40°C), headache, and severe malaise may be accompanied by lymphadenopathy, hepatosplenomegaly, and signs of meningeal irritation or mental deterioration. Involvement of the bone marrow may result in leukopenia and thrombocytopenia. The skin, along with the primary or recurrent herpetic lesion, may show a generalized vesicular eruption with a positive Tzanck test. The specific diagnosis can be made only if herpesvirus is cultured from skin, blood, or tissue.

The management of genital herpes infections is discussed in Chapter 24, page 528.

Eczema Vaccinatum

A patient with atopic dermatitis either after an inappropriately administered smallpox vaccination by a physician or after skin-to-skin contact with a recently vaccinated individual is likely to have extensive infection in the eczematous skin by the vaccinia virus, that is, eczema vaccinatum. The likelihood of this has been considerably reduced since vaccination no longer is recommended routinely for preschool children, but is recommended only for persons traveling to an endemic area of smallpox.

Vaccinia should be considered when large discrete pustules with an umbilicated center and an erythematous halo are noted in a patient with atopic dermatitis. Burned skin is also subject to vaccinia. An extensive infection in an infant carries a high probability of death since the immune system is overwhelmed. A Gram stain of the pustules should be obtained to rule out the presence of staphylococci. Skin biopsy may be helpful if cytoplasmic inclusion bodies can be demonstrated within epidermal cells. Viral cultures confirm the diagnosis. Patients with extensive cutaneous involvement and constitutional symptoms should receive vaccinia immune globulin (VIG).

Generalized vaccinia occurs in an otherwise healthy host whose vaccinial antibody response is somewhat delayed. Vaccinia virus disseminates hematogenously, resulting in a single crop of generalized vaccinial lesions, that is, umbilicated pustules. The disease is self-limited, but vaccinia immune globulin should be administered.

Rickettsial Pox

A mild, self-limited urban disease, rickettsial pox is caused by *R. akari*. The rickettsia is transmitted from its host, the mouse, to man through the bite of the mouse mite. One to two weeks after the bite, a firm papule develops at the site of inoculation. The papule enlarges to 1.0–1.5 cm in diameter and quickly undergoes central vesiculation. After crusting with eschar formation, healing with residual scar formation occurs in 3 weeks. Tender regional lymphadenitis is associated with the inoculation papule.

Three to seven days after the appearance of the inoculation papule, which may be asymptomatic but detectable in 95% of patients, systemic symptoms of temperature to 104°F (40°C), chills, sweats, malaise, and myalgia occur. A papular eruption usually accompanies the constitutional symptoms; it may be generalized, involving the palms, soles, and oropharynx. Within 24 hours, vesicles appear atop the papules. The exanthem and symptoms usually resolve in 7–10 days.

Rickettsial pox often is misdiagnosed as varicella; however, varicella can be ruled out by the absence of multinucleated giant cells in a Tzanck test. The diagnosis can be confirmed by serologic titers for specific complement-fixing antibodies.

Rickettsial pox resolves spontaneously. Tetracycline, 2 gm/day, will arrest the natural course of the disease within 24 hours of administration.

DISEASES MANIFESTED BY PURPURIC MACULES, PAPULES, OR VESICLES (Table 20.7)

Bacteremia

The presence of bacteria or bacterial products in the blood results in several types of cutaneous pathologic reaction. Some reactions are nonspecific, whereas other changes are pathognomonic of the infecting bacterium.

Meningococcemia can produce a spectrum of lesions ranging from transient petechiae to vesiculopustules on the trunk and extremities. A specific diagnosis can be made by demonstration of the organism on a Gram stain or a culture. Endotoxin from the meningococcus as well as from other gram-negative organisms can initiate disseminated intravascular coagulation. The cutaneous lesions, purpura fulminans, occur after occlusion of cutaneous blood vessels with fibrin thrombi. Hemorrhagic infarcts occur, which appear as irregular, sharply demarcated purple-to-black areas. These infarcts often are seen over pressure points and in acral areas, but may appear anywhere. The affected areas may initially be slightly raised because of hemorrhage and edema; if the patient survives, a blackened eschar develops. Penicillin is the drug of choice; chloramphenicol is used for the penicillin-allergic patient (see Table 11.2).

Gonococcemia, whether acute or subacute, produces a characteristic arthritis-dermatitis syndrome. Bacteremia occurs most frequently in menstruating women from the infected, sloughing, and denuded endometrium. About a half-dozen tender erythematous macules are noted in acral areas. During the next 24–48 hours, these lesions may evolve into hemorrhagic pustules. The cutaneous lesions are associated with tenosynovitis of the wrist or ankle, arthralgia, or frank septic arthritis. Patients should be hospitalized and treated with intravenous penicillin, approximately 10 million units/day. After the patient has been afebrile for 3 days, oral ampicillin, 500 mg every 4 hours, may be substituted for penicillin.

S. aureus bacteremia can produce metastatic cutaneous infections ranging from pustules to subcutaneous abscesses to purulent hemorrhagic lesions. *S. aureus* may be seen in a smear of the pustular aspirate and its presence confirmed by culture. An adequate number of blood cultures must be obtained, and if they are positive, the patient must be presumed to have *S. aureus* endocarditis, even in the absence of a new murmur.

Pseudomonas aeruginosa septicemia usually occurs in infants and debilitated or immunosuppressed patients. The most characteristic lesion is ecthyma gangrenosum, which appears as a gunmetal gray, indurated, relatively painless area with surrounding erythema. The lesion most frequently occurs in the axilla or anogenital area. Ulceration develops, with sloughing of the epidermis.

Subacute bacterial endocarditis caused by *Streptococcus viridans* produces several types of vascular lesion, some of which probably occur through bacterial embolization. Petechiae occur in crops on the skin or on the mucosa of the conjunctivae or palate. These lesions do not blanch with pressure, but fade in several days. The diagnostic significance of subungual splinter hemorrhages is highly overrated. Such lesions can be detected in 10% of patients admitted to a medical service, and by far the most common cause is nail trauma. Such hemorrhage in the proximal or midnail area is probably more noteworthy. Osler's nodes are tender pink papules 6–8 mm in diameter occurring on the digital pads and lasting 12–24 hours. Janeway lesions are small pink-to-slightly-hemorrhagic macules on the palms or soles. Because of the widespread use of antibiotics, these cutaneous findings are observed far less frequently as a result of the changing type of pathogenic organism.

Allergic Vasculitis

Leukocytoplastic angiitis (necrotizing angiitis) may involve only the venules in the dermal vascular plexus (allergic cutaneous vasculitis), or it may involve any organ system. The characteristic cutaneous finding is "palpable" purpura. These lesions appear first where the venous pressure is greatest, that is, on the lower legs, and they do not blanch with pressure. With sufficient vascular involvement, purpuric vesicles and even infarcts occur with formation of ulcers.

In patients with the rash of cutaneous vasculitis, the extent of systemic involvement must be determined by the history, physical examination, and laboratory studies. In patients with Henoch-Schönlein purpura, periarticular vasculitis is common with arthralgia or frank arthritis. Gastrointestinal involvement is manifested by colicky pain or, if there is intestinal obstruction, by intussusception or intramural hemorrhage. The stool specimen may be bloody or tarry, or may give a positive test for occult blood. Renal involvement with glomerulitis should be ruled out by urinalysis in which the urine is examined for erythrocytes.

Systemic corticosteroid therapy is usually not indicated for cutaneous involvement, but may be indicated with involvement of other organ systems.

Table 20.7.
Differential diagnosis for the patient with acute onset of rash and fevers: "purpuric fevers" diseases manifested by purpuric macules, papules, or vesicles.

Disease	Clinical History	Physical Examination		Diagnostic Signs	Laboratory Data Available Within 8 Hours
		General	Dermatologic		
Meningococcemia	Exposure Headache Confusion	Temperature to 104°F (40°C) Meningismis	Petechiae Scattered macules to papules to hemorrhagic vesicles Numerous large infarcts (purpura fulminans)	Rash with signs of meningeal irritation	Gram stain of pustular aspirate or cerebrospinal fluid reveals gram-negative cocci in PMN
Gonococcemia	Sexual exposure Commonly a menstruating or pregnant woman Periarticular and joint pains	Temperature to 102.2°F (39°C) Tenosynovitis Septic arthritis Possible cervicitis or pelvic inflammatory disease	Half-dozen tender macules evolving to hemorrhagic pustules	Few scattered pustules associated with tenosynovitis or arthritis Extensor areas distal extremities	Gram stain of pustular aspirate reveals gram-negative cocci
Allergic vasculitis	Drug exposure Prior streptococcal pharyngitis Arthralgia Abdominal pain	Temperature to 102.2°F (39°C) Possible arthritis Abdominal tenderness	"Palpable" purpura, most pronounced in dependent areas May become ulcerative	"Palpable" purpura	Frank or occult blood in stool Hematuria Skin biopsy

Suggested Readings

Arndt KA: *Manual of Dermatologic Therapeutics.* ed 2. Boston, Little, Brown and Co., Inc., 1978

Bruinsma W: *A Guide to Drug Eruptions.* Amsterdam, Excerpta Medica, 1973

Demis DJ, Dobson RL, McGuire J (Eds): *Clinical Dermatology.* Vols 1–4, New York, Harper & Row, 1976

Dubois EL: Results of steroid therapy in systemic lupus erythematosus. *In*: Dubois EL (Ed): *Lupus Erythematosus: A Review of the Current Status of Discoid and Systemic Lupus Erythematosus and Their Variants.* New York, McGraw-Hill, 1966, pp 388–402

Fitzpatrick TB, Walker SA: *Dermatologic Differential Diagnosis.* Chicago, Year Book Medical Publishers, 1962.

Fitzpatrick TB, Eisen AZ, Wolff K, et al (Eds): *Dermatology in General Medicine.* New York, McGraw-Hill, 1979.

Hoeprich PD (Ed): *Infectious Diseases: A Modern Treatise of Infectious Processes.* ed 2. Hagerstown, MD, Harper & Row, 1977.

Juel-Jensen BE, MacCallum FO: *Herpes Simplex Varicella and Zoster: Clinical Manifestations and Treatment.* Philadelphia, J.B. Lippincott, 1972.

Lerner AM, Klein JO, Cherry JD, et al: New viral exanthems. *N Engl J Med 269:* 678–685, 1963.

Rook A, Wilkinson DS, Ebling FJG (Eds): *Textbook of Dermatology.* ed 2, Vol 1. Oxford, Blackwell, 1979.

Rothfield NF: Lupus erythematosus. *In*: Fitzpatrick TB, Eizen AZ, Wolff K, et al (Eds): *Dermatology in General Medicine.* ed 2, New York, McGraw-Hill, 1979.

SECTION **3**

Surgery

CHAPTER **21**

Cardiovascular Emergencies

ASHBY C. MONCURE, M.D.
M. TERRY McENANY, M.D.

Editor's Note: Some of the vascular conditions involving the gastrointestinal tract are discussed in Chapter 23 (Abdominal Emergencies). These include intestinal ischemia, intestinal infarction, and ischemic colitis.

INJURIES INVOLVING THE HEART AND GREAT VESSELS

Patients with injuries potentially involving the heart and great vessels require continued vigilance on the part of the emergency physician, because failure to detect subtle evidence of anatomic or physiologic dysfunction of the great vessels or the heart can lead to catastrophically sudden death in the emergency facility. On the other hand, early detection of such injuries can set in motion the remarkably gratifying process of returning the gravely injured patient to completely normal and totally rehabilitated life. Since the incidence of blunt and penetrating injuries to the heart and great vessels appears to be increasing, early recognition of such defects has become a mandatory ability and skill for a growing number of physicians. It is of utmost importance to be continually suspicious of injuries to the heart and great vessels in the setting of seemingly innocuous blunt or penetrating injuries that appear to involve only distal sites of the body. Pericardial tamponade, unexplained hypovolemic shock, cardiac arrhythmias, ventricular dysfunction, cardiac murmurs and rubs, and radiologic evidence of a slightly widened mediastinum must alert the physician to the likelihood of a reparable and easily reversible cardiovascular catastrophe.

General Emergency Care of Major Trauma

Proper care of patients with thoracic and cardiovascular injuries begins with adequate management of the airway. Total cognizance of the presence or absence of tension pneumothorax is necessary to diagnose pericardial tamponade. The

463

importance of *correct* or *incorrect* measurement of central venous pressure is obvious, and in questionable cases, assurance must be obtained that the tip of the central venous pressure monitoring line is in the superior vena cava, because a poorly positioned line easily can lead to inappropriate therapy. Adequate monitoring of urinary output by means of an indwelling urethral catheter remains an integral part of quality emergency care.

In patients with major injuries of the heart and great vessels, access to large veins is necessary for rapid volume infusion while in the emergency ward. It is therefore of prime importance not to transfuse fluid into the pleural or peritoneal cavities. In patients with unilateral thoracic injuries, either blunt or penetrating, with or without hemothorax, large-bore intravenous cannulas should be placed in the contralateral arm or side of the neck, or in the saphenous system when injury to the inferior vena cava is unlikely. The subclavian vein can be lacerated easily in patients with blunt or penetrating thoracic trauma, and transfusion of resuscitating fluid into the ipsilateral thorax, with no contribution to intravascular space, can occur easily. Although resuscitation efforts should not be compromised, care should be taken to leave the femoral vessels free of puncture holes and cannulas, since the common femoral artery and vein are the most frequent sites of access for angiographic examination and for cannulation when cardiopulmonary bypass may be needed either for resuscitation or for repair of a major cardiovascular lesion.

Pericardial Tamponade

Pericardial tamponade is a unique concomitant of cardiac and pericardial injuries, and thorough understanding of the pathophysiology of this aberration is an absolute prerequisite to its successful management. Acute tamponade is caused by accumulation of blood or clots or both in the pericardial sac, resulting in increased intrapericardial pressure, thereby leading to decreased atrial and ventricular filling, impaired coronary blood flow, and ventricular dysfunction. The intact pericardium is a slightly expansile envelope, and even the slow accumulation of fluid can cause rapid alteration in ventricular dynamics when the "critical mass" of pericardial volume is exceeded (Fig. 21.1).

Pericardial tamponade is associated classically with elevated central venous pressure, distended jugular and peripheral veins, arterial hypotension with a narrow pulse pressure, and Kussmaul's sign (elevation of central venous pressure of more than 10 mm Hg). Pulsus paradoxus is identifiable *only* in patients breathing spontaneously. It can be so obvious as to cause obliteration of the radial pulse on inspiration; in tachypneic patients, the respiratory variations may be identifiable only with the aid of an indwelling arterial catheter. Total assurance of the absence of tamponade must be obtained *immediately* in the acutely injured patient, however, since rapid, frequently irreversible, deterioration in cardiac function frequently results. Portable chest roentgenography is rarely beneficial

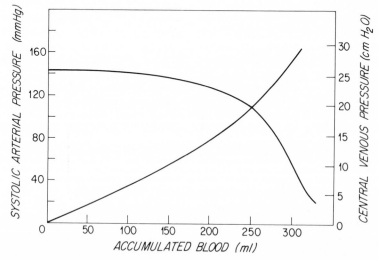

Figure 21.1. As blood accumulates in pericardial sac, pericardial and central venous pressures rise. Arterial pressure is well maintained until a critical level is reached (central venous pressure, 20 cm H₂O), after which a small increment of pericardial blood leads to arterial hypotension.

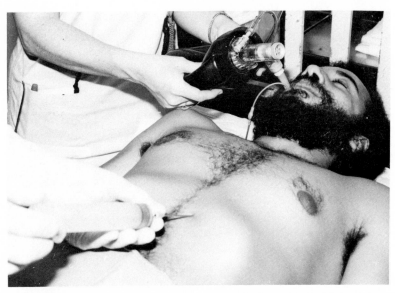

Figure 21.2. Needles (13-gauge intracath over 20-gauge spinal) are inserted into pericardial space via subxiphoid area at 30-degree angle from horizontal. Aspiration is continuous.

in the diagnosis of acute pericardial tamponade, since the pericardium usually will not have stretched enough for enlargement to be visualized radiologically before the elevated intrapericardial pressure causes circulatory embarrassment. A large pericardial silhouette frequently is associated with the more chronic causes of tamponade such as uremia, metastatic pericardial disease, and post-radiation and postpericardiotomy syndromes, but rarely is feasible with a seriously injured patient. Portable echocardiography, which is becoming more widely available and which is readily interpretable, may be helpful in diagnosing liquid pericardial collections in the patient whose condition is relatively stable.

Once pericardial tamponade is diagnosed, large volumes of intravenous fluids must be infused rapidly to resuscitate the patient while preparations for removal of the pericardial collection are made. The surgical treatment of pericardial tamponade has two phases. First, fluid must be removed from around the heart to resuscitate the dying patient; second, repair of the underlying lesion must be considered in light of any associated injury and the mechanism of trauma.

Pericardiocentesis, an emergency maneuver that effectively can relieve pericardial hypertension, is performed best through a subxiphoid approach with a large 13-gauge needle (Fig. 21.2). The subxiphoid approach is preferred to the left fourth intercostal space for safety reasons. Electrocardiographic monitoring of the probing needle, with sterile alligator clips connecting the needle to the precordial electrocardiograph lead, is ideal, but should not be a prerequisite of lifesaving pericardiocentesis. Use of a smaller spinal needle for exploration, over which the larger 13-gauge needle has been sheathed for drainage (Fig. 21.3), diminishes the chances of epicardial damage by the tap as much as does electrocardiographic monitoring. Pericardiocentesis frequently causes dramatic improvement in the patient's circulatory status with removal of as little as 40–50 ml of blood (this blood should not clot—if it quickly coagulates, it probably has been withdrawn from the right ventricle). The removal of this small amount of fluid often is sufficient to stabilize the patient's condition satisfactorily to allow the physician to proceed with other necessary diagnostic measures. However, if a significant amount of pericardial fluid reaccumulates, or if pericardiocentesis is unsuccessful in restoring cardiovascular integrity (blood *may* clot in the pericardium), thoracotomy should be performed immediately to relieve the tamponade, resuscitate the patient, and control the sites of bleeding.

Endotracheal intubation must be performed simultaneously with preparation for thoracotomy in the emergency ward or transport to the operating room. Absence of dramatic improvement with pericardiocentesis is itself a mandatory indication for endotracheal intubation.

The quickest and most flexible emergency approach to the heart and pericardium is via a left anterior thoracotomy in the fourth or fifth intercostal space, through which the pericardium can

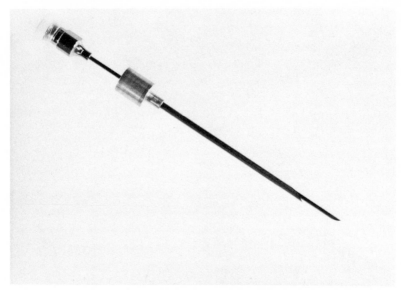

Figure 21.3.   Needle from large 13-gauge intracath is sheathed over 20-gauge spinal needle. The longer needle then is used to explore subxiphoid area. Once the spinal needle is in pericardium, as noted by aspiration of nonpulsatile, nonclotting blood, the larger needle is passed into pericardial space over the spinal needle, which then is removed.

be decompressed rapidly and most of the anterior surface of the heart exposed. Care should be taken to make the incision below the breast for better exposure and for cosmetic reasons (Fig. 21.4). This incision can be extended easily into the right side of the chest by transecting the sternum and entering the right fourth intercostal space to expose the right atrium and the intrapericardial cavae. If the sternum is transected while the patient is hypotensive, bleeding from the internal mammary arteries and veins must be expected, and must be controlled when a viable cardiac output is restored. Excellent exposure of the right side of the heart through the left anterior thoracotomy incision can be obtained by vigorous traction on the anterior aspect of the incised pericardium, rotating the heart and bringing the right atrial appendage into view without causing any mechanical cardiac impairment.

Aggressive pharmacologic therapy while these maneuvers are being carried out aids in preserving cardiovascular integrity. Reduction in cardiac output is a manifestation of depressed myocardial contractility and stroke volume. Infusion of isoproterenol (Isuprel) or dopamine quickly lowers the central venous pressure and increases arterial pressure, and rapid infusion of large amounts of crystalloid and colloid to increase filling pressures to higher than normal levels may temporarily maintain satisfactory systemic perfusion. Facilities for cardiopulmonary bypass should be available

wherever open thoracotomy may be required; impressive success has been reported regarding cardiopulmonary bypass in the resuscitation and treatment of seriously injured patients in the emergency ward (Mattox et al., 1974; Trunkey et al., 1980). However, most patients will be served better by continuous fluid and pharmacologic resuscitation and *rapid* transfer to a well-equipped operating room.

Tamponade depends, of course, on the structural integrity of the pericardial sac. A laceration more than 3 cm in length is necessary for adequate decompression of the pericardium into either pleural space. Continuous blood loss through a thoracostomy tube in a patient with possible cardiac or great-vessel injury necessitates prompt surgical intervention, since the likelihood of a cardiac wound is increased when blood loss continues unabated. The presence of only small volumes of chest-tube drainage, however, does not exclude the diagnosis of cardiac injury.

Exsanguinating Hemorrhage

Massive blood loss frequently accompanies blunt and penetrating injuries. It can occur in injuries to cardiac chambers, the aorta, the venae cavae, and the pulmonary, innominate, subclavian, internal mammary, and intercostal arteries and veins. Immediate volume replacement with crystalloid solutions is an effective, well-proved method of resuscitation, but with ongoing blood loss in the resuscitated patient, replacement of blood is required. Unfortunately, in almost all medical facilities, a lag occurs between request for and administration of blood, even in hospitals with a supply of low-titer or type-specific blood; this delay can lead to progressive homeostatic deterioration and death.

Autotransfusion

In patients with substantial hemothorax, the pleural blood is a readily available source of resuscitating fluid by means of autotransfusion. Commercial equipment is available that recovers shed blood and either (1) immediately transfuses it back into the patient's veins or (2) processes it so that the erythrocytes are concentrated and packed red blood cells can be infused. In either case, paramedical technical expertise is required that usually is not present in emergency wards. The recently introduced Sorenson system (Sorenson KGA—1900 L, Sorenson Research, Salt Lake,

City, UT 84107), however, is adapted readily to any setting and has been found to be especially effective in salvaging blood and patients after cardiac surgery (Thurer et al. 1979). In the absence of the Sorenson device, however, sterile scavenging of shed blood that has accumulated in the disposable drainage equipment used in most hospitals allows prompt reutilization of pleural blood in the resuscitation of the rapidly bleeding patient.

For collection of shed thoracic blood, a vacuum bottle such as the McGaw Empty Evacuated Standard I.V. Container (S9900) is connected either to the chest catheter or to the tap at the base of the reservoir in the drainage equipment, using large needles, stopcocks, and tubing as shown in Figure 21.5. If the chest catheter is the site of collection of reusable blood, it is clamped distally and the needle is inserted into it by sterile technique. (Collodion may be necessary to ensure an airtight fit during the scavenging maneuver and after the needle is removed.) The other end of the rigid tubing then is inserted through the administration

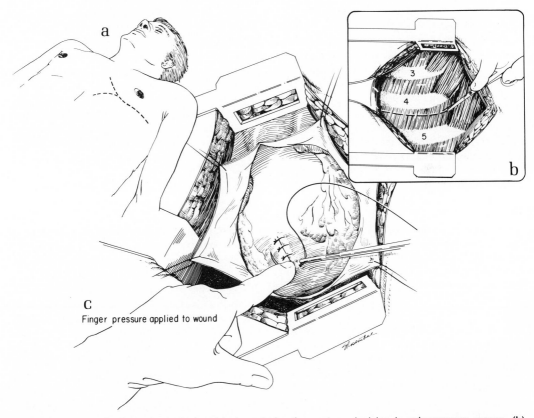

Figure 21.4. (a) Easiest access to heart is by anterior thoracotomy incision in submammary crease. (b) Intercostal incision is made in fourth or fifth interspace. (c) After pericardium is opened, most anterior knife wounds can be controlled digitally while large half-circle sutures are passed under finger to close laceration. (Note: An endotracheal tube and usually a subclavian venous catheter will have been placed before thoracotomy.)

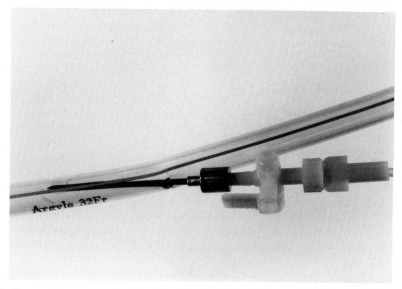

Figure 21.5. Large 13-gauge needle is inserted into intercostal chest catheter. Clamps are placed distal to insertion site and needle is connected to vacuum bottle via rigid tubing.

port of the vacuum bottle, to which heparin, 2 mg, has been added. The two stopcocks then are opened simultaneously and the shed pleural blood is collected. After the bottle fills, the stopcocks are turned off, the bottle is changed, and the procedure continues while the blood in the first bottle is transfused through an appropriate fine-screen (40 μ) filter.

No benefit can be obtained by clamping thoracostomy tubes in the presence of massive intrathoracic bleeding, in the hope of "tamponading" the injured vessel or chamber. The exception to this is when, during the insertion of a chest tube, the subclavian artery or a major pulmonary vessel is lacerated (entered) by the tube. This catastrophic complication can be avoided by not using trocar-containing thoracostomy tubes for insertion. Clamping chest tubes in other situations is detrimental because: (1) accumulation of blood in the chest collapses the lung and can cause tension hemothorax with mediastinal shift and concomitant depression of cardiac output; (2) blood in the thoracic cavity prevents full expansion of the lung, and the potential contribution of pleural symphysis to sealing any bleeding points is lost; and (3) the retained intrathoracic blood is unavailable for autotransfusion.

Blunt Trauma

Heart

Most nonpenetrating injuries are caused by motor vehicle accidents, and the steering wheel is the major offender. Compression of the mediastinal contents between the sternum and the spinal column can cause myocardial contusion; rupture of cardiac chambers; injury to coronary arteries with infarction; rupture of intracardiac septa, papillary muscles, and chordae tendineae; and rupture or laceration of cardiac valves and pericardium. Secondary rib and sternal fractures also can lacerate the pericardium and its contents. Cardiac injury must be considered in all patients with blunt chest trauma. In increasing order of importance, the signs associated with cardiac injuries are:

Fractured sternum
Tachycardia
Recurrent hemothorax
Changes in electrocardiographic pattern
Cardiac arrhythmias
Pericardial friction rub
New cardiac murmurs
Widened mediastinum
Hemopericardium

Most intracardiac injuries do not need emergency intervention in the absence of tamponade. Septal defects and valvular lesions usually do not require prompt operation. Hemopericardium unresponsive to a single pericardiocentesis, however, requires immediate intervention with the availability of cardiopulmonary bypass and repair of all identifiable lesions.

Myocardial Contusion. Blunt trauma frequently causes myocardial contusion. Many investigators have demonstrated the uniform ability of blunt trauma to cause a spectrum of insults ranging from microscopic interstitial hemorrhage to transmural necrosis and myocardial infarction (Doty et al., 1974). The increasing frequency of ventricular aneurysms occurring late after blunt trauma is testimony to the severity of direct myocardial injury that the normal heart can tolerate before fibrotic thinning with resultant ventricular failure or radiologic prominence prompts investigation and surgical therapy. Electrocardiographically diagnosed cardiac injury may occur in as many as 38% of patients who survive with major thoracic injury. Doty et al. suggest that 150,000 Americans suffer from myocardial contusion yearly; most of these lesions are misdiagnosed. Contusion of the heart has been found in 16% of all fatal thoracic injuries. The studies of Pomerantz et al. (1971) imply that myocardial contusion must be considered in patients with multiple injuries in whom cardiac output is depressed; they recommend avoidance of general anesthesia for all but lifesaving maneuvers, prolonged monitoring and treatment of arrhythmias, and anticoagulation therapy for patients with prolonged depression of cardiac output.

Chest pain is the most frequent symptom of myocardial contusion and tachycardia is the most frequent sign, but these two clinical indicators are not unique to cardiac injuries. Serial electrocardiographic examination and cardiac isoenzyme determinations are the best objective aids in making the diagnosis. Electrocardiograms routinely should be obtained in all trauma patients; in patients with thoracic trauma, electrocardiograms should be obtained daily for several days, since the electrical manifestations of the structural changes may take that long to become apparent. Technetium 99 isotope scanning and serial determinations of creatine phosphokinase isoenzymes also should be part of the routine evaluation of a patient with a suspected myocardial contusion.

Cardiac arrhythmia is the second most frequent sign of myocardial contusion, and the most common aberration is atrial flutter or fibrillation, although ventricular irritability frequently is seen. Treatment of uncomplicated contusion should be identical with that for myocardial infarction, with hospitalization, monitoring, restricted activity, and frequent examinations to detect any late complications—arrhythmias, hemopericardium, septal defect, or ventricular aneurysm—and to facilitate their early therapy.

Emergency therapy for complicated myocardial injury involves management of heart block, arrhythmias, and tamponade. Atrioventricular block should be treated by insertion of a transvenous ventricular pacemaker (see pages 931–934). Ventricular irritability usually is amenable to intravenous lidocaine hydrochloride therapy, a bolus of 3 mg/kg followed by continuous infusion of 1–4 mg/min. Infusion of more than 4 mg/min frequently is associated with seizures and should be avoided. In patients whose condition is refractory to routine doses of lidocaine, intravenous procainamide hydrochloride and bretylium tosylate should be used. Atrial arrhythmias manifested by a fast ventricular response usually can be controlled by rapid intravenous digitalization, and sinus rhythm can be maintained with quinidine. The recent introduction of verapamil has aided in the control of post-traumatic supraventricular arrhythmias; propranolol hydrochloride should not be used in patients with possible myocardial injury and depressed function (see Chapter 5 for further discussion).

Great Vessels

Blunt injury can cause disruption of the aorta, vessels to the head, and pulmonary arteries and veins; associated rib fractures also can lacerate these vessels. The clinical presentation of the patient with great-vessel injury is different from that of the patient with only cardiac injury, and includes hypovolemic shock, dyspnea, and pallor, with evidence of hemothorax. Blood loss is the major mechanical defect, and the therapy is immediate replacement. If hemothorax recurs after initial tube thoracostomy, or if considerable blood loss continues through the chest tube, thoracotomy should be performed at once.

It is rarely prudent, necessary, or successful to perform emergency thoracotomy in the emergency ward for blunt noncardiac trauma because the hypovolemic shock that is always present is treated best initially by the usual measure of massive fluid replacement. The patient should be transferred immediately to the operating room while fluid resuscitation is taking place. The rupture or laceration of a major intrathoracic vessel is best cared for by an appropriate surgical procedure in the operating room.

The forces transmitted to the thorax by deceleration injuries easily can injure the aorta and its branches. Most frequently, the isthmus of the descending thoracic aorta is involved. This is an extremely lethal injury—80% of patients so injured never will reach a medical facility alive. The injury is a fracture of the aortic intima and media with maintenance of integrity and continuity of the adventitia. This may be salvageable in young persons; the elasticity required for adventitial integrity seems to dissipate after the age of 40 years.

Disruption of the aortic wall is believed to occur because the descending aorta is fixed tightly by the intercostal arteries, ligamentum arteriosum, and subclavian artery, whereas the transverse arch is mobile and likely to move forward with sudden deceleration while the distal aorta remains stationary. The aortic tear usually is manifested by slight hypovolemia and a widened mediastinum within the bounds of an elastic, expandable adventitia. A significant proportion of patients with aortic transection have "pseudocoarctation", which is upper-extremity hypertension with diminished femoral pulses, since the hematoma surrounding the aorta at the laceration partly occludes the lumen.

A widened mediastinal shadow on a portable chest roentgenogram (Fig. 21.6) dictates urgent aortographic examination. This must be performed expeditiously even in the presence of other injuries. In the patient who arrives alive at the emergency facility, exsanguination from a torn aorta rarely occurs immediately, but in two-thirds of these patients, the aorta ruptures within 1 month. The aorta should be repaired as soon as the patient's other injuries allow; diagnosis must be immediate, however. Careful examination of the aortogram is necessary to rule out multiple sites of rupture or rupture of the proximal aorta. Lacerations of the ascending aorta and multiple tears require emergency surgical repair, other in-

juries notwithstanding. In patients with aortic transection and central nervous system injuries such as intracranial hematoma, spinal cord injury, or cerebral contusion leading to changing neurologic signs, we have tried to temporize by means of vigorous medical therapy with antihypertensive agents and propranolol, which is similar to the medical regimen for spontaneous dissection of the thoracic aorta (see pages 474–475). Postponement of repair of the aortic lesion for up to 6 weeks with maintenance of blood pressure at low normotensive levels until neurologic symptoms have stabilized or, in certain cases, until large areas of third-degree burn have been covered has been successful. All patients undergo immediate aortographic examination so that intelligent, informed decisions may be made regarding the timing of any necessary procedures. Many patients with aortic transection do have other severe injuries; however, the majority of these injuries (for example, major fractures) do not deter early surgical repair, especially with increasing use of shunts or simple aortic cross-clamping obviating cardiopulmonary bypass and systemic heparinization.

Blunt forces also can cause disruption of the intima in the proximal branches of the aorta, resulting in central nervous system symptoms or loss of pulses. The subclavian arteries especially are liable to distraction injuries with hyperexten-

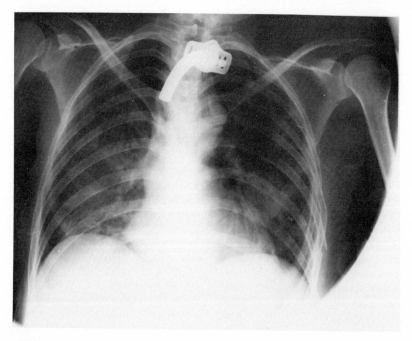

Figure 21.6.   Portable anteroposterior chest roentgenogram of patient with multiple facial fractures requiring tracheostomy. Mediastinum is widened minimally and trachea is deviated to right. Angiography demonstrated transverse rupture of descending aorta.

sion of the neck and shoulder. These injuries of the great vessels must be diagnosed by means of angiographic examination shortly after admission of the patient to the emergency ward.

Penetrating Injuries

Injuries from violent crimes occur more frequently, and as retrieval and transporting systems become more efficient, a greater number of wounded patients are being treated in civilian emergency facilities. A large percentage of penetrating cardiac wounds are still lethal (80% of all such patients are dead on arrival at the emergency facility), but earlier *correct* care can result in more survivors.

Heart

The satisfactory management of penetrating cardiac injuries requires an institutional philosophy of aggressive therapy that must be supported by investment in facilities and by an atmosphere conducive to the successful treatment of such severely injured patients. In patients with any sign of proximate life, such as a warm body, agonal breaths, or sounds in the ambulance shortly before arrival, a well-rehearsed resuscitation procedure should be instituted instantaneously. These patients should be taken either directly to an operating room or be treated by immediate pericardiocentesis and thoracotomy in the emergency facility that is prepared to carry out thoracic operations. The spectacular improvements in survival rates reported from some institutions (Mattox et al., 1974; Evans et al., 1979) attest to the validity of this approach. Ideally, cardiopulmonary bypass should be available within minutes of the patient's arrival, wherever the thoracotomy is performed.

Gunshot wounds are uniformly more damaging than knife or ice pick injuries. The magnitude of cardiac injury is usually greater, larger-caliber missiles generally are associated with massive blood loss, and spontaneous closure of a violated cardiac wall is less likely with a gunshot wound than with a knife wound. The trajectory of bullets is notoriously difficult to determine from clinical or radiologic evidence. There is no way to determine which structures a bullet has injured on its passage through the mediastinum and pleural cavities, and if there is any serious question regarding cardiac injury, thoracotomy should be performed with cardiopulmonary bypass available. Pericardiocentesis, volume replacement, and pulmonary re-expansion by tube thoracostomy are carried out immediately when the signs and symptoms of tamponade, hemopneumothorax, or low cardiac

output occur, but even if hemodynamic stabilization is obtained through these maneuvers, formal thoracotomy is advocated for these patients. Delayed pericardiotomy is seldom possible since recurrence of hemopericardium or continuous transpleural hemorrhage usually requires rapid intervention. Massive blood loss from the heart and other injured structures (aorta, venae cavae), arrhythmias from myocardial injury, and a protracted shock-like state are the major causes of death in patients whose condition is operable on arrival at the emergency ward.

Discrete ventricular wounds are the most easily reparable cardiac injuries. Blood loss must be controlled immediately, and the urgency of this requires a different philosophy of management from that usually practiced. Digital pressure on ventricular wounds often will retard the blood loss while further resuscitation procedures and fluid replacement are carried out. Then, while hemostatic control is maintained with digital pressure, mattress sutures are placed under the finger and through the myocardium. A large half-circle gastrointestinal needle with a 00 chromic catgut suture (Ethicon G-127H) buttressed with pericardium or intercostal muscle is most effective. The size and curve of this needle allow it to be passed easily under the finger, and the buttressed mattress sutures hold well in the edematous, ragged edges of a cardiac wound. In injuries adjacent to coronary arteries, the sutures should be passed under the vessel with buttresses on either side to avoid compromising the lumen. This maneuver is performed quickly, with the realization that once hemostasis is obtained and the patient is resuscitated, more formal repair of the ventricular wound should be performed using nonabsorbable sutures and Teflon felt, with the support of cardiopulmonary bypass in the operating room. Most injuries in patients who arrive alive at the emergency facility involve the right ventricle, the most anterior chamber of the heart. The entry wound does not, however, totally indicate the amount of intracardiac damage, and this should be elucidated after exsanguinating hemorrhage has been controlled.

Most ventricular lesions are approachable through a left anterolateral thoracotomy. Caval and some atrial lesions require trans-sternal bilateral thoracotomy as mentioned previously. Atrial lesions rarely can be controlled with digital pressure: the thin chamber wall provides no resistance, and partially occluding clamps usually are necessary. If these fail or are not applicable, large purse-string sutures with 00 chromic catgut frequently can help to gain control of atrial or caval lesions. Another effective maneuver in controlling atrial

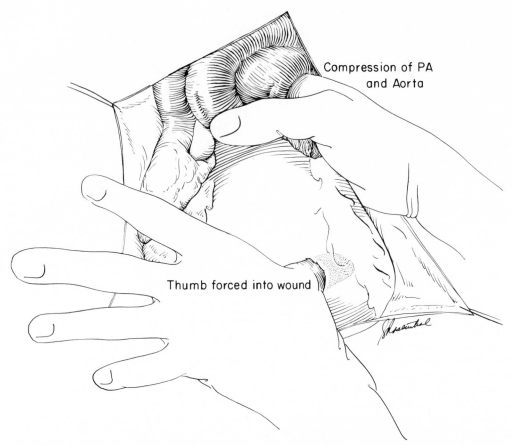

Figure 21.7. Brewer's method of "elective" cardiac arrest. With a thumb occluding the large right ventricular wound, the aorta and pulmonary artery are occluded by passing fingers of right hand through transverse pericardial sinus. With the heart arrested, large wounds may be closed quickly, after which the heart is resuscitated.

lacerations is to insert a sterile Foley catheter with a 30-ml balloon into the atrium, inflate the balloon, and with gentle traction on the catheter, occlude all but the largest atrial defects. A sterile cuffed endotracheal tube also may be effective in the management of some atrial lacerations near the inferior vena cava.

Emergency care of large ventricular lesions is difficult and frustrating, since digital control is impossible and traction sutures are ineffective because of the size of the lesion. In these instances, elective cardiac arrest may be useful (Brewer and Carter, 1968). With this technique, blood loss is controlled as well as possible by inserting the thumb into the cardiac wound and, with the other hand, gaining control of the aorta and pulmonary artery via the transverse sinus. By occluding the aorta and pulmonary artery, the surgeon can induce cardiac arrest (Fig. 21.7); the superior vena cava also may be available for pressure occlusion. Cardiac arrest makes it feasible and simple to close

the wound with carefully placed sutures that have been readied for rapid insertion. As soon as the cardiac wound is closed, heart massage and defibrillation usually return normal cardiac action. This is not preferred to cardiorrhaphy with extracorporeal support, but is extremely useful in the absence of cardiopulmonary bypass. It is important to obtain a nearly normovolemic and normotensive state before inducing cardiac arrest to afford a period of good coronary perfusion before arrest.

If control of a cardiac wound is not feasible by the previously mentioned plugging maneuver because of either size or position, other techniques of obtaining a temporarily dry field for repair of cardiac lacerations include: (1) occlusion of venous inflow, in which vascular clamps are placed across the venae cavae, resulting in an empty, collapsed heart that then can be sutured; (2) electrical fibrillation to stop the active rhythmic contraction of the ventricle (electrical fibrillation can be induced with defibrillator paddles by placing them at right angles to the epicardial surface and using an impulse of 20 watt-seconds); and (3) placement of large traction sutures on either side of the laceration and crossing them to decrease the size of the cardiotomy.

More patients with knife and ice pick wounds than gunshot wounds are treated successfully because the cardiac injury is frequently smaller, the tip of the instrument is less likely to pass completely through the heart, less soft-tissue injury occurs than is caused by the energy forces of missile passage, and the pericardial lesion more frequently is small enough to promote tamponade rather than exsanguination. The treatment of knife wounds is different also in that it is reasonable not to perform an exploratory operation immediately in a patient whose condition is hemodynamically stable or who has responded well to a single pericardiocentesis. The chances of permanently sealing the cardiac wound are greater with a knife or ice pick puncture than with a missile injury. It is also more likely for a suspected cardiac wound to be either epicardial or pericardial if caused by a knife rather than by a bullet.

Patients seen in the emergency ward with an object protruding from the chest should be evaluated and taken to the operating room with the penetrating instrument in place. If there is no radiologic or clinical evidence that the heart or great vessels have been injured, the object is removed and the patient is observed in the operating room for evidence of cardiac embarrassment or major blood loss. If the clinical course is stable, further observation without operation is indicated. However, in patients in whom penetrating cardiac injury is indicated by position, radiologic evidence, or rhythmic motion of the protruding instrument, general anesthesia should be induced (if necessary), the chest draped with the instrument in place, an ipsilateral anterior thoracotomy performed, the object removed from the heart under direct vision, and the tear immediately sutured. Satisfactory drainage of the pericardium is an important preventive measure to avoid postoperative tamponade, constrictive pericardial reaction, and other complications.

Great Vessels

Penetrating wounds of the great vessels are usually fatal more rapidly than those involving the heart alone or blunt injuries causing disruption of intimal integrity. Massive exsanguination usually ensues after a missile or knife injury of the aorta or other vessels of the thoracic outlet, the pulmonary arteries, or pulmonary veins. Cardiac wounds are protected somewhat from this fate by the pericardial envelope, which can reduce or delay blood loss. Nonpenetrating vascular injuries seen in emergency facilities are different from penetrating wounds by virtue of retention of adventitial integrity. Massive volume replacement via autotransfusion plus urgent thoracotomy and control of bleeding from the injured vessel offer the best hope of resuscitation.

Control of the brachiocephalic branches can be obtained in the emergency ward by an incision in the third intercostal space and packing of the apex of the pleural space with large packs, then transporting the patient to the operating room.

Penetrating wounds of the neck always should be suspected to involve the great vessels. Exploration of neck wounds in an operating room, not in the emergency ward, is indicated if any damage to vessels, the trachea, or the esophagus is suspected. Such suspicion should be heightened if any of the following are present:

Continued hemorrhage through entry site
Decreased or absent pulses
Hemothorax
Subcutaneous emphysema
Large or enlarging mediastinal hematoma
Neurologic deficit
Sudden hoarseness
Continuous murmur
Dyspnea
Hemoptysis or hematemesis

Emergency control of great-vessel hemorrhage frequently can be obtained by finger pressure applied through a neck wound; diffuse pressure less frequently is effective in controlling hemorrhage, but this should be attempted initially for all bleeding neck wounds.

In patients whose condition is stable or who have slowly evolving clinical signs, aortographic and selective angiographic examinations are valuable in terms of diagnosis and management. In patients who do not undergo angiographic delineation of the lesion, the entire neck and thorax must be draped for operation so that extension into the mediastinum or into either side of the thorax easily can be performed for control and repair of the innominate, carotid, or subclavian vessels (Brawley et al., 1970).

In the management of exsanguinating hemorrhage from a major arterial source, it frequently is possible to gain proximal and distal control by inserting small Foley catheters or Fogarty venous embolectomy catheters through the lumen of the vessel to occlude flow. This controls bleeding and allows careful dissection, avoiding iatrogenic injury to the trachea or esophagus. Injuries to the innominate vein can be managed by ligation of this large tributary because of the satisfactory collaterals in the upper part of the thorax.

The innovative use of internal and external arterial shunt catheters has led to spectacular success in treating patients with major vascular injury, and the flexibility of this technique warrants its consideration by all surgeons dealing with major vascular trauma in an emergency setting.

ANEURYSMS OF THE THORACIC AORTA

Aortic Dissections

Aortic dissections (dissecting aneurysms) present a medical-surgical emergency requiring urgent therapy. The lesion is caused by separation of the aortic intima and media by the progressive force of blood entering the media through a small intimal tear or through the base of an atheromatous plaque. The most common cause is hypertension, which seems to predispose the layers to the hemorrhagic separation.

Management of aortic dissections is greatly determined by the location of the intimal tear or "origin" of the dissection. The two most frequent sites of origin are the ascending aorta (60–70%) and the descending aorta just distal to the takeoff of the left subclavian artery (30%). Dissections arising in the ascending aorta can progress to involve the transverse and descending thoracic aorta and the abdominal aorta (DeBakey type I), usually either ending in an iliac obstruction or "reentering" the true abdominal aortic lumen, or they can be limited to the aortic segment proximal to the innominate artery (type II). The distally originating dissections (type III) usually progress only distally although the dissection sometimes can extend back into the transverse and ascending portions of the aorta. The location of the origin is important, since surgical therapy is directed solely to that short aortic segment. All type I and type II dissections require early surgical treatment. Type III dissections in which the false channel is thrombosed are treated satisfactorily medically, but those in which angiographic dye fills the false lumen or in which there is compromise of a major visceral or limb arterial takeoff should be treated surgically (McFarland et al., 1972).

The life-threatening characteristics of acute aortic dissections are associated with the propensity of the thinned outer investing layer (adventitia and outer third of media) to rupture, leading to acute tamponade (rupture into the pericardium),

exsanguination (rupture into a free pleural space), or a devastating aortocardiac fistula (rupture into a cardiac chamber). The course of the advancing intramedial column of blood frequently can cause obstruction of a major arterial branch of the aorta either by dissecting into the media of the branch or raising an intimal flap that then occludes the orifice of an otherwise intact major artery.

Pulse deficits—absence or diminution—occur in about 50% of proximal dissections (types I and II) and in about 15% of distal dissections. A complete check of all peripheral arteries is mandatory in any patient with severe chest pain, since the absence of a peripheral pulse may lead to the correct diagnosis of aortic dissection.

Dilation of the aortic root or dissection into the fibrous cardiac skeleton can lead to aortic regurgitation. These events can be fatal immediately. They frequently occur within hours or days of the start of dissection; therefore, prevention of the complications of aortic dissection may be possible with early treatment preceded by correct diagnosis.

Chest pain is the most frequent and most characteristic symptom of aortic dissection. It usually is described as having a catastrophic onset and a ripping or tearing quality, and it commonly migrates from front to back or vice versa. The pain may be caused by the forceful advance of the column of blood through the aortic media, or occlusion of aortic branches may lead to the sudden appearance of ischemic pain in viscera or extremities. Many patients have the symptoms and signs of a saddle or iliac arterial embolus, and the correct diagnosis is made only after an unsuccessful femoral or abdominal procedure. In most patients with major anterior pain, the origin of the dissection is proximal, while in most patients with major posterior pain, it is distal. These locations are not more than statistical probabilities, however (Slater and DeSanctis, 1976).

Auscultation may reveal the murmur of aortic insufficiency in many dissections involving the ascending aorta. It is extremely rare in type III dissections, and frequently can provide an important clue before angiographic examination as to the site of origin in anterior dissections.

Portable echocardiography can be useful in establishing the presence of a false lumen. However, the origin of the dissection cannot be determined yet by this technique.

Chest roentgenograms frequently are greatly helpful in the diagnosis of aortic dissections. Almost all patients have widened aortic and mediastinal shadows on the plain chest film. Separation of intimal calcium from the limits of the aortic shadow is an important sign in aortic injuries (Gray and Kirsh, 1975), and may be seen on the plain chest films of patients with aortic dissections.

Definitive diagnosis must be based on angiographic demonstration of (1) a dissection with a false lumen, and (2) the location of the origin of the dissection. Demonstration of the origin of the tear is necessary for appropriate medical or surgical therapy.

Angiographic examination can be performed either through a brachial or axillary approach or via the femoral artery. The advantage of the former is that the angiographic catheter does not have to pass the site of origin in distal dissections; thus, perforation of the investing adventitia is avoided. The femoral approach is usually quicker and offers the opportunity for selective visceral angiography if it is indicated by the patient's symptoms.

While clinical and angiographic diagnosis of aortic dissection is proceeding, vigorous medical therapy for the frequently associated hypertension must be instituted and carefully monitored (Wheat and Palmer, 1968). A central venous pressure monitoring line and a urethral catheter are minimal. An indwelling radial artery catheter should be used; this enhances the appropriate titration of antihypertensive medications. The radial artery catheter should be placed in the arm with the higher brachial pressure if there is a discrepancy.

The best therapy to reduce systolic hypertension and the force of ejection of blood from the left ventricle is to administer trimethaphan camsylate, 250 mg/250 ml of 5% dextrose in water, starting with 150–200 μg/min, in a continuous infusion, along with propranolol hydrochloride, 1 mg intravenously every 4 hours. Trimethaphan camsylate has the disadvantage of eliciting tachyphylaxis, and its effectiveness is usually limited to 48–72 hours. Continuous infusion of nitroprusside, 50 mg/250 ml of 5% dextrose in water, starting with 15–20 μg/min, is as effective in lowering systolic blood pressure, but it causes a reflex increase in endogenous catecholamines and thus increases ventricular contractility, which should be avoided if possible. Phentolamine, 100 mg/dl of 5% dextrose in water, also effectively lowers systemic arterial pressure, but its action is less quickly reversible than that of either trimethaphan camsylate or nitroprusside. The goal of immediate antihypertensive therapy is to lower the systolic blood pressure below 120 mm Hg.

If operation is not indicated, continued medical therapy includes: (1) propranolol hydrochloride, given to the limits of bradycardia or ventricular failure or both; (2) methyldopa; (3) reserpine; and (4) guanethidine sulfate.

Atherosclerotic Aneurysms

Atherosclerotic aneurysms of the thoracic aorta and great vessels infrequently cause acute symptoms. An insidious onset of a pressure sensation, heaviness in the chest, cough, dysphagia, or hoarseness is much more common. Sudden expansion or leakage from an aneurysm of the thoracic aorta can cause catastrophic pain and shock, and on the patient's arrival at the emergency ward the symptoms may be indistinguishable from those of acute myocardial infarction. In hypertensive patients, radiologic demonstration of the aneurysm should satisfy most criteria for vasodilator therapy. Many patients, however, are normotensive, and intravenous propranolol may be indicated even in these patients. Angiographic demonstration of the limits of the aneurysm will determine the feasibility and appropriateness of surgical therapy.

ANEURYSMS OF THE PERIPHERAL VASCULAR SYSTEM

Aneurysms commonly are caused by arteriosclerosis, although they may be secondary to trauma, cystic medial necrosis, or infection. The symptoms and signs of an arteriosclerotic aneurysm may be pain, shock, or a palpable mass. Pain may be caused by acute expansion of the aneurysm, by pressure of an expanding aneurysm against a nerve, or by free blood from a leak or rupture into a contained space such as the retroperitoneum or abdominal cavity. Hypovolemic shock is often a consequence of such a rupture. Rarely, hypertension caused by an increase in the afterload indicates thrombosis of an aneurysm. Acute arterial occlusion may be caused by emboli from laminated thrombus associated with the aneurysm. Aneurysms frequently develop near arterial bifurcations and are most commonly seen in the distal aorta, common iliac artery, common femoral artery, and popliteal artery. Aneurysms of visceral arteries are less frequently seen, the most common site being the splenic artery.

Abdominal Aortic Aneurysms

Abdominal aortic aneurysms are generally asymptomatic until they expand to 4 cm in diameter or larger. A common symptom is abdominal pain that usually is located in the middle or lower part of the abdomen, frequently to the left of the midline. Back pain is also common. Occasionally, the patient may notice a pulsatile abdominal mass

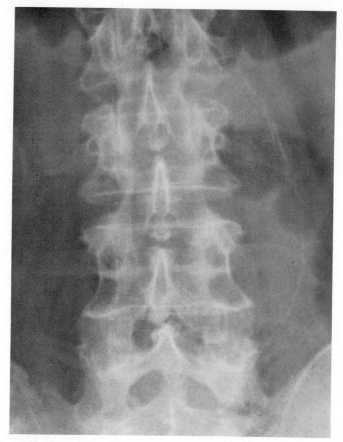

Figure 21.8. Anteroposterior roentgenogram of abdomen demonstrating calcified left lateral wall of an abdominal aortic aneurysm extending from second to fifth lumbar vertebra.

or have symptoms related to duodenal or vena caval obstruction. Thrombosis of an abdominal aortic aneurysm is rare and generally occurs to the level of the renal arteries. Symptoms include hypertension or ischemic lower extremities or both. Ischemic digits or patchy areas of ischemic skin may be due to dissemination into end-arteries of emboli from a laminated thrombus and, occasionally, cholesterol emboli from an atheroma.

The primary physical finding in a patient with an abdominal aortic aneurysm is a palpable, pulsatile, expansile, midabdominal mass that may be tender. Since the wall of such an aneurysm frequently contains calcium, an anteroposterior roentgenogram of the abdomen and a lateral projection of the lumbosacral spine may reveal its presence (Fig. 21.8). In the absence of vessel-wall calcium, echography may be helpful in assessing the size of the aorta. In a patient whose condition is stable, aortographic examination may be helpful in demonstrating the presence of a suspected abdominal aortic aneurysm and in planning its management.

Rupture of an abdominal aortic aneurysm usu-

ally is heralded by the onset of severe pain or hypotension, in which case a palpable aneurysm may not be evident. If this diagnosis reasonably can be suspected, the patient should be transported promptly to an operating room for emergency operation. The pneumatic antishock garment provides circumferential tamponade during transit. Blood for transfusion through large-bore central intravenous lines should be obtained immediately.

Abdominal or back pain associated with a palpable aneurysm but no hypotension should be ascribed to acute expansion of a known abdominal aortic aneurysm. Because the mortality from ruptured aneurysms compared with unruptured aneurysms is so high (50% and 3%, respectively), patients in whom aneurysmal expansion is suspected should be operated on immediately, although some other cause for symptoms may be found at operation in a few cases.

Iliac and Femoral Arterial Aneurysms

Common and external iliac arterial aneurysms present clinical findings similar to those of abdominal aortic aneurysms and must be dealt with promptly by operation. Internal iliac arterial aneurysms may produce symptoms due to compression of the colon, ureters, or bladder. Femoral arterial aneurysms usually do not rupture, but rather produce acute arterial occlusion. Laminated thrombus within the aneurysm may occlude the origin of the profunda femoris artery. In the presence of occlusion, the leg is more vulnerable to ischemia if there is embolization into the superficial femoral system. Prompt operation may be necessary to save the limb. Pain secondary to femoral nerve compression may be the presenting symptom. Diagnosis usually is made readily by physical examination, and early operation is necessary to retrieve emboli and to reconstruct the femoral artery. Femoral arterial aneurysms usually are present bilaterally and are seen in association with aneurysms of other arteries such as the distal abdominal aorta, iliac artery, and popliteal artery.

Popliteal Aneurysms

The symptoms of a popliteal aneurysm usually are caused either by thrombosis of the aneurysm or by distal thromboembolism. In both cases the symptoms are those of acute arterial occlusion (see pages 478–481), unless thrombosis has developed gradually enough to allow collateral circulation to bypass the block; in this instance there is only mild intermittent claudication. Occasionally, pressure from the aneurysm on a nerve or vein may produce pain or peripheral edema. A popliteal aneurysm may rupture rarely. On physical examination, this aneurysm may be diagnosed by palpation of a mass in the popliteal fossa, which need not be pulsatile. If a popliteal mass is palpated in the other leg, the diagnosis is strongly suspected, since popliteal aneurysms occur bilaterally in approximately 60% of these patients. Arteriographic examination may demonstrate the presence of a popliteal aneurysm unless it is obscured by laminated thrombus (Fig. 21.9). Prompt operation is necessary to evacuate thrombus from the peripheral arterial tree and to reconstruct the popliteal artery, usually by placement of a graft.

Visceral and Other Arterial Aneurysms

The most common visceral arterial aneurysm is that involving the splenic artery. Since this frequently is calcified, it is evident on plain roentgenograms of the abdomen. Rupture of this aneurysm is rare, but may occur, especially during the third trimester of pregnancy. Rupture into the stomach is also a rare cause of gastrointestinal hemorrhage. Renal arterial aneurysms seldom rupture, but may be associated with hypertension resulting from

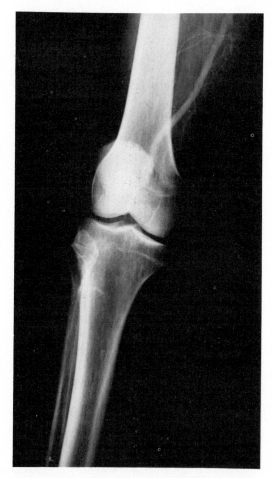

Figure 21.9. Percutaneous femoral arteriogram demonstrating occlusion of popliteal artery with absence of filling of distal vessels. Acute arterial occlusion was found to be secondary to thrombosis of a popliteal aneurysm.

distal embolization of the laminated thrombus. Aneurysms of the superior mesenteric artery are unusual, and if present, frequently are infected. Other visceral arterial aneurysms may be signaled by intra-abdominal or gastrointestinal hemorrhage due to rupture. Aneurysms of the arteries of the upper extremities are also rare and most commonly are associated with arterial trauma.

False Aneurysms

False aneurysms from infected or disrupted arterial suture lines may occur in patients who have undergone arterial reconstruction. Thus, it is critically important that the physician assessing a patient with a palpable or symptomatic aneurysm elicit a history of arterial operation. False aneurysms may also be caused by infected arterial emboli and arterial trauma.

VASCULAR TRAUMA

Trauma to a major artery can produce either immediate hemorrhage or arterial occlusion and eventual loss of function. Arterial hemorrhage is obvious and forces prompt action on the part of the physician. On the other hand, arterial insufficiency resulting from trauma may be difficult to recognize, and the examining physician must be highly suspicious of its presence to detect it promptly. Early recognition is absolutely essential to treatment, since delay may allow an irreversible ischemic injury to develop and may encourage the formation of intravascular thrombi.

With blunt trauma, the vessel can be injured in three ways: the intima can be torn, presenting a thrombogenic surface to the blood stream; the vessel can be sheared, causing a flap of intima to roll up distally and to occlude the lumen; and the vessel can be contused, causing subintimal hemorrhage and compromise of the patency of the lumen. Penetrating trauma most often is associated with hemorrhage caused by laceration, transection, or contusion of the vessel. Other consequences of penetrating trauma are false aneurysms or arteriovenous fistulas or both.

The initial response to traumatic interruption or occlusion of a major artery to a body area is vasoconstriction in that area, caused partly by a reflex mediated through the sympathetic nervous system and partly by spasm of the affected vessel. After several hours, vasodilation takes place as the point of occlusion in the artery is bypassed by means of flow through dilated collateral channels. If the patient has not suffered irreversible damage in the affected area, gradual hypertrophy of collateral channels occurs over the ensuing weeks to months. The degree of arterial insufficiency following arterial trauma depends on the site of arterial occlusion, being especially severe when bifurcations have been destroyed, and it also depends on the ability of collateral channels to deliver an adequate blood supply to the body region.

In civilian settings, penetrating trauma is the more common source of arterial injury, but arterial injury by blunt trauma does occur in about 10% of these patients. Arterial injury most frequently is overlooked in cases of blunt trauma; careful search for distal pulses in patients with musculoskeletal trauma is essential. Peripheral pulses in the extremities should be evaluated by a Doppler ultrasonic flow detector, and segmental blood pressures in the injured extremity should be measured and compared with blood pressures in the uninjured extremity.

While examining the patient with a traumatic injury, the physician may elicit a history of persistent arterial bleeding. He may find diminished or absent pulses distal to the site of injury, a bruit distal to or at the site of injury, or a large or expanding hematoma. Proximity of the wound to a major artery should bring to mind the possibility of major vascular trauma. The signs of major arterial occlusion are pain and pallor in the affected area, a lack of pulses distal to the injury, and paresthesia or paralysis or both in the affected member. Tissue sensitivity to anoxia from arterial occlusion is greater in sensory and motor nerves than in skeletal muscles, bone, and tendon.

Treatment of arterial trauma begins with management of the airway and assurance of adequate gas exchange, tamponade of hemorrhage followed by instrumental control (not with a tourniquet), and appropriate volume replacement. If hemorrhage continues, the patient should be prepared for the operating room while bleeding is controlled and transfusion is in progress. In a patient with a relatively stable condition, however, arteriographic examination should be performed to document the site of arterial injury (Fig. 21.10), only if it can be done promptly. A critical determinant of success in the management of arterial injuries is the promptness of operative management.

Although restoration of arterial inflow is of primary concern after trauma, the consequences of venous injury must not be overlooked, and injured veins initially should be dealt with as gently as the arteries. Depending on the circumstances, it may be desirable to attempt reconstruction of veins as well as of arteries.

Special emphasis is warranted concerning patients with penetrating wounds of the neck. Major vascular injury should be suspected in all such patients until the diagnosis is disproved by careful physical examination, angiography, and exploration of the wound. The tempo of the workup is dictated by the general condition of the patient. The patient with this type of injury should not be left unattended, and associated injuries to the trachea, pharynx, and esophagus always must be considered.

ACUTE ARTERIAL OCCLUSION

Acute arterial occlusion is usually caused by embolism, acute arterial thrombosis, or by thrombosis within an aneurysm (Fig. 21.11, A–C). Sudden arterial occlusion may be caused by an embolus from a central source such as the atrium (myxoma or thrombus associated with atrial fibrillation or mitral stenosis), the endocardium (mural thrombus following myocardial infarction),

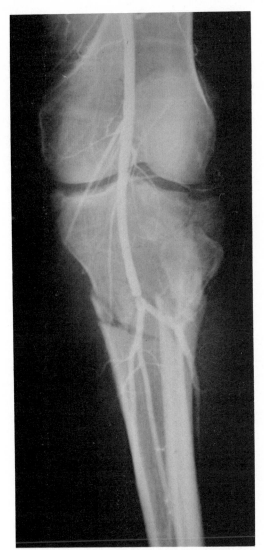

Figure 21.10. Percutaneous femoral arteriogram demonstrating intimal injury of distal popliteal artery just above its bifurcation, associated with proximal tibial and fibular fractures.

or a ventricle (aneurysm). It also may originate from a source in the arterial tree proximal to the occlusion, such as an aneurysm (laminated thrombus) or a stenotic artery (fibrin or platelet aggregates). Occasionally, trauma may produce acute arterial occlusion, and this condition may result rarely from an inflammatory process such as granulomatous arteritis or from a hematologic disorder such as a hypercoagulable state associated with infection or with a malignant condition.

Symptoms of acute arterial occlusion are determined largely by the suddenness of occlusion, the involvement of arterial bifurcations, the degree of collateral circulation, the presence of antecedent occlusive disease, and the presence of arterial spasm. The major symptom is pain, which may occur either abruptly or over a period of several hours. Paresthesia, coldness, and numbness also may be part of the symptom complex, and progressive loss of sensation and muscle function may be present. If the arterial occlusion is not relieved, the symptoms usually persist or progress. The findings of absent pulses, cool and pallid skin, and empty superficial veins even when an extremity is slightly dependent suggest the diagnosis.

It may be difficult to distinguish between thrombosis superimposed on long-standing atherosclerotic occlusive disease and an embolic occlusion. A history of intermittent claudication suggests the former, although it may be difficult to ascertain whether a patient has intermittent claudication because patients frequently attribute this symptom to musculoskeletal causes and limit their activities to prevent the onset of muscular pain. Pain caused by embolism is instantaneous and severe, as opposed to that caused by thrombosis, which may develop relatively gradually and be rather mild. If there is a recognizable probable source of embolism, and especially if there is a history of embolism, this diagnosis must be entertained strongly. The sudden appearance of cyanosis in one or more digits may be the first sign of ischemia in a previously asymptomatic extremity. In the presence of intact peripheral pulses, this finding may represent either small-vessel thrombosis, which is found most frequently in diabetic patients, or small-particle emboli to the digital vessels from a proximal source such as an aneurysm, ulcerated atheroma, or stenotic artery (Fig. 21.11D). Although symptoms produced by thrombosis of an arterial aneurysm may mimic those of embolic occlusion, the physician often may make the former diagnosis by palpating a mass in the affected extremity. In addition, since they are frequently multiple, the presence of other palpable aneurysms may suggest the correct diagnosis.

Partial or complete occlusion of the extracranial internal carotid artery may lead to transient ischemic attacks or frank strokes. After arteriographic assessment, this condition may be managed surgically. The diagnosis and treatment of this lesion are discussed in Chapter 15, pages 353–355.

Acute occlusion of abdominal visceral vessels is a result either of emboli or of thrombosis of atherosclerotic stenotic lesions that usually occur where the visceral vessels originate from the abdominal aorta. Occlusions of arteries to the digestive system are considered in Chapter 23, pages 517–519. Acute occlusion of a renal artery may produce severe flank pain and may be accompa-

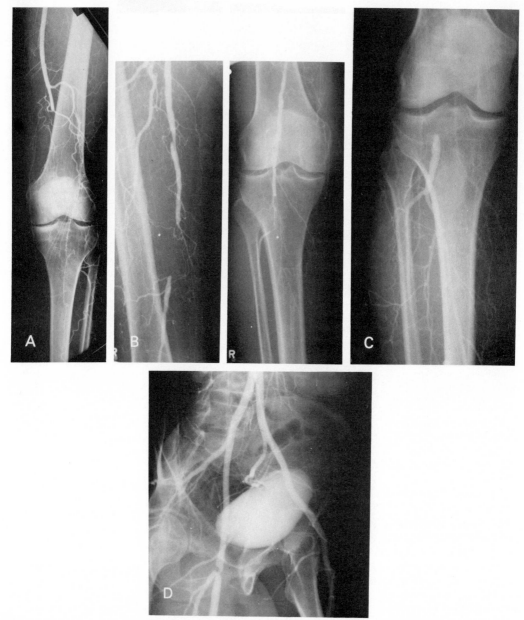

Figure 21.11. Acute arterial occlusion. **(A)** Percutaneous femoral arteriogram demonstrating occlusion of popliteal and distal superficial femoral arteries proximal to point of origin of a large side branch from the femoral artery. Acute arterial occlusion was caused by a peripheral embolus. **(B)** Percutaneous femoral arteriogram demonstrating superficial femoral occlusion (*left*) and thrombosis of terminal popliteal artery (*right*). This patient had symptoms of acute arterial occlusion superimposed on longstanding symptoms of intermittent claudication in same extremity. **(C)** Percutaneous femoral arteriogram demonstrating occlusion of popliteal artery in patient with a thrombosed popliteal aneurysm. **(D)** Oblique runoff aortogram demonstrating high-grade stenosis of right common femoral artery just above its bifurcation produced by an atheroma. Patient had ischemic digits secondary to small-particle emboli believed to be formed at site of femoral arterial stenosis.

nied by fever and hematuria or by severe hypertension or by both. A rare condition, acute occlusion of both renal arteries is associated with severe oliguria in addition to hypertension. Although viability of the kidney is threatened by severe ischemia, enough collateral circulation may exist to prevent irreversible ischemic changes, and prompt diagnosis can make successful revascularization possible. As soon as the diagnosis of renal arterial occlusion is entertained, renal perfusion should be evaluated by scintiscanning with intravenous radionuclide. If renal perfusion is not demonstrated, arteriographic assessment of the renal artery in question should be undertaken and a vascular surgeon should be consulted immediately.

In cases of acute arterial occlusion, success in restoring normal function depends on the promptness of restoration of arterial blood flow. The examining physician must deal with the problem definitively and must not consign the patient to a prolonged period of observation. When the diagnosis of acute arterial occlusion is entertained, a surgeon experienced in the management of this condition should be consulted for further therapy, and arrangements should be made for angiographic examination. In the interim, intravenous administration of heparin is advisable, unless there is a specific contraindication.

CHRONIC ARTERIAL OCCLUSION

Less frequently, patients may come to the emergency ward with chronic arterial occlusive disease, which is usually atherosclerotic. Their primary complaint is most often intermittent claudication, but they also may have other symptoms of this disease such as cutaneous ulceration or ischemic pain at rest. Recent progression of symptoms may indicate acute thrombosis superimposed on the chronic process.

The history and physical examination usually clearly suggest the diagnosis. The physician should establish the time of onset of discomfort and the progression of symptoms. The most common symptom, intermittent claudication, often is described as a cramp, an ache, tightness, or tiredness in the affected muscle. Since the patient frequently attributes this symptom to a musculoskeletal disorder, the examiner must establish carefully what aggravates and alleviates the pain. Intermittent claudication almost always occurs with exercise and usually develops after the same amount of exercise, for example, walking a certain distance. It is relieved completely by rest. Sudden progression of the symptom may indicate occlusion within the affected arterial tree.

Ischemic pain at rest usually involves the most distal parts of the affected extremity, but may be localized to an ulcer or a gangrenous digit. Often it is aggravated by cold or elevation of the limb. Pain of ischemic neuropathy, on the other hand, generally is diffuse and involves a large area of the affected extremity. It may not be aggravated by cold or elevation of the limb.

Acute deep venous thrombosis in an extremity also may cause severe pain characterized by diffuse deep aching. As in intermittent claudication, the pain may be caused by exercise. It is not relieved by rest, however, and elevation of the extremity may produce relief.

A physical abnormality elsewhere in the cardiovascular system may alert the physician to the underlying disease responsible for pain in an extremity. If a patient with such pain is found to have atrial fibrillation or mitral stenosis, for example, the physician may suspect an embolic occlusion.

Physical examination of the patient with suspected peripheral vascular disease should include assessment of the blood pressure in both arms. Determination of segmental blood pressures in the affected extremity as compared with the normal extremity may be accomplished by a blood pressure cuff and a Doppler ultrasonic flow detector. In patients with symptoms in a leg, comparison of blood pressures in the ankle in the resting state and after a standard exercise test also is helpful. The more profound the ischemia, the greater the drop in pressure recorded after exercise. If there is no drop in pressure, other causes for symptoms should be considered, such as a musculoskeletal or neurologic disorder.

The heart and origin of the great vessels, the distal abdominal aorta, and the carotid, subclavian, iliac, and femoral arteries should be auscultated to detect bruits. Pulsations in the peripheral arteries must be assessed carefully by palpation. The degree of arterial pulsation is evaluated best by someone experienced in examining for pulses in both healthy persons and those with arterial disease. Pulses are generally graded on a scale of 0–4; 0 indicates absent pulsation, and 4 is normal pulsation.

The physician should search for cutaneous manifestations of vascular disease such as xanthoma, and should note the color of the skin. Cutaneous signs may be noticeable more immediately in the acute state than in chronic arterial occlusion; in the former, the skin distal to the occlusion may be blue or white. The ischemic muscle may be tender, and there may be diminished sensation and motor function in the ischemic area.

In chronic arterial occlusion, skin and muscle atrophy may be apparent. Cutaneous ischemia may be documented by an elevation and dependency test. In a healthy person, elevation of an extremity may cause mild pallor, but in a person with significant arterial occlusive disease, the degree of pallor after 1-minute elevation is more marked. When the extremity of a healthy person is returned to the dependent position, it resumes the normal skin color in roughly 10 seconds. In patients with arterial occlusive disease, significant pallor may be evident when the affected extremity

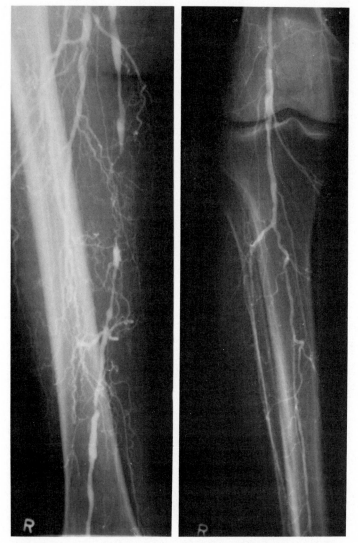

Figure 21.12.   Percutaneous femoral arteriogram demonstrating extensive atheromatous occlusive changes in superficial femoral artery (*left*) and popliteal and tibial arteries (*right*), a pattern frequently seen in patients with diabetes mellitus.

is elevated about 45 degrees, normal color returns more slowly on dependency, and the extremity may eventually assume a deep redness termed dependent rubor. The degree of ischemia is measured by the length of time prior to the appearance of rubor and its proximal extension. In the case of acute arterial occlusion with no antecedent arterial disease, rubor does not develop until ischemia has existed for more than 10 days.

Venous filling time is the time necessary to fill the superficial veins of the foot after emptying by elevation of the leg and subsequent dependency. A venous filling time longer than 15 seconds in the absence of venous varicosities is evidence of arterial insufficiency.

Patients with chronic arterial occlusion and is-

chemic ulcers should be hospitalized. If the ulcer is infected, specimens for a Gram stain and culture should be taken and the patient should be treated with antibiotics, elevation of the head of the bed, and saline dressings on the lesions if they are moist. Patients with ischemic pain at rest also should be hospitalized with the head of the bed elevated, high room temperature, and analgesics for pain. In both conditions, the feasibility of reconstruction should be assessed by arteriographic examination (Fig. 21.12).

VENOUS THROMBOSIS

Deep Venous Thrombosis

The symptoms of venous obstruction depend on the level and degree of obstruction, the available collateral venous circulation, and the underlying cause of the obstruction. The diagnosis may be obvious, as with a swollen limb that is tender from local inflammation at the point of thrombosis, or the condition may be "silent," becoming evident only when a thromboembolic event in the pulmonary circulation produces the symptoms and signs of pulmonary embolus (see Chapter 9, pages 153–158). Deep venous thrombosis frequently is associated with congestive heart failure, childbirth, operation, serious illness, and trauma. It may result from an obstruction to venous outflow such as a pelvic tumor, or in the case of the arm, impingement on the subclavian vein by thoracic outlet compression.

Thrombotic occlusion of the inferior vena cava or either common iliac vein may produce symptoms in the leg such as edema, pain, varicosities, and cutaneous signs of chronic stasis with ulceration. The patient may have intermittent episodes of thrombophlebitis. This syndrome sometimes may be seen after ligation or plication of the inferior vena cava.

Because of the risk of pulmonary embolism, it is imperative to hospitalize patients with deep venous thrombosis. Patients in whom this diagnosis is suspected should be treated initially with bed rest and heparin, 5000 units intravenously, administered in a bolus. Phlebography should then be performed to demonstrate the presence or absence of deep venous thrombosis (Fig. 21.13). If no thrombus is visualized in the deep venous system, anticoagulants should be discontinued and other causes for symptoms and signs should be considered, such as a ruptured plantaris tendon, a systemic cause for dependent edema, chronic postphlebitic state, local infection, primary lymphedema, and secondary causes of lymphatic obstruction.

If the presence of deep venous thrombosis is confirmed by phlebography, the patient should be hospitalized for an additional 7–10 days for continuous intravenous heparin therapy, during which time oral anticoagulant therapy with sodium warfarin (Coumadin) can be started. In patients in whom anticoagulation is contraindicated, such as

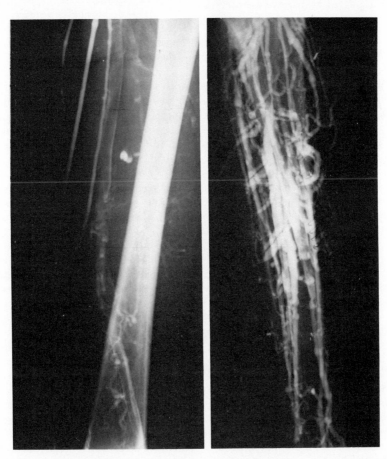

Figure 21.13.   Phlebogram of a lower extremity demonstrating extensive deep venous thrombosis in superficial femoral vein (*left*) and soleal veins (*right*).

those with an active duodenal ulcer or acute cerebrovascular accident, either ligation or plication of the vena cava, angiographic placement of an intracaval filter, or venous thrombectomy is necessary. Patients with recurrent episodes of thrombophlebitis in the leg should be treated on an outpatient basis with long-term anticoagulant therapy, elastic support when ambulatory, and elevation of the leg when at rest.

Occasionally, deep venous thrombosis progresses beyond the usual clinical phase of acute thrombophlebitis (phlegmasia alba dolens) to blue phlebitis (phlegmasia cerulea dolens). The latter condition is manifested by engorgement of the extremity with cyanosis and tenderness. If the retrograde venous pressure becomes high enough, arterial flow may cease, leading to ischemia and occasionally gangrene. The diagnosis of phlegmasia cerulea dolens is made by physical examination, arteriography, and phlebography, and most patients are treated best by anticoagulant therapy and extreme elevation of the leg. If gangrene seems imminent, venous thrombectomy and long-term anticoagulation are necessary to prevent progressive ischemia.

Superficial Venous Thrombosis

Symptoms of thrombosis of the superficial venous system include pain over the thrombosed vein and occasionally erythema. If no infection seems present, this condition can be managed on an outpatient basis with elastic compression and heat. If, however, the saphenofemoral junction seems to be involved, hospitalization and anticoagulation are advisable. If infection is present, as is often the case in sites of recent venipuncture for intravenous therapy, the patient is hospitalized, the appropriate cultures are obtained, and antibiotic therapy is instituted.

Cutaneous changes due to venous stasis, occurring primarily in the distal part of the lower leg, may lead to skin ulceration. If distal pulses are diminished or absent, the lesion must be regarded as an ischemic ulcer and treated with prompt hospitalization, conservative débridement of necrotic tissue, antibiotic therapy, and subsequent evaluation of the adequacy of arterial circulation. If pulses in the foot seem normal, the physician should ascertain whether there is invasive infection and whether treatment of the patient outside the hospital will be effective. In most cases, the patient should be hospitalized for treatment of the ulcer and instruction on how to care for it at home.

THE DIABETIC FOOT

The emergency physician frequently is called on to treat ulceration, infection, and gangrene resulting from complications of diabetes mellitus such as obliterative arterial disease and neuropathy. In a diabetic patient, obliterative arterial disease can involve both large and small arteries; thus, lesions may develop as a consequence of occlusion of either the aortoiliac or femoropopliteal systems or of the small arteries of the lower leg and foot. The progression of the obliterative process may differ in the large and small arteries, and gangrenous changes in a toe or the distal part of the foot might exist in the presence of bounding pedal pulses. In the presence of marked obliterative disease of other small vessels, infection in the soft tissue of a digit may progress to cause complete thrombotic occlusion of the arterial supply, with resultant gangrene. This condition is termed infectious gangrene of the digits. Another complication of diabetes mellitus, neuropathy is significant in that loss of sensation of pain and temperature may prevent the patient from feeling mechanical or thermal trauma, resulting in ulceration and subsequent invasive infection. Lesions in the feet of diabetic patients are more common in the presence of neuropathy.

The initial portal of entry of infection is often near a toenail or through an ulcer in a callus formed as a reaction to constant friction. These calluses ususally are located over the heads of the metatarsal bones on the sole of the foot. Progression of invasive infection depends on resistance of the host, virulence of the organism, and promptness of treatment.

All diabetic patients with foot infections should be hospitalized with bed rest. Specimens for Gram stains, cultures, and sensitivity tests should be taken, and systemic antibiotic therapy should be started on the basis of the Gram stain; antibiotics should not be withheld until return of the results of cultures and sensitivity tests. The physician should carefully ascertain whether the foot requires drainage of trapped pus and débridement of necrotic tissue. A diabetic foot threatened by sepsis frequently can be saved by early, careful débridement and drainage; thus a surgeon should be consulted early in the treatment effort. The physician should keep in mind that metabolic management of a diabetic patient may be complicated by the infection and that coexistent cardiac and renal problems often may lead to further morbidity and possibly death.

The presence of atherosclerotic occlusive disease

in the aortoiliac or femoropopliteal systems in a diabetic patient is suggested by absence of pulses and confirmed by arteriographic examination, at which time the feasibility of arterial reconstruction can be assessed. Early arterial reconstruction may save an extremity threatened by an ischemic lesion.

VASOSPASTIC STATES

Acute vasospasm leading to severe pain and ulceration and necrosis of the distal parts of the digits usually occurs in the arm and commonly is termed either Raynaud's phenomenon when it is secondary to an underlying cause (usually a connective tissue disorder) or Raynaud's disease when the underlying cause cannot be determined. This commonly occurs in young women, and there is frequently a history of pain and blanching of the fingers (and occasionally toes) associated with deep emotion or exposure to cold. The physician should search for bruits, palpate for peripheral pulses, determine segmental blood pressures, and assess whether entrapment of structures within the thoracic outlet exists.

In the differential diagnosis, the physician should consider an atherosclerotic occlusion at the origin of the brachiocephalic vessels, compression at the thoracic outlet, arterial embolism, chronic dissecting aneurysm, and arteriosclerotic changes in the digital vasculature. A chest roentgenogram to search for a cervical rib and angiograms are helpful in recognizing the cause of symptoms. If vasospasm is believed to be the primary difficulty and if these entities can be excluded, active search for collagen disease should be undertaken. Immediate relief may be produced by reserpine or papaverine administered intra-arterially or by stellate ganglionic blockade. A patient with ulceration threatening a digit should be hospitalized for local care, antibiotic therapy, and consideration for cervicodorsal sympathectomy.

COMPLICATIONS FOLLOWING ARTERIAL RECONSTRUCTION

With advances in vascular surgery leading to more operative procedures for aneurysms and arterial occlusive disease, it is inevitable that both early and late complications of these procedures will be seen more frequently. Early complications include local wound infections and hematomas, deep venous thrombosis that may lead to pulmonary embolism, thrombosis of the reconstructed arterial tree with distal ischemia, mechanical obstruction of the small intestine if the procedure involved entry into the abdominal cavity, and flare-up of an antecedent illness. A common late complication is progression of the atherosclerotic occlusive process proximally and distally to grafts, producing thrombosis of arterial grafts and of arteries on which endarterectomy has been performed. Symptoms resemble those of either acute arterial occlusion or chronic arterial occlusion with increase in ischemic manifestations. Another late complication is aneurysm at a suture line. These aneurysms usually increase in size, resulting in either a local mass with pain and venous obstruction or rupture with acute hemorrhage demanding prompt operative intervention. As with all aneurysms, laminar clot in the aneurysmal wall may break away and result in distal embolic occlusion. Thrombus formed along the wall of a previously placed graft also may cause distal embolic occlusion. A rare late complication of aortic and iliac arterial grafts is formation of a fistula to the small intestine at a graft suture line. This results in gastrointestinal bleeding that is, surprisingly, often intermittent until a major life-threatening hemorrhage occurs. Systemic infection related to this complication is common.

In any patient who has undergone an arterial reconstruction, the physician must determine what was done for the patient previously. Records of the previous hospitalization may be invaluable in this regard, and the prompt assistance of the vascular surgeon who previously cared for the patient should be sought.

Suggested Readings

Athanasoulis CA, Pfister RC, Greene RE, et al: *Interventional Radiology.* Philadelphia, W. B. Saunders, 1982

Baker CC, Thomas AN, Trunkey DD: The role of emergency room thoracotomy in trauma. *J Trauma* 20:848–854, 1980

Barker WF: *Peripheral Arterial Disease.* ed 2. Philadelphia. W. B. Saunders, 1975

Beebe HG (Ed): *Complications in Vascular Surgery.* Philadelphia, J. B. Lippincott, 1973

Blaisdell FW, Steele M, Allen RE: Management of acute lower extremity arterial ischemia due to embolism and thrombosis. *Surgery* 84:822–834, 1978

Brawley RK, Murray GF, Crisler C, et al: Management of wounds of the innominate, subclavian, and axillary blood vessels. *Surg Gynecol Obstet* 131:1130–1140, 1970

Brewer LA, III, Carter R: A rational treatment of small and large wounds of the heart. *Surg Gynecol Obstet* 126:977–985, 1968

Cranley JJ: Ischemic rest pain. *Arch Surg* 97:187–188, 1969

Crisler C, Bahnson HT: Aneurysms of the aorta. *Curr Probl Surg* 9 (no. 12), 1972

Dale WA: The swollen leg. *Curr Probl Surg* 10 (no. 9), 1973

Danto LA, Fry WJ, Kraft RO: Acute aortic thrombosis. *Arch Surg* 104:569–572, 1972

Dean RH, Yao JST: Hemodynamic measurements in peripheral vascular disease. *Curr Probl Surg* 13 (no. 8), 1976

Doty DB, Anderson AE, Rose EF, et al: Cardiac trauma: Clinical and experimental correlations of myocardial contusion. *Ann Surg 180:*452–460, 1974

Evans J, Gray LA, Rayner A, et al: Principles for the management of penetrating cardiac wounds. *Ann Surg 189:*777–784, 1979

Fairbairn JF, II, Juergens JL, Spittell JA, Jr: *Peripheral Vascular Diseases.* ed 4. Philadelphia, W. B. Saunders, 1972

Gray L, Jr, Kirsh M: A new roentgenographic finding in acute traumatic rupture of the aorta. *J Thorac Cardiovasc Surg 70:*86–88, 1975

Hight DW, Tilney N, Couch NP: Changing clinical trends in patients with peripheral arterial emboli. *Surgery 79:*172–176 1976

Imparato AM, Kim G, Davidson T, et al: Intermittent claudication: Its natural course. *Surgery 78:*795–799, 1975

Levin ME, O'Neal LW (Eds): *The Diabetic Foot.* St. Louis, C. V. Mosby, 1973

Mattox KL, Beall AC, Jr, Jordan GL. Jr, et al: Cardiorrhaphy in the emergency center. *J Thorac Cardiovasc Surg 68:*886–895, 1974

Mattox KL: Priorities in repairing a penetrated chest. *Emerg Med 14:*282–288, 1982

McFarland J, Willerson JT, Dinsmore RE, et al: The medical treatment of dissecting aortic aneurysms. *N Engl J Med 286:*115–119, 1972

Moore WS, Blaisdell FW: Diagnosis and management of peripheral arterial occlusive disease. *Curr Probl Surg 10* (no. 11), 1973

Pomerantz M, Delgado F, Eiseman B: Unsuspected depressed cardiac output following blunt thoracic or abdominal trauma. *Surgery 70:*865–871, 1971

Slater EE, DeSanctis RW: The clinical recognition of dissecting aortic aneurysm. *Am J Med 60:*625–633, 1976

Stanley JC, Thompson NW, Fry WJ: Splanchnic artery aneurysms. *Arch Surg 101:*689–697, 1970

Sugg WL, Rea WJ, Ecker RR, et al: Penetrating wounds of the heart: An analysis of 459 cases. *J Thorac Cardiovasc Surg 56:*531–545, 1968

Symbas PN, Levin JM, Ferrier FL, et al: A study on autotransfusion from hemothorax. *South Med J 62:*671–674, 1969

Thurer RL, Lytle BW, Cosgrove DM, et al: Autotransfusion following cardiac operations: A randomized prospective study. *Ann Thorac Surg 27:*500–507, 1979

Unger SW, Tucker WS, Mrdeza MA, et al: Carotid arterial trauma. *Surgery 87:*477–487, 1980

Wheat MW, Jr, Palmer RF: Drug therapy for dissecting aneurysms. *Dis Chest 54:*372–377, 1968

CHAPTER 22

Thoracic Emergencies

JOHN M. HEAD, M.D.

GENERAL CONSIDERATIONS

Many conditions related to the chest require emergency treatment because they interfere with respiration by means of the following mechanisms: (1) airway obstruction; (2) space-occupying collections of air or fluid; and (3) mechanical instability of ventilatory structures. Because the underlying mechanisms are few, the same priorities and methods of treatment can be followed in a wide variety of disorders, depending on the physiologic defect that is encountered. Accordingly, the diagnosis and treatment of the general mechanisms will be discussed first, followed by a consideration of specific injuries and diseases.

Airway Obstruction

Relief of airway obstruction takes first priority in any emergency. No resuscitation attempt is successful in the presence of an inadequate airway. The following steps should be observed:

(1) The mouth and hypopharynx should be cleared of secretions or blood by digital exploration and suction.

(2) An obstruction at the level of the hypopharynx should be relieved by an oral airway.

(3) An obstruction at the glottic or subglottic level requires tracheal intubation. The quickest method is usually passage of an orotracheal tube with the aid of a laryngoscope for visualization of the vocal cords. Alternatively, a rigid bronchoscope may be passed and left in place until it can be replaced by a nasotracheal or tracheotomy tube.

(4) An obstruction low in the trachea can be relieved only by passage of a bronchoscope, long endotracheal tube, or tracheotomy tube to the level of the carina.

All indwelling tubes used for assisted ventilation should be fitted with low-pressure, high-volume cuffs to avoid the complications of tracheal erosion, stenosis, and perforation.

In a case of extreme urgency when proper equipment is unavailable—for example, if a patient aspirates food at a restaurant—another method for relief of acute laryngeal obstruction must be used. If food aspiration is suspected, a brief attempt should be made to clear the hypopharynx with the fingers or a curved forceps. If this is unsuccessful, the Heimlich maneuver should be employed to dislodge the obstructing material. This is performed by standing behind the patient with arms around him, placing the fists one on top of the other high in the epigastrium, and forcibly squeezing. If neither of these methods is quickly effective, emergency cricothyrotomy must be performed. Insertion of a 15-gauge (1.5-inch) needle through the cricothyroid membrane will sustain life for 15–20 minutes in a vigorous person. Similarly, rapid incision of the cricothyroid membrane and insertion of the empty barrel of a ballpoint pen (Fig. 22.1) is satisfactory until intubation, formal tracheotomy, or removal of the obstruction can be accomplished. As soon as an adequate airway is established, secretions and blood should be aspirated to clear the lower respiratory tree.

All physicians engaged in emergency care should obtain instruction in emergency laryngoscopy, intubation, and bronchoscopy from an anesthesiologist or thoracic surgeon or through a course of postgraduate instruction. These techniques are the key to adequate care in thoracic emergencies. A brief discussion of endotracheal intubation and bronchoscopy is presented in the following sections. The technique of emergency cricothyrotomy detailed in Section 5, pages 920–921 and emergency tracheotomy is discussed in detail in Chapter 33, pages 755–758.

Endotracheal Intubation

Formerly considered an alternative to tracheotomy, endotracheal intubation now is preferred in the management of a wide variety of conditions manifested by obstruction or inefficient respiration or both. Upper airway obstruction in any patient

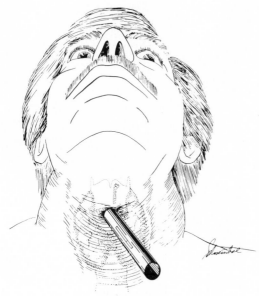

Figure 22.1. Emergency cricothyrotomy performed by rapid incision of skin with transverse stab wound of cricothyroid membrane and insertion of barrel of ballpoint pen.

can be relieved by intubation if passage of a tube is technically feasible. Likewise, an endotracheal tube will be necessary in any patient requiring positive-pressure assisted ventilation.

No absolute indications for intubation can be set forth. In general, it is indicated if severe obstruction due to hypopharyngeal or laryngeal edema is developing. It also is required when fatigue impairs ventilatory function or when respiration becomes too inefficient to maintain the arterial partial pressure of oxygen (Po_2) above 60 mm Hg or the partial pressure of carbon dioxide (Pco_2) below 50 mm Hg in an otherwise healthy patient. Arterial blood-gas values in patients with chronic pulmonary disease are discussed in Chapter 9, pages 166–168.

A nasotracheal tube is preferred to an orotracheal tube if intubation is required for more than 24 hours. It is more comfortable for the patient, and there is less motion and possibly less damage of the tracheal mucosa than with an orotracheal tube. The caliber of the tube should be as large as possible to permit adequate aspiration of secretions and to minimize plugging. A nonreactive plastic tube with a low-pressure, high-volume cuff is preferred. It may be left in place for weeks if necessary, but if intubation is required for more than 10 days, tracheotomy should be performed if the tissues of the neck are healthy. A tracheotomy tube is more easily kept free of crusts. All endotracheal tubes should be removed when they are no longer needed.

Bronchoscopy

The following tips are helpful in performing emergency bronchoscopy. If time permits, topical anesthesia can be induced rapidly by transcricoidal injection of 6–8 ml of 2% lidocaine (Xylocaine) by means of a 25-gauge (0.75-inch) needle. The patient is put in the supine position with the neck extended; this is usually the best position, although flexion provides the best access to the larynx in some patients. In patients with a short neck or a large tongue, the base of the tongue must be pulled anteriorly with a laryngoscope to expose the vocal cords. The epiglottis is lifted anteriorly with the tip of the bronchoscope until the cords are seen, and the bronchoscope is then turned 90 degrees to allow its tip to pass between the vocal cords into the trachea. The most common error is passage of the instrument too far beyond the epiglottis before lifting anteriorly, causing the instrument to enter the esophagus rather than the trachea.

Space-Occupying Collections

Collections of air or fluid frequently require removal. In the emergency setting, needle aspiration should be performed first in order to confirm the diagnosis and to determine the appropriate site for intercostal tube drainage, should the latter be necessary. If tension pneumothorax is present, needle aspiration provides temporary relief; a large-bore needle (15-gauge) left open to the air until a chest tube is inserted may be lifesaving. *Needle aspiration should always precede insertion of a chest tube* to confirm the presence of a collection. This procedure may cause pneumothorax on occasion, but it is far less dangerous than ill-advised attempts to insert intercostal catheters into nonexistent spaces, especially in the presence of pleural symphysis, since such attempts may result in laceration of the lung or pulmonary vessels.

Thoracentesis

The technique of thoracentesis depends on the location of the intrapleural collection. If possible, preliminary chest x-ray films consisting of posteroanterior and lateral views should be obtained with the patient in the upright position. Fluid collections are poorly seen in vertical projections with the patient in the recumbent position. When the upright position is not feasible, lateral decubitus and across-the-table lateral views in the supine position are helpful. The presence of pleural effusion should be confirmed, if possible, by fluoroscopic examination or by lateral decubitus films to avoid the confusion occasioned by pleural thickening.

In patients with pneumothorax, the best site for thoracentesis and subsequent thoracostomy is the second intercostal space at least 2 cm lateral to the sternum. Needle aspiration and chest tube insertion should be performed near the upper border of the rib to avoid the intercostal vessels. Unless the situation is extremely urgent, preliminary local anesthesia should be employed in which each layer, including the pleura, is anesthetized sequentially. Information gained from the infiltrating needle is useful in estimating the thickness of the chest wall and of the pleura, and air or fluid aspirated from the pleural space serves as a diagnostic aid, the latter by virtue of its appearance. If no air or fluid can be obtained through a fine-gauge (No. 22) needle, an alternative site must be considered. If air or fluid is obtained, a chest tube may be inserted safely at that site.

In the management of pleural effusion, thoracentesis or tube thoracostomy should be performed via the axilla if the patient must remain supine, or posterolaterally if he can sit up. The common error of attempting to place a needle or tube into the lowest level of an effusion often results in injury to the diaphragm, liver, or spleen. Frequently it is impossible to determine the level of the diaphragm by radiologic evaluation (Fig. 22.2) or by physical examination, whereas the upper limit of the fluid is determined easily by either method. Physical examination is the most reliable means of determining the site of aspiration; the level of dullness should be established by percussion and the interspace below this selected. As pleural fluid is removed, the lung expands and the meniscus remains at the same level, permitting removal of almost all of the fluid.

Intravenous catheters may be used for thoracentesis instead of needles; although they are less likely to injure the visceral pleura, they become plugged more easily when fibrin is present in the effusion. A large-bore (No. 14–16) needle can be used safely if a hemostat is employed as a stop to prevent insertion of the needle past the minimal distance necessary to obtain fluid (Fig. 22.3). A needle can be manipulated more easily than a catheter, and it provides more tactile information about the chest wall and the consistency of the fluid. Use of an uncontrolled suction device is unwise because rapid evacuation of a large effusion may cause excessive mediastinal shift, dyspnea, discomfort, and "pleural shock." Although it is more laborious, use of a syringe and three-way stopcock is preferable. A gentle suction system

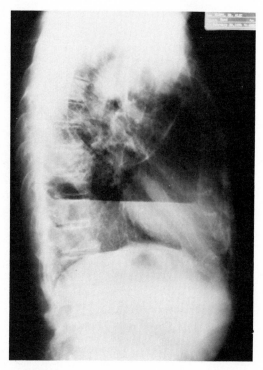

Figure 22.2.   Lateral x-ray film of chest showing that diaphragm is visible only on normal left side. A large pleural effusion completely obliterates diaphragm on affected right side.

with clamping after removal of each 400–500 ml also is satisfactory. Both of these methods allow time for expansion of the lung and equilibration of intrathoracic pressures.

Tube Thoracostomy

The two common methods of chest tube placement are by trocar and by hemostat. Although fashioning a tract by blunt dissection with a hemostat (Fig. 22.4) may be slower, this technique is safer and provides the operator with more tactile information about the thickness and consistency of the pleura. The trocars currently available are too sharp to provide a safe means of catheter placement; they lacerate the intercostal vessels or lung too easily. Tube thoracostomy can be performed painlessly if the skin, fascia, and pleura are infiltrated with lidocaine.

In the management of pneumothorax, the use of a No. 20 Foley catheter anteriorly is satisfactory. However, collections of fluid or blood should be drained by a No. 26 or 28 argyle catheter posterolaterally or low in the axilla. Both types of tube should be secured to the skin with heavy silk sutures.

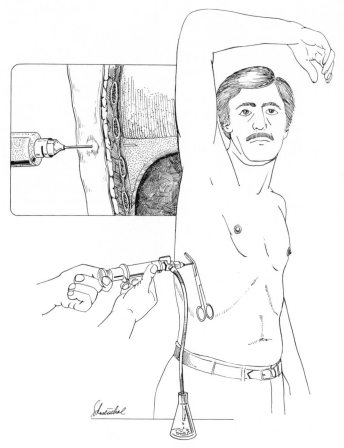

Figure 22.3.   Thoracentesis: Needle is inserted just below fluid meniscus. A hemostat prevents insertion of needle more than a few millimeters past parietal pleura.

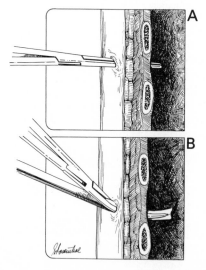

Figure 22.4.   Intercostal chest tube placement. **(A)** Formation of tract with hemostat. **(B)** Insertion of tube with hemostat.

Mechanical Instability

Although it may not be very important immediately after a chest wall injury, mechanical instability causes ventilatory inefficiency as pain and fatigue increase, and it requires specific treatment when this occurs. In the emergency ward, chest wall instability can be managed with compression bandages and administration of oxygen by endotracheal tube if necessary, while other serious injuries are evaluated. Within a few hours, however, some form of internal or external stabilization often is mandatory.

Concomitant Conditions

Pre-existent cardiopulmonary disease may cause or modify thoracic emergencies. Pulmonary emphysema, for example, greatly augments the disability produced by chest wall injuries, and it also delays the sealing of air leaks in patients with a lacerated lung or spontaneous pneumothorax. The magnitude of treatment must be gauged to the overall status of the patient, and treatment may have to be modified considerably in the presence of chronic pulmonary disease. Occasionally, therapy for the underlying illness may take precedence over treatment of the acute injury.

TRAUMA

General Considerations

Trauma causes many of the serious thoracic emergencies seen in civilian and military practice. Before appropriate therapy can be started, the mechanism of injury and the type of physiologic impairment must be determined.

Common types of blunt trauma include the following:

(1) Blast injuries, which are likely to produce cardiac and pulmonary contusion, as well as rupture of the tracheobronchial tree and of the diaphragm.

(2) Crushing injuries, which often are accompanied by disruption of the chest wall, diaphragm, or tracheobronchial tree.

(3) Deceleration, which causes injuries of the chest wall, lung, myocardium, bronchi, and aorta.

(4) Hyperextension, which occasionally disrupts the intrathoracic portion of the thoracic duct.

(5) Flexion, which produces overlapping transverse sternal fracture.

It must be remembered that most patients with major blunt thoracic injuries also have significant damage to other areas and organs. Some of the latter damage may be more serious than the thoracic disability, and its treatment may take precedence.

Penetrating chest injuries usually are produced by the following:

(1) Knife wounds, which may cause insignificant surface lacerations, but which may inflict widespread internal damage to the area reached by the blade, including pulmonary and vascular lacerations.

(2) Missile wounds, which have an unpredictable path that often is difficult to determine and which produce tissue injury along the path of the projectile, the volume of damage increasing with the velocity of the missile.

General Evaluation and Initial Treatment

In the evaluation of penetrating wounds, the location of the lesion is of paramount importance. Careful recording of entrance and exit sites and of the angle of penetration is vital. Wounds of the base of the neck and of the upper part of the thorax may involve the trachea or larynx, the great vessels, the thoracic duct, the esophagus, or a lung. Wounds of the midthorax are likely to damage the heart, the aorta, or a lung; penetrating injuries lower in the chest often involve a lung, the diaphragm, the spleen, the liver, the stomach, or the colon.

The initial physical examination is crucial to the management of thoracic trauma. It is often all that is needed to make an immediate decision regarding therapy, and it is occasionally all that is feasible. It should include careful observation of the wound at the entrance and exit sites and also of respiratory mechanics and skin color. Auscultation and percussion of the chest must be performed carefully and expeditiously, with the findings recorded for comparison with results of subsequent examinations; changes usually reveal more about the extent of injury than does the initial evaluation. The physician should inquire briefly regarding pre-existent disease. He also should note the characteristics of the sputum and of any material draining from an open wound, and should observe the patient for the development of subcutaneous emphysema.

In any patient with major thoracic trauma, treatment must be started before diagnostic tests are completed. Lines for intravenous infusion and monitoring of central venous pressure should be inserted while blood is being drawn for laboratory studies and crossmatching. Central venous pressure readings probably are more important in the management of thoracic trauma than in the management of any other injury, because they provide vital diagnostic information concerning pericardial tamponade as well as general knowledge of blood volume and circulatory dynamics.

In life-threatening situations, the following problems must be attended to before complete diagnostic evaluation:

(1) Upper airway obstruction must be relieved by whatever means required and hypoxia must be treated by administration of oxygen.

(2) Blood volume deficits should be replaced.

(3) Major chest wall instability must be partly stabilized, either by pressure dressings, sandbags, or positive-pressure assisted ventilation.

(4) Sucking wounds should be occluded by dressings.

(5) Large air or fluid collections must be evacuated.

(6) Pericardial tamponade must be relieved (see Chapter 21, pages 464–466.

After these measures are taken and the patient's clinical state is reasonably stable, the patient can undergo diagnostic testing. Roentgenographic examination of the chest is the initial step, followed by chest fluoroscopy and a barium swallow if they are indicated and feasible. If major vascular injury is suspected in a patient whose clinical condition is stable, angiographic examination should be performed early. After radiologic findings provide diagnostic information, the physician may proceed with such diagnostic and therapeutic maneuvers as nasogastric intubation, thoracentesis, and bronchoscopy. A Swan-Ganz pulmonary artery catheter inserted at this time may provide useful information in the evaluation and management of massive injuries involving several organ systems. Tetanus immunization, antibiotic therapy, and the treatment of other injuries also can be started.

Blunt Trauma

Most of the thoracic injuries seen in civilian practice result from blunt trauma, especially in a society oriented to contact sports and automobiles. Details of the traumatic event are important in determining the type of injury. For example, high-speed deceleration causes aortic transection and chest wall damage, whereas blast injuries cause serious cardiopulmonary contusion but little or no chest wall damage.

Chest Wall

Most thoracic trauma is accompanied by some degree of chest wall damage, ranging from localized contusion to extensive flail disruption. Chest wall damage itself often is severe enough to require vigorous treatment, and occasionally contributes to death of the patient. Central to proper management are recognition and correction of the impaired ventilation that frequently develops.

Contusion of the chest wall results from many domestic, athletic, industrial, and vehicular accidents. The diagnosis of rib fracture usually is ruled out by radiologic examination, but it may be impossible to exclude a fracture if the injury involves the anterior or subdiaphragmatic portions of the rib cage. Because local pain interferes with respiration and coughing, contusions should be treated in the same manner as simple rib fractures, with analgesic medications, elastic rib support, and chest physical therapy to assist in raising secretions. Contusions usually become asymptomatic in 1 or 2 weeks if there has been no disruption of bone or cartilage.

Simple rib fractures usually are caused by a direct blow to the chest wall. However, patients with osteoporosis are prone to rib fractures due to insignificant trauma or coughing. Recognition of fractures is enhanced by a careful history and

physical examination. The incident causing the fracture usually is known, pain develops abruptly and is aggravated by cough or motion, and the fracture site is always tender. Crepitation produced by motion of the bony fragments may be noted. A useful diagnostic maneuver is to apply simultaneous pressure on the sternum and back, avoiding pressure over the area of suspected fracture; resultant pain is a reliable indication of a fractured rib. Posteroanterior and lateral roentgenograms should be obtained when a fractured rib is suspected, as well as special rib views, to exclude the possibility of intrapleural collections of blood or air. Occasionally, collections are large enough to require evacuation even if only one rib is fractured.

The treatment of simple rib fractures must be adapted to individual needs. Patients in good health may need nothing more than an elastic rib belt (Fig. 22.5), preferably with a Velcro fastening to allow easy application and removal by the patient himself, and a mild analgesic. On the other hand, an elderly patient with emphysema may require hospitalization, an elastic rib belt, a narcotic analgesic, intercostal blocks, and chest physical therapy. Elastic rib belts are preferable to taping or strapping, since they are managed much more easily by the patient and seldom chafe or produce blisters. Patients recovering from a frac-

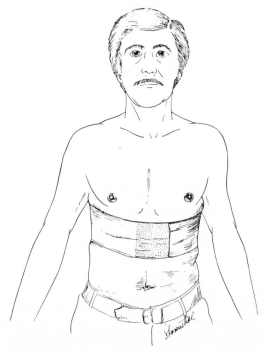

Figure 22.5. Correct placement of elastic rib belt. Belt should be placed around lower ribs, regardless of level of fracture.

tured rib are most comfortable in a semi-upright or sitting position. Those who cannot tolerate opiates because of resultant respiratory depression may require intercostal nerve block to control pain, to permit adequate ventilation, and to allow effective coughing. If repeated nerve blocks are necessary, it may be helpful to insert a series of percutaneous catheters into the intercostal spaces lateral to the spine for injection of anesthetic agents. Nerve blocks are ineffective unless they involve two intercostal nerves above and two below the injured rib. Intercostal blocks are performed by injecting 2–3 ml of 2% lidocaine or a similar agent into the appropriate intercostal spaces just below the rib and 5–6 cm lateral to the midline posteriorly.

Sternal fracture occurs in only 4% of major chest injuries. It rarely results from a direct blow to the sternum, because the sternochondral or costochondral junctions usually give way instead. Sternal fractures most often are caused by acute flexion, which results in overlapping transverse disruption with or without associated fractured ribs. The upper fragment commonly is displaced anteriorly and the lower fragment posteriorly (Fig. 22.6). This is a painful condition causing severe disability, and the fracture should be reduced and repaired by intramedullary fixation. Injury of the internal mammary vessels often accompanies sternal fractures, and surgical control of bleeding may be necessary. Widening of the mediastinum caused by mammary artery bleeding will confuse the interpretation of chest radiographs and raise the question of aortic injury. A result of major trauma, sternal fractures are usually a component of serious anterior flail injuries, and often are complicated by myocardial contusion and pulmonary laceration. Sternal fractures are visible and palpable and can be seen best on lateral x-ray views.

Flail chest typically results from fracture of at least three consecutive ribs, each in two or more places. A fracture "plate" of this type permits paradoxical motion of the chest wall of a degree that vitiates effective ventilatory effort. Nearly 65% of such injuries result from vehicular accidents, whereas about 25% are due to falls and 10% to crushing.

Posterolateral flail chest, which constitutes 55% of all flail injuries, is the result of an accident in which a force from the side is taken on the shoulder and the scapula is driven into the chest momentarily (Fig. 22.7). Anterolateral flail injury, which is seen in 35% of cases, usually occurs after impingement on a steering wheel, although it may result from crushing. This type of injury frequently is bilateral. Other types of flail injury are combi-

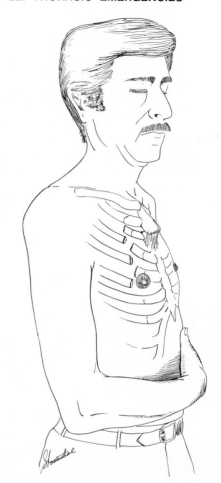

Figure 22.6. Fracture of sternum and anterior portions of ribs, showing anterior displacement of upper sternal fragment. Sternal periosteum remains intact.

nations of (1) flexion sternal fracture with rib fractures, (2) anterior and posterior rib fractures, and (3) bilateral injuries of no set pattern.

In addition to multiple rib fractures, flail chest injuries are accompanied by severe chest wall contusion, interruption of intercostal vessels and nerves, and bleeding. Contusion and laceration of the lung occur frequently, producing hemopneumothorax. The cardiovascular system may be damaged, and rupture of the diaphragm should be suspected. By itself, the injury to the chest wall interferes with ventilation of both lungs, since the flexibility of the chest wall and mediastinum prohibits transmission of normal inspiratory pressures to either lung on active ventilation (Fig. 22.8). Pain and pulmonary damage in addition to this mechanical defect make ventilation inefficient. *During the first 48 hours after injury, these problems all worsen*, with increasing displacement of rib fragments and impairment of ventilation.

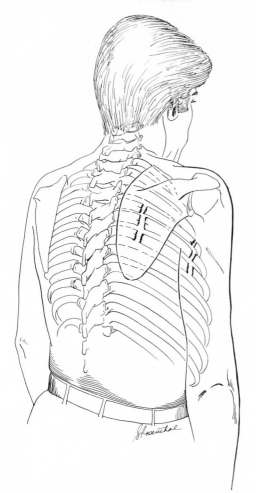

Figure 22.7.   Three-rib posterolateral flail segment caused by trauma to shoulder.

Initially, a patient with a flail chest injury is often in relatively good condition if there is no other major injury. There may be relatively little discomfort because of endorphan release. Soon, however, respiration becomes rapid, painful, shallow, and grunting in character. The flail segment is visible and palpable as it moves paradoxically with respiratory effort. Arterial blood-gas levels and vital signs are relatively normal soon after injury. However, respiratory effort becomes more labored as paradoxical motion increases with time. Arterial blood-gas values deteriorate and respiration rate and heart rate increase. The need for ventilatory assistance becomes obvious, and although positive-pressure assistance can be given by face mask in a few cases, endotracheal intubation and intermittent positive-pressure breathing (IPPB) usually are required unless pulmonary contusion is mild and unless pain can be controlled.

Some patients with small flail segments can be treated with elastic support, analgesics, intercostal blockade, humidified oxygen, and chest physical therapy. Those with underlying pulmonary disease require more effective stabilization of the flail segment by pericostal traction or direct intramedullary fixation. To apply pericostal traction, a heavy wire suture or towel clip should be placed under local anesthesia (Fig. 22.9); the amount of traction should be just sufficient to maintain the segment in position until adequate rigidity of the chest wall develops. This method is cumbersome and is appropriate only rarely.

Major flail chest injuries can cause serious respiratory disability, deformity, and death. The variables of age, vigor, concomitant injuries and preexistent disease make rigid adherence to any single management approach unwise. Control of pain by intercostal blocks often is useful. When significant pulmonary contusion exists, fluid restriction, albumin administration, and diuretics will improve respiratory exchange. (It should be noted that the radiologic diagnosis of pulmonary contusion frequently is inaccurate when there is major chest wall contusion and hemothorax.) During the past 20 years, the most common therapy has been "internal splinting" by endotracheal positive-pressure ventilation until adequate chest wall stability has been reached, usually in 10–21 days. Discontent with the complications of this method, particularly tracheal damage, has led to a resurgence of surgical stabilization of the chest wall. We believe that intramedullary fixation of disrupted bony elements within 4 days of injury is the best method of correcting deformity and achieving chest wall stability in patients who have no other potentially lethal injuries. This technique significantly improves ventilatory mechanics, shortens hospitalization, and reduces morbidity. Tracheostomy and prolonged ventilatory assistance usually are avoided.

Tracheobronchial Tree

Contusions and fractures of the *larynx* and *cervical trachea* usually are caused by direct blows and often are associated with mandibular fractures. Occasionally, the injury is so minor that the only sign of disruption is minimal subcutaneous emphysema in the neck. If air leakage is slight, careful observation may be the only management necessary. However, most major trauma to this region produces significant airway obstruction, and marked subcutaneous emphysema develops rapidly if the tracheal wall is disrupted below the vocal cords. The patient must be intubated im-

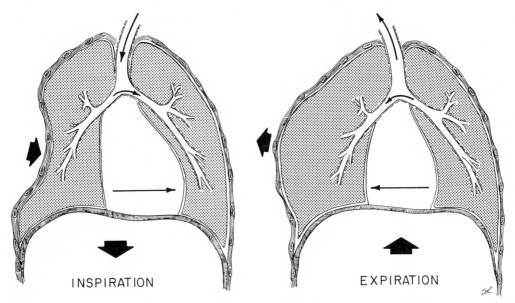

INSPIRATION   EXPIRATION

Figure 22.8. Disruption of ventilatory mechanics by flail segment on right side. Paradoxical motion of flail segment causes shift of mediastinum in same direction and affects ventilation of normal side.

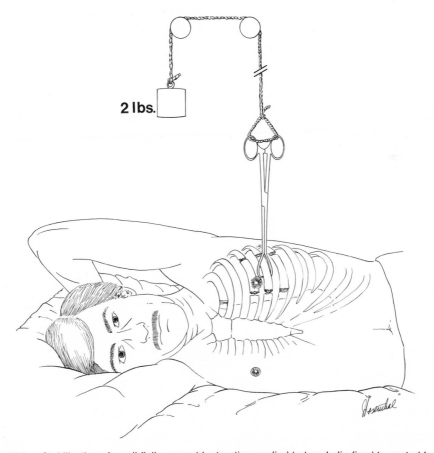

Figure 22.9. Stabilization of small flail segment by traction applied to towel clip fixed to central fragment.

mediately if possible; if it is impossible, tracheotomy must be performed immediately to restore an airway. Tracheotomy may be difficult if the cervical trachea has been completely severed, since the distal stump often retracts into the mediastinum. An adequate transverse incision with good exposure, good lighting, and ample surgical assistance is necessary for a satisfactory result. Subsequent reconstruction usually is required.

Violent deceleration occasionally disrupts the *trachea* or *major bronchi* within the thorax. The most common site of injury is a main or intermediate bronchus. The bronchial wall usually is divided completely, but the supporting loose areolar tissue and overlying pleura often remain partly intact. Mediastinal and subcutaneous emphysema develop rapidly. Occasionally, deformity of the bronchus can be visualized on the chest x-ray film. More often, the only indication of a ruptured bronchus is a large persistent air leak with failure of the lung to re-expand despite adequate suction via a large-bore intercostal tube. In this situation, bronchoscopy confirms the diagnosis by demonstrating distraction of the severed bronchus, a little local bleeding, and a bared, offset cartilaginous ring (Fig. 22.10). Early decompression with one or more intercostal catheters attached to a suction device prevents tension pneumothorax. As soon as the patient's condition permits, the bronchus

should be repaired to prevent bronchial stenosis and chronic collapse of the lung distal to the injury; it may be necessary to delay repair for a few days, because any force strong enough to avulse a bronchus almost always causes other serious injuries. On the other hand, transection of the intrathoracic trachea must be treated more aggressively, since the patient will die unless an endotracheal tube or bronchoscope can be inserted into the trachea or a mainstem bronchus below the point of severance. This permits ventilation until the trachea can be repaired at operation.

Traumatic Asphyxia

This characteristic syndrome is caused by a sustained crushing injury of the chest. Massive venous hypertension of the upper chest, neck, face, and brain is produced during crushing, resulting in typical violaceous edema, subconjunctival hemorrhages, and varying degrees of cerebral edema. Epistaxis and visual disturbances also may occur. Associated injuries of the chest wall, spine, and brain should be treated as indicated. No specific therapy for the syndrome itself is necessary.

Penetrating Injury

Penetrating injuries of the chest produce two problems: (1) a potentially open wound of the

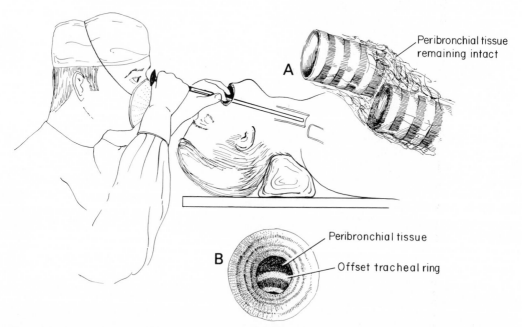

Figure 22.10.   Bronchial disruption with displacement of distal fragment. **(A)** Bronchial wall is frequently fractured completely, but peribronchial areolar tissue remains intact. **(B)** Bronchoscopic view of bared, offset tracheal ring; usually there is a little local bleeding.

chest wall; and (2) perforation or laceration of intrathoracic or intra-abdominal organs or both. The classic sucking wound of the thorax consists of a chest wall defect that admits air on inspiration but that acts as a flap valve to prevent its expulsion on expiration. The tension pneumothorax that results must be treated before management of the wound itself is even considered.

The vagaries of penetrating wounds are legendary. A stab wound of one side of the neck, for example, may lacerate the jugular vein, the esophagus, and the opposite lung. Lacerations of the midline of the neck or back may involve the spinal cord. Seemingly innocuous stab wounds of the shoulder may cause hemopneumothorax. High-speed projectiles cause the most destructive penetrating injuries; patients must be evaluated for possible injury to bones, intercostal vessels, lungs, esophagus, thoracic duct, heart and pericardium, spinal cord, diaphragm, and upper abdominal organs. It often is impossible to estimate the path of a missile except by the evidence of the injury it produces.

Sucking wounds of the chest usually are obvious. Hemothorax due to vascular injury and hemopneumothorax caused by pulmonary laceration may be suspected on the basis of chest x-ray films and confirmed by thoracentesis. The recovery of chyle from the pleural space points to thoracic duct laceration, whereas if saliva or ingested dye is recovered, esophageal injury is implicated. Bile or food recovered from the thoracic cavity signals injury to the diaphragm and an abdominal organ. Contrast studies or angiographic examination usually reveal the location of an esophageal or vascular defect. Mediastinal air seen radiologically may come from esophageal or bronchial injury; bronchoscopy and barium swallow may demonstrate the source of the leak. Fiberoptic esophagoscopy may occasionally be necessary to localize esophageal disruption.

Sucking Wound

In the emergency ward, a sucking wound of the chest wall should be occluded with a dressing of petrolatum gauze and Elastoplast to prevent further entry of air, and the pneumothorax should be evacuated with a chest tube. If tension pneumothorax is causing acute respiratory distress, the chest tube can be inserted through the wound and left in place until definitive treatment is undertaken. After collections of blood and air have been evacuated and the patient's condition is stable, the chest wall wound either should be debrided or excised and then sutured. If continued bleeding,

serious leakage of air, or major visceral injury becomes evident, early operative repair of the implicated organs is imperative.

Occasionally, the chest wall wound itself is a major problem. If a large defect exists after debridement of devitalized tissue, it may be necessary to swing muscle flaps to achieve adequate closure.

Most penetrating thoracic wounds are complicated by hemothorax; this condition usually is managed adequately by intercostal catheter drainage. There is little evidence that administration of fibrinolytic agents is effective. Only occasionally is pulmonary decortication indicated to prevent crippling fibrothorax.

Visceral Injury

Penetrating wounds are more likely than blunt injuries to damage blood vessels, pulmonary tissue, the tracheobronchial tree, the esophagus, the thoracic duct, and the abdominal viscera. When massive bleeding indicates a serious vascular or cardiac injury, immediate thoracotomy is necessary to prevent death. A lung shattered by a high-velocity projectile may require resection, but in the treatment of most contusions and lacerations of the lung, excision of tissue should be avoided. Lacerations of the esophagus and trachea or major bronchi must be repaired without delay. Division of the thoracic duct as indicated by chylothorax can be managed initially by insertion of a chest tube for drainage. Since persistent leakage of chyle eventually produces severe malnutrition, thoracotomy with ligation of the duct may be necessary later. Injury to abdominal organs and the diaphragm is frequent, and surgical repair commonly is indicated.

Burn Injury

A vague and poorly defined term, "smoke inhalation" refers to inspiration of a variety of gases as well as soot. The products of combustion depend on the material burned: wood releases irritating aldehydes and resins, wool produces cyanides, and some plastics release phosgene. Most fires generate carbon monoxide, and exposure to it must be assumed in any fire victim. Certain combustible agents such as hydrazine are toxic and can be inhaled in gaseous form at temperatures below their ignition points. The result of smoke inhalation is direct irritation of the mucosa of the airway that causes injury ranging from edema to necrosis, with or without damage to the alveolocapillary membranes. Systemic absorption of toxic substances can also occur.

The term respiratory or pulmonary "burn" is used even more loosely, since thermal injury of the intrathoracic airway never occurs unless the victim inhales gas containing steam or heated carbon particles or has no laryngeal reflexes. Laryngospasm normally prevents the passage of dry air that is hot enough to produce significant subglottic trauma. If a fire victim sustains injury to the respiratory tract, the damage is produced largely by the toxic products of combustion and is augmented by a thermal component only if steam or hot soot is inhaled. Severe thermal burn of the subglottic airway (Fig. 22.11) is seen in less than 5% of cases, and usually is present only in a comatose patient. We therefore use the term "inhalation injury" to describe the results of inhalation of the products of combustion.

Inhalation Injury

Inhalation injury should be suspected in a fire victim under any of the following conditions:

(1) The burn occurred in an enclosed space.

(2) The fire involved toxic chemicals or plastics (this includes many synthetic materials used in clothing and in home furnishings).

(3) The patient has an extensive facial burn.

(4) There is soot in the patient's sputum.

(5) Erythema and edema of the oropharynx are noted.

(6) The patient's voice is hoarse.

In general, the diagnosis of inhalation injury is made by history and physical examination rather than by laboratory or radiologic assessment. The pulmonary interstitial tissue and the small airways are affected before radiologically visible changes develop. If inhalation injury has occurred, tachypnea and agitation heralding respiratory deterioration always develop within the first few days, preceding the appearance of abnormal arterial blood-gas measurements and x-ray findings. The effects of inhalation injury are usually at their worst on the fourth or fifth day and subside within 14 days in survivors.

Erythema, edema, and soot seen on examination of the hypopharynx, larynx, and trachea reliably indicate inhalation injury. The severity of mucosal changes, however, can be either more or less than the severity of physiologic damage. Laryngoscopy and bronchoscopy can be useful in guiding treatment. Chest x-ray films almost always are normal for 24–48 hours and, therefore, are seldom helpful.

Edema of the upper portion of the airway may cause obstruction that is suggested by labored respiration with the use of accessory respiratory

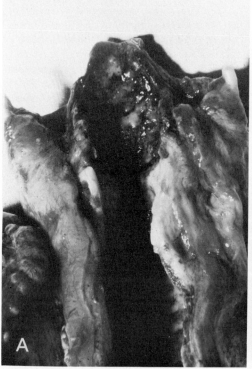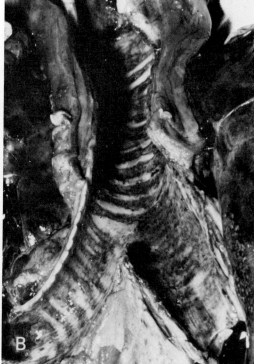

Figure 22.11.   Severe thermal injury of airway. **(A)** Necrosis of epiglottis and larynx. **(B)** Denudation of mucosa of tracheobronchial tree in same patient.

muscles and by sternal retraction. The clinical signs of respiratory insufficiency caused by damage to the lower airway, however, resemble those of pulmonary edema.

When inhalation injury is suspected, treatment should be started immediately. A short-term (12-hour), high-dose course of a corticosteroid compound should be instituted without delay, since these agents are ineffective unless started within a few hours of injury. They are given to reduce the tissue damage caused by toxic inhalation, although clinical and laboratory proof of their efficacy is incomplete. We recommend intravenous administration of methylprednisolone sodium succinate, 10 mg/kg initially, possibly repeating it 12 hours later. Tapered doses thereafter are unnecessary.

Airway obstruction and failing respiration as evidenced by deteriorating arterial blood-gas values are managed best by nasotracheal intubation, although orotracheal intubation may be used if necessary. Tracheotomy should be performed initially only if intubation from above is impossible. Since most of these patients have burns of the face and neck, tracheotomy usually is followed by the development of cervical wound sepsis and bacterial invasion of the tracheobronchial tree, and death from bronchopneumonia usually results. Tracheotomy may be performed safely later if prolonged ventilatory support is required and if there is no local burn. After intubation, a warm mixture of humidified oxygen (usually 40–50%) is administered.

Reluctance to use indwelling nasotracheal tubes for long periods is understandable. In the treatment of a potentially lethal burn injury, however, fear of laryngeal damage by a tube must not interfere with administration of lifesaving support. Plastic endotracheal tubes can be used for 6–8 weeks in most patients without serious permanent laryngeal damage. After long periods of intubation, endoscopic examination of the larynx and trachea should be performed at the time of extubation to assess the adequacy of the upper airway and the need for tracheotomy or reconstruction.

In patients with deteriorating arterial blood-gas values from either alveolocapillary diffusion block or inefficient ventilatory mechanics, assisted ventilation with IPPB is indicated. Positive end-expiratory pressure (PEEP) often is needed as respiratory failure and interstitial pulmonary edema develop. Careful monitoring of central venous pressure during and after fluid replacement is essential to avoid overload and the superimposition of left heart failure and pulmonary edema on the inhalation injury.

A difficult problem encountered frequently is the management of a person brought to the hospital because of "smoke inhalation." Usually the patient recovers after receiving humidified oxygen for 1–2 hours. However, those who show visible evidence of upper airway injury and those injured in fires involving chemicals or plastics should receive corticosteroids and should be hospitalized for short-term observation in case they have been exposed to a potentially lethal agent such as phosgene. Rarely does the inhalation injury syndrome develop later than 2 days after exposure.

With the fact in mind that exposure to carbon monoxide occurs in most fires, management of inhalation injury may be summarized as follows:

(1) Humidified oxygen (100%) should be administered on admission and for 4 hours thereafter.

(2) The patient and the circumstances of the injury should be evaluated.

(3) Laryngoscopic and bronchoscopic examination should be performed if diagnosis is in doubt.

(4) Corticosteroids should be given if inhalation injury is confirmed or strongly suspected.

(5) Nasotracheal intubation should be performed for upper airway edema, plus IPPB and PEEP if respiratory failure develops.

Thermal Injury

In patients with thermal injury to the airway, maximal damage is to the pharynx, larynx, and trachea. Swelling of the hypopharynx and larynx may cause upper airway obstruction. Thermal damage to the tracheobronchial tree is seen occasionally as the result of inhalation of steam or of superheated air by a comatose patient. Tracheal injury that is visible on bronchoscopic examination usually terminates at the level of the carina. Most of these injuries are manifested by erythema and edema; occasionally, necrotic mucosa may slough and produce obstruction unless it is removed endoscopically or by coughing. Severe thermal damage predisposes the airway to invasive sepsis that is rapidly fatal if it is not controlled. Even mild degrees of thermal injury to the trachea lower mucosal resistance to the effects of indwelling tubes and suction catheters.

It may be difficult to determine whether tracheobronchial injury is caused by heat or by toxic gases; often there is a mixture of the two. Bronchoscopic examination is the best method of differentiation. Toxic inhalation injury produces redness and edema to all bronchial divisions, most marked in the lower lobes, whereas thermal injury causes uniform, continuous redness and swelling to a demarcated level that is usually in the trachea (Fig. 22.12). Both findings may be evident in the

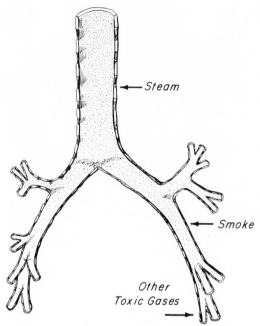

Figure 22.12. Sites of inhalation and thermal injuries. Thermal damage—by steam, for example—involves only the trachea and mainstem bronchi. Smoke damages the entire bronchial tree. Some toxic products of combustion, such as phosgene, produce injury primarily at alveolar level.

same patient. Rarely is the treatment substantially affected by confusion between the two conditions. If there is any evidence of toxic inhalation, corticosteroids should be given.

Management of thermal injury may be summarized as follows: (1) administration of humidified oxygen; (2) evaluation of the patient and the circumstances of the injury; (3) laryngoscopic and bronchoscopic assessment if indicated, obtaining specimens for cultures; (4) nasotracheal intubation if significant edema of the hypopharynx and larynx develops; tracheotomy only if the neck is not burned; (5) administration of broad-spectrum antibiotics intravenously for severe injuries; (6) repeated bronchoscopic removal of mucosal sloughs if needed; (7) extubation as soon as possible; (8) later tracheal reconstruction if indicated.

Other Injuries

Three other respiratory problems can result from major burns: aspiration of vomitus, ventilatory restriction due to circumferential deep burns of the thorax, and early respiratory failure without inhalation injury.

Vomiting occurs after any major trauma and burns are no exception. In approximately 1% of patients with extensive burns, death results from vomiting and aspiration. Gastric dilation and paralytic ileus frequently follow burns, particularly in children. Routine introduction of a nasogastric tube on admission prevents this complication.

Deep circumferential thoracic burns (en cuirasse) restrict ventilation in the same manner that circumferential burns of an extremity impair the circulation. Restricted respiratory motion is visible, and double or triple vertical escharotomies may be needed to release the constriction interfering with motion of the chest wall (Fig. 22.13).

Rarely, early respiratory failure develops after cutaneous burns when there is no inhalation injury. Usually the patient is elderly and the burn is extensive. This phenomenon is poorly understood in humans, although alveolocapillary hyperpermeability and interstitial pulmonary edema readily develop after cutaneous wounds in laboratory animals. The syndrome is similar to shock lung and may be caused by a circulating burn toxin. These patients require the same treatment as do those with inhalation injury.

Pulmonary Aspiration of Gastroesophageal Contents

Despite recognition by Hippocrates more than 2000 years ago and classic descriptions by Hunter, Simpson, Mendelson, and Teabout during the past two centuries, and despite numerous studies during recent years, bronchopulmonary aspiration is still a vexing problem. The setting, risks, methods of prevention, and treatment are known and are not controversial for the most part. Constant attention to detail is required for success; and even then aspiration cannot always be prevented.

The precise frequency of gastropulmonary aspiration is unknown, but some generalities are well documented. After surgery, some degree of gastroesophageal regurgitation occurs about 26% of the time, and pulmonary aspiration may occur in as much as 16% of the time.

About 40% of intubated patients develop some degree of aspiration. Endotracheal cuff inflation can reduce this to 20%, but even careful use of high-volume, low-pressure cuffs on endotracheal tubes does not guarantee protection against aspiration.

The clinical setting in which aspiration occurs is well known. Especially prone are patients with: (1) neurologic and seizure disorders, particularly when consciousness and cough reflex are depressed; (2) drug and alcohol overdosage and anesthesia; (3) poor gastric or esophageal emptying or induced gastric distention (i.e., use of esophageal obturator airways).

Aspiration of solid material causes an entirely

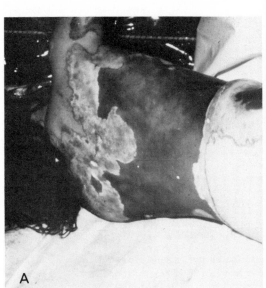
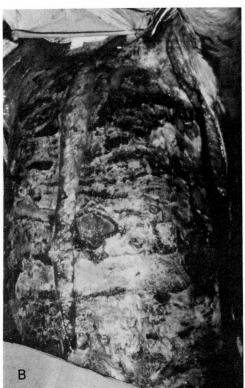

Figure 22.13. **(A)** Deep, circumferential thoracic burn of type that restricts ventilatory motion. **(B)** Vertical escharotomies to release constriction that has persisted after primary excision and skin grafting.

different syndrome from that of inhalation of gastric juice. The former causes airway obstruction manifested by cyanosis, stridor, and labored respiration. It often follows trauma or overindulgence at banquets. The response to the inhalation of gastric contents depends on the pH of the aspirate. It is estimated that 0.3 ml/kg of gastric juice with a pH below 2.5 is needed to produce serious pulmonary damage. This is a chemical injury, clinically identical to the inhalation injury associated with major burns. Massive acid aspiration causes pulmonary edema within minutes, accompanied by bloody bronchorrhea, hypotension, and low cardiac output. Atelectasis, shunting, and infiltrates visible by x-ray develop within 8 hours, the radiologic abnormalities becoming fully developed by 24 hours. Major pathology usually is in the lower lobes. Clinical deterioration (and hypovolemia) continues for 48 hours, with 60% mortality. Aspiration of smaller quantities of acid gastric juice produces a more leisurely, less severe course. The basic pathology is capillary endothelial injury with interstitial edema, surfactant inhibition, reduced compliance, elevated airway pressures, and vascular shunting. In severe cases, thrombosis of segmental pulmonary artery

branches occurs. When ischemia develops in areas of damaged lung, shunting will diminish. Therefore, reduction of the initial degree of shunting after serious aspiration injury actually may be an ominous sign.

The role played by bacterial invasion is variable. Acid gastric juice usually has a sparse bacterial flora. However, patients taking cimetidine or suffering from small bowel obstruction have a rich intestinal flora in their stomachs. In this case, bacterial pneumonia frequently occurs after the initial injury.

The emergency treatment of gastropulmonary aspiration should be keyed to the pathology. When aspiration of particulate matter causes tracheobronchial obstruction, bronchoscopic clearing of the airway is indicated. Laryngeal obstruction may require immediate tracheostomy. When aspiration of liquid gastric contents occurs, thorough endotracheal suctioning should be performed, followed by intubation and intermittent positive-pressure ventilation.

Ventilator therapy probably prevents irreversible pulmonary vascular spasm and thrombosis and thereby reduces mortality. Intravenous restoration of intravascular volume is important; albumin administration is particularly effective, as most of it is retained in the intravascular space. Ventilator therapy should be continued for at least 12 hours. Immediate administration of steroids is beneficial in the laboratory, though unproved clinically. Steroid dosage should be large and brief. Bronchopulmonary lavage is more damaging than helpful. There is experimental evidence that prostacyclin and ibuprofen are beneficial, perhaps because they block release of capillary permeability factors. This information may point the way to future therapy for this type of pulmonary inhalation injury.

A word about prevention in the emergency setting is in order. Trauma victims often have full stomachs and often vomit while partially conscious or during induction for emergency surgery. Prompt insertion of a properly functioning nasogastric tube will prevent needless deaths. The current use of the esophageal obturator airway in resuscitation not only increases the risk of aspiration, but also necessitates gastric deflation afterwards. The administration of intravenous cimetidine to patients prior to emergency surgery will reduce the severity of subsequent aspiration by controlling the gastric pH.

Injury From Ingestion of Caustic Material

Ingestion of a caustic agent results in a series of injuries beginning in the mouth. When a large quantity of caustic material is swallowed, the most severe damage is to the hypopharynx, the middle and lower portions of the esophagus, and the antrum of the stomach.

Although little can be done to counteract the caustic effects of the ingested material except immediate administration of milk or water, several additional emergency measures are necessary. Damage to the mouth and pharynx must be evaluated; since spillover often occurs, injury to the epiglottis and laryngeal structures should be sought and the possibility of aspiration considered. Kerosene frequently produces significant pneumonia. Early visualization of the esophagus and stomach by means of barium contrast study is essential, and the radiologic findings should be confirmed directly by gentle esophagogastroscopy with a minimum of insufflation of air. The latter procedure is accomplished most safely during the first 36 hours, before the danger of perforation becomes maximal; it is essential because the operator can note areas of necrosis heralding impending perforation that may not be apparent radiologically.

Patients who have ingested a caustic agent

should be given antibiotics directed against oral gram-positive organisms and corticosteroids to minimize possible esophageal scarring. In mild to moderately severe cases, good parenteral nutrition is essential while the patient is being observed for evidence of upper gastrointestinal perforation. If endoscopy unequivocally reveals necrosis, the patient should be operated on promptly to resect necrotic segments and to anastomose healthy tissue if possible or to exteriorize the gastrointestinal tract in discontinuity if necessary.

Patients showing no evidence of sepsis or esophageal perforation should swallow a heavy silk or linen thread to enable safe, controlled bougienage to be performed periodically during the first 3–4 weeks. Bougienage will maintain an adequate lumen during the healing period and possibly prevent the need for later resection because of cicatricial stenosis.

NONTRAUMATIC EMERGENCIES

Respiratory Tract

Respiratory failure may be caused by many infectious, inflammatory, neoplastic, and neuromuscular diseases, as well as by drugs and nonspecific processes. The approach to management should be guided by the physiologic defect involved. Respiratory emergencies secondary to alveolocapillary diffusion block caused by pulmonary edema, pneumonia, or other inflammatory disease are discussed elsewhere, along with those due to obstructive airway disease and hypoventilation (see Chapter 9, pages 166–175). If tidal volume falls too low in a patient with a neuromuscular disease such as myasthenia gravis, poliomyelitis, or acute idiopathic polyneuritis, ventilatory assistance may be required.

Mechanical obstruction of the upper airway may be caused by a variety of diseases ranging from infections such as diphtheria to tracheal neoplasms. Emergency treatment depends on the level of obstruction; most patients can be managed by endotracheal intubation or by tracheotomy. Obstruction by a tumor low in the trachea (Fig. 22.14) may necessitate intubation of a mainstem bronchus for acceptable ventilation. Inflammatory obstruction of the larynx can be treated successfully with humidified oxygen in many instances, reserving endotracheal intubation or tracheotomy for severe cases.

Tumors of the trachea or major bronchi may occur at any level, and usually are manifested by a characteristic syndrome consisting of some degree of respiratory obstruction and an audible

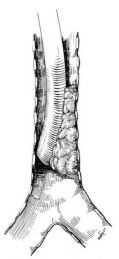

Figure 22.14.   Relief of obstruction caused by tracheal tumor by passage of endotracheal tube down to or past lower limit of tumor.

wheeze; chest x-ray findings often are normal. The proper diagnosis is suggested by radiologic visualization of the trachea, preferably by tomography. Since the airway of these patients is often marginal, any manipulation such as bronchoscopy should be performed only under full operating room conditions with an anesthesiologist available and a long endotracheal tube at hand to pass into a mainstem bronchus, should total obstruction result from bleeding or edema. Bronchoscopic removal of as much tumor as possible to restore an adequate airway is sometimes the best emergency treatment in this difficult situation, allowing time for evaluation and planning of definitive radiation or surgical therapy.

Non-neoplastic stenosis of the trachea causes problems similar to those caused by neoplastic occlusion. Patients who have had tracheotomy or endotracheal intubation may return to the hospital within the year after these events because of progressive stridor due to obstruction. A wheeze usually is audible, and obstruction is frequently more severe than the patient's physician suspects. Obstruction can result early from formation of tracheal granulation tissue or late from cicatricial stenosis after damage from the cuff of an endotracheal tube. When tracheal narrowing is caused by granulations, the diagnosis may be suggested by the irregular contour of the stenotic segment that can be demonstrated by tomographic examination of the trachea and confirmed by bronchoscopy. Emergency treatment consists of bronchoscopic removal of the granulations with cauterization when this is feasible, or passage of an endotracheal

tube through the obstructed zone to relieve acute obstruction, if necessary. Cicatricial stenosis of the trachea is suggested by tapered narrowing that is demonstrated by tomography and confirmed by bronchoscopy. Bronchoscopy should be attempted *only* in the operating room with inhalation anesthesia expertly achieved without intubation. Frequently, this type of stenosis can be dilated somewhat through or by a rigid bronchoscope; this relieves the obstruction and gains time for evaluation and for planning tracheal resection. Fiberoptic bronchoscopy is contraindicated in the presence of tracheal obstruction.

Tracheal obstruction by a foreign body may be an acute emergency, whereas a foreign body in a distal bronchus often causes collapse of the lung distal to it with subacute infection. Foreign bodies should be removed endoscopically as soon as the diagnosis is suggested by history or demonstrated radiologically. After a foreign body has been lodged in a bronchus for more than a few hours, edema forms around it, atelectasis occurs distal to the obstruction, and pneumonitis quickly develops. Endoscopic removal of a chronically impacted foreign body obscured by granulations may be exceedingly difficult; early removal of bronchial foreign bodies will avoid the need for thoracotomy and bronchotomy later.

Occlusion of the superior vena cava by carcinoma, lymphoma, or thrombus brings about a progressive state characterized by edema of the face and neck and often by dyspnea that is the result of tracheal edema. Severe superior vena caval syndrome results in serious ventilatory impairment and requires immediate treatment with humidified oxygen and elevation of the head of the bed, administration of diuretics and corticosteroids. If the obstruction appears to be neoplastic, radiation treatment should begin before histologic confirmation. If these measures fail, intubation and ventilatory assistance may be necessary.

It should be apparent from the foregoing discussion of respiratory emergencies that bronchoscopic instruments are essential in any emergency facility. A rigid bronchoscope saves lives in true emergencies. Most endoscopic examinations for diagnosis and therapy, however, should be performed in the operating room.

Massive Hemoptysis

Although uncommon, massive hemoptysis can be a difficult problem with serious implications. Mortality rates vary with the rapidity of bleeding and often reach 75% if blood loss exceeds 600 ml in 6 hours; asphyxia is the usual cause of death.

Tuberculosis, mycetoma, abscess, bronchiectasis, arteritis, vascular anomalies, and carcinoma are among the causes; thus, serious bleeding may occur at any age, usually from bronchial vessels.

A poor outcome can be avoided only by prompt assessment and vigorous management and by the use of all available techniques. Early steps in management should include crossmatching of several units of blood, placement of a reliable infusion line, and measurement of blood loss as well as vital signs. The patient should lie on the affected side, if known, and should be encouraged to clear the airway by gentle coughing. The cough reflex should not be abolished by sedation. When possible, careful radiographic study is important, because it may outline the diagnosis and localize the source.

Early bronchoscopy is vital. A rigid bronchoscope should be used to clear the bronchial tree of blood and clots and to localize the source, if possible. The fiberoptic bronchoscope is less effective for the removal of large amounts of liquid and clotted blood, but is more likely to permit localization of the source after clearing of the airway. If the source cannot be identified, angiography is indicated.

Control of bleeding must then be obtained. There are three methods available; the proper choice will depend on accuracy of localization, the underlying disease process, and the condition of the patient. The approaches available are (1) endobronchial balloon tamponade, (2) arterial embolization, and (3) surgical resection.

Endobronchial tamponade can be performed by inserting a Fogarty catheter through either rigid or flexible bronchoscopes into the (preferably segmental) bronchus from which the bleeding occurs. If this is the primary method of treatment (as in a poor-risk patient with diffuse lung disease), the balloon should remain inflated for 24 hours. If there is no further bleeding after deflation, the catheter is removed several hours later. In case the primary lesion is surgical and resectable, preliminary balloon tamponade with a Fogarty (for a peripheral lesion) or unilateral endotracheal tube intubation (for a more central lesion) should be used to control the airway during preparation for surgery.

Arterial embolization is an attractive approach in certain situations. When localization of the bleeding site is possible only by bronchial or intercostal angiography, especially in the presence of diffuse pulmonary disease, therapeutic embolization may be done at the same sitting if it will not damage the spinal circulation. This technique also is useful in treatment of recurring hemoptysis in patients who have diffuse benign disease or untreatable tumor.

The key to the management of severe hemoptysis is recognition of its lethal nature and prompt intervention centered on endoscopic localization and/or control.

Pleural Space

A common thoracic emergency, *spontaneous pneumothorax* usually results from rupture of a superficial apical bleb. This may occur at any time; often it occurs in healthy young adults, but it also can be found in middle-aged or elderly patients who have chronic pulmonary disease. Pneumothorax frequently occurs without warning or a predisposing incident, and is manifested by sudden chest pain with varying degrees of dyspnea. Healthy persons may experience relatively little disability, since the leak seals quickly; patients with asthma or emphysema are more severely disabled and often respond to treatment slowly. In either type of patient, initial treatment is the same. A small pneumothorax (less than 20%) either can be observed closely or be managed by anterior needle aspiration if there is no evidence of continuing air leakage. A larger collection of air or pneumothorax with persistent air leakage should be treated by intercostal catheter suction; tube thoracostomy is performed easily by an anterior approach. In the long term, this procedure will shorten the hospital stay. *Tension pneumothorax* (see page 488) is an urgent emergency requiring immediate pleural decompression, often prior to confirming x-ray.

Usually the bleb seals and stable expansion of the lung occurs within a few days. When there is underlying emphysema, however, it is common for air leakage to continue for 7–12 days. If a significant leak persists with no sign of impending closure, active measures must be taken to close it, especially if there have been previous episodes of pneumothorax. Permanent protection against recurrence is particularly necessary in patients who have had contralateral pneumothorax, because spontaneous bilateral pneumothorax can be fatal. Thoracotomy and resection of blebs, along with pleural poudrage or pleurectomy, is an effective therapeutic and preventive measure. There is increasing evidence that intrapleural instillation of topical inflammatory agents such as tetracycline is equally effective. In patients who have serious pulmonary disease, chemical pleurodesis may be much better tolerated than open thoracotomy.

Large *pleural effusions* often require emergency

treatment, whether they are caused by benign or malignant disease. Thoracentesis just below the fluid level that is determined by physical examination usually resolves the urgent problem. "Pleural shock" caused by mediastinal shift can be avoided if the fluid collection is withdrawn slowly. In patients with recurrent malignant pleural effusion, an intercostal thoracostomy tube should be inserted laterally or posterolaterally to permit gradual evacuation of the fluid, followed by intrapleural instillation of an agent such as tetracycline to produce permanent pleural symphysis.

An uncommon emergency, *spontaneous hemothorax* may result from rupture of a bleb or may be caused by systemic disease such as uremia, hemophilia, or a connective-tissue disorder such as rheumatoid disease or lupus erythematosus. Aspiration by needle or catheter should be employed when possible, although thoracotomy may be necessary in cases of clotted and loculated hemothorax. Since fatal hemorrhage is likely if thoracotomy is performed in a hemophilic patient, operation should be avoided if at all possible in the treatment of hemophilic hemothorax.

Empyema also can result in a true emergency. Pleural space collections of purulent material may be caused by hematogenous infection of a pre-existent effusion, by pneumonia or tuberculosis, by perforation of an organ, or by contamination due to a ruptured subphrenic abscess. Regardless of the cause, acute empyema should be confirmed by needle aspiration and drained by intercostal catheter suction, concomitant with antibiotic therapy. If the physician is certain that adjacent pleural symphysis already has occurred, rib resection and open drainage are the proper emergency measures. The timing of open drainage, however, depends largely on the causative organism. In infections caused by streptococci or pneumococci, firm adhesions are slow to develop because of the bacterial production of hyaluronidase, whereas many staphylococcal and mixed infections produce adhesions more rapidly. In the former instance, open drainage must be delayed for 2 weeks to prevent a major collapse of the lung and massive empyema. Open drainage may be performed 1 week after onset of a fibrogenic empyema without fear of pulmonary collapse.

Esophagus

Obstruction

Esophageal obstruction is a fairly common manifestation of a variety of mechanical and motor problems such as strictures, webs, lower esophageal rings, tumors, diverticula, and achalasia. In most cases, the acute incident is precipitated by eating. In children, the usual cause of obstruction is a foreign body such as a coin, usually unaccompanied by esophageal disease. Emergency treatment depends on the nature of the obstructing object, its location as confirmed by barium swallow, and the type of any underlying esophageal disease. An ingested foreign body should be removed promptly. If gentle traction employing a balloon-tipped catheter under fluoroscopic control is unsuccessful, endoscopic removal is indicated. When a bolus of food is producing obstruction, dissolution should be attempted by ingestion of 5 ml of a 1–4% solution of papain every half hour for a total of six doses. If this fails to clear the obstruction, esophagoscopy with mechanical extraction of the bolus is necessary. When the cause of acute esophageal obstruction is unknown, radiologic and endoscopic examinations should be performed, and bougienage may be necessary. Obstruction caused by achalasia or stricture yields temporarily to the passage of a Hurst or Maloney mercury bougie. However, most patients who seek attention for obstruction caused by intrinsic esophageal disease should be admitted for intravenous hydration, diagnostic studies, and appropriate treatment. It should be stressed that obstructive dysphagia does not occur without cause, and it is the duty of the physician to demonstrate that cause.

A few patients seek emergency care because of a large esophageal diverticulum that has progressed to severe, unremitting obstruction. This diagnosis can be suspected by the patient's history, and often is confirmed by gurgling in the neck on palpation and by barium contrast study. Unwise attempts at instrumental manipulation often result in perforation of the diverticulum. Curative operation should be performed after dehydration and malnutrition have been corrected intravenously.

Acute esophagogastric obstruction is sometimes the result of an incarcerated hiatal hernia. This emergency is discussed with other conditions related to the diaphragm (see page 507).

Perforation

Acute perforation of the esophagus may be caused by peptic ulcer, tumor, an ingested sharp object, instrumental manipulation, or trauma. So-called spontaneous perforation of the normal esophagus may occur after retching, usually with an overfilled stomach; the likely mechanism is transmission of elevated intragastric pressure into the esophagus while the glottis and the cricopharyngeal sphincter are closed. By the same mechanism, blunt trauma to the upper part of the abdomen can tear the esophagus; this also commonly occurs proximal to the esophagogastric junction. All types of perforation cause pain, fever, and toxic malaise. Subcutaneous emphysema commonly but not invariably is present, and some bleeding often occurs. The pain may be felt in the upper part of the abdomen, the back, the substernal region, or the neck, depending on the level of perforation. Pleural effusion with subsequent empyema frequently accompanies perforation of the intrathoracic esophagus. The diagnosis can be made if air is visualized in the mediastinum, upper retroperitoneum, or neck on x-ray films. Water-soluble contrast studies should be performed to demonstrate the site of the leak.

The level of perforation is an important determinant of prognosis and treatment. Leaks in the neck have a better prognosis than those located more distally. Frequently they can be treated by antibiotics and observation until the resultant cervical abscess is localized well enough for incision and drainage. Oral feeding must be withheld until the fistula is closed. If perforation is noted during or immediately after instrumentation, however, it is safer to proceed with immediate surgical closure.

Intrathoracic perforation of the esophagus still produces significant mortality and, therefore, is a surgical emergency. Prompt recognition and operative closure are the keys to a successful outcome. The clinical improvement seen after preliminary chest tube drainage of an esophagopleural fistula should not delay operation. Closure is accomplished best while the tissues in the region of the perforation are still reasonably healthy, so it must be done as soon as the diagnosis is confirmed. Location of the leak and the presence of underlying disease dictate the details of the method. If carcinoma is associated with the perforation, emergency esophagectomy may be necessary.

The sharp distinction between the prognosis and treatment of perforations at different levels points out the need for prompt suspicion of and confirmation of the diagnosis, along with precise radiologic location of the perforation. Location by means of endoscopy is not very reliable because the site of perforation often is not visible.

Occasionally, esophageal leaks become evident several days or more after they have occurred. Empyema in the right hemithorax, for example, may develop a week after endoscopic examination, and the barium swallow may or may not demonstrate a leak. Sometimes a dye such as methylene blue that is ingested and then recovered from the pleural space confirms the presence of a small fistula. These subacute situations can be managed conservatively by treatment of the empyema, since mediastinitis has not progressed and since the fistula has closed spontaneously. If mediastinitis is progressive or if the fistula has not closed, these patients also require operation.

Hemorrhage

Esophageal hemorrhage is a relatively uncommon complication of esophagitis, achalasia, and tumor, but is a regular result of gastroesophageal mucosal tears of the Mallory-Weiss type and of esophageal varices (see Chapter 23, page 521). A rare cause of bleeding and partial obstruction is "esophageal apoplexy" which is spontaneous intramural bleeding in the presence of hypertensive arteriosclerotic disease with perforation through the mucosa into the esophageal lumen and decompression of the intramural hematoma.

In most cases, esophageal bleeding subsides without surgical treatment. Persistent, rapid bleeding, however, requires prompt investigation and active management. Gentle nasogastric intubation and iced saline lavage to clear the stomach and esophagus of clots will aid subsequent endoscopic attempts to visualize the bleeding site. Endoscopy should be performed before a barium swallow, because coating of the esophagus with barium obscures the mucosa for at least 24 hours. Should the cause and site of hemorrhage still be unknown after these maneuvers, angiographic demonstration is required. This is a valuable diagnostic aid because uninformed exploration and resection of the esophagus is unacceptable. After the defect is located by angiography, the patient may be treated with injection of vasospastic drugs by way of the feeding vessels if surgical resection is contraindicated. In patients with massive bleeding due to achalasia or esophagitis, however, resection may be lifesaving. In cases of persistent bleeding from Mallory-Weiss or other lacerations, early surgical repair is the treatment of choice.

Acute Esophagitis

A common condition, *reflux (peptic) esophagitis* is sometimes severe, causing pain, esophagospasm, and dysphagia, with occasional perforation or bleeding. In the absence of bleeding or perforation, emergency treatment consists of elevation of the head of the bed, frequent administration of antacids, cimetidine, and antispasmodic agents, and bougienage if there is a stricture. If the diagnosis is suspected, it should be confirmed by esophagoscopy.

Bleeding usually subsides after this conservative regimen. If it does not, a course of vasoconstrictor drugs should be administered by angiographic techniques, and if this fails, emergency esophagectomy must be performed. Perforation at the site of ulceration must be treated by surgical repair or resection as soon as the diagnosis is made.

Infectious esophagitis is an uncommon condition that may be caused by a variety of organisms. In the past, bacteria were the usual infecting agents, but at present the most common organisms are yeasts and fungi that multiply in the esophagus if esophageal bacteria are suppressed by antibiotic therapy for other infections or during chemotherapy or immunosuppressive therapy for malignant conditions. Inflammatory edema and esophagospasm produce pain and dysphagia. The diagnosis is usually evident on examination of the mouth, although esophagoscopy occasionally is necessary for confirmation. Treatment consisting of oral and intravenous fluids and frequent ingestion of antifungal solutions such as nystatin usually brings relief in a few days.

The rare case of bacterial esophagitis requires prompt diagnosis by esophagoscopy and culture, and necessitates early treatment with appropriate antibiotics while parenteral nutrition is maintained.

Esophagospasm

The pain of esophagospasm is a common cause of admission to an emergency facility because of its similarity to cardiac pain. The history is usually diagnostic when there is no conclusive evidence of cardiac disease, and the patient should be asked about the relation of the pain to swallowing and posture and about any history of gastroesophageal disease or emotional tension. Occasionally, formal esophageal manometric studies and acid-perfusion testing are necessary to differentiate esophagospasm from cardiac disease.

A few patients show remarkably obstructive dysphagia due to esophagospasm. Severe motility disorders manifested by tertiary contractions occasionally may be seen in elderly patients. These are caused presumably by a neurologic deficit. No emergency treatment is needed. Also, muscle spasm with intraluminal pressures as high as 200 mm Hg causes obstruction and severe substernal pain in patients with muscular hypertrophy of the esophagus. This diagnosis can be suspected after barium swallow, but must be confirmed by manometric study. Other than reassurance, no emergency treatment is necessary. The symptoms can be relieved only by extensive esophagomyotomy.

Diaphragmatic Hernia

Any type of diaphragmatic herniation may cause a true emergency. Hernias at the foramina of Bochdalek and Morgagni may lead to incarceration and strangulation of upper abdominal viscera. Hiatal hernias cause several types of serious problems:

(1) Paraesophageal hernias, commonly involving incarceration of the gastric fundus, cause bleeding and occasional strangulation.

(2) Large axial hernias may admit small intestine or colon into the intrathoracic sac, where it is obstructed and/or strangulated.

(3) Large axial hernias containing more than one-half of the stomach are subject to the development of gastric volvulus; this often produces complete obstruction with occasional bleeding and gangrene.

All large diaphragmatic hernias usually are suspected first if an air-fluid level is demonstrated on a chest x-ray film. In the absence of pain, fever, leukocytosis, or obstruction, satisfactory emergency treatment may consist of elevation of the head of the bed, administration of intravenous fluids, and gastrointestinal decompression, with repair to follow within a few days. However, persistent obstruction, pain, or bleeding requires early operation. In the case of the large incarcerated axial hiatal hernia, pain and obstruction may be relieved quickly by nasogastric intubation. If this fails or if there is fever, leukocytosis, or reactive pleural effusion indicating gastric necrosis, immediate surgical intervention is mandatory to prevent ischemic perforation, pleuritis, and peritonitis. Because gastric volvulus in huge hiatal hernias usually occurs in elderly patients, it commonly is fatal if operative treatment is delayed.

Suggested Readings

Broe PJ, Toung TJK, Cameron JL: Aspiration pneumonia. *Surg Clin North Am 60*:1551–1564, 1980

Burke JF, Salzman EW: Spontaneous hemopneumothorax in a hemophiliac. *JAMA 169*:623–625, 1959

Culver GA, Makel HP, Beecher HK: Frequency of aspiration of gastric contents by lungs during anesthesia and surgery. *Ann Surg 133*:289–292, 1951

Dor V, Noirclerc M, Chauvin G, et al: Les traumatismes graves du thorax: Place de l'osteosynthese dans leur traitement. *Nouvelle Presse Med 1*:519–523, 1972

Editorial: Massive hemoptysis. *Br Med J 17*:1570, 1978

Garzon AA, Gourin A: Surgical management of massive hemoptysis. *Ann Surg 187*:267–271, 1978

Love JW: Chest injuries. *JAMA 232*:385–387, 1975

Malt RA, Head JM, Sweet RH: Knife wound of the neck, with

transection of the esophagus and contralateral hemopneumothorax. *N Engl J Med 268*:1353, 1963

Moore BP: Operative stabilization of nonpenetrating chest injuries. *J Thorac Cardiovasc Surg 70*:619–630, 1975

Naclerio EA: *Chest Injuries: Physiologic Principles and Emergency Management.* New York. Grune & Stratton, 1971

Shackford SR, Virgilio RW, Peters RM: Selective use of ventilator therapy in flail chest injury. *J Thorac Cardiovasc Surg 81*:194–201, 1981

Strain JD, Moore EE, Markovchick VJ, et al: Cimetidine for the prophylaxis of potential gastric acid aspiration pneumonitis in trauma patients. *J Trauma 21*:49–51, 1981

Swersky RB, Chang JB, Wisoff BG, et al: Endobronchial balloon tamponade of hemoptysis in patients with cystic fibrosis. *Ann Thorac Surg 27*:262–264, 1979

Toung TJ, Cameron JL, Kimura T, et al: Aspiration pneumonia: Treatment with osmotically active agents. *Surgery 89*:588–593, 1981

Trinkle JK, Richardson JD, Franz JL, et al: Management of flail chest without mechanical ventilation. *Ann Thorac Surg 19*:355–363, 1975

Utsunomiya T, Krausz MM, Valeri CR, et al: Treatment of aspiration pneumonia with ibuprofen and prostacyclin. *Surgery 90*:170–176, 1981

CHAPTER 23

Abdominal Emergencies

ASHBY C. MONCURE, M.D.
LESLIE W. OTTINGER, M.D.

The first task of an emergency physician caring for a patient with an abdominal complaint is to arrive at a working diagnosis as promptly as possible. The diagnosis then must be refined on the basis of a complete history, thorough physical examination, and evaluation of laboratory tests and roentgenograms. Valid clinical judgment requires accurate information; inaccurate or incomplete information can be disastrously misleading. Even if a specific diagnosis is not immediately achievable, the physician should be able to ascertain whether a potentially life-threatening condition such as hemorrhage, visceral perforation, or advancing infection seems likely, and consult with a surgeon accordingly.

Since the patient with an abdominal complaint is frequently so uncomfortable and lethargic as to be inaccurate in responding to the examiner's questions, the examiner must compensate for this by being as thorough and specific as possible. If it is feasible, the examiner should ask the patient for a chronologic narrative of his difficulty. Information should include the mode and site of onset of the symptom; the character of any pain, including its extension; the presence or absence of nausea, vomiting, constipation, obstipation, or diarrhea; the character of the vomitus or stool; the presence or absence of fever or chills; previous occurrence of the symptom as well as its constancy or intermittence; and maneuvers employed by the patient to gain relief. Accompanying relatives or friends, as well as previous medical records, can be invaluable in leading the physician to a correct diagnosis. A thorough medical history including previous operations, medications, allergies, and diseases may provide significant information regarding the present illness.

Acute abdominal disease in the elderly may have an atypical presentation, and awareness of this may permit earlier diagnosis. Far-advanced disease may be indicated by only subtle symptoms or signs, presumably due to altered pain threshold and bodily responses. In these patients, repeated abdominal examination may be necessary to diagnose a significant, possibly life-threatening intra-abdominal process.

After the patient is completely disrobed, physical examination should begin with careful evaluation of the vital signs. The physician should ascertain the blood pressure, the presence or absence of fever, and the character and rate of the pulse and respirations. At any point, he may need to establish an adequate airway or to start blood replacement or both before continuing with the examination. He also should note the general appearance of the patient—whether he appears ill, icteric, diaphoretic, or pallid—and his position. If the patient is lying on his back with flexed knees, it may indicate peritoneal irritation.

After the vital signs are evaluated, the physician should examine the skin, head, neck, breasts, chest, abdomen, groins, rectum, pelvis, and extremities. A physical abnormality far from the abdomen may alert the physician to the underlying disease responsible for the patient's abdominal complaint. For example, a patient with abdominal pain who is found to have atrial fibrillation or mitral stenosis may have an embolus in a visceral vessel.

During auscultation, the character of peristalsis should be noted. Peristalsis may be increased in acute gastroenteritis and mechanical intestinal obstruction, and it is commonly diminished or absent in the presence of peritoneal irritation. Audible, normal peristalsis does not exclude the possibility of intra-abdominal inflammation.

Before palpating the abdomen, the examiner should elicit a cough to locate the site of pain; thus he may choose to palpate this area after examining the remainder of the abdomen. The most reliable physical finding indicating peritoneal irritation is the presence of voluntary or involuntary spasm or both. Spasm only can be determined accurately by gently placing the palm of the hand on an abdominal quadrant over the rectus muscle, asking the patient to breathe deeply, and gently depressing the examining hand with the other hand. Voluntary spasm of the rectus muscle will disappear as the patient exhales, whereas involuntary spasm will not. In the latter instance, the muscle will feel tense and boardlike.

The exact area of tenderness should be noted by gentle palpation with one finger. This may suggest the viscus affected by the intra-abdominal process. On removal of the hand pressing near the tender area, rebound tenderness may be felt in the primary site of pain, providing further evidence of peritoneal irritation. The flanks should be carefully palpated along with the lower part of the chest wall. An inflammatory process adjacent to the retroperitoneum is suggested by pain elicited on extension of the iliopsoas or obturator muscle.

The patient should be examined for masses, hepatosplenomegaly, and free fluid within the abdominal cavity. If dullness and tenderness coincide on gentle percussion, a mass should be sought in this location. Herniation through a previous abdominal incision also should be sought.

The groins must be examined carefully and gently in all patients. The scrotum is invaginated with the index finger to permit palpation of the external inguinal ring and the inguinal canal, where a mass usually indicates a hernia. An indirect inguinal hernia is palpable as an elliptical mass descending along the cord, usually descending further with cough or Valsalva's maneuver. A direct inguinal hernia is palpable as a globular mass close to the pubis. A femoral hernia is more difficult to outline because the empty space of the femoral canal, where the herniation occurs, is not distinctly palpable. The readily identifiable structure in the femoral canal is the pulsating femoral artery as it emerges from under the inguinal ligament. Therefore, after identifying the femoral artery, the examiner should search for the hernia two fingerbreadths medial to this structure.

The inguinal region is more difficult to assess in women because the labia cannot be invaginated. It is examined by placing the finger in the area of the external ring and then the palm of the hand over the area of the internal ring and having the patient cough as each area is examined. The femoral region is examined as in men. If at all possible, the examination should be conducted with the patient in both supine and standing positions.

Pelvic and rectal examinations must be carried out to evaluate the patient's condition completely. Pelvic examination is described in Chapter 24, page 526. To inspect the anus and rectum thoroughly, they must be palpated and endoscopic examination of the rectum must be performed. Extreme pain on introduction of the palpating finger usually indicates acute inflammation or stenosis of the anal canal, and further efforts to examine this area should be postponed. Usually, after moderate resistance, the sphincter relaxes and the finger can be advanced to examine the rectum circumferentially. The prostate gland or the area of the pouch of Douglas also should be palpated. Sigmoidoscopic examination may provide further information.

Laboratory tests should include a complete blood cell count, urinalysis, examination of the stool specimen for occult blood, and determination of the blood glucose, blood urea nitrogen, and serum amylase levels. Hematocrit determinations can be repeated easily and frequently. Although the hematocrit value cannot be employed as the sole guide to suspected blood loss or changes in plasma volume, it frequently is used in conjunction with blood pressure, pulse, urinary output, and central venous pressure. A low initial hematocrit reading suggests an antecedent chronic illness, chronic gastrointestinal blood loss, or acute hemorrhage.

The white blood cell count usually is elevated in inflammatory conditions, although it occasionally may be normal early in the course of acute disease. In the elderly, it may be within normal limits even in the presence of marked intra-abdominal inflammation. If the white blood cell count is normal, an abnormal differential may suggest an inflammatory process. In the presence of inflammation, there is usually an increased number of polymorphonuclear leukocytes and band forms as well as toxic granulation within leukocytes.

Determination of the platelet count, prothrombin time, and partial thromboplastin time is necessary in patients with hemorrhage. Measurement of serum electrolyte levels is valuable in patients with gastrointestinal losses either from vomiting, diarrhea, or intraluminal sequestration accompanying intestinal obstruction. In all patients with abdominal pain, even children, the serum amylase and lipase levels should be determined.

In patients with abdominal pain or trauma, paracentesis may rapidly alert the physician to the presence of free blood, bile, or purulent material. A negative tap, however, does not exclude the presence of abdominal fluid. Paracentesis may be performed with a long, 19-gauge needle on a small syringe passed through a locally anesthetized area lateral to the rectus muscle in each abdominal quadrant. It also may be accomplished by percutaneous placement of a polyethylene catheter through the midline in the lower abdominal area in patients who have not undergone any previous abdominal operation. This should be done after the patient has voided. Gram staining and culture of the obtained fluid should be done, the fluid should be examined for amylase content and red and white blood cell counts should be performed.

Roentgenographic examination of the patient with an abdominal complaint is essential, and should include abdominal films with the patient both supine and upright; both diaphragms should be shown in the latter position. If the patient cannot be upright, a left lateral decubitus film should be obtained. If an intravenous pyelogram is indicated, it may be obtained while the plain films are being taken. A chest film is essential, since lower thoracic processes can cause abdominal pain. Angiographic examination may be used to evaluate patients with trauma and those in whom an occluded visceral vessel or a dissecting aneurysm is suspected. Radioactive scanning may be helpful in evaluating the liver and spleen after trauma. Barium or water-soluble contrast examination of the intestine may be necessary to define suspected disease further. Since coronary thrombosis occasionally may cause upper abdominal pain, an electrocardiogram should be recorded in patients more than 25 years old.

As stated previously, after collecting all pertinent information, the clinician must establish a working diagnosis by weighing probabilities. If he or she thinks that the patient's life is threatened, consultation with a surgeon to decide whether operation is necessary is advisable. If he or she does not suspect a serious intra-abdominal process, a plan must be formulated for further diagnosis and for treatment. Therapy may involve hospital admission or outpatient care with follow-up evaluation. In the latter case, if the patient is seen later with the same complaint, he probably should be hospitalized for further diagnostic studies.

ACUTE ABDOMEN

General Considerations

In almost all nontraumatic abdominal emergencies, the correct diagnosis can be established with a detailed history and careful physical examination alone, laboratory tests usually being needed only for diagnostic confirmation. In many instances of acute abdominal pain, however, the patient may require supportive therapy before a diagnosis can be made. For example, as soon as the presence of diffuse purulent peritonitis is detected and before the surgeon establishes the cause at laparotomy, the physician should start intravenous antibiotic therapy, volume replacement, and other supportive measures. The management of the painful acute abdomen, therefore, requires a two-fold approach. On the one hand, the physician must protect against the hazards of the underlying pathologic process. On the other hand, he cannot treat the patient definitively until the diagnosis is established. Diagnostic and therapeutic procedures in many instances must proceed simultaneously, each giving way to the other under appropriate circumstances. Because of these dual considerations—diagnosis and therapy—it is important that the overall responsibility for treatment of the patient be delegated to one person. Transfer of responsibility to another individual must follow a formal procedure, and all those caring for the patient must know whom to consult for decisions relating to priority of therapeutic and diagnostic measures.

In taking the patient's history, the physician should give special attention to the onset and character of the pain. Time of onset, the quality and site of the pain at onset, changes in its site and character, whether it has interrupted or prevented sleep, and any exacerbating or relieving factors should, if possible, be determined. Such factors can include eating, defecation, micturition, walking, coughing, and changes in truncal position. Although some patients may be unable to describe the pain clearly, the physician should try to determine the degree of localization of the pain, its sharpness or dullness, its periodicity, whether it has been uniform since onset, or whether it has diminished or even disappeared.

Types of Pain

Abdominal pain can be characterized as visceral or somatic, that is, originating from a viscus or from parietal peritoneum, abdominal wall, or retroperitoneal tissues. Although it is clear that these dissimilar types of pain result from a difference in distribution of pain receptors, the neurologic pathways for transmission of each type are not understood fully.

The surfaces of the abdominal viscera contain pain receptors similar to those in the skin, but in the viscera, these receptors are widely spaced. Thus, these organs are relatively insensitive to localized stimuli, such as cutting or crushing. Diffuse stimulation of nerve endings such as that caused by forceful contraction of the smooth muscle or occlusion of the blood supply is the usual cause of visceral pain. On the other hand, tissues of somatic segments contain a higher concentration of pain receptors, and stimuli of many types evoke pain in these areas.

Visceral pain is typical of such conditions as acute obstruction of the small intestine, passage of a calculus through the urinary tract, and acute obstruction of the common bile duct. As a result of its diffuseness and other characteristics, patients sometimes have difficulty in describing visceral pain clearly. Afferent nerve fibers traverse the intestinal ganglia and enter the spinal cord in such a way that it is usually impossible for the patient with an intestinal condition to discern whether the course of pain is on the right or the left side; for example, pain arising from either the right or the left colon usually is perceived in the midline of the lower part of the abdomen. This principle does not apply to the urinary tract, however. Even though visceral pain of gastrointestinal origin usually is referred to the midline, the level in the longitudinal axis often does reflect the source. Pain from the biliary tree or duodenum may be felt in the epigastrium, that from the small intestine in the umbilical region, and that from the colon inferior to the umbilicus. Visceral pain often has a gripping or cramping quality because it usually is produced by rhythmic peristaltic spasms. It can, however, be due to severe intestinal ischemia, in which case the precise mechanism of pain stimulation is unclear. Although severe spasm of intestine deprived of its arterial blood supply sometimes may provide the stimulus, ischemic abdominal pain can last long after the intestinal spasm, and in fact, ischemia alone may cause the pain. Severe, diffuse, anterior abdominal distress unrelieved by narcotics is characteristic of visceral ischemia; unfortunately, the symptoms are too nonspecific to allow quick diagnosis.

Somatic pain usually is differentiated easily from visceral pain. The patient can specify its location fairly accurately, and will describe it as sharp, burning, or tearing. Since somatic pain is the result of irritation or injury to a specific area of tissue, it can be exacerbated by pressure or change in position.

Referred pain more often is misleading than helpful in making a diagnosis, since visceral pain may be perceived as if it originated from a somatic segment because of crossover between visceral and somatic afferent nerve pathways. On the body surface, referred pain is located at the dermatome of the segment from which the viscus developed in the embryo. A striking example of referred pain is that which accompanies the passing of a renal calculus. Pain appears in the right flank, and moves obliquely across the flank into the groin and even into the labium or testis before it is relieved by passing of the calculus into the bladder. Gallbladder discomfort can be referred to the middle and lower regions of the right scapula. Frequently, somatic pain from the diaphragm is referred to the posterior aspect of the ipsilateral shoulder down to the middle of the scapula. Referred diaphragmatic pain is particularly important in the early detection of upper abdominal peritoneal irritation.

Causes of Peritoneal Irritation

Inflammatory reactions such as perforation of the appendix, perforation of a colonic diverticulum, and cholecystitis irritate the parietal peritoneum, resulting in somatic pain. Local irritation due to a well entrenched infectious process rather than the mere presence of bacteria seems to produce this symptom. For example, when perforation of the colon occurs and large numbers of bacteria escape into the peritoneal cavity, signs of peritoneal irritation do not appear until the infection is established.

Several types of fluid may cause somatic pain when released into the peritoneal cavity. Blood may or may not evoke such pain. For example, in the case of a hemorrhaging ectopic pregnancy, the patient either may have signs and symptoms suggesting severe, diffuse peritonitis or have a distended but otherwise normal abdomen. The fluid from a tumor can be exceedingly irritating to parietal peritoneum; such irritation occurs most commonly with ruptured ovarian cysts, and patients may have the symptoms of acute, diffuse peritonitis. Bile and urine usually cause severe peritoneal irritation.

The most acid contents of the digestive organs are the most irritating. Gastric acid evokes immediate and severe symptoms, whereas the intestinal contents, with a more neutral pH, cause symptoms only after the onset of bacterial peritonitis. Because there are few bacteria in the small intestine, such a perforation may not cause signs of peritoneal irritation for many hours.

Specific Conditions

Noninflammatory Perforations

Distal Esophageal Perforation. Spontaneous perforation of the distal portion of the esophagus usually is not associated with preceding pathologic esophageal changes. Since the perforation, which is usually a linear tear, occurs near the stomach, gastric contents and gas are released into the mediastinum and the left or, occasionally, the right pleural space. Onset of pain is sudden, and symptoms resemble those of a perforated peptic ulcer; in some patients perforation occurs soon after a heavy meal or forceful vomiting. Severe epigastric pain is the most typical feature. On physical examination there is little evidence of peritoneal irritation in the upper part of the abdomen. This combination of severe pain and absent physical signs should alert the physician to the diagnosis. Thoracic symptoms related to the presence of infected pleural fluid appear late. A chest roentgenogram showing fluid and possibly gas in the pleural space adds additional support to the diagnosis (Fig. 23.1); an early film may show only mediastinal air. If the diagnosis remains obscure, contrast studies may be employed, but a water-soluble contrast solution should be used in place of barium. The physician should immediately administer antibiotics and start volume replacement. It is important to diagnose this condition early, since mortality increases in accordance with delay in operation.

Gastric Ulcer or Tumor. In patients with a perforated gastric ulcer or tumor, symptoms often develop gradually because these lesions frequently occur in the presence of a low level of gastric acid secretion. The patient experiences epigastric pain with occasional referral to the shoulders. There may be a history of the rather nonspecific symptoms of gastric ulcers and tumors: changes in tolerance for food, gnawing visceral pain in the upper part of the abdomen, and weight loss. Except when a tumor is strongly suspected, laparotomy should take precedence over contrast studies.

Duodenal Ulcer. Because a duodenal ulcer usually is associated with normal or high levels of gastric acid secretion, its perforation is frequently accompanied by the dramatic onset of symptoms. Key information in the history may be either longstanding duodenal ulcer disease or recent epigastric distress and heartburn. Upper abdominal, peritoneal, and diaphragmatic irritation is common, producing prominent findings on palpation. Conversely, if the amount of escaped gastric contents and acid is small, the entire presentation may be surprisingly subtle. The first strong evidence of such a perforation may be free air under the diaphragm on roentgenographic examination. Contrast studies of the upper part of the gastrointestinal tract may not demonstrate a peptic ulcer perforation if it has been sealed off by adjacent structures. If the physician suspects a perforation

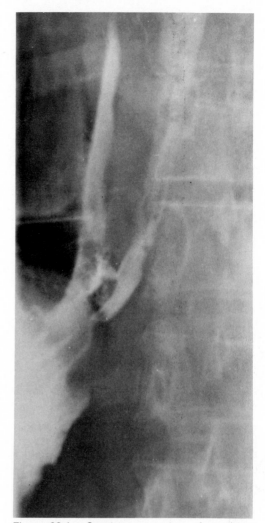

Figure 23.1. Spontaneous rupture of esophagus (Boerhaave's syndrome) confirmed by water-soluble contrast study (lateral view).

nasogastric decompression should be started. Colloid loss from peritoneal surfaces injured by released acid may be very high, and the physician should anticipate the need for replacement.

Meckel's Diverticulum. Although perforation of a Meckel's diverticulum may occur, this happens so rarely that preoperative establishment of the diagnosis is unusual. Perforation often results from ulceration related to heterotopic gastric mucosa within the diverticulum.

Colonic Perforation. When unrelated to inflammatory conditions, most perforations of the colon occur in the cecum. Obstructing carcinoma in the left colon or severe impaction can cause dilatation and perforation with release of gas and other colonic contents. Since these do not cause much irritation to peritoneal surfaces, signs of peritonitis develop gradually as bacterial infection becomes established. Decompression of the colon is not a necessary sequel to perforation; often a colon dilated with gas is noted on the plain roentgenogram despite the presence of free gas. As a rule, perforation should be considered imminent when the diameter of the cecum exceeds 12 cm. Parenteral antibiotics should be administered immediately. A contrast study of the left colon can guide the surgeon in correct management, but contamination of the peritoneal cavity with barium may result.

Pelvic Conditions. The contents of a perforated ovarium tumor, especially of an endometrioma, may prove strongly irritating to peritoneal surfaces. Sudden onset of severe lower or diffuse abdominal pain is the first sign of such a perforation. Bleeding from an ectopic pregnancy may produce the same symptom. However, since the peritoneum is not necessarily sensitive to the presence of blood, somatic pain may be absent and hypovolemic shock may ensue without warning. The character of preceding menstrual periods often suggests either an endometrioma or ectopic pregnancy; this is not true with most ovarian cysts.

Inflammatory Conditions

Cholecystitis. The precise mechanism of mild attacks of cholecystitis is unclear. In some patients, obstruction of the cystic duct by a calculus generates visceral symptoms of upper abdominal discomfort and fullness. In others, an inflammatory reaction occurs that causes somatic pain. In severe episodes of cholecystitis, inflammation of the parietal peritoneum over the gallbladder causes characteristic sharp, burning distress in the right upper abdominal quadrant. Referral of pain to the right scapular region sometimes occurs in mild episodes, and is common in severe attacks.

Most mild episodes of cholecystitis are of short duration, and the patient usually attributes them to indigestion. An atttack severe enough to cause a patient to seek emergency care is likely to be different. Often it will have started a few hours after a meal. The pain may have wakened the patient during the night and then intensified, reflecting an increasingly inflammatory component with resultant somatic signs. Plain roentgenograms show gallstones in only about 20% of patients. The oral cholecystogram is also of limited value in the diagnosis of acute cholecystitis. If normal gallbladder function is demonstrated, cholecystitis can be excluded. The converse is not true, however, since abnormal or absent function can occur in several other disorders besides cholecystitis, such as pancreatitis and acute gastroenteritis.

Imaging techniques utilizing ultrasound or computed tomography can reliably demonstrate the presence of gallstones. Radioisotope scanning techniques may also be used to evaluate gallbladder function. These diagnostic tools must be used in the proper context, and over-reliance on them can lead to serious errors in management.

An attack of cholecystitis lasting longer than a few hours can lead to such complications as gangrene, perforation, and empyema. The patient should be hospitalized and treated with parenteral antibiotics, nasogastric decompression, and operation when appropriate.

Cholangitis. This is a bacterial infection within the hepatic ducts associated with partial obstruction of the common hepatic duct either by calculus, stricture, or less commonly, tumor. The gallbladder sometimes is involved. A careful history may elucidate the cause of the obstruction. The patient complains of gradually increasing discomfort in the epigastrium and back. This pain has both visceral and somatic components, and often is deceptively mild. Tenderness in the right upper abdominal quadrant is a sign of accompanying inflammation of the gallbladder. Scleral icterus sometimes is present, a finding seldom seen with uncomplicated cholecystitis. The physician often can demonstrate tenderness of the liver by gentle percussion with the fist over the right hepatic lobe. Because the bacteria in the biliary radicles are disseminated readily into the bloodstream, a high incidence of septicemia occurs as a complication of cholangitis. The physician should immediately start antibiotic therapy and prepare the patient for surgical decompression of the obstructed biliary tree.

Pancreatitis. The diagnosis of acute pancreatitis is one of the most difficult to make on the basis of history and physical findings alone. The patient with an acute attack usually can give a specific time that symptoms began. Pain commonly is experienced in the upper part of the abdomen, and may extend to the back. Nausea, anorexia, and vomiting are frequent. On examination, upper abdominal tenderness is ordinarily deeper than that caused by a perforated peptic ulcer, for example. Sometimes the examiner can palpate a tender mass in the upper part of the abdomen. If pancreatitis is suspected, confirmation by laboratory tests is essential. Fortunately, the serum amylase determination is a fairly reliable test for acute pancreatitis. Early management includes nasogastric decompression, colloid replacement, and antibiotic therapy.

Patients with chronic or relapsing pancreatitis often have a history suggesting the diagnosis. Each attack may mimic acute pancreatitis, but there are usually fewer physical findings. The serum amylase level is frequently normal. Recurrent attacks sometimes may be caused by a chronic pseudocyst that may be palpable in the upper part of the abdomen.

Duodenal Ulcer. Unless perforation occurs, duodenal ulcers seldom cause sufficiently intense symptoms to be abdominal emergencies. A posterior perforation may result in pancreatic inflammation that in its early stages cannot be distinguished from pancreatitis due to other causes. This type of attack, however, tends to be mild.

Regional Enteritis. This chronic disease, distinguished by long-standing symptoms of intermittent abdominal cramps, diarrhea, and weight loss, is seldom an acute condition. Occasionally, perforation of the small intestine occurs, and the resultant abscess may dissect along tissue planes and emerge at a remote location such as the femoral area or the flank. The physician should suspect the diagnosis from the history and the presence of these abscesses.

Some attacks involving the terminal portion of the ileum are not preceded by chronic symptoms, and may be indistinguishable from acute appendicitis. A mass in the right lower abdominal quadrant frequently is palpable; this alone does not confirm the diagnosis. Since barium studies are contraindicated in the possible presence of appendicitis, the diagnosis is usually established at operation.

Colitis. Patients with ulcerative colitis are less likely than those with regional enteritis to be seen initially with acute abdominal pain. Many days of increasingly severe cramps, nausea, and diarrhea customarily precede the somatic pain caused by toxic dilatation and perforation of the intestine. Usually the patient's chief complaint is bloody diarrhea. Sigmoidoscopic examination often strongly suggests the diagnosis. Sometimes the disease may have progressed to the toxic stage, with fever and abdominal distention, but not pain, being the distinguishing signs.

Patients with granulomatous colitis have the same general symptoms and signs as patients with regional enteritis or ulcerative colitis, and abdominal pain without a suggestive history is unusual.

Appendicitis. Perhaps more has been written about acute appendicitis and its diagnosis than about any other process causing abdominal pain. The diagnosis, however, frequently is missed, especially in very young and very old patients. Typically, the patient describes recent revulsion to food and visceral pain in the middle of the abdomen as the initial symptoms. Symptoms of non-

specific gastroenteritis such as diarrhea and vomiting sometimes may precede appendicitis. As local peritoneal irritation develops, the patient experiences sharp somatic pain in the right lower abdominal quadrant. The local inflammatory process, particularly in the presence of an abscess, sometimes forms a palpable tender mass. It is important to remember that with acute appendicitis a completely typical presentation is the exception.

Mesenteric Adenitis. An inflammation of the lymph nodes in the mesentery of the terminal portion of the ileum, mesenteric adenitis may simulate appendicitis, although the history is likely to be less precise and the physical findings are usually less well localized. Unless improvement is observed within a few hours, laparotomy is necessary to establish the diagnosis.

Carcinoma of the Cecum. The neoplasm sometimes results in perforation because of necrosis or because of cecal dilatation behind the tumor. A palpable mass and positive stool guaiac test may indicate the correct diagnosis, but often the signs resemble those of appendicitis. If a perforated malignant lesion of the cecum is suspected, laparotomy without roentgenographic studies other than plain films is preferable in most patients.

Colonic Diverticulum. If a diverticulum of the right colon becomes perforated, the symptoms also may mimic those of appendicitis. Diverticula of this type are most common in patients of Oriental extraction. Again, laparotomy is preferable to roentgenographic studies in establishing the diagnosis.

Perforation associated with a diverticulum is more likely to occur in the distal portion of the sigmoid colon than in the transverse or right colon. Occasionally, the perforation occurs without chronic symptoms. Patients have a recent history of obstipation or diarrhea, along with increasingly severe somatic pain in the left lower part of the abdomen, the pelvis, and the perineum. Left lower abdominal and suprapubic tenderness is typical. The involved segments occasionally may lie so deep within the pelvis that only on vaginal and rectal examination can tenderness be appreciated. Edema and abscesses associated with perforated sigmoid diverticula produce a boggy and often ill-defined mass whose size and discreteness may indicate the severity of the septic process. Abscesses usually are contained by contiguous structures, but occasionally may rupture into the peritoneal cavity, causing symptoms and signs of diffuse peritonitis in the lower part of the abdomen. In patients in whom the sigmoid colon lies to the right of the midline, signs of perforation may be confused with those of appendicitis, although the history is usually different. Since barium studies frequently are deceptively normal in patients with perforating sigmoid diverticulosis, they should not be relied on in making the diagnosis.

Pelvic Inflammatory Disease. Acute paracervicitis, salpingitis, and tubo-ovarian abscesses with contiguous inflammatory changes, which usually are categorized together as pelvic inflammatory disease, may simulate most of the aforementioned inflammatory conditions of the lower part of the abdomen. A careful history is the chief means of establishing the diagnosis. Pelvic inflammatory disease usually occurs in young, sexually active women. Frequently, the patient reports previous similar episodes. The physical findings are diffuse lower abdominal tenderness, fever, and higher white blood cell count than would be associated with other suspected diagnoses. Laparoscopic examination is sometimes of great value when the diagnosis is in doubt. Response to antibiotics may be dramatic. Surgical exploration, however, is sometimes necessary to drain an abscess or to exclude the presence of a septic process unrelated to the pelvic genital structures.

Perihepatitis (Fitz-Hugh-Curtis syndrome) is an unusual complication of gonococcal pelvic inflammatory disease characterized by upper abdominal peritonitis, especially on the right, with somatic pain. On auscultation, a rub may be heard over the liver. Unless the pelvic symptoms and signs are florid, the condition is likely to be confused with acute cholecystitis. It responds rapidly to antibiotics.

Gastroenteritis. Acute gastroenteritis is common among younger patients, and may be confused with many of the conditions previously discussed. Causes include bacteria, enteric viruses, amoebae, and other gastrointestinal irritants. Recent nausea, vomiting, diarrhea, and cramping visceral pain are typical complaints. The physician may elicit a description of similar symptoms among the patient's acquaintances. Tenderness may be found on abdominal examination, but is usually minimal and poorly localized. A few hours of observation often confirm the diagnosis.

Obstruction

Gastric Obstruction. Acute gastric obstruction usually occurs at the pylorus. It is most often the result of scarring from chronic peptic ulcer disease, but also may be produced by pyloric edema and spasm. The patient commonly gives a history of peptic ulcer symptoms and recent vomiting. He or she may have acute abdominal pain. A hugely dilated stomach may be noted, and diagnosis can be confirmed by aspiration of gastric contents. Gastric tumors and bezoars rarely lead to acute obstruction, tending instead to produce chronic partial obstruction.

A rather unusual cause of acute gastric obstruction is incarceration of a large paraesophageal hiatal hernia. These hernias may not be associated with a history of esophageal reflux, although the patient may experience postprandial discomfort due to distention of the herniated portion. Physical findings usually are lacking, although bleeding can suggest strangulation. Diagnosis may be suggested by a chest roentgenogram, especially if a nasogastric tube has been inserted.

Intestinal Obstruction. In its early stages, obstruction of the small intestine is associated with anorexia and intermittent visceral pain. In its acute stage, it usually provokes forceful peristaltic contractions proximal to the block, which lead to intense cramping pain. As the obstructed loops dilate, peristalsis ceases. Pain may subside and be replaced by the sensation of abdominal distention. Since some episodes of obstruction of the small intestine are spontaneously relieved, a history of prior similar attacks may be elicited.

In most patients, vomiting occurs. If the upper portion of the small intestine is obstructed, it may begin within 1 or 2 hours of the onset of pain. If the site is more distal, many hours may elapse before vomiting begins. The vomitus is initially light brown and thin, being the contents of the stomach and duodenum. Later, as contents of the small intestine reflux into the stomach, the vomitus becomes more viscid and opaque, and is often dark brown and foul smelling. As the intestinal muscular layers proximal to the obstruction become stretched and flaccid, vomiting may cease. Distal to the obstruction there is still active peristalsis, so it is common for defecation to occur after the onset of pain. However, obstipation eventually develops.

Physical examination in the early stages of obstruction reveals no tenderness, and bowel sounds may seem normal. Later, as loops of intestine become dilated, the tone of peristalsis becomes cavernous or high pitched. Borborygmi, frequently described but seldom observed vigorous rushes of peristaltic sound, are probably present only during the earliest stages of obstruction.

Postoperative adhesions are the most common cause of obstruction of the small intestine in adults, and the history often includes a previous abdominal operation. Another cause of obstruction is abdominal hernia. The physical examination should include a search for a hernia in the umbilical region, at previous abdominal incisions, and in the inguinal and femoral regions. A femoral hernia in an obese patient easily may be overlooked. When intestine incarcerated in a hernia is the cause of obstruction, the hernial mass is almost always tender, even after long-standing incarceration. Obstruction also may be caused by intussusception due to an intraluminal lesion such as a polyp. In the case of intussusception, the resultant mass is sometimes palpable. Bleeding from vascular compromise of the intussuscipiens may occur.

Less common causes of obstruction of the small intestine are metastatic peritoneal implants and incarceration of intestinal loops in internal hernias. The former diagnosis often is established by the history. Volvulus involving the cecum, the sigmoid colon, the small intestine around an adhesion, or the midportion of the ileum about the superior mesenteric artery is another cause of mechanical obstruction. Plain abdominal roentgenograms with upright and supine views are usually all that is needed to confirm the diagnosis of intestinal obstruction (Fig. 23.2), regardless of the cause.

The presence of severe, steady pain in a patient with intestinal obstruction suggests vascular compromise of a segment of intestine, which may occur with volvulus of any kind, intussusception, or strangulation of an incarcerated hernia. In the presence of pain of this type, the potential for infarction dictates urgent surgical management.

Mechanical obstruction of the colon is a treacherous condition ordinarily caused by a left-sided carcinoma. Malignant lesions in the colon tend to spread circumferentially through the lymphatics, narrowing the lumen so that it tends to become blocked by fecal material. Fecal impaction can also cause colonic obstruction.

If the ileocecal valve does not permit reflux of colonic contents into the small intestine, the colon may become greatly distended while the small intestine remains normal, in which case there is no vomiting to indicate blockage. Perhaps because peristaltic activity in the colon is less vigorous than in the small intestine, the patient may report very little pain. Passage of a small, often watery stool at the onset of symptoms is common, and is followed by obstipation. Abdominal examination may reveal minimal distention, although cavernous bowel sounds are usually detected on auscultation. It is necessary to establish an early diagnosis because spontaneous perforation may occur if the colonic contents cannot reflux into the small intestine.

Plain roentgenograms with the patient in the supine and upright positions are a mainstay in the diagnosis of obstruction. Expert interpretation is essential, since obstructed loops may be filled with fluid rather than gas. Confirmation of the diagnosis of colonic obstruction may be obtained by sigmoidoscopic examination and barium studies.

Initial treatment of any patient suspected of intestinal obstruction should include the placement of a nasogastric tube to prevent aspiration of vomitus. The physician should anticipate loss of large amounts of fluid high in protein and electrolytes into obstructed loops of intestine and arrange for fluid replacement. Although long tubes may be used for intestinal decompression, surgical exploration is the primary form of treatment in all but a few cases.

Ischemia

Although abdominal pain due to intestinal ischemia is seen infrequently in the emergency facility, it deserves stress for two reasons. First, the signs and symptoms are so nonspecific that the diagnosis is exceedingly elusive. Second, salvage of a sufficient length of intestine for normal long-term survival may depend on early diagnosis and operative intervention.

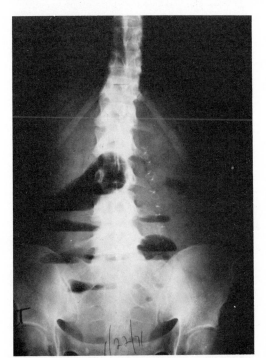

Figure 23.2. Plain roentgenogram of abdomen in patient with ileal obstruction secondary to postoperative adhesion (upright view).

Intestinal Infarction. Regardless of the cause, intestinal infarction is a surgical emergency. The major causes of intestinal infarction are arterial thrombosis and embolization, venous occlusion, occlusion of small arteries resulting from arteritis, and occlusion of the major visceral arteries resulting from dissection of the abdominal aorta. Intestinal infarction also can develop in patients without any discoverable obstruction of a major vein or artery.

Whatever the cause, the initial response of ischemic intestine and the symptoms are the same. Submucosal edema occurs first, followed by mucosal infarction that produces intraluminal bleeding. The muscular layers respond initially with intense spasm and then with loss of tone and dilatation. Spasm often leads to vomiting and diarrhea. Perforation follows after a variable length of time.

As has been noted, all patients with intestinal infarction have pain as a presenting symptom. Although pain is visceral because it results from muscular spasm, it persists even after the intestine becomes dilated, tending to be intense, poorly localized, and steady rather than cramping. Onset of pain may be gradual or abrupt; sudden onset is typical of pain caused by an embolus. Intestinal infarction may develop in some patients with a history of episodic intestinal angina, which is characterized by postprandial abdominal pain and weight loss over the period of the attacks.

In the early stages of intestinal infarction, nothing unusual can be found on abdominal examination. Except for occult blood in the gastric and rectal contents, there is a puzzling absence of abnormal physical findings in these patients, who appear to be suffering from a major abdominal catastrophe.

Leukocytosis is a common but not invariable sign of intestinal infarction. In many instances, the higher the white blood cell count, the more extensive the infarction. The serum amylase level usually is elevated somewhat. Plain abdominal roentgenograms may show characteristic signs of infarction, but usually do not. Early selective angiographic examination is sometimes diagnostic when the infarction is caused by an arterial thrombus or embolus.

Ischemic Colitis. This process perhaps is associated with both impaired vascular supply and bacterial invasion of colonic segments, and it must be differentiated from colonic infarction resulting from major arterial or venous occlusion. The patient usually describes left-sided abdominal pain and bloody diarrhea without previous episodes.

On physical examination, there is tenderness in the region of the involved colonic segment, which is almost invariably the descending colon from the splenic flexure to the middle of the sigmoid. Contrast studies usually demonstrate characteristic "thumbprinting" (Fig. 23.3), indicating pseudopolyposis caused by submucosal edema and hemorrhage. Sigmoidoscopic examination reveals no mucosal abnormalities, whereas in instances of infarction resulting from occlusion of the inferior mesenteric artery, the injury extends low enough to involve the rectal mucosa. Since many patients with ischemic colitis recover without surgical intervention, it is important to differentiate between

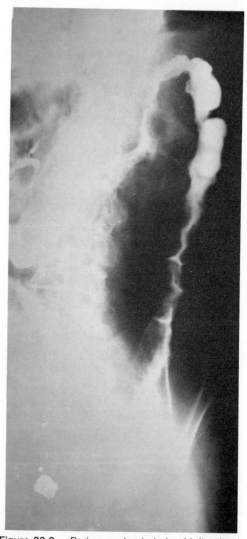

Figure 23.3. Barium contrast study of left colon in patient with ischemic colitis. Nodular submucosal edema ("thumbprinting") is present in nondistensible descending colon.

this disease and infarction caused by major vascular occlusion.

Retroperitoneal Processes

Infection, calculus, and obstruction of the urinary tract are discussed in other chapters. Of the other retroperitoneal causes of abdominal pain, the only one that merits emphasis is rupture of an abdominal aortic or iliac arterial aneurysm. Almost one-half of patients with ruptured aneurysms complain primarily of abdominal pain, although back pain is more characteristic of this catastrophe. The pain is sometimes one-sided. An initial step in the evaluation of any patient complaining of abdominal or back pain should be palpation of the abdominal aorta. In a few patients with ruptured aneurysms, only a mass will be palpated, but in most cases the pulsatile aneurysm easily is detected on abdominal examination. Any patient with a previously diagnosed abdominal aortic aneurysm who complains of either abdominal pain or back pain must be considered to have retroperitoneal leakage from the aneurysm. Emergency operative intervention offers the only chance of survival. If operation precedes the development of hypotension, hypotensive renal injury, and cardiac arrest, the patient usually recovers.

Unusual Causes of Acute Abdominal Pain

Acute abdominal pain can be caused by conditions unrelated to the abdominal organs themselves. For example, when diabetes mellitus escapes control, it sometimes causes diffuse, nonspecific abdominal pain as well as elevation of the serum amylase level. Porphyria, sickle cell disease, tabes dorsalis, and spinal osteomyelitis also may lead to abdominal symptoms. Patients with pulmonary tuberculosis may have a history of episodes of abdominal pain that can be associated with enteric tuberculosis. Pleural conditions such as pleurodynia or pneumonia sometimes produce pain in the adjacent somatic segments that is felt in the abdomen; this is a reason for a routine chest roentgenogram in patients with abdominal pain. Finally, abdominal pain is a common symptom in patients with acute myocardial infarction. In some instances it is referred pain, but in others it is caused by intestinal ischemia.

Systemic Factors Influencing Intra-abdominal Emergencies

Several systemic factors may influence the occurrence, presentation, and management of some of the conditions that have been discussed. Among these is diabetes mellitus. In the diabetic patient, infection seems less well contained by the normal tissue response. Cholecystitis in the diabetic, for example, tends to progress more frequently and more quickly to gangrene, empyema, and perforation.

Patients receiving long-term corticosteroid therapy exhibit a less dramatic response to many of the conditions discussed. Because these drugs suppress inflammation, signs and symptoms tend to be less intense and slower to develop. For example, it is more difficult to judge the severity of peritonitis resulting from perforation in a patient receiving corticosteroids.

General obtundation, such as that which may accompany hypotension, hypoxemia, or septicemia, also tends to obscure abdominal symptoms. In such cases, the physician must consider the possibility that abdominal disease may be the underlying cause of the patient's abnormal signs and symptoms.

The patient with a neurologic lesion blocking the sensation of pain over the abdominal wall presents an especially difficult problem. The physician must depend on what few findings can be elicited by history and physical examination, and must repeat laboratory tests frequently. In some patients, local peritoneal reflexes will persist, so muscle spasm may develop despite the fact that the abdomen is generally flaccid.

The patient who is readmitted to an emergency facility soon after being discharged following an abdominal operation deserves brief comment. By far the most frequent reason for such a readmission is the development of an abdominal wall or intra-abdominal abscess, which sometimes represents an impending fistula. Intelligent management begins with obtaining the details of the operative procedure. Septicemia, bleeding or obstruction, requires the usual treatment.

Finally, no better advice could be offered to those interested in this subject than to become familiar with *The Early Diagnosis of the Acute Abdomen* by Sir Zachary Cope. This small volume is probably the most informative source available on abdominal emergencies.

GASTROINTESTINAL HEMORRHAGE

General Considerations

The emphasis in this section is on the patient whose life is threatened by hypovolemia due to rapid blood loss. Most patients who are evaluated by the emergency physician are not in this category, however, having either less severe hemorrhage or chronic intestinal blood loss. All the lesions that are to be discussed can lead to either of these forms of bleeding. It should be emphasized that the initial responsibility of the emergency physician pertains to the life-threatening aspects of the hemorrhage. The earliest possible estimate of quantity and rate of blood loss, rather than the exact diagnosis, is the key to initial management of massive hemorrhage.

Both the duration and the rate of blood loss affect the emergency presentation of the patient with gastrointestinal bleeding. Occasionally, prolonged losses at a relatively slow rate result in severe anemia and precipitate such secondary problems as congestive heart failure. At the other end of the spectrum is the acutely exsanguinating hemorrhage, typically from esophageal varices or a duodenal ulcer. Site also determines the symptoms and findings. Esophageal bleeding, as from varices, frequently leads to vomiting of almost all the blood lost. Bleeding from the stomach may be manifested by hematemesis, but most of the blood lost may pass into the distal portion of the gastrointestinal tract. Sometimes, when the site of origin is the duodenum, all blood passes distally in this way. When the upper gastrointestinal losses are slight or moderate, the blood is changed in its passage and melena results. With massive bleeding, maroon stools and even unchanged blood clots are passed rectally. Likewise, lesser degrees of bleeding from the small intestine and even from the right side of the colon can be manifested by melena. Finally, blood lost from the rectum or anus is usually unchanged and obvious to the patient even when the loss is slight.

A careful history obtained from both the patient and his relatives often indicates the source of bleeding. Chronic alcoholism with attendant portal hypertension and symptoms suggesting long-standing peptic ulcer disease are both significant in establishing the diagnosis. The physician also should inquire about the recent use of aspirin, aspirin-containing drugs, and other upper gastrointestinal irritants.

It is necessary both to assess the quantity of blood lost and to determine the origin in the gastrointestinal tract. In an episode of acute hemorrhage, stabilization of the hematocrit may take several hours, so an abnormal hematocrit value may not be an accurate guide to the quantity of blood lost. Vital signs provide a more valid index. The observation that tachycardia and hypotension in the seated patient disappear in the supine position serves as a warning that although the patient's condition appears stable, vascular collapse is impending.

Before bleeding stops, passage of a nasogastric tube may confirm that the source of hemorrhage is in the esophagus, stomach, or duodenum. In the patient with red rectal bleeding, sigmoidoscopic examination provides information as to whether the blood is originating from above the lower part of the rectum. Both of these measures should be initiated as soon as possible. Screening tests to exclude a prothrombin or platelet deficiency also should have early priority.

Whatever the cause of bleeding, initial management must be directed toward preventing hypovolemia and its complications. This includes placement of large intravenous catheters for rapid infusion of fluids, crossmatching of whole blood, and monitoring of vital signs. Every patient with gastrointestinal bleeding should be treated as if hypovolemic shock were about to develop. Once sufficient data have accumulated to justify a less urgent approach, such emergency measures can be modified or discontinued. Unfortunately, it is all too common to treat the patient conservatively until hypotension unexpectedly signals massive hemorrhage.

Fiberoptic esophagogastroscopy and selective angiography are major recent contributions to the management of profuse gastrointestinal bleeding. Barium studies are less valuable, and usually should be deferred until the patient's condition has become stabilized and the bleeding has been controlled.

The specific sequence in which various diagnostic maneuvers are employed depends on several factors, such as the rapidity of blood loss, the most likely source of bleeding, and the availability of skilled endoscopists and angiographers. As in other emergencies, it is important that one person have responsibility for the overall integration of diagnostic and therapeutic steps. Although the identity of this individual will change as the patient is transferred from the emergency facility, there should be no doubt at any time as to who is responsible.

Major Causes of Massive Gastrointestinal Hemorrhage

Upper Gastrointestinal Hemorrhage

The management of exsanguinating hemorrhage from any source in the upper part of the gastrointestinal tract is a challenge. Bleeding may be exacerbated by any of the three diagnostic measures now commonly employed—barium studies, endoscopy, and angiography, The benefits of immediate operative intervention must be weighed against the increased risk of delay and diagnostic tests. The mounting availability of selective angiography, not only for diagnosis but also for therapy, has given the physician a new option, and in institutions where it is available, it has caused a shift of emphasis away from immediate surgical treatment.

Esophageal Varices. The esophagus and esophagogastric junction are seldom sources of exsanguinating hemorrhage except under two circumstances. The first of these is the presence of esophageal varices associated with portal hypertension. Because bleeding occurs directly into the esophagus, copious hematemesis is common. The patient often describes the major symptom as blood welling up in the mouth, rather than forceful vomiting. Most patients have a history of previous episodes of upper gastrointestinal bleeding and of either heavy, prolonged alcohol usage or an episode of hepatitis or jaundice. If hemorrhage is continuing and varices are the suspected source, the physician should pass a Sengstaken-Blakemore tube or similar device designed to tamponade the distal portion of the esophagus. Cessation of bleeding indicates that the blood is coming from the esophagus rather than from a more distal site. The physician must remember that a tube for tamponade will obstruct the esophagus, so blood and oral secretions must be removed. If there is any cerebral obtundation, an endotracheal tube should be placed to prevent the common complication of aspiration pneumonitis. Vitamin K and fresh-frozen plasma may help to shorten a prolonged prothrombin time when this contributes to continued bleeding.

Mallory-Weiss Tears. These short, linear mucosal lacerations at the esophagogastric junction are the other source of copious esophageal hemorrhage, and they sometimes are associated with a history of violent vomiting. The bleeding is from small arteries that have been torn, and pain is not a usual complaint. The diagnosis can be established only by endoscopy, angiography, or laparotomy. A tube for the tamponade of varices does not always control this arterial hemorrhage.

Hiatal Hernia. A large paraesophageal or axial hiatal hernia may manifest its presence by upper gastrointestinal hemorrhage. Endoscopic examination and barium studies of the stomach provide the diagnosis. Once the diagnosis is established, urgent operative intervention is necessary, since bleeding raises the possibility of incarceration with strangulation.

Esophagitis. Massive bleeding is uncommon in the patient with chronic esophagitis secondary to gastroesophageal reflux, although oozing may result in chronic anemia. The rare exception occurs in the presence of a deep esophageal ulcer. The history and early endoscopic examination are important aspects of the diagnosis.

Gastric Conditions. Hemorrhage from the stomach can be caused by gastritis or superficial stress ulceration. Gastric ulcers and ulcers in tumors are not so common a cause of massive gastric hemorrhage. Angiographic examination and laparotomy provide the diagnosis, whereas barium studies frequently do not. Whatever the source, gastric bleeding is less likely to stop so long as the stomach is distended with clot. Passage of a large orogastric tube for iced saline lavage and evacuation of clots occasionally stops the bleeding, and also provides a means of measuring the rate of hemorrhage.

Peptic Ulcer. The most common cause of copious upper gastrointestinal bleeding is peptic ulcer disease. Because of erosion of the ulcer into the gastroduodenal or pancreaticoduodenal arteries, which are large vessels, the amount of blood lost can be massive. Although most patients with a bleeding peptic ulcer have long-standing symptoms and possibly a previous diagnosis revealed by an upper gastrointestinal series, some, particularly older patients, have no such history.

If there is a large amount of bleeding into the proximal portion of the duodenum, blood usually refluxes into the stomach and is vomited or recovered on aspiration of the gastric contents. Occasionally, however, the blood is lost entirely into the distal portion of the gastrointestinal tract, and is manifested by black or maroon stools and sometimes by blood clots. If bleeding is ongoing, angiographic or esophagogastroscopic examination either will establish the diagnosis or provide sufficient information that the physician may infer the presence of a bleeding ulcer. An upper gastrointestinal series almost always shows either an active ulcer or a deformity of the duodenum, but it cannot establish this as the bleeding site. As in the case of gastric bleeding, lavage of the stomach is useful in clearing blood clots and in judging the rate of blood loss. Recovery of only small amounts of blood from the stomach does not, however, exclude extensive ongoing loss into the distal portion of the gastrointestinal tract. Signs of hypovolemia and increased vigor of peristaltic activity provide additional evidence of continuing blood loss. The decision whether to operate or to persist with medical management must be made quickly when hemorrhage is massive.

Rare Causes of Upper Gastrointestinal Hemorrhage. Other interesting but exceedingly rare causes of major upper gastrointestinal bleeding are hepatic injury leading to hematobilia, duodenal tumors, and aortoenteric fistulas. Hematobilia is associated with colicky pain, intermittent jaundice, and profuse hemorrhage. The diagnosis is established on angiographic examination.

Because of the vascularity of the duodenum, duodenal tumors tend to bleed when they become necrotic. The presence of such a tumor usually is suggested by a history of weight loss and partial obstruction of the duodenum or biliary tree. An upper gastrointestinal series reveals the diagnosis. Tumors arising from adjacent retroperitoneal structures, such as the kidney, also may cause duodenal bleeding.

Aortoenteric fistulas are almost always a complication of an implanted graft after aortic resection. The diagnosis should be considered in any patient with gastrointestinal bleeding and previous operation on the aorta or iliac vessels. Surprisingly, bleeding from such fistulas is not always profuse. Aortic aneurysms can give rise spontaneously to fistulas into the duodenum, but these are exceedingly rare.

Lower Gastrointestinal Hemorrhage

Lesions of the Small Intestine. The small intestine is rarely the source of massive bleeding. Three unusual exceptions are bleeding from an ulcerated Meckel's diverticulum, bleeding from hamartomatous tumors in patients with Peutz-Jeghers syndrome, and bleeding from jejunal diverticula similar to that seen in patients with bleeding colonic diverticula. Rarely, arteriovenous malformations and leiomyomata may also lead to bleeding from the small intestine. Angiographic examination is the most accurate and often the only method by which the site of bleeding can be established other than laparotomy.

Diverticulosis. Any major bleeding in the colon usually leads to the passage of maroon and red stools, although slow bleeding from the right colon and right portion of the transverse colon may be manifested by melena only. Massive colonic bleeding almost always originates from diverticula. Many diverticula arise at sites where major blood vessels perforate the muscle wall, and bleeding is usually the result of erosion into one of these vessels. A typical history of bleeding diverticulosis includes passage of a huge, bloody stool without preceding symptoms, followed by faintness. Angiographic examination provides the only specific means of diagnosis; if it cannot be employed, barium studies must be performed to assist the surgeon in planning a possible emergency operation, despite the fact that such studies increase the likelihood of recurrent bleeding.

Other Colonic Lesions. Copious colonic bleeding also may arise from cecal ulcerations and vascular malformations. Tumors of the colon, including polyps, bleed routinely, but seldom enough to provoke hypovolemia, chronic anemia being the usual presentation. Ischemic and ulcerative colitis are two other causes of bleeding; they usually are suggested by a characteristic history.

Hemorrhoids. Hemorrhoidal bleeding may occasionally be profuse enough to be frightening. In this instance, sigmoidoscopic examination is of obvious importance. Portal hypertension or some form of bleeding dyscrasia should be suspected in the patient whose bleeding is voluminous enough to constitute a serious, acute problem.

ABDOMINAL TRAUMA

General Considerations

Successful treatment of the severely injured patient requires frequent examination by the physician in charge, who must be alert to the possibility of multiple covert injuries in the presence of major trauma.

Abdominal trauma, particularly when it is blunt, frequently is associated with injuries to the head, chest, and extremities. The clinician's immediate priorities are to establish an airway with effective gas exchange and to control bleeding. Resuscitation is discussed in Chapter 2. Immediate laparotomy may be necessary to control hemorrhage.

The largest group of patients with penetrating or blunt abdominal trauma consists of those whose condition is stable on admission to the emergency facility. When treating such a patient, the physician first should draw blood for typing and cross-matching and place intravenous lines for transfusion, and then assess the patient's condition to determine the extent of the injury and to plan the protocol for diagnosis and treatment. A patient with a traumatic abdominal injury should be closely attended at all times, and if his condition deteriorates, he should be treated promptly—by operation if necessary.

If the patient is unconscious, the physician first must assess the status of gas exchange and ensure an adequate airway. Care must be taken to avoid complicating a possible cervical spinal injury. If there is evidence of shock, hypovolemia should be considered as the probable cause, and crystalloid and colloid replacement should be started. The physician then should investigate the possibility of an injured intra-abdominal or retroperitoneal structure by physical examination and paracentesis. An unconscious patient must be watched closely for signs of deterioration even if he is considered to be without significant intra-abdominal injury.

The patient who is seen initially with unstable vital signs and one or more obvious sites of abdominal trauma must be treated more urgently with prompt airway control, volume replacement, and operative assessment of the injury. The operating room must be alerted on admission of the patient, and the patient should be cared for initially in a special area within the emergency facility containing equipment for venous cutdown, endotracheal intubation, tracheotomy, closed tube thoracostomy, and even pericardiotomy. The physician promptly should place large intravenous lines, draw blood for typing and crossmatching, and then infuse a balanced salt solution such as Ringer's lactate. Hypotension from moderate hemorrhage (500 ml) usually can be corrected with rapid administration of several liters of a balanced salt solution in the course of 15 minutes. Blood loss exceeding 500 ml requires infusion of whole blood. If hypotension does not respond promptly to crystalloid infusion, uncrossmatched type-specific blood should be administered until crossmatched type-specific blood becomes available. The patient who responds initially to crystalloid by elevation of blood pressure to a nearly normal level but who subsequently becomes hypotensive will require administration of whole blood and probably prompt exploration if other injuries cannot be implicated as a source of the blood loss.

Penetrating Trauma

Penetrating abdominal wounds in civilian settings usually are not associated with injuries to other systems. Although much has been written about injection of wound tracts with water-soluble contrast material to determine depth and about following the patient with interval examinations without exploration, a simpler treatment plan is probably more desirable. If it cannot be determined whether a stab wound has penetrated the peritoneal cavity, the wound should be extended under local anesthesia to determine its depth. If the patient's condition is stable and the wound involves only the abdominal wall, local management and follow-up evaluation are recommended. However, if it appears that the peritoneum has been penetrated, the patient should be prepared for surgical exploration of the abdominal cavity. All gunshot wounds of the abdomen should be explored, whether or not penetration is evident, because shock waves may have injured intra-abdominal structures. If missile injury has occurred and the patient's condition permits, biplane abdominal roentgenograms should be obtained before laparotomy to determine the probable trajectory of the missile. Laparotomy also is indicated when there is a missile injury of the lower thoracic region.

If a patient with penetrating trauma has profound hypovolemia, prompt, massive, intravenous administration of a buffered salt solution, colloid, and type-specific blood should be carried out as the patient is taken to the operating room for control of hemorrhage. Support of blood pressure during transit may be assisted by circumferential tamponade to the abdominal cavity provided by a G-suit or MAST trousers. Airway intubation and assisted ventilation may also be necessary.

Blunt Trauma

Blunt abdominal injuries frequently are associated with injuries to other organ systems that may obscure the diagnosis and complicate the treatment, and physical findings often are not marked until long after the injury has been sustained. The physician must suspect major injury even though the patient has few symptoms or signs. He must evaluate carefully the patient's condition on admission and at subsequent intervals if the condition appears stable.

The most frequent complaint of a patient with blunt abdominal trauma is abdominal pain; the most common physical findings are tenderness with rigidity and involuntary guarding of the abdominal wall. If the patient is hypotensive, but has no demonstrable source of blood loss, intra-abdominal or retroperitoneal bleeding should be presumed and exploration should promptly be performed.

Specific Organ Injuries

Spleen. The abdominal organ most frequently injured by blunt trauma is the spleen. A ruptured spleen is suggested by a history of trauma to the left upper abdominal quadrant or left lower portion of the rib cage resulting in pain with or without free blood in the abdominal cavity on paracentesis. Radioisotope scanning and arteriographic examination of the spleen may be useful in patients in whom the diagnosis is suspected (Fig. 23.4); the treatment is prompt splenectomy. In pediatric patients, special attempts are advisable to preserve part or all of the damaged spleen. Occasionally, a subcapsular splenic hematoma

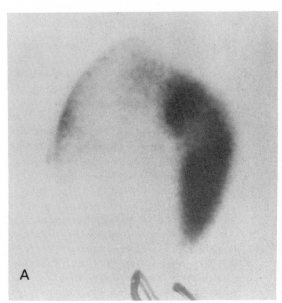
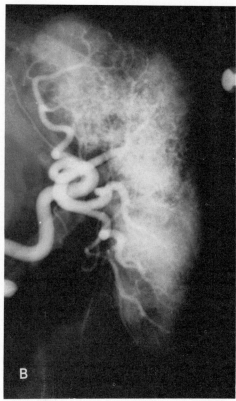

Figure 23.4. (A) Radioisotopic scan of spleen showing bandlike defect in upper portion. Confirmation that the defect was caused by traumatic fracture was obtained by means of the angiogram (B) and at subsequent laparotomy.

may rupture days to weeks after the traumatic event. The history of previous trauma and evidence of intra-abdominal hemorrhage should suggest the diagnosis.

Kidney. The kidneys frequently are injured in blunt trauma to the abdomen. Hematuria, which may be gross or microscopic, suggests the diagnosis. Further discussion occurs in Chapter 25, 538–540 pages.

Liver. The liver frequently is fractured during blunt abdominal trauma, with associated injuries to neighboring structures almost always occurring. The usual manifestation of hepatic trauma is intra-abdominal bleeding with hypovolemia, and suspected injury dictates abdominal exploration.

Duodenum. The duodenum occasionally is injured in blunt abdominal trauma, but because of its retroperitoneal position, abdominal signs may be minimal initially. Retroperitoneal air may be demonstrated on abdominal roentgenograms. Water-soluble radiopaque dye administered orally may reveal a duodenal extravasation. Since injury may be isolated to the duodenum and not involve the pancreas, serum amylase levels may be normal.

If a duodenal injury is suspected, laparotomy is indicated.

An uncommon lesion resulting from blunt abdominal trauma is intramural hematoma of the duodenum, which usually is manifested as an obstruction high in the small intestine. The diagnosis is made on contrast examination of the upper part of the gastrointestinal tract, which reveals obstruction at the third portion of the duodenum. Treatment consists of nasogastric aspiration with intravenous replacement of fluid and electrolytes and elective evacuation of the intramural hematoma.

Small Intestine. The small intestine frequently is injured from blunt trauma either by being pressed against the vertebral column, by being torn by forces applied to the abdomen, or by bursting from sudden high pressure. Because of the nearly neutral pH and low number of bacteria in the small intestine, the diagnosis at first may not be readily apparent, but will be elucidated gradually over a period of hours as the abdomen is examined at intervals. On development of signs of peritonitis, exploratory operation should be performed.

Stomach. Injuries to the stomach usually are due to penetrating wounds, and often are associated with injuries to the surrounding viscera. A gastric injury usually is obvious on admission because of the trajectory of the missile or the path of the instrument. Blunt injury may result from a direct blow to the epigastrium. However the trauma occurs, blood usually is present in the nasogastric aspirate, and signs of peritoneal irritation develop early. Prompt abdominal exploration is indicated.

Large Intestine. Blunt injury to the large intestine usually is associated with massive peritoneal contamination. The rectum rarely is injured in blunt abdominal trauma, even in severe pelvic fractures. Both the colon and the rectum occasionally are injured in penetrating trauma, frequently in association with injuries to other structures. Peritoneal signs, as well as evidence of blood loss, along with the trajectory of the missile or path of the instrument usually suggest the diagnosis. Prompt operation is necessary.

Pancreas. The pancreas may be fractured bluntly over the vertebral column near the superior mesenteric artery, or it may be injured by penetrating trauma. As in injuries to the duodenum, physical findings may be few at first, but signs of peritoneal irritation gradually develop. The serum amylase level usually is elevated. Abdominal exploration should be performed when the condition is strongly suspected, even if there are few indications other than evolving peritoneal signs.

Pelvis. A fractured pelvis frequently is associated with disruption of the membranous urethra as well as with major injuries to the liver, spleen, and other intra-abdominal viscera. Because bleeding from a fractured pelvis can occur both in the retroperitoneum and in the abdomen, neither site can be excluded without laparotomy. Arterial hemorrhage from a pelvic fracture is controlled best by arteriographic demonstration of the source of hemorrhage and occlusion of the vessel by the angiographic catheter. Exploration of the abdominal cavity before angiographic control of pelvic hemorrhage is recommended to ensure that major abdominal visceral injury has not occurred. Circumferential tamponade with a G-suit or the MAST trousers may be helpful in this situation.

Suggested Readings

Athanasoulis CA, Waltman AC, Novelline RA, et al: Angiography: Its contribution to the emergency management of gastrointestinal hemorrhage. *Radiol Clin North Am* 14:265–280, 1976

Ballinger WF, II, Rutherford RB, Zuidema GD (Eds): *The Management of Trauma.* ed 2. Philadelphia, W. B. Saunders, 1973

Botsford TW, Wilson RE: *The Acute Abdomen. Major Problems in Clinical Surgery.* Vol 10. Philadelphia, W. B. Saunders, 1969

Byrne JJ, Moran JM: The Mallory-Weiss syndrome. *N Engl J Med* 272:398–400, 1965

Cope Z: *The Early Diagnosis of the Acute Abdomen.* ed 14. London, Oxford University Press, 1972

Crook JN, Gray LW, Jr. Nance FC, et al: Upper gastrointestinal bleeding. *Ann Surg* 175:771–782, 1972

Dunphy JE, Botsford TW: *Physical Examination of the Surgical Patient.* ed 4. Philadelphia, W. B. Saunders, 1975

Lewis T: *Pain.* New York, Macmillan, 1942

Malt RA: Control of massive upper gastrointestinal hemorrhage. *N Engl J Med* 286:1043–1046, 1972

Palmer ED: The vigorous diagnostic approach to uppergastrointestinal tract hemorrhage: A 23-year prospective study of 1,400 patients. *JAMA* 207:1477–1480, 1969

Shires GT: *Care of the Trauma Patient.* New York, McCraw-Hill, 1966

Simeone JF, Ferrucci JT: New trends in gallbladder imaging. *JAMA* 246:380–383, 1981

Welch CE: *Intestinal Obstruction.* Chicago, Year Book, 1958

CHAPTER 24

Gynecologic and Obstetric Emergencies

DAVID S. CHAPIN, M.D.

Emergencies involving the female reproductive organs present the physician with a double challenge—treatment of the condition and, in some cases, prevention of permanent psychologic damage. This chapter provides a practical approach to these emergencies that will allow the emergency physician to meet this challenge.

PELVIC EXAMINATION

The hallmark of the gynecologic evaluation is the pelvic examination. It is essential that the emergency facility have a proper table with comfortable stirrups, a spotlight, and a movable headrest, and specula of all sizes. If possible, the patient should urinate before the examination to empty the bladder. The examination begins with the patient supine on the table with her heels in the stirrups and her knees as far apart as possible. Women find this an extremely uncomfortable position. Gentleness of voice, manner, and touch, and constant eye contact will reduce the patient's anxiety, allowing a more informative examination. Draping of the patient's knees and abdomen is a common custom to preserve a modicum of modesty.

The external genitalia are observed for swellings, lesions, and inflammation. The size of the clitoris should be noted as well. Lacerations and gland secretions about the hymen are visualized when the labia are gently spread apart with the fingers. The patient is asked to strain down to evaluate the support of the vaginal wall, and the physician notes prolapse of the uterus or urinary incontinence.

Speculum examination is then performed. The proper size of speculum should be selected. For most women, a medium-sized Graves speculum is appropriate; for virginal women, a Pedersen's speculum is narrower and more comfortable.

Obese women require a large Graves speculum. The speculum should be inserted slowly and gently, and it should be aimed toward the sacral promontory since the axis of the vagina has a posterior tilt. Because surgical lubricant will invalidate Papanicolaou smears, Gram stains, and cultures, only warm water should be used to lubricate the speculum. The vaginal wall and cervix can be evaluated visually after the speculum has been opened and the set screw adjusted. Smears for exocervical cytologic examination are taken by scraping around the cervical os with a spatula. Swabbing inside the cervical canal provides specimens for cytologic smears as well as cultures.

After gentle removal of the speculum, the bimanual examination is begun. Two fingers of the gloved hand are coated with surgical lubricant and inserted slowly into the vagina while the other hand palpates the suprapubic region. As the fingers in the vagina are moved anteriorly and posteriorly and from left to right around the cervix, the uterus and adnexa are felt between the two hands of the examiner. The size, shape, mobility, and tenderness of these organs should be noted, as well as the presence or absence of abnormal masses. Finally, the examiner places one finger in the rectum and one in the vagina. Sweeping the finger in the rectum from left to right allows complete evaluation of the cul-de-sac.

The pelvic examination is the most important technique for evaluation of such gynecologic signs and symptoms as vaginal discharge, vaginal bleeding, and pelvic pain.

VAGINAL DISCHARGE

Although vaginal discharge usually presents a minimal threat to health, it is a nuisance and sometimes a threat to emotional stability and family well-being. After he makes a diagnosis, the emergency physician must take care to explain to the patient what was found and how it arrived there, that the condition can be cured, and that the genital organs will function normally again without permanent damage.

Fungal and Parasitic Disease

The most common cause of vaginal discharge, is *Candida albicans*. This yeast-like fungus, commonly part of the normal vaginal flora, can overgrow after or during a course of antibiotics, after menses, or after a change in diet, climate, or sexual partner. Pregnancy, diabetes, and birth control pills are common predisposing factors. Infection occurs most often in the summer, when wet bathing suits and perspiration-soaked underclothes are worn for extended periods of time. The patient complains of an irritating itch, most often associated with a thick, cheesy discharge. Dysuria may occur. The labia may be red and edematous, but the vagina usually appears normal except for the discharge. If a drop of discharge is placed in potassium hydroxide solution and smeared, microscopic examination will reveal budding mycelia. However, the itch can be so severe and the discharge so characteristic that it is improper to withhold treatment even if mycelia are not seen. Culture on Nickerson's medium or Sabouraud agar confirms the diagnosis. Treatment consists of insertion of nystatin vaginal suppositories twice a day for 10 days or miconazol nitrate cream (Monistat) at bedtime for 1 week. A 3-day course of miconazol or clotrimazole (Gyne-Lotrimin) has become an acceptable alternative. A nystatin corticosteroid cream may be applied to the labia to relieve symptoms.

Trichomonas vaginalis is another common cause of vaginal discharge. A protozoon that lives in the genital tracts of both men and women, it is probably transmitted by sexual contact, which may not necessarily be recent. The patient usually complains of recent onset of a copious, odorous vaginal discharge and an intermittent itch. Her sexual partner has no related physical complaints. Examination reveals red, edematous labia and a reddened, roughened vaginal wall. The cervix often is covered with punctate red spots. The discharge is classically greenish and frothy; when a drop is mixed with an equal part of physiologic saline solution and examined microscopically, motile trichomonads can be seen. Flagellated protozoa, they are slightly smaller than the white blood cells that also are present. Treatment consists of administration of metronidazole (Flagyl), 250 mg orally three times a day for 7 days. The sexual partner(s) must be treated with 250 mg orally twice a day for

7 days to minimize recurrence. Alternatively, treatment of both partners with 2 gm over 24 hours is equally effective. The patient must be warned that alcoholic beverages will cause gastrointestinal upset while metronidazole is being taken. In resistant cases, a vinegar douche can be used—2 tablespoons of white vinegar to 1 quart of warm water twice a day.

Bacterial Infection

Gonorrhea, caused by *Neisseria gonorrhoeae*, is presently the second most common infectious disease in the United States, after the common cold. Discharge that is most often green and unpleasant smelling may be the only symptom, although dysuria often is present as well. Vaginal inflammation is minimal, but potential for involvement of the pelvic genital organs is great. Gram-negative intracellular diplococci are the hallmark of gonorrhea; diagnosis may be suggested by a Gram stain of the discharge and confirmed by culture on Transgrow or Thayer-Martin medium. If gonorrhea is suspected, the physician should ask the patient whether her sexual partner or partners have urethral discharge or dysuria. Blood should be drawn for serologic testing for syphilis. The patient should be treated with procaine penicillin G, 4.8 million units intramuscularly, and probenecid, 1 gm orally. In the penicillin-allergic patient, tetracycline, 1.5 gm orally followed by 0.5 gm orally four times a day for 4 days, or spectinomycin, 2 gm intramuscularly, will suffice. The patient should not be told that she has gonorrhea or be reported to public health authorities until the cultures become positive, since the diagnosis can have a disruptive effect on family relationships.

Gardnerella vaginalis (formerly *Hemophilus vaginalis*) appears to be a common pathogenic factor in vaginitis. The discharge usually is white or yellow and thick, and is more bothersome in its volume than in the irritation it causes. On microscopic examination of the discharge mixed with saline, it contains "clue" cells, epithelial cells with dots of bacterial matter clinging to the cell membrane. Final diagnosis is by culture on blood agar. Treatment has been controversial, but recent literature suggests that metronidazole, 500 mg twice a day for 5–7 days, is the only reliable regimen. Other systemic antibiotics cure less than 50% of patients. The partner(s) should also be treated for this sexually transmitted disease.

Nonspecific Causes

If a patient complains of vaginal discharge and if none of the mentioned pathogens is identified, a diagnosis of nonspecific discharge must be made. It is likely that such discharge is caused by streptococci, staphylococci, or another vaginal inhabitant, but neither wet microscopic preparations, cultures, nor Gram stains are diagnostic. This type of discharge must be treated with one of the many available nonspecific vaginal creams, liquids, or douches, and the patient should be told at the outset that more than one such medication may be necessary before the condition is alleviated.

VULVOVAGINAL LESIONS

A Bartholin's cyst often appears after an episode of vaginitis, especially gonorrheal vaginitis, but it also may appear without preceding infection. Located just under the skin at the lateral border of the vaginal fourchette, the swollen gland may produce mild symptoms or none at all, requiring no treatment except explanation and reassurance. If the cyst is red, tender, and fluctuant, making intercourse and sitting impossible, incision and drainage under general anesthesia are indicated. If it is not yet fluctuant, hot sitz baths, antibiotics, and analgesics are the usual temporizing measures. General anesthesia is advised for surgical drainage since local anesthesia is rarely adequate. After incision and drainage of a Bartholin's gland abscess, a large asymptomatic cyst may remain. Elective marsupialization or excision of this lesion prevents recurrent abscess.

Herpetic vulvovaginitis recently has increased in incidence concomitantly with other sexually transmitted diseases. Herpes simplex virus type II is the usual infecting agent, but type I is isolated in 10–15% of cases. In primary cases, herpetic vesicles form in clusters on the perineal skin and labial mucosa. They commonly rupture after 12–36 hours, leaving small grouped ulcerations. Usually, by the time the patient seeks medical attention, the ulcers are extremely painful. The patient may be unable to sit, and the ulcers burn on urination. On physical examination, the physician usually sees grouped ulcerations 2–3 mm in diameter on the labia and perineum and occasionally in the vagina or on the cervix. Inguinal lymph nodes commonly are enlarged and tender on palpation. The diagnosis usually can be made by inspection and can be confirmed by culture of the virus or biopsy.

Many methods of treatment, including photoinactivation, ether, acetone, corticosteroids, and antimetabolites, have been tested by several investigators; they are all either unreliable or of no benefit. A new drug, acyclovir (Zovirax), has been approved for use in immunosuppressed patients. A 5% ointment has recently been approved by the FDA for topical application. When applied in a first episode of herpes, it reduces both severity of symptoms and the time to crusting of vesicles, but it does not prevent recurrence. Fortunately, the disease is self-limited. The first attack usually lasts 10–14 days, and the patient may be unable to work or attend school during the first week—in this case, a medical excuse is appropriate. Analgesics and frequent sitz baths relieve symptoms until the disease subsides. Attacks may recur months or even years later, but these episodes are usually both shorter in duration and less uncomfortable. Since there may be a causal relationship between genital herpetic infection and cervical cancer, these patients should have a Papanicolaou smear every 6 months after the diagnosis is made.

VAGINAL BLEEDING

Sudden severe vaginal bleeding can be one of the most frightening occurrences in a woman's life. The physician is obligated not only to diagnose and to treat the cause of the bleeding but also to meet the patient's related emotional needs.

The physician must first assess the extent of bleeding, institute supportive measures, and begin laboratory evaluation before establishing the definitive diagnosis by means of the history and physical examination. A calm, reassuring manner is essential. The physician can estimate the amount of bleeding by examining clothing and pads and by obtaining vital signs. Intravenous infusion for volume replacement should be started immediately, and specimens for a complete blood cell count, sedimentation rate determination, serologic test for syphilis, urinalysis, and urine pregnancy test should be sent to the laboratory. Blood is drawn at the same time for typing and crossmatching. While waiting for the results of laboratory tests, the physician can take the history and perform further physical examination.

Diagnostic Procedures

The diagnostic possibilities in patients with vaginal bleeding severe enough to be classified as an emergency include complications of pregnancy such as incomplete abortion (possibly septic), ectopic pregnancy, placenta previa, abruptio placentae, and postpartum hemorrhage. Vaginal trauma, cervical or endometrial carcinoma, and menstrual dysfunction also can cause bleeding.

Complications of Pregnancy

History. As in all gynecologic evaluations, a complete menstrual history including menarche, periodicity, duration, and amount of regular flow is obtained. The date of the last period and whether it was normal constitute the most important data to be determined. Pregnancy should be suspected whenever a period is delayed or scanty. Spontaneous abortion can be suspected if the last period was 6–8 weeks previously; ectopic pregnancy usually results in mild bleeding after 5–6 weeks of amenorrhea.

The physician should ask the patient if she has had intercourse recently. Since patients may deny sexual activity if they think the physician will disapprove, he should ask the question in a kind, matter-of-fact way, with the same tone as other questions. He also should determine whether birth control was utilized, and if so, which method. Use of contraceptive pills makes the possibility of pregnancy unlikely, whereas an intrauterine device can suggest the possibility of an ectopic pregnancy.

If the patient is bleeding and reports symptoms of early pregnancy such as nausea, fatigue, breast tenderness, and urinary frequency, and if the menstrual history suggests pregnancy, spontaneous abortion is suggested. This condition also may be suspected if the symptoms of pregnancy disappeared a day or two before the bleeding began.

If the patient has abdominal pain, its location, duration, mode of onset, and persistence afford diagnostic clues. Crampy midline pain beginning after onset of vaginal bleeding suggests spontaneous abortion, whereas constant pain that may precede the bleeding can signal ectopic pregnancy. If pelvic infection is present, the pain is more likely to be constant and bilateral.

If the patient is in the 26th week of pregnancy or beyond and is bleeding, two serious conditions are possible—abruptio placentae and placenta previa. In the former condition, the placenta separates prematurely. Indications are usually pain, which is either rhythmic or steady, and a tense uterus. The major complications of abruptio placentae are excessive blood loss, disseminated intravascular coagulation, and fetal death. Placenta previa is a condition in which the placenta covers the cervix below the head of the fetus. Blood loss is usually slow and unaccompanied by pain, but hypovolemic shock occasionally can occur. Because pelvic examination of bleeding patients in the third trimester of pregnancy can cause sudden massive hemorrhage by dislodging the placenta, it should be performed only in the operating room. Heavy bleeding after delivery or therapeutic abortion usually results from retained products of conception, as is the case in incomplete abortion.

Physical Examination. In addition to performing a general physical examination, the emergency physician should pay careful attention to the following:

(1) Temperature. A temperature of 100°F (37.8°C) may be present with either incomplete abortion or ectopic pregnancy; a higher fever strongly suggests infection complicating one of these conditions or pelvic inflammatory disease (PID).

(2) Abdomen. The signs of peritonitis, such as localized tenderness, rebound tenderness, and guarding, accompany ectopic pregnancy, septic abortion, and PID, but usually do not accompany uncomplicated incomplete abortion. Bowel sounds are often normal. A mass in the midline is consistent with second-trimester abortion.

(3) Cervix. If blood is coming from the cervical os and if no tumor is seen, the endometrium is the source of bleeding. If the cervix appears dilated on either speculum or digital examination, abortion is either complete, incomplete, or about to begin. The physician should look for signs of induced abortion such as tenaculum marks or lacerations. Placental tissue in the cervical os or vagina indicates abortion; it should be removed and sent for pathologic examination. Bleeding often decreases after removal of this tissue. Pus in the opening or cervical tenderness or both indicate sepsis; specimens for culture should be taken during the speculum examination, before lubricant has been introduced into the vagina. Warm water usually suffices as a speculum lubricant.

(4) Uterus. Enlargement usually indicates pregnancy, either aborted or intact. Tenderness on palpation suggests sepsis, and crepitation signals clostridial infection. The incidence of this complication, commonly seen in criminal abortion, fortunately has declined since the legalization of therapeutic abortion.

(5) Adnexa. Unilateral tenderness or enlargement or both suggest ectopic pregnancy, whereas bilateral tenderness or enlargement or both are more consistent with either PID or septic abortion.

(6) Cul-de-sac. Bulging into the posterior part of the vaginal fornix signifies intraperitoneal hemorrhage, as in ectopic pregnancy.

Laboratory and Radiologic Findings. The hematocrit value will be low whatever the cause of bleeding, but will not reflect sudden recent blood loss. A white blood cell count of 12,000–15,000 cells/cm^3 may reflect incomplete abortion or ectopic pregnancy; a higher count indicates sepsis. A sedimentation rate more than 20 mm/hr (Wintrobe) is consistent with chronic infection. Clotting studies should be performed and fibrin split products should be measured if abruptio placentae is suspected.

The urine pregnancy test is positive in approximately 95% of women in whom the pregnancy is normal but in only 50% with an ectopic pregnancy, and is therefore of little diagnostic value. The serum test for the β subunit of human chorionic gonadotropin will aid greatly in the diagnosis because it is positive in normal pregnancy even before the missed period, and is also positive even when there is minimal functioning trophoblastic tissue, as in ectopic pregnancy.

In many diagnostic dilemmas of early pregnancy, ultrasonography is extremely helpful in locating trophoblastic tissue in the Fallopian tube or uterus, as well as in delineating placenta previa in late pregnancy.

An x-ray film of the chest with the patient upright may reveal air under the diaphragm if the uterus has been perforated, and an anteroposterior x-ray film of the abdomen may show gas in the uterus if clostridia are present.

Definitive Diagnosis. The diagnosis of postpartum hemorrhage is usually obvious by the history; other serious vaginal hemorrhage, such as bleeding due to either an aborting, aborted, or ectopic pregnancy, can be more difficult to diagnose.

Abortion. When patients in the first trimester of pregnancy have vaginal bleeding without pain, the diagnosis of threatened abortion can be made. This situation occurs in 20–25% of all pregnancies, but only 40–50% of these result in complete abortion. Cramps, extremely heavy blood loss, passage of tissue other than blood clot, or an effaced or dilated cervix indicates incomplete or inevitable abortion. The patient has had a complete abortion if the entire conceptus has been expelled, the uterus has returned to normal size, and cramps and bleeding have subsided. Septic abortion is any abortion, induced or spontaneous, in which infection is present, in which case septic shock may be more life-threatening than bleeding.

Ectopic Pregnancy. Since it has myriad manifestations, ectopic pregnancy must be suspected in any patient with a recently irregular menstrual pattern, lower abdominal pain of any type, signs and symptoms of recent blood loss, or a pelvic mass. Only one of these factors need be present to raise the suspicion, and neither the patient nor the physician should sleep until the diagnosis is excluded. Culdocentesis—insertion of a 20-gauge spinal needle on a large syringe into the cul-de-sac through the posterior vaginal wall and withdrawal of peritoneal fluid—can be performed without anesthesia in the emergency ward to determine the presence of hemoperitoneum and thus ectopic pregnancy or ruptured ovarian cyst (Fig. 24.1). Negative results do not exclude these diagnoses, however, and laparoscopy in the operating

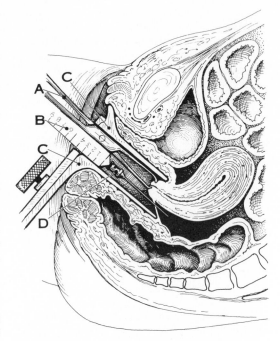

Figure 24.1. Culdocentesis. The instruments are (*A*) tenaculum, (*B*) syringe, (*C*) speculum, and (*D*) 20-gauge spinal needle. (Reproduced by permission, from *Stedman's Medical Dictionary*. ed. 23. Baltimore, Williams & Wilkins, 1976.)

room may be necessary to make the final diagnosis.

Vaginal Trauma

When the history is taken, the patient should be questioned about the possibility of vaginal trauma. Accidental impalement on fences, sticks, and bicycle seats occurs frequently in children. Chemicals such as lye and potassium permanganate that are instilled in attempts at abortion can cause multiple bleeding ulcerations. Sexual abuse of children also should be considered.

Carcinoma

If carcinoma is visualized in the cervix or if endometrial carcinoma is suspected because of postmenopausal bleeding, it is possible to confirm the diagnosis in the emergency ward with cervical or endometrial biopsy. However, bleeding is usually slow enough for the patient to be admitted for colposcopic biopsy and perhaps dilatation and curettage.

Dysfunctional Bleeding

Dysfunctional or anovulatory uterine bleeding occurs in women ranging in age from the teens to the forties. It consists of irregular periods that are either too frequent, too long, or both. Bleeding is usually not excessive, but the patient often seeks emergency care. If the results of pelvic examination are normal and if abortion is ruled out, an endometrial biopsy specimen demonstrating proliferative endometrium will confirm the diagnosis. Biopsy is not usually part of the emergency ward workup, however, and may be postponed.

Therapy

The therapy for both spontaneous and induced abortion as well as for postpartum hemorrhage is dilatation and curettage. Although curettage is not mandatory in the small percentage of apparently complete abortions, it is usually safest to perform this procedure since curettage ensures completion. In many cases, dilatation and curettage may be performed under local anesthesia, and it should be performed immediately unless bleeding is minimal enough that it may be done later. If the abortion is septic, intravenous broad-spectrum antibiotics should be given before the procedure. The drugs of choice presently are penicillin, 1–5 million units every 4 hours, and chloramphenicol, 500–750 mg every 6 hours, given in combination. As an alternative to chloramphenicol, clindamycin, 600 mg every 8 hours, is gaining in popularity, since it is an excellent antibiotic with an anaerobic spectrum. It usually is safe to operate after the second dose of intravenous penicillin has been administered. Oxytocin may be given intravenously, 10–20 units/liter, to reduce bleeding before the operative procedure, and if hypovolemic or septic shock is present, it also must be treated before operation (see Chapter 3, pages 41–47 and 51–56).

The patient needs repeated reassurance that spontaneous abortion was not brought on by anything she did or did not do and that it will have no effect on future pregnancies. Almost all patients feel guilty in such a situation and require psychologic support.

The treatment of ectopic pregnancy is immediate laparotomy and removal of all trophoblastic tissue. If possible, the Fallopian tube should be preserved by salpingostomy or segmental resection, but salpingectomy is often necessary. Ipsilateral oophorectomy is advocated by some, but this procedure remains controversial.

In patients in the third trimester of pregnancy who are bleeding and who have pain suggesting abruptio placentae, hypovolemic shock should be treated and blood clotting studies begun immediately. If there is no evidence of disseminated intravascular coagulation (that is, if partial thrombo-

plastin time, platelet counts, and fibrinogen level are normal) and if the fetus demonstrates a normal heart rate on monitoring, normal labor can be anticipated and observed, at least temporarily. If, however, the fetus is in distress or the clotting factors are depressed, whole blood, fresh-frozen plasma, or cryoprecipitate should be administered and caesarean section performed immediately. Delivery is the ultimate treatment of abruptio placentae. In patients with painless bleeding, in whom placenta previa is more likely, ultrasonography will confirm the diagnosis. Bed rest usually will slow the bleeding, and delivery can be postponed to a more elective time. Occasionally, however, severe blood loss persists and warrants immediate caesarean delivery. The physician should remember that pelvic examination in the third-trimester bleeding patient should be performed only in the operating room.

Patients with anovulatory bleeding do not require immediate therapy. Dilatation and curettage at a later time is indicated to exclude carcinoma in patients more than 35 years old. An injection of progestin or oral progesterone to stop the bleeding is undesirable not only because of the heavy withdrawal flow a few days later but also because it renders the results of subsequent endometrial biopsy invalid. Reassurance and short-term follow-up care constitute better emergency treatment.

Bleeding from traumatic lesions of the vagina and vulva usually can be controlled by suturing under local anesthesia; children require general anesthesia.

Since most carcinomas bleed slowly, admission to the hospital for exact diagnosis and a staging procedure is more important than emergency therapy. If bleeding from a cervical lesion is excessive, vaginal packing usually decreases the flow; occasionally, an endometrial lesion requires immediate admission for curettage to minimize loss of blood.

PELVIC PAIN

Lower abdominal pain in women presents a difficult diagnostic problem requiring the expertise of the general surgeon, internist, and gynecologist. Chapters 12, 23, and 25 treat the causes of abdominal pain unrelated to the genital tract.

Pelvic Inflammatory Disease

Acute PID and ectopic pregnancy are the two emergency conditions of greatest concern to the gynecologist. The classic history and physical findings of the latter have been described; the former is at least as protean in its aspects.

History

Commonly manifested by dull, continuous, worsening bilateral pain in the lower part of the abdomen, PID often begins after a menstrual period. The pain usually has been present a day or two before the patient seeks help, and she complains that activity, especially running and sitting, aggravates the pain. Intercourse may be impossible because of deep dyspareunia. Bleeding and discharge may be present. Nausea, a common symptom of developing appendicitis, is not a feature of PID, nor is a change in bowel habit. Previous venereal disease or a partner with urethral discharge suggesting the same, infertility, recent abortion or delivery, and use of an intrauterine device are factors predisposing to pelvic infection, and the patient should be asked about them.

Physical Examination

On physical examination the physician commonly elicits bilateral lower abdominal tenderness, often with marked rebound tenderness and guarding. Bowel sounds are normal, neither hypoactive as in peritonitis caused by appendicitis, intestinal perforation, or pancreatitis, nor hyperactive as in gastroenteritis. Extension of the iliopsoas and obturator muscles is not painful. In severe cases, tenderness is elicited when the patient's torso is shaken or when the patient coughs. Temperatures as high as 104–105°F (40–40.6°C) are seen, although some patients with severe infection can be afebrile.

If PID is suspected, the pelvic examination should be modified to provide the maximal amount of information with minimal discomfort. Speculum examination should be performed without lubricant, and specimens of blood and pus should be taken for cultures and Gram stains. In the bimanual examination, slow, gentle motion of the fingers is essential. Tenderness of the uterine fundus on compression and bogginess and tenderness of the adnexa on palpation confirm the diagnosis of PID, whereas enlargement and tenderness of the adnexal structures are signs of tuboovarian abscess. Manipulation of the cervix stretches the intensely inflamed parametrial tissues, causing severe pain that can make the patient jump for the ceiling. This "chandelier" sign is pathognomonic of acute PID, but it also destroys all hope of further meaningful evaluation, so it should be elicited last in the bimanual examination.

If the fundus and adnexa are not tender but cervical manipulation elicits pain, a less severe episode of PID may exist. Ectopic pregnancy always must be considered when diagnosing pelvic infection. The benefits of laparoscopy for definitive diagnosis make it well worth the risks, and its more frequent use by emergency physicians undoubtedly will result in delivery of proper treatment to more patients. The emergency physician should remember that pelvic examination often exacerbates symptoms and increases fever, and he should keep the number of examinations to a minimum.

Laboratory Findings

Laboratory findings consistent with the diagnosis of PID are an elevated white blood cell count (often more than 25,000 cells/mm^3), elevated sedimentation rate, normal hematocrit value, and a Gram stain revealing *N. gonorrhoeae*.

Therapy

Once PID has been diagnosed, it should be treated with bed rest and antibiotics. Intrauterine devices should be removed. If the patient is afebrile and the white blood cell count is low, procaine penicillin G, 4.8 million units intramuscularly, should be administered and then repeated 2 days later. In addition, bed rest at home, no intercourse, and frequent follow-up visits are necessary. A 10-day course of oral penicillin, ampicillin, or tetracycline is sufficient for patients who can be relied on to take medication regularly, but follow-up examination in 3 or 4 days is essential nonetheless. If the patient has a temperature above 101°F (38.3°C) or a white blood cell count more than 20,000 cells/mm^3 or both, hospitalization and parenteral administration of antibiotics will effect a more rapid cure and result in less permanent damage. Antibiotics with a gram-negative and anaerobic spectrum such as intravenous chloramphenicol, intramuscular gentamicin, and intramuscular clindamycin should be administered along with intravenous penicillin for the first few days. Inactivity is at least as important as antibiotic therapy. Fowler's position with the pelvis as dependent as possible aids in keeping the infectious process localized. The patient can be discharged after she has been afebrile for 48 hours, and she should be followed for a short time.

If fever persists or tubo-ovarian abscess develops or both, laparotomy with excision or drainage of the abscess is necessary. The treatment of tuboovarian abscess that is present on admission is controversial. Some authorities prefer immediate laparotomy. We recommend at least 48 hours of therapy with antibiotics, reserving laparotomy for those patients whose condition either fails to respond or worsens. If laparotomy for appendicitis reveals pelvic infection instead, the physician should remove nothing, but merely drain the abscesses and rely on intravenous administration of antibiotics postoperatively.

If the diagnosis is definite and if there has been no recent pregnancy, a gonococcal infection is the most likely cause, and pending culture reports, this possibility should be mentioned to the patient. Recent laparoscopic studies suggest that gonococci account for only 30–40% of all PID cases, with gram-negative bacilli, anaerobes, and chlamydiae accounting for the rest. The patient should be informed of the possibility of tubal damage from gonococcal PID and of the necessity for vigorous treatment and avoidance of repeated infection. The physician should not lead the patient to believe that she is sterile, however; many unwanted pregnancies have resulted from attempts to prove the physician wrong.

Ovarian Cyst

Cysts of the ovary, both benign and malignant, rarely cause pain, being more commonly discovered during a routine pelvic examination. Occasionally, however, a corpus luteum cyst ruptures spontaneously, causing hemoperitoneum; symptoms and physical findings are similar to those of ectopic pregnancy. An uncommon condition, a twisted ovarian cyst causes pain, leukocytosis, and even fever, but rarely causes peritonitis or hemorrhage. The presence of a unilateral tender mass on pelvic examination suggests the diagnosis, but unilateral PID should also be considered. Occasionally an asymptomatic ovarian mass is found in a patient with unrelated symptoms and signs. These lesions require no therapy or evaluation in the emergency ward; if they persist, the patient will require elective laparotomy.

Laparoscopy is an excellent low-risk procedure that usually allows the emergency physician to differentiate between ruptured or twisted ovarian cyst and ectopic pregnancy or to exclude them. If physical examination, laboratory tests, and laparoscopy are not diagnostic, the physician should reassure the patient that the pain does not represent significant disease, and should examine her again in 2 or 3 days. He should discuss and explore emotional factors contributing to the patient's condition, but should not imply that the pain is "all in the head," since she then will lose confidence in him and go to another physician.

TOXEMIA OF PREGNANCY

Toxemia of pregnancy, a syndrome of the second half of pregnancy, is characterized by hypertension and proteinuria. In its more severe form, convulsions (eclampsia), fetal death, disseminated intravascular coagulation, hepatic failure, and maternal death can occur. Usually, patients are seen with preeclampsia, the preconvulsive, less severe form. The diagnosis is made on the basis of systolic pressure over 140 mm Hg or diastolic pressure over 90 mm Hg or both in a pregnant woman or in a woman who has recently given birth. Proteinuria of 1^+–2^+ in a randomly taken urine specimen corroborates the diagnosis. Edema, hyperreflexia, and retinal arteriolar spasm may be present, but are not essential to diagnosis. The patient often reports headache, visual disturbances, and epigastric pain.

Treatment depends on the severity of the disease, but all patients should be hospitalized and the fetus appropriately monitored. Mild preeclampsia with blood pressure 150/100 mm Hg or less, less than 5 gm of protein in the urine per 24 hours, and normal reflexes can be treated initially with bed rest. Severe preeclampsia, with blood pressure 160/100 mm Hg or greater, more than 5 gm of protein per 24 hours, oliguria, visual disturbances, epigastric pain, pulmonary edema, or disseminated intravascular coagulation should be treated aggressively to prevent convulsions, lower blood pressure, and correct clotting defects. Delivery then should take place promptly. Magnesium sulfate, 4 gm at once, followed by 1 gm/hr intravenously, is the treatment of choice for severe preeclampsia and eclampsia. Hydralazine hydrochloride is the usual choice for lowering systolic blood pressure if it is greater than 180/120 mm Hg. The lower pressure probably prevents cerebral hemorrhage and improves renal blood flow, but it also lowers placental blood flow, and lowering the diastolic pressure below 100 mm Hg is not recommended.

In patients with eclampsia, the treatment above follows control of convulsions with magnesium sulfate or intravenous diazepam. Delivery should be accomplished within 6–12 hours.

MANAGEMENT OF EMERGENCY STATES IN THE PREGNANT WOMAN

Pregnant women are seen in emergency facilities with almost all of the diseases they may contract when not pregnant, from the common cold to a ruptured cerebral aneurysm. Each condition must be evaluated and treated while paying extra attention to the presence of the fetus and the altered physiologic state of the mother.

Diagnostic procedures such as physical examination, cardiograms, and blood tests are easy to perform and no more harmful to the pregnant patient than to the nonpregnant patient. The appendix moves higher as pregnancy progresses, and a white blood cell count of 12,000–15,000 cells/mm^3 may be normal during pregnancy, but in general, diagnostic tests are interpretable in their usual way. Use of diagnostic x-ray examination commonly leads to controversy, however. No threshold dose of radiation has been established beyond which there is risk to the fetus. Excessive radiation, as in radiation therapy for a malignant condition or in a nuclear holocaust, has been shown to be teratogenic. Therefore, while unnecessary x-ray examination is to be avoided, concern for safety should not prevent its proper use in the pregnant patient. Prior consultation with a radiologist should keep exposure to a minimum. Chest x-ray films when pneumonia is suspected, an intravenous pyelogram when a renal calculus is suspected, and a lung scan when pulmonary embolism is suspected should not be avoided merely because the patient is pregnant.

Treatment of shock in pregnant patients differs little from standard treatment. Rapid fluid replacement to restore intravascular volume is essential to preserve uterine blood flow as well as flow to the maternal kidneys and brain. It is important to place the patient in the left lateral position or at least to displace the uterus to the left, since uterine pressure on the inferior vena cava accentuates the effects of hypovolemia.

Surgical treatment for unrelated acute conditions such as appendicitis, cholelithiasis, trauma, penetrating injury, intestinal obstruction, or recurrent pulmonary emboli should be performed as indicated. Maternal death may result from failure to perform these necessary procedures. Although operation in the first trimester may cause abortion, the pregnancy usually is unaffected and the fetus unharmed, especially if teratogenic drugs are avoided. Operation in the second trimester rarely interrupts the pregnancy unless sepsis is involved. Although operation in the third trimester may trigger premature labor, it can be temporarily stopped by ritodrine or other β-sympathomimetic drugs.

USE OF DRUGS IN PREGNANCY

The use of drugs in pregnancy presents the physician with a large and confusing body of knowledge and misinformation. The reader should remember that there is a difference between the failure of evidence to find an association of drug use with malformation or disease, and the presence of evidence that there is no association. A few drugs are proved teratogens or are otherwise dan-

gerous, and many presently have no defined danger. As a result of this confusion, the general rule should be to avoid all drugs if possible and to use those of no proved danger when necessary.

The first trimester is, of course, the time when drugs have the most potential to interfere with embryogenesis and organogenesis. Table 24.1 lists proved and suspected teratogens; they should all be avoided unless they are absolutely necessary and the risks are explained to the patient. For example, a woman requiring phenytoin for epilepsy may be willing to take the 4–5% chance of bearing an infant with heart disease or cleft palate; this is approximately double the risk in the general population. Common drugs that appear to be safe in the first trimester include antibiotics of the penicillin family, analgesics including aspirin, and doxylamine succinate (Bendectin), although doxylamine has been subject to recent controversy.

After the first trimester, drugs still pose a threat to the fetus. Most groups of drugs have apparently safe members and demonstrably risky members. Analgesics of all types can be used until the last month or two, when salicylates and prostaglandin inhibitors must be discontinued. Their anticoagulant properties pose a threat of intracranial hemorrhage to the fetus. They also may be associated with premature closure of the ductus arteriosus and with delayed and prolonged labor. Acetaminophen and narcotics (used for acute problems only) are not associated with these dangers. Antibiotics can be given readily to pregnant women when necessary, with the exceptions of tetracycline and erythromycin estolate. Sulfonamides also should be avoided in the third trimester since they

Table 24.1.
Proved and suspected teratogenic agents.

Proved teratogens
   Synthetic progestins
   Diethylstilbestrol (DES)
   Androgens
   Chemotherapeutic agents
   Organic mercury
   Sodium warfarin
   Trimethadione
   Hydantoins
   Thalidomide
Suspected teratogens
   Antihistamines
   Tetracycline
   Lysergic acid diethylamide (LSD)
   Marihuana
   Diazepam (Valium)
   Chlordiazepoxide hydrochloride (Librium)
   Hexachlorophene

compete with bilirubin for binding sites in the fetal liver, and can lead to increased neonatal jaundice. Psychotropic drugs such as barbiturates and tricyclic antidepressants can be used if absolutely necessary, but their safety is no better established than their dangers. Adrenal corticosteroids were thought to be dangerous in the past, but it now appears that chronic use in diseases such as asthma, severe allergy, and Addison's disease results in no damage to the fetus. In fact, these drugs are now of proved benefit when given to the mother to mature the fetal lungs when premature delivery is imminent. Anticoagulants pose a special problem. Sodium warfarin crosses the placenta, causes malformations in the developing embryo, and causes anticoagulation in the fetus later in pregnancy. Heparin does not cross the placenta. Consequently, when treating a pregnant woman for thrombophlebitis or pulmonary embolus, the physician must provide long-term parenteral anticoagulation with heparin.

The most common environmental hazards to the fetus in our society are tobacco, alcohol, and caffeine. Neonates born to smokers on average weigh 200 gm less than those born to nonsmokers. The incidence of obstetric complications is also higher in smokers. Intake of more than eight cups of coffee a day also is associated with decreased birth weight and an increased fetal mortality rate. Alcohol intake of more than 3 oz/day is associated with a group of anomalies called the fetal alcohol syndrome. Minimal alcohol consumption is not associated with anomalies, but since the maximum safe level is not known, the Food and Drug Administration recently has advised pregnant women to consume no alcohol at all.

During lactation, most drugs appear in the milk in quantities equal to amounts in the plasma. Consequently, drugs that should be avoided in the third trimester also should be avoided during lactation, if possible.

PRECIPITATE DELIVERY IN THE EMERGENCY WARD

Occasionally, women arrive at the emergency ward in the second stage of labor, fully dilated and pushing, and the receiving physician has no time in which to transfer her to the labor area or to an obstetric hospital. Delivery is imminent when the fetal scalp is showing at the introitus, the rectum is dilated, and the perineum is bulging. After these observations, another contraction or two is all that is necessary. The patient should be placed on an examination table or stretcher and allowed to assume either a supine or a lateral recumbent posi-

tion. Her knees should be bent and the upper leg supported by an attendant if she chooses the lateral position. No attempt should be made to prevent the head from emerging. The patient should be encouraged to push gently and slowly if possible, and to concentrate on the attendant's words. As the patient pushes the fetal head out, gentle pressure on the head by the attendant's hand toward the patient's rectum will prevent periurethral injury and put more stretch on the perineum. If the perineum is not stretching sufficiently so that a crack appears in the skin, or if blood from inside the vagina is noted, episiotomy can be performed while the patient is pushing. This procedure consists of a 3–4 cm (or less) scissors-cut posterior from the fourchette toward the rectum. The patient will not feel it if it is done at the height of a push, and anesthesia is unnecessary. During this entire process, it is essential to communicate to the patient what is happening and to instruct her when to push more slowly and when to stop pushing. As soon as the head emerges, she should stop pushing for a few seconds while the infant's mouth is suctioned free of mucus with a bulb syringe and the umbilical cord is doubly clamped and cut if around the infant's neck. Gentle posterior pressure on the head will then allow the infant's anterior shoulder to pass under the pubic symphysis. When this stage has been completed, anterior pressure will help the posterior shoulder over the perineum or episiotomy. The remainder of the infant usually slips out quickly without much pushing after delivery of the shoulder. The slower the delivery, the less tearing or episiotomy extension will occur.

The baby will be slippery and easily could be dropped. He or she should be placed slightly downward on the bed or table and the throat suctioned until clear crying is heard. The infant delivered this easily usually will cry well without much external stimulation. If respiration does not begin in 30 seconds (remember that flow through the umbilical cord is still oxygenating the baby somewhat), gentle stimulation such as striking the soles with a finger or rubbing the back usually will suffice. Do not strike the baby on the buttocks.

After good respiration is established, the cord should be doubly clamped about 3–6 cm from the baby and cut between the clamps. The baby then can be given to the mother. The placenta will separate in 2–10 minutes and usually can be removed from the vagina by gentle traction on the cord or pressure on the uterine fundus. Once the placenta has been delivered, it should be inspected to be sure all the cotyledons are present, and the uterine fundus should be massaged to minimize bleeding. The episiotomy or lacerations then should be sutured under local anesthesia, with the patient supine.

Good verbal control of the mother, with proper positioning of the staff, is more important than preparation of the skin or draping of the patient. Delivery is an imperfectly sterile procedure at best, and to lose control of the birth process by observing the formalities of sterile precautions serves no one's best interest.

Precipitate deliveries frequently are associated with cervical tears, postpartum hemorrhage, and amniotic fluid embolism. Therefore, the vagina and cervix should be inspected carefully, and an intravenous infusion containing oxytocin, 10–20 units/liter, should be started as soon as feasible.

Most quick deliveries proceed easily, and by following these guidelines the emergency staff will avoid panic, minimize the mother's anxiety, and allow the baby to emerge into an atmosphere of calm and tenderness.

RAPE

Rape is a serious medical, legal, and social problem, discussion of which has been avoided for too long. According to the Federal Bureau of Investigation, a rape was reported to the police once every 9 minutes in 1973. It is probable also that many more were reported only to hospitals or were not reported at all. FBI statistics indicate that rape in the United States increased by more than 60% between 1968 and 1973.

Medical education and literature have not dealt sufficiently with this subject; consequently, physicians are less well informed about rape than about most other medical topics. Also, the physician needs to deal with his own feelings about rape and sexuality before the patient can be treated adequately. In general, the raped patient has been mistrusted and neglected by male-dominated institutions that seem to be more concerned with the rights of the accused. It is essential that the physician realize that a male has committed a serious physical crime against the victim. The assumption that the rape victim was in some way a willing partner usually is incorrect.

History

The physician should question the patient sympathetically, openly, and respectfully. The chief complaint "I've been raped" should be accorded the same credibility as any other chief complaint. It is difficult and painful for the patient to talk about the details of the rape, since under normal circumstances they would be considered too intimate for discussion. She should, however, be en-couraged to discuss the assault and the events preceding it to help her integrate this shocking reality. Most often the patient will feel guilty, and she should be told that this is normal.

The physician should evaluate the patient's emotional state, noting responses to certain topics of discussion. These notes can be helpful to the victim at a later court action and also to a psychiatrist or social worker attempting to evaluate her emotional needs. While taking the patient's history, the physician should ascertain the date of her last menstrual period, whether she uses birth control methods, and whether she has had PID, keeping in mind that her past sexual behavior has no bearing on whether or not she was raped.

Physical Examination

The patient probably will not be hysterical, although this is a common belief. Instead, she probably will be calm and inquisitive and will need to know what is going to happen during examination to be able to differentiate it from the rape itself.

A general physical examination should be performed. All unusual findings should be noted, such as scratches, bruises, friction burns, lacerations, disheveled appearance, and torn clothing. Most raped patients do *not* fight back so that they may get out of the situation alive. The threat of force leads to rape as well as does force itself.

The pelvic examination should focus on vaginal lacerations, secretions, cervical trauma, and uterine and adnexal tenderness. Specimens from the cervix and rectum should be cultured for gonococci; vaginal secretions should be saved for microscopic and laboratory examination. The patient's clothing, properly labeled, should be saved for the police to examine. Proper labeling includes the names of personnel who received the articles and the place of storage. The patient's pubic hair should be combed and the products saved in a similar manner. The importance of keeping the patient's confidence during the examination by answering all her questions cannot be emphasized enough.

Laboratory Findings

A wet preparation of vaginal secretions should be examined promptly for sperm and the results recorded. Mucus from the cervix should be cultured on either Thayer-Martin or Transgrow media, and a Gram stain should be performed in a search for gram-negative intracellular diplococci. A specimen of vaginal secretion or a scraping from underclothing or both should be sent to the chemical laboratory for an acid phosphatase test, which may be available only at the police laboratory. A pregnancy test using urine or serum should be performed to exclude conception previous to the rape. Blood should be drawn for a serologic test for syphilis; this test should be repeated 1 month after the rape.

Therapy

All rape patients should be treated as venereal disease contacts. Procaine penicillin G, 4.8 million units intramuscularly, should be administered with probenecid, 1 gm orally. In penicillin-allergic patients, tetracycline, 250 mg orally four times a day for 10 days, or spectinomycin, 2 gm intramuscularly, can be substituted.

Diethylstilbestrol (DES) has been advocated for use as a postcoital contraceptive measure. The side effects and possible long-term complications are sufficiently undesirable that its use should be restricted to those patients who are likely to be ovulating; administration should begin within 48 hours of the assault. The recommended dosage, 25 mg twice a day for 5 days, may cause enough nausea and vomiting that the patient will discontinue the pills. Prochlorperazine (Compazine) rectal suppositories should be provided for this eventuality. Recently, DES has been implicated in malignant lesions of the vagina in female offspring of women who took it during pregnancy. Also, the long-term effects on the patient of the recommended high dosage have not been established. In most large cities, therapeutic abortion also is available should the patient wish to terminate a pregnancy resulting from rape. These two alternatives should be discussed with the patient so that she may make an informed choice. If she elects to take DES, she must be advised that an abortion will be recommended should pregnancy occur and also that the date of her next period cannot be predicted.

Diazepam (Valium), 5 mg four times a day for 5 days, or another tranquilizer should be offered to the patient, since it is our experience that almost all rape victims will require it within a short time. The physician also may prescribe a sleep medication, such as flurazepam hydrochloride (Dalmane), 30 mg as required.

The patient's need for emotional support should be obvious. She must deal with the crisis, not avoid it, and must be encouraged to do so. Resources capable of providing this support vary from community to community. Ideally, a rape crisis center, known to police and health care facilities, exists in the area, or the police department has a rape unit. A rape crisis center provides support, counseling, and exposure to groups of other women who have been raped. It also can help the patient in her interactions with police, lawyers, courts, family, and friends, and refer her to professional groups for psychotherapy if necessary. The support of the rape crisis center should be solicited as soon as possible, preferably at the time of the initial examination.

The physician's legal responsibilities in cases of rape are not defined clearly nationwide. In most states, only the physical findings are admissible as evidence in court. In some states, however, the physician's testimony may be allowed for corroboration if he was the first person to hear the details of the assault. In any event, accurate records are of the utmost legal importance (see Chapter 39, pages 902–906). The physician's participation in legal procedures after a rape depends on his willingness to help the patient's cause. It is incumbent on him to learn the local statutes pertaining to rape and the locations of supporting resource facilities.

Suggested Readings

Amir M: *Patterns in Forcible Rape.* Chicago, University of Chicago Press, 1971

Buchsbaum HJ (Ed): *Trauma in Pregnancy.* Philadelphia, W.B. Saunders, 1979

Diagnostic x-rays are no cause for abortion—but caution is advised. *JAMA 236*:2269, 1976

Green R (Ed): *Human Sexuality: A Health Practitioner's Text.* Baltimore, Williams & Wilkins, 1975

Jones GS, Jones HW, Jr: *Novak's Textbook of Gynecology.* ed 10. Baltimore, Williams & Wilkins, 1981

Medea A, Thompson K; *Against Rape.* New York, Farrar, Straus, Giroux, 1974

Pritchard JW (Ed): *William's Obstetrics.* ed 7. Baltimore, Williams & Wilkins, 1981

Schwarz RH, Yaffe SJ: *Drug and Chemical Risks to the Fetus and Newborn.* New York, Alan R. Liss, 1980

J Obstet Gynecol 58 (suppl 5):1–105, 1981

CHAPTER 25

Urologic Emergencies

STEPHEN P. DRETLER, M.D.
ERIC J. SACKNOFF, M.D.
ROBERT J. BATES, M.D.

The emergency physician should be acquainted fully with the various acute and chronic urologic conditions seen daily in the emergency ward. This chapter is divided into major sections on traumatic injuries and nontraumatic emergencies, and conditions requiring immediate surgical attention are distinguished from those necessitating more conservative treatment. The hope is that all physicians—whether surgeons, internists, or pediatricians—may identify clearly the clinical problem by the history, physical examination, radiologic evaluation, and laboratory analysis, and then may make the appropriate judgment for surgical consultation or medical care.

TRAUMATIC INJURIES

Injury to the genitourinary tract may result from trauma to the chest, flank, abdomen, pelvis, or perineum. If the patient has gross hematuria or obvious perineal injury, the presence of genitourinary damage will be apparent. In the absence of immediately recognizable signs, however, the recognition and treatment of genitourinary injury requires knowledge of the anatomy of the structures involved, the circumstances in which damage to these organs may occur, the signs and symptoms of injury, the available methods of diagnostic evaluation, and the general principles of management.

Upper Urinary Tract

The kidneys and their vascular pedicles are located in the retroperitoneum behind the 12th rib, overlying the transverse processes of the upper lumbar vertebrae. The left kidney and upper ureter with their enveloping fascia (Gerota's fascia) lie adjacent to the spleen, separated only by peritoneum. The kidney lies in contact with the posterolateral chest wall (the 10th, 11th, and 12th ribs), the diaphragm and overlying pleura, and the tail

of the pancreas at its superomedial margin, and is posterior to the descending colon. The right kidney and upper ureter are 1–2 cm lower, and also are protected by the diaphragm and the 11th and 12th ribs. The right renal pelvis is adjacent to the duodenum, and its upper pole, which is separated from the liver by peritoneum, is posterior to the hepatic flexure of the colon. The fascia of each kidney includes an adrenal gland.

Despite the protection given the kidneys by their anatomic position, traumatic injuries are not uncommon and are accompanied by injury to other organ systems in 60–80% of cases.

Penetrating renal injuries most commonly result from gunshot and stab wounds. On the right, they may be associated with injuries to the lung, diaphragm, pleura, liver, colon, and duodenum, and on the left, the diaphragm, pleura, spleen, lung, pancreas, and colon. Any penetrating injury in these regions suggests involvement of a kidney or its pedicle. *Blunt injuries* to the chest, flank, or abdomen may cause renal damage by: (1) direct compression of the kidney against the vertebrae and paraspinal muscles; (2) laceration by a fractured rib or fractured transverse vertebral process; or (3) tearing or avulsion of the pedicle. Renovascular injury may result from acceleration-deceleration forces that produce partial or complete avulsion of the renal pedicle or disruption of the intima with subsequent thrombosis. In addition, ureteral injury may occur from blunt or penetrating trauma to the upper part of the abdomen or the flank. Stab and gunshot wounds commonly cause ureteral and renal pelvic lacerations, and severe hyperextension may cause ureteropelvic avulsion, especially in children. Relatively minor trauma may produce renal pelvic rupture in a congenitally deformed kidney.

Signs and Symptoms. Because other organ injuries often are associated with renal trauma and require emergent therapy, renal injuries often are overlooked. A high index of suspicion must be maintained in evaluating all patients with blunt or penetrating injury. The most common sign of renal injury is hematuria. Other signs and symptoms include manifestations in the flank, such as localized pain or colic with the passage of blood clots or kidney fragments, ecchymosis, or a mass caused by blood or urine or both; pain referred to the testis, groin, or shoulder; and hemorrhagic shock. Transient hypertension may occur from segmental injury and ischemia or from compression by a perirenal hematoma (Page kidney). Absence of hematuria or of a mass or pain in the flank does not exclude the possibility of renal injury. Lacerations may occur without hematuria, especially if the ureter or renal pelvis is avulsed. Shock may decrease renal blood flow in such a way that neither hematoma nor extravasation of urine will be immediately obvious, and vascular thrombosis may cause total loss of renal function without signs of flank hemorrhage, hematuria, or urinary extravasation. Hematuria is absent in 65% of patients with major renal vascular injuries. Therefore, even in the absence of obvious signs and symptoms of renal injury, trauma to the lower part of the chest, the abdomen, or the flank necessitates complete renal evaluation.

Diagnostic Studies. The patient who has sustained multiple injuries without obvious perineal injury or pelvic fracture should undergo urethral catheterization with a No. 18 French Foley catheter unless blood at the urethral meatus suggests urethral damage. If perineal, pelvic, or lower abdominal injury has occurred, retrograde urethrography should be performed before urethral catheterization. Urine obtained by catheterization often contains 5–10 red blood cells in each microscopic high power field, and does not necessarily indicate genitourinary tract injury. If possible, the patient should void a specimen for accurate determination of hematuria. Reflex urethral catheterization in patients with multiple injuries without proper evaluation of the lower urinary tract is to be condemned, since it may convert partial urethral injuries to complete disruptions.

All patients with significant blunt or penetrating injury to the lower part of the chest, the flank, or the abdomen should undergo radiologic kidney-ureter-bladder (KUB) examination and drip infusion nephrotomography. The KUB film may demonstrate a fractured rib or transverse process, obliteration of the psoas margins or of the renal outline by extravasated blood or urine, scoliosis to the side of renal injury resulting from ipsilateral psoas muscle spasm, displacement of bowel loops,

elevation of the diaphragm, or foreign bodies in the area of the kidney. The KUB film is usually normal, however, and the absence of these findings does not exclude renal injury. Drip infusion nephrotomography with 120 ml of a 50% solution of meglumine or sodium diatrizoate (Hypaque) over 5 minutes is required to rule out urinary tract damage in the presence of any of the following: hematuria; flank tenderness or mass; evidence of a fractured 10th, 11th, or 12th thoracic vertebra or transverse vertebral process; or signs of other intra-abdominal injury, such as air under the diaphragm or positive results of abdominal paracentesis. The nephrotomogram will demonstrate penetrating renal injury, renal fracture, urinary extravasation, areas of segmental destruction, and loss of function, and is accurate in 95% of cases. Renal arteriography is indicated if the patient has any of the above findings or an enlarging flank mass or continued blood loss. If the nephrotomogram reveals only minor injury, such as contusion, arteriographic examination may be deferred until the clinical course is more defined.

Renal scanning with technetium compounds may be used to determine whether the kidney is injured in patients allergic to dyes containing iodine. Furthermore, this is a noninvasive method of monitoring the function of an injured kidney that is under observation.

Retrograde pyelography is indicated only if extravasation noted on a drip infusion pyelogram suggests damage to the renal pelvis or the ureter.

Treatment. The major indications for surgical exploration and repair of an injured kidney are: (1) loss of function confirmed by arteriography; (2) massive or continued blood loss; (3) significant extravasation; (4) evidence of major injury, such as a laceration or fracture; and (5) penetrating injury—from a stab or gunshot wound, for example. Total loss of function indicates avulsion of the pedicle or intimal tearing and arterial thrombosis. If the pedicle is avulsed, bleeding is usually so massive that immediate surgical intervention is necessary. Before exploration, however, it is essential to demonstrate the presence of a contralateral kidney; this may be done in the operating room by infusing 120 ml of a 50% solution of meglumine or sodium diatrizoate and then obtaining a KUB film. Thrombosis of the renal artery without avulsion also requires immediate surgical treatment. The salvage rate of kidneys in this circumstance is low, however. Therefore, if other serious life-threatening injuries have occurred, such as multiple chest and head injuries, renal arterial thrombosis may be treated conservatively. In the case of continued blood loss or extravasation with an expanding flank mass, arteriographic examination must be performed before exploration to define the extent of injury. Failure to do this preoperatively may result in unnecessary nephrectomy. Major renal lacerations or fractures must be debrided, drained, and repaired. However, partial loss of renal function is unlikely to improve with surgical repair if it is due to intrarenal damage. Penetrating renal injuries must be explored to debride necrotic tissue and to drain septic material.

Most renal injuries result from blunt trauma, and although the aforementioned injuries require surgical repair, 85% of renal injuries can be managed nonoperatively. Contusions and minor lacerations in kidneys that function during infusion pyelography are treated best by hospitalization and observation to monitor renal function, urinary extravasation, blood loss, and hematuria.

The principles of management of renal injuries in children are similar to those in adults. In children, however, the kidneys are even more susceptible to injury since they are proportionally larger and have a minimal protective layer of fat. Moreover, Gerota's fascia, which provides a protective cover around the adult kidney, is poorly developed until the child is 10 years old. Approximately 20% of renal injuries in children occur in the presence of pre-existent disease such as hydronephrosis or Wilms' tumor.

Ureteral laceration usually is managed by surgical exploration after identification by retrograde urography. When shock has occurred, renal blood flow decreases and urinary extravasation from ureteral injury may be unrecognized. Therefore, the course of the ureters should be observed carefully on the urogram and questionable areas should be examined with a retrograde ureteropyelogram. Renal salvage depends on early recognition of the injury and repair during the initial abdominal exploration. Delayed recognition of ureteral injuries often results in otherwise avoidable nephrectomy.

Lower Urinary Tract

Bladder

The urinary bladder is protected anteriorly and laterally by the pubic arch, supported inferiorly by the pelvic diaphragm, and covered superiorly and posteriorly by the peritoneum and intraperitoneal structures. Bladder injuries are classified as contusion, intraperitoneal rupture, extraperitoneal rupture, and combined intraperitoneal and extraperitoneal rupture. Injury results from blunt or penetrating trauma to the lower part of the abdo-

men or the pelvis, and commonly occurs when the bladder is distended. Blunt trauma accounts for at least 80% of all bladder injuries. Although 70% of patients with blunt injuries to the bladder have an associated pelvic fracture, only about 15% of pelvic fractures have an associated bladder injury.

Long-distance runners may be seen in the emergency ward with gross hematuria and suprapubic pain secondary to continuing blunt trauma of the empty bladder against the bladder base. An area of contusion at the bladder base and posterior wall on cytoscopy confirms the diagnosis.

Pressure necrosis of the bladder base with tissue slough and a vesicovaginal fistula may occur after childbirth as a result of prolonged pressure of the fetal head on the bladder base during a difficult delivery.

In children, the bladder is abdominal, not pelvic; hence, even when not distended, it is susceptible to injury when lower abdominal trauma occurs.

Signs and Symptoms. Bladder injury may be unrecognized when other major trauma has occurred. The first sign of rupture, whether intraperitoneal or extraperitoneal, may be a nonpalpable bladder and the absence of urine in the bladder after placement of a Foley catheter. Intraperitoneal rupture with extravasation of blood and urine may cause peritoneal irritation, guarding, tenderness, and lower abdominal rigidity. Blood and urine under the diaphragm may cause pain referred to the shoulder. If uninfected, however, intraperitoneal urine may be well tolerated. Extraperitoneal rupture usually occurs on the anterolateral wall near the neck of the bladder, and most often results from perforation by bony segments of a fractured symphysis or pubic arch. Lower abdominal pain, tenderness, and guarding may occur, but are more localized than in patients with intraperitoneal rupture. All degrees of bladder injury may result in either gross or microscopic hematuria. Incontinence may occur suggesting a vesicovaginal fistula.

Diagnostic Studies. When lower abdominal or pelvic trauma has occurred, a Foley catheter should not be inserted until an x-ray film has established whether the pelvis is fractured. If the patient has a fractured pubic arch or symphysis, a urethrogram must be obtained to exclude the possibility of urethral rupture before passage of a catheter. If no evidence of pelvic fracture exists, a Foley catheter may be placed. The presence of urine in the bladder does not rule out perforation. Cystography with anterior, posterior, and right and left oblique views should be performed. The bladder should be filled under gravity with

300–400 ml of radiopaque contrast material, and the dye should be left in the bladder for 10 minutes since small perforations may not be visible immediately. Since a filled bladder may obscure small areas of extravasation, a drainage film is taken after washing out residual contrast material with saline solution. Intraperitoneal rupture causes dye to outline the loops of intestine or to accumulate in the dependent portions of the peritoneal cavity, especially the paracolic recess (Fig. 25.1A). In patients with extraperitoneal rupture, dye is confined to the perivesical area (Fig. 25.1B). After cystography, an intravenous urogram should be obtained to confirm the integrity of the upper urinary tract. If extravasation of dye visualized on the cystogram is so massive that it obscures the lower portions of the ureters, retrograde ureterograms may be necessary to exclude injury.

Treatment. Suspected bladder contusions with pelvic trauma, hematuria, and no extravasation seen on the cystogram may be treated nonoperatively with or without a Foley catheter.

Extraperitoneal bladder injuries should be treated surgically unless the injury is small and single, the urine is uninfected, and the injury is recognized within several hours of occurrence. All other injuries need exploration, drainage of the perivesical space, a suprapubic catheter, and antibiotic coverage.

Similarly, intraperitoneal bladder rupture may be treated with catheter drainage and antibiotics. However, it has been our policy to explore and close the majority of these injuries unless the leak is small and the urine uninfected.

Urethra

The anatomic location and extent of a urethral injury determines its presentation and treatment. Injury may result in partial transection of the urethral mucosa or total disruption, with considerable differences in therapy and eventual outcome.

A urethral injury should be sought when blood is present at the meatus or in the voided specimen obtained after trauma, or if the patient is unable to void. In addition, urethral injuries should be suspected in patients with pelvic fractures or perineal or "straddle" injuries.

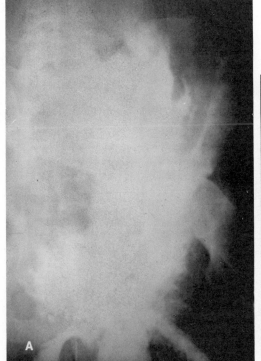 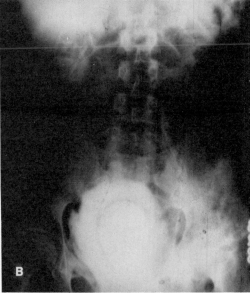

Figure 25.1. Bladder rupture. **(A)** Intraperitoneal bladder rupture with total extravasation of dye causing sunburst effect. **(B)** Extraperitoneal bladder rupture with extravasated dye confined to perivesical space, producing halo effect.

The key to the diagnosis of urethral injury is urethrography. Catheters should not be passed before urethrography in any patient suspected of having a urethral injury, since partial disruptions can be transformed into complete disruptions. Urethrography should be performed fluoroscopically, with the patient placed in a 45-degree right oblique position with the hips flexed. Water-soluble nonviscous radiopaque contrast material, 10–20 ml, should be instilled through a No. 12 French Foley catheter inserted into the fossa navicularis of the penis located just inside the meatus. Generally, partial ruptures will be characterized by periurethral extravasation at the site of injury with contrast material present in the bladder, whereas complete disruption will show only periureteral extravasation. We have seen patients with partial disruption and no flow of contrast material into the bladder because of edema obstructing the proximal portion of the urethra.

Anterior Injury. The male urethra is divided into anterior and posterior portions. The anterior urethra is located distal to the urogenital diaphragm, which surrounds the external spincter, and includes the bulbous and pendulous segments of the urethra. It is contained by the corpus spon-

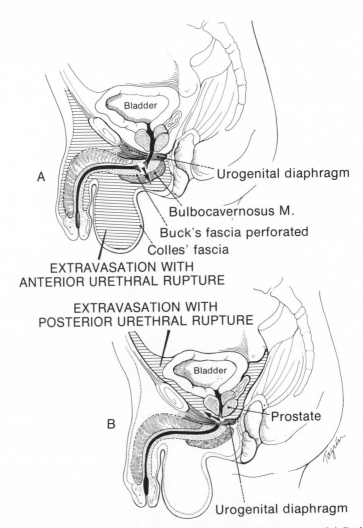

Figure 25.2. Urethral rupture. **(A)** Anterior rupture of bulbar urethra distal to urogential diaphragm. Typically, there is extravasation of blood and urine through Buck's fascia into perineum, scrotum, and anterior abdominal wall. **(B)** Posterior urethral rupture demonstrating prostate sheared proximal to urogenital diaphragm and elevated cephalad in pelvis. Characteristically, because of the intact fascial plane of the urogenital diaphragm, extravasated blood and urine are contained within anterior and posterior retroperitoneum of pelvis. Ecchymosis of the perineum or scrotum would not be found unless this fascial plane were torn.

giosum and corpora cavernosa, which are enveloped by Buck's fascia. Posteriorly Buck's fascia attaches to the urogenital diaphragm, and anteriorly it extends to the abdominal wall. Buck's fascia must be perforated for blood and urine to extravasate into the perineum or scrotum where it will be contained by Colles' fascia (Fig. 25.2A).

There are four general types of injury to the anterior urethra: (1) blunt trauma as seen in the classic straddle injury; (2) injury secondary to instrumentation or probing; (3) penetrating trauma; and (4) injury as the result of indwelling catheters. The most common is the straddle injury in which the bulbous segment is crushed against the undersurface of the pubic rami, resulting in contusion or laceration of the urethra and corpus spongiosum. A fall on a crossbar of a ladder, the top of a fence, or the horizontal bar of a bicycle is a classic example of a straddle injury. Probing injuries usually result from self-inflicted trauma or attempts to pass catheters, whereas penetrating injuries generally occur from gunshot and stab wounds. Injuries due to instrumentation occur at fixed portions of the urethra: the meatus and the suspensory ligament. Indwelling catheters block secretions and promote infection, scarring, and pressure necrosis with subsequent formation of fistulas.

A foreign body in the urethra may cause symptoms of lower urinary tract irritation. Sometimes, but not always, a history of insertion of the foreign body is obtained. Frequently, the diagnosis is made only after x-ray examination of the lower part of the abdomen reveals the offending agent. Admission and urologic evaluation by endoscopic techniques are necessary for removal of the object.

Signs and Symptoms. The history of a blow to the perineum or of a straddle injury should alert the physician to the possibility of anterior urethral injury, especially if blood is found at the urethral meatus or the patient is unable to void. Hematuria may be present, but the urine may become clear as blood is washed from a damaged urethra. Extravasation of blood and urine into the perineum or scrotum indicates urethral injury with perforation of Buck's fascia. Since Buck's fascia extends over the anterior abdominal wall, extravasated urine may migrate cephalad. Anterior urethral injury without disruption of Buck's fascia will confine blood and extravasated urine to the penile shaft.

Urethrography will confirm the diagnosis and define the extent of injury (Fig. 25.3).

Treatment. Partial disruptions of the anterior urethra can be treated with one of two methods, depending on the extent of injury and the degree

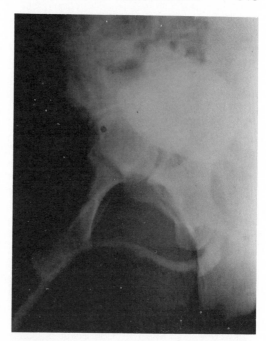

Figure 25.3. Anterior urethral rupture. Retrograde urethrogram shows extravasation of dye from bulbar urethra.

of hematoma and extravasation. If the associated hematoma and urinoma are extensive, local drainage is advocated. Suprapubic urinary diversion is instituted by percutaneous cystotomy (see Section 5, p. 920–921) or formal operative cystotomy. One method of treatment involves only suprapubic drainage and later assessment of urethral healing, whereas the second method involves gentle passage of a urethral catheter to stent the injury during healing. Using the latter method, Pontes reported that 15 of 16 patients had excellent results. We prefer to insert a percutaneous suprapubic catheter initially and to drain any large fluid collections. Later, if there is a question regarding the extent of urethral injury, a cystogram with voiding films (if possible) is obtained, and one week after injury, urethroscopy is performed and a urethral catheter placed. Secondary repair of urethral strictures may be necessary.

Complete anterior urethral disruptions should be treated similarly. Some authorities advocate immediate repair, and others delayed repair. We have followed the latter course without difficulty, repairing the urethra after resolution of all periurethral reaction.

Posterior Injury. The posterior portion of the urethra includes the membranous segment, which traverses the urogenital diaphragm, and the prostatic segment. Ruptures of the posterior urethra usually are not associated with extravasation of blood or urine to the perineum, scrotum, or anterior abdominal wall (Fig. 25.2B) because of the strong fascial planes that attach the urogenital diaphragm laterally to the inferior ischiopubic rami, anteriorly to the pubic symphysis, and posteriorly to the ischial tuberosities and the perineal body. The prostate gland is held in position primarily by the puboprostatic ligaments. Distortion of the pelvic girdle during trauma shears these ligaments, with resultant avulsion of the urethra at the prostatomembranous junction. Around the entire posterior urethra run the parasympathetic and sympathetic nerves responsible for erection and ejaculation. Injury to this area, therefore, may result in impotence, whereas injury to the urinary sphincter, which lies in the urogenital diaphragm, may result in incontinence. Shearing forces that avulse the puboprostatic ligaments produce complete detachment of the prostate gland and bladder from the urogenital diaphragm, resulting in cephalad migration of these structures. Hemorrhage results from tears of pelvic veins, fragmentation of bone, and lacerations of the obturator artery.

Trauma to the membranous and prostatic portions of the urethra carries a high and often permanent morbidity, frequently resulting in severe obliterative scarring of the urethra, impotence, and incontinence. If unnecessary manipulation is avoided at the time of injury, however, these complications can be minimized.

Signs and Symptoms. When pelvic trauma has occurred, posterior urethral injury should be suspected. The patient will be unable to void, and blood may be visible at the urethral meatus. Abdominal examination may show a distended bladder palpable well out of the pelvis, especially after fluid replacement. This occurs when the bladder and prostate gland are detached from the pelvic diaphragm and migrate cephalad. The internal sphincter of the bladder neck prevents urine from leaking into the retroperitoneal space. Rectal examination may reveal cephalad migration of the prostate gland and periprostatic hematoma. Shock may be present if laceration of a pelvic vein or of the obturator artery has resulted in massive retroperitoneal bleeding. Unless the urogenital diaphragm is ruptured, blood will not appear in the scrotum or perineum.

Diagnostic Studies. A KUB film should be obtained whenever pelvic injury is suspected. If it reveals a pelvic fracture or diastasis of the pubic symphysis, retrograde urethrography should be performed. If urethral laceration is apparent on the urethrogram (Fig. 25.4), suprapubic drainage of urine is necessary since introduction of a catheter into an open retropubic space may result in infection of the retroperitoneal hematoma. An enlarging hematoma elevates the bladder further out of the pelvis and compresses its sides, giving the diagnostic inverted teardrop shape seen in the cystographic phase of an intravenous urogram or on a cystogram performed via a cystostomy tube. We consider transfemoral arteriography to be the best technique to locate the source of retroperitoneal bleeding.

Treatment. Laceration of the posterior urethra is best treated with immediate suprapubic cystostomy, blood replacement, and control of pelvic hemorrhage, which is accomplished by injection of Gelfoam or autologous clot during arteriography to occlude the bleeding site. If pelvic bleeding requires continued blood replacement or causes hypotension, temporary tamponade may first be achieved by means of external counterpressure with a G-suit or MAST trousers. The ruptured urethral segments are best approximated 3–6 months after injury.

External Genitalia

Penis

Elastic bands, bottles, rings, nuts, and other constricting objects may cause severe penile edema. In some cases, swelling may be so great that the band causing the constriction is obscured, but careful examination of the penis will reveal such a foreign body. Removal of the object requires anesthesia by penile nerve block and possibly the combined ingenuity of both the emergency physician and the hospital maintenance personnel, who may be called on to supply the proper tools.

Penile lacerations should be treated with the same attention to preserve tissue and function as lacerations in other areas. If the ventral surface is lacerated, the examiner particularly should be cognizant of the possibility of urethral injury, and a urethrogram should be obtained. If any doubt exists, endoscopic examination should be performed. Despite the apparent severity of the laceration, repair of the corpora, the urethra, and the skin can provide excellent functional and cosmetic results. If skin has been lost from the shaft, the injury is debrided with preservation of as much tissue as possible; skin grafting may be performed later.

Testes

Scrotal trauma may result in contusion, laceration, destruction, or dislocation of a testis. Contusion of a hydrocele may cause a hematohydrocele, but hemorrhage usually is tamponaded within the hydrocele sac. Testicular laceration may result in extravasation of blood into that side of the scrotum. Surgical repair with drainage of the severely lacerated testis decreases morbidity. Unless the testis is destroyed, orchiectomy is rarely necessary. When the testis is dislocated from forceful trauma to the scrotum, it may be displaced into the inguinal canal, in which case exploration and fixation are imperative.

Autonomic Dysreflexia

Patients with acute or stable spinal cord injuries may have autonomic dysreflexia in response to various nociceptive and proprioceptive stimuli applied below the level of the specific spinal cord lesion. This syndrome is characterized by severe headache, paroxysmal elevation of systolic and diastolic blood pressure, reflex bradycardia, convulsions, and possibly, cerebral hemorrhage. Flushing and excessive sweating of the face, neck, and dermatomes above the level of the cord lesion, nasal congestion, and a pilomotor response occur. The most common stimuli for this condition are

urinary retention and rectal dilation. Autonomic dysreflexia occurs in patients with spinal cord lesions above the 6th thoracic vertebra with intact distal spinal cords.

Treatment should be directed at prompt relief of the inciting stimulus and physiologic supportive therapy. It should be emphasized that this is a life-threatening condition that requires prompt, thorough evaluation.

NONTRAUMATIC EMERGENCIES

Colicky Flank Pain

Flank pain of urinary tract origin, whether colicky or noncolicky, results from stretching of the renal capsule, and is referred along the 8th, 9th, and 10th thoracic nerve roots. It may be due to obstructed urinary outflow, intrarenal swelling, or alterations in renal blood flow. The character of the pain, medical history, physical examination, laboratory data, and radiologic studies are all important in the differential diagnosis.

Acute, colicky flank pain suggests partial or complete obstruction of urinary outflow, which usually is due to one or more calculi. The colic results from smooth muscle spasm and intermit-

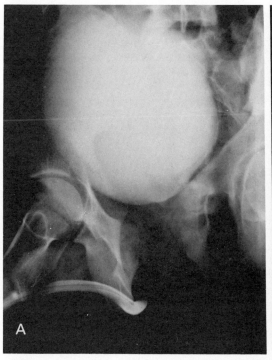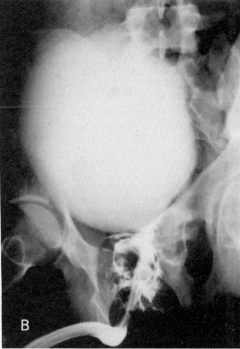

Figure 25.4. Posterior urethral rupture. **(A)** Early phase of retrograde urethrogram showing cephalad elevation of bladder with retained dye from intravenous pyelogram. **(B)** Later phase of retrograde urethrogram showing misplaced Foley catheter resulting from posterior urethral rupture. Note extravasation of dye into periprostatic tissue.

tent distention of the proximal portion of the ureter and the renal pelvis that occurs with each peristaltic wave. If obstruction is at the uretero-pelvic junction, the pain is referred only to the flank. Upper ureteral obstruction may cause referral of pain to the testis along the 11th and 12th thoracic nerve roots because of the similar origin of the nerve supply. Obstruction in the middle of the ureter causes pain referred to the ipsilateral lower abdominal quadrant, and may mimic appendicitis or diverticulitis, but without localized point tenderness or rigidity. Lower ureteral pain from the intravesical ureter may cause symptoms of an irritated bladder.

Causes

A history of renal calculi is suggestive, but conditions other than calculi also may cause colic, such as blood clot from a renal or pelvic tumor or a sloughed renal papilla. Sloughing of a papilla is particularly likely in diabetic patients and in patients with a history of acute or chronic urinary tract infection.

Physical Examination

The patient with colic is agitated, diaphoretic, and in excruciating pain. In contrast with the immobilized patient who has peritoneal irritation, he often thrashes about the bed trying to find a comfortable spot to relieve the colic. Physical examination reveals tenderness at the costovertebral angle, but minimal evidence of abdominal guarding and no rigidity or rebound tenderness. Nausea and vomiting often are prominent acute symptoms. Fever occurs if infection is present proximal to the site of obstruction; gram-negative septicemia may accompany colic, especially if urinary tract infection was present before the onset of acute obstruction.

Diagnostic Studies

Urinalysis usually reveals red blood cells, but rarely reveals clots. Traces of albumin are commonly present when the urine contains many red blood cells. If total unilateral obstruction has occurred, it is possible that the urine will contain no cells at all. Pyuria will be present if infection accompanies the obstruction, and urinary cultures should be obtained. A urinary pH of approximately 8.5 suggests urea-splitting organisms (usually *Proteus* species) and the presence of struvite (magnesium-ammonium-phosphate) calculi. Examination of the urine for crystals of uric acid, calcium oxalate, and cystine helps establish a diagnosis before a KUB film or an intravenous

urogram is taken. Slight elevation of the white blood cell count may occur during colic; more than 15,000 white blood cells/mm^3 suggests active infection.

The KUB film may reveal radiopaque calculi, such as calculi composed of calcium oxalate, cystine, calcium phosphate, or magnesium-ammonium-phosphate. Since uric acid calculi, papillae, and blood clots are radiolucent, they cannot be seen on the KUB film. Approximately 85% of renal calculi are radiopaque, however. Confusion may occur in the presence of calcified mesenteric lymph nodes or if there are phleboliths in the pelvic veins. Phleboliths are spherical and have a hollow center, whereas calculi usually are irregularly shaped and have an eccentric depression on one surface, which was their site of attachment to the renal papilla. Staghorn and branched calculi are likely to be visualized on the KUB film at the calyceal infundibulum and at the ureteropelvic junction.

Intravenous urography is essential as an emergency procedure in the patient with colic if he has severe, unremitting pain or fever. Patients whose pain has diminished and who are afebrile may be treated with analgesics, and a urogram may be obtained on the following day; if x-ray facilities are available in the emergency ward, however, it is reasonable to obtain an intravenous urogram at the time of the colicky episode. During an episode of renal colic, the urogram shows a delay in function of the ipsilateral kidney as a result of distal obstruction. This delay may be 5 or 10 minutes in the presence of acute or partial obstruction, or it may be several hours in total or chronic obstruction. The dye eventually will fill the ureter to the site of the obstruction, but several films may have to be obtained before this is visualized. Persistence on the part of the radiologists, with delayed films at regular intervals, may be necessary for satisfactory anatomic detail eventually to be obtained. In acute obstruction, small amounts of urine and dye may extravasate around the renal pelvis. This is due to the higher osmotic pressure of the dye within the obstructed urinary tract, which increases the volume in the renal pelvis and ruptures the calyceal fornix (Fig. 25.5). Such extravasation is not an indication for surgical intervention, but is an indication for close clinical observation.

If a calculus is suspected on the KUB film, the urogram will confirm its presence and position. Small, irregular calcifications in the pelvis may be suspected to be calculi, but a column of dye must end at the calculus to confirm this initial impression. Oblique films always are necessary to demonstrate that the calcification seen on the KUB film remains within the contrast-filled ureter. If the patient has a calculus at the ureterovesical junction, an oblique film obtained after the patient has voided may demonstrate the calculus at the apex of the ureter.

Treatment

The ureteropelvic junction, the middle of the ureter at the site of the iliac vessels, and the intramural portion of the ureter are the narrowest segments of the ureter, and it is usually at one of these three sites that the calculus lodges and causes symptoms. The decision to be made in the emergency ward is whether the calculus is small enough to pass through the ureter spontaneously.

Calculi lodged at the ureteropelvic junction usually are too big (more than 8 mm in diameter) to pass down the length of the ureter. Symptoms often subside as the calculus becomes dislodged and floats back into the pelvis. If the calculus is smaller than 8 mm in diameter and is not causing

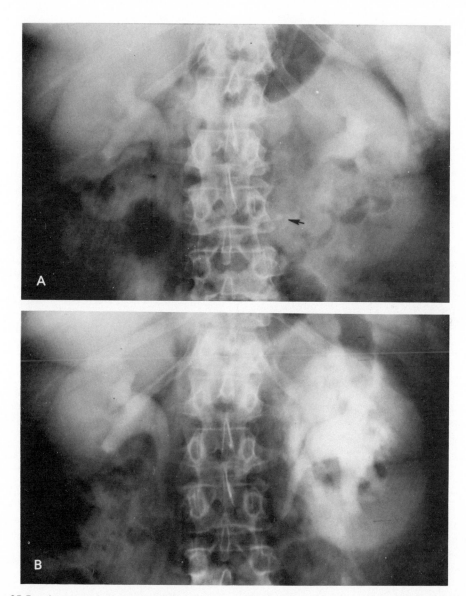

Figure 25.5.   Acute renal obstruction with extravasation. **(A)** Intravenous pyelogram 10 minutes after injection of dye. Note calcified stone (*arrow*) at tip of left transverse process of third lumbar vertebra and delayed function of left kidney. **(B)** Forty minutes after injection, excretion of dye ends at level of calculus with peripelvic extravasation of contrast material. Note acute dilatation of calyces and general swelling of left kidney.

sepsis or total obstruction or both, conservative management with hydration, analgesics, and antibiotics usually promotes spontaneous passage. If the calculus is larger, surgical intervention is usually necessary. However, in the case of uric acid calculi, medical therapy may be tried initially. Since uric acid calculi usually will dissolve in alkaline urine, raising the urinary pH with either sodium bicarbonate or potassium citrate may be successful. However, in the presence of sepsis, some form of surgical intervention is necessary, regardless of the type of calculus.

In patients who have a calculus in the ureter, the indications for surgical removal or extraction with a stone basket are sepsis, persistent pain, fever, or total obstruction. Lower ureteral calculi more than 8 mm in diameter usually require surgical management.

If colic is caused by a sloughed papilla or a blood clot, treatment must be directed toward the primary cause—diabetes, acute infection, or neoplasm.

Noncolicky Flank Pain

Causes

Noncolicky flank pain of renal origin may result from several conditions. Acute onset of noncolicky pain usually is caused by changes in blood flow that may be due to a renal arterial embolus, renal venous thrombosis, dissection of the renal artery, or rupture of a renal arterial aneurysm. The most common cause of a renal arterial embolus is atrial fibrillation, but emboli may occur in patients with a mural thrombus after myocardial infarction and in patients with an atrial or ventricular septal defect.

Nonacute, noncolicky flank pain of renal origin usually results from intrarenal changes or perinephric infection. The conditions most commonly causing this type of pain are acute pyelonephritis, renal abscess, perinephric abscess, bleeding into a renal tumor, and nonobstructive renal calculi.

Acute pyelonephritis is more common in women and may occur in an otherwise normal urinary tract, but it usually is due to an underlying disorder such as vesicoureteral reflux, obstruction at any level of the urinary tract, diabetes mellitus, or hematogenous embolization. In patients with urinary tract obstruction, the obstructive process may be within or outside the tract. Pyelonephritis may be unilateral or bilateral, with flank pain, fever, and chills. High fever is common. Associated symptoms such as urinary frequency, urgency, and dysuria may precede other symptoms. In severe cases, nausea and vomiting may occur. Induced

abdominal pain, rather than flank pain, is common.

Renal abscess may occur from intrarenal obstruction or hematogenous spread. Suppuration caused by intrarenal obstruction usually results from gram-negative organisms, whereas abscesses arising from hematogenous spread are often staphylococcal. The clinical signs and symptoms are indistinguishable from those of pyelonephritis.

Nonacute, noncolicky flank pain of renal origin must be distinguished from many nonurologic conditions that cause pain in the back or at the costovertebral angle. An inclusive list would be encyclopedic. The most common nonurologic conditions include musculoskeletal and duodenal disorders, cholecystitis, pancreatitis, pneumonitis, and pulmonary infarction.

Diagnostic Studies and Treatment

In patients with a renal arterial embolus, urinalysis reveals albuminuria (2+ to 3+) and microscopic hematuria. An intravenous urogram may show partial or total loss of function, depending on the site at which the embolus has lodged. If confusion exists regarding whether delayed function is due to ureteral obstruction or vascular obstruction, renal scanning may be employed for clarification. If loss of function is seen on the urogram and if calculus is not the cause, a renal arteriogram is obtained as soon as possible and surgical treatment is instituted. Embolization may be differentiated from renal venous thrombosis by renal arteriography. In renal venous thrombosis, the arteriogram shows a patent artery with only a nephrogram to represent function. In the presence of embolization, however, the arteriogram reveals arterial obstruction with nonfunction of the affected kidney or segment (Fig. 25.6). Renal venous thrombosis may be either unilateral or bilateral, and usually is associated with severe albuminuria. Diagnosis is confirmed by cavography or by selective renal venography. Treatment requires anticoagulation with high doses of heparin and often includes management of an underlying associated disorder such as a malignant condition, thrombophlebitis, or nephrotic syndrome. Renal arterial embolectomy has been successful in well-selected patients with obstruction of the main renal artery or of one of the primary branches.

Patients with aortic dissection and renal arterial involvement have pain in both the flank and the back; urography shows no function on the affected side. Therapy is directed toward the aortic dissection (see Chapter 21, pages 474–475). Rupture of a renal arterial aneurysm is rare, and is manifested by the acute onset of flank pain and hemorrhagic shock. Seldom does a patient with this condition live long enough to arrive at an emergency facility for treatment. Small leaks, however, may be demonstrated on an arteriogram.

In patients with acute pyelonephritis caused by a urea-splitting organism, the urinary pH will be more than 8.5. Mild proteinuria is common in patients with renal infection. Microscopic examination of urine reveals abundant white blood cells, and the presence of white blood cell casts indicates a renal origin. Bacteria may be identified on the Gram stain of unspun urine. If a single organism is identified in each high power field of Gram-stained uncentrifuged urine, culture of that specimen is usually associated with a count of more than 100,000 organisms/ml and therapy should be started. Leukocytosis usually is present.

The treatment of patients with acute pyelonephritis is determined by the degree of sepsis and the presence of underlying disorders. Patients who do not appear severely ill and who have a temperature less than 101°F (38.3°C) may be given oral antibiotics and followed as outpatients. Elderly persons, those with chills and a temperature of more than 101°F, and those with a known underlying disorder should be hospitalized for parenteral treatment with antibiotics and immediate urographic examination to identify the underlying disorder. The management of gram-negative sepsis is discussed in Chapter 11.

In patients with a renal abscess caused by hematogenous spread, urinalysis may show no cells. If high fever is present, the urogram is obtained immediately. The presence of a mass and fever should lead the examiner to suspect abscess. Tomographic sections of the kidney may reveal the fluid-filled cavity (Fig. 25.7), and should be obtained if available on an emergency basis. Ultrasound studies also may demonstrate a fluid-filled cavity with thickened walls, which is consistent with abscess. A gallium scan may confirm the presence of leukocytes in an abscess cavity. Renal arteriography performed to differentiate abscess from tumor will reveal a relatively avascular mass. If septicemia persists despite antibiotic treatment, surgical intervention is necessary.

Perinephric abscess is difficult to distinguish from pyelonephritis and renal abscess. Perinephric inflammation leads to loss of the psoas shadow on the KUB film, and nephrotomography may reveal a thickened Gerota's fascia lifted away from the renal shadow. Inspiratory and expiratory films may show failure of the kidney to move with respiration because of the inflammatory adhesions. Ultrasound studies demonstrating a perinephric fluid collection may be the only absolute evidence. Chest x-ray films may show an ipsilateral pleural effusion or elevation of the ipsilateral diaphragm. The underlying cause of the abscess should be determined. Treatment consists of intramuscular or intravenous administration of antibiotics and incisional or percutaneous drainage.

Bleeding into a renal tumor may cause noncolicky flank pain. Flank tenderness, hematuria, and mild leukocytosis may be present, but pyuria and other indications of sepsis are absent. The intravenous urogram should suggest the diagnosis, ultrasound studies will support the presence of a solid lesion, and angiographic examination or computed tomography will best confirm a tumor of the renal parenchyma. A tumor of the renal pelvis, however, may not be visualized with angiography, and requires retrograde pyelography and cytologic study of the urine for delineation.

Hematuria

Hematuria may occur as a manifestation of many primary and secondary diseases of the upper and lower portions of the urinary tract (Fig. 25.8). The character of the bleeding may suggest the site and cause.

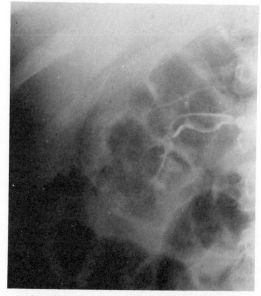

Figure 25.6. Renal artery embolus. Arteriogram shows nonfunction of right kidney with intraluminal filling defect outlined by contrast medium.

Description

Gross hematuria refers to obviously bloody urine, whereas *microscopic* hematuria denotes ostensibly clear urine with red blood cells seen only with a light microscope. Hematuria noted only at the beginning of urination is termed *initial* and is caused by a urethral condition. Blood appears in the first portion of the urinary specimen as the clear urine from the bladder washes the bleeding area. Unless urethral bleeding is brisk, only microscopic hematuria occurs in the remainder of the specimen. Hematuria occurring only at the end of urination is termed *terminal* and the blood usually comes from the prostate gland, bladder neck, or trigone as a result of contraction of the bladder neck as voiding ceases. *Total* hematuria, or urine that is blood-tinged throughout urination, may occur with active bleeding anywhere in the urinary tract, but usually indicates a site above the prostate gland. The passage of long, stringy, or vermiform clots suggests bleeding above the bladder with formation of a ureteral cast. Large, fresh clots most often occur when bleeding is from the bladder or prostate. Painless bleeding is characteristic of tumors; it also may occur, however, in hemorrhagic disorders, benign prostatic hypertrophy, and other nonmalignant conditions. Painful hematuria is common in inflammatory diseases, most notably cystitis and urinary calculus disease.

History

In addition to the descriptive character of the hematuria, other facets of the patient's medical history may indicate the cause. Cyclophosphamide (Cytoxan) may produce hemorrhagic cystitis. Anticoagulant therapy and platelet disorders may result in hematuria not only by causing abnormal blood clotting but also by stimulating an asymptomatic tumor to manifest itself. Even if the character of the bleeding suggests a site or cause and the bleeding is self-limited, every patient with hematuria requires thorough investigation consisting of a history, physical examination, urinalysis, blood studies, urography, and cystoscopy for precise identification of the bleeding point.

Physical Examination

A patient with atrial fibrillation, flank pain, and hematuria should be suspected of having an embolic renal infarct. A palpable flank mass suggests a renal tumor. Flank tenderness may indicate a ureter blocked by a calculus, clot, or tumor; glomerulonephritis; or papillary necrosis due to diabetes, acute pyelonephritis, or phenacetin therapy. In patients with cystitis, suprapubic or bladder tenderness is common. Prostatic tenderness often is elicited in the presence of acute prostatitis, and a hard, nodular prostate gland may indicate carcinoma. Commonly, total gross hematuria in older men is secondary to benign prostatic hypertrophy. Urethral tumors are commonly palpable. In women, a urethral caruncle or prolapsed urethra may be the site of bleeding, and may easily be

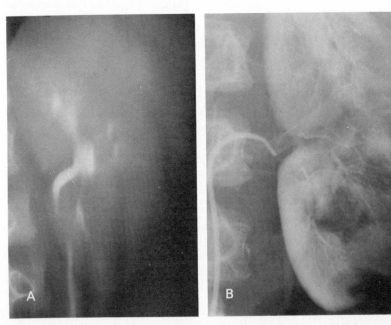

Figure 25.7.   Renal abscess. **(A)** Intravenous pyelogram shows calyces of left lower pole to be splayed and flattened, suggesting a mass. **(B)** Arteriogram shows poor function in left lower pole with draping of tertiary vessels around abscess wall.

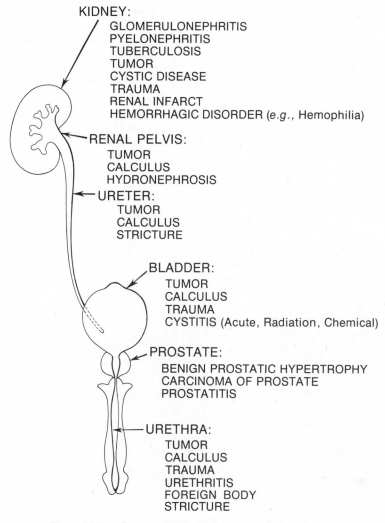

KIDNEY:
GLOMERULONEPHRITIS
PYELONEPHRITIS
TUBERCULOSIS
TUMOR
CYSTIC DISEASE
TRAUMA
RENAL INFARCT
HEMORRHAGIC DISORDER (*e.g.*, Hemophilia)

RENAL PELVIS:
TUMOR
CALCULUS
HYDRONEPHROSIS

URETER:
TUMOR
CALCULUS
STRICTURE

BLADDER:
TUMOR
CALCULUS
TRAUMA
CYSTITIS (Acute, Radiation, Chemical)

PROSTATE:
BENIGN PROSTATIC HYPERTROPHY
CARCINOMA OF PROSTATE
PROSTATITIS

URETHRA:
TUMOR
CALCULUS
TRAUMA
URETHRITIS
FOREIGN BODY
STRICTURE

Figure 25.8.   Causes of gross and microscopic hematuria.

visualized during pelvic examination. Although infiltrating carcinoma of the bladder may be palpated on bimanual examination, the absence of a palpable mass does not exclude the possibility of carcinoma as a source of bleeding.

Diagnostic Studies

Urinalysis. Even in the presence of gross hematuria, red blood cells must be identified under the microscope in all instances of apparent urinary tract bleeding. Red urine without blood cells may occur after eating beets, after ingestion of laxatives containing phenolphthalein, and in hemolytic syndromes that result in hemoglobinuria. Red cell casts may accompany red blood cells in patients with acute or focal glomerulonephritis. Obvious bacterial cystitis in women accompanied by gross hematuria should be confirmed with urinalysis

and urinary culture and appropriate follow-up studies planned.

Blood Studies. An hematocrit will indicate possible chronic blood loss and provide baseline information for the management of severe bleeding. The prothrombin time, partial thromboplastin time, and platelet count are necessary to exclude a coagulation defect. Immediate blood typing and crossmatching are necessary in patients with heavy bleeding. Serum creatinine and blood urea nitrogen levels indicate the degree of renal function. Since elevations of serum calcium may occur in patients with renal cell carcinoma, the serum calcium, phosphorus, and alkaline phosphatase are measured when this diagnosis is suspected. Similarly, the serum acid phosphatase should be measured in patients in whom a diagnosis of prostatic carcinoma is a possibility.

Intravenous Urography. An intravenous pyelogram should be obtained in the emergency ward or as soon as possible in all patients with gross or microscopic hematuria. Delay may be hazardous if severe bleeding starts abruptly, followed by shock, gram-negative sepsis, or acute clot retention. The urogram may be helpful in identifying renal masses (Fig. 25.9A), ureteral obstruction, and complete or partial loss of function associated with emboli, and may suggest the presence of a bladder tumor (Fig. 25.9B). Often the cystographic phase of the intravenous pyelogram may show unsuspected clot retention. In patients allergic to the dye used, a radioisotopic scan of the kidney may be obtained to visualize and to quantitate renal function.

Cystoscopy. Cystoscopic examination is necessary in all but the most obvious cases of hematuria—for example, in the presence of urethritis, obvious cystitis, or a previously identified cause. Although it is most effective in identifying the site of bleeding if performed during acute bleeding, emergency cystoscopy is not always possible. Patients with recurrent bleeding from an unidentified source, however, should undergo immediate cystoscopy to identify the bleeding site. Fulguration of bleeding points, biopsy of tumors, and retrograde studies also may be performed at the time of cystoscopic examination.

Urinary Cytology. Urinary specimens for cytologic examination should be obtained in all pa-

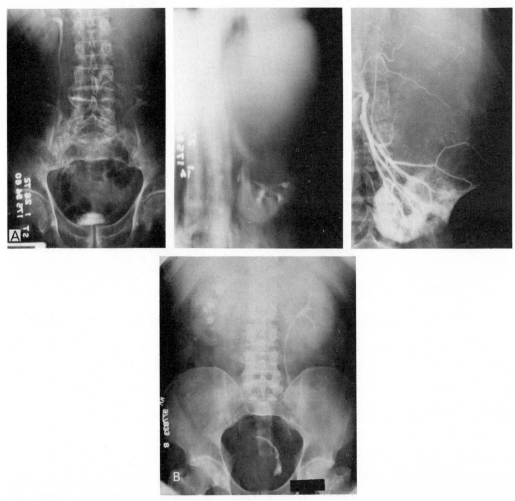

Figure 25.9. **(A)** Renal cell carcinoma. *Left,* Intravenous pyelogram shows left upper pole mass compressing left lower pole with flattening of calyces and nonfunction of upper pole. *Middle,* Tomographic cut of intravenous pyelogram confirms left upper pole mass. *Right,* Arteriogram confirms huge left upper pole mass compressing hilar structures and renal parenchyma downward. **(B)** Bladder tumor. Huge intravesical filling defect causing right renal obstruction and hydronephrosis.

tients in whom a neoplasm is suspected. However, identification of malignant cells in the sediment is hampered by the presence of many red blood cells, and more accurate cytologic examination is possible when active bleeding has ceased.

Treatment

The emergency treatment of patients with hematuria should be directed at replacing blood, preventing or treating clot retention, and gaining as much information as possible about the cause so that specific therapy may be instituted promptly. If the urine is darker than rosé wine or contains clots, a whistle-tip catheter is placed into the bladder and saline solution is infused by hand with an irrigating syringe. Parenteral administration of analgesics may be necessary when the bladder is vigorously irrigated. The bladder should be free of clots and the urine should be almost clear before irrigation by hand is stopped and a No. 22 French three-way Foley catheter with a 5-ml balloon is inserted with continuous normal saline irrigation. When the clots have been irrigated from the bladder, bleeding often ceases. A bladder distended with clots does not allow vessel contraction. After clot retention has been relieved, further evaluation may be carried out.

If attempts to free the bladder of clots by hand irrigation are unsuccessful or if clots plug the catheter, it may be necessary to evacuate the clots under anesthesia with a cystoscope.

If the patient has had a prostatectomy recently and if irrigation fails to keep the urine clear, or if for other reasons bleeding is suspected from the prostatic fossa, the three-way catheter with a 30-ml balloon is placed on traction to occlude and to tamponade the bladder neck. Although a small amount of oozing may occur around the catheter, the main source of prostatic bleeding will be compressed by balloon pressure.

In the absence of trauma, uncontrollable bleeding from the upper urinary tract rarely occurs. A blood clot ususally blocks the ureter and urinary output proximal to the obstruction tamponades the bleeding. If continuous, uncontrollable hemorrhage occurs from the upper tract, emergency evaluation including intravenous urography and arteriography is necessary. In isolated instances, transarteriographic embolization of renal bleeding points may be used to stop hemorrhage. Otherwise, surgical exploration may be necessary.

In patients with massive bleeding from prostatic carcinoma, fibrinolysis may be the cause. This occurs when fibrinolysins are released from the carcinoma either locally in the gland or systemically to promote conversion of plasminogen to the proteolytic enzyme plasmin, which destroys fibrin. When this diagnosis is suspected, the levels of serum fibrinogen and fibrin split products must be determined. If the fibrinogen level is below normal limits and if fibrin split products are increased, intravenous therapy with ε-aminocaproic acid is instituted, 5 gm in 250 ml of dextrose in water over 1 hour, followed by 1 gm/hr thereafter during acute bleeding.

All patients with gross hematuria and patients passing blood clots, except perhaps women with symptoms of acute cystitis, should be hospitalized for thorough urologic evaluation. If hematuria has ceased, the patient must be impressed with the necessity of having a complete investigation to uncover the source of the problem. Too often, patients who are seen with one epiosde of bleeding and who are discharged from the emergency ward fail to return because no further bleeding occurs. It is the responsibility of the emergency physician to see that this does not happen.

Lower Tract Irritation and Inflammation

Symptoms

The onset of urinary frequency, urgency, or dysuria indicates either primary or secondary irritation of the lower urinary tract, that is, the bladder, prostate gland, seminal vesicles, or urethra. Voluntary voiding usually does not occur until urinary volume in the bladder reaches 350–400 ml and the stretch reflex along the 2nd, 3rd, and 4th sacral nerves is activated. This reflex is mediated by the cerebral cortex. When voiding is incomplete, the critical volume that initiates the voiding reflex is reached rapidly and urinary frequency occurs. Irritation of the lower tract by infection or a foreign body causes the bladder to contract at lower volumes, and frequent voiding and dysuria then develop. The dysuria that accompanies inflammation may be felt as a pressure sensation in the suprapubic area, but is experienced more often as pain in the urethra.

Primary infections of the kidneys and ureters may result in secondary irritation of the lower urinary tract and symptoms of frequency and dysuria. In addition, calculi lodged in the intramural portion of the ureter may mimic lower tract inflammation. Frequency also may result from reduction in bladder volume caused by extravesical masses, and without dysuria it may result from glycosuria, diabetes insipidus, and renal concentrating defects such as chronic pyelonephritis, potassium depletion nephropathy, uric acid nephropathy, and sickle cell disease. In addition, diuretics may result in frequency. Upper tract disease as a cause of urinary frequency and dysuria usually may be ruled out by: (1) a careful history that excludes renal defects associated with frequency; (2) the absence of glycosuria; (3) a urinary specific gravity greater than 1.010; and (4) the absence of flank pain and tenderness.

Conditions and Treatment

Cystitis. As an isolated condition, cystitis occurs almost exclusively in women. Although acute infection of the bladder may develop in men, it is almost always a secondary manifestation of upper tract disease or mechanical obstruction. In women, acute cystitis may be bacterial or nonbacterial; the symptoms of each, however, are similar: frequency, urgency, dysuria, and suprapubic discomfort. Hematuria is common, but is not always present. The symptoms of cystitis often occur after sexual intercourse, since vaginal and perirectal intestinal organisms may be introduced into the urethra, where they multiply. Although the patient may seek emergency care for the initial episode, the natural history of cystitis is to have frequent recurrences. Unless pyelonephritis is also present, flank pain, high fever, and elevation of white blood cell count do not occur.

Physical examination reveals urethral and suprapubic tenderness, especially during bimanual examination. Pressure on the urethra frequently causes small droplets of pus to exude from the infected periurethral glands. The urethral meatus may be strictured. Meatal stenosis may be congenital in younger women, whereas in older women the urethral meatus may be scarred sufficiently from atrophic vaginal mucosa to be almost pinpoint.

Urinalysis usually reveals bacteriuria and also may show significant hematuria. If a Gram stain of the uncentrifuged urine shows organisms, it can be assumed that culture of that specimen will reveal more than 100,000 organisms/ml. A "midstream" urinary specimen is collected for culture before antibiotic therapy is given. Intravenous urography is unnecessary as an emergency procedure unless upper tract disease is suspected. Similarly, voiding cystourethrography should not be performed on an emergency basis, since inflammation of the bladder may cause small amounts of reflux, which disappear when the inflammation subsides. Lower urinary tract infections in men require thorough evaluation including cystoscopy if indicated.

Oral administration of antibiotics should be started on an outpatient basis without waiting for urinary culture results. Most intestinal bacteria that invade the urinary tract respond to commonly used antibiotics. The most common organism to cause cystitis in women is *Escherichia coli*. For uncomplicated cystitis the sulfonamides are recommended—sulfisoxazole 2 gm initially followed by 1 gm every 6 hours for 7–10 days, or nitrofurantoin macrocrystals, 100 mg initially followed by 50 mg every 6 hours for 7–10 days. Other antibiotics, including ampicillin and tetracycline, may be equally effective. If sulfonamides are chosen, the urinary specimen should be tested for sensitivities. The patient should be instructed about the need for another urinary culture 1 week after drug therapy is stopped. Except when cystitis is associated with gram-negative sepsis, these patients usually are treated as outpatients.

Nonbacterial cystitis may be caused by tuberculosis, schistosomiasis, or interstitial cystitis (Hunner's ulcer). Tuberculosis of the bladder may occur without a history of pulmonary disease, and typically produces sterile pyuria. The symptoms are usually severe and unremitting, and the diagnosis frequently is made only on cystoscopic examination of the bladder wall following failure of the usual antibiotic treatment for bacterial cystitis. Cultures take 6 weeks for positive results, and rarely is this diagnosis made in the emergency ward. Schistosomiasis may cause severe nonbacterial bladder symptoms, and the diagnosis depends on eliciting a history of residence in an endemic area. Interstitial cystitis is characterized by extremely painful, frequent voiding, and its onset is rarely acute. The absence of pyuria in a patient with severe urgency, frequency, and dysuria should lead the examiner to suspect this diagnosis. Confirmation is possible only on cystoscopic examination.

Emphysematous cystitis occurs when gas-producing bacteria colonize in the bladder and infiltrate the bladder wall, causing air bubbles that are visible on radiologic examination. Patients usually have signs of gram-negative sepsis as well as symptoms of lower tract infection. Treatment includes drainage of the bladder, administration of antibiotics, and correction of the causative factor, which is usually obstruction.

Bladder Calculi. Calculi in the bladder may cause irritative symptoms manifested by frequency, urgency, and dysuria. They rarely occur spontaneously, and are usually the result of chronic infection or bladder outlet obstruction. The history of a neurogenic bladder, an indwelling urethral catheter, chronic urinary tract infection, or symptoms of outlet obstruction suggests this diagnosis. Physical examination is usually uninformative. Urinalysis reveals both red and white blood cells and bacteria when infection is present. A urinary pH greater than 8.5 suggests urea-splitting infection, which creates the alkaline medium necessary for precipitation of magnesium-ammonium-phosphate complexes, the most common type of "infection" calculus. Calculi associated with outlet obstruction and no infection are usually composed of uric acid, and are not visualized on the KUB film. However, if intravenous urography is performed, the uric acid calculi may appear as filling defects in the bladder. Other causes of radiolucent filling defects include an enlarged median lobe of the prostate gland, bladder tumor, blood clots, a Foley catheter balloon, and ureterocele. Treatment of bladder calculi consists of removing the stones, correcting the primary problem, providing urinary drainage, and treating infection. These patients usually need to be admitted for cystoscopic examination and urologic investigation.

Acute Prostatitis. This disease usually occurs in men between the ages of 20 and 40 years. In addition to urinary frequency, urgency, and dysuria, symptoms may include fever, suprapubic discomfort, perineal pain, referred pain in the testes, initial or terminal hematuria, and hemospermia. The patient may have a urethral discharge of a thin, white, watery consistency, which increases in the morning and with a Valsalva maneuver. Frank urinary retention may occur if prostatic swelling is severe enough to cause total outlet obstruction. A history of nonspecific urethritis or gonorrhea is common; however, neither of these is necessary for prostatitis to occur.

Physical examination may reveal suprapubic discomfort, epididymitis, and a tender boggy prostate gland. If a prostatic abscess is present, one segment of the prostate may be exquisitely tender or may feel fluctuant.

Urinalysis may show red blood cells or white blood cells or both. The three-glass urinary test may be used to differentiate the site responsible for the pyuria or hematuria. In this test, the patient is asked to void the first 10 ml of urine into the first container. This washes the anterior urethra. He then is instructed to void most of the remaining urine into the second container and the last few milliliters into the third container. If the first specimen contains the largest number of blood cells, the disease process is localized to the anterior urethra. If the largest number of cells is in the third specimen, this indicates disease of the prostate gland, bladder neck, or posterior urethra, since contraction of the bladder neck as voiding ceases

forces cells into the urine. If the number of blood cells is the same in all specimens, the site of disease is usually above the bladder neck.

A Gram stain and culture of urethral discharge should be obtained to rule out gonorrhea. Although systemic bacterial infection may be localized to the prostate gland and although infections from common urinary pathogens such as *E. coli*, the enterococci, and Klebsiella may occur, in most instances of acute prostatitis no bacterial pathogen is identified. Prostatic massage to obtain secretions should be avoided in patients with acute prostatitis since this manipulation may induce retrograde seeding of bacteria via the vas deferens to the epididymis, resulting in acute epididymitis or septicemia.

If the diagnosis is established by the aforementioned means, emergency urography is unnecessary. If a KUB film is obtained, prostatic calcifications may be noted; these indicate a chronic inflammatory process, but prostatitis may occur in their absence.

If the gonococcus is not implicated, the most effective antibiotics for the treatment of acute prostatitis are the tetracyclines, 500 mg four times a day for 10 days. The other agent useful in this situation is a combination of sulfamethoxazole and trimethoprim, both of which act as folic acid antagonists. Trimethoprim is able to cross the cell barrier and to enter the prostatic secretions. Bed rest and hot tub baths also may be helpful in relieving symptoms. Instrumentation with a urethral catheter should be avoided, since the presence of a catheter in the prostatic fossa will cause an inflammatory reaction around the orifices of the prostatic ducts, impede drainage, and aggravate the condition. Urinary retention in the presence of acute prostatitis should be treated with percutaneous suprapubic drainage.

Palpable prostatic abscesses require systemic antibiotic therapy and may need drainage by needle aspiration, transurethral unroofing, or perineal exploration.

Seminal Vesiculitis. This condition is almost impossible to distinguish from acute prostatitis unless a discrete tender mass is palpable above the prostate gland. Seminal vesiculitis rarely occurs as an isolated phenomenon and usually accompanies prostatitis. The treatment is identical.

Acute Urethritis. This condition is manifested by urinary frequency, dysuria, and urethral discharge, alone or in combination. The discharge can be thick, yellow, and purulent when caused by *Neisseria gonorrhoeae* or thin, white, and watery when caused by Trichomonas, Chlamydia, or other nonbacterial organisms.

The symptoms of gonococcal urethritis usually begin 3–10 days after sexual exposure. Except for a discharge, the findings on physical examination may be normal. The anus and mouth should always be examined for signs of extragenital involvement. A Gram stain of urethral secretions may reveal gram-negative intracellular diplococci, and even if the smear is negative a specimen should be cultured. A serologic test for syphilis always should be performed before antibiotic treatment, and should be repeated 2 weeks and 3 months after contact if the proper incubation period has not been reached.

Acute gonococcal urethritis is best treated with penicillin, 4.8 million units intramuscularly, together with probenecid, 1 gm orally to prolong the blood level of penicillin by blocking renal tubular excretion. This treatment is successful in most patients. Persons allergic to penicillin should be given tetracycline, 500 mg four times a day for 10 days, with the expectation of a 96% success rate. Follow-up outpatient treatment should be arranged.

Nonspecific urethritis shows no evidence of gram-negative intracellular diplococci on the Gram stain, and cultures may not reveal a urinary pathogen. Tetracycline, 500 mg four times a day for 10 days, is the most effective treatment. Recurrences are frequent.

Strains of Chlamydia recently have been associated with nonspecific urethritis. They do not grow on ordinary commercial culture media and can be cultured only under special sophisticated laboratory conditions. These strains seem to be responsive to the tetracyclines, which is probably why most cases designated as nonspecific urethritis respond well to these agents.

Urethritis caused by Trichomonas is distinguished from nonspecific urethritis by the presence of flagellated protozoa seen during examination of the discharge by the hanging-drop technique. Identification of these organisms is an indication for simultaneous treatment of both sexual partners with metronidazole (Flagyl) for 10 days.

Periurethral Abscess. The symptoms of periurethral abscess are those of lower urinary tract irritation. Pain and a palpable mass at the penoscrotal junction, along the course of the urethra in women, or in the perineum should alert the examiner to the possibility of this diagnosis. Communication between the urethra and the abscess cavity may result in intermittent discharge of purulent material via the urethra. Another symptom suggesting this diagnosis is the complaint of dribbling after voiding. This occurs in both men and women as the abscess cavity fills and then empties after urination.

In the past, this condition most often was seen as a result of gonococcal infection with stricture, urethral perforation, subsequent abscess formation, and multiple fistulization (watering-pot perineum). Today, periurethral abscess more commonly is found at the penoscrotal junction as a result of pressure necrosis from an indwelling urethral catheter and at sites of urethral perforation from instrumentation or trauma.

Physical examination shows a tender, fluctuant mass, and pressure on the mass may cause pus to exude from the urethra. Treatment is accomplished with systemic antibiotics and temporary suprapubic urinary diversion by either a percutaneous technique or formal cystostomy, depending on the period of drainage required. Local incision, drainage, and urethroplasty may be necessary. Admission and urologic consultation are required.

Acute Urinary Retention

The adult patient with acute urinary retention seeks emergency care because of suprapubic discomfort, the inability to void, dribbling, or severe urinary frequency. The most common causes of acute urinary retention are listed in Table 25.1. The history and physical examination aid in determining the cause of retention and, therefore, the treatment.

History

Progressive symptoms of decrease in urinary stream, nocturia, urinary frequency, or dysuria in an elderly man suggest benign prostatic hypertrophy. A history of urologic procedures, including prostatectomy, catheterization, or endoscopic examination, may indicate bladder neck contracture or urethral stricture, whereas prior prostatic carcinoma suggests obstruction at the bladder neck from growth of the neoplasm. Inflammatory diseases of the urethra, especially gonorrhea, predispose to urethral strictures. In young men with prostatitis and posterior urethritis, urethral discharge, fever, and perineal pain precede acute urinary retention. Acute episodes of herpes progenitalis may result in retention, and a history of ulcers should be sought. Urethral bleeding (initial hematuria) may suggest a urethral tumor or foreign body as the cause of retention. A history of neurologic disease may indicate that the patient has an incompetent, flaccid neurogenic bladder. If the patient recently has ingested drugs—specifically, antihistamines, atropine compounds, or α-

Table 25.1.
Causes of acute urinary retention in adults.

Penis	Neurologic causes
Phimosis	Motor paralytic
Paraphimosis	Spinal shock
Meatal stenosis	Spinal cord syndromes
Foreign body constriction	Sensory paralytic
Urethra	Tabes dorsalis
Tumor	Diabetes
Foreign body	Multiple sclerosis
Calculus	Syringomyelia
Urethritis (severe)	Spinal cord syndromes
Stricture	Herpes zoster
Meatal stenosis (female)	Miscellaneous
Hematoma	Drugs
Prostate gland	Antihistamines
Benign prostatic hypertrophy	Anticholinergic agents
Carcinoma	Antispasmodic agents
Prostatitis (severe)	Tricyclic antidepressants
Bladder neck contracture	α-adrenergic stimulators
Prostatic infarction	"Cold" tablets
	Ephedrine derivatives
	Amphetamines
	Psychogenic problems

adrenergic stimulators—this may be the cause of acute retention. Sudden interruption of the urinary stream followed by inability to void implies a urethral calculus. The diagnosis of psychogenic urinary retention is a diagnosis of exclusion, but this condition commonly is encountered in young hospital-associated women who have no history to suggest another cause.

Causative Factors and Treatment

Penis. Phimosis, or adherence of the prepuce, may be found during physical examination. This causes retention by obstructing the flow of urine. Relief of obstruction in the emergency ward is accomplished by instillation of a local anesthetic and either dilation of the pinpoint meatus or performance of a dorsal slit procedure. Paraphimosis may cause constriction of the urethra and vascular insufficiency because of the circumferential obstructing bands, and therefore requires immediate reduction (see pages 561–562). Meatal stenosis is obvious as the examiner tries to separate the glans to visualize the urethral orifice; this condition may follow circumcision, indwelling catheterization, or a urethral procedure, or may occur without an obvious cause. Meatotomy under local anesthesia in the emergency ward provides immediate relief of obstruction (Fig. 25.10).

Urethra. Palpation of the urethra may reveal a tumor, foreign body, or calculus, In men, obstructing tumors of the urethra usually occur in the distal third. Relief of obstruction requires proximal urinary drainage by cystostomy or suprapubic placement of a catheter. Removal of foreign bodies is discussed on page 543. A calculus lodged in the urethra is usually palpable at or just distal to the penoscrotal junction. Since the urethra narrows proximal to this point, the force of the urinary stream usually wedges the calculus in this area. A gentle attempt to "milk" the calculus the remaining length of the urethra may be made after instillation of anesthetic jelly. However, this is usually unsuccessful because the jagged edges of the calculus snag and macerate the urethral mucosa. The calculus that is too large to be removed in this manner requires cystoscopic or operative removal.

Urethritis, whether nonspecific, trichomonal, or gonococcal, may cause copious urethral discharge or meatal swelling with associated urinary retention. Although passage of a urethral catheter may be possible, an inwelling foreign body will exacerbate the urethritis. Temporary urinary diversion by means of a suprapubic catheter with appropriate antibiotic therapy is the treatment of choice.

Unless the patient has a history of urethral stricture or urethral instrumentation, a stricture may not be recognized unless the examiner is unable to pass a catheter to the level of the prostate gland. The most common sites of stricture formation are the submeatal area and the bulbous urethra just distal to the urinary sphincter. Before urethral dilation is attempted, the physician should

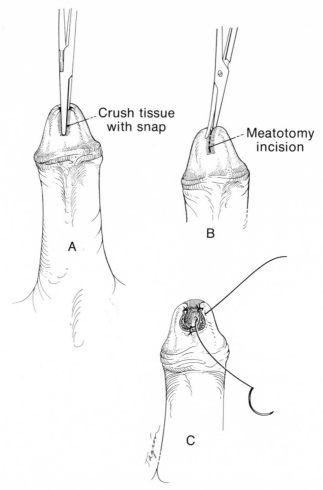

Figure 25.10.   A difficult catheterization because of meatal stenosis may be simplified with meatotomy. **(A)** A straight clamp is placed into the urethra, and meatal tissue is crushed at 6 o'clock to prevent bleeding. **(B)** Meatotomy is performed with scissors along crushed tissue. **(C)** Cut edges of urethra and glans penis are approximated with interrupted 4–0 chromic absorbable sutures.

try to insert a No. 12 French Foley catheter or a No. 10 straight infant feeding tube. If one of these is successfully passed through the strictured area, it should be left in place, and then, in the course of the next few days, progressively larger catheters may be passed as the stricture softens. A stricture should not be dilated progressively in the emergency ward since sepsis and urethral injury too often ensue. Under no circumstances should anyone other than a urologist attempt to dilate a stricture with urethral sounds or stylets in the emergency ward.

Failure to pass a small catheter beyond the strictured area traditionally has necessitated the use of a filiform and a follower (Fig. 25.11). After instillation of anesthetic jelly, a filiform is inserted gently into the urethra until it passes the point of obstruction. It is then advanced into the bladder and a well-lubricated No. 10 or No. 12 French follower is screwed to the outside end, advanced into the bladder, and secured with tape. The follower, not the filiform, has an orifice to provide urinary drainage. The filiform stays curled within the bladder. Even if the filiform cannot be passed, it should be left in place since it will fill the small pits and false passages that may surround a stricture. The physician should continue to pass filiforms until all the false passages are filled and one filiform finally is passed through the strictured orifice. This filiform then should be advanced into the bladder and the remainder of the filiforms should be removed. The follower then may be attached and advanced. Once obstruction has been relieved by this method, the follower should not be removed, nor should progressive dilation be performed in the emergency ward since attempts to insert the next larger size may be unsuccessful. Progressive dilation with successively larger followers may be achieved over the next few days with the patient in the hospital. Endoscopic examination and dilation may be performed under spinal or general anesthesia. The presence of a large amount of blood after seemingly successful placement of a follower may result from false passage or from perforation of the median lobe of the prostate gland. Passage of filiforms and followers should be accompanied by intramuscular injection of broad-spectrum antibiotics to prevent septicemia, and should be performed by experienced physicians.

Our preferred treatment of urethral obstruction that cannot be overcome with gentle attempts at passing a urethral catheter is to use one of the many percutaneous suprapubic tubes now available. With appropriate preparation of the suprapubic skin, local anesthesia, and sterile technique, this method causes minimal discomfort and trauma, and leaves the urethra unscathed so that thorough radiologic and endoscopic evaluation may be performed later under optimal conditions.

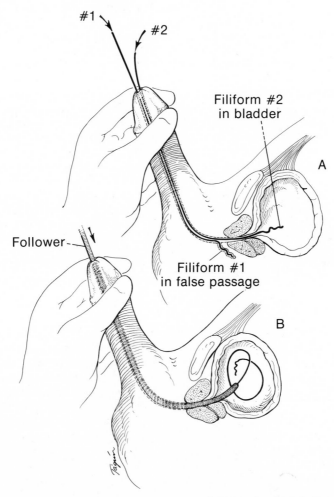

Figure 25.11. Technique of passing filiforms and followers. **(A)** With the penis held upright to make the urethra straight, the filiform is passed gently through the urethra with a fine, light touch. If obstruction is encountered, the filiform is usually lodged in a small, periurethral false passage. In order that the false passage will not be entered again, filiform #1 is left in place while filiform #2 is passed gently into the blader. **(B)** A No. 10 or No. 12 French follower then is screwed into end of filiform. After additional lubricating jelly is applied to the follower, it is passed directly and smoothly into the bladder. The follower may be taped securely to the penis and attached to gravity drainage until further treatment by the urologist.

Prostate Gland. A history of progressive urinary outlet obstruction (hesitancy, nocturia, and diminished stream) preceding acute urinary tract obstruction in an elderly patient suggests prostatic disease. The most common condition is benign prostatic hypertrophy. Rectal examination reveals a prostate gland that may or may not feel enlarged. However, the size of the prostate has no relation to the degree of obstruction. The anatomic problem in benign prostatic hypertrophy is compression of the urethral lumen by the lateral lobes of the prostate gland or obstruction of the proximal end of the urethral lumen by an enlarged median lobe (Fig. 25.12).

When benign prostatic hypertrophy is suspected, the urethra is anesthetized with lidocaine jelly and a No. 16 French Foley catheter with a 5-ml balloon is inserted (larger balloons cause bladder spasms). If it cannot be passed into the bladder, a smaller-caliber Foley catheter or a coudé catheter may be used. The deflection in the distal 3 cm of the coudé catheter allows it to be passed over an obstructing median lobe. Failure to pass a coudé catheter successfully may be due to either total obstruction of the bladder neck by median lobe elevation or bladder neck contracture so severe that only a pinpoint orifice is present. Filiforms, followers, sounds, and stylets should be avoided in this situation, since the median lobe may be perforated easily, resulting in uncontroll-able bleeding and sepsis. Suprapubic catheter placement is the treatment of choice.

When drainage is established successfully, the bladder is decompressed slowly—300–400 ml initially, followed by 200 ml/hr. Rapid decompression of a chronically distended bladder may lead to severe mucosal hemorrhage and clot retention. During the first few hours after decompression of a chronically distended bladder, postobstructive diuresis may develop. Urine may be passed at a rate of up to 1000 ml/hr, resulting in hypotension and shock unless fluid is replaced. Postobstructive diuresis may be caused by one or more of the following: (1) an increased concentration of blood urea nitrogen secondary to obstructive renal failure and acting as an osmotic diuretic; (2) damage to the proximal and distal renal tubules by hydronephrosis, resulting in a renal concentrating defect; (3) failure of the damaged distal tubule to respond to endogenous or exogenous antidiuretic hormone; and (4) total body water overload. If this syndrome occurs, an intravenous line should be placed so that fluid volume may be restored. Replacement needs may be determined by frequent urinary and serum electrolyte determinations.

Once a catheter has been placed, its function should be tested by instillation and withdrawal of irrigating solution to ensure that it is in the bladder and not curled in the prostatic fossa. Oral antibiotics and attention to asepsis at the penile meatus

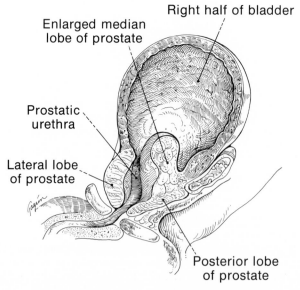

Figure 25.12.   In addition to prominent lateral lobes, enlarged median lobe of prostate contributes to marked bladder outlet obstruction. In such instances, a curve-tipped coudé catheter may negotiate channel of prostastic urethra more easily than a standard straight-tipped Foley catheter.

reduce the incidence of catheter-induced infection. Asepsis is maintained with applications of an antibiotic ointment (Neosporin) and frequent washings with benzalkonium chloride (Zephiran). The patient is admitted and further diagnostic workup is then performed.

Neurologic Causes. Many neurologic conditions may result in acute urinary retention. Spinal shock and spinal cord syndromes are easily recognizable, as are some of the other neurologic diseases that are accompanied by obvious neurologic signs. However, the neurogenic bladder resulting from tabes dorsalis, diabetes, multiple sclerosis, and syringomyelia may be difficult to recognize when urinary retention is the primary manifestation of the disease. The physician particularly should be aware of these possibilities in younger patients who do not have any signs or symptoms of outlet obstruction. In patients in whom neurologic impairment is recognized as causing urinary retention, a catheter should be passed to empty the bladder and to relieve obstruction, but it should not be left in place. Patients with neurologic bladder disease despite adequate treatment continue to have residual urine after voiding that is much greater than normal, and any infection in the bladder is difficult to eradicate. Therefore, these patients should be hospitalized and catheterized every 6 hours or more often if bladder distention causes pain. This decreases the incidence of urinary tract infection and calculi. Bladder function studies should be performed and a program developed for improving emptying of the bladder.

Pharmacologic Causes. Medications may cause acute urinary retention in patients with no history or only mild symptoms of obstructive uropathy. Drugs that cause bladder atony include antihistamines (Benadryl), anticholinergic and antispasmodic agents (Donnatal, Lomotil, and Pro-Banthine), and tricyclic antidepressants (Tofranil and Elavil). Drugs that cause bladder neck closure by their action as α-adrenergic stimulators include "cold" tablets, ephedrine derivatives, and amphetamines.

Patients with urinary retention who have been exposed recently to these agents should be catheterized and then the catheter should be removed. The offending agent should be discontinued. Hospitalization is necessary unless the patient lives near enough that he can return to the emergency ward if retention recurs.

Psychogenic Origin. Urinary retention in young women in the absence of outlet obstruction or neurologic incompetence should suggest the possibility of a psychogenic source. This rarely occurs in males, but may occur in a young man who has had prostatitis and who is concerned about his urinary tract. When a psychogenic origin is suspected, treatment should consist of catheterization for the isolated episode of retention without use of an indwelling Foley catheter. Follow-up psychiatric consultation should be encouraged when the urologic workup has established the absence of an organic cause.

Penile Edema

Conditions and Treatment

Balanitis and Posthitis. Inflammation of the glans penis (balanitis) and inflammation of the foreskin (posthitis) commonly occur together and may result from poor hygiene or phimosis. The foreskin becomes edematous, erythematous, and tender, and in severe circumstances the inflammatory response may progress proximally on the penile shaft. Bullous edema, local ulcers, and drainage may occur. In less severe cases, foreskin retraction, cleansing with soap and water, and application of an antibiotic ointment (Neosporin) may be sufficient treatment. Severe or recurrent inflammation or inability to retract the foreskin necessitates circumcision after local swelling has diminished.

Phimosis. In this condition, the meatus of the foreskin is too narrow to permit retraction over the glans. Phimosis may be congenital or acquired, the latter being common in diabetes. If the meatus of the foreskin is adherent, urinary retention may occur. In this circumstance a probe may not even fit into the orifice. Dilation with a hemostat may provide immediate relief of urinary obstruction. An emergency dorsal slit procedure (Fig. 25.13) may be necessary; dilation of the orifice, however, usually suffices in the emergency situation, after which circumcision may be carried out as an elective procedure.

Paraphimosis. Paraphimosis is the condition in which the foreskin becomes permanently retracted behind the corona of the glans penis. There is a proximal and a distal contraction ring. As a result, the tissue between the rings becomes edematous and tender, sometimes progressing to infarction. This may occur spontaneously after masturbation, intercourse, or failure to reduce the foreskin following catheter insertion. This swelling should not be confused with angioneurotic edema of the foreskin, which may occur as a localized phenomenon in response to allergy, especially in children. In angioneurotic edema, the constriction bands are absent. The treatment of paraphimosis should be

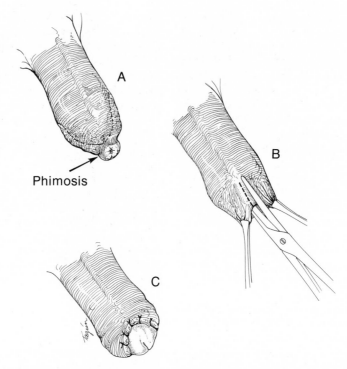

Phimosis

Figure 25.13.   Dorsal slit procedure. **(A)** Phimotic foreskin. **(B)** After foreskin is crushed with a straight clamp at 12 o'clock, it is incised with scissors. **(C)** Cut edge of foreskin should be hemostatically sutured with interrupted 4–0 chromic absorbable sutures. Formal circumcision may be performed as an elective procedure when patient's condition has stabilized.

directed toward immediate reduction of the fore-skin. If gentle pressure on the glans penis with simultaneous traction on the foreskin is unsuccess-ful, the base of the penis may be infiltrated with local anesthetic without epinephrine, the edema fluid may be squeezed from the foreskin between the constriction bands, and the prepuce may then be pulled over the glans. Both constriction rings must be reduced. Partial reduction is common, but if reduction is incomplete, total paraphimosis may recur within minutes. Failure to reduce the fore-skin manually necessitates an emergency dorsal slit procedure.

Lymphedema. Penile lymphedema almost al-ways is accompanied by scrotal swelling. The lym-phatic vessels of the scrotal halves freely anasto-mose with those of the penis and drain into the superficial and deep inguinal lymph nodes, which then drain into the iliac node chains. Lymphedema of the penis and scrotum may be caused by ob-struction due to tumor or by inguinal adenitis, as in filariasis or lymphogranuloma venereum. Pelvic tumors involving the iliac node chains may block the lymphatics to the genitalia resulting in penile and scrotal lymphedema, and x-ray treatment to pelvic lymph nodes also may result in this condi-

tion. Lymphedema must be differentiated from other causes of penile and scrotal swelling, such as tuberculosis, anasarca, deep pelvic venous throm-bosis, a large pelvic tumor, or urinary extravasa-tion due to trauma. The treatment of penile lymphedema should be directed toward the pri-mary cause and should not involve compression dressings.

Local Infection. An abrasion or skin disorder may result in local infection and lead to penile swelling. Infection of the suture line after circum-cision is one of the most common causes of penile edema. Treatment consists of local dressings and appropriate antibiotic therapy if cultures are pos-itive.

Priapism. In this condition the penis becomes uncontrollably erect for a prolonged period be-cause the venous drainage of the corpora caver-nosa fails. It may be isolated (idiopathic), or it may be secondary to a variety of disorders, includ-ing sickle cell disease or trait, trauma, instrumen-tation, tumor, or leukemia. In many instances the condition may be spontaneously reversed, but if it persists, it ultimately results in fibrosis of the cor-pora cavernosa and impotence. Since the advent of surgical methods for correction of priapism, this condition has been categorized as a surgical emergency.

The diagnosis of prolonged erection is recognized easily, but unfortunately, the nature of the disorder encourages procrastination that frequently results in a decreased chance of surgical success. The examiner must try to determine the primary underlying disease, and examination should include a complete blood cell count with differential, a sickle cell preparation, hemoglobin electrophoresis, and careful evaluation for an underlying malignant condition.

Treatment has included several conservative measures, such as intracorporeal instillation of heparin, fibrinolytic therapy, local application of ice, ice water enemas, and drainage of the corpora with a large-bore needle; with few exceptions, however, the results have been poor. If erection has persisted for more than a few hours, a corpus cavernosum-corpus spongiosum shunt should be performed under local anesthesia by a urologic surgeon. Since the venous drainage of the corpora cavernosa has been impaired and since the corpus spongiosum rarely is affected, this shunt provides the easiest and most successful method of drainage of the obstructed corpora cavernosa. Immediate consultation and treatment are essential for these patients.

Scrotal Masses

History and Physical Examination

The recognition of a scrotal mass, even in the absence of pain, may be sufficient cause for an anxious patient to seek emergency care. Most scrotal masses may be differentiated by history and physical examination; some, however, may require surgical exploration for confirmation and diagnosis. A history of associated trauma, urinary tract infection, urinary tract instrumentation, systemic associated diseases such as mumps and syphillis, the mode of onset, and the presence or absence of pain aids in the differential diagnosis of the scrotal mass. Physical examination must be performed with the patient both standing and supine to determine the site of the mass and its relation to the testis, the epididymis, the spermatic cord, and the inguinal canal. Transillumination of the mass should be attempted either with a two- or three-cell flashlight with a flange or with the light cord from a fiberoptic light source.

Conditions and Treatment

Hydrocele. A nontender, fluid-filled mass that surrounds the testis and that may be transilluminated is termed a hydrocele. It results from the accumulation of fluid between the two layers of the tunica vaginalis. Most hydroceles occur in older patients and are idiopathic and asymptomatic. An acute, symptomatic hydrocele is frequently a complication of orchitis, epididymitis, trauma, or a malignant tumor. A hydrocele in a younger patient, especially if the onset is acute, suggests the possibility of underlying disease and the need for further investigation. Methods of investigation include ultrasonography, testicular scanning, and surgical exploration.

Testicular Tumor. Although a testicular neoplasm usually is manifested as a painless mass palpable in the body of the testis, acute pain due to necrosis and hemorrhage may precipitate a visit to the emergency ward. Except in the case of a large tumor, the epididymis is normal and is separate from the testicular mass. Pain may be elicited on palpation. The mass cannot be transilluminated, although the presence of a secondary hydrocele may cause confusion. Physical examination may reveal gynecomastia due to chorionic gonadotropins if choriocarcinoma is present. The absence of gynecomastia does not exclude the presence of choriocarcinoma. If a testicular tumor is suspected, the patient should be admitted for transinguinal exploration as soon as feasible.

Torsion. Torsion of the spermatic cord is common in young men, as well as in children. It is characterized by the acute onset of testicular pain, either during physical activity or at rest, and the involved testis immediately swells. Physical examination reveals an exquisitely tender mass in which the epididymis and testis cannot be distinguished. A secondary hydrocele may be present, and transillumination may demonstrate fluid. With the examiner facing the patient, the torsion occurs counterclockwise in the left testis and clockwise in the right. The twist initiates cremasteric muscle spasm and causes the affected testis to become elevated in the scrotum. The rapid onset and the absence of pyuria aid in distinguishing torsion from epididymitis. Prehn's sign also may be helpful: elevation of the testis relieves the pain of epididymitis, but increases that of torsion. The distinction, however, is difficult, and exploration of the scrotum often is necessary to substantiate the diagnosis. Recently, testicular scanning has helped in the differentiation by showing an absent blood supply in the testis that has undergone torsion. In addition, use of a Doppler probe may be helpful in distinguishing spermatic cord torsion from epididymitis and orchitis.

Treatment of suspected torsion is immediate surgical exploration with untwisting and fixation.

The opposite testis also is fixed with sutures because of the high incidence of later torsion in the opposite side. Emergency treatment is of utmost necessity, since failure to restore the blood supply to a testis within 4–6 hours results in a high incidence of testicular infarction. Even if several hours have passed, however, and infarction of the seminiferous cells has occurred, exploration and detorsion are warranted to attempt to preserve the more hardy testosterone-producing interstitial cells.

Epididymitis. In patients with epididymitis the onset of pain is usually gradual, and pain peaks after several hours or days. Epididymitis often is manifested initially simply by epididymal tenderness without a palpable mass, and frequently it is associated with a history of urinary tract infection, prostatitis, gonorrhea, or instrumentation. Retrograde passage of bacteria down the vas deferens is postulated as the means by which the epididymis is seeded with pathogens.

Physical examination may show only a slight induration or a tender nodule, which is usually in the most inferior and dependent portion of the epididymis; in other patients, however, the entire epididymis may be involved or an associated hydrocele may be present. This makes the distinction between epididymitis, orchitis, tumor, and torsion difficult. Urinalysis may reveal pyuria if there is an associated urinary tract infection. A urinary specimen should be cultured when the diagnosis of epididymitis is suspected. The white blood cell count often is elevated.

Treatment includes bed rest, ice packs applied to the scrotum, scrotal support, an anti-inflammatory agent such as indomethacin (Indocin), and antibiotics. Unless a specific pathogen is known, any of the broad-spectrum antibiotics is a good choice for initial therapy. Unless the patient is febrile, antibiotics may be given orally. If the patient has a temperature greater than 101°F (38.3°C) or a tender, fluctuant mass, hospitalization with intramuscular or intravenous administration of antibiotics is necessary. Persistent fever or temperature spikes during antibiotic therapy necessitate surgical exploration and excision of the abscessed epididymis.

Orchitis. Orchitis is rare, but may occur secondary to epididymitis or a viral infection. Mumps is the most common cause. Orchitis parotidea ("mumps" orchitis) is usually unilateral. The onset of pain is sudden and difficult to distinguish from that of torsion. The testis becomes enlarged, congested, and tender, probably because of infarction necrosis of the seminiferous tubules. The overlying scrotum may become erythematous and edema-

tous. The absence of pyuria or any other urinary tract symptoms and the presence of parotitis may aid in distinguishing this condition from epididymitis. In orchitis associated with mumps, microhematuria and proteinuria may be present. The virus is recoverable in the urine, but not by routine methods.

Treatment is directed toward relief of pain. Infiltration of the spermatic cord with a local anesthetic may provide considerable relief. Bed rest, analgesics, and ice packs may be helpful. Mumps orchitis results in loss of spermatogenesis in 25–35% of patients, although androgenic function usually remains. Hospitalization is recommended.

Varicocele. Insufficiency of the left spermatic vein may result in an ill-defined scrotal mass. This is usually a chronic process associated with discomfort or heaviness in the affected side of the scrotum. Approximately 15% of men have a left varicocele to some degree, which is most often asymptomatic. The acute onset of a varicocele on the left or right side may be the first symptom of a retroperitoneal mass. On the right side, the testicular vein empties into the inferior vena cava. A right varicocele is always the result of obstruction of the right spermatic vein at this level. Vena caval thrombosis or an extrinsic mass such as carcinoma, lymphoma, or sarcoma is usually the cause.

The left spermatic vein empties into the left renal vein. The acute onset of a left varicocele with pain localized to the scrotal area is most often due to renal cell carcinoma with propagation of a tumor thrombus in the left renal vein, resulting in obstruction of the drainage of the left spermatic vein. Renal venous thrombosis and, more rarely, lymphoma also may cause this problem.

Intravenous urography, ultrasonography, vena caval angiography with selective catheterization of the renal vein, and transfemoral angiography are often necessary for the identification of any underlying condition. Treatment should be directed toward the underlying cause, not toward the varicocele itself. A scrotal support will relieve symptoms. However, persistent pain and swelling despite conservative care may be relieved by inguinal exploration and ligation of the veins of the spermatic cord at the internal inguinal ring.

Other Scrotal Masses. Other than the masses already discussed, the most common scrotal mass is probably the inguinal hernia that descends into the scrotum. Careful examination usually defines the limits of the hernia in the scrotum and its extension into the inguinal canal. The testis can be palpated as distinct from the mass. Unless examination is conducted carefully, an incarcerated hernia may be confused with a mass of testicular or epididymal origin. Other lesions, including spermatocele, epididymal tumor, and mesenchymal tumor of the cord structures, may all be palpated as scrotal masses, but are not usually seen as acute problems.

Suggested Readings

Bright TC, Peters DC: Ureteral injuries due to external violence: Ten years' experience with 59 cases. *J Trauma* 17:616–620, 1977

Devine CJ, Jr, Devine DC, Horton CE: Anterior urethral injury: Etiology, diagnosis and initial management. *Urol Clin North Am* 4:125–131, 1977

Dowd JB: Flank pain in nonurologic disease. *Med Clin North Am* 47:437–445, 1963

Emanuel B, Weiss H, Collin P: Renal trauma in children. *J Trauma* 17:275–278, 1977

Garrett RA: Pediatric urethral and perineal injuries. *Pediatr Clin North Am* 22:401–406, 1975

Griffin WO, Jr, Berlin RD, Ernest CB, et al: Intravenous pyelography in abdominal trauma. *J Trauma* 18:387–392, 1978

Gross M: Rupture of the testicle: The importance of early surgical treatment. *J Urol* 101:196–197, 1969

Hai MA, Pontes JE, Pierce JM, Jr: Surgical management of major renal trauma: A review of 102 cases treated by conservative surgery. *J Urol* 118:7–9, 1977

Kerr WS, Jr: Injuries to the genitourinary tract. *In* Cave EF, Burke JF, Boyd RJ (Eds): *Trauma Management*. Chicago, Year Book, 1974, pp. 1071–1086

Margolies MN, Ring EJ, Waltman AC: Arteriography in the management of hemorrhage from pelvic fractures. *N Engl J Med* 287:317–321, 1972

Masters FW, Robinson DW: The treatment of avulsions of the male genitalia. *J Trauma* 8:430–438, 1968

McDougal WS, Persky L: *Traumatic Injuries of the Genitourinary System*. Baltimore, Williams & Wilkins, 1981

McLaughlin AP, III, McCullough DL, Kerr WS, Jr: The use of external counterpressure (G-suit) in the management of traumatic retroperitoneal hemorrhage. *J Urol* 107:940–944, 1972

Morehouse DD, MacKinnon KJ: Urological injuries associated with pelvic fractures. *J Trauma* 9:479–496, 1969

Persky L, Hoch WH: Genitourinary tract trauma. *Curr Probl Surg* Year Book. Medical Publishers, Inc., Chicago, September, 1972

Pontes JE, Pierce JM, Jr: Anterior urethral injuries: Four years' experience at the Detroit General Hospital. *J Urol* 120:563–564, 1978

Richardson JR, Jr, Leadbetter GW, Jr: Non-operative treatment of the ruptured bladder. *J Urol* 114:213–216, 1975

Robards VL, Haglund RV, Lubin EW, et al: Treatment of rupture of the bladder. *J Urol* 116:178–179, 1976

Scott R, Carlton CE, Goldman M: Penetrating injuries of the kidney: An analysis of 181 patients. *J Urol* 101:247–253, 1969

Turner-Warwick R: A personal view of the immediate management of pelvic fracture urethral injuries. *Urol Clin North Am* 4:81–93, 1977

Tynberg D, Hoch WH, Persky L, et al: The management of renal injuries coincident with penetrating wound of the abdomen. *J Trauma* 13:502–508, 1973

Waterhouse K, Gross M: Trauma to the genitourinary tract: A five year experience with 251 cases. *J Urol* 101:241–246, 1969

Weems WL: Management of genitourinary injuries in patients with pelvic fractures. *Ann Surg* 189:717–723, 1979

Wein AJ, Murphy JJ, Mulholland SG, et al: A conservative approach to the management of blunt renal trauma. *J Urol* 117:425–427, 1977

CHAPTER **26**

Orthopaedic Emergencies

JOSEPH S. BARR, JR., M.D.
EDWIN T. WYMAN, JR., M.D.

Persons with traumatic and nontraumatic musculoskeletal conditions constitute a significant proportion of emergency ward patients. This chapter outlines the diagnosis and treatment of uncomplicated orthopaedic emergencies and the initial care of patients with more serious conditions who will be referred to the orthopaedic surgeon.

Emergency medical technicians usually are well trained in extrication and splinting techniques, and patients should arrive in the emergency ward with fractures well splinted. Physician review of splinting techniques with nonhospital paramedical personnel will help improve early patient care, and a manual such as the American Academy of Orthopaedic Surgeons' *Manual on Emergency Care and Transportation of the Sick and Injured* is most useful for this purpose.

History

The physician should question the patient about the mechanism and severity of the trauma, the mode of onset of a nontraumatic condition, and whether there had been previous injury to the affected part of a similar nontraumatic episode. The possibility of referred pain should be considered as well; for example, knee pain may be the only indicator of a hip problem.

Physical Examination

Physical examination should enable the physician to reach an accurate diagnosis in most cases; knowledge of topographic anatomy is essential in this regard. Early, accurate evaluation of neurovascular function is important, and the examiner should document it carefully, noting motor and sensory deficits indicating partial or complete injury to peripheral nerves or nerve roots (see Figs. 26.1 and 26.2 and Fig. 27.8). In the severely injured limb, distal pulses and capillary filling must be

evaluated. If vascular injury is suspected, arteriographic examination may be indicated. Compartment syndromes may be subtle, or they may present with the classic signs of muscle ischemia—pain, pallor, paralysis, pulselessness, and paresthesias—particularly when associated with a fracture of the tibia, radius, ulna, or distal part of the humerus. Pain on passive extension of the fingers or dorsiflexion of the ankle is the best early clinical sign of an impending compartment syndrome. Repeated readings of fascial compartment pressures or Doppler changes may be helpful. Compartment pressures may be measured easily with an 18-gauge needle and saline manometer, or if available, a wick catheter and pressure transducer. Normal tissue pressure is 12–20 cm H_2O. When tissue pressure exceeds diastolic pressure (cm H_2O - mm Hg), fasciotomy should be considered immediately. Effective treatment of compartment syndromes depends totally on *early recognition*, through tissue pressure measurement and monitoring.

Splints and Dressings

After physical examination but before x-ray films are taken, fractures should be splinted for immobilization (Fig. 26.3). In general, if there is enough concern to order an x-ray film, the extremity should be splinted. Splints need not be complicated. The requirements are that they (1) immobilize the part, (2) do no further damage (such as cause excess pressure on the skin), (3) are comfortable, and (4) are transportable. Splints prevent bone ends from doing further damage and provide more comfort than any amount of pain medication alone. They may be improvised easily, and in only one case (the Thomas' splint for a femoral shaft fracture, Fig. 26.3B) is a specific splint always needed. Neurovascular function dis-

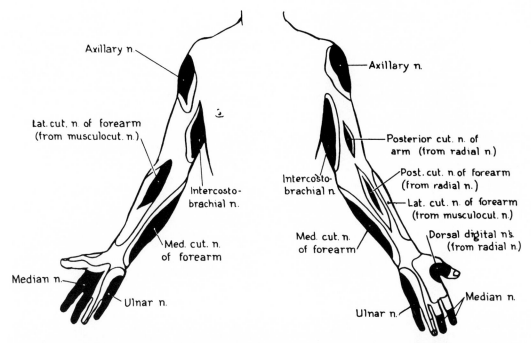

Figure 26.1. Map showing typical distribution of major peripheral nerves in upper limbs (from Foerster O: Die Symptomatologie der peripheren Nerven, in Lewandowsky MH: *Handbuch der Neurologie* [Berlin: J. Springer, 1929], Erganzungsbd. 2. Teil, pp. 975–1508).

tal to the fracture should be evaluated. Gentle traction and realignment of a badly displaced fracture often restore distal circulation. After specimens are taken for culture, open (compound) fractures should be cleansed of gross debris, dressed, and splinted. Loose pieces of bone and traumatized skin should *not* be discarded. Broad-spectrum antibiotics should be started and tetanus prophylaxis given as indicated (see Chapter 11, page 242). The cast or splint should be checked a day after application to assess circulation of the limb. Persistent pain, especially if in one area, requires that the part be evaluated in detail to rule out circulatory compromise or excessive skin pressure. Evaluation will involve cast adjustment or removal, and should be done by the physician responsible for the treatment of the fracture.

Orthopaedic Injuries in Multiple-Trauma Patients

In patients with multiple system injuries, life-threatening emergencies often require such immediate evaluation and treatment that significant orthopaedic injuries may be overlooked for an extended time. To avoid this, within the first half-hour that the patient is in the emergency ward, a member of the emergency ward team should perform a brief but complete examination of all bony

parts. Examination should include observation of deformity; palpation for edema, crepitation, or pain; and passive and active range of motion of all joints. Suspicious areas should be evaluated first for distal neurologic change and circulatory state and then splinted.

SPINAL INJURIES

Cervical Spine

Remember:

(1) Unconsciousness may indicate a cervical spine injury.

(2) A scalp laceration also may indicate a cervical spine injury.

(3) X-ray films must show the entire cervical spine.

Fracture and Dislocation

Injury to the cervical spine should be presumed, until proved otherwise, in any patient who is unresponsive and unconscious after a fall, a diving injury, or a motor vehicle accident. An adequate airway must be established and the patient's neurologic status evaluated. Tracheal intubation may be performed if the physician is careful not to hyperextend the patient's neck. The patient's head and neck should be immobilized temporarily with

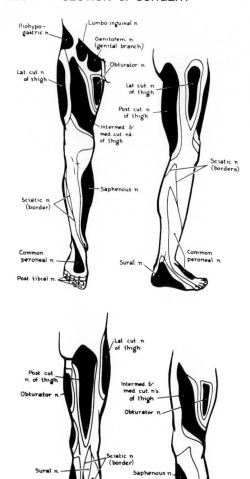

Figure 26.2. Map showing typical distribution of major peripheral nerves in lower limbs (from Foerster O: Die Symptomatologie der peripheren Nerven, in Lewandowsky MH: *Handbuch der Neurologie* [Berlin: J. Springer, 1929], Erganzungsbd. 2. Teil, pp. 975–1508).

a collar, sandbags, or four-poster brace, and x-ray films should be obtained as soon as possible.

In addition to anteroposterior and lateral views, oblique and open-mouth views are necessary. Facet fractures or dislocations can be seen in oblique views, whereas the open-mouth view shows the odontoid process. Since the cervicothoracic junction is difficult to visualize in muscular persons, either the patient's shoulders must be pulled down or an oblique ("swimmer's") view taken, with one arm up and one arm down. The physician must not dismiss the possibility of a dislocation or fracture until the cervical spine has been visualized completely (Fig. 26.4).

If dislocation or fracture is diagnosed, definitive immobilization with skull tongs or a halo device is carried out. Dislocations may be reduced by either manipulation or gradually increased skull traction. Patients with undisplaced fractures, such as mild compression fractures, may wear a Thomas collar, a "Philadelphia" collar, or a four-poster brace until further treatment decisions are made.

Soft-Tissue Injury

Sprain. The neck frequently is injured in rear-end automobile collisions. The occupants are suddenly accelerated which causes hyperextension of the head and neck beyond normal physiologic limits. The resultant condition has been called "whiplash" injury; more appropriate terms are either acute cervical sprain or acceleration-extension injury of the cervical spine. Properly adjusted head restraints on car seats prevent or minimize this injury.

Patients with acute cervical sprain may have some limitation of neck motion and muscle tenderness, although in the first hours after the injury the physical findings may be minimal. Later, conspicuous muscular spasm and tenderness may occur in all the cervical musculature. Abnormal neurologic findings are uncommon.

X-ray films of the cervical spine are usually normal in patients with acute cervical sprain, although a small chip or avulsed fragment occasionally is seen along the anterior edge of a vertebral body. The space between the spine and the larynx may be widened by retropharyngeal hematoma.

A soft collar, analgesic medications, and muscle relaxants, alone or in combination, usually are sufficient for treatment of this injury. Some common muscle relaxants are diazepam (Valium), methocarbamol (Robaxin), carisoprodol (Soma), and orphenadrine citrate (Norgesic). In severe cases, bed rest for several days or longer may be needed. Traction usually increases the discomfort.

Radicular Pain. Neck pain unrelated to traumatic injury may be caused by a number of conditions affecting nerve roots, and the onset may be sudden or gradual. The physician sometimes can establish which nerve root is involved by determining whether pain extends to the interscapular area, shoulder, arm, or fingers. During physical examination he should elicit muscle or nerve

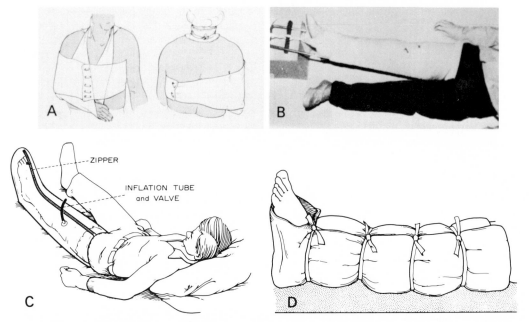

Figure 26.3.   Temporary fracture immobilization. **(A)** Velpeau's bandage (sling and swathe) for shoulder and humeral injuries. (Reproduced by permission, from Rowe CR: Shoulder girdle injuries, in Cave EF, Burke JF, Boyd RJ (Eds): *Trauma Management*. Copyright © 1974 by Year Book Medical Publishers, Inc., Chicago.) **(B)** Thomas' splint for hip and femoral fractures. **(C)** Air splint and **(D)** pillow splint for tibial, ankle, and foot injuries.

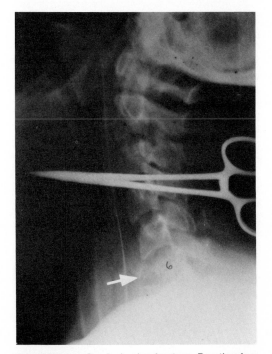

Figure 26.4.   Cervical spine fracture. Bursting fracture (*arrow*) of body of sixth cervical vertebra resulting in quadriplegia (earlier radiograph only showed down to fifth vertebra).

tenderness and test sensation, reflexes, and muscular strength.

Anteroposterior, lateral, and oblique x-ray films may show cervical spondylosis due to degenerative changes with narrowing of the intervertebral spaces and osteophytes in the neural foramina. On the other hand, such films may be normal in the patient with an acute cervical disc condition.

Radicular pain may be relieved with hot packs, muscle relaxants, analgesics, and a cervical collar. Head halter traction of 3–4 kg with the neck slightly flexed is recommended, and is most effective with the patient lying down rather than sitting. Patients with severe pain should be hospitalized and may require narcotic analgesics.

Thoracic and Lumbar Spine

Remember: Fracture of the thoracic or lumbar spine may cause significant ileus.

Fracture and Dislocation

The patient with a suspected fracture or dislocation of the thoracic or lumbar spine should be transported on a spinal board or other firm surface (see Chapter 27, page 608). The physician should turn the patient with a "logrolling" technique and examine the back for bruises and tenderness to ascertain the level of injury. Spinal cord injury necessitates careful neurologic examination, with special attention to the presence or absence of sacral sparing.

Anteroposterior and lateral films are usually adequate for initial evaluation. Laminagraphy and myelography may be used in some instances to evaluate compromise of the neural canal by bone or disc fragments. The patient may be placed on a turning frame (Stryker frame) or a firm mattress. Frequent changes in position are essential, since pressure sores over bony prominences can appear within 4 hours. General supportive measures such as intravenous fluid administration and insertion of a Foley catheter are carried out, and the patient is evaluated for other injuries. Since retroperitoneal hematoma may cause ileus lasting several days, a nasogastric tube may need to be introduced. Patients with minimal compression fractures of the thoracic or lumbar vertebrae may not require hospitalization.

Soft-Tissue Injury

A patient with pain in the lower part of the back from a fall or from lifting a heavy object may have a lumbar soft-tissue injury; this often is superimposed on a chronic back problem. In making the diagnosis, however, the physician also should consider other possibilities such as renal calculi or infection, a gynecologic condition, a leaking aortic aneurysm, or herpes zoster.

In the orthopaedic workup, the physician should test the range of motion of the patient's lumbar spine. Muscle spasm may cause sciatic scoliosis. The physician can evaluate the strength of the patient's leg muscles by having him walk on heels and tiptoes. Limited passive straight leg raising on the affected side indicates irritation of the sciatic nerve. Palpation over the lumbar area and the sciatic nerve in the buttock and posterior part of the thigh often elicits tenderness. Weakness of the quadriceps muscle and a decreased knee reflex indicate involvement of the 3rd and 4th lumbar nerve roots. If the 5th lumbar nerve root is involved, there may be weakness of the extensor hallucis longus, tibialis anterior, or peroneal muscles and decreased sensation over the dorsum of the foot. A lesion of the root of the 1st sacral nerve may cause weakness of the gastrocnemius muscle, sensory loss over the lateral aspect of the foot, or decreased ankle jerk. Differentiation between acute lumbar sprain and disc injury may be difficult or impossible on initial physical examination.

Roentgenographic findings are often normal in patients with acute back pain. Spina bifida occulta is usually an incidental finding. About 5% of the population have either spondylolysis, a defect in the pars interarticularis that is best seen on oblique views (Fig. 26.5), or spondylolisthesis, a forward slip of the 5th lumbar vertebra onto the 1st sacral vertebra. These conditions are often symptomatic. Narrowed interspaces, which occur as intervertebral discs degenerate, may also be visualized. Droplets of myelographic dye seen on the x-ray film testify to prior back problems.

Treatment of pain in the lower part of the back includes analgesic medications, hot packs, muscle relaxants, and bed rest in the lateral position or supine with pillows under the knees. A lumbar corset may be helpful. Patients with severe pain may require hospitalization for nursing care and further evaluation.

INJURIES OF UPPER EXTREMITIES

Shoulder

Remember:

(1) X-ray examination is not complete unless an axillary or tangential scapular (Neer) view is obtained.

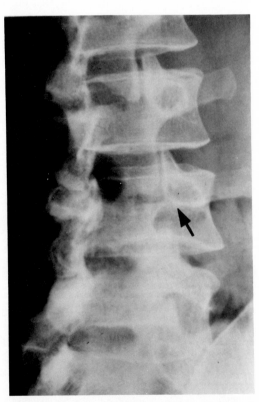

Figure 26.5. Spondylolysis. Oblique radiograph showing defect (*arrow*) in pars interarticularis of fourth lumbar vertebra.

(2) Shoulder pain after convulsion may indicate posterior dislocation.

(3) Shoulder pain with lack of passive external rotation also may indicate posterior dislocation.

(4) An anteroposterior x-ray view of the shoulder with a posterior dislocation may appear normal.

(5) Inability to actively initiate abduction may indicate rotator cuff tear.

(6) Shoulder pain with normal x-ray findings may indicate rotator cuff injury.

Brachial Plexus

Severe depression or hyperabduction of the shoulder girdle can stretch or tear the brachial plexus. On physical examination, the physician may palpate fullness and elicit tenderness from the hematoma in the supraclavicular fossa. Neurologic examination reveals the extent of damage. Horner's syndrome may be evident if the cervical sympathetic chain is damaged.

Sternoclavicular Joint

The sternoclavicular joint rarely is injured, but when the shoulder is struck hard from the side, the inner end may be dislocated upward or retrosternally. Pressure on the trachea by the clavicle in a retrosternal dislocation may cause acute, life-threatening dyspnea. The diagnosis is made best by physical examination. Palpation reveals the absence of the head of the clavicle just lateral to the sternal notch. Upward dislocation can be seen on anteroposterior and oblique x-ray views; laminagrams may be needed to demonstrate retrosternal dislocation.

Closed reduction of a retrosternal dislocation may be done by placing a tightly rolled towel between the shoulders and applying firm pressure backward on both shoulders. It may be possible to grasp the inner end of the clavicle and pull up. Closed reduction usually is successful if the dislocation is recent; open reduction may be necessary otherwise, although many chronic dislocations are relatively asymptomatic. Upward dislocation is reduced easily, but is difficult to immobilize effectively.

Clavicle

Fracture of the clavicle results commonly from a fall on the extended arm or on the shoulder. Clavicular deformity may be visible. Tenderness over the fracture site is elicited on palpation, and anteroposterior and oblique x-ray films usually demonstrate the fracture.

A soft figure-of-eight bandage padded in the axillae usually is effective and comfortable; it should be tightened every few days to keep the shoulders abducted. Open reduction rarely is indicated.

Acromioclavicular Joint

Injury to the acromioclavicular joint results from a fall on or a blow to the tip of the shoulder. Three types of injury can be distinguished:

(1) *Strain.* The patient has tenderness over the joint without displacement visible on x-ray films.

(2) *Subluxation.* Less than 1 cm of upward displacement of the distal clavicle is apparent on physical examination and x-ray film.

(3) *Dislocation.* There is more than 1 cm of upward displacement, which is caused by the upward pull of the trapezius muscle. X-ray views with the patient holding 2-kg weights in both hands help demonstrate the deformity (Fig. 26.6).

Patients with strains and subluxations may be treated with a sling for 1–2 weeks. Reduction of a complete dislocation by downward pressure on the distal clavicle is easy to achieve, but difficult to maintain by closed means. For younger, athletic patients, operative repair may be indicated.

Glenohumeral Joint

Dislocation. The glenohumeral joint frequently is dislocated from a fall or abduction of the arm. In a patient with a previous dislocation, minimal trauma may cause recurrence. It may be difficult or impossible to reduce a dislocation more than a few days old. The physician should be aware of this, particularly in patients such as chronic alcoholics. In an anteroinferior dislocation, the humeral head is palpable in the anterior part of the axilla. The patient should be examined for evidence of axillary nerve injury (lack of sensation over the lateral part of the shoulder and deltoid muscle palsy). Occasionally, pressure of the humeral head on the axillary structures may cause distal neurovascular compromise.

Posterior dislocations (Fig. 26.7) are uncommon and may go unrecognized. *Inability to rotate the arm externally* is the principal diagnostic sign. If the physician stands behind the seated patient, he may see that the affected shoulder is flat anteriorly and full posteriorly. In roentgenographic examination, at least two views are necessary for accurate diagnosis, an anteroposterior view and either a Neer view or an axillary view. Transthoracic views are difficult to interpret in heavy patients, and should not be obtained in these cases.

There are several techniques for reducing an anterior dislocation (Fig. 26.8), all of which de-

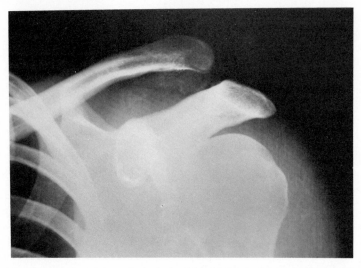

Figure 26.6.   Dislocation of acromioclavicular joint. Distal clavicle is displaced upward 1 cm.

pend on relaxing the shoulder muscles, particularly the subscapularis and pectoralis major. Muscle relaxation may be potentiated with intravenous analgesics or drugs such as diazepam. Occasionally, general anesthesia may be necessary. Traction on the wrist with the arm somewhat abducted, together with countertraction using a sheet passed under the axilla, often is successful. The Kocher maneuver involves slowly and gently flexing the patient's arm and applying traction to the elbow with abduction and external rotation, followed by adduction and internal rotation. The Stimson method involves use of a weight tied to the wrist of a prone patient with the arm hanging over the side of the stretcher. The elevation method uses traction to pull the arm almost directly overhead, followed by thumb pressure under the humeral head to lift it into the glenoid fossa.

A sling and swathe, or Velpeau's bandage (Fig. 26.3A), should be maintained for 3 weeks in the case of an anterior dislocation to allow the articular capsule of the glenohumeral joint to heal. An x-ray film should be obtained after reduction to confirm the reduction and to ascertain that no fractures occurred during manipulation or were unrecognized in the original films.

Fracture. Many types of fracture and fracture-dislocation occur in the head and neck of the humerus. If the humeral head or neck is fractured,

there is local pain, swelling, and ecchymosis. The physician often can elicit crepitation on moving the arm. Anteroposterior and axillary films are essential for diagnosis and to determine whether the humeral head is dislocated. Most patients can be treated nonoperatively with immobilization or closed reduction and immobilization. Severely comminuted and displaced fractures may require open reduction or prosthetic replacement.

Humeral Shaft

Remember:

(1) Fracture of the humeral shaft requires check of radial nerve function before and after reduction.

(2) In patients with a humeral supracondylar fracture a compartment syndrome (Volkmann's ischemia) may develop.

Especially in the presence of a fracture of the middle or distal part of the humerus, the patient should be tested for injury to the radial nerve. Radial nerve sensation can be tested at the dorsum of the first web space, and motor function can be ascertained by asking the patient to extend the wrist *and metacarpophalangeal joints.* The interphalangeal joints are extended by the lumbrical and interosseus muscles, which are innervated by the median and ulnar nerves.

Anteroposterior and lateral films should be ob-

Figure 26.7.   Posterior dislocation of shoulder. **(A)** Patient is unable to externally rotate left shoulder that has posterior dislocation. **(B)** Viewed from above, left shoulder is prominent posteriorly. **(C)** Anteroposterior radiographs of right and left shoulders show some asymmetry, but diagnosis of posterior dislocation is not obvious. **(D)** Axillary radiographs (*right and left*) show left humeral head posterior to glenoid fossa. **(E)** Technique of axillary radiographic view. (Parts **A, B,** and **E** all reproduced by permission, from Rowe CR: Shoulder girdle injuries, in Cave EF, Burke JF, Boyd RJ (Eds): *Trauma Management.* Copyright © 1974 by Year Book Medical Publishers, Inc., Chicago.)

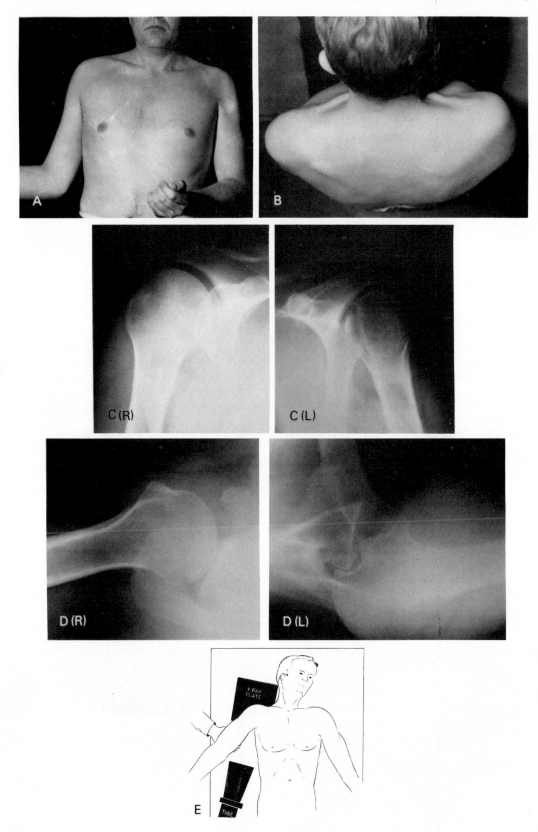

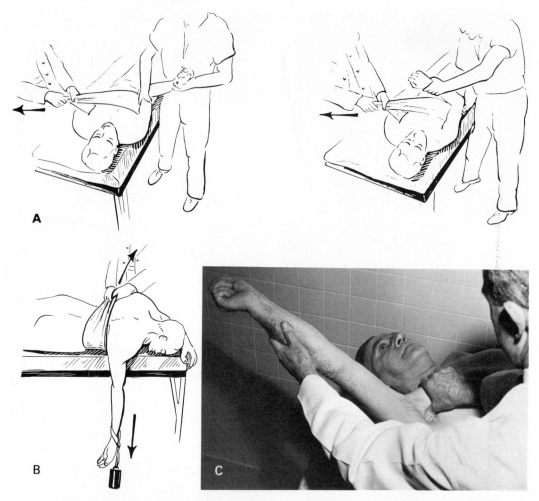

Figure 26.8.   Reduction of anterior shoulder dislocation. **(A)** Kocher method. **(B)** Stimson method. **(C)** Elevation method. **(A–C** reproduced by permission, from Rowe CR: Shoulder girdle injuries, in Cave EF, Burke JF, Boyd RJ (Eds): *Trauma Management*. Copyright © 1974 by Year Book Medical Publishers, Inc., Chicago.)

tained to confirm the diagnosis. Gentle traction usually produces good alignment of the humeral shaft. The reduction can be maintained by coaptation plaster splints placed medially and laterally and snugly wrapped on from axilla to elbow with the forearm supported by a collar and cuff at the wrist (Fig. 26.9). A hanging plaster cast may produce distraction or angulation at the fracture site.

Elbow

Remember:

(1) Elbow pain with negative x-ray findings may indicate radial head fracture.

(2) Elbow injuries in children less than 10 years old require films of *both* elbows for comparison.

(3) A line on any x-ray film of the elbow drawn through the center of the radius always meets the

center of the capitellum if the radius is not dislocated.

If the physician suspects a fracture or dislocation of the elbow, he should palpate the bony prominences—medial and lateral epicondyles, olecranon, and radial head—for tenderness and crepitation. Neurovascular evaluation of the forearm and hand should be carefully carried out.

Anteroposterior and lateral x-ray films are obtained. If the physician suspects a fracture of the radial head, he can order several rotational views. The radial head normally points at the capitellum in all views; if it does not, it is dislocated (Fig. 26.10). In children, the multiple secondary ossification centers are confusing, and films of the opposite normal elbow are often helpful for comparison.

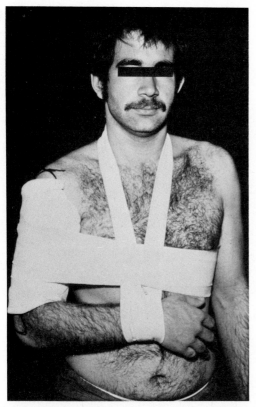

Dislocation

Dislocations of the elbow usually are reduced easily and are immobilized in a posterior splint and sling with the elbow flexed 90 degrees. Range-of-motion exercises should be started as soon as the swelling begins to subside. Isolated radial head dislocations do occur and must be recognized; this injury occurs more commonly, however, with a fracture of the proximal part of the ulna (a Monteggia fracture, Fig. 26.11). In a young child, a sudden pull on the arm by a strong child or by an adult may cause subluxation of the radial head, commonly called pulled elbow or nursemaid's elbow. The patient refuses to use the arm, and physical examination reveals resistance to full supination. X-ray films are normal. Firm supination of the forearm produces a palpable click over the radial head, and the child is usually asymptomatic within a few minutes.

Fracture

In adults, displaced olecranon fractures require excision or repair of the bony fragment. Radial head fractures with minimal disruption of the articular surface respond to conservative measures such as aspiration of accompanying hemarthrosis. Gentle testing of pronation and supination is carried out. If this results in less than 60 degrees of

Figure 26.9. Coaptation splints with collar and cuff for humeral fracture.

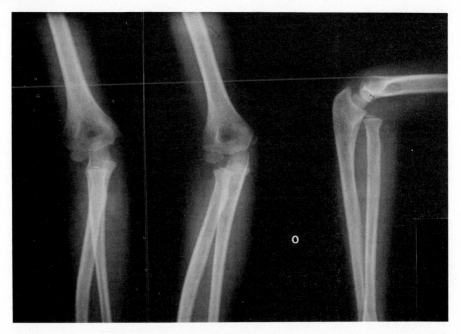

Figure 26.10. Three x-ray views of dislocated radial head in right arm of 6-year-old child (*left to right:* anteroposterior, oblique, and lateral). Radial head does not point to capitellum.

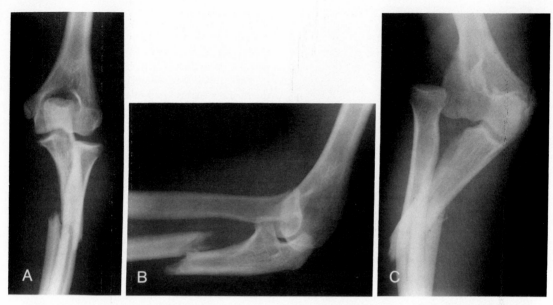

Figure 26.11. Monteggia fracture. **(A)** Anteroposterior view and **(B)** lateral view. Radial head subluxation is subtle, but it is apparent on both views that a line drawn up the center of the radius would not bisect the capitellum. **(C)** Oblique view. On this view, dislocation is obvious.

each motion, or if a loose body is present on x-ray examination, operation probably will be required. Adult patients with supracondylar fractures of the humerus require hospitalization for traction or operative repair. In children, since a supracondylar fracture may compromise circulation and lead to muscle ischemia and eventually Volkmann's contracture, the radial pulse must be monitored carefully after closed reduction. If the circulatory status is uncertain, treatment in traction is the safest course.

Forearm

Remember:

(1) Displaced forearm fractures in adults usually require open reduction.

(2) Reduced green-stick fractures in children may angulate again, even in a cast.

(3) Compartment syndromes can occur in patients with forearm fractures.

Obvious angular deformity accompanies fracture of the forearm. Immediate, careful evaluation of neurovascular function is essential. X-ray films should include anteroposterior and lateral views from the wrist to the elbow.

In children, green-stick fractures of the forearm must be bent the other way to fracture the opposite cortex, or angulation will recur; surgical repair is rarely necessary. In adults, closed reduction when both the radius and the ulna are fractured often fails to produce good alignment, particularly in rotation. The usual treatment, therefore, is open

reduction and fixation with rods or plates. On the other hand, isolated fractures of one bone may at times be treated with closed reduction. Compartment syndromes also can occur in patients with these fractures.

Wrist

Remember:

(1) Wrist pain with normal x-ray findings may indicate navicular fracture.

(2) Navicular fracture or rupture of thumb abductor tendon can occur with Colles' fracture.

(3) Always check the position of the lunate bone to rule out perilunate dislocation.

(4) Wrist pain with negative x-ray findings may indicate intercarpal subluxation.

Injuries to the distal part of the radius and ulna are common and usually are caused by a fall on the outstretched hand. Colles' fracture, a term mistakenly used for wrist fractures in general, refers to a dorsally displaced fracture of the lower end of the radius with accompanying fracture of the ulnar styloid process (Fig. 26.12). Dorsal displacement of the hand and wrist produces the silver-fork deformity. Tenderness over the anatomical snuffbox suggests a navicular fracture.

X-ray films should include anteroposterior and lateral views, with navicular views if a navicular fracture is suspected. Comparison views of the other wrist are helpful in evaluating other carpal fractures and dislocations.

Local, regional, or general anesthesia is used in

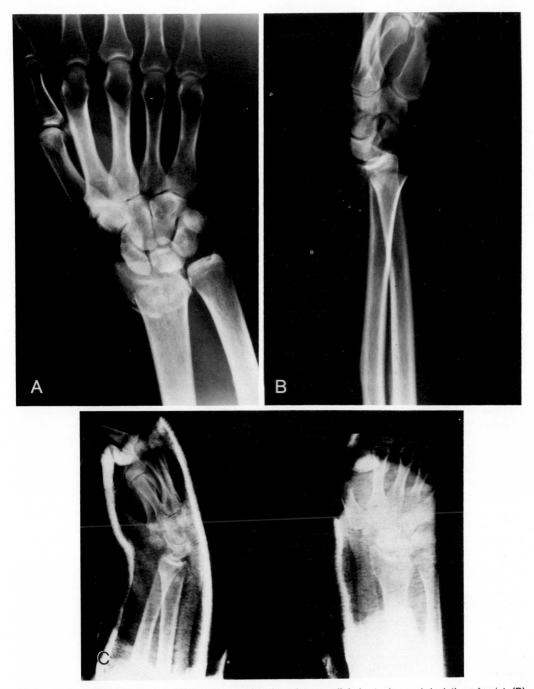

Figure 26.12.   Colles' fracture. **(A)** Anteroposterior view shows radial shortening and deviation of wrist. **(B)** Lateral view shows dorsal angulation. **(C)** Postreduction films obtained after reduction show restoration of anatomic position.

the repair of displaced fractures of the wrist. Strong traction and countertraction are applied to disengage and to disimpact the bony fragments, which then are pushed into place and maintained in a stable position. The hand and wrist after a Colles' fracture usually are held in pronation, with ulnar deviation and some wrist flexion. Smith's fracture, or reverse Colles' fracture, is best held in supination with slight wrist flexion. Either a gutter splint open on the ulnar side or volar and dorsal plaster splints are applied, wrapping them on carefully to avoid wrinkles. The elbow then is immobilized to prevent forearm rotation. A cast circling the wrist should be avoided because of soft-tissue swelling, and volar plaster splints should not go beyond the midpalmar crease to allow full metacarpophalangeal flexion. The patient should be seen on the following day to assess reduction and circulation, tightening or loosening the splints as indicated. Finger and shoulder exercises should be encouraged to prevent later complications such as causalgia and Sudeck's atrophy. In elderly patients, the fracture may not be reduced in order to regain early function. This will result in permanent cosmetic deformity, however. Median nerve compression is also a possibility with this fracture, and nerve function should be evaluated.

In an adult patient, the diagnosis of "wrist sprain" should be made only after navicular fracture has been excluded. If there is any tenderness of the navicular bone, a case that includes the thumb as well as the wrist should be applied even if x-ray films do not demonstrate a fracture. Films should be repeated in 2 weeks with the cast removed. If a navicular fracture has occurred, it will be visualized and the cast should be replaced. If no fracture is seen, the definitive diagnosis of wrist sprain can be made and the cast can be left off.

Wrist trauma may include dislocation or subluxation of the proximal or the distal carpal row. These injuries, which may be subtle and which may occur without visible fracture, require detailed study of intercarpal relationships and comparison with the normal wrist. A common injury of this type is perilunate dislocation, in which hyperextension of the wrist occurs with dislocation of the distal carpal row dorsally. Return of the hand to the neutral position then flexes the lunate bone 90 degrees. Even though the lunate is now rotated to this degree, the x-ray film looks deceptively normal unless the examiner looks carefully at the lunate itself (Fig. 26.13).

In older children, displacement of the distal part of the radial epiphysis is common, and requires accurate reduction to avoid growth retardation. A torus fracture of the distal radius (buckling of the dorsal cortex), commonly seen in children, requires only a splint or a light cast for 2–3 weeks.

INJURIES OF LOWER PART OF TRUNK

Pelvis

Remember:

(1) Pelvic fracture may cause fatal retroperitoneal bleeding.

(2) Pelvic fracture also may cause significant injury to the urethra and bladder.

(3) Fractures of the acetabulum may disrupt hip function or injure the sciatic nerve.

(4) Fractures through the sacral foramen may damage bowel and bladder function.

(5) A catheter should not be introduced if there is blood at the penile meatus.

Patients with a pelvic fracture may have local tenderness over the pubic or ischial rami, iliac wings, or sacrum. Diastasis of the pubic symphysis may be palpable, and compression of the ilia may cause pain in the pelvis or sacroiliac region. Hypotension and a decreased hematocrit may provide evidence of blood loss; an increase in abdominal girth indicates retroperitoneal hemorrhage. Pelvic or rectal examination also may reveal bony tenderness or the presence of hematoma. Injuries to the femoral, obturator, or sciatic nerves may accompany pelvic fractures. Identification and early documentation of nerve injuries are important.

An anteroposterior film of the pelvis and lateral films of the sacrum and coccyx are necessary for diagnosis. Anteroposterior films with the tube tilted 30 degrees caudad and cephalad, as well as films taken in 45-degree internal and external oblique projections, provide additional information about the displacement of complicated pelvic fractures.

The physician must be aware that significant or even fatal hemorrhage can follow a pelvic fracture (see Chapter 35, pages 794–796). Even seemingly minor fractures to the pubic rami, for example, can result in major retroperitoneal bleeding, and with severe pelvic fractures, exsanguination may occur. Adequate intravenous fluid and blood replacement is essential; an external pressure device (G-suit or MAST trousers) may save the patient's life by providing a temporary means of tamponade.

Injuries to the bladder and urethra often are associated with pelvic fractures (Fig. 26.14). In the presence of such a fracture, the emergency physician should consult a urologist before performing any procedures involving these structures, particularly if there is blood at the penile meatus (see Chapter 25, pages 541–544). Catheters are to be avoided in patients with urethral perforation. A retrograde urethrogram is therefore necessary before attempts to pass a catheter. If extravasation is demonstrated, suprapubic drainage of the bladder is indicated.

Hip

Remember:

(1) If the leg is flexed, adducted, and internally rotated, the hip is posteriorly dislocated.

(2) If the leg is shortened and externally rotated, the hip is fractured.

(3) Hip dislocation may cause sciatic nerve injury.

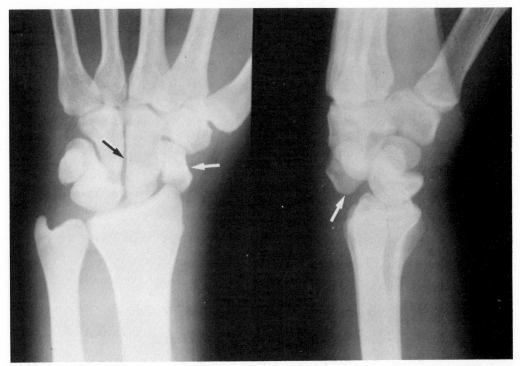

Figure 26.13. Perilunate dislocation. (*Left*) Anteroposterior view. *Arrows* indicate abnormalities of navicular and lunate configurations. (*Right*) Lateral view. The lunate bone does not articulate with distal carpal row (*arrow*).

(4) Ability to walk and move the hip does *not* prove that the femoral neck is not fractured.

Hip fractures occur primarily in elderly patients. If the patient has a displaced fracture of either the femoral neck or the intertrochanteric region, the affected leg is shortened and externally rotated, and attempts to move the leg are painful. Severe trauma may cause dislocation of the hip posteriorly. In this situation the leg is adducted, flexed, and internally rotated. Injury to the sciatic nerve occurs in about 15% of posterior dislocations, and function of the peroneal and posterior tibial divisions of the nerve should be evaluated. Rarely, anterior and obturator dislocations occur; the patient's leg is rotated externally and the femoral head may be palpable.

Anteroposterior and lateral x-ray films are necessary. The examiner should remember that the farther a structure is from the film, the more it is magnified. Thus, in the anteroposterior film, the affected femoral head will appear larger than the normal femoral head if the dislocation is anterior and smaller if it is posterior. Undisplaced fractures of the femoral neck, greater trochanter, and acetabulum may be difficult to visualize, and the films must be examined carefully.

Fractures of the femoral neck may be strongly impacted in a slightly valgus position (Fig. 26.15).

This may result in enough stability for the patient to move the hip moderately comfortably and even walk, although with a limp. These fractures may be hard to outline on x-ray films, and often are not diagnosed, with the patient discharged from the emergency ward with crutches. They can, however, become fully displaced later. Therefore, any patient with a painful hip after a fall, even if able to walk and with negative x-ray findings, should be admitted and placed on bedrest until *repeated* x-ray films and absence of symptoms on rest prove there is no fracture.

In patients with a hip fracture, Buck's extension should be applied with traction straps below the knee and 2 kg of weight. Hip dislocations require immediate reduction, usually under general or spinal anesthesia. Intertrochanteric fractures and comminuted acetabular fractures may cause significant hemorrhage. All patients with hip fractures and dislocations should be hospitalized for definitive treatment.

INJURIES OF LOWER EXTREMITIES

Thigh

Remember:

(1) The patient may lose 4–6 units of blood into the surrounding tissue.

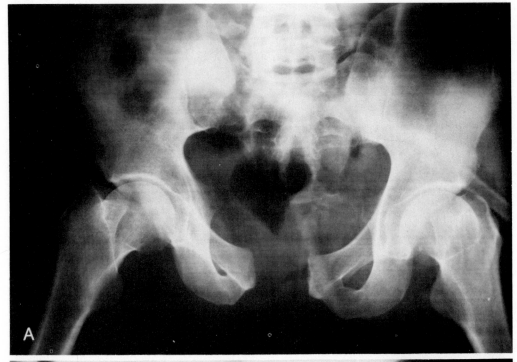

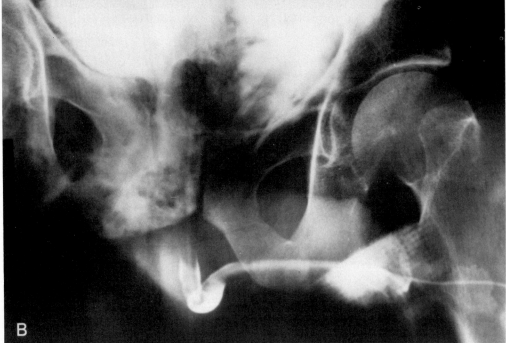

Figure 26.14.   Pelvic fracture. **(A)** Disruption of pubic symphysis and sacroiliac joint with wide displacement. **(B)** Urethrogram confirms urethral injury.

(2) Femoral fractures require traction with a Thomas' splint in the emergency ward, or preferably at the scene of the accident.

(3) This injury may occur with hip dislocation, so x-ray films of the pelvis and hip are always necessary.

Fracture of the femur is diagnosed easily. The leg should be splinted at the scene of injury, and

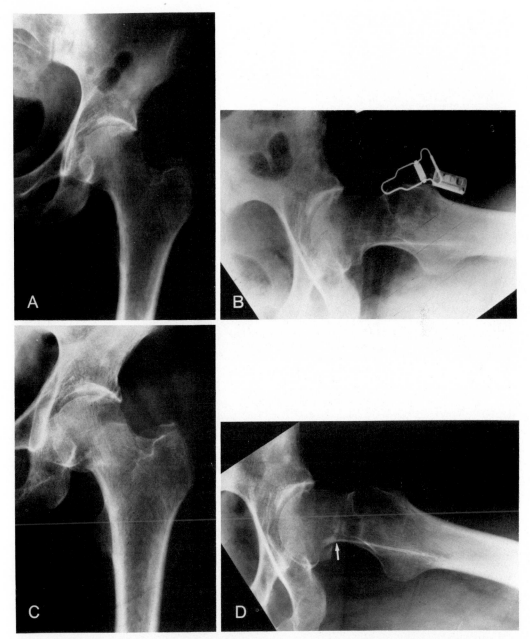

Figure 26.15. **(A)** Anteroposterior view and **(B)** lateral view of normal hip. **(C)** Anteroposterior view of undisplaced, slightly impacted femoral neck fracture. Note appearance of fracture line at superior femoral neck and area of sclerosis (impaction) and trabecular irregularity medially just beneath femoral head. **(D)** Lateral view of same fracture. Note overlap of trabecular lines (*arrow*) and cortical break posteriorly just below femoral head.

immobilization and traction should be applied in the emergency ward with a Hare traction splint or a Thomas' splint (Fig. 26.3B). The status of distal neurovascular structures must be ascertained. Anteroposterior and lateral x-ray films are taken, including the entire femur and hip in case an ipsilateral hip fracture or dislocation has occurred simultaneously (Fig. 26.16). Since a closed femoral fracture can cause loss of 4–6 units of blood into the tissues of the thigh, blood should be replaced as indicated.

Knee

Remember:

(1) Patellar fractures may be associated with hip dislocation.

(2) Knee dislocations commonly occlude or divide the popliteal artery.

(3) The presence of pedal pulses in a young person with knee dislocation does *not* rule out arterial injuries.

Fractures of the patella often can be palpated. If the fracture is complete, it prevents active knee extension by inhibiting quadriceps activity. Fractures of the distal femur or tibial plateau may rapidly cause tense, painful hemarthrosis. Aspiration of the hemarthrosis under sterile conditions will relieve symptoms. If the aspirate contains fat globules floating on top of the blood, communication between the marrow canal and the joint is proved. The extremity is immobilized or placed in traction as indicated.

Ruptures can occur within the quadriceps muscle above the patella or in the patellar tendon below. These usually can be palpated and, if complete, will not allow the patient to lift his leg with the knee extended. The patella may be seen as too high or too low on the lateral x-ray film. Complete ruptures of this type require surgical repair.

Dislocation or subluxation of the patella is common, occurring frequently in obese women who have genu valgum (knock-knee). The dislocated patella sometime can be palpated lateral to its normal position; more often, subluxations of the patella reduce spontaneously, and the diagnosis can be made if the patient complains of pain when the patella is pushed laterally.

Soft-tissue injuries around the knee joint frequently are seen. Squatting and twisting may damage the medial or lateral meniscus. A torn meniscus may cause the knee to lock in flexion or may prevent its full extension. Palpation of the joint line usually elicits tenderness over the affected meniscus. Sprains and tears of the collateral ligaments can be diagnosed by careful palpation and by causing pain or instability on application of varus or valgus stress to the extended knee. Injury to a cruciate ligament causes anteroposterior instability, which is best demonstrated with the knee flexed.

In the case of a knee injury, anteroposterior and lateral x-ray films are ordered routinely. A tangential view is helpful in patellar injuries, and stress films should be obtained to evaluate injured ligaments and fractures of the tibial plateau (Fig. 26.17).

A result of severe trauma, true dislocation of the knee is rare. All ligaments are torn, rendering the

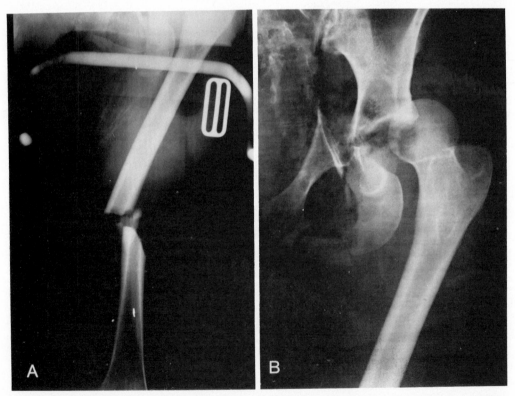

Figure 26.16.   Femoral shaft fracture. **(A)** Anteroposterior view reveals adducted proximal fragment. **(B)** Hip film reveals concomitant posterior fracture-dislocation.

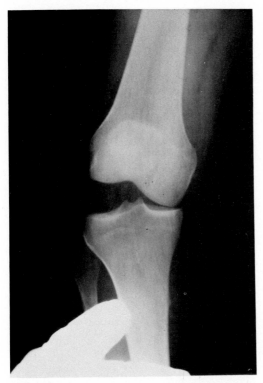

Figure 26.17. Stress radiograph of knee. Application of varus stress reveals complete disruption of lateral ligaments.

knee completely unstable. Anterior dislocation (tibia dislocated forward) is liable to stretch or tear the popliteal artery, and the peroneal nerve also is often stretched.

A true orthopaedic emergency, the dislocated knee should be reduced immediately. Peripheral pulses should be evaluated after reduction, and if compromise of the popliteal artery is suggested, arteriographic examination should be carried out promptly and the injured vessel repaired, since collateral circulation in the popliteal area is insufficient to nourish the distal part of the leg. Pedal pulses may be present because of excellent collateral circulation about the knee, particularly if the patient is a teenager. Often this is not sufficient, however, to prevent eventual distal circulatory compromise as swelling occurs in the injured area. Therefore, arteriograms commonly are needed to define the exact status of the popliteal artery.

Dislocation of the patella can be reduced by extending the knee and flexing the hip (straight leg raising) to relax the quadriceps muscle. It is treated with a compression dressing composed of multiple layers of either sheet wadding or Webril and an Ace bandage wrapped from ankle to groin. Crutches that are adjusted to leave 2.5 cm between

the top of the crutch and the axilla should also be used, taking care that weight is borne on the hands, not on the axillae.

If the physician diagnoses patellar fracture, a partial or complete ligamentous tear, or injury to a meniscus, the patient may be admitted to the hospital for definitive treatment.

Lower Leg

Remember:

(1) Fracture of the neck of the fibula may damage the peroneal nerve.

(2) Fracture of the proximal third of the tibia may cause circulatory impairment.

(3) In fractures of the fibular shaft, treatment of symptoms is sufficient.

Intra-articular fractures of the proximal part of the tibia usually occur on the lateral side ("plateau" fracture) because of a valgus knee injury. Aspiration of blood from the knee that contains fat globules will indicate this. Significant depression of fragments into the metaphysis of the tibia may require open reduction.

Fractures of the shaft of the fibula (except for those within 3 inches of the lateral malleolus) occur from direct blows and may be treated symptomatically, since this part of the fibula does not take part in weight-bearing. Although fibular neck fractures do not require significant treatment, they may be accompanied by injury to the peroneal nerve.

Fractures of the proximal third of the tibia may cause vascular compromise because of their approximation to the trifurcation where the blood vessel is significantly tethered (Fig. 26.18).

Because of its subcutaneous position, the tibia frequently is involved in open fractures. The wound may range in size from a pinpoint opening due to a sharp piece of bone that pierces the skin from within (grade 1) to a large area involving skin and muscles that is a result of severe external trauma (grade 3). Neurovascular status distal to the wound must first be evaluated carefully; gentle traction with alignment often restores distal circulation. Open fractures are inspected, specimens are taken for culture, and the wound is cleansed of debris. A sterile dressing is then applied, and the limb is splinted in an air or pillow splint (Fig. 26.3, C and D). If the wound is large and is bleeding briskly, it is best to control the bleeding with pressure dressings, since attempts to clamp the vessel under emergency conditions may damage the adjacent nerves.

Anteroposterior and lateral x-ray films are taken with the leg splinted and should include both the

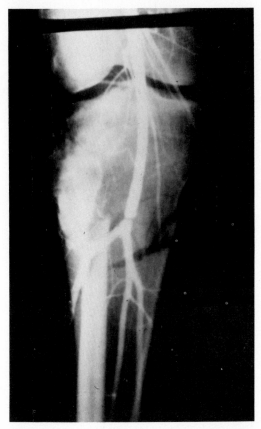

Figure 26.18. Fracture of proximal tibia with intimal tear of popliteal artery proximal to its trifurcation, where artery is tightly fixed.

knee and the ankle. In open fractures, antibiotics and tetanus prophylaxis are administered, and the patient is admitted for further treatment. Most patients with closed tibial fractures should be admitted for elevation of the leg and observation of the circulation. Patients with isolated fibular fractures or, occasionally, undisplaced tibial fractures may be treated on an outpatient basis with immobilization of the leg in a cast.

Ankle

Remember:

(1) The mortise view is the most important x-ray view.

(2) A widened mortise without fracture may indicate a Maisonneuve fracture of the fibula.

Twisting injuries of the foot can produce sprains and fractures of the ankle. Ligamentous injuries should be tested as soon as possible before swelling occurs. The most commonly injured ligaments in the body are the lateral ligaments of the ankle (Fig. 26.19A), which are stretched or torn when the foot is inverted. Careful palpation reveals the site of damage. Stressing the foot and ankle demonstrates whether the tear is complete, since complete ligamentous tears are less painful to stress than partial tears. Injuries of the deltoid (medial) ligament are less common, but must be recognized since the deltoid ligament is important for ankle stability.

Fractures of the ankle also are evaluated by palpation and stressing. A displaced medial malleolus often can be diagnosed before x-ray examination by the presence of a palpable fracture line over the distal and medial portions of the tibia. Until definitive treatment is undertaken, the ankle should be treated with ice packs, splints, and elevation. In general, it is best to "overtreat" ankle sprains. Immobilization in a plaster cast provides the best environment for healing of ligaments. The cast should be continued, allowing weight-bearing as tolerated, until the patient has been bearing full weight without pain for 1 week. This usually takes 3–4 weeks, but may take as long as 8 weeks. Minimal sprains may be treated with adhesive strapping or Ace bandages and crutches.

Fractures of the ankle may involve the lateral malleolus alone, the lateral and medial malleoli (bimalleolar), or the lateral, medial, and posterior malleoli (trimalleolar) (Fig. 26.20). They occur usually from an internal rotation force of the body on the fixed foot. Complete or partial dislocation of the talus can occur, and treatment is directed at restoration of the mortise to provide stability to the ankle. Significant loss of fibular length requires correction also. Widening of the mortise may be apparent on x-ray films without a visible fracture. Palpation of the side of the calf usually will elicit tenderness over the middle and upper part of the fibula. The Maisonneuve fracture (Fig. 26.21) is a rupture of the deltoid ligament with a high fibular fracture allowing lateral displacement of the talus and a widened mortise without visible fracture on x-ray films of the ankle. It is a commonly undiagnosed injury in emergency wards.

Anteroposterior and lateral views as well as a mortise view should be routinely obtained. The mortise view (Fig. 26.19B) is similar to the anteroposterior view, but the leg is internally rotated about 30 degrees. A distance larger than 5 mm between the medial malleolus and the talus is evidence of injury to the deltoid ligament. In a normal ankle, the tibia and fibula should overlap. If they are separated, the tibiofibular ligament has been torn (Fig. 26.22). The posterior malleolus of the tibia can be evaluated on the lateral view. Stress views can be taken for full evaluation of ligamentous injury and stability (Fig. 26.19C).

In a fracture-dislocation of the ankle, with the talus displaced laterally or posteriorly, it often is

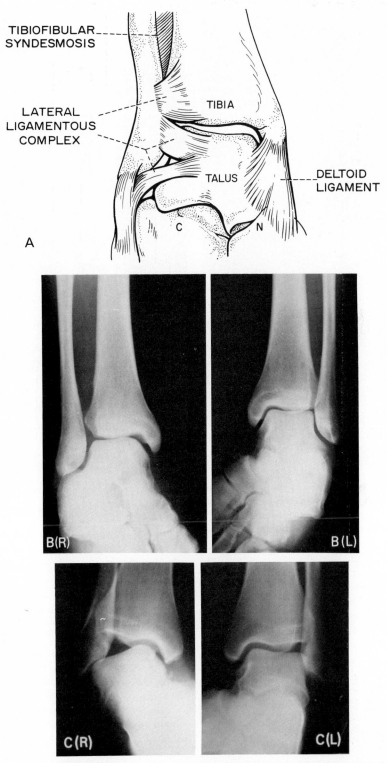

Figure 26.19. Ligamentous injuries of ankle. **(A)** Major ligaments of ankle; *N* = navicular bone, *C* = calcaneous bone. **(B)** Mortise views of injured (*right*) and normal (*left*) ankles; in right ankle note increased space between talus and tibia medially (torn deltoid ligament) and widening of interval between tibia and fibula (torn syndesmosis). **(C)** Inversion stress views of injured (*right*) and normal (*left*) ankles in another patient; in right ankle note marked tilting of talus resulting from complete tear of lateral ligaments.

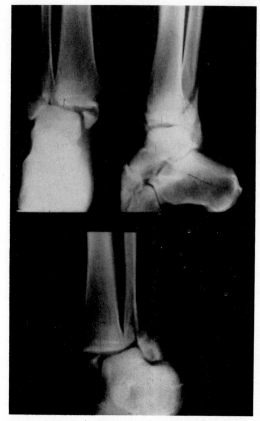

Figure 26.20. Trimalleolar fracture-dislocation of ankle. Note fractures of medial, lateral, and posterior malleoli, and disruption of ankle mortise.

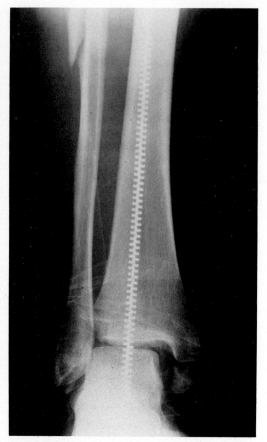

Figure 26.21. Maisonneuve fracture. Note widening of mortise and high fibula fracture that may easily be missed on films of the ankle only.

possible to reduce the talus back under the tibia without anesthesia. This should be done as quickly as possible to minimize swelling and neurovascular compromise. An undisplaced or minimally displaced fracture can be treated with a cast. X-ray films should be taken after the cast is applied to be sure that the position remains satisfactory.

Malleolar fractures also may occur in conjunction with severe shattering of the distal tibia in an intra-articular fracture. This is the so-called pilon fracture, which often results in late post-traumatic osteoarthritis.

Ankle sprains may be associated with osteochondral fractures of the talus, which may be seen as small flecks near the medial or lateral portion of the tibial articulation of the talus. These injuries are more severe than sprains and may require surgical intervention.

Foot

Remember:

(1) Significant midfoot pain and swelling may indicate metatarsal-tarsal (Lisfranc) dislocation.

(2) Metatarsal neck fractures require lateral x-ray films (plantar angulation).

(3) Fractures of the neck of the talus and talar dislocations may result in avascular necrosis.

(4) Os calcis fractures may be accompanied by spinal compression fractures.

Fractures of the talus usually involve the talar neck and can compromise the bony circulation, leading to avascular necrosis. Displacement of the fragment seen on the lateral x-ray film must be corrected accurately. Dislocations of the talus from the tibia above or the os calcis below may also occur, with or without accompanying fractures. These injuries also are prone to later avascular necrosis to the talus. Reduction commonly can be accomplished by closed methods, but requires general or spinal anesthesia.

Fractures of the os calcis usually result from falls and commonly are work related. The fracture may be an avulsion of a large piece of the posterior part of the os calcis by the gastrocnemius tendon attachment, which usually requires open reduction to restore effective lengths of the involved muscle.

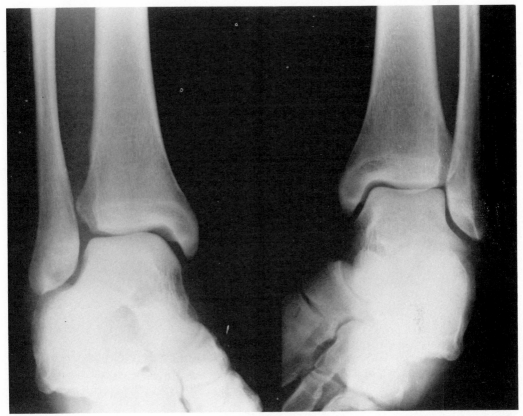

Figure 26.22.   Tear of tibiofibular ligament. (*Left*) Mortise view demonstrates that fibula and tibia do not overlap and that there is increased space between them.(*Right*) Mortise view of normal ankle for comparison. Stress views would confirm the diagnosis.

However, it is more often a crush injury, with decrease in the height of the bone, lateral protuberance, and severe involvement of the subtalar joint (Fig. 26.23). The injury commonly is accompanied by a lumbar compression fracture; therefore, the presence of an os calcis fracture requires examination of the back. Functional recovery is long, and return to work usually is slow. Early treatment consists of splinting with a compression dressing, plaster, and elevation. Hospital admission usually is indicated. Intra-articular fractures of the os calcis in its articulation with the cuboid bone also can occur and are commoniy undiagnosed because they are only obvious on oblique films of the foot.

The midfoot (navicular and cuneiform bones on one end and metatarsal bases on the other) is an area of great stress at the apex of the arch of the foot. Dislocations in this area can occur with or without fractures of the metatarsal bones (Lisfranc fractures), with the metatarsals usually moving as a unit on the midtarsal bones (Fig. 26.24). Closed reduction may be unstable, and surgical fixation may be required. These injuries may be difficult

to interpret on x-ray examination, but should be suspected whenever there is considerable swelling and pain in the midfoot. Since compromised circulation is a definite danger in these fractures, admission with close observation is mandatory.

Fractures of the metatarsal shaft usually occur from direct blows (when not associated with Lisfranc type injuries), and conservative management with a cast is sufficient. Fractures of the metatarsal neck, however, present a different problem because they often angulate in a plantar direction and present weight-bearing problems later if allowed to heal in that position. Recognition of this fracture may be difficult since lateral x-ray films are required to show the deformity and these are not obtained routinely in most radiology departments. Simple closed manipulation to correct the plantar angulation together with cast immobilization is all that is needed. The most common metatarsal fracture is an avulsion fracture of the base of the 5th metatarsal bone by the peroneus brevis in inversion injury. Treatment of symptoms without cast immobilization is usually sufficient. A fracture more distal in the 5th metatarsal (Jones'

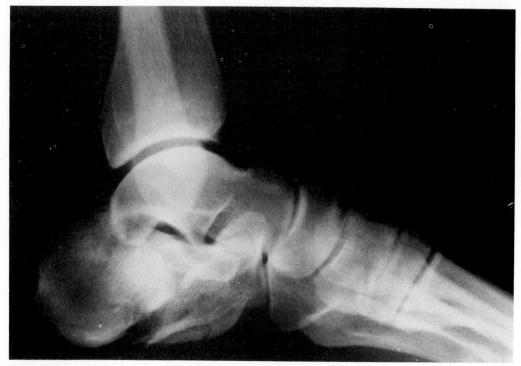

Figure 26.23.   Os calcis fracture. Note decrease in height of heel, as well as comminution and disruption of subtalar joint anatomy.

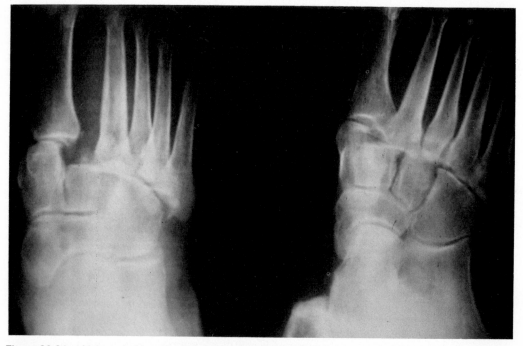

Figure 26.24.   Lisfranc fracture. (*Left*) Anteroposterior view and (*right*) oblique view. Note lateral dislocation of 2nd through 5th metatarsals, best seen on anteroposterior view.

fracture) can occur in the proximal cortical portion of the metatarsal shaft. This fracture heals slowly and requires cast immobilization for many weeks and occasionally operative correction.

Metatarsophalangeal dislocations occur with the phalanx dislocated dorsally. Although closed reduction usually is accomplished easily, at times the capsule or flexion tendon will prevent closed reduction, and open reduction will be required.

Fractures of the phalanges of the toes occasionally are angulated enough to require manipulative reduction, but more commonly they require only taping to the neighboring toe for support. The proximal phalanx of the great toe bears much greater stress, however, and often requires support by a splint or a cast.

Stress Fractures

Remember:

(1) Pain without injury but with prior unusual activity may indicate stress fracture.

(2) Stress fracture can occur in any weight-bearing long bone.

(3) Stress fracture will not show on x-ray films for 2–4 weeks.

Although stress fractures most commonly occur in the second metatarsal shaft, they can occur in any weight-bearing long bone, including the femoral shaft or neck. The patient has no history of injury, but usually has participated in some unusual activity such as a long walk or a stressful athletic event. There is tenderness over the involved part, but x-ray findings are negative. Only after some external callus has formed in 2–4 weeks is the diagnosis assured. Since treatment is applied according to symptoms, the emergency physician needs only to suspect the diagnosis, treat the part to protect weight-bearing, and obtain more x-ray films later to confirm the diagnosis (Fig. 26.25).

Avulsion Fractures

These injuries usually occur in athletic events, often in sports that require sudden stops and starts, such as basketball, sprinting, and hockey. They are basically tendon or muscle "pulls", but instead of the muscle failing, its insertion to bone is pulled away. The diagnosis may be made on x-ray examination by observation that the location of the avulsion is the same as the location of muscle insertion. Common sites are the anterosuperior iliac spine (sartorius muscle), the anteroinferior spine (rectus femoris), the lesser trochanter (psoas), the ischial tuberosity (adductors), and so on. Displacement may look significant on x-ray films, but

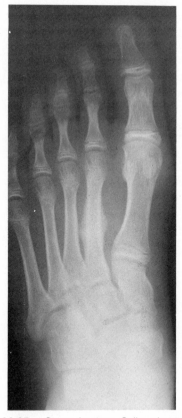

Figure 26.25. Stress fracture. Callus about second metatarsal bone in cross-country runner indicates healing stress or fatigue fracture.

treatment of symptoms is usually all that is needed. Symptoms may be intense, however, and brief hospitalization for control of pain may be required.

PEDIATRIC INJURIES

Remember:

(1) Fractures rarely are treated by open reduction.

(2) Remodeling depends on growth potential, and rotational malalignments remodel poorly.

(3) Supracondylar humeral fractures are dangerous because of the frequency of compartment syndromes.

(4) Lateral condylar humeral fractures in young children may be difficult to recognize because of unossified epiphyses.

(5) Repeated fractures or unusual mechanisms of injury may indicate child abuse.

(6) Anteroposterior subluxations of up to 4–5 mm in the midcervical spine in young children

may occur normally or with upper respiratory tract infections.

Fractures in children almost always are treated conservatively. Depending on the child's age and potential for growth, a considerable degree of malalignment is remodeled within the first year after fracture. Angular deformities are remodeled better if they occur near a joint. Rotational deformities are remodeled poorly. Thus, in many fractures, less satisfactory reductions are accepted than would be the case in adults. Because the child's periosteum is thicker and more active, and because of the child's growth potential, healing times are usually much shorter than in adults. However, for the same reasons, the extra blood flow to the fractured extremity that is needed to heal the fracture may cause general overgrowth of the bone for 1 year afterward. In the lower extremities, this may cause a significant discrepancy of leg lengths.

Green-stick fractures commonly occur in children. These fractures splinter rather than break cleanly, and they may angulate even though close contact of the fragments is maintained by the thick periosteal tube. The least significant of these fractures is the torus or "buckle" fracture, most commonly seen in the radius. There is no angular deformity or displacement, and x-ray films will show only a small cortical buckling on one side of the bone. The injury, which often is unrecognized, is treated according to symptoms. If angular deformity occurs in more extensive green-stick fractures, and if correction is carried out, it is desirable to break the opposite cortex during reduction to prevent the angular deformity from recurring. X-ray films should be repeated over the next 4 weeks to evaluate maintenance of the reduction.

In growing children, the epiphyseal plate is often the point of least resistance to the force of trauma, and it may "slip" with or without some attached epiphyseal or metaphyseal bone. These injuries are classified by Salter (Fig. 26.26). They commonly occur at the wrist, shoulder, and ankle. Grade 1 injuries of the distal femur easily may be mistaken for knee ligament injuries in young football players. Acute epiphyseal slips usually are reduced easily by closed methods. Since the injury is essentially through soft tissue (the epiphyseal plate), healing times are even less than for fractures, and reduction is difficult if it is delayed for even a few days. Later growth disturbance because of arrest of the injured epiphyseal plate is uncommon in grades 1, 2, and 3 injuries. It can occur, however, particularly in grades 4 and 5 injuries, and parents should be advised of this at the time

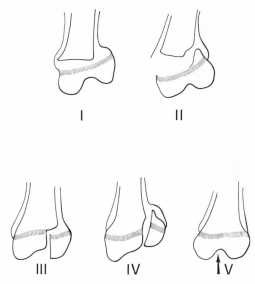

Figure 26.26. Salter classification of epiphyseal plate injuries. I, Injury includes epiphyseal plate only. II, Injury includes epiphyseal plate and metaphysis. III, Injury includes epiphyseal plate and epiphysis. IV, Injury includes epiphyseal plate, epiphysis, and metaphysis. V, Compression injury to epiphyseal plate only. (Since there is no displacement, x-ray findings are negative.)

of injury. All patients with epiphyseal plate injuries should have x-ray films 1 year later to evaluate the condition of growth.

Two fractures about the elbow should be mentioned specifically. Fractures through the lateral epicondyle of the humerus almost always extend through the capitellum, which in younger children remains largely uncalcified and therefore invisible on x-ray films. The pull of the extensor muscles can rotate this large intra-articular fragment as much as 180 degrees *without* showing wide displacement of the ossification center of the capitellum. For this reason, it is imperative that if this injury is suspected, *both* elbows be carefully x-rayed in the same projection, followed by comparison of the relative position of the capitellar ossification centers on both sides. If there is any difference in their position, this fracture is likely. Open reduction is usually necessary. If significant displacement is not recognized, permanent and irreparable damage to the elbow will occur.

Supracondylar fractures of the humerus commonly occur in falls on the outstretched arm. Whereas these may be undisplaced and may heal in 3–6 weeks with splinting only, wide displacement may be present in anteroposterior, mediolateral, and rotational planes. Closed reduction may be unstable, and often the fracture is treated by traction or pinning. If rotational reduction is not well achieved, unsightly varus deformity with decreased carrying angle will occur. Proper treatment requires meticulous and constant orthopaedic judgment and care. This fracture may damage the brachial artery or cause significant swelling and ischemia within the deep volar compartment of the forearm, leading to Volkmann's contracture if unrecognized. This compartment syndrome is the most common encountered in childhood fractures and its onset can be insidious. The earliest sign of Volkmann's contracture is increasing volar forearm pain on passive finger extension, rather than the absence of radial pulse, blueness of fingers, or motor loss. All patients with displaced supracondylar humeral fractures must be admitted to the hospital, and most patients with undisplaced or minimally displaced fractures should also be admitted for observation.

Cervical spine injuries can occur in children, but it should be remembered that, in the young child, inflammatory conditions in the throat or even normal anatomy will allow up to 4–5 mm of forward subluxation of one cervical vertebra on another, particularly in the midcervical spine. If a child is seen after injury with a fixed rotatory deformity of the head, the examiner should remember that rotatory subluxation of the 1st cervical vertebra on the 2nd can occur and that the deformity may not be due to muscular spasm only.

Avulsion fractures can occur in teenagers as in young adults, and are treated in a similar manner (see page 589). Some avulsion fractures, however, include part of an adjacent epiphysis, as in the case of avulsion of the tibial tubercle. If displaced, these fractures may require open reduction and fixation.

Fractures of the femoral neck either through bone or epiphyseal plate do occur in children, and nearly always require open or closed reduction and internal fixation. A good result is even less likely than in the elderly because of the high incidence of avascular necrosis of the femoral head.

Fractures that seem to have an unusual mechanism of injury should alert the examiner to the possibility of child abuse, particularly when evidence of a prior fracture is apparent from history or x-ray findings. The examiner and other members of the emergency staff such as pediatricians and social service personnel should thoroughly investigate the possibility of child abuse if it is suspected, using as much tact and gentleness as possible.

OTHER CONDITIONS OF SOFT TISSUES AND JOINTS

Bursitis and Tendonitis

Severe discomfort can occur within a few hours of onset of bursitis or tendonitis. Areas commonly affected include the shoulder, elbow, hip, and knee. If the shoulder is involved, glenohumeral motion may be limited or nonexistent because of pain. Gentle palpation may elicit point tenderness over the supraspinatus tendon, subacromial bursa, or bicipital groove. At the elbow, the olecranon bursa or the lateral epicondyle may be involved, inflammation of the latter being known as "tennis elbow." Inflammation of the bursa over the greater trochanter of the hip may be painful enough to limit or prevent walking. Four bursae of the knee are affected similarly: the prepatellar, infrapatellar, Voshell's, and anserine. Voshell's bursa lies between the superficial and deep layers of the medial collateral ligament at the joint line, and the anserine bursa lies beneath the tendons of the sartorius and gracilis muscles near their insertion to the tibia. With the exception that calcification may be present in the supraspinatus tendon, subacromial bursa, or Voshell's bursa, x-ray findings are usually normal.

Treatment consists of anti-inflammatory medications given orally, locally by injection, or in combination. The most effective drug administered orally is phenylbutazone, 100 mg three or four times a day for 5–7 days. Phenylbutazone should be taken with meals or with an antacid to help prevent gastric irritation, and is contraindicated in patients with active ulcer disease. Temporary relief can be gained by local infiltration of the painful area with a mixture of an anesthetic and a corticosteroid preparation; the corticosteroid usually quiets the inflammation within 1 or 2 days. Narcotic analgesics often are necessary also.

In olecranon and prepatellar bursitis, the physician must determine whether the inflammation is sterile or septic. Fluid is aspirated from the bursa for a Gram stain and culture; if infection is present, hospitalization for surgical drainage and antibiotic therapy is necessary.

Joint Pain

The sudden onset of pain in a joint may arise from such conditions as internal derangement (loose body or torn meniscus), infection, gout, or pseudogout (chondrocalcinosis). The physician examines the joint for erythema, tenderness, and effusion, and tests it for range of motion. Some infections, such as those caused by the gonococcus, may affect more than one joint. Fluid should be aspirated under sterile conditions (see pages 955 to 958) and the following laboratory procedures performed: white blood cells count and differential, glucose determination (with blood glucose measured at the same time), mucin test, Gram stain, culture in aerobic and anerobic media, and examination for crystals. Under polarized light, urate crystals have strongly negative birefringence, but calcium pyrophosphate crystals have weakly positive birefringence; the former are diagnostic of gout, the latter of pseudogout. Anteroposterior and lateral x-ray films of the joint are examined for a loose body. Calcification of menisci or articular cartilage suggests pseudogout.

Infectious arthritis is treated by drainage of the joint and administration of antibiotics. Gout responds well to colchicine, indomethacin, or phenylbutazone. Pseudogout is best treated with phenylbutazone.

Ruptured Tendons

The shoulder, knee, and leg are the most common sites of ruptured tendons; rupture often occurs during strenuous activity. At the shoulder, inability of the patient to abduct the glenohumeral joint may signal rupture of the rotator cuff. Unusual fullness of the biceps muscle when it is tensed suggests rupture of the tendinous attachment of the long head of the biceps. At the knee,

rupture of the quadriceps or patellar tendon results in inability to extend the knee actively, and a defect above or below the patella usually can be palpated. In the leg, a sudden push-off can rupture a tendon; the patient usually reports a sharp snap or a sensation like being hit in the back of the calf with a rock. In diagnosing this injury, the physician should differentiate between three conditions: (1) rupture of the plantaris tendon, which causes tenderness and swelling, followed by ecchymosis primarily in the upper part of the calf; (2) partial tear of the musculotendinous junction of the gastrocnemius muscle, termed "tennis leg", which is diagnosed by eliciting point tenderness of the medial calf at the inferior edge of the muscle belly; and (3) rupture of the Achilles tendon, which is indicated by weakness of plantar flexion, a palpable gap just above the os calcis, and a positive squeeze test. For the squeeze test the patient kneels with the feet hanging free, the calf musculature is squeezed, and plantar flexion results if the Achilles tendon is intact; there will be no motion of the ankle if it is ruptured (Fig. 26.27). X-ray findings are usually normal in tendon injuries.

Surgical repair usually is indicated for complete ruptures of the rotator cuff in the shoulder and the quadriceps and patellar tendon at the knee. Ruptures of the biceps tendon at the shoulder usually are treated according to symptoms. Achilles tendon ruptures may be treated by open repair or cast immobilization with the foot in the equinus position for 8 weeks.

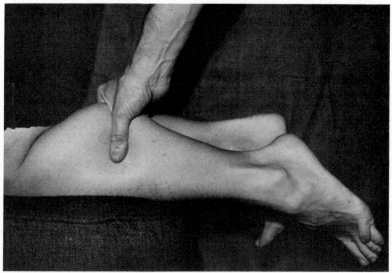

Figure 26.27.   Squeeze test for Achilles tendon injury. If tendon is ruptured, plantar flexion will *not* occur; this tendon is intact.

Suggested Readings

Blount WP: *Fractures in Children.* Baltimore, Williams & Wilkins, 1954

Cave EF, Burke JF, Boyd RJ (Eds): *Trauma Management.* Chicago, Year Book, 1974.

Charnley J: *The Closed Treatment of Common Fractures.* ed 3. Baltimore, Williams & Wilkins, 1961

Crenshaw AH (Ed): *Campbell's Operative Orthopaedics.* ed 5. St. Louis, C.V. Mosby, 1971

De Palma A: *The Management of Fractures and Dislocations: An Atlas.* Philadelphia, W.B. Saunders, 1970

Emergency Care and Transportation of the Sick and Injured. Committee on Allied Health, American Academy of Orthopaedic Surgeons, Chicago, 1977

Harris JH, Jr, Harris WH: *The Radiology of Emergency Medicine.* Baltimore, Williams & Wilkins, 1975

Heppenstall C (Ed): *Fracture Treatment and Healing.* Philadelphia, W.B. Saunders, 1980

Rang M: *Children's Fractures.* Philadelphia, J.B. Lippincott, 1974

Rockwood CA, Jr, Green DP (Eds): *Fractures.* Philadelphia, J.B. Lippincott, 1975

Watson-Jones R: *Fractures and Joint Injuries.* ed 4. Baltimore, Williams & Wilkins, 1952 (Vol 1), 1955 (Vol 2)

Whitesides TE, Jr, Haney TC, Morimoto K, et al: Tissue pressure measurements as a determinant for the need of fasciotomy. *Clin Orthop 113:*43–51, 1975

CHAPTER 27

Neurosurgical Emergencies

EDWARD P. BAKER, Jr., M.D.
JAMES G. WEPSIC, M.D.

Most neurosurgical emergencies that confront the emergency physician involve trauma to the brain, spinal cord, or peripheral nerves. These injuries are common—approximately 70% of all serious accidents involve injury to the central nervous system and about the same percentage of all trauma fatalities result from injury to the brain or spinal cord. There are, however, numerous other catastrophic disorders of the brain that are acute emergencies and that require early involvement of the neurosurgeon, including occlusive carotid artery disease, acute subarachnoid hemorrhage from aneurysm or vascular malformation, spontaneous intracerebral hemorrhage, brain tumor, brain abscess, subdural or epidural empyema, and acute hydrocephalus. The initial management of these conditions is discussed in Chapter 15, whereas this chapter is mainly concerned with neurosurgical emergencies of traumatic origin.

HEAD INJURIES

Transportation, Evaluation, and Initial Treatment

The first priority in treating a patient with a head injury is the maintenance of a satisfactory airway during every phase of treatment. Since the comatose patient is likely to vomit and aspirate, particularly if he has been drinking alcoholic beverages, placing him on his side will allow drainage of oral contents by gravity. This is the best position for transportation if the patient's head and neck can be secured appropriately. Properly equipped ambulances have facilities for strapping the patient in this position to a firm board, and contain suction devices to maintain an oral airway as well as equipment to deliver oxygen. Insertion of a nasotracheal or endotracheal tube to guarantee a patent airway and to prevent aspiration may be lifesaving if the patient must be transported a considerable distance. Extremes of flexion and extension of the neck during intubation must be avoided.

Hypoxia and hypercapnia greatly exacerbate the brain swelling commonly seen with major intracranial trauma, and correction of these abnormalities takes precedence over all other considerations. Hypotension, if present, is likely to be due to extensive blood loss, and patients in shock are likely to have surgical problems involving other areas in addition to head injuries. In children, however, this rule may not apply, since significant blood loss with respect to blood volume can occur with serious head injuries and scalp lacerations. Hypotension with warm extremities because of a sympathectomy effect may be the first sign of a significant spinal cord injury in the comatose patient in whom neurologic evaluation of motor strength and sensation is limited.

The immediate concern of surgical treatment is to preserve life, and in these patients, many of whom have sustained injury to many body systems, the diagnosis and treatment of those injuries not posing an immediate threat to survival should be deferred until the neurologic status has been clarified and the necessary therapeutic measures instituted. Narcotics and sedatives should not be given to the patient with a head injury until the diagnosis is clear, because they may modify the neurologic findings and because they usually are unnecessary.

All too often, an accurate history concerning the mechanism of injury, the patient's condition at the scene, his previous neurologic and medical status, handedness, allergies, medications, and habits of drug and alcohol use cannot be obtained from the victim and should be sought from rescue workers, friends, and relatives. Appropriate laboratory examinations to determine the presence and amount of alcohol and illicit drugs in the blood are in order if there is any possibility that these substances may be contributing to the patient's condition.

Experience in this country and in wartime has demonstrated that the overall mortality and morbidity from serious head injuries is substantially lowered when the patient is transported directly to a complete facility that will provide the appropriate diagnostic studies and definitive treatment. If the receiving hospital lacks an experienced neurosurgical trauma team, operative and postoperative facilities, and the capability of computed tomography (CT) scanning and angiography, it is best to consider immediate transfer to a neurosurgical trauma center. Patients to be transported should be intubated, and hypoxia, hypercapnia, and hypotension should be corrected. A loading dose of corticosteroids may be administered.

The initial neurologic examination should be recorded carefully, since it represents the baseline from which subsequent departures will be measured. The single most important factor in determining the diagnosis and prognosis at any stage of the illness is the patient's level of consciousness, especially when compared with a previously established level of function. Orientation and ability to speak are assessed easily in awake patients, who should also be asked about headache, vision, hearing, and pain in the neck, back, or elsewhere. In patients not responding to voice, the response to pain is noted. Inspection of the scalp, nares, mouth, and external auditory canals for local signs of trauma yields valuable clues regarding the site and nature of the injury, and may reveal foreign bodies, depressed fractures, cerebrospinal fluid (CSF) leaks, and blood within the middle ear.

Motor function is evaluated by observation of the posture and tone of the extremities and by appraisal of movement, either voluntary or spontaneous, or in response to noxious or painful stimulation in comatose patients. Decerebrate posturing may be due to physiologic or anatomic transection of the midbrain, or it may be the result of direct primary midbrain contusion or secondary to midbrain compression by an expanding mass; regardless of the cause, the prognosis is grave. Persons in a decerebrate attitude exhibit rigid extension of the neck and the extremities on one or both sides. The ankles are plantar flexed, the wrists pronated with thumbs clenched in the palms. Less commonly seen, decorticate posturing also is caused by brainstem injury and is similar except that the arms are flexed at the elbows, the dystonic thumb-in-palm held closely against the chest.

The size of the pupils and their reaction to light should be noted and charted periodically; a dilated, fixed pupil in a comatose patient indicates transtentorial herniation until proved otherwise, and usually is due to an expanding hematoma. Bilateral fixed dilated pupils occur with rostral midbrain injuries and in the terminal phase of tentorial herniation, whereas pinpoint unreactive pupils indicate a lesion of the pontomedullary junction. The roving side-to-side eye movements frequently seen in unconscious patients are nonspecific, but their presence indicates that the extensive brainstem pathways for extraocular movements are intact. Eye movement on head turning (the so-called doll's eye movements tested for only after inspection of cervical spine films) and nystagmus after cold-water irrigation of the tympanic membrane are normal responses and have the same significance; conversely, the absence of these reflexes implies brainstem injury. Forced conjugate deviation of the eyes indicates damage to either the ipsilateral frontal eye field or the contralateral portion of the medulla.

Babinski's sign may be present; if it is bilateral, it is not particularly informative, but if it is unilateral, it may indicate the side of the lesion. Alterations in the vital signs—slowing of the pulse rate, widening of the pulse pressure with increasing systolic and decreasing diastolic pressures, and slow, irregular respirations—constitute the classic Cushing's triad. They occur late in the course of patients with increasing intracranial pressure, and if treatment is delayed until these alterations develop, the outcome is almost always fatal.

Diagnostic Studies

Plain x-ray films of the skull demonstrate most linear and depressed fractures of the convexities, foreign bodies, and occasionally, pre-existent pathologic lesions. Depressed fractures often are better demonstrated by oblique views taken with the injured portion of the skull positioned tangentially to the x-ray beam. The pineal gland, calcified in about 55% of patients more than 20 years of age serves as a valuable midline indicator, and its position should be carefully measured. Before victims of high-velocity trauma are moved, lateral cervical spine films (as a minimum) should be obtained, including the 6th and 7th cervical vertebrae; these films should be examined to determine whether an unsuspected fracture is present.

Since the introduction of CT scanning by Hounsfield in 1973, the widespread availability of this technique has revolutionized the diagnosis of craniocerebral trauma. A good CT scan clearly will demonstrate hematomas anywhere within the cranial contents, foreign bodies, the presence of edema, the size, position, and configuration of the ventricular system, displacements of the midline, air-fluid levels within the paranasal sinuses, and many fractures of the skull and facial bones not apparent on conventional radiographs. It is the study of choice for any patient with a serious head injury, and is so superior to any other method of diagnosis that patients with these injuries should not be taken to hospitals not having immediate access to a scanner unless there are no alternatives. Examination takes only a few minutes and is without risk, if care is taken to maintain the airway of comatose patients during positioning and scanning. It is expensive, however, and patients with *minor asymptomatic head injuries* not accompanied by abnormal neurological signs *do not require CT scans.*

Before CT scanning was available, cerebral angiography by either direct carotid puncture or retrograde femoral catheterization was the mainstay of diagnosis. Neurosurgical trauma centers maintain this capability for use in special cases and during periods that the scanner is "down." Angiography reliably demonstrates significant extracerebral hematomas and most intracerebral clots (the latter less accurately than does CT scanning). The technique is relatively time-consuming, however, and not without risk.

Lumbar puncture is not a useful technique in the acute setting because the information derived seldom influences treatment and because the risk of precipitating fatal transtentorial herniation or a foramen magnum pressure cone by disturbance of intracranial dynamics is substantial. Electroencephalography, ultrasound, and radioisotope scanning do not usually provide definitive information in acute trauma victims, although these studies may be extremely useful during later phases of management.

Just as CT scanning has relegated cerebral angiography to a position approaching obsolescence, the new technique of nuclear magnetic resonance may someday be even better, and may reshape completely the diagnostic approach to patients with head trauma.

SCALP AND SKULL INJURIES

Scalp Lacerations

Because of its luxuriant blood supply, the scalp shares with the face the distinction of being the most rapidly healing, infection-resistant tissue in the human body. This vascularity can be a liability, however, in that extensive scalp lacerations can result in major shock-producing blood loss. Bleeding is controlled easily by digital pressure or by application of fine hemostats to the arterial bleeders with eversion of the galea aponeurotica while the initial neurologic and general medical appraisal proceeds. Repair of lacerations should await examination of skull x-ray films to determine whether a more serious injury requiring operation is present.

If the injury is limited to the scalp, the surrounding hair should be shaved, the skin "prepped," and the scalp about the wound infiltrated with lidocaine hydrochloride with epinephrine injected through healthy scalp rather than through the edges of the wound. Satisfactory anesthesia can be achieved by field block if the physician is familiar with the innervation of the scalp. The area then is prepped again, drapes are applied, and the wound is irrigated with saline solution to remove hairs and other foreign material such as road dirt or gravel. If the laceration is full thickness, the underlying skull should be inspected visually and digitally for fracture. Any fracture is, by definition, compound, and should be repaired in the operating room. If no fracture is found, contused devitalized skin, galea, and periosteum are trimmed to viable tissue and the wound is closed without drainage. Regardless of the method chosen, the integrity of closure rests on the strength of the galea. These wounds can be closed with either a layer of absorbable sutures in the galea plus nylon or polyester sutures in the skin or by full-thickness sutures of wire, nylon, or polyester, taking care to include the galea.

Lacerations involving the loss of small areas of scalp often can be closed as described above if tension-free apposition of the wound edges can be obtained by undermining the surrounding scalp in the subgaleal plane. Larger areas of scalp loss require advancement or rotational scalp flaps, and plastic surgical assistance should be sought.

In infants, cephalhematoma often occurs as a consequence of birth trauma or after minor injury. Usually subgaleal, the swelling may dissect over wide areas of skull; if it is subperiosteal, expansion of the clot is limited by the joints of the skull, and the configuration of the mass conforms with the anatomy of the underlying bone. In these small patients, the mass may become alarmingly large, but the temptation to aspirate these clots should be resisted since they eventually undergo spontaneous resorption. Occasionally, a cephalhematoma will become calcified, but the resultant cosmetic defect is rectified later by natural remodeling.

Linear Skull Fractures

The finding of a linear skull fracture on x-ray examination serves as an indicator of the force and locus of the blow to the head, and should alert the physician to the possibility of a serious underlying brain lesion. Many simple linear fractures are unaccompanied by structural brain damage, but they may occur with any combination or degree of intrinsic brain injury or intracranial hematoma. Conversely, some patients with devastating brain injuries have no fracture. Most convexity fractures are diagnosed easily on plain x-ray films, but fractures of the base of the skull extending into the paranasal sinuses or orbits of the middle ear are usually demonstrated only by special views or on a CT scan. Some basal fractures are indicated by the clinical signs of blood behind the tympanic membrane (fracture of the petrous pyramid) or CSF leakage (fracture into paranasal sinus or middle ear); some are indicated by associated x-ray findings such as intracranial air or opacification or air-fluid levels within the sinuses.

The fracture itself requires no treatment. Most acute epidural hematomas and almost all posterior fossa hematomas, however, occur with fractures crossing the vascular grooves of the middle meningeal vessels or extending into the foramen magnum, respectively. In addition, some of the complications of linear skull fractures discussed later are delayed in appearance or in recognition. For these reasons, in-hospital observation for at least 24 hours is advisable.

Depressed Skull Fractures

For depression to occur, a greater force or a more sharply focused blow is required than that ordinarily resulting in linear fracture; the bone is comminuted and splits in the plane of the middle table as it is driven inward. The brain may escape injury with minor degrees of depression, but dural and cortical laceration-contusion is common and may give rise to subdural or intracerebral hemorrhage in about 30% of cases. The extent and location of the focal brain wound and the presence of associated hematoma determine the nature of the resultant neurologic deficit. These fractures are diagnosed on plain x-ray films (Fig. 27.1), often with supplementary tangential views, by noting the deformity of the calvarium or the increased density in regions of bone fragment overlap; the degree of depression and comminution usually is underestimated by this method. CT scans almost always reveal these fractures, and they often are detected by visual or digital examination of scalp lacerations.

Surgical elevation is indicated for fractures depressed by more than the thickness of the skull, particularly if they lie adjacent to the motor strip or speech cortex. Small depressions over the cerebellum do not require repair, and those over dural

venous sinuses are best left undisturbed unless sinus obstruction or hemorrhage is indicated. Compound depressed skull fractures should be repaired as early as possible to lessen the risk of wound infection leading to meningitis or brain abscess. The infection rate in promptly treated cases should be well under 5%, with a concomitant decrease in the incidence of post-traumatic epilepsy.

The surgical approach to these lesions is through a scalp flap placed about the circumference of the depressed area. These fractures usually are impacted tightly and a burr hole at the perimeter usually is required to gain access to the epidural space. Sometimes the depressed fragments can be levered gently into place with a periosteal elevator; more often, portions of the depression must be removed with a ronguer before this can be done. If dura and cortex are lacerated, they are suitably debrided and hemostasis is obtained before dural closure. Underlying cortical markings are usually visible through intact dura, but if they are not seen unmistakably, the dura should be opened to exclude the presence of subdural hematoma. Larger bone fragments can be wired into place, and residual gaps in the skull can be filled with bits of bone laid in as a mosaic graft; they will usually incorporate well if postoperative protection is provided, and thus eliminate the need for cranioplasty.

Compound depressed fractures are treated in essentially the same manner with the addition of careful debridement of the scalp wound. They are approached through the laceration, which may be extended for adequate exposure. Experience has shown that bone fragments can be replaced safely in wounds less than 24 hours old that are not grossly contaminated if meticulous attention is paid to the other surgical principles of wound care. This tactic is especially useful in treating frontal fractures, where secondary cranioplasty may not yield a satisfactory cosmetic result.

Depressed fractures in infants, often called ping-pong fractures, rarely undergo spontaneous resolution and usually require elevation. Unlike adults, the flexible bone of infants usually can be reduced by a periosteal elevator placed through an adjacent burr hole that is then filled with bone dust.

Complications of Skull Fractures

Carotid-Cavernous Fistula

Basal fractures of the sphenoid bone and missile injuries may cause carotid-cavernous fistulas, which result from laceration of the internal carotid artery as it courses within the cavernous sinus. The syndrome also is produced by spontaneous rupture of an intracavernous carotid artery aneurysm.

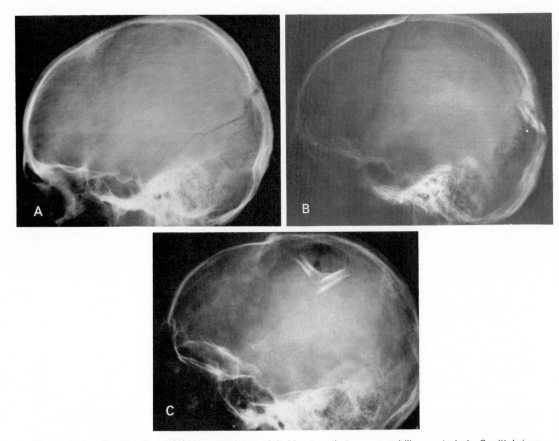

Figure 27.1. Skull fractures. **(A)** Linear parietooccipital fracture that crosses midline posteriorly. Sagittal sinus laceration may occur with this fracture. **(B)** Depressed occipital fracture with associated sinus laceration. **(C)** Depressed parietal fracture with cerebral laceration by bony fragments.

Blood perfuses the cavernous sinus under arterial pressure, and causes extreme dilation of tributary veins and retrograde flow into the orbits; intracranial rupture seldom occurs. Massive conjunctival injection, chemosis, scleral hemorrhage, and bilateral pulsating exophthalmos follow. A bruit may be audible over the orbits, temple, or forehead. Continued progression results in extraocular palsies and loss of vision.

Obliteration of the fistula is accomplished by occlusion of the intracavernous carotid artery with an intra-arterial balloon passed under fluoroscopic control, or by muscle embolization combined with cervical and intracranial carotid ligation.

Cranial Nerve Injury

Injury to a cranial nerve usually results from fracture through the foramen of exit at the base of the skull. The olfactory nerve is the most commonly affected, and may be damaged either by cribriform plate fracture or by the shearing action of the brain at the moment of a blow to the occiput, which can avulse the olfactory filaments as they pass through the cribriform plate. The resultant anosmia is permanent, but rather than complaining of loss of smell, patients tend to complain more of distortion or loss of taste, since appreciation of flavor is mediated largely by olfactory perception. True ageusia (loss of taste perception) does not occur with trauma.

Injury to the optic nerve from fracture through the optic foramen is rare; since this nerve develops embryologically as a fiber tract of the brain, regeneration does not occur and surgical decompression of the optic foramen has been unsuccessful in restoring lost vision.

Partial or complete oculomotor palsy may be an element of transtentorial herniation; the nerve is compressed at the tentorial notch by the medial temporal lobe displaced by an expanding intracranial mass. These patients are comatose, and other grievous signs of hemispheral and brainstem dysfunction are present. Oculomotor nerve palsy in a conscious patient with signs of trauma to the face or front of the head is likely to be due to injury within the orbit. Trochlear and abducens nerves also may be injured in the orbit or from fracture through the superior orbital fissure. Occasionally, isolated abducens nerve palsy occurs as a false lateralizing sign with diffuse brain injury of any degree or with raised intracranial pressure.

Intracranial injury to the trigeminal nerve is uncommon, but sensory loss due to division of its peripheral branches is frequent with facial lacerations and fractures; rarely, painful facial dysesthesias are a late sequela. Facial lacerations should be closed carefully to avoid further injury to the nerve or its inclusion in the suture. The prognosis for regeneration of the nerve with restoration of sensation is excellent.

Fractures through the petrous portion of the temporal bone may injure the facial nerve or the auditory or vestibular branches (or both) of the acoustic nerve. Peripheral facial palsies are characterized by paralysis of the ipsilateral side of the face, including the forehead, whereas central facial palsies of cortical origin spare the forehead because of the bilateral innervation of this muscle. Facial palsies may be immediate or may occur days after injury—the so-called tardy facial palsy. Neither type requires operation, but the chances of recovery are much better with the delayed type. Function cannot be recovered after acoustic nerve injury, but patients with post-traumatic hearing loss should undergo otologic evaluation, lest potentially treatable causes of conduction deafness such as ossicular disruption be overlooked.

Injuries to the lower cranial nerves are usually the result of penetrating wounds outside the skull.

CSF Rhinorrhea and Otorrhea

About 5% of patients have CSF rhinorrhea or otorrhea after closed head injury. CSF leakage requires a pathway of communication from the subarachnoid space into the sinuses, nasopharynx, or middle ear through a dural tear, fractured bone, and lacerated mucosa. Fractures into the ethmoid sinus through the cribriform plate or into frontal or sphenoid sinuses are the most common avenues of rhinorrhea. CSF in the middle ear will result in otorrhea if the tympanic membrane is ruptured; if not, CSF may flow through the eustachian canal into the nasopharynx and give rise to an interesting variety of rhinorrhea. The fluid is identified as CSF by testing for glucose and chloride content. Saliva and nasal secretions contain negligible amounts of glucose whereas the glucose level in CSF is about two-thirds of that in blood, and the CSF chloride concentration is approximately 120 mEq/liter.

Patients with CSF leakage are treated with bed rest with the head elevated, and are instructed not to blow their nose or attempt to stem the flow of fluid, lest they cause retrograde flow of contaminated debris into the subarachnoid space. Otorrhea usually stops within 1–3 days, and operative treatment seldom is required. In about 85% of patients with rhinorrhea, the leak closes spontaneously, but a small percentage of patients may return months or even years later with delayed meningitis.

The value of prophylactic antibiotics remains unsettled, but since the most common organism resulting in meningitis secondary to rhinorrhea is *Streptococcus pneumoniae*, many surgeons advocate their use in this group of patients and in patients with pre-existent sinusitis or ear infection.

If the fracture is complex, identification of the pathway of the CSF fistula may be difficult and may require CT scanning in both axial and coronal planes, conventional tomography, and various dye or radioisotope studies in conjunction with careful ear-nose-and-throat examination.

Generally accepted indications for surgical repair include persistent rhinorrhea, meningitis, and cerebral herniation into the fracture. Surgical repair is accomplished after brain swelling has subsided and after any overt infection has been eradicated.

Intrinsic Brain Injuries

Cerebral Concussion

The clinical correlates of cerebral concussion include (1) amnesia—retrograde amnesia for events immediately preceding injury, and a usually longer period of anterograde amnesia for happenings after injury, and (2) a period of unconsciousness lasting up to 20 minutes. Longer periods of unconsciousness are likely to be related to at least minor degrees of brain contusion. Young children occasionally manifest generalized seizures or transient cortical blindness after concussion; these are alarming phenomena, but are not necessarily of unfavorable prognostic importance.

These patients should be admitted for overnight observation unless a responsible family member is willing and able to waken the patient hourly and return him to the hospital promptly if deterioration occurs. X-ray films of the skull should be obtained, but CT scans or other diagnostic studies ordinarily are not required.

In uncomplicated cerebral concussion, neurologic deficit is maximal at the time of injury and is followed by rapid and steady improvement. Variations from this course should alert the physician to the possibility of a more serious head injury. Prolonged hospitalization or enforced invalidism is not in the best interest of the patient, and the common post-traumatic sequelae of headache, psychologic dysfunction, and memory disorders seem to be less pronounced in those who resume their normal pursuits as soon as possible.

Cerebral Contusion and Laceration

Mechanical damage to the brain at the moment of impact results from the linear and rotational forces imparted by the blow, which disrupts axons and nerve cell bodies and frequently lacerates the cerebral cortex. Coincident vascular damage may give rise to acute subdural or intracerebral hematoma or traumatic subarachnoid hemorrhage, depending on the size and location of the injured vessel. The area of structural injury may be limited to the cortex and adjacent white matter directly beneath the blow, or in the case of contrecoup contusion, it may be limited to the opposite side of the brain, with the tips and undersurfaces of frontal and temporal lobes the sites of predilection. With larger impact forces, extensive disruption of white matter occurs deep within the cerebral hemispheres and brainstem. The clinical spectrum of patients with brain contusion ranges from those with minor damage and a neurologic syndrome only slightly more severe than cerebral concussion to those having devastating brain destruction with decerebration and irreversible coma. Brain contusions are common in the absence of either fracture or significant hematoma, and are a major cause of death or lasting neurologic disability.

The syndrome of primary brainstem injury deserves special mention because of the frequency with which it is encountered in clinical practice. These patients present with signs of midbrain injury: deep coma with bilaterally dilated fixed pupils and decerebrate rigidity followed shortly by hypothalamic signs of disordered thermoregulation and diabetes insipidus. A reliable history that the midbrain signs were present in the seconds or minutes after injury helps differentiate this entity from the otherwise clinically indistinguishable syndrome of midbrain compression due to tentorial herniation. Survivors of the injury are few and they are likely to be left in a persistent vegetative state. Skull x-ray films, intracranial pressure, and CT scans may all be normal, although sometimes, small midbrain hemorrhagic lesions or associated hemispheral injury are seen on the scan. Brain contusions always cause cerebral edema, and if the volume of damaged brain is large enough, increased intracranial pressure. Unless there is an associated intracranial clot to be evacuated, surgical therapy has little to offer these patients, and treatment is limited to the various medical methods of managing brain edema and increased intracranial pressure.

Traumatic Intracranial Hematomas

Acute Epidural Hematoma

Rapidly evolving and often lethal, acute epidural hematomas are formed by laceration of a dural vessel, which produces a clot between the skull and the dura. Most commonly, hemorrhage originates from a branch of the middle meningeal artery that has been lacerated by a fracture, although bleeding from meningeal veins, dural sinuses, or emissary veins can also produce less rapidly evolving clots. In 90% of adult patients with an epidural hematoma, skull fracture is demonstrated by x-ray examination, at operation, or at autopsy. Only about 50% of children, however, have skull fractures associated with this lesion. When a linear fracture crosses the grooves of the meningeal vessels or dural sinuses, the physician should suspect such a clot.

The classic history is that of an injury resulting in brief loss of consciousness from which the patient wakens and is comparatively well—the so-called lucid interval—followed in a few hours by expansion of the clot, compression of the brain surface, cerebral edema, and an increase in the overall intracranial pressure. The increased pressure results in headache, vomiting, weakness of the contralateral limbs, and deterioration of the patient's state of consciousness. With further enlargement of the clot, transtentorial herniation occurs. The temporal lobe is displaced inward until its most medial portion, the uncus, is forced down over the free edge of the tentorium, compressing the brainstem and the adjacent ipsilateral oculomotor nerve (Fig. 27.2). Unless the brainstem compression is relieved quickly, death results. As the medial portion of the temporal lobe herniates, it displaces the oculomotor nerve, first paralyzing the pupilloconstrictor fibers; as a result, the ipsilateral pupil becomes widely dilated and unreactive to light. Further displacement of the temporal lobe compromises the blood supply to the midbrain, and the midbrain itself is compressed with displacement against the contralateral tentorial edge and, finally, compression of the opposite oculomotor nerve. As these events occur, the hemiparesis becomes a hemiplegia, coma deepens, decerebrate rigidity develops, the opposite pupil becomes dilated and fixed to light, midbrain hem-

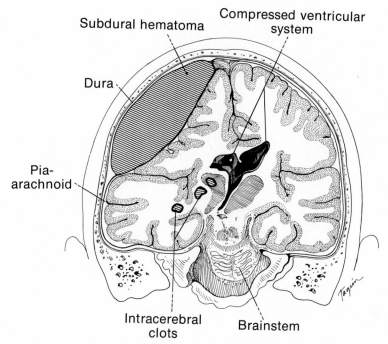

Figure 27.2.   Temporal lobe hematoma displacing brainstem against edge of tentorium and compressing 3rd nerve.

orrhages develop, the centers for cardiorespiratory regulation cease functioning, and death follows. Although this pattern is classic and occurs in most patients with a temporal extracerebral hematoma, one phase in the evolution of the midbrain compression may occur more quickly than another, and progressive neurologic worsening may be subtle. Careful observation of the patient's level of consciousness and neurologic status is imperative if an epidural hemorrhage is considered.

Early removal of the hematoma before transtentorial herniation is essential for a favorable outcome. In one large series, 77% of patients died who were decerebrate before operation, whereas only 1 patient died of 74 who were conscious before operation.

If time permits, a CT scan should be obtained since it is confirmatory (Fig. 27.3A), but patients arriving in the emergency ward with clear-cut signs of an evolving epidural hematoma or in whom the signs develop after arrival should be intubated, crossmatched for blood, and taken directly to the operating room for exploratory burr holes without further diagnostic studies. Although there are more than 2000 board-certified neurosurgeons in the United States, the urgency of these lesions occasionally requires the general surgeon to intervene while awaiting neurosurgical assistance; it therefore behooves surgeons in training to

prepare themselves for this contingency. Emergency physicians should not sit by while the deadly events of transtentorial herniation unfold to a fatal conclusion, and if a neurosurgeon is not at hand, they must proceed with operation (Fig. 27.4).

Aside from timeliness, the two essential ingredients of a successful procedure are (1) the removal of the clot to relieve brain compression, and (2) securing of the source of bleeding to prevent recurrence. The initial burr hole should be placed over the laceration or fracture. If none is obvious, the burr hole is made over the temporal area on the side of the dilated pupil. A vertical scalp incision is first made 2 cm anterior to the ear and carried down to the zygoma to allow access to the temporal bone. The temporalis fascia and muscle are divided, preferably with a cautery, and the muscle is retracted and stripped from the outer table of the skull. Frequently, a fracture line is noted at this stage. The burr hole is placed with a standard drill and burr, and as the blood clot extrudes, the craniectomy is enlarged with rongeurs. This relieves the pressure and allows further time for more extensive neurosurgical intervention, which may include conversion of the craniectomy to a temporal craniotomy utilizing a standard bone flap.

As the clot is removed, hemostasis is achieved by electrocoagulation or ligation of the main

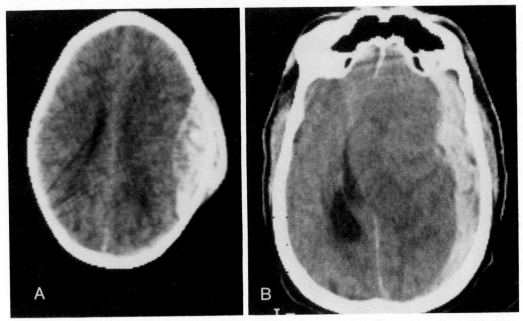

Figure 27.3. **(A)** Acute epidural hematoma in 8-month-old infant who underwent scanning 30 minutes after a fall. Clot is 2 cm thick. Note swelling of overlying scalp. En route to operating room, the child showed early signs of tentorial pressure cone. Immediate evacuation of clot was followed by complete neurologic recovery within a few hours. **(B)** Acute subdural hematoma with compression and displacement of ventricles. Subdural blood is free to spread over the convexity, but extension of epidural clot is restricted by attachments of dura to skull and these hematomas tend to be thick relative to the area of brain covered.

trunks of the middle meningeal vessels as they appear on the dura; occasionally, the middle meningeal artery must be dissected to its origin at the foramen spinosum and ligated there. Any obvious dural bleeding is coagulated and dural tenting sutures are placed between the outer layer of dura and the inner layer of temporalis muscle or pericranium to control dural venous oozing. Once the clot has been removed and extradural hemostasis is absolute, the presence of a coexistent subdural hematoma can be determined by opening the dura and examining the underlying cortical surfaces. There is often little obvious brain damage. If the patient's postoperative progress is not satisfactory, a CT scan is in order to determine whether any other treatable lesion is present.

Acute Subdural Hematoma

Acute subdural hematoma (Fig. 27.3B) is over 30 times more common than epidural hematoma, and is the lesion most frequently associated with death or morbidity in most reported series of head injuries. Usually the result of vehicular accident, assault, or a fall, most of these lesions are accompanied by severe impact-produced intrinsic brain injuries, such as laceration-contusion (often bilateral), intracerebral hemorrhage, and primary brainstem contusion. For years, the reported mortality ranged from 70–90%. In one series, 89% of

patients with decerebrate rigidity died; if dilated fixed pupils were also present, the mortality rose to 95%. Recently, however, Seelig et al. (1981) reported a remarkable reduction in mortality to 30% in patients undergoing operation within 4 hours of injury, as compared with 90% in those operated on after 4 hours. Improved functional recovery also occurred in the first group. These are the best results that have been reported, and they were achieved by effective triage and CT-scan diagnosis, followed by immediate evacuation of the clot and the aggressive use, during every phase of treatment, of all medical measures to control intracranial hypertension.

Surgical removal is accomplished by a rapid subtemporal craniectomy with partial evacuation of the clot to effect at least some degree of decompression, followed by craniotomy sufficient to provide exposure to remove the rest of the clot and to secure the source of the bleeding. Intracerebral hematoma, if present, is removed and obviously devitalized brain tissue debrided. Because of the consistency of rapidly clotted blood, these lesions cannot be adequately treated by multiple burr holes.

Chronic Subdural Hematoma

Often the result of minor trauma that cannot be recalled, this lesion occurs mainly in those with

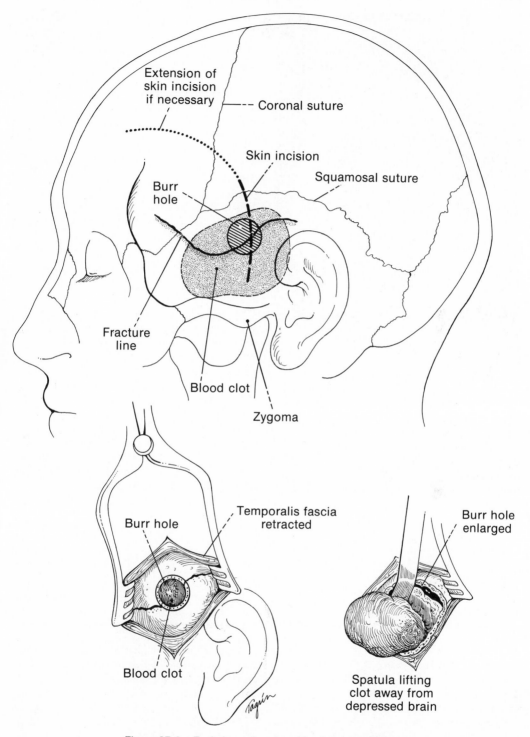

Figure 27.4.   Technique of acute epidural clot evacuation.

some degree of brain atrophy due to either normal aging or the chronic cytotoxic effects of alcohol. Chronic subdural hematoma is also one of the common major complications of long-term anticoagulant therapy (Fig. 27.5) The current mortal-

ity approaches 20%, and reflects the difficulties in diagnosis and treatment of this disorder in an elderly population with major diseases in other body systems.

Bleeding usually originates from a cortical vein

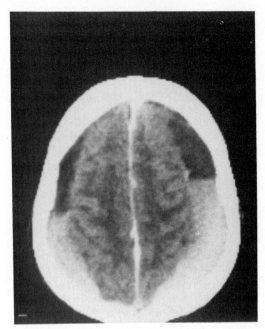

Figure 27.5. Bilateral chronic subdural hematomas in patient receiving anticoagulants. With the patient's head in the usual supine position for scanning, the heavier particulate matter in this liquefied clot has settled posteriorly; the serum component of low attenuation value is layered over the more anterior convexity.

that has been lacerated near its entry into the superior sagittal sinus by shearing movement at the moment of impact. After clotting, the blood becomes sequestered by the formation of subdural membranes; as time passes, the volume of the hematoma increases, probably by the inflow of water to equalize the increasing osmotic pressure created by the breakdown of hemoglobin molecules within the clot. The initial gradual enlargement of the mass is well tolerated, but when compensatory displacement of the brain and ventricular system begins to fail, clinical signs and symptoms appear. The patient may complain of headache, and relatives note changes in mentation accompanied by psychomotor slowing. As brain compression slowly increases, the patient becomes dull and focal neurologic changes appear. Because these presenting complaints are nonspecific, chronic subdural hematomas are often misdiagnosed as stroke, tumor, metabolic derangement, dementia, or even senility, unless a high index of suspicion is maintained in evaluating each of these illnesses.

Shift of the pineal gland on plain skull films is common unless the hematoma is bilateral, as occurs in about 20% of cases. Chronic subdural hematomas are readily diagnosed by CT scanning, and should be surgically evacuated without delay. Completely liquefied hematomas can be evacuated through burr holes, but solid clot requires the wider exposure of a bone flap. The major postoperative problem in these patients with pre-existent loss of brain substance is failure of the brain to re-expand and fill the cavity formerly occupied by the hematoma. Brain expansion is encouraged by the use of subdural drains, generous hydration, and nursing care with the patient in the head-down position. Despite these measures, recurrent subdural collections are common. Recurrence is suggested by the postoperative clinical course, and is confirmed by CT scanning. The collection should be removed either by needle aspiration through the original burr holes or by actually reopening the burr holes in the operating room.

Posterior Fossa Hematoma

Hematomas in the posterior fossa are 20 times less common than supratentorial hematomas; they are more often extradural than subdural, and if extradural, they may extend upward over the occipital lobes. More than 50% of these hematomas occur in children. Most cases result from a direct blow to the occiput, and a fracture extending into the foramen magnum or across the transverse sinus is nearly always present. The hematoma compresses the cerebellum and medulla, and obstructs the outflow of CSF from the 4th ventricle, producing acute hydrocephalus. Besides signs of local trauma, the clinical findings include altered consciousness, severe headache, gaze palsies, and papilledema. These clots were difficult to diagnose before CT scanning; most were located by exploratory burr holes placed for clinical reasons, and it may be that they are much more common than previously thought. Immediate suboccipital craniectomy with removal of the clot is the treatment of choice.

Intracerebral Hemorrhage

Acute intracerebral hematoma frequently occurs as an element of a high-velocity acceleration-deceleration injury in association with acute subdural hematoma and cerebral laceration-contusion. The devastating effects of an expanding clot within the white matter of the cerebral hemisphere are compounded by the compressive effects on adjacent brain tissue, with resultant edema and ischemia, intracranial hypertension, and displacement-compression of brainstem structures. The CT scan (Fig. 27.6) provides accurate localization and permits the surgeon to approach the mass through the most expendable portion of the brain surface.

Delayed intracerebral hematoma can occur days or even weeks after injury, and is being increasingly recognized as a cause of deterioration after initial neurologic stabilization.

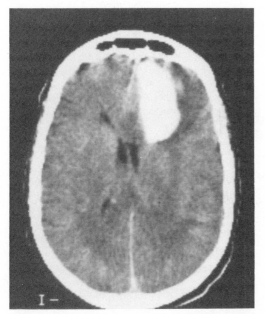

Figure 27.6. Acute intracerebral hematoma. This contrecoup lesion followed a blow to the occiput.

Penetrating Brain Injuries

The extensive experience of military neurosurgeons in Vietnam resulted in reduction in the mortality of missile-produced brain wounds to just under 10%. This figure is not usually matched in civilian practice, where most gunshot wounds are self-inflicted and the weapon is perhaps better aimed. A bullet striking the calvarium shatters the bone locally and usually fragments, driving pieces of bone and metal into the brain as secondary missiles. Sometimes a bullet fragment traverses the brain, but lacks the energy to exit through the opposite side of the skull and ricochets back into the brain, producing even more extensive destruction (Fig. 27.7). To understand the anatomic structures traversed by the missile, the physician must first study the position of the entry and exit wounds and the trajectory of the projectile as seen on radiographs, including stereoscopic views. He or she must then correlate this information with the neurologic findings. CT scanning may provide more precise information regarding the proximity of the track to the ventricular system and major vascular structures, as well as delineate secondary intracerebral hemorrhage.

The principles of treatment are well known from military experience. They consist of early débridement with removal of in-driven bone fragments, hematoma, and devitalized brain tissue, followed by watertight dural closure with pericranial or

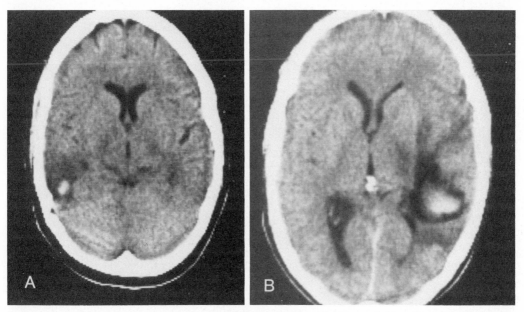

Figure 27.7. **(A)** Hemorrhagic contusion of posterior left temporal lobe seen 8 days after injury. This lesion was not visible on initial scan. **(B)** Right parietal contusion with computer-measured 6-mm shift of midline. Extensive edema of adjacent white matter and deformity of ventricle may be seen.

fascial graft if necessary to lessen the probability of postoperative infection from without and to prevent CSF leakage or local cerebral herniation. The decision to search for an isolated piece of metal outside the main track is difficult, especially if it lies in an important, otherwise uninjured sector of brain, and sometimes these fragments are best left in place.

Medical Adjuncts to Treatment

All mechanisms producing structural brain damage by either compression or contusion result in some degree of cerebral edema. Since the total volume of the intracranial contents is fixed by the skull, small increases in volume produce disproportionately large rises in intracranial pressure. Lesser volumes of brain swelling are initially accommodated by a decrease in volume of the venous side of the cerebrovascular bed and by displacement of CSF from the subarachnoid space and ventricle. Once the limits of these compensatory actions are reached, however, further increments of swelling markedly increase intracranial pressure. Cerebral perfusion pressure (mean arterial pressure − intracranial pressure) then decreases and irreversible cerebral ischemia and cell death follow.

The complex pathophysiologic processes implicated in brain swelling are incompletely understood, but some of the components believed to be important include the following: loss of autoregulation of the cerebral vasculature with consequent vasodilation, passive congestion, and increased cerebral blood volume; loss of water and plasma constituents into the extracellular space through damaged capillaries; and breakdown of the blood-brain barrier and ischemia-induced intracellular edema with swelling of neuron and astrocyte cell bodies.

Since the mortality and morbidity resulting from major head injuries relate directly to the presence, severity, and duration of increased intracranial pressure, medical control of cerebral swelling and intracranial pressure plays a central role throughout the active treatment phase of all patients. Measurement of intracranial pressure by one of the many implantable monitoring devices available permits adjustment of medical therapies to the changing needs of the patient. At the same time, it provides valuable prognostic information and often warns the surgeon of impending deterioration before worsening neurologic signs become apparent.

Controlled Hyperventilation

Normally, cerebral blood flow adjusts automatically in response to arterial P_{CO_2} and, to a lesser degree, P_{O_2} to maintain cerebral perfusion despite variations in systemic blood pressure; the relationship is roughly linear over a wide range of P_{CO_2} values. Hyperventilation reduces the partial pressure of carbon dioxide and therefore the volume of the vascular bed in uninjured portions of the brain that have not lost autoregulation and thus remain responsive to carbon dioxide.

After intubation, hyperventilation with a volume respirator is used to achieve an arterial P_{CO_2} from 26–30 mm Hg and a P_{O_2} of 80 mm Hg or greater. Pancuronium or morphine is given if necessary to control ventilation. The frequent blood-gas determinations needed to monitor this treatment require insertion of an arterial line.

Osmolar Diuretics

Intravenous hyperosmolar agents create an osmotic gradient that draws extracellular water across the semipermeable membrane known as the blood-brain barrier into the bloodstream. Their effect in lowering intracranial pressure is therefore limited to decreasing the extracellular volume of those uninjured areas of the brain that still have an intact blood-brain barrier. Mannitol is the most widely used osmotic diuretic, and is available as a 20% solution; the usual dose for maximal effect is 1–1.5 g/kg given by rapid infusion with an indwelling catheter in place. Reduction in intracranial pressure is usually evident within 30 minutes and the effect may last for 3–6 hours. When mannitol is used in conjunction with intracranial pressure monitoring for prolonged treatment of intracranial hypertension, much smaller doses are given periodically to maintain intracranial pressure below the normal level of 15 mm Hg.

Mannitol-induced hypervolemia may precipitate congestive heart failure in patients with impaired cardiac reserve, and pretreatment with furosemide should be considered in these patients. Derangements of serum osmolarity and electrolyte concentrations are common and appropriate laboratory monitoring is essential.

Corticosteroids

There is no conclusive evidence that corticosteroids reduce traumatic brain edema. However, their unquestioned beneficial effects on the cerebral edema associated with brain tumors, and a strong clinical impression that they have a favorable effect in some trauma victims has led to their widespread use in many trauma centers. The precise mode of action of corticosteroids in the trauma setting is unknown. Adult dosages of the two commonly used agents are as follows: dexamethasone, 20 mg as a loading dose followed by 4–20 mg every 6 hours, and methylprednisolone, 100 mg initially and 40–100 mg at 6-hour intervals. Some physicians advocate much higher doses, but the therapeutic advantages of such "megadose" therapy remain to be demonstrated. Duration of treatment is determined by the clinical response or the course of intracranial pressure monitoring or both.

The major complication of corticosteroid therapy is gastrointestinal bleeding, and patients receiving high doses should have the pH of gastric contents titrated to neutrality with antacids and cimetidine. Electrolyte abnormalities and exacerbation of diabetes are also encountered.

High-Dose Barbiturate Therapy

Despite aggressive treatment with hyperventilation, mannitol, corticosteroids, and fluid restriction, severe uncontrollable intracranial hypertension develops in a substantial percentage of patients, terminating in brain death as intracranial pressure reaches systemic arterial levels and cerebral perfusion pressure decreases to zero. High doses of barbiturates are effective in controlling intracranial pressure in some patients, and good functional recovery from an otherwise untreatable and hopeless situation may follow. Pentobarbital and thiopental are the agents currently used, and their principal mode of action is presumably a direct constrictor effect on cerebral vasculature with reduction of cerebral blood volume. Barbiturate-induced coma requires administration of anesthetic doses of barbiturates for days or weeks, and has potential for serious cardiovascular complications. Continuous monitoring of intracranial pressure, intraarterial pressure, and other parameters of cardiovascular function, and the direction of a surgeon experienced with the technique are prerequisites for its use.

Although the early data appear promising, controlled randomized studies are in progress to determine the usefulness of barbiturate therapy in the overall management of increased intracranial pressure.

Anticonvulsant Medications

Patients with structural brain injury of any degree are potentially likely to have grand mal or partial seizures. Since a major seizure may impair ventilation, exacerbate other injuries (especially spinal and long-bone fractures) and becloud the neurologic findings by introducing confusing postictal phenomena, prophylatic anticonvulsant medication is advisable. Phenytoin is the drug of choice, and is given intravenously as a separate infusion of 0.5–1.0 gm for adults at a rate not to exceed 20 mg/min. Phenobarbital is an equally effective rapid-acting anticonvulsant. Treatment after the initial loading dose is determined by the clinical course and is guided by serum levels of the drug chosen. Patients with simple cerebral concussion do not need anticonvulsants.

Temperature Control

Since elevated body temperature increases the rate of cerebral metabolism and intensifies brain edema, these patients are kept normothermic by the use of acetaminophen administered rectally or hypothermia equipment or both. Traumatic subarachnoid hemorrhage may cause low-grade temperature rises for several days after brain injury, but this is a diagnosis of exclusion, tenable only after other more likely causes of fever such as atelectasis, pneumonia or urinary tract infection have been excluded. Disordered thermoregulation of hypothalamic origin is manifested by high fever unaccompanied by sweating or by subnormal temperature without piloerection or shivering; frequently, there are wide swings between these extremes and diabetes insipidus is usually present.

Fluid Requirements

Overzealous administration of hypotonic intravenous fluids is likely to occur during the early triage phase of patient evaluation. This should be avoided since excess water exacerbates cerebral edema and further increases intracranial pressure. Overhydration is particularly irrational if the physician is attempting to achieve the opposite effect with osmotic diuretics. These patients are best managed with mild dehydration, and 0.45% normal saline in 2.5% dextrose in water infused at 60–75 ml/hr will provide adequate fluid replacement for an adult for many days. Careful measurement of water balance and monitoring of serum electrolyte levels and renal function will detect metabolic abnormalities before they become serious. If prolonged coma is likely, nutritional support through a gastric feeding tube should be started as early as possible.

Traumatic diabetes insipidus results from injury to the hypothalamic-posterior pituitary axis, and is characterized by urine output in excess of 200 ml/hr for several hours with specific gravity less than 1.005. Polyuria may be intermittent and is intially best managed by fluid replacement. If projected urinary output exceeds 10 liters within 24 hr, 3–5 units of pitressin tannate in oil will stop the polyuria, but intravenous fluids must then be reduced sharply to match the reduced output, lest dilutional hypotonicity and iatrogenic water intoxication occur.

Diagnosis of Brain Death

The diagnosis of irreversible coma and brain death can seldom be made in the emergency ward because most criteria for brain death specify a time interval over which the listed neurologic signs must be present. However, careful recording of a detailed neurologic examination of patients with the clinical manifestations of brain death allows a final determination to be made as early as is consistent with the criteria chosen. After final consultation with the family, the patient can then be pronounced dead and the supportive effort discontinued; preferably, permission to remove transplantable organs will have been obtained.

There are many sets of acceptable criteria for brain death, but those formulated by the Ad Hoc Committee of the Harvard Medical School seem to have the most widespread acceptance. These criteria are paraphrased as follows. There is no spontaneous activity, decerebrate or otherwise, and no response to external stimuli, including intense pain. Respiratory effort is absent during a 3-minute trial off the respirator after arterial P_{CO_2} has been normalized and the patient ventilated with room air for 10 minutes. The pupils are dilated and fixed to light; ocular movement in response to head turning and ice-water irrigation of the ears is absent. Corneal and pharyngeal reflexes cannot be elicted, and "as a rule" tendon reflexes are also absent. An isoelectric electroencephalogram is confirmatory evidence of brain death. All findings must be present on repeated examination 24 hours later. Hypothermia (temperature below 90°F [32.2°C]) and central nervous system depressants such as barbiturates must be excluded.

These criteria are under revision, and many believe that neither the presence of preserved deep tendon reflexes (which are segmentally mediated spinal cord reflexes) nor the absence of dilated pupils (as long as the pupils are fixed to light) should prevent a diagnosis of brain death.

SPINAL INJURIES

Transportation and Preliminary Evaluation

Transportation of the patient with a spinal cord injury must be carefully planned and well organized. The patient should not be moved until sufficient trained persons are available to lift him as a unit, maintaining the head, neck, and thorax in the position in which the patient was found. Jostling or other motion of the neck may dislocate the fracture and produce an increase in neurologic deficit. The patient who is to be transported a significant distance should be placed on a firm board or stretcher with pillows or blanket rolls under the normal cervical and lumbar curvatures. If neck injury is suspected, sandbags should be placed against both sides of the head or a Mixter four-poster or Philadelphia collar applied. The patient should be treated with minimal amounts of analgesics, since these may interfere with respiratory function and neurologic evaluation.

A thorough, detailed history of the injury should be obtained, including whether motor movement was immediately impaired. A complete general physical examination should be performed, maintaining the patient in a neutral position with the head and spine aligned.

Respiratory embarrassment often accompanies spinal cord injuries. Lesions from the 5th cervical vertebra to the midthoracic region interfere with intercostal and abdominal breathing. The cell bodies for the phrenic nerves lie at about the level of the fourth cervical vertebra, and cord injury at or above this level interferes with diaphragmatic breathing. Arterial blood gases, tidal volume, and vital capacity should be measured early. If necessary, nasotracheal intubation may be carried out to maintain adequate oxygenation, taking care not to move the neck. If intubation is not possible, tracheostomy may be performed. Adequate spontaneous respiration can often eventually be established once the acute effects of the injury subside. Therefore, early support of ventilation is essential. Hypotension may develop as a result of the functional sympathectomy produced by the spinal cord injury, and may be difficult to diagnose in the patient with multiple lesions. However, the presence of warm extremities and significant neurologic deficit should alert the examiner to the possibility of sympathetic injury, and treatment with vasopressor agents, fluids, and wraps of the extremities should be instituted accordingly. Frequently, head injuries and cervical spine injuries are present together. Examination of the front and the back of the head for evidence of trauma may provide some clue as to the nature of the spinal injury—whether it be extension or flexion.

The motor and sensory systems should be evaluated completely. It is crucial that a sensory examination with charting of findings be carried out as soon as possible after the injury so that documentation of progression or regression of deficit can be established. This is important in deciding on surgical treatment as well as prognosis. The dermatome level of the sensory loss should be estimated (Fig. 27.8). Muscle strength and tone should be evaluated carefully and the deep tendon

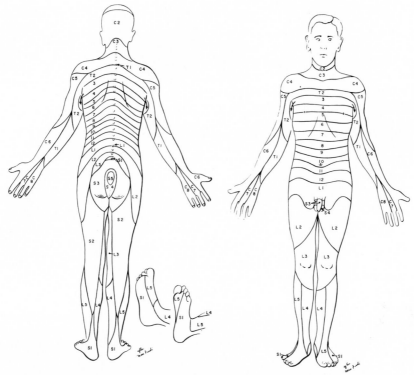

Figure 27.8. Dermatome map of human body. Note position of cervically innervated skin on anterior portion of chest as well as high thoracic innervation of inner aspect of arm. Reproductions of this map should be available in areas caring for patients with spinal cord injuries so that sensory findings can be charted daily. (Reproduced by permission, from Wepsic JG: Injuries to the spinal cord and cauda equina, in Cave EF, Burke JF, Boyd RJ (Eds):*Trauma Management.* Copyright © 1974 by Year Book Medical Publishers, Inc., Chicago.)

reflexes noted. Reference to a motor function and reflex chart may be useful to those who are not routinely involved with the care of neurologic patients (Table 27.1).

Anatomy

In adults, the spinal cord extends from the foramen magnum to the second lumbar vertebra, suspended by the dentate ligaments, nerve roots, and supplying blood vessels within an arachnoid sac containing shock-absorbing CSF (Figs. 27.9 and 27.10). It is covered by tough, fibrous dura that is hydraulically buffered by the surrounding epidural fat and blood vessels, and it is enclosed within the bony confines of the spinal canal. This structural and buffering arrangement makes the spinal cord one of the body's most well-protected organs. Not only does it have a firm bony covering, constructed to allow maximal movement, but also the hydraulic system within the subarachnoid space provides excellent shock absorption. The cauda equina begins approximately at the interspace of the first and second lumbar vertebrae and extends to the sacrum. The lower part of the spinal

canal with its enclosed nerve roots is less sensitive to injury than the upper portion housing the cord.

The cord receives its blood supply from a network of extensive collaterals that enter the spinal canal with the nerve roots (Fig. 27.11). In most persons, one ventral radicular artery is usually considerably larger than the others; this artery originates from the aorta between the eighth thoracic and third lumbar vertebrae, and provides the blood supply for most of the thoracic section of the cord. Paraplegia can result from occlusion of this artery by traumatic or iatrogenic dissection. The arterial supply of the more rostral part of the cord is derived from the vertebral arteries. As the vessels terminate within the cord, they are end-arteries that provide little collateral circulation within the gray matter of the cord itself.

The spinal cord is almost cylindrical, with its width always greater than its dorsoventral diameter. It noticeably enlarges at the regions of innervation of the upper extremities as well as at the lumbosacral region. There are usually 31 pairs of spinal nerves in man. The first pair originates from the vertebral column between the first cervical

Table 27.1.
Motor function chart.

Cord Segment	Muscles	Action to be Tested	Nerves
		Shoulder Girdle and Upper Extremity	
C1–4	Deep neck muscles (sternomastoid and trapezius also participate)	Flexion of neck Extension of neck Rotation of neck Lateral bending of neck	Cervical
C3–4	Scaleni Diaphragm	Elevation of upper thorax Inspiration	Phrenic
C5–T1	Pectoralis major and minor	Adduction of arm from behind to front	Thoracic anterior (from medial and lateral cords of plexus)
C5–7	Serratus anterior	Forward thrust of shoulder	Long thoracic
C5(3–4)	Levator scapulae	Elevation of scapula	Dorsal scapular
C4–5	Rhomboids	Medial adduction and elevation of scapula	Dorsal scapular
C5	Supraspinatus	Abduction of arm	Suprascapular
C5–6	Infraspinatus	Lateral rotation of arm	Suprascapular
C5–8	Latissimus dorsi, teres major and subscapularis	Medial rotation of arm Adduction of arm from front to back	Subscapular (from posterior cord of plexus)
C5–6	Deltoid	Abduction of arm	Axillary (from posterior cord of plexus)
C5	Teres minor	Lateral rotation of arm	Axillary (from posterior cord of plexus)
C5–6	Biceps brachii	Flexion of forearm Supination of forearm	Musculocutaneous (from lateral cord of plexus)
C6–7	Coracobrachialis	Adduction of arm Flexion of forearm	Musculocutaneous (from lateral cord of plexus)
C5–6	Brachialis	Flexion of forearm	Musculocutaneous (from lateral cord of plexus)
C6–8	Triceps brachii and anconeus	Extension of forearm	
C5–6	Brachioradialis	Flexion of forearm	
C5–7	Extensor carpi radialis	Radial extension of hand	Radial (from posterior cord of plexus)
C6–8	Extensor digitorum communis	Extension of phalanges of index finger, middle finger, ring finger, little finger	
C6–8	Extensor digitorum communis	Extension of hand	
C6–8	Extensor digiti quinti proprius	Extension of phalanges of little finger Extension of hand	Radial (from posterior cord of plexus)
C6–8	Extensor carpi ulnaris	Ulnar extension of hand	
C5–7	Supinator	Supination of forearm	
C6–7	Abductor pollicis longus	Abduction of metacarpal of thumb Radial extension of hand	
C6–7	Extensor pollicis brevis and longus	Extension of thumb	Radial (from posterior cord of plexus)
C6–8	Extensor pollicis brevis and longus	Radial extension of hand	
C6–8	Extensor indicis proprius	Extension of index finger Extension of hand	
C7–T1	Flexor carpi ulnaris	Ulnar flexion of hand	

Table 27.1.—*continued*

Cord Segment	Muscles	Action to be Tested	Nerves
C8-T1	Flexor digitorum profundus (ulnar portion	Flexion of terminal phalanx of ring finger, little finger	
C8-T1	Flexor digitorum profundus (ulnar portion)	Flexion of hand	
C8-T1	Adductor pollicis	Adduction of metacarpal of thumb	Ulnar (from medial cord of plexus)
C8-T1	Abductor digiti quinti	Abduction of little finger	
C8-T1	Opponens digiti quinti	Opposition of little finger	
C8-T1	Flexor digiti quinti brevis	Flexion of little finger	
C8-T1	Interossei	Flexion of proximal phalanx, extension of two distal phalanges, adduction and abduction of fingers	
C6–7	Pronator teres	Pronation of forearm	
C6–7	Flexor carpi radialis	Radial flexion of hand	
C7-T1	Palmaris longus	Flexion of hand	
C7-T1	Flexor digitorum sublimis	Flexion of middle phalanx of index finger, middle finger, ring finger, little finger	Median (C6–7 from lateral cord of plexus; C8-T1 from medial cord of plexus)
C7-T1	Flexor digitorum sublimis	Flexion of hand	
C6–7	Flexor pollicis longus	Flexion of terminal phalanx of thumb	
C7-T1	Flexor digitorum pro-fundus (radial portion)	Flexion of terminal phalanx of index finger, middle finger	
C7-T1	Flexor digitorum pro-fundus (radial portion)	Flexion of hand	
C6–7	Abductor pollicis brevis	Abduction of metacarpal of thumb	
C6–7	Flexor pollicis brevis	Flexion of proximal phalanx of thumb	
C6–7	Opponens pollicis	Opposition of metacarpal of thumb	Medial (C6–7 from lateral cord of plexus; C8-T1 from medial cord of plexus)
C8-T1	Lumbricals (the two lateral)	Flexion of proximal phalanx and extension of the two distal phalanges of index finger, middle finger	
C8-T1	Lumbricals (the two medial)	Flexion of proximal phalanx and extension of the two distal phalanges of ring finger, little finger	
		Trunk and Thorax	
	Thoracic, abdominal, and back	Elevation and depression of ribs	Thoracic and posterior lumbo-sacral branches
		Contraction of abdomen Anteroflexion and lateral flexion of trunk	
		Hip Girdle and Lower Extremity	
T12–L3	Iliopsoas	Flexion of hip	Femoral
L2–L3	Sartorius	Flexion of hip (and eversion of thigh)	

Table 27.1.—*continued*

Cord Segment	Muscles	Action to be Tested	Nerves
L2–L4	Quadriceps femoris	Extension of knee	
L2–3	Pectineus	Adduction of thigh	
L2–3	Adductor longus	Adduction of thigh	
L2–4	Adductor brevis	Adduction of thigh	
L3–4	Adductor magnus	Adduction of thigh	Obturator
L2–4	Gracilis	Adduction of thigh	
L3–4	Obturator externus	Adduction of thigh	
L3–4	Obturator externus	Lateral rotation of thigh	
L4–5,S1	Gluteus medius and minimus	Extension of thigh	
L4–5,S1	Gluteus medius and minimus	Medial rotation of thigh	Superior gluteal
L4–5	Tensor fasciae latae	Flexion of thigh	
S1–2	Piriformis	Lateral rotation of thigh	
L4–S1	Gluteus maximus	Abduction of thigh	Inferior gluteal
L5–S2	Obturator internus	Lateral rotation of thigh	Muscular branches from sacral plexus
L4–S2	Gemelli	Lateral rotation of thigh	Muscular branches from sacral plexus
L4–S1	Quadratus femoris	Lateral rotation of thigh	Muscular branches from sacral plexus
L4–S2	Biceps femoris	Flexion of leg (assists in extension of thigh)	
L4–S1	Semitendinosus	Flexion of leg (assists in extension of thigh)	Sciatic (trunk)
L4–S1	Semimembranosus	Flexion of leg (assists in extension of thigh)	
L4–5	Tibialis anterior	Dorsal flexion of foot	
L4–5	Tibialis anterior	Supination of foot	
L4–S1	Extensor digitorum longus	Extension of toes II–V	
L4–S1	Extensor digitorum longus	Dorsal flexion of foot	
L4–S1	Extensor hallucis longus	Extension of great toe	Deep peroneal
L4–S1	Extensor hallucis longus	Dorsal flexion of foot	
L4–S1	Extensor digitorum brevis	Extension of great toe and the three medial toes	
L5–S1	Peronei	Plantar flexion of foot in pronation	Superficial peroneal
L5–S2	Tibialis posterior and triceps surae	Plantar flexion of foot in supination	
L5–S2	Flexor digitorum longus	Plantar flexion of foot in supination	
L5–S2	Flexor digitorum longus	Flexion of terminal phalanx, toes II–V	
L5–S2	Flexor hallucis longus	Plantar flexion of foot in supination	Tibial
L5–S2	Flexor hallucis longus	Flexion of terminal phalanx of great toe	
L5–S1	Flexor digitorum brevis	Flexion of middle phalanx, toes II–V	

Table 27.1.—*continued*

Cord Segment	Muscles	Action to be Tested	Nerves
L5-S2	Flexor hallucis brevis	Flexion of proximal phalanx of great toe	
S1–2	Small muscles of foot	Spreading and closing of toes	Tibial
S1–2	Small muscles of foot	Flexion of proximal phalanx of toes	
S2–4	Perineal and sphincters	Voluntary control of pelvic floor	Pudendal

(Reproduced by permission, from Wepsic JG: Injuries to the spinal cord and cauda equina, in Cave EF, Burke JF, Boyd RJ (Eds): *Trauma Management.* Copyright © 1974, by Year Book Medical Publishers, Inc., Chicago.)

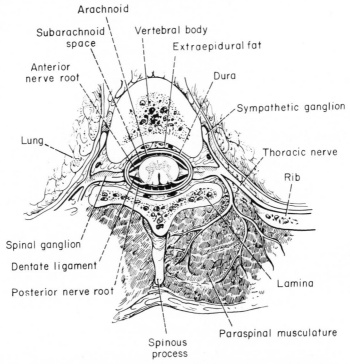

Figure 27.9. Transverse section through a thoracic vertebra and the spinal cord. Excellent protection of cord is apparent when relationships of surrounding musculature, bony canal, epidural fat, and cerebrospinal fluid are considered. Relation of dorsal root to spinal cord is shown. (Reproduced by permission, from Wepsic JG: Injuries to the spinal cord and cauda equina, in Cave EF, Burke JF, Boyd RJ (Eds): *Trauma Management.* Copyright © 1974 by Year Book Medical Publishers, Inc., Chicago.)

vertebra and the skull, with each of the remaining pairs of cervical nerves leaving *above* the vertebra of the corresponding number. Since there are eight pairs of cervical nerves and only seven cervical vertebrae, the 8th cervical nerve leaves the spinal column between the 7th cervical and 1st thoracic vertebrae. Beginning with the 1st thoracic nerve, all the remaining spinal nerves pass from the vertebral column below the vertebra of the corresponding number (Fig. 27.12).

The effects of spinal cord trauma are expressed as motor, sensory, and visceral deficits distal to the site of injury. Usually, the major effect is interruption of the descending or ascending white matter tracts, and although gray matter lesions are extremely important in the midcervical region in patients with "central cord injury," the vital motor and sensory deficits noted on first examination are due to tract interruption (Fig. 27.13).

Motor impulses descend in three corticospinal tracts: the crossed lateral tract, the uncrossed lateral tract, and the ventral tract. These originate

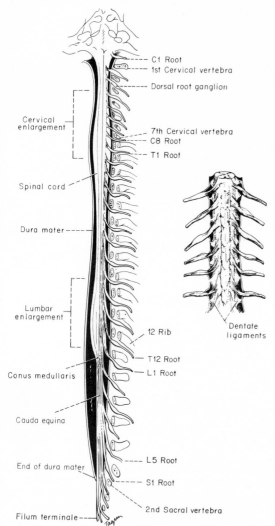

Figure 27.10. Spinal cord and surrounding structures. Note position of 1st, 7th, and 8th cervical roots with respect to vertebral level at which they emerge. Cervical and lumbar enlargements are depicted as well as relationship of dentate ligaments to the cord, posterior rootlets, and dura mater. (Reproduced by permission from Wepsic JG: Injuries to the spinal cord and cauda equina, in Cave EF, Burke JF, Boyd RJ (Eds): *Trauma Management*. Copyright © 1974 by Year Book Medical Publishers, Inc., Chicago.)

mainly in the precentral gyrus and descend from the cortex via the internal capsule and cerebral peduncle, crossing to the opposite side along the ventral aspect of the medulla. The fibers terminate on cells in posterior, intermedullary, and ventral gray matter, and their interruption produces voluntary motor paralysis. The reticulospinal tracts originate in the pontine and medullary reticular formations. Interruption of or injury to these fibers in the upper cervical region may result in apnea while the patient sleeps. Visceral activity is modulated by the reticulospinal fibers, as well as by other multisynaptic chains of neurons that terminate on both preganglionic autonomic and somatic efferent neurons. "Automatic" visceral activity is usually eventually possible in the absence of descending impulses if the relevant nerve roots and segmental cord levels are preserved in the face of higher transection of the cord.

Ascending pathways carry information about distal visceral and cutaneous sensibilities. The spinothalamic tracts related to pain and temperature sensibilities arise from cells in the dorsal gray matter, cross the midline via the ventral commissure, and ascend in the lateral portion of the anterior quadrant to terminate in the medullary and thalamic nuclei. Touch and vibration sensibilities are served by the posterior columns. The more lateral group of fibers, the fasciculus cuneatus, originates from dorsal horn cells of the first cervical vertebra to the 6th thoracic vertebra, whereas the more medial group, the fasciculus gracilis, originates from cells below the 6th thoracic vertebra. They terminate in the nucleus cuneatus and nucleus gracilis and then project rostrally via the medial lemniscus.

Diagnostic Studies

When a spinal cord injury is suspected, anteroposterior, lateral, and open-mouth x-ray films of the neck, as well as standard views of the thoracic and lumbar sections of the spine, are mandatory if the patient's life is not otherwise threatened. The head and neck should be maintained in good position with manual or halter traction. Good views of the lower cervical vertebrae should be obtained, since these are frequently the site of fracture-dislocation and are also the most difficult areas to visualize because of the superimposed radiodensity of the shoulders. Visualization is facilitated by drawing down the arms and shoulders while the head is supported. Oblique or "swimmer's" views can be taken if this tactic fails to demonstrate the junction of the seventh cervical and first thoracic vertebrae.

X-ray study can give information regarding fractures or dislocations of the major bony elements, the presence of osteoarthritis, and the presence of foreign bodies or bone within the spinal canal (Fig. 27.14). Although the x-ray findings are informative, they never reveal the total extent of clinical disruption; at operation the extent of frac-

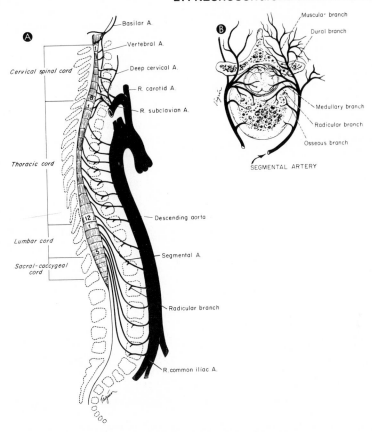

Figure 27.11. **(A)** Blood supply of spinal cord in human fetus arising from subclavian artery, iliac artery, and aorta. Note that the vertebral artery supplies segmental arteries in upper cervical region whereas more direct branches from the deep cervical artery supply mid- and lower cervical cord. Variability in this supply is great, and the most consistent feature of detailed examination of the blood supply to the cervical cord, in particular, is its variability. The number of important large radicular branches varies, as does the level of entry or position of the vessel with respect to anterior or posterior roots. In general, a large radicular branch arising from the aorta between the 8th thoracic and 3rd lumbar vertebrae provides largest amount of blood to thoracic cord. This is the artery of Adamkiewicz. **(B)** Spinal anatomy of a large segmental and radicular artery. Supply to dura mater, muscles, and bone arises from these vessels. As noted above, entry of medullary arteries through the intervertebral foramen is variable. Microscopic dissection during operation on posterior or anterior roots is often necessary to preserve this important blood supply. (Reproduced by permission, from Wepsic JG: Injuries to the spinal cord and cauda equina, in Cave EF, Burke JF, Boyd RJ (Eds): *Trauma Management.* Copyright © 1974 by Year Book Medical Publishers, Inc., Chicago.)

ture and dislocation usually considerably exceeds that seen on the films. In addition, neural damage may be severe even when x-ray findings do not indicate serious injury.

Blockage of the spinal subarachnoid space has been used as one criterion for surgical intervention. If the space is compressed because of dislocation or impingement of bony elements on the spinal cord, operation has been suggested. The most satisfactory method of demonstrating the subarachnoid space is myelography. More centers are performing emergency myelographic examination to demonstrate the exact nature and level

of a compressive lesion that may or may not be evident from clinical observation and plain x-ray films. With the patient in the prone position, the radiopaque oil is placed in the lumbar subarachnoid space and the patient is then positioned with the upper part of the spine dependent, allowing the dye to run into the upper cervical region. When this is not practical, the spinal needle can be introduced with the patient supine, placing the needly laterally through the foramen between the first and second cervical vertebrae.

Emergency air or metrizamide myelographic studies augmented by tomography or CT scanning

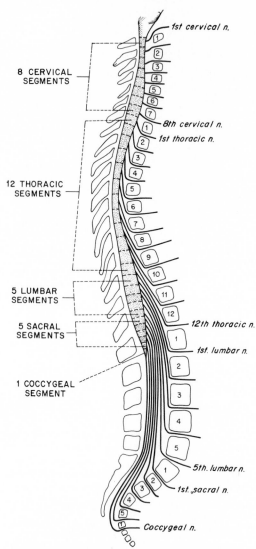

1st cervical n.

8 CERVICAL
SEGMENTS

8th cervical n.
1st thoracic n.

12 THORACIC
SEGMENTS

5 LUMBAR
SEGMENTS

12th thoracic n.

5 SACRAL
SEGMENTS

1st. lumbar n.

1 COCCYGEAL
SEGMENT

5th. lumbar n.

1st. sacral n.

Coccygeal n.

Figure 27.12. Relation of bony vertebral level to spinal cord level and nerve root exit. (Reproduced by permission, from Wepsic JG: Injuries to the spinal cord and cauda equina, in Cave EF, Burke JF, Boyd RJ (Eds): *Trauma Management.* Copyright © 1974 by Year Book Medical Publishers, Inc., Chicago.)

have recently allowed more detailed evaluation of lesions in centers specializing in acute spinal cord injury.

Once the nature of the injury has been established, the neurologic deficit determined, and the anatomic substrate demonstrated with plain x-ray films or myelograms, further therapy must be considered.

Immobilization

With any significant dislocation of the neck, it is best to immobilize the head and neck to prevent further dislocation. Several devices for skeletal traction are available. The simplest are those that can be screwed into the calvarium in a position to provide traction along the longitudinal axis of the spinal canal. Gardner-Wells tongs are the most satisfactory device now available for skeletal traction; these allow simple fixation without drilling into the calvarium by using a sharp screw-in pin that can be controlled by a built-in torque indicator. In children, in whom the calvarium is thin, and in adults with a bony disorder of the skull or a skull fracture, skeletal traction can be applied to the head by placing heavy wires in the epidural space and by bringing them out through burr holes in the parietal area. Emergency application of a halo device—a body cast with an attachment for skeletal fixation of the head—is also useful for cervical immobilization.

After x-ray films have been obtained and an airway established, skeletal traction can be applied to patients with a cervical fracture or dislocation. The patient is placed supine with a small roll beneath the normal cervical curvature and sandbags against both sides of the head. The skin above the ear is shaved and cleansed. Care is taken to mark where the tongs are to be inserted so that the ends are symmetrically placed. In general, placement directly above or slightly posterior to the pinna allows traction along the axis of the spine. If realignment is necessary, the spine may be slightly flexed or extended by adjusting the direction of force and the level of the thorax; placement of tongs need not be based on such considerations. After the skin over the site of installation is infiltrated with an anesthetic agent, the Gardner-Wells tongs are screwed into the scalp and outer table of the skull. The depth of screw insertion is indicated by the automatic protrusion of a pressure-sensitive pin at the hub end of the screw on one side. The Gardner-Wells tongs hold securely with little danger of inner table penetration.

For traction to be effective, the upper portion of the body must be elevated slightly so that the body serves as counterweight. Correct skeletal alignment during traction should be checked repeatedly and x-ray films obtained to be sure that the pull of the tongs is along the axis of the spinal canal. The rope connecting the tongs to weights can be fed through the center hole of a Stryker frame or kept in place with a Rogers frame, which permits a constant angle of traction yet allows the patient to turn from side to side in a standard hospital bed. When the patient lies on his side, a small pad should be placed beneath the dependent ear and cheek to maintain a neutral position of the cervical spine. In the average adult, 7–10 pounds of traction can be applied to maintain stability. If a

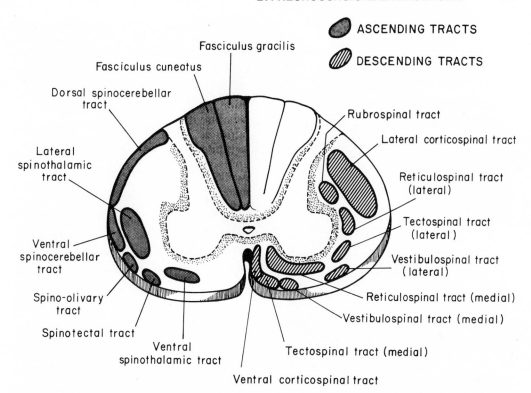

Figure 27.13. Cross-section of low cervical spinal cord showing ascending and descending tracts. (Reproduced by permission, from Wepsic JG: Injuries to the spinal cord and cauda equina, in Cave EF, Burke JF, Boyd RJ (Eds): *Trauma Management.* Copyright © 1974 by Year Book Medical Publishers, Inc., Chicago.)

dislocation is present, a large amount of weight should be placed on the tongs initially to fatigue the paraspinal musculature, allowing reduction to take place. A common error is to begin with small amounts of weight and to increase the weight gradually, hoping that realignment will result. If there is a significant dislocation, it is usually wisest to begin with 30–40 pounds. If it becomes apparent that the facets are locked in a dislocated position, operative reduction may be required. Closed manipulative reduction of cervical fractures carries an extremely high risk and should not be done. Asepsis should be maintained in the area of the tongs, and the patient should be sedated for comfort.

Traction is unnecessary in the treatment of thoracic and lumbar fractures, but the patient should be nursed on a frame that permits frequent change of position without manipulation of the spinal alignment. All bony prominences must be protected from pressure.

Later immobilization is possible utilizing a halo device.

Fractures and Dislocations

Although contusions and temporary dislocations of the spinal cord without a bony abnormality may be common, injuries associated with bony fractures and dislocations are the most serious spinal injuries, since moderate to severe cord damage usually results. Fractures or dislocations of any type from the second cervical vertebra to the 1st thoracic vertebra carry the most guarded prognosis. If the dislocation is between the 2nd and 4th cervical vertebrae, the patient may die immediately or have complete quadriplegia. If respiratory function is adequate initially, it may rapidly deteriorate as intercostal and phrenic muscles fail with progressive cord edema. Fractures and dislocations below the 4th cervical vertebra may produce quadriplegia with sparing of some arm muscles. In this area of cervical cord enlargement, dislocation of a few millimeters may produce a total permanent distal deficit.

Fracture-dislocations in the thoracic region may be radiographically more impressive, yet spare some distal neurologic function. Fractures at the thoracolumbar junction are almost always compression fractures and may result in injury to the distal part of the cord or the cauda equina. The bony deformity produced by these fractures is often pronounced enough to warrant operation to stabilize the spine. If the lesion is distal to the 1st lumbar vertebra with compression of elements of

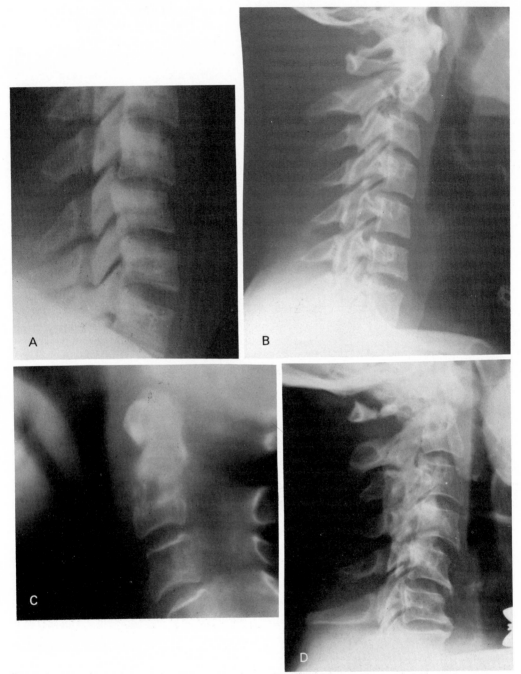

Figure 27.14. Spinal fracture-dislocations. **(A)** Posterior dislocation of 6th cervical vertebra producing quadriplegia. **(B)** Fracture-dislocation of 2nd and 3rd cervical vertebrae without neurologic deficit. **(C)** Fractured odontoid process (tomogram). **(D)** Fractured arch of 1st cervical vertebra.

the cauda equina, prognosis is better. Compressed nerve roots are more likely to recover after decompression; we therefore believe that traumatic lesions of the conus medullaris and cauda equina should be explored as early as possible.

Although hemorrhage within the spinal canal is usually not a major problem in patients with a spinal injury, the special case of patients with rheumatoid arthritis should be considered. These patients have a higher incidence of subdural and epidural clots associated with fracture-dislocations; this is thought to be due to the structural abnormalities of the bones and joints. Early exploration and clot evacuation in these patients may be extremely gratifying.

Linear fractures without dislocation are relatively mild injuries and may involve only the transverse or spinous processes. If no neurologic deficit is present, the patient may be treated with collar immobilization; there is usually no lasting disability.

Compression fractures usually result from hyperflexion. The anterior surface of the vertebra is pinched, so the centrum gives way laterally or posteriorly into the spinal cord. This type of fracture occurs frequently in the cervical region as the result of a diving accident, but is most common at the thoracolumbar junction in patients who have fallen onto the buttocks or feet. A profound deficit often immediately results.

Atlanto-occipital dislocations are rare and most often result in immediate death. *Atlantoaxial dislocations* are usually caused by a sudden jerk backward of the head and neck and are associated with fracture of the odontoid process and rupture of the cruciate ligaments. In patients who do not die immediately, this lesion is usually not attended by a neurologic deficit. Treatment consists of immobilization, with stabilization occurring over a 6- to 8-week period. At that point, fluoroscopic examination of head motion should cautiously be carried out to see whether fusion of the first and second cervical vertebrae and the occiput is necessary.

"Hangman's fracture" is a bilateral avulsion fracture through the arch of the axis without injury to the odontoid process that results from sudden severe hyperextension of the head and neck. This type of injury may be seen in victims of motor vehicle accidents. If the patient survives, there is usually no associated neurologic deficit. This is thought to be due to increased space in the upper cervical canal as compared with the size of the cord and the fact that decompression occurs during the injury by avulsion of the neural arches. These fractures heal spontaneously and are usually best treated by prolonged immobilization.

Teardrop fractures are cervical fractures produced when extreme flexion causes the body of the involved vertebra to be compressed, with the anteroinferior fragment displaced downward and forward and the posteroinferior portion projected into the spinal canal. The posteroinferior portion can injure the anterior portion of the spinal cord. When such a condition occurs, especially in the

presence of neurologic deficits and myelographic indications of a block, early operative decompression and removal of bone and herniated disk material are indicated. The custom has been to employ a posterior approach, since an anterior approach risks pressing the bony fragments into the cord. Recent use of the operating microscope and halo fixation have led some surgeons to favor an early anterior approach, however, with excellent results.

Neurologic Syndromes Associated with Spinal Cord Injury

The degree of injury to the spinal cord can vary from rapidly reversible concussion, in which there is no neuroanatomic lesion, no blood in the CSF, and no subarachnoid block, to complete transection of the cord with loss of all neurologic function below this level. Bruising of the cord with subpial hemorrhage and usually blood in the CSF indicates spinal cord contusion, which is always accompanied by a neurologic deficit. The cord may be lacerated or contain hemorrhages. These findings are similar to those noted in the contused brain.

Anterior spinal cord injury results from acute impingement of bone or herniated disc fragments on the anterior portion of the cord. Corticospinal and spinothalamic functions are immediately interrupted, with some preservation of touch, position, and vibration sense. Early operation is indicated, and patients often make an exceptional recovery if the cord has not been lacerated.

Central cervical spinal cord injury usually results from hypertension of the cervical spine in patients with significant cervical spondylosis. It is characterized by considerable impairment of motor movement in the upper extremities and frequently less severe impairment of the lower extremities. Sensory loss and bladder dysfunction occur as well. The mechanism of this injury remains unclear; some believe it is due to contusion, whereas others believe it is caused by ischemia. Such a lesion does not require operation, and patients frequently experience a significant degree of recovery with immobilization and corticosteroids.

Brown-Séquard's syndrome with loss of motor function on one side and loss of sensory function on the other is not commonly seen in spinal fracture-dislocations because it requires the presence of a unilateral cord injury that completely spares the opposite side. This syndrome is produced by interruption of the corticospinal tracts supplying the ipsilateral musculature and the spinothalamic tracts receiving sensibility impulses from the contralateral side. A traumatic lateral disc herniation or epidural clot may produce such a finding, and surgical decompression may be necessary if myelographic examination demonstrates such a lesion.

Operative Indications

Worsening neurologic signs, a complete block of the subarachnoid space on manometric or myelographic testing, a compound fracture, a penetrating wound of the spine, a foreign body within the spinal canal, and the syndrome of acute anterior spinal cord injury are indications for immediate surgical decompression. Later operations to prevent deformity, achieve stability, and realign dislocated fragments are also important.

The operative approach for emergency neurosurgical decompression or débridement is to perform a total posterior laminectomy of the involved area, taking care not to dislocate fragments that may be impinging on the spinal cord. Fusion may be performed at the initial decompression, should instability or dislocation be obvious. After all bony fragments are removed from the spinal canal, the dura is opened and the spinal cord is visualized. The dentate ligaments may be sectioned if there is evidence of a herniated mass anterior to the cord, but manipulation of the injured spinal cord or myelotomy to decompress the swollen cord has not been satisfactory.

Prognosis

One of the most difficult areas to face in caring for acute quadriplegic patients involves evaluating their prognosis. In a recent report on a large group of patients, all patients who were cognitively intact with complete quadriplegia 72 hours after injury failed to walk 1 year afterward. Of those with incomplete sensory loss 72 hours after injury, 47% walked at 1 year, and in those with incomplete motor loss, 87% walked at 1 year. These figures should provide a guide in discussing prognosis with the patient and his family.

The Acute Back

The emergency ward is often where patients who have experienced sudden back pain associated with exertion seek treatment. Many patients state that on lifting an object they had sudden, severe, incapacitating back pain, muscle spasm, and varying amounts of pain into the lower extremities, and in addition, were unable to straighten up. The differential diagnosis includes many possibilities, from simple muscle spasm and strain to acute ruptured intervertebral disc. Al-

though most patients have a minor condition and can be treated effectively with muscle relaxants and bed rest, patients with reflex changes, sensory loss, motor weakness, or difficulties with bowel or bladder function require special attention. The acute presentation of patients wtih neurologic loss associated with motion-induced back pain is usually due to posterior protrusion of the herniated or ruptured nucleus pulposus into the intervertebral foramen, which causes compression of the exiting nerve roots (Fig. 27.15). The first sacral nerve root between the 5th lumbar vertebra and the sacrum is compressed the most frequently, producing loss of the ankle jerk, sensory abnormalities on the lateral aspect of the foot and on the sole, and weakness of the gastrocnemius and soleus muscles. Less frequently, disc protrusion occurs between the 4th and 5th lumbar vertebrae with compression of the 5th lumbar nerve root, resulting in no change in reflexes but loss of sensation over the dorsum of the foot and great toe with weakness of the foot and toe dorsiflexion muscles. Large midline disc protrusions that may initially fill the spinal canal are occasionally seen between the 5th lumbar and 1st sacral vertebrae and between the 4th and 5th lumbar vertebrae. These protrusions may result in compression of the entire cauda equina below this level, producing sacral sensory loss and urinary retention. They are neurosurgical emergencies that require immediate operation.

After neurologic examination has established the degree of neural involvement, lumbosacral spine films can be obtained to document the presence or absence of bony abnormalities. Narrowing of the relevant interspace is often observed.

Hospitalization with complete bed rest for 2 weeks often results in significant alleviation of low back pain and muscle spasm, and even reversal of neurologic deficit. Myelographic examination (Fig. 27.16) is recommended only after a regimen such as this, and it should be followed by surgical correction of the nerve root compression if one is demonstrated. All too often, patients with a slight neurologic deficit and minimal symptoms are subjected to myelographic examination and operation when a more progressive conservative approach could yield more favorable long-term results. To facilitate bed rest, adequate analgesia and sedation should be provided; muscle relaxants such as diazepam (Valium) are helpful in addition to bed rest.

Body scanning of the lumbar spine may also yield an accurate diagnosis without the need to introduce contrast material into the spinal canal. This study has the advantage of also demonstrat-

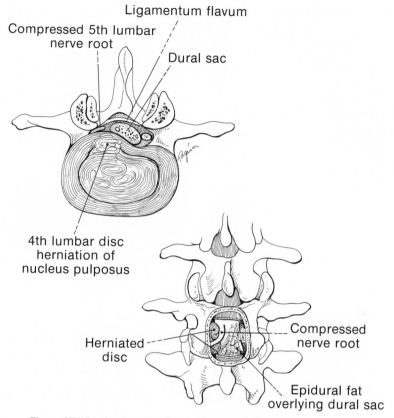

Figure 27.15.   Lumbar disc fragment compressing exiting nerve root.

ing the lateral recesses and neural foramen. Abnormalities in these areas may also contribute to the clinical findings in addition to an acute ruptured disc.

Neck pain is a frequent complaint of patients who suffer an acceleration-deceleration injury. The extent of injury may range from muscle spasm and pain—"whiplash"—to severe fracture-dislocation that may not have an associated neurologic deficit. Caution should be exercised in evaluating this type of condition in the emergency ward. Fracture-dislocation should be assumed until proved otherwise. Only then is it reasonable to treat the patient conservatively with collars and muscle relaxants. Usually, a period of immobilization with liberal use of analgesics decreases the muscle spasm. Persistent neck pain and occipital pain after accidents of this type are often difficult to treat, and patients may complain of pain for several months or even years. A conclusive pathologic study of this entity has never been done, since patients rarely have a neurologic deficit and seldom undergo special diagnostic studies. When

neurologic loss is present, hospitalization is indicated; if improvement does not occur, myelograms may be required to demonstrate the presence of cervical disc herniation. When large disc herniation is present, spinal cord compression may occur, producing quadriparesis and other long-tract signs. These signs are indications for immediate decompression either anteriorly by resection of the disc and fusion or posteriorly with laminectomy.

Thoracic disc rupture, although extremely rare, can be manifested by paraplegia, and immediate attention to the patient with a history of heavy lifting, sudden pain in the middle of the back, and bilateral lower extremity paresthesias or weakness is essential. Emergency myelographic examination should be carried out and surgical decompression performed if the myelogram reveals spinal cord compression. Delay may result in an irreversible neurologic deficit.

Suggested Readings

Ad Hoc Committee of the Harvard Medical School: A definition of irreversible coma: Report of the Ad Hoc Committee of the Harvard Medical School to examine the definition of

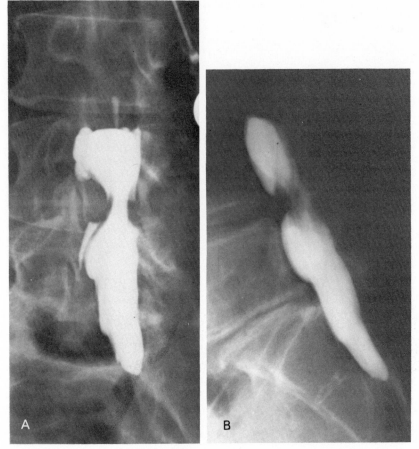

Figure 27.16.   Myelograms demonstrating herniated lumbar disc. **(A)** Oblique view showing large defect with compression of exiting root. **(B)** Lateral view showing posterior dislocation of dural sac by disc fragment.

brain death. *JAMA 205:*337–340, 1968

Austin G (Ed): *The Spinal Cord: Basic Aspects and Surgical Considerations,* ed 2. Section VI, Spinal trauma. Springfield, Ill, Charles C Thomas, 1972, pp. 227–278

Black, PM: Brain death. *N Engl J Med 299:*338–344, 393–410, 1978

Caveness WF: Onset and cessation of fits following craniocerebral trauma. *J Neurosurg 20:*570–583, 1963

Comarr AE, Kaufman AA: A survey of the neurological results of 858 spinal cord injuries: A comparison of patients treated with and without laminectomy. *J Neurosurg 13:*95–106, 1956

Crosby EC, Humphrey T, Lauer EW: Spinal cord, in *Correlative Anatomy of the Nervous System.* New York, Macmillan, 1962, pp. 56–111

Gallagher JP, Browder EJ: Extradural hematoma: Experience with 167 patients. *J Neurosurg 29:*1–12, 1968

Gurdjian ES: Recent advances in the study of the mechanism of impact injury of the head—a summary. *Clin Neurosurg 19:*1–42, 1972

Guttmann L: *Spinal Cord Injuries: Comprehensive Management and Research.* Oxford, Blackwell, 1973

Hammon WM: Analysis of 2187 consecutive penetrating wounds of the brain from Vietnam. *J Neurosurg 34:*127–131, 1971

Harwood-Nash DC, Hendrick EB, Hudson AR: The signifi-

cance of skull fractures in children. A study of 1,187 patients. *Radiology 101:*151–155, 1971

Joyner J, Freeman LW: Urea and spinal cord trauma. *Neurology 13:*69–72, 1963

Langfitt TW, Gennarelli TA: Can the outcome from head injury be improved? *J Neurosurg 56:*19–25, 1982

Langfitt TW, Tannanbaum HM, Kassell NF: The etiology of acute brain swelling following experimental head injury. *J Neurosurg 24:*47–56, 1966

MacGee EE, Cauthen JC, Brackett CE: Meningitis following acute traumatic cerebrospinal fluid fistula. *J Neurosurg 33:*312–316, 1970

Marshall LF, Smith RW, Shapiro HM: The outcome with aggressive treatment in severe head injuries. Part I: The significance of intracranial pressure monitoring. *J Neurosurg 50:*20–25, 1979

Marshall LF, Smith RW, Shapiro HM: The outcome with aggressive treatment in severe head injuries. Part II: Acute and chronic barbiturate administration in the management of head injury. *J Neurosurg 50:*26–30, 1979

Matson DD: Spinal cord injury, in *Neurosurgy of Infancy and Childhood,* ed 2. Springfield, Ill, Charles C Thomas, 1969, pp. 359–375

Maynard FM, Reynolds GG, Foutain S, et al: Neurological prognosis after traumatic quadriplegia. *J Neurosurg 50:*611–616, 1979

McKissock W: Subdural haematoma: A review of 389 cases. *Lancet 1*:1365–1369, 1960

Miller JD, Butterworth JF, Gudeman SK, et al: Further experience in the management of head injury. *J Neurosurg 54*:289–299, 1981

Munro D: Cord bladder—its definition, treatment and prognosis when associated with spinal cord injuries. *N Engl J Med 215*:766–777, 1936

Munro D, Merritt HH: Surgical pathology of subdural hematoma based on a study of one hundred and five cases. *Arch Neurol Psychiatry 35*:64–78, 1936

Rosenbaum WI, Greenberg RP, Seelig JM, et al: Midbrain lesions: Frequent and significant prognostic feature in closed head injury. *Neurosurgy 9*:613–620, 1981

Rossier AB, Berney J, Rosenbaum AE, et al: Value of gas myelography in early management of acute cervical spinal cord injuries. *J Neurosurg 42*:330–337, 1975

Schneider RC: The syndrome of acute anterior spinal cord injury. *J Neurosurg 12*:95–122, 1955

Schneider RC: Craniocerebral trauma, in *Correlative Neurosurgery,* Kahn EA, Crosby EC, Schneider RC, et al (Eds). ed 2. Springfield, Ill, Charles C Thomas, 1969, pp. 533–596

Schneider RC: Trauma to the spine and spinal cord, in *Correlative Neurosurgery,* Kahn EA, Crosby EC, Schneider RC, et al (Eds). ed 2. Springfield, Ill, Charles C Thomas, 1969, pp. 597–648.

Schneider RC, Kahn EA: Chronic neurological sequelae of acute trauma to the spine and spinal cord. Part 1. The significance of the acute-flexion or "tear-drop" fracture-dislocation of the cervical spine. *J Bone Joint Surg 38A*:985–997, 1956

Seelig JM, Becker DP, Miller JD, et al: Traumatic acute subdural hematoma: major mortality reduction in comatose patients treated within four hours. *N Engl J Med 304*:1511–1518, 1981

Talalla A, Morin MA: Acute traumatic subdural hematoma: A review of one hundred consecutive cases. *J Trauma 11*:771–777, 1971

Tarlov IM: Spinal cord compression studies: Time limits for recovery after gradual compression in dogs. *Arch Neurol Psychiatry 71*:588–597, 1954

Taveras JM, Wood EH: *Diagnostic Neuroradiology,* ed 2. Baltimore, Williams & Wilkins, 1976

Wagner FC: Management of acute spinal cord injury. *Surg Neurol 7*:346–350, 1977

Wallis W, Kutt H, McDowell F: Intravenous diphenylhydantoin in treatment of acute repetitive seizures. *Neurology 18*:513–525, 1968

Wise BL, Chater N: The value of hypertonic mannitol solution in decreasing brain mass and lowering cerebrospinal fluid pressure. *J Neurosurg 19*:1038–1043, 1962

Wright RL: Traumatic hematomas of the posterior cranial fossa. *J Neurosurg 25*:402–409, 1966

CHAPTER 28

Thermal Injuries

MICHAEL B. LEWIS, M.D.
NICHOLAS E. O'CONNOR, M.D.

More than 70,000 burned patients are admitted to hospitals in the United States each year. Although the figure is unknown, a greater number of burned patients are seen in the emergency ward, treated, and released. These patients together constitute a large group who by the very nature of their injury are first seen by the emergency physician.

The severity of the burn injury can vary from a mild sunburn requiring no treatment to a major full-thickness burn whose treatment requires the extensive resources of modern medicine. Although many factors will determine the final outcome, proper emergency care is the first step toward satisfactory recovery.

As with any injured patient, the first priority is to ensure an adequate airway and to stop hemorrhage. These topics are discussed elsewhere and will not be dealt with in this chapter, except that some respiratory problems unique to the burned patient will be pointed out.

One of the initial responsibilities of the physician is to stop the burning process. Burning has usually stopped before the patient's arrival in the emergency ward, but occasionally, bits of smouldering clothing are still attached to the skin. The glowing fiber is extremely hot and must be removed to prevent further injury.

For clarity of presentation, the emergency care of the burned patient has been divided into the following topics:

(1) determination of the cause of the burn;

(2) determination of the extent and depth of the burn;

(3) evaluation of the patient's general health status and the presence or absence of coexistent injuries;

(4) determination of the need for hospitalization;

(5) initiation of the necessary resuscitative measures, including fluid replacement, respiratory care, and general treatment;

(6) initiation of burn wound care.

By no means should the order of presentation of this material be interpreted as implying priorities. In fact, in the actual care of the burned patient, many different aspects of management can and should be carried out simultaneously.

Electrical burns, chemical burns, and frostbite are discussed separately at the end of the chapter.

ETIOLOGY

Many agents can cause burns. These include ultraviolet light, scalding liquids and steam, flash explosions, flame, electricity, and certain chemicals. Most burns necessitating hospital admission result from flash or flame injury, whereas many of the more minor burns not requiring admission result from contact with scalding material or hot metal.

The causative agent is important because it often suggests the depth of the burn and the presence of coexistent injuries. For instance, a scald due to a hot liquid most often will be a partial-thickness burn that is not associated with other lesions. On the other hand, a flame injury sustained in a closed space will most likely be a full-thickness burn that is probably accompanied by respiratory injury.

As many details as possible about the accident should be obtained. The time that the burn occurred as well as any previous treatment should be noted.

EXTENT AND DEPTH OF THE BURN

Knowledge of the extent of the body surface involved and the depth of the burn is necessary to determine the prognosis, the need for hospitalization, the resuscitative measures indicated, and the proper treatment of the burn wound.

The "rule of nines" (Table 28.1), which is probably the simplest method for determining the body surface area burned in an adult patient, divides the surfaces of the body into units that are multiples of nine. By determining the portion of each unit involved, the examiner quickly can estimate the body surface area burned. Since the percentage of the body surface area represented by the different anatomic units varies with age, a different system is needed for infants and children. The "rule of fives" (Table 28.2) is a reasonably accurate system that is similar to the rule of nines in design and use except that each of the body units is a multiple of five.

In discussions of the burn wound, the terms first-, second-, and third-degree burn are used to indicate the depth of injury to the skin. The terms partial-thickness burn and full-thickness burn are used interchangeably with second-degree burn

and third-degree burn, respectively. All full-thickness burns and some partial-thickness burns will require skin grafting for definitive wound closure. Although no completely reliable method exists for determining the depth of a burn in the emergency ward, there are many clues available. The most helpful diagnostic considerations are the type of burning agent, the appearance of the burn, and the presence or absence of sensation. The relationships of these factors to the depth of the burn are outlined in Table 28.3.

All this information should be recorded accurately and completely. This is most readily done and the information most easily interpreted at a later time if a diagram is used (Fig. 28.1).

GENERAL EVALUATION

All pertinent information should be gathered, including the patient's age and weight, allergies to drugs, medications being taken, tetanus immunization status, and acute or chronic medical illnesses. A rapid but thorough physical examination should include the recording of pulse rate, blood pressure, respiration rate, temperature, and level of consciousness. Examination of the internal nares for singed vibrissae and the posterior oropharynx for soot may suggest an inhalation respiratory injury. Judicious use of a laryngoscope is helpful in examining the pharynx.

The physician should examine the patient carefully for other trauma sustained at the time of the burn injury; coexistent injuries are not at all uncommon, but often are missed. Respiratory damage and long bone fractures occur frequently, but central nervous system, chest, and abdominal trauma may also occur. These injuries must be sought and given appropriate priority in treatment.

In the more seriously burned patient requiring hospitalization, the following laboratory and x-ray studies are necessary: complete blood cell count; urinalysis; measurement of serum electrolytes, blood urea nitrogen, and serum proteins; prothrombin time; typing and crossmatching of blood; and chest x-ray films.

When the history and physical examination suggest the presence of concomitant disease or injury, the following tests may be indicated: liver chemistries; measurement of serum creatinine and blood glucose; stool guaiac test; arterial blood-gas analysis; skull, facial, long bone, and abdominal x-ray films; and an electrocardiogram.

NEED FOR HOSPITALIZATION

The decision to hospitalize a patient is based on many factors, including age, concomitant disease

Table 28.1.
Rule of nines: rapid means of estimating body surface area burned in adult patients.

Area	Percent
Head and neck	9
Arm	
Right	9
Left	9
Torso	
Front	18
Back	18
Leg	
Right	18
Left	18
Genitals and perineum	1
Total	100

Table 28.2.
Rule of fives: rapid means of estimating body surface area burned in infants and children.

Area	Infant	Child
	%	
Head and neck	20	15
Arm		
Right	10	10
Left	10	10
Torso		
Front	20	20
Back	20	20
Leg		
Right	10	15
Left	10	15
Totals	100	105

Table 28.3.
Depth of burn injury.

Depth or Classification	Structural Damage	Causal Agent	Clinical Appearance	Sensation
First-degree	Only superficial layers of epidermis devitalized; dilation of intradermal vessels	Ultraviolet exposure Very short flash	Erythema; blanches with pressure	Present
Second-degree (partial-thickness)	Destruction of epidermis to basal layer; deeper skin appendages preserved in dermal layer; clefting of epidermis with fluid collection	Spillage of scalding material Flash Some chemicals	Blister formation, erythema, weeping; superficial skin can be wiped away; erythematous areas should blanch with pressure	Present
Third-degree (full-thickness)	Destruction of all skin elements, epidermal and dermal; coagulation of subdermal blood vessels	Flame Immersion Some chemicals	Dry, pale white, charred, leathery, inelastic, visible thrombosed vessels; sometimes red from fixed hemoglobin and will not blanch	Absent
Fourth-degree (involvement of muscle, bone, and other deep structures)	Destruction of all skin elements along with necrosis of deeper structures	Electricity Flame occasionally	Deeply charred, shrunken, often with exposed bones; explosive appearing	Absent

or injury, and most importantly, the extent, depth, and location of the burn. Although each case differs, certain guidelines for admission have been found helpful (Table 28.4). In addition, all patients suspected of having an inhalation injury and patients with small burns but with other associated severe injuries should be admitted.

RESUSCITATIVE MEASURES
Prevention of Shock

In patients requiring hospitalization because of the extent of the burn injury, the accumulation of edema fluid (water, crystalloid, and protein) in the burn wound is of such magnitude that if it goes untreated hypovolemic shock will occur. Classically, burn wound edema has been thought to develop progressively during the first 48 hours after injury, but more recent evidence suggests that the accumulation of edema fluid is complete within 24 hours. Fluid replacement should begin immediately. Most methods of determining the initial fluid requirement are based on the patient's body weight and the percent of the body surface area burned. The most commonly used formulas for fluid replacement are the Brooke, Evans, and Baxter formulas (Table 28.5). It is standard not to use a figure greater than 50% body surface area in these formulas even though the actual percentage may be higher.

It is important to realize that these formulas should be used only as a guide to begin fluid replacement. Alterations in the rate of fluid administration must be made frequently, depending on the adequacy of treatment as determined by careful monitoring of the following: (1) urinary output (40–60/ml/hr in the adult) and specific gravity; (2) vital signs (blood pressure, pulse rate, and respiration rate); (3) central venous pressure; and (4) hematocrit (a minor degree of hemoconcentration is acceptable). Two intravenous catheters should be placed, one with its tip centrally located so that central venous pressure may be determined. No indwelling venous catheters should be inserted in lower extremity veins because of the high incidence of resultant thrombophlebitis. An indwelling urinary catheter should be inserted to allow recording of urinary output. These variables are all easily monitored and should carefully be recorded every half-hour or every hour. Changes will suggest the need for altering the rate of fluid administration. The use of flow sheets (Figs. 28.2 and 28.3) allows these decisions to be made more rapidly and more accurately. In patients with more serious burns and in those with coexistent cardiac or pulmonary disease or injury, monitoring of the arterial blood gases (P_{O_2}, P_{CO_2}, and pH) can be helpful (Fig. 27.2).

Date Burned _____ —

Date of Evaluation _____ —

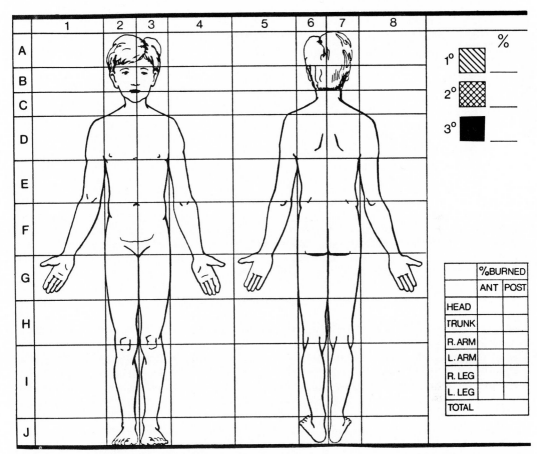

Figure 28.1. Burn diagram. This allows quick, accurate, and reproducible recording of surface area and depth of burn; it should become a permanent part of the patient's record.

Inhalation Injury (see also Chapter 22, pages 498–499)

Injury to the respiratory tract is one of the most dangerous and most frequent complications of burns and is the leading cause of death in fire victims. More than one-half of the 12,000 annual fire deaths in the United States are caused by inhalation injury. There are three kinds of inhalation injury: upper airway damage, pulmonary parenchymal injury, and carbon monoxide poisoning.

Upper airway and laryngeal edema result from the inhalation of hot gases and the irritating chemicals in smoke. The tissue damage caused by these agents leads to upper airway edema and laryngeal spasm and edema usually within 3–6 hours after

Table 28.4.
Admission guidelines for burned patients.

Age	Burn Depth	Body Surface
<10 yr >65 yr	Second-degree	10% or more
10–65 yr	Second-degree	20% or more
All ages	Third-degree	>5%[a]
All ages	Deep second- or third-degree	Face, perineum, hands, or feet

[a] In many cases, these patients are best treated with primary excision and grafting of the burn wound.

injury. Increasing hoarseness, inability to swallow secretions, and an increased respiration rate are signs of impending upper airway obstruction.

On examination, burns of the face or neck,

Table 28.5.
Fluid replacement formulas for first 24 hours.

Source	Colloid	Electrolyte Solution	Water	Rate
			ml	
Brooke[a]	0.5 ml/kg/% BSA burned	1.5 ml/kg/% BSA burned	2000	¹/₂ first 8 hr
				¹/₄ second 8 hr
				¹/₄ third 8 hr
Evans[a]	1 ml/kg/% BSA burned	1 ml/kg/% BSA burned	2000	¹/₂ first 8 hr
				¹/₄ second 8 hr
				¹/₄ third 8 hr
Baxter[b]		4 ml/kg/% BSA burned		¹/₂ first 8 hr
				¹/₄ second 8 hr
				¹/₄ third 8 hr

BSA = body surface area.
[a] Approximately one-half the amount estimated for the first 24 hours is given the second 24 hours.
[b] Only maintenance fluids are given the second 24 hours; colloid is given as necessary.

singed nasal hairs, inflamed or swollen posterior pharyngeal mucosa, and edema of the glottis suggest potential airway difficulty. Such patients should be considered for immediate endotracheal intubation. If the airway edema has progressed too far, intubation may be impossible, and tracheotomy will be necessary. Humidified air should be provided through the endotracheal tube.

Pulmonary parenchymal injury should be suspected with a history of fire in a closed space (the fire being associated with copious smoke production), and if other victims of the same fire have inhalation injury. The same irritating chemicals (aldehydes and nitrates in wood smoke, cyanides and phosgene in smoke from synthetic materials) that cause airway damage are toxic to the pulmonary parenchyma and may lead to necrotizing bronchiolitis, intraalveolar edema, and hyaline membrane formation. Soot particles in the sputum and an elevated carboxyhemoglobin concentration warn of possible pulmonary injury. The injury produces the pathophysiologic changes seen with bronchopneumonia. These changes usually are not manifest for 12–24 or as much as 48 hours. The patient may then have an increased respiration rate, auscultatory signs of bronchospasm, a chest x-ray appearance compatible with congestion and edema or bronchopneumonia, and a falling arterial Po_2. The chest x-ray signs usually lag behind the clinical signs. Early fiberoptic bronchoscopic examination is helpful in determining the extent of the damage to the lower part of the airway. Patients with this injury are treated for its complications, namely, hypoxemia and infection. Corticosteroids to be effective must be administered within the first hour; prophylactic antibiotics are not recommended. Careful monitoring of fluid administration to prevent pulmonary overload is especially important.

Carbon monoxide poisoning, the most common single cause of death in burn victims, is separate from upper airway or pulmonary injury in its pathophysiology. Carbon monoxide is a colorless, odorless, tasteless, nonirritating gas liberated from incomplete combustion of carbon compounds. Carbon monoxide combines with hemoglobin to form carboxyhemoglobin. The affinity of hemoglobin for carbon monoxide is approximately 250 times greater than its affinity for oxygen and, therefore, even a small amount of carbon monoxide in the atmosphere successfully competes with oxygen for the binding sites of hemoglobin. The resultant carboxyhemoglobin besides rendering the patient functionally anemic, shifts the oxyhemoglobin dissociation curve to the left, making the patient even more hypoxic. Death is due to hypoxia, hypercapnia, and acidosis.

Carbon monoxide poisoning is suggested by any of the signs associated with inhalation injury, but can be confirmed by determining the level of carboxyhemoglobin in an arterial or venous blood sample. A carboxyhemoglobin level from 15–25% suggests mild carbon monoxide poisoning. A level greater than 25% suggests serious poisoning, especially if the injury occurred more than 1 hour before testing. Patients with mild poisoning are treated with oxygen administered by face mask. Those with serious poisoning are intubated and placed on assisted ventilation with 100% oxygen. Administration of 100% oxygen is continued for several hours until the carboxyhemoglobin level is below 10%.

General Treatment

Most burned patients requiring hospitalization have some degree of reflex ileus. Oral feedings of both liquids and solids should be withheld until proper function of the gastrointestinal tract has

PERMANENT RECORD COPY
MASSACHUSETTS GENERAL HOSPITAL

CRITICAL CARE DATA SHEET

#	Time	Conditions (spont/Vent type/O2 Flow)	FiO2	pO2	pCO2	pH	Na	K	Hct.	TP	OSM	C.I.	O2 Cont.	VENTILATION TV	RR	IP	PEEP
1																	
2																	
3																	
4																	
5																	
6																	
7																	
8																	
9																	
10																	
11																	
12																	
13																	
14																	
15																	
16																	
17																	
18																	

BLEEDING STUDIES						RENAL							
Time	PT	PTT	Plats.	Fibrin	Other	Time	Na	K	OSM	BUN	Creat.	pH	Analysis/Other

X-Rays Results	Miscellaneous	
Time	Time	Result

Figure 28.2. Critical care data sheet. A flow sheet like this to record electrolytes, arterial blood gases, and hematocrit in early resuscitative phase facilitates interpretation of data. This should be readily available at bedside.

		FLUID INTAKE							OUTPUT				
DATE	HOUR INTERVAL	TOTAL	PLASMA	WHOLE BLOOD	SALINE SOLS. IV	SALINE SOLS. PO*	OTHER FLUIDS IV	OTHER FLUIDS PO*	TOTAL	URINE Vol.	URINE S.G.	VOM-ITUS	DIARRHEA	EXUDATE
	m to m													
	m to m													
	m to m													
	m to m													
	m to m													
	m to m													
	m to m													
	m to m													
	m to m													
	m to m													
	m to m													
	m to m													
12 hour total														
24 hour total														

DATE OF BURN:
HOUR OF BURN (H.B.):
DATE OF ENTRY:
HOUR OF ENTRY:
NAME
UNIT NO.

* SALINE SOLS. = any fluid containing salt.
* OTHER FLUIDS = fluids which do not contain salt, such as milk, fruit juices, broth not containing salt, bottled beverages, tea, coffee.

Figure 28.3. Fluid balance sheet. Knowledge of exact intake and output is critical to management of the acutely burned patient. A flow sheet such as this should be used and be readily available at bedside.

returned. This could take only 1–2 hours or as long as several days.

In severely burned patients and in patients whose level of consciousness is altered, insertion of an indwelling nasogastric tube for immediate gastric emptying and constant suction drainage is indicated to prevent regurgitation and vomiting with possible aspiration. This is especially important if the patient is to be transported to another hospital or to a different area in the same hospital.

Most burned patients have some discomfort and apprehension requiring analgesia and sedation. It must be remembered that agitation may be a sign of cerebral hypoxia, not of discomfort, and medication might only aggravate the situation. When sedation and analgesia are necessary in the hospitalized patient, a small dose of morphine sulfate, 1–3 mg intravenously, is usually satisfactory. The oral, subcutaneous, or intramuscular route should not be used, since absorption cannot be predicted. On an outpatient basis, oral analgesics and sedatives can be given safely.

A standard set of admission orders should be established for burned patients requiring hospitalization (Table 28.6).

Table 28.6.
Typical admission orders for burned patients requiring hospitalization.

Nothing by mouth
Intake and output every hour (record)
Vital signs every hour (record)
Urinary output and specific gravity every hour (record)
Central venous pressure every hour (record)
Fluid orders (Brooke, Evans, or Baxter formula)
Wound care specifics
Nasogastric tube, gravity or low suction (record output)
Humidified oxygen by face mask
Aqueous penicillin, 600,000 units intravenously twice a day for 48 hr
Morphine sulfate, 1 mg/15 kg body weight intravenously every 3 hours as needed
Wound care
Daily weight

BURN WOUND CARE
Cleansing and Débridement

Most burns require little cleansing and débridement. Blisters should be left intact. Adherent clothing, dirt, and other foreign material should be removed. A mild nondetergent soap and warm water rinse may be helpful; strong detergent soaps and those containing hexachlorophene should be avoided.

Sterile precautions should be taken when burn wounds are handled. A cap, mask, sterile gown, and sterile gloves should be worn. Wound specimens for culture should be taken before initiating topical treatment. The burned areas should be elevated several centimeters above heart level if possible.

Specific Wound Care and Topical Agents

First-Degree Burns

Most of these injuries result from excessive exposure to the ultraviolet rays of the sun or a sunlamp. Topical and oral analgesics are usually all that is necessary. Occasionally, in patients with very extensive sunburn, significant edema develops, together with malaise, easy fatigability, anorexia, and nausea. Except in very young and very old patients, this situation can still safely be managed on an outpatient basis.

These patients must be examined carefully for ocular injuries and ophthalmologic consultation should be obtained as indicated.

Second-Degree Burns

Most isolated partial-thickness or second-degree burns result from scalding. Although immediate immersion of the burn in cold water is effective in limiting the depth of the injury and in controlling edema, immersion is of little benefit after the first few minutes except to relieve pain. Since most patients arrive in the emergency ward several minutes to several hours after the injury, immersion is probably not indicated.

Both open and closed methods of treatment are acceptable, but for reasons of comfort and convenience the closed method is preferable. This is especially true for outpatients. Dressings should be applied under sterile conditions. A single layer of nonadherent fine-mesh gauze placed immediately next to the wound should be covered by several layers of multiple-ply, coarse-mesh gauze without cotton filling. This is then secured by an elastic wrap or bias stockinette applied firmly but not tightly. The dressing should be changed under sterile conditions every 4–5 days. Temperature elevation above 100.4–101.3°F (38–38.5°C), purulent drainage, and other signs of infection are reasons for more frequent dressing changes.

The burned parts should be immobilized and kept elevated, if possible, with bed rest for lower-extremity burns, an arm sling for upper-extremity burns, and elevation of the head of the bed for head and neck burns. If the hand is burned, it should be splinted with the wrist extended, the metacarpophalangeal joints flexed, and the interphalangeal joints extended. After the dressing has been applied, a plaster or isoprene splint should be molded and secured to the burned hand (Fig. 28.4). At each dressing change, the joints of the hand should be put through active and passive range-of-motion exercises. As soon as the wound is healed, which usually requires less than 2 weeks, the splint is discarded.

Partial-thickness burns of the face and neck often are treated more easily by the open technique, since bulky dressings are difficult to manage around the eyes, nose, and mouth. In the open method, the wound should be rinsed gently twice a day with sterile physiologic saline solution, followed by application of an antibiotic ointment such as bacitracin, neomycin, or polymyxin B.

Partial-thickness burns should heal spontaneously. Depending on the depth of the burn, it may take from 5 days to 3 weeks for a complete epithelial cover to develop. Dressings should be continued throughout this period. Table 28.7 summarizes the outpatient management of partial-thickness scalds.

Patients with partial-thickness burns in combination with full-thickness burns are best treated with the technique used for the latter (see below).

Third-Degree Burns

Most full-thickness burns result from flame injury or immersion in a hot liquid. Unless the wound is very small, these patients require hospitalization. The emergency ward treatment of such patients is summarized in Table 28.8.

During the past few years, several topical agents have been developed that decrease bacterial proliferation in the burn wound and thereby prevent some secondary septic complications. These agents have been most beneficial in increasing survival in those patients with full-thickness burns covering 40–60% of the body surface area, but they are routinely used in all full-thickness burn injuries. The four most common agents are 0.5% silver nitrate solution, 10% mafenide acetate cream (Sulfamylon), 1% silver sulfadiazine cream (Silvadene), and povidone-iodine ointment (Betadine). Techniques of application, advantages, and disadvantages of these four agents are given in Table 28.9. No one agent is clearly superior to the others,

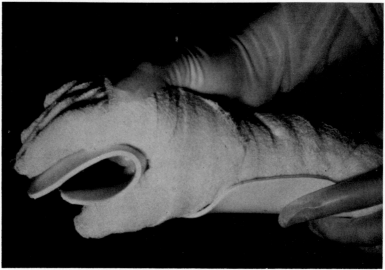

Figure 28.4. Isoprene splint for hand and forearm is depicted with wrist extended, metacarpophalangeal joints flexed, and interphalangeal joints extended. This facilitates return of good function.

Table 28.7.
Outpatient management of partial-thickness scald.

Historical and physical findings related to burn
    injury
    Cause
    Time
    Pictorial description of extent and depth of burn
    Related injuries
Pertinent past medical history
    Chronic illnesses
    Medications
    Allergies
    Status of tetanus prophylaxis
Sterile burn wound care
    Minimal cleansing and débridement; blisters are
      left intact
    Application of dressing
    Elevation of burned parts; splints
    Dressing change in 4–5 days
Tetanus prophylaxis
Low-dose penicillin therapy for 5 days

and which is used should be determined by familiarity and availability. The agents should be applied as soon as possible after cleansing the wound, and the patient should be covered with sterile sheets to maintain sterility and to provide warmth.

The concept of early or primary burn wound excision that is applied to the management of small, full-thickness burns has been expanded to include more extensive full-thickness burns as well. Reports indicate that this can decrease morbidity, mortality, and length of hospitalization. This does not change the initial wound care that is necessary in the emergency ward, however.

Escharotomy

In circumferential full-thickness burns of the extremities or torso, escharotomy may become an urgent necessity. The constriction resulting from this type of burn injury can lead to circulatory compromise in the extremities, manifested by peripheral cyanosis, edema, and later ischemic changes that are limb-threatening if not treated adequately and promptly. Circulation in the hands and feet should be assessed every few hours by feeling for peripheral pulses, observing capillary refill, and if possible, checking arterial pulse volumes and flows with Doppler recorders.

A circumferential burn of the thorax associated with an inelastic eschar can seriously limit respiratory motion, increase the work of breathing, and lead to respiratory failure, manifested by rapid and labored respirations, cyanosis, irritability, and inability to ventilate even after intubation and ventilatory support. Although escharotomy rarely requires anesthesia, since the eschar is insensate, it is best performed in the operating room where adequate sterility, lighting, instruments, and assistance are available.

Tetanus Prophylaxis

All partial-thickness and complete-thickness burns result in necrotic tissue. Under these conditions, the possibility of tetanus exists, and although this disease is rare, adequate prophylaxis should be carried out (see Table 11.6), since tetanus in the burned patient is almost always fatal. Toxoid booster injections should be given to those already

Table 28.8.

Emergency ward treatment of partial-thickness and full-thickness flame burns requiring hospitalization.

Initiate any emergency airway measures necessary
  Humidified oxygen
  Be alert for respiratory distress and treat appropriately
Elicit historical and physical findings related to burn injury
  Cause
  Time
  Prior treatment
  Pictorial description of extent and depth of burn
  Related injuries
Elicit pertinent past medical history
  Chronic illnesses
  Medications
  Allergies
  Status of tetanus prophylaxis
Obtain necessary laboratory and radiologic studies
Insert the following catheters:
  Intravenous
  Central venous pressure
  Indwelling urinary
  Nasogastric
Initiate fluid replacement with electrolyte-containing solution
Calculate expected fluid requirements
Start flow sheet of vital data
Begin local wound care
Administer tetanus prophylaxis
Give first dose in penicillin therapy

immunized; injections for passive immunization must be given to those without a previous history of active immunization, and must be repeated during the course of treatment.

Systemic Antibiotic Therapy

Although the most common cause of morbidity and mortality in burned patients is infection, the intensive use of systemic antibiotic prophylaxis has been ineffective in decreasing the incidence of invasive sepsis. During the first few days after a burn injury, the eschar seems to be a barrier to invasive organisms, except for the virulent β-hemolytic streptococcus. Since this organism is so common in the upper part of the respiratory tract, especially in children, routine low-dose penicillin prophylaxis is indicated. Usually, 600,000 units of penicillin G twice a day for 2 days is sufficient.

ELECTRICAL BURNS

Although electrical burns are truly thermal injuries since they result from the conversion of electrical energy to thermal energy, they often differ in their presentation and treatment sufficiently to require separate consideration. For descriptive and clinical purposes, these injuries are usually divided into those of high voltage (more than 1000 volts) and low voltage (fewer than 1000 volts) and into flash injuries and actual contact or arc injuries.

Table 28.9.

Comparison of available topical agents for burn management.

Agent	Technique of Application	Advantages	Disadvantages
0.5% silver nitrate solution	2.5 cm thick coarse-mesh gauze dressing soaked every 2 hr with solution; dressing changed every 12 hr	Only minimal pain with application; occlusive dressing comfortable; decreased evaporative losses; easily used in grafted and ungrafted areas	Delays eschar separation; electrolyte abnormalities—hyponatremia, hypokalemia, hypocalcemia; discolors everything; does not penetrate eschar
10% mafenide acetate cream (Sulfamylon)	Apply every 24 hr and replenish as needed; dressing usually not used	Penetrates eschar; easy to apply; nonstaining	Acidosis; burning pain with application; delays eschar separation; sensitivity reactions (10–15%); inhibits epithelialization
1% silver sulfadiazine cream	Apply every 12 hr and replenish as needed; dressing of fine-mesh gauze may be used	Easy to apply; nonstaining; minimal pain; no electrolyte or acid-base problems	Does not penetrate eschar well; delays eschar separation; occasional suppression of white blood cell count
Povidone-iodine ointment (Betadine)	Apply every 8 hr; dressing of fine-mesh gauze usually used	Easy to apply; minimal pain	Increases serum iodine levels; occasional burning pain; delays eschar separation

Flash burns result from the heat generated by a nearby electrical flash or "explosion." The current of electricity does not contact or arc to the body surface. In low-voltage flash burns the injury is usually a first- or second-degree burn. The skin surface may appear charred, but this blackening of the epidermis resulting from the explosion usually is cleansed away easily. High-voltage flash burns can lead to more extensive second- and third-degree burns, which should be managed like any other second- or third-degree burn.

It is the actual contact or arc electrical burn that results in a different type of injury. The lesion is almost always full-thickness or greater, and in high-voltage injuries, damage to muscle, blood vessels, nerves, tendons, fat, and bone commonly occurs. The proportions of the deep wound and necrosis in high-voltage injuries are often much more extensive than the surface necrosis might indicate; this can be suggested by signs of ischemia, cyanosis, edema, and anesthesia in a limb. Whereas high-voltage contact or arc injuries are extensive, low-voltage burns are usually localized. A common low-voltage arc injury in small children is the full-thickness lesion of the oral commissure or lip sustained when a child chews through an electrical cord or sucks on an extension cord outlet (110-volt household current). This injury is discussed more fully in Chapter 29, page 648.

Much of the discussion on the emergency evaluation and treatment of the more usual thermal burns applies to electrical burns as well. In addition, the following should be noted:

(1) The voltage of the current contacted and the points of entrance and exit should be determined. These two areas are usually the most extensively damaged, since the current accumulates at these points. If these two points are known, the approximate pathway of most of the current can be established.

(2) Early fasciotomy of the extremities is often necessary, since intense muscular swelling in confined fascial compartments occurs. This is an operating room procedure, but impending ischemia of the limb should be sought carefully in the emergency ward.

(3) Because these burn injuries are often deep, the usual topical methods of treatment are inadequate. Surgical débridement is necessary; however, these wounds can be dressed temporarily in the emergency ward under sterile conditions with one of the topical agents mentioned earlier.

(4) Myoglobinemia and severe acidosis commonly occur as a result of extensive muscle damage. If these are inadequately treated, renal failure quickly results. Treatment depends on recognition

and careful monitoring. Myoglobin manifests itself by imparting a port-wine color to the urine. Laboratory tests are available for confirmation, but are rarely necessary. Acidosis is best diagnosed and monitored by means of arterial blood-gas determinations. For this, an indwelling arterial line is helpful. Treatment is based on adequate hydration to maintain a good urinary output and alkalinization of the serum and urine. Vital signs should be monitored to prevent overhydration and pulmonary edema. Enough electrolyte-containing solution should be given to maintain a urinary output of 100 ml/hr or greater. Sodium bicarbonate should be added to the intravenous solutions in sufficient amounts to keep the urine alkaline and the serum pH within the normal range. Myoglobin casts cannot precipitate so readily if the urinary output through the renal tubules is rapid and alkaline.

(5) Damage to internal organs has been reported; when the entrance and exit points suggest a pathway through the thoracic or abdominal cavity, the area must be evaluated carefully to rule out the possibility of internal injuries.

(6) Myocardial damage can result from high-voltage electrical injuries. In its most severe form, immediate ventricular fibrillation and death occur. An electrocardiogram should be obtained immediately on arrival of the patient in the emergency ward. The myocardial injury can be an infarct or an arrhythmia, and should be treated accordingly.

(7) Late development of cataracts and neurologic sequelae has been reported, and initial examination should note the status of the eyes and nervous system. Proper consultation should be obtained as indicated.

(8) Because of the violent muscle contractions that occur with high-voltage contact and the frequency of an associated fall, long bones are sometimes fractured.

(9) Damage to the spinal cord may occur and may not be apparent on initial examination. A demyelinating lesion may develop. Since this injury can be progressive, daily neurologic assessment is necessary.

CHEMICAL BURNS

These injuries, which are infrequent, may result from contact with a wide variety of chemical agents. The degree of injury depends on the chemical, its concentration, duration of contact, and the natural penetrability and resistance of the tissues involved. Chemicals do not usually "burn" in that they do not cause destruction by hyperthermic activity. Rather, they damage tissue by causing

Table 28.10.
Methods of treatment for "burns" from chemical agents.

Employ water lavage		Special methods
Chromic acid	Na metal	—excision
Potassium permanganate	Lyes	—weak acid lavage
Cantharides	Hydrofluoric acid	—boric acid or $NaHCO_3$ wash
Dimethyl sulfoxide	Chromic acid	—dilute Na hyposulfite wash
Lyes	Chlorox	—milk, eggwhite, starch paste, or
KOH		1% Na thiosulfate
NaOH	Phenol (cresol)	—avoid alcohol
NH_4OH	White phosphorus	—1:5000 $KMNO_4$ or 2% $Cu(SO_4)$
LiOH	Dichromate salts	—(a) 2% hyposulfite wash
$Ba(OH)_2$		(b) monobasic/dibasic K-Na
$Ca(OH)_2$		HPO_4 solution 7%/18% in wa-
Chlorox		ter buffer wash
Phenol (cresol)	Alkyl mercury agents	—debride and remove blister fluid
Dichromate salts	Lewisite	—British anti-Lewisite
Tungstic acid	H_2SO_4,HCL (muriatic acid)	—soda lime, soap as magnesium
Picric acid		hydroxide washers
Tannic acid		
Sulfosalicylic acid		
Trichloroacetic acid	Avoid oils	
Cresylic acid	Cantharides	
Acetic acid		
Formic acid	Avoid water lavage	
	Na metal	
Give calcium salts	H_2SO_4	
Oxalic acid	HCL (muriatic acid)	
Hydrofluoric acid		
Cover with oil		
Na metal		
Phenol (cresol)		
White phosphorus		
Mustard gas		

(Reprinted by permission from Jelenko C III: Chemicals that "burn." *J Trauma 14:* 65–72, 1974.)

coagulation of protein by one of several processes—reduction, oxidation, desiccation, corro-
sion, or vesication.

It is important to determine which chemical
agent has caused the injury, since treatment varies
(Table 28.10). The immediate treatment for most
chemical burns is irrigation of the surface with
copious amounts of water to dilute and to remove
the offending agent. Standing in a shower or holding the injured part under a water spigot is the
easiest means of doing this. If the eyes are involved, they should be irrigated with copious
amounts of sterile physiologic saline solution or
water and ophthalmologic consultation obtained.

In injuries resulting from some chemical agents,
water lavage is contraindicated, since it will cause
additional ionization, heat, and further damage.
In these few cases, neutralization with the appropriate agent is indicated (Table 28.10).

Of special interest are those injuries caused by
hydrofluoric acid, commonly used in the semicon-
ductor industry and in rust-removing agents, as
well as for etching glass. The fluoride ion is more
harmful than the hydrogen ion and tends to penetrate deeply, causing necrosis and painful ulceration unless neutralized. The best method of neutralization is direct injection of 10% calcium gluconate solution into the involved areas. This often
immediately relieves the pain.

Once the initial stage of treatment is completed,
be it irrigation, neutralization, or other means,
further wound management depends on the degree
of injury and does not differ from the management
of burns caused by the more usual agents.

COLD INJURY

There are basically two kinds of cold injury,
hypothermia and cold-induced tissue injury. The
three categories of tissue injury are frostbite, trench
foot, and immersion foot. Hypothermia may be
associated with tissue injury and vice versa. Hypothermia is also discussed in Chapter 10.

Hypothermia

Accidental hypothermia, whether from exposure to cold air or cold water, reflects an imbalance between the heat produced by the body and the heat lost from it. By adjusting rates of heat production and heat loss, humans maintain a stable core body temperature range for optimal enzyme functioning. For example, for each centigrade degree of temperature drop, biochemical activity decreases about 10%. The normal core body temperature is in a narrow range from 97.5–99.5°F (36.4–37.5°C). Heat may be convected, conducted, and radiated from the body surface and released by evaporation of sweat. Control of the environment and use of protective clothing is the major defense against heat loss. Physiologic adjustments to protect against loss of body heat include exercise, shivering, basal thermogenesis under the control of the hypothalamus, and peripheral vasoconstriction. For example, shivering can increase the basal metabolic rate 4–5 times that of normal.

There are three types of accidental hypothermia: acute, subacute, and chronic. An individual who is plunged into cold water that causes his core body temperature to decrease swiftly experiences *acute* immersion hypothermia. A person exposed much of the night to snow or rain in the cold with insufficient clothing or shelter to maintain body core temperature may suffer from *subacute* hypothermia. *Chronic* hypothermia, in which cooling occurs over several days, is usually the result of drugs, disease, or failure of the body's temperature-regulating mechanism, perhaps combined with age that causes a slow but nonetheless potentially lethal cooling. This might occur indoors without the individual's ever leaving his living quarters if room temperatures are lower than the person can safely tolerate. Patients with chronic hypothermia almost always have some associated serious disease.

Accidental hypothermia is defined as the pathologic state occurring after core body temperature is reduced below 95°F (35°C) as a result of accidental cold stress. With continued stress the condition may be progressive and fatal unless body temperature is restored and concomitant metabolic aberrations are corrected. The diagnosis is made by taking a rectal temperature reading with a low-reading thermometer. Axillary and oral temperatures are misleading. With the rectal temperature below 95°F (35°C), shivering and vasoconstriction become intense, and the patient loses manual dexterity but is still relatively well oriented. At this stage, hypothermia is easily reversible. Below

89.6°F (32°C), hypothermia becomes severe; shivering is replaced by marked muscular rigidity and stiff movement. The patient is obtunded and is progressing to full stupor. The blood pressure may not be detectable, but a strong carotid or femoral pulse can be palpated. Breathing becomes shallow and irregular and the heart rate begins to slow. Below 80.6°F (27°C), hypothermia is profound with deep coma and rigidity. Pulmonary edema can occur and there is great risk of ventricular arrhythmia.

The most devastating effect of hypothermia occurs when the core temperature drops below 77°F (25°C). Below this temperature, ventricular fibrillation usually develops, and as the temperature gets below 68°F (20°C), asystole occurs. If hypothermia is acute, there may be only relatively mild associated acidosis. If it is chronic, more serious acidosis may accompany cardiac arrest.

As soon as hypothermia is recognized, action must be taken to prevent further cooling. Wet clothing is removed and the patient is placed in a dry blanket. Rewarming should begin as soon as possible, but only in facilities where medical resources are available to deal with resultant complications. This is especially true for patients with severe and profound hypothermia. Individuals with mild hypothermia can have external heat sources applied, (such as the bodies of warm companions), can be given hot drinks, and can be encouraged to do isometric exercises.

In the rewarming of patients with severe or profound hypothermia, it is important, if possible, to warm the core of the body before the periphery. If the periphery of the body is warmed first (as when a patient is immersed in warm water), peripheral vasodilation quickly occurs, allowing the previously trapped cool blood to return centrally and causing the core body temperature to decrease further. This leads to rewarming shock, in which the supercooled heart cannot return the amount of blood that the rewarmed skin demands. The most effective way of rewarming the patient's body core is to use peritoneal, gastric, or colonic lavage. Peritoneal lavage is carried out by insertion of a catheter and use of isotonic peritoneal dialysate heated by a blood-warming coil to 95–98.6°F (35–37°C). Every 20–30 minutes, 2 liters of dialysate are exchanged with the object of raising the rectal temperature above 86°F (30°C) as soon as possible to avoid refractory ventricular fibrillation. At the same time, an endotracheal tube should be inserted to protect the airway since vomiting may ensue with central rewarming. Once the rectal temperature exceeds 86°F (30°C), a hypothermia pad or warm-water bath can be used to raise the temperature more slowly. The patient will require an infusion of saline solution to support blood pressure as the periphery becomes rewarmed. Furthermore, any associated acidosis should be corrected carefully, and overcorrection with resultant alkalosis should be avoided. There are many case reports of patients with profound hypothermia and cardiac arrest who have been successfully treated with prolonged cardiopulmonary resuscitation and rewarming.

Frostbite

In the United States, most cases of frostbite occur in persons who have become comatose from injury or alcohol. Except in rare instances, frostbite is restricted to the extremities of the body or to areas such as the chin, cheeks, nose, and ears. The severity of injury is influenced by the intensity of the initial exposure (that is, type and duration of contact) and the length of time before adequate circulation is restored.

Two types of reaction occur when tissue comes in contact with cold. First, the superficial tissue at the site of contact freezes to a depth dependent on the degree of cold and the duration of contact. With freezing, ice crystals grow between cells, and if the source of cold is not removed, the crystals continue to grow, dehydrating and severely damaging the adjacent cells. Intense freezing causes crystals to form within the cells, damaging them immediately.

Second, arteriolar vasocontriction occurs in the tissue adjacent to the frozen layer, rapidly reducing the blood flow in this zone. With arteriolar constriction, shunts occur that allow blood to bypass the affected capillary bed, and if the source of cold is not removed, the whole area begins to freeze.

The following retrospective classification designed by the United States Army during the Korean War divides frostbite injury into four stages: (1) erythema and edema with no blister formation; (2) erythema and edema with blisters; (3) full-thickness injury with gangrene and no loss of part; and (4) complete necrosis with loss of part. This classification is useful in reporting frostbite injuries, but it is more helpful to the clinician to divide frostbite injuries into superficial and deep, before the injured part has been thawed.

Superficial frostbite involves only the skin or the tissues immediately beneath it. The frozen part is white and firm on the exterior, but soft and resilient below the surface when depressed gently and firmly. After rewarming, the frostbitten area

will first become numb and mottled blue or purple; it will then swell, sting, and burn. In more severe cases, blisters will occur beneath the epidermis in 24–36 hours. These slowly dry and become hard and black in about 2 weeks. General swelling of the injured area occurs and subsides in the same period. After edema subsides, the skin peels and remains red, tender, and extremely sensitive even to mild cold. It may also perspire abnormally for a long time.

In deep, unthawed frostbite, a much more serious injury, the injured part is hard and solid and cannot be depressed. Damage not only involves the skin and subcutaneous tissues but also goes deep into the tissue beneath (even including bone). Deep frostbite is usually accompanied by huge blisters that may take from 3 days to 1 week to develop. Swelling of the entire hand or foot takes place and lasts for 1 month or more. After rewarming, the frostbitten area becomes blue, violet, or gray, and throbbing pains may occur that lasts up to 8 weeks. The blisters eventually dry, blacken, and slough, leaving beneath an exceptionally sensitive thin, red layer of new skin that takes months to return to a normal state.

In extreme cases of deep frostbite, the frostbitten part turns gray and remains cold when thawed. If edema and blisters develop, they appear along the line of demarcation between the severely frostbitten area and the remainder of the limb. From 1–2 weeks after injury, the tissue becomes black, dry, and shriveled to the beginning of the healthy tissue. Eventually it falls off. If the dead tissue becomes infected, it will become wet, soft, and inflamed, the remainder of the limb will become painful and swollen, and the eventual loss of tissue will increase.

The first and most important principle in the treatment of frostbite is rapid rewarming of the injured part. The injured part should be immersed in water kept between 98.6–104°F (37–40°C); warmer water can be harmful. Rewarming at this temperature usually takes only 20 minutes; longer periods are not thought to be helpful. Rewarming is painful and if the patient's condition is otherwise good, he may be given an analgesic. After the injured part is warmed, it should be covered with sterile bandages carefully to minimize friction or trauma. It is critically important to protect the injured tissue at all times. A frozen part should never be rubbed before, during, or after rewarming.

Other measures in the treatment of frostbite are similar to those used for patients with burn injuries. The patient should be given tetanus prophylaxis, placed on a penicillin regimen for several days, and given intravenous fluids if needed.

Administration of low-molecular-weight dextran to help improve circulation to the injured part and heparin to prevent further thrombosis of small vessels in the injured area is sometimes carried out and depends on the condition of the patient. Once the patient is admitted to the hospital, the use of α-adrenergic blocking agents and sympathectomy may be considered. Finally, *the physician should never débride or amputate any tissue* because it is very difficult in the early stages of frostbite to determine eventual viability of the injured part.

Trench foot and *immersion foot* are the subacute and chronic variations of frostbite. The eventual tissue injury can be as severe as with frostbite, and therefore, these injuries should be treated in the same way. Trench foot and immersion foot are rare in civilian life.

Suggested Readings

Baxter CR: Crystalloid resuscitation of burn shock, in *Contemporary Burn Management*. Polk HC, Jr, Stone HH (Eds). Boston, Little, Brown, 1971, pp. 7–32

Burke JF, Quinby WC, Jr, Bondoc C, et al: Patterns of high tension electrical injury in children and adolescents and their management. *Am J Surg 133:* 492–497, 1977

Iverson RE, Laub DR, Madison MS: Hydrofluoric acid burns. *Plast Reconstr Surg 48:*107–112, 1971

CHAPTER 29

Maxillofacial and Soft-Tissue Injuries

MICHAEL B. LEWIS, M.D.

Injuries to maxillofacial structures and soft tissues occur all too frequently, constituting the largest group of injuries seen in many emergency wards. These injuries can result from a variety of causes, including motor vehicle and home accidents, athletic and occupational accidents, animal bites, and intentional trauma. They are discussed in one chapter because of their many similarities, but they are separated into maxillofacial and soft-tissue injuries because of some important differences.

MAXILLOFACIAL INJURIES

The face is a person's most important physical characteristic, and as such, great emphasis has been placed on it by society. When the face is injured, the goals of treatment must include not only return of function but also restoration of appearance. This requires a thorough understanding of the anatomy and function of the tissues involved and also an absolute insistence on excellence of work. The specialty of plastic and reconstructive surgery was founded and developed on this recognition and need.

Maxillofacial trauma can be classified as soft-tissue injury and facial bone fractures. It is important to classify all facial trauma not only for statistical and medicolegal reasons but also for proper treatment, which depends on recognition of the differences between the types and locations of these injuries.

The mechanism of injury should be determined, since it often suggests the presence of other injuries or the need for special treatment; for example, the patient with facial trauma resulting from an automobile accident is more likely to have associated serious injuries and to require immediate emergency measures than the patient who has been injured in a minor accident in the home.

Many of these injuries have medicolegal sequelae, and the attending physician, who often is asked to provide information or to give a deposition, must be able to supply factual data regarding the injury, treatment, and prognosis. It is mandatory, therefore, that accurate, complete records be kept. Diagrams and photographs are excellent means of recording the injury.

Anatomy

It is essential that basic facial anatomy be understood before undertaking the treatment of facial injuries, and a textbook of anatomy should be available in every emergency ward. An understanding of the relations of the facial bones to the skull bones is particularly important (Fig. 29.1), as is knowledge of the facial and trigeminal nerves.

The facial nerve (cranial nerve VII) exits from the stylomastoid foramen at the base of the skull and turns immediately downward and laterally to enter the parotid gland, where it divides into multiple branches that supply the muscles of facial expression in the ipsilateral half of the face (Fig. 29.2). Because it is relatively deep throughout most of its course, especially the proximal portion, it is not often injured. Deep lacerations in the region of the parotid gland, however, can injure the facial nerve as well as the parotid duct. The parotid (Stensen's) duct usually lies deep to the middle third of an imaginary line extending from the middle of the upper lip to the tragus, and is closely accompanied by the buccal branch of the facial nerve (Fig. 29.2).

Most of the sensation on the face is provided by the sensory branches of the trigeminal nerve (V). Injury to the arborizing branches of this nerve rarely results in permanent anesthesia because of regeneration of the nerve and the overlapping sensory pattern. It is not necessary to repair these

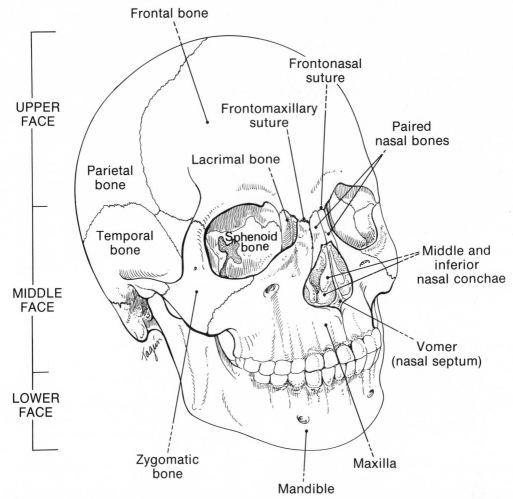

Figure 29.1. Facial bones. For descriptive purposes, the face is divided into upper, middle, and lower regions.

small sensory nerves. Knowledge of the pertinent anatomy (Fig. 29.3) is helpful since specific patterns of decreased sensation often result from certain facial fractures.

The arterial blood supply to the face is derived from branches of the external carotid arteries, and venous drainage is accomplished through the internal and external jugular system. Rarely, massive hemorrhage occurs when one or more of the major branches are injured.

Immediate Treatment

Airway

As with any injured patient, establishment of an adequate airway is of first priority. An obstructed airway is manifested by rapid and labored respirations, tachycardia, cyanosis, lethargy, and often, extreme agitation. Breath sounds are decreased

and rhonchi are present. The possible causes of airway obstruction in maxillofacial injuries are multiple:

(1) Facial fractures (maxilla and mandible) can result in posterior displacement of these bones and their attached soft tissues, obstructing the upper part of the airway.

(2) Hemorrhage into the soft tissues can lead to progressive swelling and airway obstruction.

(3) Foreign bodies such as teeth, dentures, glass, and clothing can become lodged in the airway.

(4) Hemorrhage sufficient to "drown" the patient can occur.

(5) Direct laryngeal or tracheal injury can collapse and obstruct that portion of the airway.

Emergency tracheotomy is rarely needed in cases of airway obstruction accompanying maxillofacial injuries except in the unusual instance of direct laryngeal injury. If the airway appears ob-

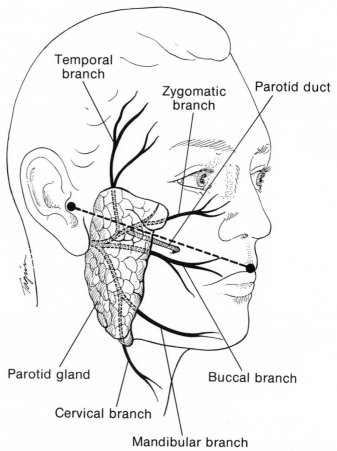

Figure 29.2. Facial nerve and its branches in relation to parotid gland and duct. Facial nerve lies deep in gland substance.

structed, a quick digital search for a foreign body lodged in the upper airway should be carried out. If the airway is being obstructed by intraoral and pharyngeal bleeding, the patient usually struggles to sit up if he is conscious, since it is easier to expectorate the blood and to clear the airway in the upright position. The patient should be helped in this effort and should be provided with suction.

Obstruction caused by displacement of soft tissues posteriorly in mandibular and maxillary fractures can be alleviated immediately by grasping the tongue or jaw and pulling it forward. If the patient is conscious and alert, placing him on his side to prevent posterior displacement is often sufficient to maintain an airway. In the unconscious or semiconscious patient with an obstructed airway, oral endotracheal intubation is necessary. This is preferable to emergency tracheotomy for several reasons: it is quicker, it may make tracheotomy unnecessary, and it is safer—in emergency tracheotomies there is a high incidence of inadvertent injury to important neighboring structures.

Hemorrhage

Because of the rich blood supply to the face from the external carotid arteries, a certain amount of bleeding accompanies most injuries. Massive bleeding, however, is rare. Most external bleeding can be controlled with pressure. When this is inadequate, the lacerated vessels must be clamped and ligated, being careful to avoid injury to branches of the facial nerve. Excessive bleeding from lacerations of the oral mucosa is best controlled by closing the lacerations with sutures. Intranasal hemorrhage from branches of the internal maxillary artery, when it is persistent, must be controlled by packing. Placement of a postnasal pack against which the anterior packing is done is necessary to control this type of hemorrhage (see Chapter 33, pages 744–747).

Shock

Hemorrhagic shock is rare from maxillofacial injuries alone. When shock is present, even when

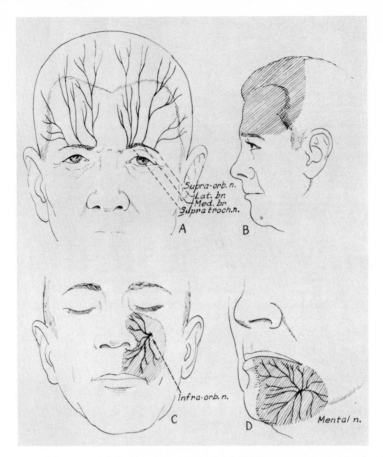

Figure 29.3. Sensory nerves of facial region (trigeminal origin). **(A)** Sensory nerves of forehead often injured in frontal sinus-supraorbital rim fractures. **(B)** Resultant area of anesthesia. **(C)** Area of anesthesia resulting from injury to infraorbital nerve common in zygomatic fractures. **(D)** Area of anesthesia resulting from injury to inferior alveolar nerve common in fractures of mandibular body. (Reproduced by permission, from Converse JM: *Kazanjian & Converse's Surgical Treatment of Facial Injuries*, ed. 3. © 1974, Baltimore, Williams & Wilkins.)

the patient has a severe maxillofacial injury, some other cause must be sought and is often found.

Associated Injuries

Most major maxillofacial injuries result from motor vehicle accidents and are frequently accompanied by other major injuries. Fractures of the skull, cervical portion of the spine, and long bones are common, and thoracic and abdominal organs can also be injured. A quick but thorough examination is mandatory to establish treatment priorities. Special care is necessary in handling patients who might have a cervical spinal injury, since improper handling of such an individual may result in quadriplegia (see Chapter 26, pages 567–568).

Wound

Although definitive treatment of soft-tissue injuries can be delayed, it is important to unravel all distorted flaps of skin, tacking them in place with a single stitch, when necessary, to avoid vascular compromise. A dry sterile dressing can be placed temporarily over the wound to prevent further contamination.

Diagnosis

The three techniques used in diagnosing facial injuries are inspection, palpation, and x-ray examination.

Inspection

Soft-tissue injuries are usually readily visible. The type of injury should be noted and foreign bodies sought. The eyelids should be separated and the globe examined. If ocular injury is suspected, ophthalmologic consultation should be obtained. The mouth should be opened and the mucosal surface examined for laceration and hematoma. Missing teeth should be noted and accounted for. Function of the facial musculature should be determined.

Inspection alone often suggests facial fractures. Facial asymmetry, localized hematoma or ecchymosis, disturbances in ocular movement, diplopia, anesthesia of areas innervated by the terminal branches of the trigeminal nerve, epistaxis, malocclusion, sublingual hematoma, limitation of mandibular excursion, and buccal sulcus lacerations all suggest underlying fracture (details are given later with specific injuries).

Palpation

Palpation of known bony prominences on both sides often suggests asymmetry when swelling and ecchymosis prevent this determination from inspection alone. Tenderness, crepitation, sharp "step-offs," angulation, and abnormal movement are further signs of facial fractures.

X-ray Examination

For confirmation of suspected facial fractures and delineation of unrecognized fractures, x-ray examination is necessary. X-ray films of the cervical spine and skull should also be obtained in all cases of severe facial fracture. The most useful views for the facial bones are:

(1) Waters' view (occipitomental)—for fractures of the middle of the face involving the maxilla, the zygomatic bone, or the nasal or orbital regions;

(2) posteroanterior view—for mandibular, frontal, and zygomatic fractures;

(3) Towne projection view—for fractures of the mandibular rami and condyles;

(4) lateral oblique views of the mandible—for fractures of the mandibular body, angles, and rami;

(5) submental vertex (jug-handle) view—for fractures of the zygomatic arches;

(6) nasal views (lateral and occlusal).

Preliminary Considerations Before Treatment

Priorities

Except for the emergency measures previously described, the treatment of facial injuries is not lifesaving and should be deferred until more immediately threatening injuries have been treated. Although soft-tissue closure can be postponed up to 24 hours with the use of sterile saline dressings and antibiotics, it should be delayed this long only when absolutely necessary. With coordination between specialists, soft-tissue damage can be repaired simultaneously with surgical treatment of other regions.

Except for nasal fractures, the treatment of facial fractures can be delayed several days without affecting the final result. In fact, this often is preferred since the early swelling and ecchymosis make accurate fracture reduction and placement of incisions more difficult.

Transportation

Before the patient with severe facial injuries is transported to another hospital or to another area within the same hospital, several precautionary measures should be taken. A good airway must be present. The stomach should be emptied by means of an indwelling nasogastric tube. If there has been an associated cervical spinal injury, the head and neck must be stabilized with sandbags or a four-poster brace. An intravenous line should be placed, and basic laboratory studies such as a complete blood cell count and typing and cross-matching of blood should be performed.

Tetanus Prophylaxis

Patients with facial injuries should receive tetanus prophylaxis (see Table 11.6). The removal of all devitalized tissue is equally important in preventing tetanus, which has an extremely high mortality.

Anesthesia

General anesthesia is necessary when repair is extensive and complicated, when severe intraoral lacerations have occurred (especially in children), and in most facial fractures. If general anesthesia is being used for the correction of other conditions, it may be convenient to repair the facial injuries concomitantly.

Most minor soft-tissue injuries can be repaired under local anesthesia. The preferred anesthetic is a 1% solution of lidocaine with epinephrine (1:100,000). In small lacerations, local infiltration of these agents through the wound edges minimizes the pain and the amount of agent required. Although anesthesia occurs rapidly after infiltration, the beneficial vasoconstrictive effect of epinephrine takes approximately 10 minutes, and debridement and suturing should be delayed for this period.

In infants and children, sedation and restraint are often necessary. The following combination is effective: meperidine hydrochloride, 25 mg/ml; promethazine hydrochloride, 8 mg/ml; and chlorpromazine hydrochloride, 5 mg/ml. The dosage is

1 ml/25 lb to a maximum of 2 ml. Morphine, 0.1 mg/kg, is an alternative, but should not be given to infants less than 6–8 months old. These agents must be given adequate time to take effect (45 minutes) before restraining the patient and repairing the injury.

Wound Preparation, Healing, and Postoperative Care

Except for superficial abrasions that heal by epithelialization alone, leaving no scar, wounds heal by one of the following methods:

(1) primary intention—direct approximation of wound edges;

(2) delayed primary intention—wound closure by approximation of wound edges or grafting *after* the wound has been allowed to develop early granulation tissue;

(3) secondary intention—wound closure by granulation, contraction, and epithelialization. Since skin is an organ and unable to regenerate completely, all these methods of wound healing leave scars that are composed primarily of collagen.

In general, the most aesthetically acceptable scars result from healing by primary intention. Anything that interferes with primary healing, even in a portion of the wound, causes additional scarring and a less acceptable result. Proper wound preparation, débridement, suturing, and postoperative management are the prerequisites for primary healing.

The skin around the wound should be prepared with a bland nondetergent soap, and the wound itself should be irrigated with sterile physiologic saline solution and all foreign material removed. Obviously devitalized tissue should be débrided. Excision of large amounts of questionably viable tissue is not recommended; later revisional operation is preferable to the unnecessary sacrifice of viable tissue. Repair should be carried out meticulously and skillfully with minimal and delicate handling of tissue. Postoperatively, wounds should be protected by occlusive dressings that provide some pressure and immobilization. Pressure can help prevent hematoma and excessive swelling, both of which can interfere with primary wound healing. Constant and excessive motion of a wound after repair can cause additional inflammation, promote "suture marks," and lead to unnecessary scar tissue.

An effective means of providing pressure and immobilization for smaller wounds is the cocoon tape dressing (Fig. 29.4A). A single layer of fine-mesh gauze is placed next to the wound, reinforced

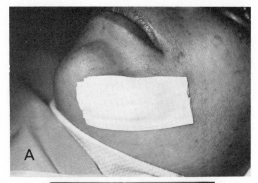

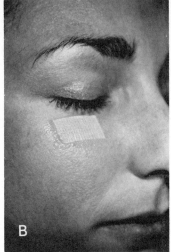

Figure 29.4. **(A)** Cocoon dressing. **(B)** Fine-mesh gauze/collodion dressing.

by several layers of coarse gauze, all held in place by multiple layers of 0.5-inch adhesive tape. In areas where this type of dressing is difficult to place, a dressing of fine-mesh gauze and collodion is a good substitute (Fig. 29.4B). Larger and multiple wounds are best protected with a circumferential head dressing. Excessive talking and chewing are discouraged to avoid unnecessary motion at the wound site. The head should be kept elevated. Sutures should be removed within 3–5 days and the wound dressed again for an additional 7–10 days.

The final aesthetic result in wound healing depends on many factors, some of which are beyond the surgeon's control. The relation of the final scar to the relaxed skin tension lines is extremely important (Fig. 29.5). Scars that are parallel or nearly parallel to these lines usually look better. The degree of crush and contusion plays an important role, as does the age of the patient and the location of the injury. In discussing the prognosis with the patient or his family, the physician must point out these factors.

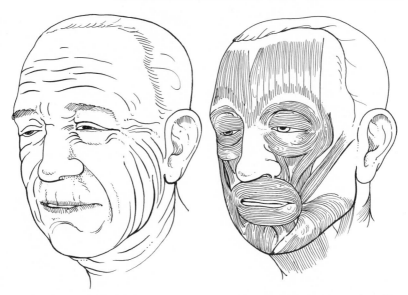

Figure 29.5.   Relaxed skin tension lines (wrinkle lines) and underlying facial muscles. (Reproduced by permission, from McGregor IA: *Fundamental Techniques of Plastic Surgery and Their Surgical Applications*, ed. 6. © 1975, Edinburgh, London, and New York, Churchill Livingstone.)

Treatment

General Management of Soft-Tissue Injuries

Most soft-tissue injuries result from relatively minor trauma and can effectively be treated in the emergency ward. Extensive injuries and those involving specialized areas of the face, however, require special expertise, time, and assistance not usually available in the emergency facility. These patients should be referred to the plastic surgeon for care; they often require hospitalization and surgical repair in the operating room.

Simple Laceration. This is probably the most common facial injury encountered. Repair should be carried out under local anesthesia. After the surrounding skin is prepared and the wound irrigated, devitalized tissue is very conservatively débrided. Ragged and contused wound edges should be excised to provide healthy, perpendicular skin margins. When it is necessary, hemostasis should be achieved by fine catgut ligatures or cautery. Slight undermining of the wound margins at the subdermal plane allows more accurate suture placement and relieves some tension from the wound margins.

Interrupted loop sutures are probably the most accurate means of closing a laceration (Figs. 29.6 and 29.7). If correctly placed, the sutures provide good approximation with just the proper amount of wound edge eversion without leaving any dead space. Equal "bites" with a perpendicular course of the needle ensure level wound edges. Any fine adjustments can be made by knot placement. Suture material should be 5–0 or 6–0 monofilament nylon swaged on a cutting needle, and sutures should be placed every 2–3 mm. It is important to tie the sutures just tightly enough to approximate the wound edges. Some postoperative wound edema should be considered when determining the tightness of each suture.

In deeper lacerations, multilayered closure is indicated to eliminate dead space, to ensure proper alignment of deeper structures, and to prevent a depressed, widened scar. Muscle should be approximated with interrupted absorbable sutures of either 4–0 chromic catgut or polyglycolic acid (Dexon). Subcutaneous or subcuticular suturing should be performed with interrupted sutures of polyglycolic acid or 5–0 plain catgut (Fig. 29.8).

Intraoral lacerations of the tongue or mucous membranes should be closed with interrupted 4–0 chromic catgut or black silk sutures. Catgut has the advantage of not having to be removed, but its knot-holding ability is much less than that of silk.

A number of other suture techniques are available (Fig. 29.8). The vertical mattress suture is helpful in everting wound edges when this is a problem. Continuous sutures can save time, but offer less edge and tension control. A continuous subcuticular (intradermal) suture has the advantage of not leaving suture marks even when left in

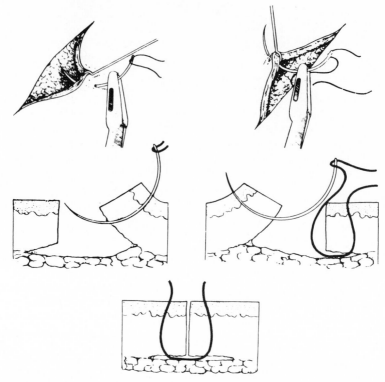

Figure 29.6.   Simple loop suture, with perpendicular course of needle through everted skin edge. (Reproduced by permission, from McGregor IA: *Fundamental Techniques of Plastic Surgery and Their Surgical Applications,* ed. 6. © 1975, Edinburgh, London, and New York, Churchill Livingstone.)

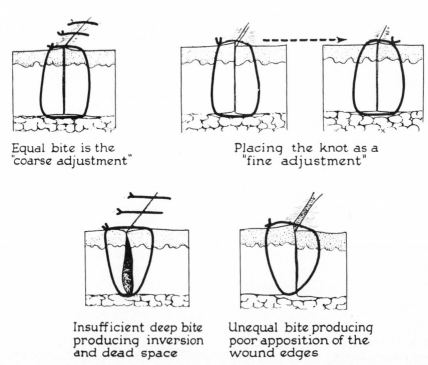

Equal bite is the
"coarse adjustment"

Placing the knot as a
"fine adjustment"

Insufficient deep bite
producing inversion
and dead space

Unequal bite producing
poor apposition of the
wound edges

Figure 29.7.   Correct adjustments and possible errors in placement of simple loop sutures. (Reproduced by permission, from McGregor IA: *Fundamental Techniques of Plastic Surgery and Their Surgical Applications,* ed. 6. © 1975, Edinburgh, London, and New York, Churchill Livingstone.)

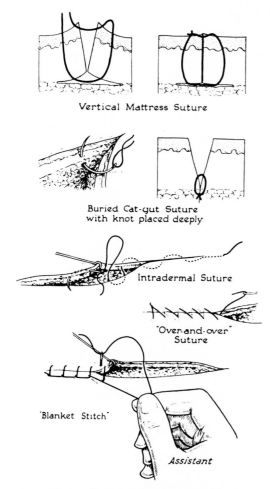

Vertical Mattress Suture

Buried Cat-gut Suture
with knot placed deeply

Intradermal Suture

"Over-and-over"
Suture

"Blanket Stitch"

Assistant

Figure 29.8. Other commonly used skin suture techniques. (Reproduced by permission, from Mc-Gregor IA: *Fundamental Techniques of Plastic Surgery and Their Surgical Applications*, ed. 6. © 1975, Edinburgh, London, and New York, Churchill Livingstone.)

place for 10–12 days. Accurate skin apposition is more difficult, however.

Complicated Laceration. Included are those lacerations that are irregular or stellate or that contain partly avulsed tissue (flaps). These injuries are generally more difficult to treat, and result in a less than ideal scar deformity. If the wound is small enough that it can be completely excised and the resultant defect closed primarily without distortion, this should be done. Otherwise, a conservative approach to débridement should be taken. Distorted tissue should be returned to its appropriate place. Where several lacerations meet, a single buried stitch is helpful in bringing the points together. Severely beveled skin edges, which are frequently seen in partial avulsion injuries, should be excised sharply.

Avulsion Injury. When a significant amount of

tissue has been lost, some form of local flap or free skin graft is often necessary. This requires the skill of a specialist and is best performed in the operating room. However, if the area of tissue loss is small and primary closure can be obtained without undue tension, the wound should be converted to a lenticular shape with freshened, undermined edges and closed primarily.

Human and Animal Bites. Puncture wounds of the face resulting from human or animal bites should not be closed. After they are carefully cleansed, irrigated, and débrided, *no* suturing should be undertaken. Lacerations resulting from animal bites, however, should be sutured. Special attention to irrigation, débridement, and tetanus prophylaxis is required, and antirabies precautions should be taken (see Table 11.7). Broad-spectrum antibiotics should be administered for 1 week. When substantial tissue has been avulsed, more complicated reconstruction is necessary and a plastic surgeon should be consulted.

Human bites are potentially more dangerous because of the associated introduction of many types of pathogenic bacteria. Admission to the hospital for systemic antibiotic administration and wet dressings is often necessary. The wound should be cleansed and débrided thoroughly when first seen and closed a few days later with nylon sutures loosely approximating the skin. Deep sutures should be avoided. Later scar revision may be necessary. Tetanus prophylaxis should be carried out.

Abrasion. This injury, which implies partial-thickness damage, heals spontaneously by epithelialization. The wound should be cleansed with a bland soap and water solution and protected by frequent applications of an antibiotic ointment or covered with a single layer of a nonadherent petrolatum-impregnated gauze.

Accidental Tattoo. In certain types of injuries, small foreign particles can become imbedded in the dermis. The particles are usually obvious because of the color they impart to the area after cleansing and irrigation have removed all the foreign material. If left untreated, accidental tattoo results in permanent discoloration of the area.

These particles are best removed within the first 12 hours before they become fixed in the tissue. Scrubbing with a stiff, sterile brush is the best method of doing this. Grease or oil in a wound can usually be dissolved and removed by using small amounts of ether or acetone as a solvent. The treated areas are dressed with an antibiotic ointment or covered with a single layer of petrolatum-impregnated gauze.

Only small, easily accessible areas are amenable to this treatment under local anesthesia. General anesthesia is usually necessary to treat larger areas adequately.

Foreign Bodies. In general, all foreign bodies should be removed at the time of initial treatment. Despite meticulous attempts to completely remove very small foreign bodies such as multiple glass splinters, these patients often require additional removal of foreign bodies later.

Small metal fragments from missiles that are located deeply in noncritical locations are often best left alone. More harm can be done by attempting removal than by leaving them in place.

Soft-Tissue Injuries to Specific Regions

Eyelids. Eye examination for corneal abrasion, anterior chamber hemorrhage, laceration of the globe, and visual disturbance should precede any repair in this area. Simple lacerations of the eyelid skin present no special problem, especially if oriented transversely. Careful suturing usually results in an inconspicuous scar. If the eyebrow is involved, it should be cleansed but *never* shaved. If the laceration goes through it, the eyebrow must be aligned properly during suturing. In more complicated lacerations of eyelid skin in which small flaps have resulted, minimal débridement should be carried out. Careful salvage and placement of each flap can produce an excellent result in many cases. Lacerations in this region are often associated with multiple imbedded foreign particles, and care should be taken to remove these before suturing. Lacerations involving the full thickness of the eyelid, the medial canthal region with its nasolacrimal apparatus, or the lateral canthus require repair by a specialist.

Nose. Full-thickness lacerations of the nose that enter the vestibule require layered closure. Because of the bony character of the upper part of the nose, these lacerations usually occur in the lower half (Fig. 29.9). The nasal mucosa or vestibular lining is closed with 5–0 catgut interrupted sutures, placing the knots so they face into the nasal cavity. It is usually unnecessary to suture the nasal cartilage, but if its alignment is difficult, a few very fine catgut sutures can be placed in the perichondrium. The skin of the nose is ideal for the continuous subcuticular (intradermal) suture technique. A 5–0 nylon is recommended. This relieves tension on the 6–0 nylon interrupted simple loop cutaneous sutures that are then placed, and allows their early removal. In the fleshy tip of the nose, with its numerous sebaceous glands and pores, cutaneous sutures tend to cut in and to leave marks, so their early removal is important.

Avulsion injuries of the nose require grafting,

and the patient should be referred to a specialist.

Lip. Lacerations of the lip that cross the vermilion-cutaneous junction or "white roll" (Fig. 29.10A) require accurate alignment of this anatomic landmark (Fig. 29.10B). Full-thickness lip lacerations should be closed in three layers. The mucosal layer should be closed with interrupted sutures of 5–0 catgut with the knots placed on the mucosal surface. Since these knots tend to untie, two or three extra "throws" should be placed and the ends cut long. The muscular layer of the lip should carefully be approximated with interrupted 4–0 chromic catgut or polyglycolic acid sutures. The skin should be closed with 6–0 nylon, taking care to align the vermilion-cutaneous junction accurately.

Avulsion injuries of the lip, which most frequently result from dog bites, require complicated reconstruction, either immediately or later, and the patient should be seen by a plastic surgeon as early as possible. This also applies to electrical burns involving the lip. This injury is common in toddlers who inadvertently place a live extension plug into the mouth or chew through a "hot" cord. As the current arcs through the saliva at the corner of the mouth, extremely high temperatures develop, destroying the full thickness of the lip and commissure (Fig. 29.11). Controversy exists concerning the need for early débridement of this necrotic tissue. Many surgeons prefer to allow the tissue to slough spontaneously. This can result in late hemorrhage from the labial artery, and if this course is chosen, the parents and nursing staff should be cautioned. Tetanus immunization and a clear liquid diet are recommended.

Intraoral Injury. Lacerations of the mucous membranes and the tongue should be closed primarily with interrupted 4–0 chromic catgut or black silk sutures.

Parotid Duct and Facial Nerve. Deep lacerations in the cheek can injure the parotid duct and facial nerve, but as stated previously, this happens only infrequently because of their relatively deep location (see page 639 and Fig. 29.2). A high index of suspicion is necessary to diagnose injuries to these structures. Weakness of some or all of the ipsilateral facial musculature indicates injury to the facial nerve. Leakage of clear fluid from a laceration of the cheek suggests injury to the parotid duct or the gland substance. A fine polyethylene catheter or lacrimal probe passed into the oral opening of the parotid duct, opposite the upper second molar, that emerges in the cheek wound indicates division of the duct.

The small peripheral branches of the facial nerve (anterior to an imaginary vertical line from

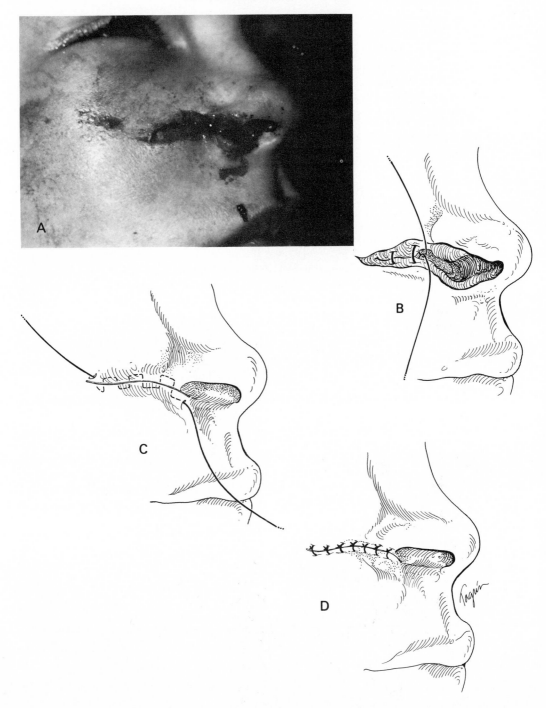

Figure 29.9.   **(A)** Full-thickness nasal laceration. **(B)** Closure of vestibular lining with 5–0 catgut interrupted sutures, followed by **(C)** a 5–0 nylon continuous subcuticular suture, followed by **(D)** 6–0 nylon interrupted simple loop skin sutures.

the lateral canthus of the eye) do not require neurorrhaphy. However, the divided deep soft tissue must be approximated accurately. This usually results in restoration of function after a period during which nerves regenerate. Injury to the more proximal portions of the facial nerve or parotid duct requires more sophisticated repair by a specialist.

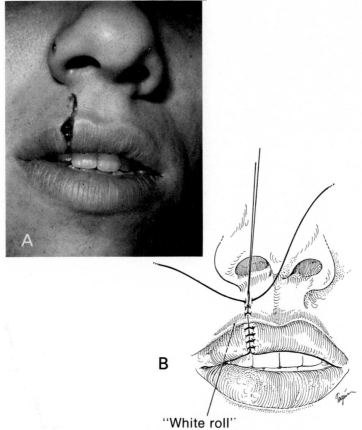

Figure 29.10. **(A)** Lip laceration through vermilion-cutaneous junction ("white roll"). **(B)** Repair of lip laceration demonstrating accurate placement of suture to align "white roll."

Ear. Injuries to the ear often result in jagged lacerations and partial avulsions. The ear is extremely vascular, and flaps based on very small pedicles often survive and should not be excised during débridement. Because of its vascularity, precise hemostasis is necessary if hematomas are to be avoided.

Lacerations involving only the skin of the ear can be managed satisfactorily in the emergency ward. Field block anesthesia can be obtained easily by the injection of a 1% lidocaine solution with epinephrine (1:100,000) around the ear where it attaches to the head. This avoids the need for difficult, painful injection of the anesthetic agent into the ear itself. Fine 6–0 nylon interrupted sutures should be used.

If the cartilaginous framework of the ear has been lacerated, it is usually necessary to trim the cartilage along the wound so that the skin can be approximated over it without tension and without buckling of the cartilage. A few absorbable 5–0

interrupted sutures in the perichondrium are used to hold the cartilage together.

Subperichondral hematoma resulting from blunt trauma can cause cauliflower ear if not immediately and adequately treated. Needle aspiration of all blood should be carried out after preparing the skin with an antiseptic solution. If this is impossible or if hematoma recurs, hospitalization and surgical intervention will be required.

After repair of these injuries, a conforming compression dressing is necessary. Slightly moistened pieces of cotton should be placed behind the ear and within the contour of the anterolateral surface. The ear is then covered with fluffed gauze and a circular head dressing is applied.

In more severe avulsion injuries, everything possible must be done to save all exposed cartilage, since later reconstructive duplication of this intricate structure is impossible. The remaining portion of the ear is usually buried in the adjacent mastoid or temporal skin, followed later by reconstructive

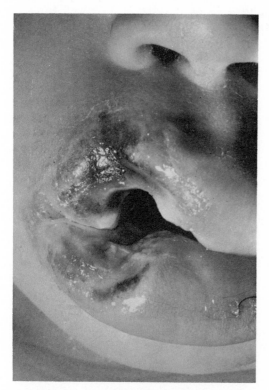

Figure 29.11. Severe full-thickness electrical burn involving oral commissure and upper and lower lips.

operation by a plastic surgeon. Early referral to the specialist is highly recommended.

Facial Fractures

Most facial fractures require reduction and fixation under general anesthesia. Because of this and because of the frequency of associated injuries, hospitalization is necessary. The emergency measures sometimes needed have already been discussed. In open fractures communicating with the oral, nasal, or sinus cavities or to the skin surface, broad-spectrum antibiotic prophylaxis is preferred. This is especially important when a dural tear has occurred, resulting in cerebrospinal fluid rhinorrhea. Definitive treatment of all but simple nasal fractures requires specialized training, and will not be dealt with here. However, diagnosis of these fractures is discussed, since the emergency physician must be able to recognize these injuries.

The most commonly fractured facial bones are the nasal bones, the zygomatic bones, and the mandible. This is so because of their relative prominence on the face. Facial fractures are much less common in children because the relatively greater

size and prominence of the cranium affords protection to the smaller facial bones.

Nasal Fracture. Isolated nasal fracture is common, frequently resulting from intentional or athletic trauma. The diagnosis of nasal fracture is made clinically, and the usual signs include:

(1) depression or deviation of the nasal pyramid;

(2) epistaxis;

(3) periorbital ecchymosis and edema;

(4) tenderness;

(5) crepitation and abnormal motion of the nasal bones on palpation;

(6) obstruction of the airway by a buckled or deviated septum.

X-ray films of the nasal bones should be obtained to document the injury and for medicolegal purposes, but should not dictate treatment. Treatment should be undertaken on the basis of the clinical appearance of the nose (Fig. 29.12). Undisplaced nasal fractures diagnosed by x-ray findings alone do not need treatment except for splinting. In children, a seemingly insignificant nasal injury or undisplaced fracture can result in later deformity due to altered growth, and parents should be cautioned about this possibility.

The results of treatment of nasal fractures are all too frequently poor. It is a difficult problem to deal with, even for extremely experienced physicians. If possible, nasal fractures should be treated by surgeons familiar with nasal surgery and corrective rhinoplasty. Treatment is best undertaken

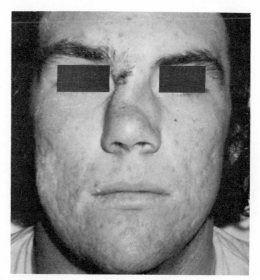

Figure 29.12. Nasal fracture with obvious deformity.

early, before swelling and fixation of a buckled septum take place.

Since many nasal fractures are managed in the emergency ward, a detailed description of the technique follows:

The first step is to determine exactly which deformity is present, namely, depression, angulation, or septal distortion. Then, after the face is washed with soap and water, local anesthesia is attained. Cotton applicators soaked in a 10% cocaine solution provide topical anesthesia to the mucous membranes. The infraorbital nerves (Fig. 29.3) are blocked with a 1% lidocaine solution with epinephrine (1:100,000) and field block anesthesia is accomplished by infiltration of the same agent across the glabellar region and the base of the columella. It takes 10–15 minutes for anesthesia to be complete, and reduction should not be carried out until this time has passed.

A closed Kelly clamp covered with a thin piece of rubber tubing is effective for disimpacting, mobilizing, and reducing the nasal fracture if the other hand simultaneously palpates and molds the nose. Walsham forceps are also used for this maneuver. An Asch forceps is the best instrument available to reposition and to mold the deviated nasal septum (Fig. 29.13).

An external splint of plaster of Paris is used to protect the nose and to control edema. Internal packing is rarely necessary; when it is used, it should not block the airway or be placed so that it displaces the nasal bones laterally.

Nasal fractures in children require brief general anesthesia for reduction, and hospitalization is therefore necessary.

Naso-orbital-ethmoidal Fracture. These fractures usually occur in conjunction with other fractures of the middle of the face. In addition to the signs usually seen in the simple nasal fractures, lateral displacement of the medial canthi is noted (traumatic telecanthus). The Waters' view is a helpful x-ray film in confirming this injury. Treatment is complex and often involves open reduction and internal fixation.

Zygomatic Fracture. There are usually three points of fracture and some degree of separation in fractures of the zygomatic bone—along the inferior orbital rim, at the frontozygomatic suture region, and at the junction with the temporal bone in the arch (Fig. 29.14). The following clinical signs usually are present:

(1) periorbital ecchymosis and edema;

(2) anesthesia in the distribution of the infraorbital nerve (Fig. 29.3);

(3) flattening of the "cheekbone" eminence;

(4) Angulation and tenderness of the infraorbital rim;

(5) trismus.

Diplopia and limitation of external ocular movements because of involvement of the orbital floor and muscle entrapment are less frequently seen.

The Waters' x-ray view is best for demonstrating the fractures, and usually shows clouding of the maxillary antrum as well. The submental vertex (jug-handle) view demonstrates the fracture line in the zygomatic arch.

Several different procedures have been described to reduce and to immobilize the depressed zygomatic bone. Many fractures can be reduced by the semi-open technique described by Gillies and colleagues without internal fixation. Experience is necessary to know which fractures are correctable by this approach. The remainder must be repaired by direct open reduction with internal interosseous wire fixation. General anesthesia is necessary for these operations.

Isolated fracture of the zygomatic arch results from a direct blow with a relatively narrow object. Fractures usually occur simultaneously in three places along the arch, and depression results. The clinical signs for diagnosis include:

(1) swelling and tenderness in the region of the zygomatic arch;

(2) interference with mandibular movements from impingement on the coronoid process;

(3) periorbital ecchymosis and edema.

The submental vertex x-ray view best demonstrates this fracture. It usually can be elevated by the semi-open technique described by Gillies and colleagues (1927). Only rarely is internal fixation necessary.

Maxillary Fracture. These fractures result from a direct force applied to the middle of the face or from beneath the lower jaw. When severe, they are often associated with mandibular fractures, naso-orbital-ethmoidal fractures, basilar skull fractures, and cerebrospinal fluid rhinorrhea. It is this group of patients that is most likely to have problems with hemorrhage and airway obstruction. LeFort classified maxillary fractures in three groups (Fig. 29.15): I (transverse), II (pyramidal), and III (craniofacial disjunction). Fractures of the maxilla are not always so isolated as LeFort implied, but this classification is a useful aid in thinking about these injuries. Clinical and x-ray findings depend on the location of the fracture, but the following clinical findings are often present:

(1) malocclusion;

(2) elongation of the middle of the face;

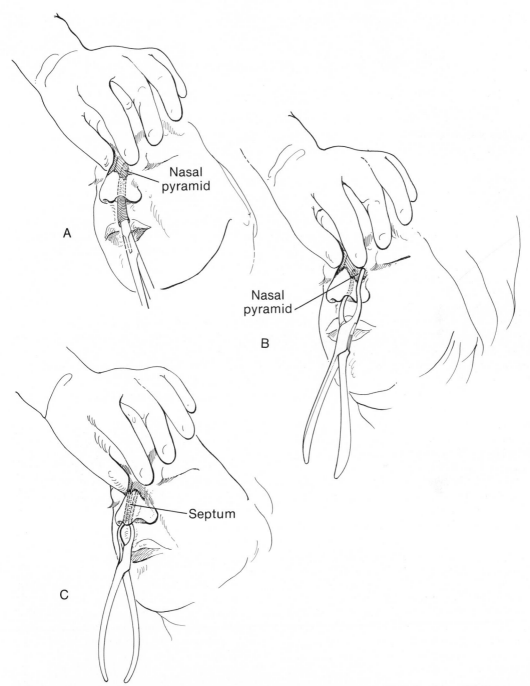

Figure 29.13. Instruments and techniques used in treating nasal fractures. **(A)** Kelly clamp. **(B)** Walsham forceps. **(C)** Asch forceps.

(3) periorbital ecchymosis and edema;

(4) abnormal mobility of the maxilla when grasped between the examiner's thumb and forefinger and forceful motion is attempted, causing pain as well as abnormal motion;

(5) mucosal lacerations in the upper buccal sulcus.

The Waters' view is the most helpful x-ray film. Treatment of these complex fractures is based on the goals of restoration of normal occlusion, ceph-

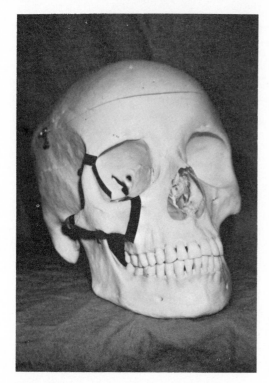

Figure 29.14.   Lines of usual zygomatic fracture.

alad fixation to a stable foundation, and use of aesthetically acceptable incisions.

Orbital Floor (Blow-out) Fracture. The pure blow-out fracture involves only the thin orbital floor, sparing the orbital rim, and it usually results from a direct force applied to the globe itself. Instead of causing eye injury, the force is transmitted to the orbital floor, which fractures into the maxillary sinus. The usual findings include:

(1) periorbital ecchymosis and edema;

(2) limitation of external ocular movements because of muscle entrapment (inconsistent);

(3) enophthalmos and diplopia before swelling compensates for the displacement of the orbital contents into the maxillary sinus;

(4) discrepancy of eye level;

(5) hypesthesia over the distribution of the infraorbital nerve (inconsistent).

The examiner must be alert to avoid missing this injury. Waters' view usually shows only clouding of the maxillary antrum. Tomograms of the orbital floor are necessary to confirm the diagnosis.

Muscle entrapment, enophthalmos, and persistent diplopia are indications for surgical correction to free the muscles and to replace the intraorbital contents. Blepharoplasty or a conjunctival incision is used, and often a small disc of autologous tissue or silicone is required to reconstruct the floor of the orbit.

Mandibular Fracture. The mandible is probably the most frequently fractured facial bone in children, but mandibular fracture is seen much more commonly in adults. Fracture results from a direct blow to the mandible, and often it occurs in more than one site. The common clinical findings include:

(1) malocclusion;

(2) limitation of mandibular movement;

(3) abnormal motion;

(4) ecchymosis, swelling, and tenderness near the fracture site;

(5) mucosal lacerations of the lower buccal sulcus;

(6) missing or loose teeth;

(7) anesthesia of the ipsilateral region of the lower lip because of injury to the inferior alveolar nerve (Fig. 29.3);

(8) sublingual hematoma.

Fractures of the mandible are best demonstrated by posteroanterior, lateral oblique, and occlusal views. The Towne projection view is helpful in demonstrating fractures of the mandibular rami and condyles. Treatment almost always requires intermaxillary fixation, often augmented by open reduction and internal fixation.

Frontal Sinus-Supraorbital Rim Fracture. This is an unusual fracture resulting from a direct blow, and is frequently associated with skull fracture. Possible signs include:

(1) periorbital ecchymosis and edema;

(2) local tenderness and depression;

(3) anesthesia of the forehead (Fig. 29.3);

(4) commonly a bursting type of laceration over the fracture;

(5) epistaxis.

The x-ray films that demonstrate these fractures best are the Waters' and posteroanterior views and lateral views of the skull.

SOFT-TISSUE INJURIES

The types of soft-tissue injury that occur elsewhere on the body are, in general, similar to those that occur in the facial region, and in many respects their treatment is also similar. However, because of the less abundant blood supply and differences in function and in the time required for the healing wound to attain adequate strength, the specific management of these lesions varies. This is especially true with soft-tissue injuries of the lower extremities. Discussions of electrical burns and frostbite are found in Chapter 28, pages 633–634 and 637–638.

Minor Injuries

Minor abrasions, contusions, and lacerations can be managed under local anesthesia in the

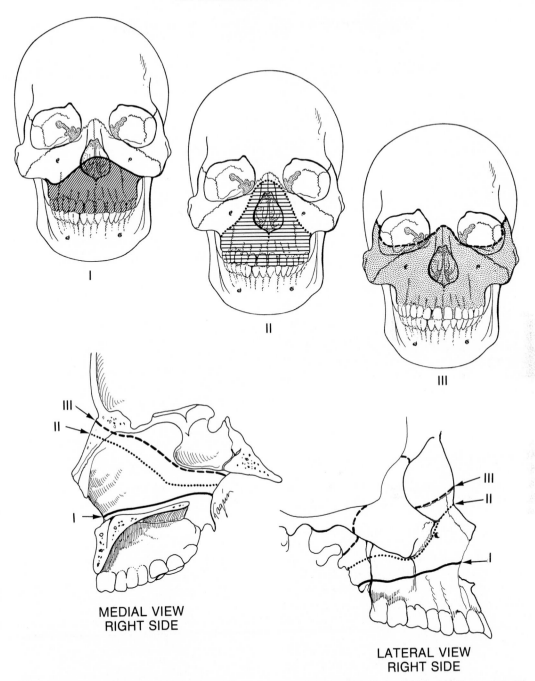

Figure 29.15. LeFort classification of maxillary fractures. *I*, transverse; *II*, pyramidal; and *III*, craniofacial dysjunction.

emergency ward. The skin should be prepared with bland soap and water and the wound irrigated with sterile physiologic saline solution. All foreign bodies should be removed and any necrotic tissue débrided. Tissues should be handled atraumatically with delicate forceps and skin hooks. Needless crushing of tissue delays healing and increases the chance of infection and the amount of scar

tissue. Hemostasis should be accomplished with catgut ligatures. The subcutaneous tissues should be approximated with absorbable sutures of 3–0 or 4–0 catgut, depending on the strength required. The skin is closed with 4–0 or 5–0 nylon sutures spaced at 3- to 5-mm intervals and at equal distances from the wound margin. The wound should then be protected with a dressing that applies light pressure and offers some immobilization. Excessive motion at the wound site increases the inflammatory response, causes unnecessary oozing of blood, increases the possibility of infection, and affects the final aesthetic result. The injured areas are best kept elevated. Tetanus prophylaxis should be given. Antibiotics are not routinely administered to patients with minor lacerations and abrasions.

Clean lacerations may be closed safely up to 8 hours after injury. After this time and in extremely untidy wounds, a delayed primary technique should be considered.

Major Injuries

Most severe soft-tissue injuries are associated with other critical injuries, including fractures and intrathoracic, intra-abdominal, and head injuries. Initial care includes the resuscitative measures necessary to establish an airway, stop hemorrhage, and treat shock if present. Hemorrhage from major soft-tissue wounds can be controlled by local pressure or by a properly placed tourniquet when an extremity is involved. This allows time for evaluation and resuscitative measures to be carried out before transfer to the operating room, where these wounds are treated in conjunction with other emergency surgical procedures.

Tetanus prophylaxis is extremely important, and systemic administration of broad-spectrum antibiotics should be started before operation.

Lower Extremity Soft-Tissue Injuries

Because of their unique position and function for weight-bearing and ambulation and secondary to a relative lack of anastomosing blood vessels in the skin, the lower extremities are vulnerable to some unusual manifestations of soft-tissue injuries. All the injuries to be described require hospitalization and general anesthesia for definitive treatment. Bed rest with the legs elevated is also necessary to aid healing.

Contusion. Blunt trauma that does not disrupt the skin can injure blood vessels of varying sizes. If only smaller, superficial vessels are damaged, a relatively innocuous ecchymosis (bruise) results. However, if one or more larger blood vessels are damaged, a large collection of blood (hematoma) results. Smaller hematomas can be expected to resolve spontaneously, but rest, elevation, and mild compression of the area are necessary. An enlarging hematoma requires incision, evacuation of the blood, and ligation of the offending vessel.

Hematoma between the muscular fascia and overlying subcutaneous fat usually occurs as a result of a shearing or degloving force, and often results in necrosis of the overlying skin and subcutaneous tissue. This is common in the pretibial region (Fig. 29.16). Excision of necrotic skin, evacuation of the blood, and skin grafting are required.

Laceration. Deep lacerations, that is, lacerations extending beneath the skin and superficial subcutaneous tissue, require that distal motor and sen-

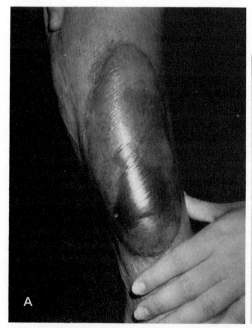

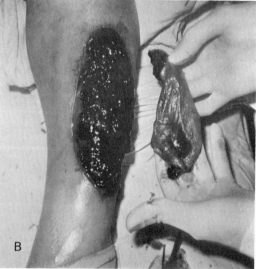

Figure 29.16.   **(A)** Large hematoma in pretibial region. **(B)** Necrosis of overlying skin.

sory function be examined thoroughly; the possibility of injury to a major vessel must also be considered. Adequate knowledge of the regional anatomy is necessary to evaluate these injuries properly. Since repair is often complicated, surgical and orthopaedic consultations are required.

An unusual type of injury is the pretibial laceration. Because the cortex of the tibia is so close to the skin surface and subcutaneous fat is minimal, injuries that appear to be only lacerations are often partly avulsing or degloving as well. Suturing alone does not suffice since necrosis of all the degloved or partly avulsed tissue often occurs (Fig. 29.17).

Although this type of injury may appear innocuous, skin grafting is usually required and patients often must be hospitalized for several weeks for complete healing.

Degloving Injury. In this common injury, the skin and subcutaneous tissue are separated from the underlying fascia. This occurs as a result of a shearing force, and is most often seen when a leg has been run over by the tires of a motor vehicle. Degloving of a large portion of the leg can occur without any disruption of the skin, although there are usually breaks in the skin that result in avulsion flaps. Because of the poor circulation and as a result of the associated crush injury, much of the degloved skin and subcutaneous tissue will not survive, and proper treatment might include débridement followed by skin grafting.

Crush Injury. Fractures of the long bones of the leg and of the foot are commonly associated with crush injuries. In addition, if a leg has been crushed under a considerable weight for a relatively long period, serious closed injury, primarily to muscle, is likely. After the pressure has been removed, the leg swells because of extravasation of red blood cells and plasma through damaged vessels and capillaries. Myoglobin and other products of damaged tissue leak into the general circulation. The combination of these events can cause the crush syndrome, which if untreated leads to shock and renal insufficiency.

Treatment includes the prompt restoration of blood volume with blood, plasma, and electrolyte solution sufficient to maintain a good urinary output (75–100 ml/hr). The urine usually has a port-wine color owing to the heme pigment of myoglobin and hemoglobin. Alkalinization of the urine with sodium bicarbonate is important to prevent precipitation of the pigment in the renal tubules. The legs should be immobilized, slightly elevated, and left uncovered. Because of the frequency of circulatory impairment resulting from swelling, careful and frequent evaluation is necessary. Extensive fasciotomy of all muscle compartments is often required and should be carried out early.

The crush syndrome is an extremely serious injury, and the early resuscitation and treatment are similar to what is required for the patient with a major electrical burn (see Chapter 28, pages 633–634).

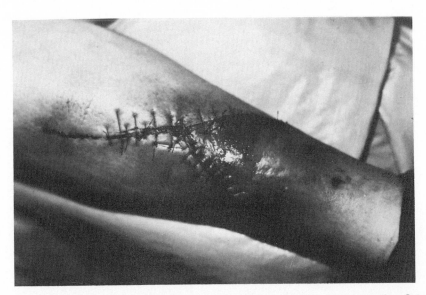

Figure 29.17.   Impending necrosis of skin flaps around unwisely sutured pretibial laceration. Suturing under tension actually increases amount of tissue loss.

Stab Wounds

Deep injury to nerves, major blood vessels, and tendons can result from a stab wound. Careful neuromuscular and vascular examination is required. Excessive bleeding from the wound or an unusually large hematoma suggests injury to a major vessel. A surgeon should see these patients in the emergency ward.

Missile Wounds

Bullets or shotgun blasts usually cause the missile wounds that are seen in civilian hospitals. The degree of injury depends on the caliber, the velocity, and the distance that the missile traveled. Emergency measures include controlling hemorrhage by direct pressure or a tourniquet, treating shock if present, covering the wounds with a sterile dressing, and evaluating the extent of the deep injury. All but the most superficial wounds require operative débridement. When a major vessel is injured, immediate reconstruction is necessary. Nerve repair is usually delayed. The wounds are closed by a delayed primary technique or are allowed to close by secondary intention. It is unnecessary to remove all metal fragments ("shot"), and attempted removal can, at times, cause more harm than good.

Suggested Readings

Converse JM: *Kazanjian & Converse's Surgical Treatment of Facial Injuries*, ed 3, vols 1 and 2. Baltimore, Williams & Wilkins, 1974

Dingman RO, Natvig P: *Surgery of Facial Fractures*. Philadelphia, WB Saunders, 1964

Gillies HD, Kilner TP, Stone D: Fractures of the malarzygomatic compound: With a description of a new x-ray position. *Br J Surg 14*:651–656, 1927

McGregor IA: *Fundamental Techniques of Plastic Surgery and Their Surgical Applications*, ed 6. Edinburgh, London, and New York, Churchill Livingstone, 1975

Schultz RC: *Facial Injuries*. Chicago, Year Book, 1970

CHAPTER 30

Oral Surgical Disorders

WALTER GURALNICK, D.M.D.
R. BRUCE DONOFF, D.M.D., M.D.

Oral surgical emergencies range from toothache to severe facial bone fractures. Within this broad spectrum are a variety of problems commonly seen in the emergency ward, such as postextraction hemorrhage, salivary gland afflictions, acute dental infection with accompanying cellulitis, dislocated jaws, and avulsed teeth. Since the emergency ward serves as the primary care facility for a large number of patients, diagnosis and management of oral surgical emergencies is important to all emergency physicians.

POSTEXTRACTION HEMORRHAGE

Bleeding from a tooth socket is not usually a serious problem, but it is frightening for the patient and it can be frustrating and difficult to control. It is therefore a common reason for seeking emergency treatment. Bleeding results most frequently from lack of compression of the clot, which appears as a protruding gelatinous mass extending from the socket over the adjacent teeth. As long as the clot remains, bleeding will continue. The clot should be removed with a sponge or suction tip, and a tight gauze wad large enough to create pressure should be placed over the socket. If pressure for 20–30 minutes does not stop the bleeding, other measures should be taken. Bleeding most frequently occurs from either of two sites—the edges of the socket or the interdental papilla. Therefore, if bleeding persists, sutures of 3–0 catgut on a cutting needle should be placed across the socket after injection of a local anesthetic agent. Profound anesthesia is easily obtained in the mouth by proper use of a local anesthetic. As a general rule, the upper jaw is anesthetized by infiltration, the lower jaw by blocking the appropriate inferior alveolar nerve. For those unacquainted with intraoral injection techniques, several texts are available, such as *Pain Control* by Trieger (1974). If bleeding is still uncontrolled, an absorbable hemostatic agent such as Gelfoam or Surgicel can be put in the socket after debriding the clot, and sutures can then be placed again.

If bleeding continues, the possibility of a hemorrhagic disorder should be considered. Persistent unexplained bleeding may be a symptom of a severe hemorrhagic condition such as hemophilia, or it may be the initial indication of acute leukemia. Also, in patients receiving anticoagulants, bleeding may persist after an extraction if the prothrombin time is greater than 1½ times the control value. In such cases, appropriate laboratory studies are necessary before effective treatment can be given.

FRACTURED AND AVULSED TEETH

Another common problem in the emergency ward is a fractured tooth or avulsion of one or more teeth. If the crown of the tooth is fractured without exposure of the pulp, immediate treatment is unnecessary. The patient can be advised to see a dentist as soon as possible, preferably within a few days. If the fracture transects the pulpal tissue, however, pain is intense, and emergency treatment consisting of extirpation of the pulp should be rendered. If a dentist is not available within the hospital, the patient should be referred to one immediately. Local dental societies usually maintain an on-call list of practitioners available for emergency needs.

In cases of avulsion, the patient is frequently a child who has fallen and knocked out an incisor. A tooth that has been avulsed and brought with the patient usually survives if it is replanted within a few hours. It should be washed with sterile saline, immersed in a penicillin-streptomycin solution, and inserted into the socket under local anesthesia. The tooth may be stabilized after replantation by suturing medially and distally to it or by using periodontal packing as a cementing device. An-

659

other technique is to wire the replaced tooth to firm adjacent teeth; this is a quick, simple way of effecting good stabilization (Fig. 30.1). The patient should take antibiotics for 7–10 days and should be restricted to a soft diet. In about 3 weeks, the replanted tooth should be firm. Replantation should always be attempted if the tooth is available, although the prognosis becomes poorer the longer the tooth has been out of the mouth. Lacerations of the mucosa and through-and-through lacerations should be closed with sutures as carefully as the skin surface.

Occasionally, a group of teeth with attached alveolar bone is dislodged. In such cases, reduction to proper anatomic position is accomplished by manual manipulation under local anesthesia. The prognosis for both bone and teeth is surprisingly good after such manipulation. As with avulsed teeth, some form of immobilization must be provided for several weeks.

ACUTE ALVEOLAR ABSCESS

Patients with an acute alveolar abscess, with or without cellulitis, are frequently seen in the emergency ward. Such patients are in severe pain, and if the infection is severe, as in Ludwig's angina (Fig. 30.2), the patient may be in serious trouble. As with any other abscess, the treatment is drainage if there is fluctuation, removal of the offending agent (a tooth in this instance) if it is necessary and if it can be done atraumatically, and finally,

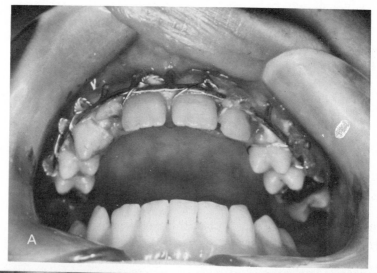

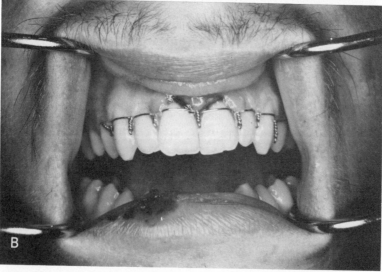

Figure 30.1.   Stabilization of avulsed teeth. **(A)** Arch bar technique. **(B)** Wiring.

antibiotic therapy and supportive care. If either intraoral or extraoral fluctuation exists (Figs. 30.3 and 30.4), incision and drainage should be accomplished with appropriate anesthesia. In some cases, the procedure can be performed on an outpatient basis, but in many instances, admission is warranted. The choice of antibiotic depends on the patient's history of drug sensitivity and the fact that the predominant organism in odontogenic infections is a penicillin-sensitive streptococcus. Nonallergic patients with severe cellulitis should be given 10 million units/day of aqueous penicillin in divided doses via an open intravenous line. For less severe infections, particularly in ambulatory patients, oral penicillin should be prescribed; 500

mg of penicillin V four times a day is a suggested regimen. For penicillin-allergic patients, erythromycin, clindamycin, and ampicillin are possible alternatives. In all cases of acute odontogenic infection, the possibility of admission should seriously be considered.

PERICORONITIS

A common odontogenic infection is pericoronitis, inflammation of the gingiva surrounding an impacted wisdom tooth. Facial swelling, painful swollen gingiva in the mandibular retromolar area, submandibular adenopathy, and trismus are typical findings. Emergency treatment consists of application of heat to the face, warm saline rinses, antibiotics, and analgesics. Penicillin V, 250 mg orally four times a day, is the drug of choice if not contraindicated by allergic or idiosyncratic reaction. Symptoms usually resolve significantly in 48 hours, and definitive treatment—removal of the impacted tooth—can be undertaken thereafter.

SALIVARY GLAND INFECTION

The differential diagnosis of facial swellings must include infections of the parotid and submandibular glands. These conditions are usually manifested by tender preauricular and submandibular swellings. Diagnosis is often made by intraoral examination of the parotid (Stensen's) or submandibular (Wharton's) duct. The opening of the parotid duct is on the buccal mucosa adjacent to the maxillary molar teeth; the opening of the submandibular duct is in the anterior floor of the mouth. The area of the opening is dried with a

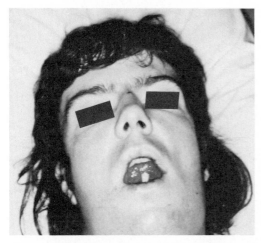

Figure 30.2. Ludwig's angina. Note protrusion of tongue resulting from elevation of floor of mouth.

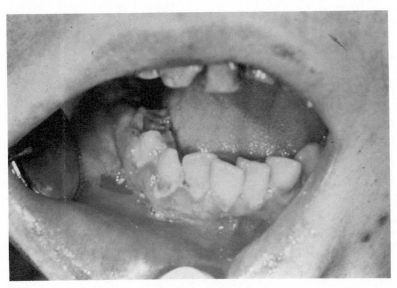

Figure 30.3. Fluctuation in buccal sulcus.

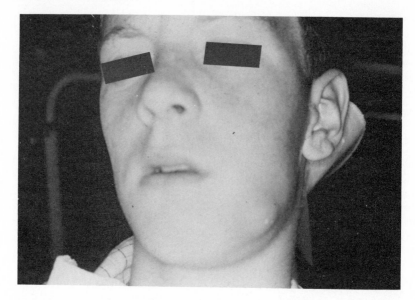

Figure 30.4.   Extraoral fluctuation.

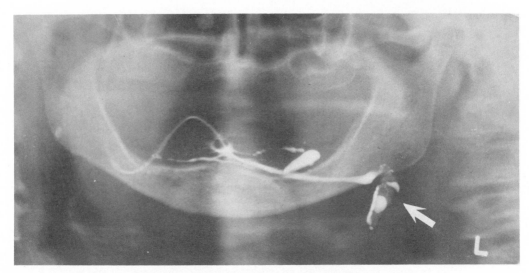

Figure 30.5.   Stone in submaxillary gland (*arrow*).

gauze sponge, and pressure is then applied repeatedly from back to front along the course of the duct. The examiner may find diminished salivary flow, inspissated saliva, or pus, all of which suggest a pathologic process. Palpation may reveal the presence of a calculus, which can be confirmed by radiologic examination, using an occlusal view for the submaxillary gland (Fig. 30.5) and a lateral jaw film or panoramic view for the parotid duct and gland.

The condition of patients with parotitis, particularly older patients, may be extremely toxic. Fever, dehydration, and an elevated white blood cell count are usual. Hospitalization with supportive care, intravenous fluids, and antibiotics is required. In contrast with other oral infections, *Staphylococcus aureus* is the usual pathogen. Intravenous oxacillin, 6–8 gm/day, is the drug of choice in the nonallergic patient. Ampicillin, clindamycin and cephalexin (Keflex) are alternatives. Stimulation with heat and lemon drops is a useful adjunct. If present, pus should be cultured; failure to respond to treatment within 48 hours raises the possibility of an abscess requiring surgical drainage. Fortunately, this is uncommon, and resolution usually occurs with conservative but vigorous measures.

Submandibular glands more commonly become

infected because of calculus formation or duct stricture. Calculi should be removed intraorally if possible, preferably after infection has been controlled. Calculi in the gland, however, necessitate excision of the gland. Sialography is useful in both parotid and submandibular gland infections. Irregularities of the main duct system or calculi may be revealed, and the procedure has a useful dilating effect. Sialography should not be performed until the infection has been controlled.

If salivary gland infection is eliminated in the differential diagnosis of such facial swellings, other possibilities must be considered, including mumps, drug-induced "mumps," mononucleosis, cat-scratch fever, and cellulitis of the external auditory canal. Parotid tumors are usually not tender. Systemic lupus erythematosus and sarcoidosis may cause unilateral enlargement of the parotid gland; Sjögren's syndrome is usually bilateral. Tuberculosis and some fungal diseases may also mimic salivary gland infections.

ACUTE MUCOUS MEMBRANE DISEASE

Patients with acute Vincent's disease (trench mouth, Vincent's infection, Vincent's angina) or other lesions of the mucous membranes such as herpes or aphthobullous stomatitis are often seen in the emergency ward. All these mucosal diseases cause considerable pain, bleeding gums, and occasionally an elevated temperature and generalized malaise. They also produce understandable anxiety. They may be symptomatic of underlying disease ranging from benign mononucleosis to such serious conditions as leukemia and pemphigus. Treatment in the emergency ward is primarily directed at alleviating pain. This can be accomplished by prescribing topical anesthetics such as lidocaine (Xylocain Viscous) or diclonine hydrochloride (Dyclone), as well as analgesics. A complete blood cell count may be advisable as a preliminary screening test, and in all instances, follow-up treatment should be advised and appropriate arrangements made for such care.

FACIAL FRACTURES AND DISLOCATIONS

Traumatic lesions constitute a large percentage of the conditions seen in the emergency ward. The patient's survival may depend on initial evaluation and treatment, long before a specialist or team of specialists is called on for definitive repair of injuries. Although it is preferable to repair facial fractures promptly, definitive treatment need not be compromised if it is deferred for as long as 7–10 days because of a concomitant life-threatening

condition. Initial attention is focused on patency of the airway, control of hemorrhage, neurologic abnormalities, and internal injuries.

Respiratory embarrassment is common in patients with mandibular and midface fractures. It may be caused by mechanical obstruction if the tongue has fallen back into the oropharynx because of fracture at the symphysis with resultant release of the genial attachments. In such cases, bringing the tongue forward with a ligature tied extraorally relieves the obstruction promptly. Occasionally, foreign bodies such as fragments of dentures or teeth may also mechanically occlude the airway. Suspicion of such obstruction calls for rapid but careful inspection of the mouth and throat. Dentures are constructed of acrylic and are not radiopaque; missing fragments should carefully be sought. Respiratory embarrassment may also be caused by severe hemorrhage from a lacerated tongue or other lacerations, nasal bleeding, and through-and-through wounds that have severed large vessels. Control of bleeding sites must be accomplished quickly or an alternate airway provided by either endotracheal intubation or emergency tracheotomy.

After an airway is established and hemorrhage is arrested, the patient's neurologic status should be assessed. If it is indicated by the history and the examination, neurosurgical consultation takes precedence over treatment of facial fractures. At the same time, possible thoracic and abdominal injuries must be considered before proceeding with extensive examination of facial injuries.

Mandible

In the management of facial fractures, the findings derived from careful clinical examination are confirmed by certain specific x-ray views. It is important to understand the value of each type of view that may be ordered. Diagnosis of a mandibular fracture usually requires several views. A panoramic film is an excellent initial screening view and may occasionally be all that is necessary. Other views include the lateral oblique, which is particularly useful in visualizing the body of the mandible, and the posteroanterior, which is helpful in assessing the condition of the symphysis and the condyles, as well as in visualizing lateral displacement of the body and fractures of the rami. In addition, an occlusal view is helpful in elucidating a suspected fracture of the symphysis. Condylar fractures that are not readily seen are best diagnosed by means of the Towne's projection view or a panoramic film (Fig. 30.6).

Emergency treatment of mandibular fractures is

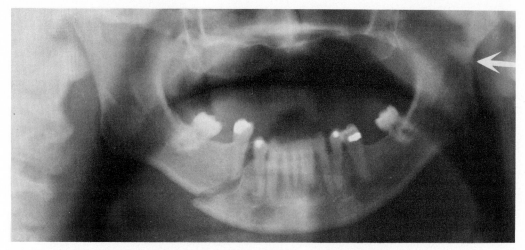

Figure 30.6. Typical fracture of body of mandible and contralateral condylar fracture (*arrow*).

usually definitive except in the presence of hemorrhage or an airway blocked by a posteriorly displaced fractured lower jaw. If definitive closed or open reduction must await treatment of other injuries or neurologic clearance, the mandible should be stabilized temporarily with wire, either alone or in conjunction with an arch bar.

Since condylar fractures often present a problem in management, recognition is important. A blow on the chin often produces no injury other than fracture of a mandibular condyle. Clues to diagnosis include (1) malocclusion because of premature molar contact resulting from a decrease in the height of the mandibular ramus; (2) inability to palpate the condylar head as the patient opens and closes his mouth (palpation can be attempted either anterior to the ear or with a finger in the external auditory meatus); (3) pain in the preauricular area on opening the mouth; and (4) deviation to the fractured side when the mouth is opened. Careful radiologic assessment is imperative since condylar fractures are often subtle and can be overlooked because of more obvious injuries. The Towne's projection view and the panoramic view offer the best means for radiologic diagnosis.

Diagnostic failure can lead to disturbing symptoms of pain and deviation of the jaw. In children, the condylar region is extremely vascular until the age of about 6, and during these years injury may cause extensive hematoma, ankylosis, and growth impairment. Treatment is therefore directed to early mobilization. If necessary, short-term intermaxillary fixation is employed to establish occlusion; if occlusion is normal, fixation is not used.

Although a condylar fracture in a patient with massive maxillofacial injury such as a LeFort III

fracture (see Fig. 29.15) may seem trivial, ability to restore the normal appearance of the face rests on alignment of the maxilla against an intact mandible. This is difficult to achieve if there are no posterior teeth or if the mandible has "gagged open" because of collapse on the side of the condylar fracture. In the management of these fractures in adults, basic principles include the following: (1) if there is malocclusion, intermaxillary fixation for 10–21 days is required to establish proper occlusion in either unilateral or bilateral fractures; (2) if there is no malocclusion, a soft diet and limited jaw motion are recommended; and (3) if an open bite exists and particularly if the patient has no posterior teeth, open reduction (Fig. 30.7) of at least one side in bilateral fractures should be considered.

Zygomaticomaxillary Complex

Assessment of the zygomaticomaxillary complex is somewhat more complicated than assessment of the mandible. Extensive edema occurs rapidly and makes it difficult to diagnose the underlying skeletal injuries. Careful physical and radiologic examination provides accurate diagnosis from which appropriate surgical treatment can be planned.

On inspection, an elongated face and bilateral circumorbital ecchymosis are noted in midface fractures—the result of dropping of the maxilla. At the same time, in LeFort II and III fractures the posterior teeth often cause "gagging" of the occlusion, preventing closure, and the patient appears to have an open bite. If the patient is seen shortly after injury, flattening of the upper part of the cheek indicates a zygomatic fracture; this can

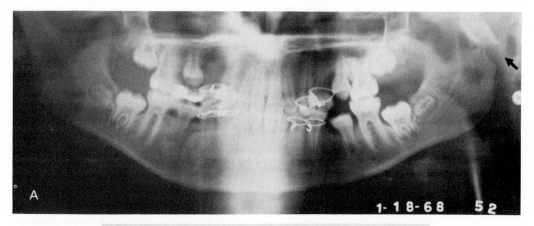

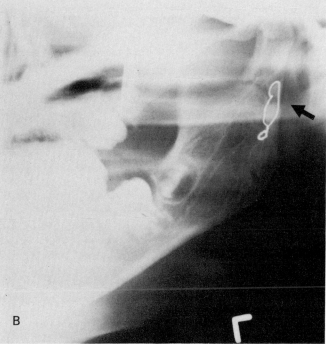

Figure 30.7. **(A)** Fractured (totally distracted) condyle (*arrow*). **(B)** Open reduction and interosseous wiring of condyle (*arrow*).

be observed by standing behind the patient and sighting the superior orbital margin from above. Bleeding from the nose or ears or both should be sought, particularly to determine whether there is cerebrospinal fluid leakage—a finding that is sometimes difficult to confirm, but that suggests a LeFort II or III fracture.

Other important findings may be noted from inspection of the eyes. Discrepancy of ocular levels, as determined by a line projected between the pupils, may result from a blow-out fracture with herniation of the orbital contents through the fractured floor into the antrum. Subconjunctival

ecchymosis may indicate fracture of the lateral orbital wall, part of a typical tripod fracture of the zygomaticomaxillary complex. Restriction of ocular movements is diagnostic of muscle entrapment in orbital floor injury, and diplopia suggests disruption of the orbit by a zygomaticomaxillary fracture.

Visual inspection should be followed by palpation. The index finger should be moved over the entire orbital rim to note both tenderness and step defects. Particular attention should be given to the zygomaticofrontal and zygomaticomaxillary sutures. In addition to step defects, crepitation is often detected. If the patient is conscious and responsive, anesthesia of the cheek, nose, and lips should be investigated, its existence being very suggestive of a fracture through the infraorbital or zygomatic branch of the trigeminal nerve.

Intraoral examination follows manual inspection of the face. First, mobility of the maxilla should be tested by holding the bridge of the nose with one hand while grasping the upper anterior teeth with the other hand. Movement can be seen and felt as it is transmitted to the firmly grasped nasal bones. There may be ecchymosis of the upper buccal sulcus, as well as anesthesia of the gingiva and teeth in the area. Fractures of the lateral antral wall and zygomatic buttress can sometimes be palpated. At the same examination, gagging due to displacement of the maxilla may be observed; limitation of mandibular movement may result from impingement of a fractured zygomatic arch on the coronoid process of the mandible.

On the basis of clinical findings, certain x-ray views are indicated. The Waters' view (also known as the occipitomental projection) is the most useful film for demonstrating fractures of the zygomaticomaxillary complex. The orbital rims, zygomatic arches, and antra are all visualized. In addition, a submental vertex (jug-handle) view will demonstrate fractures of the zygomatic arch that other films might not. No radiologic examination of a patient with multiple facial fractures is complete without posteroanterior and lateral skull films to investigate possible cranial injury. The usefulness of tomography is probably limited to cases of questionable blow-out fractures, in which it may confirm what was suggested in a Waters' view.

Temporomandibular Joint

Another distressing jaw problem seen in the emergency ward is dislocation of the temporomandibular joint (Fig. 30.8). It demands prompt reduction and careful explanation and follow-up care. In this type of dislocation, which may result from trauma or sudden stretching of masticatory muscles as in excessive yawning, the condylar head is held anterior to or on the articular eminence by myospasm. The dislocation is treated by simple manual reduction, although spontaneous reduction may occur if the patient is sufficiently relaxed. The use of meperidine hydrochloride (Demerol) or a muscle relaxant such as diazepam (Valium) can facilitate either spontaneous or manual reduction. Reduction is performed by standing in front of the patient and placing the index fingers in the buccal mandibular sulci, applying pressure inferiorly and posteriorly over the retromolar pads; at the same time, thumb pressure is directed superiorly at the symphysis. Firm pressure is applied gradually and consistently until the condyle is repositioned in the glenoid fossa. A sponge is useful as a finger cushion. To prevent recurrent dislocation, it is necessary to restrict opening of the mouth for several hours and to restrict mandibular movement for 2–3 weeks.

Occasionally, a dislocation cannot be reduced without general anesthesia and muscle relaxants. Repeated injection of a local anesthetic into the masseter muscle or joint space is usually unsuccessful and unpleasant for the patient; it is not ordinarily an alternative to general anesthesia. If dislocation occurs frequently, intermaxillary fixation may be necessary until definitive treatment

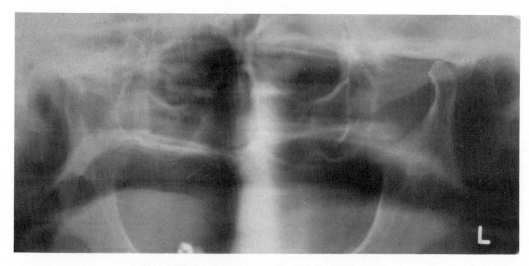

Figure 30.8.   Temporomandibular joint dislocation.

can be given, but only for a short period. Patients with habitual dislocation may have to be told to bury the chin in the chest during yawning.

The extrapyramidal neuromuscular effects of phenothiazine derivatives such as prochlorperazine maleate (Compazine) are well known. Diagnosis is based on the history and clinical findings. Symptoms may include agitation, spasm of neck muscles sometimes progressing to torticolis, carpopedal spasm, trismus, and dislocation of the jaw. Treatment includes reassurance and discontinuance of the drug. Barbiturates and diphenhydramine hydrochloride (Benadryl), 50 mg intramuscularly, are helpful.

INJURY TO PAROTID GLAND AND DUCT

Soft-tissue injuries are dealt with in Chapter 29. However, injury to the parotid gland and duct, a significant and unique injury occasionally found accompanying facial trauma, deserves emphasis. Primary recognition and treatment of this class of injury prevents complications of fistula, sialocele, and infection. Careful clinical examination should be conducted in cases of laceration of the cheek. Although hemostasis must be obtained for direct visualization into the wound, blind clamping in this region is inadvisable and primary examination may be better carried out in the operating room.

If parotid duct injury is suspected and the duct cannot be visualized within the wound or if a severed end is not visible, the duct should be probed. A lacrimal duct probe can usually be passed via the oral opening of the parotid duct. This makes it easier to locate the duct in the wound to determine if it has been transected or lacerated; in such a case the probe will emerge in the wound. If the probe does not exit into the wound, it can be palpated through the wound and the location of the duct in relation to the injury can be ascertained. If there is still a question as to duct injury after probing, two choices exist: methylene blue can be injected into the duct and its presence in the wound observed, or a sialogram

can be obtained. These studies are useful to determine whether the parotid gland has been injured and its capsule violated. Facial nerve function must also be carefully evaluated.

The lacerated parotid duct is best treated by direct anastomosis, using 6–0 silk sutures over a plastic catheter; No. 16 or No. 18 Intracath tubing works well. The catheter is left sutured to the buccal mucosa for 10–14 days. Antibiotics should be administered prophylactically; penicillin is recommended if the patient is not allergic to it. Gland stimulation with lemon drops and dilation of the duct are useful.

If the damage to the duct prevents direct anastomosis, the proximal portion of the duct must be found and ligated. Gland atrophy will ensue. Direct damage to the capsule and gland demands meticulous closure of the capsule and closure of the wound in layers. This is of paramount importance to recovery of distal facial nerve function as well. Usually, facial nerve injuries distal to a line projected from the outer canthus of the eye to the gonial notch of the mandible (about 2 cm from the angle of the jaw) do not require anastomosis.

Suggested Readings

Epker BN, Burnette JC: Trauma to the parotid gland and duct: Primary treatment and management of complications. *J Oral Surg* 28:657–670, 1970

Guralnick WC (Ed): *Textbook of Oral Surgery.* Boston, Little, Brown, 1968

Hötte HH: *Orbital Fractures.* Springfield, Illinois, Charles C Thomas, 1970

Irby WB (Ed): *Facial Trauma and Concomitant Problems: Evaluation and Treatment.* St. Louis, CV Mosby, 1974

Kelly JF (Ed): *Management of War Injuries to the Jaws and Related Structures.* Department of the Navy, 1978

McCarthy PL, Shklar G: *Diseases of the Oral Mucosa: Diagnosis, Management, Therapy.* New York, McGraw-Hill, 1964

Pozatek ZW, Kaban LB, Guralnick WC: Fractures of the zygomatic complex: An evaluation of surgical management with special emphasis on the eyebrow approach. *J Oral Surg* 31:141–148, 1973

Rowe NL, Killey HC: *Fractures of the Facial Skeleton*, ed 2. Edinburgh, Livingstone, 1968

Trieger N: *Pain Control.* Berlin, Buch- und Zeitschriften-Verlag Die Quintessenz, 1974

CHAPTER 31

Emergency Care of the Injured Hand

RICHARD J. SMITH, M.D.

The initial treatment of an injured hand often determines the nature of further reconstructive surgical procedures, the duration and severity of disability, and the ultimate function of the entire limb. To restore its versatility and strength, the surgeon must provide smoothly gliding muscle-tendon units and a stable skeletal framework, minimize contractures and adhesions of skin, tendons, and joints, and preserve sensation. Complications such as subcutaneous hematoma, edema, and superficial infection, which often resolve without sequelae if they occur elsewhere, may result in permanent restriction of motion if they occur in the hand. The appearance of the hand is also of great importance; a self-conscious patient may not use a limb that is badly scarred or mutilated. Although hand injuries are common in busy emergency wards, this in no way lessens their importance or the responsibilities of the physician treating them.

GENERAL CONSIDERATIONS

History

The proper evaluation and treatment of the patient with a wounded hand requires adequate knowledge of both the injury and the patient's previous medical history. Information concerning allergies to antibiotics and other drugs and the history of previous tetanus immunization are essential for planning medical therapy. Did the patient sustain other injuries at the time of the accident? Although the victim of an assault, for example, may be concerned about a stab wound of the palm, he may also have injuries to the chest wall that have caused pneumothorax. The history should also include the occupation and dominant hand of the patient, since the prognosis is often influenced by these factors.

Details of the mechanism of the injury are often crucial to treatment. If the hand has been cut by glass, the type of glass is important since tinted bottles and fine glassware frequently contain lead that may be visible on x-ray examination. A hand injured in a press may have a thermal injury as well as a crush injury. The physician should ask if the press was hot and if the hand was exposed to its repeated action. Although machine oil at the edges of a wound may make the wound look dirty, it may be innocuous. Air bubbles deep in a wound may appear ominous on x-ray examination, but may merely be the result of irrigation with hydrogen peroxide solution before arrival at the emergency ward. Small, seemingly harmless lacerations, however, may actually harbor spirochetes, streptococci, and clostridia if they are the result of a human bite.

If an amputated portion of the hand has been retrieved, its history must also be noted. Where was it found? Was it subjected to heat or repeated trauma? Was it washed, cooled, or treated with antiseptics? These questions must be asked as part of the complete history before the patient is anesthetized, since surgical decisions may depend on the patient's responses.

A standard hand injury history form is often valuable in rapidly obtaining a complete, relevant record that is useful in evaluating the injury and in planning treatment. This form should be brief but comprehensive.

Preliminary Examination and Evaluation

Before the injured hand is examined, the entire limb should be inspected. The patient, a coworker, or a family member may have applied a tourniquet to stop the bleeding and the sleeve may then have been rebuttoned, concealing it. All bracelets, rings, and other jewelry must be removed from the hand, regardless of the patient's sentiments, since such objects may act as tourniquets as the limb swells.

Except for the most minor lacerations, all wounds of the hand should be examined radiologically. If the films can be taken without delay and if the patient's general condition is stable, it is usually advisable to perform x-ray examination before other examination of the hand. With more serious injuries, however, excessive delay in rendering primary wound care should be avoided.

Severe crush and explosion injuries and burns need not be inspected in the emergency ward, since such an examination would be painful and would cause unnecessary contamination. Less severe wounds may be examined in the emergency ward under aseptic conditions. The patient should be calmed and should preferably be placed in the supine position. The examiner should wear a mask and sterile gloves. After the injured hand is placed on a sterile field, all dressings are cut down to the bottom layer, which is soaked loose in a pan of sterile saline if it is adherent to the wound. The wound should not be probed. Coagulated blood is gently removed with a sponge soaked in hydrogen peroxide solution. Superficial foreign material should be cleansed from the wound, although it is not necessary to remove all ingrained dirt or grease from the surface of the skin. Benzene is an excellent and painless solvent for many types of grease, ink, and paint. The wound is then gently lavaged with sterile saline or Ringer's lactated solution and a sterile sponge is applied until definitive care can be rendered.

Inspection of the cleansed hand lying at rest is probably the most valuable part of the hand examination. With the wrist in mild dorsiflexion, any irregularity in the normal curve of the semi-flexed fingertips is immediately apparent, calling attention to a flexor tendon injury. With the forearm in pronation and the wrist in palmar flexion, a lag of extension at a metacarpophalangeal joint signals an extensor tendon injury. Malrotation of a fingernail usually indicates a rotated fracture of a tubular bone, either phalanx or metacarpal. Depression of a metacarpal head suggests a fracture of the metacarpal neck. If the thumb is supinated and adducted against the index finger, injury to the median nerve should be suspected.

The color, temperature, and moisture of the fingertips are also noted. With laceration of a sensory nerve, normal perspiration in the corresponding part of the finger stops at once. A finger in which both neurovascular bundles are lacerated is likely to be pale and cool, and its viability is precarious.

Tests of tendon and nerve function are performed simply and painlessly. Alternate flexion and extension of the fingers, thumb, and wrist, active adduction and abduction of the thumb and index finger, and a brief sensory examination often provide most of the information required for neuromuscular evaluation (Tables 31.1 and 31.2, Fig. 31.1). Nothing can more rapidly distress an alarmed child than use of a pin or needle for pinprick evaluation. To test sharp-dull discrimination, the examiner should touch, but not jab, the skin with a pinpoint, and the patient should be allowed to watch. A more sensitive test is to ask a patient to differentiate between the milled edge of a quarter dollar and the smooth edge of a nickle. To diagnose major nerve injuries, the physician should test the autonomous zones of the radial, median, and ulnar nerves at the dorsum of the first web, the tip of the thumb, and the tip of the little finger, respectively.

The anatomic diagnosis and the extent of all injuries are recorded, preferably with a sketch of the hand wounds. Photographs should be taken. The physician then decides whether to treat the injury in the emergency ward or in the operating room. The limb is splinted and elevated until definitive treatment is given. The patient and his family are told of the general plan of treatment and the expected prognosis.

Débridement and Cleansing

Thorough cleansing of the wound is most important in the treatment of an injured hand. The uninjured portion of the hand may be washed and shaved in the emergency ward to permit proper examination. Complex wounds should not be cleansed deeply without regional or general anesthesia, and cleansing must be done in a sterile field. Most bleeding can be controlled with gentle pressure. It is unnecessary to attempt total hemostasis before débridement and lavage.

After the patient has been brought to a sterile area, a pneumatic tourniquet is padded with sheet cotton and applied to the upper arm. The limb is exsanguinated by elevation and the tourniquet cuff is inflated to a pressure of 100–150 mm Hg above systolic pressure. A rubber band tourniquet around the base of a finger or a catheter tourniquet wrapped around the wrist or forearm may cause damage to nerves or blood vessels since the pressure is unchecked. Even without anesthesia, almost all patients can tolerate a properly applied pneumatic tourniquet for at least 20–30 minutes if the arm has been exsanguinated.

With sterile technique, the skin around the

Table 31.1.
Intrinsic muscle innervation and function to the hand.

Muscle	Function	Innervation	Test or Observation
Thenar muscles (abductor pollicis brevis, flexor pollicis brevis, opponens pollicis)	Abduction, pronation, flexion—first metacarpal; abduction, flexion—proximal phalanx of thumb; extension—distal phalanx of thumb	Median nerve, with occasional ulnar nerve contribution	Compare abduction of both thumbs from palmar plane; have patient oppose thumb tip to tip of little finger; with paralysis, thenar atrophy, poor thumb abduction from palm, poor thumb rotation
Adductor pollicis	Adduction—first metacarpal and proximal phalanx of thumb in palmar plane; flexion—proximal phalanx of thumb; extension—distal phalanx of thumb	Ulnar nerve	Have patient pull sheet of paper from examiner—interphalangeal joint of thumb will acutely flex (Froment's sign) if adductor is weak
Hypothenar muscles (abductor digiti quinti, flexor digiti quinti, opponens digiti quinti)	Flexion, pronation—fifth metacarpal; flexion—metacarpophalangeal joint of little finger; extension—interphalangeal joints of little finger	Ulnar nerve	Have patient oppose tip of little finger to thumb tip (little finger abduction possible through extensor digiti quinti proprius)
All interosseus muscles	Flexion—metacarpophalangeal joints; extension—interphalangeal joints	Ulnar nerve	No active abduction or adduction of involved fingers; ring and little fingers clawed (lumbricals of index and middle fingers, supplied by median nerve, prevent clawing)
Dorsal interossei	Abduction of fingers from middle finger		
Palmar interossei	Adduction of fingers to middle finger		
Lumbrical muscles	Flexion—metacarpophalangeal joints; extension—interphalangeal joints	Median nerve—index and middle fingers; Ulnar nerve—ring and little fingers	Difficult to test if interossei are intact; if interossei are paralyzed, lack of metacarpophalangeal flexion with interphalangeal extension of index and middle fingers indicates lumbrical paralysis

wound is washed thoroughly and the hand is sponged gently with soapy water. Coagulated blood is removed. The wound is lavaged with 4 liters of either sterile saline or Ringer's lactated solution, and the hand is placed on a sterile towel. The surgeon then puts on new gloves, cleanses the wound with an antiseptic solution such as povidone-iodine and drapes the limb for operation.

The depths of the wound are now explored, and foreign bodies are extracted. The edges of the wound are held back by blunt rakes for thorough exposure and débridement. Splinters of bone that are not attached to soft tissue are removed. Muscle that is dark, not contractile, and obviously not viable is excised. Lacerated tendons and nerves are identified and tagged with sutures. Surgical reconstruction of deeper tissues and skin grafting are then performed (details are given in later sections).

After the operation is completed, the wound is again copiously irrigated, the arm is elevated, and the tourniquet is released and removed. Gentle pressure is applied to the wound for 4 or 5 minutes. Hemostasis is usually obtained more quickly and less traumatically with cautery than with large numbers of ligatures. The edges of skin and subcutaneous tissue should not be excised unless they are ragged, necrotic, or crushed.

Table 31.2.
Extrinsic muscle innervation and function to hand.

Muscle	Function	Innervation
Flexor carpi ulnaris	Flexion, ulnar deviation—wrist	Ulnar nerve
Palmaris longus	Flexion—wrist (weak)	Median nerve
Flexor carpi radialis	Flexion, radial deviation—wrist	Median nerve
Flexor pollicis longus	Flexion—distal phalanx of thumb	Median nerve (anterior interosseous branch)
Flexor digitorum profundus	Flexion—distal phalanges of fingers	Median nerve (anterior interosseous branch)—index and middle fingers Ulnar nerve—ring and little fingers
Flexor digitorum superficialis (sublimis)	Flexion—middle phalanges	Median nerve
Abductor pollicis longus	Extension—first metacarpal	Radial nerve (dorsal interosseous branch)
Extensor pollicis brevis	Extension—proximal phalanx of thumb	Radial nerve (dorsal interosseous branch)
Extensor pollicis longus	Extension—distal phalanx of thumb	Radial nerve (dorsal interosseus branch)
Extensor carpi radialis longus	Extension, radial deviation—wrist	Radial nerve
Extensor carpi radialis brevis	Extension—wrist	Radial nerve (dorsal interosseous branch)
Extensor digitorum communis, extensor indicis proprius, extensor digiti quinti proprius	Extension—proximal phalanges of fingers	Radial nerve (dorsal interosseous branch)
Extensor carpi ulnaris	Extension, ulnar deviation—wrist	Radial nerve (dorsal interosseous branch)

Dressings

Properly applied hand dressings serve several purposes. They protect the wound from contamination, absorb drainage, provide even pressure, and close potential dead spaces. Many dressings also serve as splints. A hand dressing must be comfortable, and should not cause maceration or tissue strangulation. Tight compression dressings are never indicated for hand wounds.

While dressings are applied to the hand, an assistant usually holds the hand by the tips of the index and middle fingers to preserve the width and concavity of the palm and to prevent the first, fourth, and fifth metacarpal bones from being squeezed together or flattened. In a typical hand dressing, one layer of petrolatum gauze covers the wound to prevent the skin from adhering to the dressing. Loosely packed fluffs of gauze that do not contain cotton are then placed in the natural concavities of the hand, with one or two thicknesses of gauze between the fingers. Volar and dorsal strips of sheet cotton are placed on the hand and forearm, and the wrist is supported with a plaster splint. A layer of springy gauze and a nonrubberized elastic bandage complete the dressing. If the fingers do not need to be immobilized, the dressing should end at the distal palmar crease

to allow full mobility of the metacarpophalangeal joints. If the thumb does not need to be immobilized, it is freed to the carpometacarpal joint. After the dressing is completed, the arm is elevated so that the fingers are higher than the level of the heart. A stockinette that is cut to expose the fingers and thumb may be applied over the dressing and attached to an intravenous pole. If the patient is discharged, he is instructed to suspend the arm by tying the stockinette to a bedpost or a high-backed chair. With infants and young children, hand dressings are always extended above the elbow and the elbow is flexed to 70 degrees to prevent the child from slipping the dressing off the arm.

After operation, a hand that has been severely crushed may exhibit borderline viability because of edema, capillary sludging, and poor venous blood flow. The fingers may remain cool and blue. Enzymes administered orally or parenterally do not appear to be effective in preventing or decreasing edema. Sluggish circulation may be improved with plasma expanders, anticoagulants, or cervical sympathetic blockade. Such treatment, of course, is influenced by the general condition of the patient and the presence of associated injuries. In a healthy patient, 500–1000 ml of dextran 40 given at a rate of 30–50 ml/min expand plasma volume and decrease platelet aggregation and fluid tran-

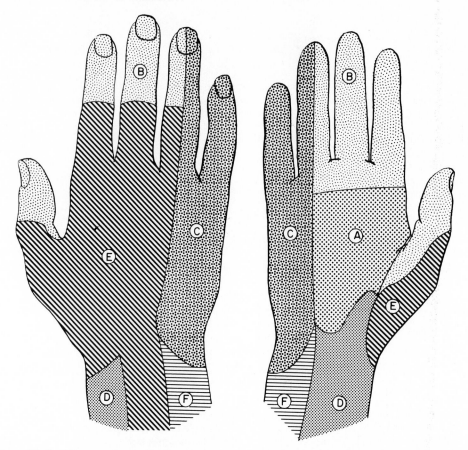

Figure 31.1. Diagram of normal sensory distribution of the hand indicates areas supplied by (*A*) palmar cutaneous branch of the median nerve, (*B*) digital branches of the median nerve, (*C*) superficial branches of the ulnar nerve, (*D*) lateral antebrachial cutaneous branch of the musculocutaneous nerve, (*E*) superficial branches of the radial nerve, and (*F*) medial antebrachial cutaneous nerve.

sudation into soft tissues. If the hand remains dusky, intravenous heparin or oral salicylates are administered for anticoagulation unless there are severe wounds elsewhere. If hematuria, hematoma, ecchymosis, or petechiae develop, anticoagulants are discontinued.

Continuous sympathetic blockade frequently relieves pain in the limb, and may help prevent small-vessel shutdown due to arteriolar spasm in the injured, edematous hand. Under local anesthesia a 16-gauge polyethylene catheter approximately 12.5 cm long is inserted into the region of the cervical sympathetic chain at the level of the cricoid cartilage. A 10-ml syringe is attached to the tube and taped to the neck. Every 8–12 hours, 10 ml of a 0.5% bupivacaine hydrochloride solution with epinephrine (1:200,000) is injected into the catheter. The sympathetic blockade is continued for about 5 days.

Antibiotic and Tetanus Prophylaxis

Antibiotics are administered routinely to patients with severely contaminated, deep, or contused open wounds; a history of antibiotic allergy influences the choice of medication. Oxacillin, cephalothin, or lincomycin is preferred, and is administered intravenously for 3 or 4 days. If the patient is afebrile after this time and if the wound appears to be healing normally, intravenous administration is discontinued and the patient is given antibiotics orally for another week. Outpatients with dirty or edematous wounds are treated with oral oxacillin, cephalexin, or lincomycin. Local irrigation with a bacitracin-neomycin solution is employed for severe wounds and for wounds entering a joint. A tetanus toxoid booster dose and human immune globulin are also given unless the patient has had a full course of tetanus immunization within 10 years. Immune globulin is unnecessary in the treatment of clean, minor wounds if the patient has had complete tetanus immunization. In such cases, the patient is given a tetanus toxoid booster dose (see Table 11.6).

SOFT-TISSUE INJURIES

Primary or Secondary Wound Closure— General Considerations

Whether a wound should be closed primarily or secondarily is a serious decision. Inappropriate primary wound closure may jeopardize the function of the hand if edema, necrosis, and infection supervene. However, appropriate primary closure will prevent continued contamination, desiccation, and drainage of the deep tissues. The decision for or against primary closure depends on the following factors:

(1) *Degree and type of contamination* at the time of injury. Hand wounds in persons working in bacteriology and autopsy laboratories and in dirty areas such as barnyards, as well as injuries from human and animal bites, are notorious for the virulence of the bacterial contaminants. Rarely should such wounds be closed.

(2) *Time since injury.* Since the bacterial count increases geometrically within hours after injury, primary closure of a badly contaminated wound more than 24 hours old is rarely justified.

(3) *Type of wound.* Rank and Wakefield have differentiated between "tidy" and "untidy" wounds. In tidy wounds, such as those caused by a knife, glass edge, or razor blade, foreign material is not ground into the deeper tissues or pushed through fascial or synovial planes. Only the local tissues are injured, tissue viability is determined easily, and edema is minimal. In untidy wounds, tissues are crushed, torn, burned, or ripped, and it is often impossible to assess the extent of venous thrombosis, edema, deep tendon injury, necrosis, and contamination on initial examination. If an untidy wound is treated late, it may be wiser to débride and to lavage the wound and to close it secondarily in order to minimize the possibility of necrosis or infection.

(4) *Other factors.* There are many types of injuries such as snakebites, injection injuries, close-range gunshot wounds, and thermal injuries that require special treatment. These wounds are often best left open.

If careful evaluation of the degree and type of contamination, the time since injury, the tidiness of the wound, and other factors raise doubt about the wisdom of primary closure, the physician should leave the wound open for delayed closure and should apply wet dressings.

Skin Grafts

Split-Thickness Skin Grafts

A thin split-thickness skin graft has an excellent chance of "taking" over virtually any tissue bed on the surface of the hand with the exception of cortical bone and bared tendon. At the dorsum of the hand, loss of skin and subcutaneous tissue is preferentially treated with split-thickness skin grafting. Small fingertip losses with intact subcutaneous pulp may also be managed with a split-thickness graft. These grafts should not be used to treat a partly amputated finger with exposed bone, since dysesthesia and a tender finger tip frequently result.

Split-thickness skin grafts often contract as much as 75%. To prevent joint contracture the surgeon should design the edges of the recipient area so that the edges of the graft are not perpendicular to skin creases. Since thin split-thickness grafts are somewhat friable, they are not recommended in the gripping areas of the hand such as the palm and the volar aspects of the fingers and thumb. Either a thick split-thickness graft or a full-thickness graft is preferable in these areas.

Small split-thickness skin graft may be removed from the medial aspect of the arm several centimeters above the elbow, or from the thigh or buttock. Since grafts from the volar aspect of the forearm may cause a hyperpigmented, readily visible scar, this region is not a preferred donor site. Multiple postage-stamp-sized grafts leave unsightly donor and recipient sites and are not used.

In adult patients the graft is taken 0.018 inch thick, and is held to the recipient site with interrupted sutures of 5–0 nylon. In children, a graft 0.014-inch thick is used and may be sutured in place with absorbable catgut. Opening numerous drainage holes by means of small incisions in the graft, known as "piecrusting," appears of little value. The graft is covered with a single thickness of petrolatum gauze, which is held snugly to the graft with interrupted catgut sutures. The gauze must not be applied circumferentially. We have found this technique to be preferable to use of a stent for holding the graft evenly over the convex areas of the hand. Several thicknesses of wet sheet cotton are placed over the gauze and held in place with dry dressings. The recipient area is splinted.

Unless drainage, pain, or signs of infection develop, the dressing is not disturbed for 5 days.

Full-Thickness Skin Grafts

A full-thickness skin graft contracts less than a split-thickness graft, and is better able to resist friction and pressure. Thus these grafts are preferred to split-thickness grafts for the gripping surfaces of the hand when the patient has a good graft bed of viable and vascular tissue. Full-thickness skin grafts should not be placed over bone or tendon sheath; without a good vascular bed, these grafts may fail to become revascularized fast enough to maintain viability. As with split-thickness grafts, the recipient site is designed so that the edges of the graft are not perpendicular to flexion creases.

Small grafts may be removed from the medial aspect of the arm. In patients with dark skin, grafts to the fingertips may be taken from the arch of the foot or adjacent to the medial malleolus to minimize hyperpigmentation of the graft. Larger grafts are removed from the inguinal crease. No subcutaneous tissue is transferred with the full-thickness graft. The thickness of the donor skin is carefully trimmed so that it has an "orange-peel" appearance. Like the split-thickness graft, after the full-thickness graft is sutured to the donor site, it is held in place with a sutured petrolatum gauze dressing.

Composite Grafts

Some surgeons have used the composite graft of skin and subcutaneous tissue to cover a deep soft-tissue defect of a fingertip of an infant or child. The surgical technique is similar to that used with partial-thickness and full-thickness skin grafts. We have not found such grafts necessary.

Flaps

If skin with subcutaneous tissue is transferred to a recipient area with its viability maintained through a vascular stalk, the transfer is considered a flap. Frequently, flaps of skin and subcutaneous tissue may be advanced, transposed, or rotated in such a manner that the vascular pedicle can remain permanently undisturbed. These one-stage *local flaps* retain sensation, contract little, and do not become hyperpigmented as do many split-thickness and full-thickness skin grafts. Pedicle flaps may be transferred to any clean tissue bed, and thus provide ideal coverage for exposed bone and tendon.

Frequently, large areas cannot be covered by shifting adjacent skin, and pedicle flaps must be constructed from a more remote region such as the opposite arm, the chest, the inguinal region, or the abdomen. *Remote flaps* must be detached from the donor site after they have become revascularized from the recipient area. Although they provide excellent coverage, such flaps do not retain sensation since nerves and vessels are transected when the flap is detached. Remote flaps shrink little, but do become somewhat hyperpigmented. Pedicle flaps from the abdomen tend to become more adipose when the patient gains weight, and often appear bulky. For these reasons, local flaps are preferred when possible.

Free vascularized tissue transfers may be used to cover relatively large skin defects in one stage. These *free flaps* may be removed from any one of several regions where the skin and subcutaneous tissue are well perfused by a vascular stalk. The vein, artery, and occasionally the superficial nerve of the flap are joined to the recipient vessels and nerves.

Local Flaps. Fingers with amputated tips in which several millimeters of the distal phalanx are exposed are often best treated with a *V-Y advancement flap* (Fig. 31.2). Use of a lateral V-Y flap (Kutler flap) results in a longitudinal scar at the fingertip, which may be tender and dysesthetic. For that reason, we prefer volar V-Y advancement. A V-shaped incision is made *through the skin only*, with its apex at about the level of the distal flexion crease of the finger. Incisions are *not* made through the subcutaneous tissue. A triangle is formed with the amputation site as the base. The scalpel blade is then inserted through the amputation site adjacent and parallel to the volar cortex of the remaining portion of the distal phalanx. The subcutaneous tissue is separated from the phalanx and from the insertion of the flexor digitorum profundus tendon. The flap then is advanced distally to cover the defect. The base of the V is sutured to the nailbed and to the dorsal skin of the fingertip. The defect left at the apex of the triangle by advancing the flap is closed side to side, forming the stem of the Y. Contour, padding, and excellent sensation are usually restored with this flap.

With avulsion of the skin of the thumb tip, a *quadrangular volar advancement flap* (Fig. 31.3) has proved to be safe and versatile. Longitudinal midaxial (dorsolateral) incisions are made through the skin and subcutaneous tissue on both sides of the thumb from the wound to the proximal flexion crease. The skin, subcutaneous tissue, and both neurovascular bundles are elevated with the flap from the underlying bone and from the pulleys and sheath of the flexor pollicis longus tendon. The thumb tip is flexed and the flap is advanced

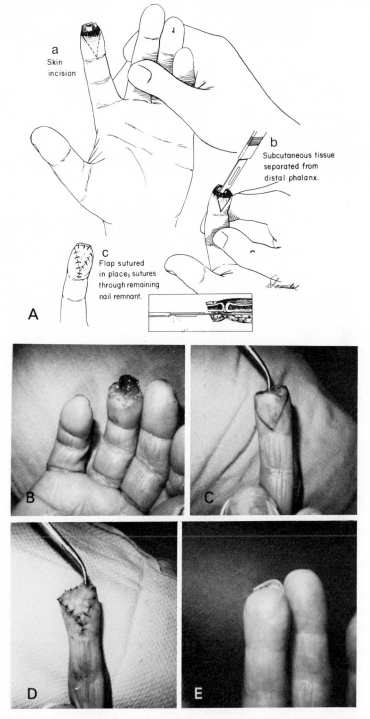

Figure 31.2. Volar V-Y advancement flap. **(A)** Technique. (*a*) Skin incision extends to defect. Its apex lies at level of distal flexion crease. (*b*) Subcutaneous tissue is separated from distal phalanx by transecting longitudinal septa just superficial to the periosteum. Care should be taken not to detach the insertion of the flexor digitorum profundus tendon. (*c*) The triangular flap is advanced distally and sutured to the dorsal skin or nail. This leaves a proximal defect that is closed side to side. In the dissection, subcutaneous tissue is not incised, but is drawn distally with the skin flap. **(B)** Avulsion of ring fingertip has left 1.5 cm of distal phalanx protruding from site of injury. **(C)** Outline of skin incision is drawn. **(D)** After the skin has been incised and subcutaneous tissue freed from the volar aspect of the distal phalanx, the flap is advanced distally and sutured in place. **(E)** Four weeks later, appearance of fingertip is good. Sensibility and circulation to the flap have remained intact.

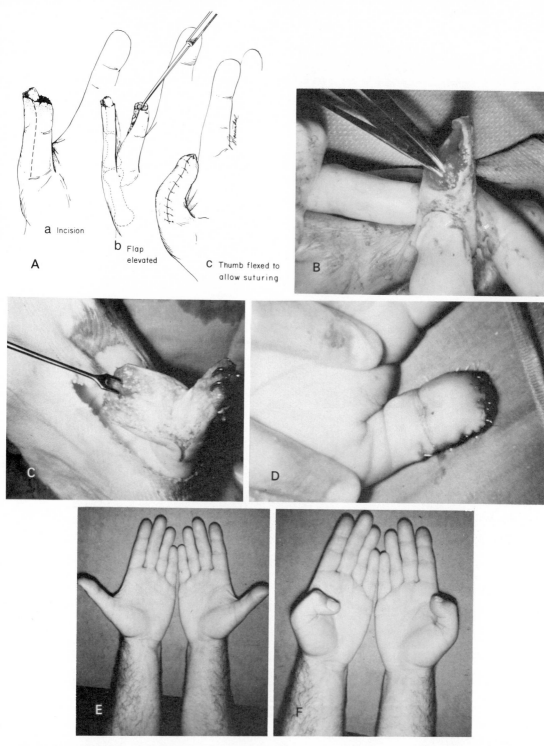

Figure 31.3. Quadrangular volar advancement flap. This should only be used for the thumb and not for the fingers. **(A)** Technique. (*a*) Longitudinal midaxial incisions are made on either side of thumb to proximal flexion crease. (*b*) Skin, subcutaneous tissues, and neurovascular bundles are elevated. (*c*) Interphalangeal joint of thumb is flexed and flap is advanced distally. **(B)** Volar avulsion injury of thumb tip sustained an hour previously. **(C)** Volar flap is developed with subcutaneous tissues and neurovascular bundles freed with flap from phalanx. **(D)** Flap is advanced and sutured in place. **(E)** Two months postoperatively there is complete extension of thumb tip and good thumb tip padding with skin of normal sensibility. **(F)** There is mild loss of interphalangeal flexion of thumb because of initial injury.

676

distally to be sutured to the nailbed and dorsal skin. Such flaps can be advanced up to 2.0 cm. The thumb tip is kept partly flexed for 3 weeks while the advanced skin heals in its new position. Although the ability to hyperextend the interphalangeal joint of the thumb may be lost after this procedure, flexion contracture is rare. An excellent aesthetic and functional result is usually achieved. This procedure should only be used for the thumb and should *not* be used to cover defects in the fingers. Quadrangular advancement flaps in the fingers often cause flexion contracture of the interphalangeal joints and may jeopardize the venous drainage and arterial supply or the dorsal skin. These problems are rarely encountered in the thumb.

Z-plasty (Fig. 31.4) may be used to prevent flexion contractures in fingers with a longitudinal volar wound that crosses flexion creases. Oblique incisions are made at 60-degree angles to the skin laceration to form the letter Z. Each of the three limbs of the Z should be equal. The midpoint of the longitudinal limb of the Z (the laceration) should fall at a flexion crease. With the two flaps transposed, the longitudinal incision is rotated 90 degrees so that the scar lies in the line of the flexion crease. Skin length is increased about 50%. To prevent excessive tension on the apex of each flap, sutures should be inserted obliquely to advance each flap toward its apex.

The *neurovascular island pedicle flap* (Fig. 31.5) is rarely used in emergency operations. Occasion-

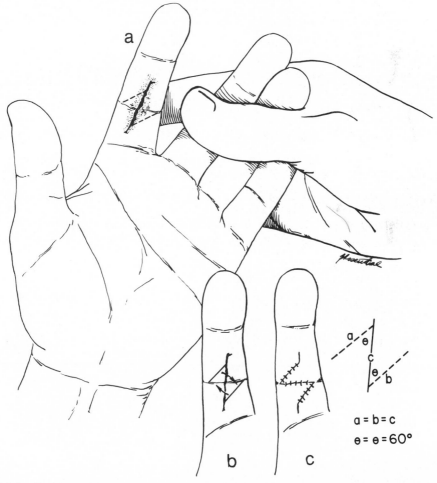

$$a = b = c$$
$$\theta = \theta = 60°$$

Figure 31.4. Z-plasty may be used to transpose a longitudinal scar so that it does not cross a flexion crease. If a scar is perpendicular to a flexion crease, it is likely to cause flexion contracture. (*a*) Oblique limbs, usually drawn 60 degrees to the longitudinal scar, are placed equidistant from the flexion crease. Each limb should equal the length of the longitudinal scar between them. (*b*) The triangular flaps are transposed. (*c*) The transposed flaps are sutured in place. This increases the length of the injured skin by about 50%, but may cause some narrowing in the area of flap transposition. For large wounds, multiple Z-plasties are therefore recommended.

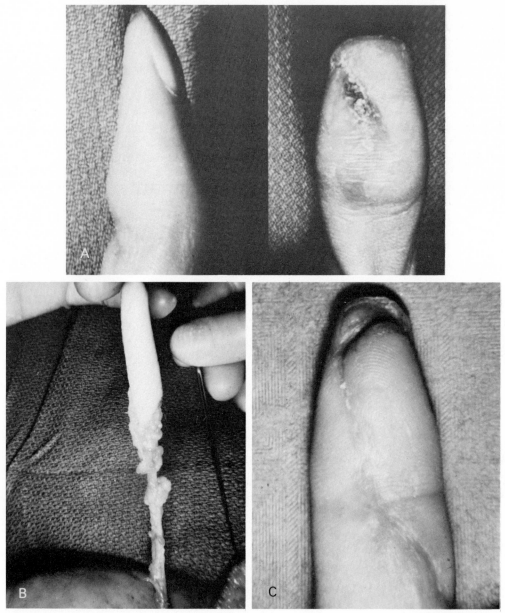

Figure 31.5. Neurovascular island pedicle flap. **(A)** Planing injury to volar aspect of thumb tip covered with split-thickness skin graft. Without padding, the thumb tip is tender and dysesthetic. Subcutaneous tissue, blood supply, and sensibility are required. **(B)** Skin and subcutaneous tissue have been transposed with neurovascular bundles from middle finger to thumb tip. Donor site was covered with full-thickness skin graft. **(C)** Two months after transposition of neurovascular island pedicle flap, there is excellent two-point discrimination and good padding to thumb tip. The patient was able to return to his job as a carpenter.

ally, however, if there is extensive soft-tissue loss on the volar side of the thumb and associated severe injury to an adjacent finger requiring amputation, a primary neurovascular island pedicle flap is indicated. The volar skin and subcutaneous tissue of the donor finger are elevated with its neurovascular bundle. The neurovascular bundle is carefully traced into the palm. The proper digital nerve to the adjacent finger is identified, and its fibers are preserved and separated from the donor nerve in the common digital nerve stem. Communicating and perforating branches of the donor digital artery and vein are ligated distal to the superficial palmar arch. The donor flap is then transferred with its neurovascular pedicle by tunneling it to the recipient site at the thumb tip. Although excellent sensation and circulation are restored to the thumb by this procedure, the patient usually continues to perceive the thumb as the donor finger. It usually is best to transfer this type of flap as a secondary procedure.

Rotation and *transposition flaps* may be swung from the dorsum of the finger to cover a volar defect. The donor area is covered by a split-thickness skin graft. Occasionally, large defects in the skin and subcutaneous tissue at the dorsum of the hand overlying the tendons or joints may also be covered by rotation or transposition flaps (Fig. 31.6). If properly designed, the donor tissue should move readily and without tension to fill the defect.

The surgeon should cut a pattern of the proposed flap from a rubber glove or sponge and plan the design of the flap carefully before making any incision.

Remote Pedicle Flaps. A large soft-tissue defect on the volar side of the finger or thumb can often be covered with a *cross-finger pedicle flap* (Fig. 31.7). This is particularly useful when the flexor tendons are exposed. The margins of the recipient area are enlarged, if necessary, so that the borders of the flap are not perpendicular to finger flexion creases. An appropriately shaped flap of skin and subcutaneous tissue is elevated from an adjacent finger with its uncut base at the side of the recipient finger. The donor flap should be made approximately 15% larger than the measured recipi-

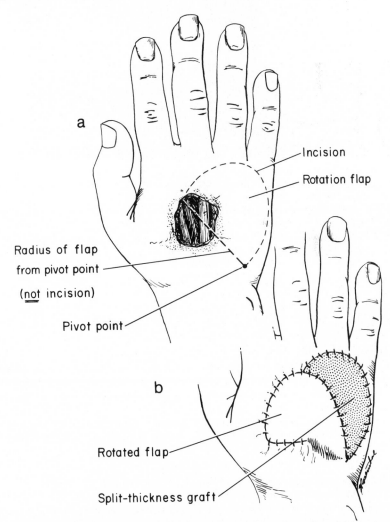

Figure 31.6.   With an avulsion injury to the dorsum of the hand, skin with subcutaneous tissue and excellent blood supply can be provided over tendons and bones by means of a rotation flap. (*a*) The pivot from which the flap is rotated should be selected so as to leave a wide base to the flap and to provide sufficient skin to cover the defect. (*b*) Flap is rotated to cover defect. Donor site is covered with split-thickness skin graft.

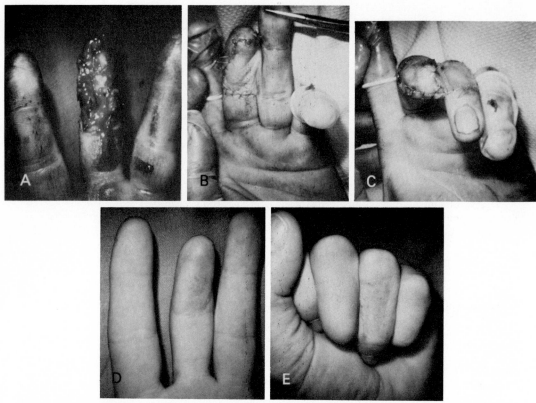

Figure 31.7. Cross-finger pedicle flap. **(A)** Volar aspect of middle finger was severely injured in a press machine. The distal phalanx was amputated, and flexor tendons were exposed throughout the remaining stump. Skin with subcutaneous tissue is required. **(B)** A cross-finger flap is elevated from dorsum of ring finger. The flap is freed volar to skin ligaments (Cleland's ligaments) to radial side of ring finger. The flap is made 15% larger than the defect so that it can be sutured without tension. **(C)** Donor site of cross-finger flap is covered with split-thickness graft. **(D)** Six months later, durable skin covers recipient site of middle finger. **(E)** Donor site has healed with slight discoloration but no functional disability.

ent area to ensure adequate skin coverage. The flap is elevated to include the soft tissue over the dorsal tendon aponeurosis of the donor finger. As the flap is freed, it is brought to the volar side of the recipient finger as one would turn the page of a book. Lateral skin ligaments (Cleland's ligaments) at the hinge ("bridge") side of the flap anchor the skin to the deep fascia in the region of the proximal interphalangeal joint, and must be divided to ensure adequate freedom of the flap with transfer. The donor site and the flap bridge are covered with a split-thickness skin graft that is covered with petrolatum gauze and a sterile dressing. A sponge is placed between the bridge and the web of the involved fingers, and the fingers are held together with soft dressings of sheet cotton and springy gauze. Plaster of Paris is rarely necessary. The cross-finger flap is detached after 3 weeks. The donor site will appear depressed, but will gradually fill in. Within 3–6 months, normal

flexion creases will appear within the flap at the recipient site. The donor site will usually become hyperpigmented. With circumferential loss of skin from a thumb or finger, the volar side may be covered with a cross-finger flap, and the dorsum of both the recipient and donor fingers may be covered with a split-thickness skin graft.

The *thenar flap* (Fig. 31.8) is useful for covering a large avulsion injury of the fingertip with bone exposed in a young patient in whom a V-Y advancement flap would not provide sufficient tissue for coverage. The immobilization that is necessary after a thenar flap is applied risks flexion contracture in the recipient finger, and this operation should be avoided in patients with small-joint arthritis or stiffness. Two quadrangular flaps are elevated from the thenar eminence in the form of the letter H. The proximal flap is sutured to the dorsum of the recipient finger; the distal flap is sutured to the volar side of the fingertip. The bases

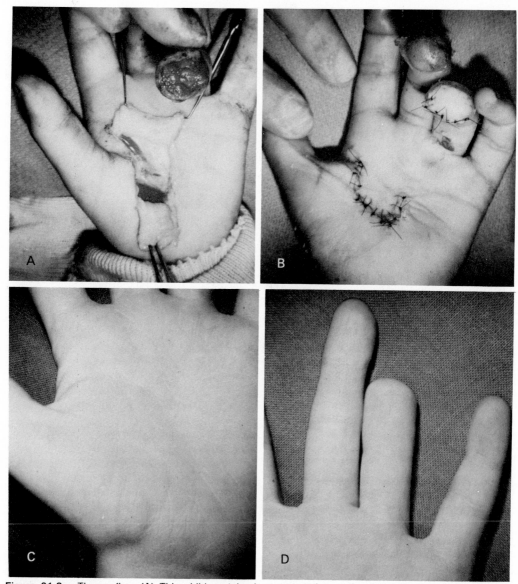

Figure 31.8.   Thenar flap. **(A)** This child sustained an amputation at the tip of the ring finger. Bone is protruding. An H-flap is elevated from the thenar eminence. The distal thenar flap is sutured to the volar aspect of the fingertip and the proximal thenar flap to its dorsum. This creates a closed system. **(B)** The finger is detached from the palm 17 days later. The distal thenar flap is used to close the donor site. The proximal thenar flap remains attached to the finger and is sutured to close the defect. **(C)** Six months later, the donor site is virtually invisible. **(D)** Recipient site is healed with well-vascularized, well-padded skin.

of the two flaps are then advanced and sutured to each other, creating a completely closed system. At 14–17 days, one flap—usually the distal one—is detached from the finger, and the other—usually the proximal flap—from the thenar eminence. The donor and recipient sites are closed by advancing each of the flaps. The finger is held in complete extension for several days with an aluminum splint

padded with foam rubber, after which time range-of-motion exercises are begun.

Major loss of skin and subcutaneous tissue such as occurs after a severe avulsion or explosion injury is best treated in the operating room with coverage by a *remote flap. Axial pattern flaps* derive their circulation from a vascular pedicle that provides robust circulation through a narrow base.

Random flaps, such as the cross-finger pedicle, cross-arm, and abdominal flaps, are perfused diffusely and must be elevated on a broad base if they are to survive. The *groin tube flap* is one of several versatile axial pattern flaps that may be used to replace major skin defects in acutely injured patients. The groin tube is elevated from the inguinal region and is based on the superficial circumflex iliac vessels as they exist from the femoral vessels. Because of the excellent blood supply, relatively long tubes may be raised and applied in one stage. This permits considerable mobility of the recipient limb, and generous amounts of skin and subcutaneous tissue are available for soft-tissue cover.

If the volar skin has been lost from several digits, the *cross-arm flap* should be considered. Immobilization of the hand to the medial aspect of the opposite arm for 3 weeks allows complete mobility of the elbow and hand on the donor side and is relatively comfortable. The skin is of good quality and less fatty than skin from the abdomen or groin.

If other donor sites are available, we avoid using pectoral skin as a flap. Scarring at the donor site is often distressing. *Abdominal flaps* provide excellent coverage of broad areas. They should be defatted at the time of application, and they should be based on a broad pedicle, preferably no smaller than the length of the flap.

NERVE INJURIES

Peripheral nerve injuries are of three major types: neurapraxia, axonotmesis, and neurotmesis. *Neurapraxia** may result from contusion, ischemia, or local pressure on a nerve, and causes functional interference with impulse transmission. As the effects of contusion subside or the source of pressure is relieved, the nerve recovers spontaneously and often quite rapidly. For example, neurapraxia of the radial nerve may result from a patient's sleeping with his head resting on his arm. The hand is numb and has "fallen asleep." The extensors of the fingers and wrist are weak. Speed of recovery depends on the duration and severity of the injury. With mild neurapraxia, the patient may recover completely within a few minutes. In other cases, recovery may take days or weeks. Return of sensibility and muscle function occurs diffusely and not proximally to distally.

---

*Neurapraxia is often misspelled "neuropraxia." Derivation is neur, nerve; a, without; praxia, working. The term neuropraxia would mean "nerve working" and, therefore is incorrect.

If a nerve has been damaged more severely as the result of a traction injury or prolonged or severe compression or contusion, anatomic interruption of the axons or *axonotmesis* can occur. The supporting structures of the nerve, including the Schwann cells, endoneurium, perineurium, and epineurium, remain intact. If the cause of axonotmesis is eliminated, the nerve recovers as the axons regenerate at the rate of 1–2 mm/day. *Neurotmesis* represents complete anatomic interruption of axons and supporting neural structures, either as a result of division of the nerve or severe traction or compression. Patients with neurotmesis require operation for restoration of function.

If a hand has been severely injured, it may be difficult to determine whether the abnormality of nerve function is due to neurapraxia, axonotmesis, or neurotmesis. Neurotmesis may be suspected if the patient has total anesthesia in the autonomous sensory distribution of the nerve, an open wound over the suspected area of nerve injury, or Tinel's sign (paresthesia in the sensory distribution of the injured nerve on percussion at the site of injury). Irregular distribution of hypesthesia, rapid improvement of the sensory deficit, or continued perspiration in the sensory areas supplied by the involved nerve suggests neurapraxia or axonotmesis, and operation may often be deferred or may prove unnecessary.

Following World War II, many surgeons advocated secondary repair of nerve lacerations. After reviewing the long-term results of battle injuries, they concluded that better restoration of function and sensation was achieved if nerve repair was delayed for at least 3–4 weeks. Several factors may have influenced the results: a less hurried and better equipped operating staff at the time of elective reconstruction, clearer visualization of the extent of nerve injury, a thicker epineurium better able to hold sutures, and a lower incidence of wound infection. We believe, however, that in the case of a cleanly lacerated wound with relatively little contusion, traction, or tearing, primary neurorrhaphy performed by a competent, well equipped staff is preferred to delayed nerve repair. Primary repair is the treatment of choice in cleanly incised wounds treated within 24 hours because the nerve ends are more easily oriented, nerves and tendons can be repaired during one operation, and the patient usually recovers more quickly. If the nerve cannot be repaired primarily, the ends of the lacerated nerve should be sutured side to side to prevent retraction and to facilitate secondary repair.

Group fascicular repair is often used for the

larger nerves, and is performed in the operating room. Under magnification the cut ends of the nerve are oriented by matching the location of the vasa nervorum on either cut end and by matching groups of fascicles according to their size and shape. Each group of fascicles is then repaired with 10–0 nylon sutures. With smaller nerves, 8–0 or 9–0 interrupted nylon epineurial sutures provide neat closure.

VASCULAR INJURIES

Diagnosis and treatment of major arterial injuries to the upper limb are discussed in Chapter 21, pages 478–481. The viability of the hand is endangered only rarely by ligation of either the radial artery or the ulnar artery, and the viability of a finger is seldom threatened by ligation of one or even both digital arteries. It has been suggested, however, that the high incidence of sensitivity to cold in previously injured limbs may be lessened by primary vascular repair of injured arteries in the fingers or wrist. Although it is not always necessary to repair these vessels if the hand is pink and clearly viable, such repairs should be considered by surgeons familiar with microvascular techniques.

Volkmann's Contracture

Ischemic contracture of the muscles of the forearm or the intrinsic muscles of the hand can be an alarming sequel to many injuries of the upper limb. The soft tissues of the forearm are subdivided into anterior and posterior compartments by the radius, ulna, and interosseous membrane and are encased by a circumferential investing fascia. Fractures about the elbow and forearm, direct trauma to the forearm, and constrictive dressings and pressure to the limb each may cause edema of the volar compartment of the forearm. As the muscles swell, venous outflow is further impeded and edema increases. Since the anterior compartment is a closed space, any pressure on the arterioles and capillaries will result in ischemia with necrosis of muscle cells. Within a few hours, tissue pressure in the anterior compartment can rise dramatically. The patient will complain of severe, increasing pain exacerbated by any attempt to extend the wrist or fingers passively. The hand becomes pale and cyanotic. As the pressure within the forearm builds, compressive neuropathy develops, first affecting the median nerve and then the ulnar nerve. The deepest muscles of the forearm are affected earliest and most severely. The

flexor digitorum profundus, flexor pollicis longus, and later the flexor superficialis and the wrist flexors gradually lose their power to contract. Ulnar and radial pulses may disappear.

If the compression is not released promptly, irreversible changes may occur in these muscles and nerves. As the muscle cells become necrotic, they are replaced by yellow fibrous tissue. The nerves are enveloped by a thickened constricting epineurium. The contracted joints become fibrotic and resist any attempt at passive motion. An established Volkmann's contracture (Fig. 31.9) causes severe deformity and disability. The forearm is thin and atrophic, the wrist is in acute palmar flexion, the palm is flattened, and the fingers are clawed. There is atrophy of the thenar and interosseus muscles and hypesthesia of the entire palm. Active flexion of the interphalangeal joints is markedly limited because of loss of muscle substance. Passive correction of joint contraction may be impossible.

If this tragic progression is to be avoided, an impending Volkmann's contracture must be treated promptly and vigorously. A flexed elbow must be extended even if it jeopardizes fracture reduction. All tight restrictive bandages should be released. The limb should be elevated. Measuring intracompartmental tissue pressure by means of a needle attached to a manometer or a wick catheter has been useful in evaluating the severity of the deep edema. When intracompartmental pressure exceeds 40 mm Hg, operation is usually indicated. Clinical signs, however, are often more useful in evaluating whether conservative measures are effective in stopping the increasing edema. If any of the signs of impending Volkmann's contracture persist, such as sluggish capillary refill, absent radial or ulnar pulses, continuing or increasing pain about the forearm, persistent hypesthesia in the median and ulnar nerve distribution, and pain on passive extension of the fingers, the investing fascia of the forearm should be surgically released.

Operating should be performed promptly, before muscle necrosis has begun. The lacertus fibrosus is transected when the volar antebrachial fascia is released. Each of the muscle compartments of the volar side of the forearm must be freed. Once the muscles are freed, they often bulge volarly well past the level of the skin. In these cases the skin should be allowed to remain open, and secondary closure should be performed several days later. If a serpiginous skin incision has been made, portions of the wound may be closed after the primary operation.

Use of intra-arterial tolazoline (Priscoline), sym-

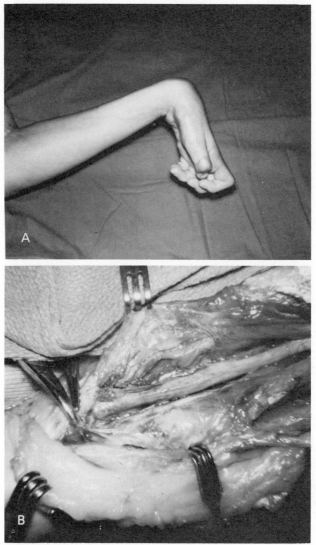

Figure 31.9.   Volkmann's contracture. **(A)** Supracondylar fracture resulted in severe vascular compromise of the forearm. Fascial release had not been performed and Volkmann's contracture developed. The wrist is acutely palmar-flexed, the fingers are in the claw position, and the thumb is flexed at the interphalangeal joint. This deformity can be avoided by prompt fascial release and revascularization of the forearm. **(B)** Exploration of forearm reveals fatty necrosis of muscle and compression of ulnar nerve (seen here) and median nerve with constricting scar. Nerve function can usually be restored if neurolysis is performed promptly.

pathetic nerve block, anticoagulants, and plasma expanders has been suggested for the treatment of impending Volkmann's contracture. However, since the penalties of delay are irreversible changes in muscles, joints, and nerves, if there is any serious doubt regarding the vascular status of a limb 30–60 minutes after all external pressure has been removed, this is sufficient indication for operation.

Occasionally, ischemic contracture of the dorsal compartment of the forearm may occur after a serious injury to the forearm. These patients have pain with attempts at passive flexion of the meta-carpophalangeal joints. Under these circumstances the dorsal compartment should be released down to the interosseous fascia.

Late treatment of Volkmann's contracture consists of excision of the infarct, neurolysis of the involved nerves, and occasionally tendon transfers and nerve grafts.

Ischemic Contracture of the Intrinsic Muscles of the Hand

The interosseus muscles of the hand lie in a closed compartment bounded by the volar and dorsal interosseous fascia and the four metacarpals. Rapidly increasing edema may initiate a cycle of ischemia, muscle necrosis, and further edema. Any attempt to flex the interphalangeal joints while the metacarpophalangeal joints are held in extension will be painful and limited. If untreated, ischemic contractures of the interosseus muscles (Fig. 31.10) will cause an "intrinsic-plus" deformity. The fingers stiffen in flexion at the metacarpophalangeal joints and in extension at the interphalangeal joints. Although the pathologic process that causes ischemic contracture of the interosseus muscles is identical to that of Volkmann's contracture of the forearm, the resultant deformity is the reverse. The deformities of Volkmann's contracture are due to fibrosis of the extrinsic flexor muscles combined with ulnar and median nerve palsy; this causes clawhand. The metacarpophalangeal joints are hyperextended and the interphalangeal joints are flexed. With ischemic contracture of the interossei, however, imbalance is due to excessive intrinsic muscle tone.

With signs of impending ischemic contracture of the interossei, all interosseus muscle compartments should be released. Through a dorsal transverse incision, the dorsal interosseous fascia proximal to each of the four web spaces is divided. The muscles are permitted to expand freely. If necessary, skin closure may be delayed. If the adductor pollicis appears tight, its fascia may be released through a dorsal or palmar skin incision. If edema has caused interosseus muscle compartment syndrome, it may well have caused constriction. Postoperatively, the hand should be immobilized with the thumb in abduction and the metacarpophalangeal joints in extension for 1 or 2 weeks. Active and passive flexion exercises of the interphalangeal joints are begun immediately after operation.

TENDON INJURIES

Flexor Tendons

Laceration

Probably no topic causes more controversy among hand surgeons than the treatment of flexor tendon lacerations. Because of the tight area in which the tendons must glide and the restricted tendon excursion caused by peritendinous adhesions, loss of mobility is common after primary tendon repair. The results of operation depend on which tendon is injured and when, where, and how the tendon was injured, as well as the age of the patient and the operative technique. Our criteria for choosing the plan of primary care of

cleanly lacerated flexor tendons are given in Table 31.3; sites of injury are illustrated in Figure 31.11.

The treatment of flexor tendon injuries varies with different surgeons. Some prefer primary repair of both the flexor digitorum profundus and the flexor digitorum superficialis regardless of the site of injury; others, however, never repair flexor tendons in zone 2 primarily since tendons repaired in this area have the highest risk of failure due to adhesions. If the wound is grossly contaminated or if there are signs of severe contusion, tendon avulsion, severe joint injury, or a badly comminuted fracture adjacent to the tendon injury, we do not repair the tendons primarily, and prefer an early secondary flexor tendon graft instead.

It has been contended that with laceration of both flexor tendons in "no-man's-land" (zone 2) the risks of tendon rupture and peritendinous adhesions are lessened if the superficialis and profundus tendons are both repaired. The theoretical advantages of repairing the superficialis tendon are that (1) repair preserves the blood supply of the profundus tendon through the vinculum longus and (2) the superficialis provides a good sliding bed for the repaired profundus. However, when two tendons are repaired rather than one, there is twice the tendon bulk and twice the amount of suture material; this increases the mass of collagen that must glide through the tight digital canal. Profundus tendon blood supply through the vinculum longus and the flattened insertion of superficialis can be preserved without suturing both tendons. With laceration of both flexor tendons in zone 2, if the nature of the wound suggests a high risk of postoperative adhesions, we resect 2 cm of the proximal cut end of the superficialis and leave the distal end undisturbed.

Motion is achieved early after operating, without tension to the repaired profundus tendon, by protecting the hand with a dorsal plaster splint that maintains the wrist and metacarpophalangeal joints in 30 degrees of palmar flexion. The repaired finger is flexed further by rubber band traction to a small hook cemented to the fingernail or to a suture placed through the fingernail (Fig. 31.12, B and C). The patient is encouraged to extend the finger actively to the limits of the splint after the first day. Flexor tendon lacerations in no-man's-land in infants and children up to 3 or 4 years old are difficult to treat by this method, and the fingers should be immobilized in moderate flexion for 4 weeks after injury.

Avulsion

Closed avulsions of the flexor digitorum profundus are most common in the ring finger, and they

Table 31.3.
Evaluation and primary care of flexor tendon lacerations.

Tendon	Site of Injury[a]	Other Considerations	Treatment
FDP and FPL	1		Advancement
FDP	Between 1 and 2		Suture; advancement if 0.5 cm or less
FDP	2	Fracture, contused tissues, untidy injury	Tenodesis at distal interphalangeal joint
		No bone injury, clean, sharp wound	Suture; early motion with rubber band flexion splint
FDP and FDS	2	Comminuted fracture, badly contused tissue, untidy injury	Close wound; secondary tendon graft
		No bone injury, clean, sharp wound	Suture FDP; may suture FDS or excise proximal cut end; early controlled motion with rubber band flexion splint
FPL	2, 6	Clean, sharp wound	Suture primarily
FDP and FDS	3	1 finger involved	Suture both tendons
		>1 finger involved	Suture both tendons to index finger; suture FDP only, to other fingers in untidy wounds
FDS	3	Child or 1 or 2 tendons in adult	Suture
		3 or 4 tendons in adult	Suture index only
FDP and FDS	4	Median nerve almost always injured	Suture FDP and nerve; excise segment of FDS of ulnar fingers; close carpal canal if "bowstringing"
FDP and FDS	5	Nerves usually involved, FCU and FCR frequently involved	Suture all structures in tidy injuries; in adults with untidy wounds, do not suture FDS of ulnar 3 fingers; ? suture of FCU if ulnar nerve injured
FCU or FCR	5		Repair
PL	5		None

FDP = flexor digitorum profundus; FPL = flexor pollicis longus; FDS = flexor digitorum superficialis; FCU = flexor carpi ulnaris; FCR = flexor carpi radialis; PL = palmaris longus.
[a] See Figure 31.11.

frequently result from a football injury when a player's finger is caught on an opponent's jersey. The patient notices swelling of the proximal segment of the finger and is unable to flex the distal joint. There is often limited flexion of the proximal interphalangeal joint as well because of both incarceration of the ruptured profundus tendon at the insertion of the superficialis tendon and retraction of the lumbrical muscle along with the ruptured profundus. Proximal retraction of the lumbrical origin on the flexor digitorum profundus causes increased tension on the lumbrical tendon. This results in hyperextension of the middle phalanx known as "lumbrical-plus" deformity. If the profundus tendon is to be repaired, treatment must be prompt since a delay of more than 1 or 2 days is likely to cause irreparable contraction of the end of the tendon. X-ray examination usually reveals a small avulsed fragment of the volar lip of the distal phalanx lying near the neck of the proximal phalanx. At operation the tendon is threaded back to its insertion and held there with a pullout suture. The hand is immobilized in mild flexion for 3½ weeks.

Extensor Tendons

Laceration

Most extensor tendon lacerations may be repaired primarily, regardless of the site of injury.

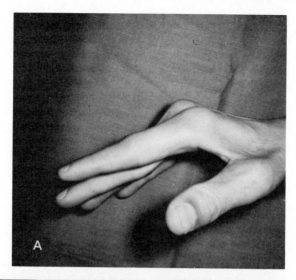

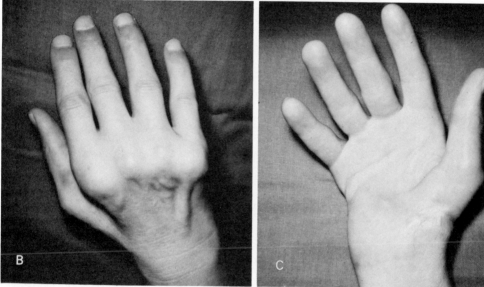

Figure 31.10.   Ischemic contracture of intrinsic muscles caused by cast compression. **(A)** Ischemic contracture of intrinsic muscles of the hand will occur if there is severe vascular embarrassment of the hand subsequent to injury. In this case, a tight cast had been applied to treat a fracture of both bones of the forearm. This led to severe venous engorgement and intrinsic muscle contracture. The metacarpophalangeal joints were acutely flexed and interphalangeal joints extended. This deformity can be prevented in most cases by release of tight constricting casts and dressings. If there is severe edema of the hand after injury, the intrinsic muscles should be decompressed by interosseous fasciotomy before necrosis has occurred. **(B)** Interosseus muscle atrophy may be associated with intrinsic contracture if there is muscle necrosis. **(C)** Severity of cast compression is suggested by scarring secondary to cutaneous necrosis at thumb base.

Whereas the flexor tendons lie within synovial sheaths in the fingers and palm, the extensor tendons are surrounded by a specialized connective tissue called paratenon at the dorsum of the metacarpal bones and fingers. Thus, repair is less likely to be complicated by restrictive adhesions. Although flexor tendon repairs should be performed in the operating room, a well-equipped emergency ward may be a suitable place to repair a cleanly lacerated extensor tendon. The lacerated ends are approximated with either a buried figure-of -8 suture or a horizontal mattress suture of 4–0 nylon. Several 7–0 nylon interrupted sutures may be used to smooth the juncture site. After repair, a volar plaster splint is applied to support the wrist in 30 degrees of dorsiflexion with the metacarpo-

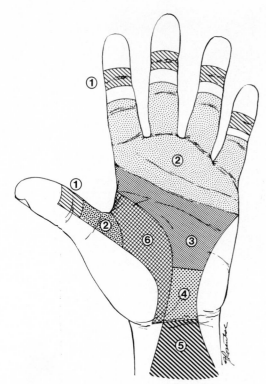

Figure 31.11. Diagram of zones of potential tendon injuries to the hand.

If a tendon has been lacerated in zone 1, it may be advanced to its insertion and reattached.

If lacerated between zones 1 and 2 and if less than 0.5 cm of tendon stump remains, the tendon should be advanced and sutured to bone. If injury occurred with the finger in extension and if more than 0.5 cm of tendon stump remains, tendon repair is indicated.

In zone 2, if only the flexor digitorum profundus has been lacerated, it may be repaired primarily and early controlled motion instituted. If both the flexor digitorum profundus and the flexor digitorum superficialis have been lacerated, primary repair of one or both tendons may be performed for clean injuries. For dirty or untidy wounds, a secondary tendon graft may be planned.

Tendon advancement is preferred if the flexor pollicis longus is lacerated in zone 1. For injuries to the flexor pollicis longus in zone 2, primary repair is advised. In zone 6, the flexor pollicis longus should be repaired primarily in tidy injuries.

In zone 3, the flexor digitorum profundus should be repaired primarily. The flexor digitorum superficialis may also be repaired if the injury is relatively clean.

Injuries in zone 4 can be dangerous. If several profundus and superficialis tendons have been transected, scarring is minimized by excision of the superficialis and repair only of the flexor digitorum profundus, particularly with untidy injuries.

Proximal to the hand, in zone 5, both the flexor digitorum profundus and the flexor digitorum superficialis may be repaired in tidy injuries.

phalangeal and interphalangeal joints in about 15 degrees of flexion. All four fingers are immobilized even if only one has been repaired. If an extensor tendon of the thumb has been repaired, a splint is applied to hold the thumb abducted from the plane of the palm with the metacarpophalangeal and interphalangeal joints in 15 degrees of flexion. The physician should avoid splinting the metacarpophalangeal joints in full extension or hyperextension because of the risk of extension contractures. Immobilization should be continued for approximately 4 weeks.

Rupture

Closed avulsion of the extensor tendon at its insertion on the distal phalanx produces a mallet finger. Operation is infrequently indicated. The finger should be immobilized for at least 5 weeks in full extension at the distal joint and in mild flexion at the proximal interphalangeal joint. Premade plastic splints are available to hold this position. One may prefer a circular plaster cast applied around a layer of tubed gauze held to the finger with tincture of benzoin. Some physicians insert a Kirschner wire through the distal joint to maintain the immobilization; however, we do not recommend this since the distal joint may become infected or stiff.

Rupture of the central slip of the extensor tendon and of the triangular ligament that holds the lateral bands dorsally results in volar subluxation of the lateral bands and retraction of the central slip proximally. This produces the boutonnière deformity, in which the distal interphalangeal joint gradually becomes hyperextended and the proximal interphalangeal joint is swollen and flexed. Surgical repair is not the proper primary treatment for such injuries. A volar splint or circular cast is applied to the finger while the proximal interphalangeal joint is held in full extension. Active and passive flexion of the distal joint is encouraged. Immobilization must be continued for 5 weeks. If active extension of the proximal interphalangeal joint is not regained by this treatment, operation is then required.

FRACTURES

Most fractures of the hand can be treated by simple reduction and immobilization. Open reduction and internal fixation may be required for phalangeal and metacarpal fractures with rotational deformity or excessive angulation, for irreducible Bennett's fractures, and occasionally for fractures of the carpal bones. Use of pulp traction, skeletal traction, or banjo splints is contraindicated

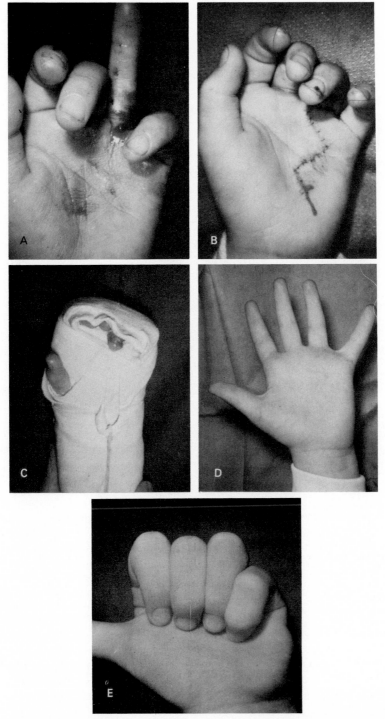

Figure 31.12.   Repair of lacerated flexor tendons in "no-man's-land." **(A)** Laceration of flexor digitorum profundus and flexor digitorum superficialis in zone 2 of ring finger by a piece of glass several hours previously. **(B)** Primary repair of flexor digitorum profundus was performed. Three cm of proximal cut end of flexor digitorum superficialis was excised. A suture is passed through nail to be attached to rubber band flexion device. A small hook can be cemented to fingernail for rubber band flexion rather than placing a nail suture. **(C)** A dorsal plaster splint is applied to the wrist and finger in mild flexion. The finger is further flexed with rubber band traction attached to a safety pin in the dressings. **(D)** Two months after operation there is full extension. **(E)** Excellent flexion has been restored.

since such methods of reduction and immobilization are more hazardous to the skin and joints than are open reduction and internal fixation.

The only treatment required in fractures of the tuft of the distal phalanx is treatment of symptoms, such as drilling holes in the base of the fingernail to relieve pain by decompression of a subungual hematoma. Nondisplaced fractures at the interphalangeal joints may be immobilized for 3 weeks with a volar splint. A nondisplaced fracture of the volar lip of the middle phalanx should be treated with a dorsal splint in 30 degrees of flexion. Active proximal interphalangeal flexion is encouraged. Extension past 30 degrees is prevented for 3 weeks. If a large articular fracture is displaced, it is treated with open reduction and fixation with a Kirschner wire. Angulated fractures of the proximal and middle phalanges can usually be reduced by gentle traction under local anesthesia and immobilized in semiflexion over a plaster or aluminum splint. Persistent angulation of up to 30 degrees is acceptable in children, and usually causes little disability or deformity. Indeed, in children up to the age of 10 years, open reduction of such fractures is rarely necessary except in cases of rotational malalignment.

Fracture of the metacarpal neck is one of the most common fractures in the hand, and is often the result of a fight. If the volar angulation of the distal fragment is more than 30 degrees, closed reduction may be attempted under local anesthesia by flexing the entire finger acutely and pushing the proximal phalanx dorsally to extend the metacarpal head. Once the fracture is reduced, the finger must not be immobilized in this acutely flexed position. If the deformity recurs with relaxation of the pressure and extension of the finger, open reduction and internal fixation should be performed if there is more than 20 degrees of volar angulation of the second or third metacarpal bone, since these bones are relatively immobile at their bases, or if there is more than 40 degrees of angulation of the fourth or fifth metacarpal bone, which are quite mobile at the carpometacarpal joints.

Compound fractures should be opened, debrided, and lavaged. If necessary, they should be fixed with nonthreaded crossed Kirschner wires passed through the fracture site in a retrograde, oblique direction. The wires are removed in 6–8 weeks. We rarely employ cerclage bands or wires. Recently, we have used compression plates and screws to maintain reduction of unstable fractures and to permit early active motion. They are used in only a small percentage of the patients we see.

To manage metacarpal bone loss following a machine accident or gunshot wound, the fractured metacarpal bones are aligned with longitudinal Kirschner wires and their length is maintained with transverse wires holding them to adjacent uninjured metacarpal shafts. After operation the metacarpophalangeal joints are held in 70 degrees of flexion to prevent joint contracture, and the thumb is held abducted from the palm.

A Bennett's fracture is a fracture of the ulnar base of the first metacarpal bone. It is usually associated with subluxation or dislocation of the metacarpal on the trapezium. To reduce this fracture the thumb is placed in traction and immobilized in opposition. If the dislocation is reducible but the metacarpal tends to slip out of position, percutaneous Kirschner wires are passed through the trapeziometacarpal joint and between the first and second metacarpals. If reduction cannot be achieved by closed methods, open reduction and internal fixation of both the fracture and the dislocated bone are usually indicated. We expose the fracture site by making a J-shaped incision at the dorsal base of the first metacarpal bone that curves volarly across the thenar eminence. The surgeon must be careful not to injure the superficial nerves of the thenar eminence. The origins of the thenar muscles are retracted distally and Kirschner wires are drilled retrograde through the metacarpal and across the fracture site. The fracture is reduced, the wire is drilled proximally, and a second wire maintains reduction of the dislocation by passing from the first to the second metacarpal bone.

Fractures of the carpal bones may usually be reduced and held in a plaster cast without difficulty. A scaphoid fracture should be suspected after a fall on the outstretched hand with tenderness in the anatomical snuff-box even if x-ray findings are normal. In such a case, immobilization of the thumb and wrist for 2 weeks with a plaster splint is wise. A second x-ray film should then be obtained and the splint removed if no fracture is seen. Scaphoid fractures usually require prolonged immobilization of 3 months or more for healing. When the plaster cast is applied, the thumb tip is left free, with the thumb placed in opposition and the wrist immobilized in 20 degrees of palmar flexion and radial deviation. With vertical scaphoid fractures and fractures of the proximal pole of the scaphoid bone, we recommend immobilization of the elbow for the first 3 weeks to prevent forearm rotation, since these fractures are particularly slow to heal.

JOINT INJURIES

Dislocations of the interphalangeal joints usually are readily reduced by traction; in fact, many patients report spontaneous reduction that occurs immediately after the injury. In all cases the joint should be immobilized for 3 weeks and active and passive exercises encouraged thereafter. With dorsal subluxation or dislocation of the middle phalanx, a small avulsed fragment of the volar lip is frequently seen on x-ray examination. In these patients a dorsal splint preventing extension past 30 degrees should be applied after reduction. The patient is allowed to flex his fingers actively, but hyperextension is prevented; this maintains the mobility of the joint while allowing the fracture and avulsion to heal.

Occasionally, dorsal dislocation of the metacarpophalangeal joint may be irreducible by closed means; this is especially true in the index finger. In this instance the head of the second metacarpal bone is trapped between the lumbrical muscle, the flexor tendons, the volar plate, and the superficial palmar ligaments. Dorsal dislocations of the proximal phalanx of both the thumb and the little finger may also be irreducible by closed means because of interposition of the volar plate or entrapment of the metacarpal head by the flexor tendons. In all such cases, open reduction is required promptly to free the incarcerated tendons or ligaments.

Gamekeeper's thumb refers to a deformity caused by gradual stretching of the ulnar collateral ligament of the metacarpophalangeal joint of the thumb, although the term has been extended to include acute ruptures of this ligament. These injuries heal poorly if there is extreme instability of the proximal phalanx to passive radial stress. If deviation of more than 45 degrees is produced, if the proximal phalanx is subluxated volarly, or if there is a grossly displaced fracture fragment, primary operative repair of the avulsed ligament and of any associated fragment of bone with imbrication of the adductor tendon is indicated. The reverse deformity, rupture of the radial collateral ligament, is also repaired by operation if the joint exhibits extreme instability. A sprained thumb with less than 45 degrees of lateral instability rarely requires operation, and is usually treated with immobilization in plaster for 3 weeks.

Dislocation of one or more carpal bones is frequent after severe injuries to the wrist. X-ray films should always be examined carefully to determine whether the capitate fits well into the distal concavity of the lunate; anterior dislocation of the lunate and perilunar dislocation are frequently overlooked. On an anteroposterior x-ray film of the wrist, the lunate should appear quadrangular. If it is triangular and overlaps the capitate, intercarpal dislocation should be suspected.

These dislocations require immediate closed reduction, which is usually achieved by traction, flexion, and digital pressure on the lunate bone followed by restoration of the neutral position. After reduction, another x-ray film should be obtained and examined carefully for widening between the scaphoid and lunate bones; an abnormally large space signals probable rotatory subluxation of the scaphoid bone. This injury usually requires open reduction, repair of the torn intercarpal ligaments, and internal fixation (Fig. 31.13).

TRAUMATIC AMPUTATIONS

The treatment of amputated fingertips is discussed earlier. In the case of a more proximal amputation of a finger, primary closure is preferred after a clean injury. If disarticulation through the proximal or distal interphalangeal joint has occurred, the tendons should be advanced distally, severed, and allowed to retract. They should not be sutured to each other over the end of the bone. Nerves should be cleanly transsected so that they do not lie adjacent to the amputation stump. When there is disarticulation at the distal interphalangeal joint, the lumbrical tendon is transsected proximal to the proximal interphalangeal joint to prevent development of a lumbrical-plus deformity. The end of the amputated bone is rounded to avoid bony "dog ears" but it is not necessary to remove the articular cartilage.

The amputation stump should be left as long as is possible with adequate coverage of skin. There are two exceptions to this: (1) For both aesthetic and functional reasons, amputation through the proximal phalanx of either the index finger or the little finger is probably best treated by resection at the base of the corresponding metacarpal bone (ray resection). The age and occupation of the patient must be considered in making the decision whether to amputate the entire finger. (2) In ring avulsion injuries, amputation is the preferred procedure, although exceptions may be made for children, particularly if the ring finger of the left hand is involved. We believe that better functional and aesthetic results are achieved in adults if the finger is amputated at the site of injury as a primary procedure, followed by ray resection and transfer of the fifth metacarpal to the fourth metacarpal base (Fig. 31.14). This is not an emergency procedure; it may be performed at the patient's convenience.

Replantation

Few events in reconstructive surgery related to the hand have received more public attention than

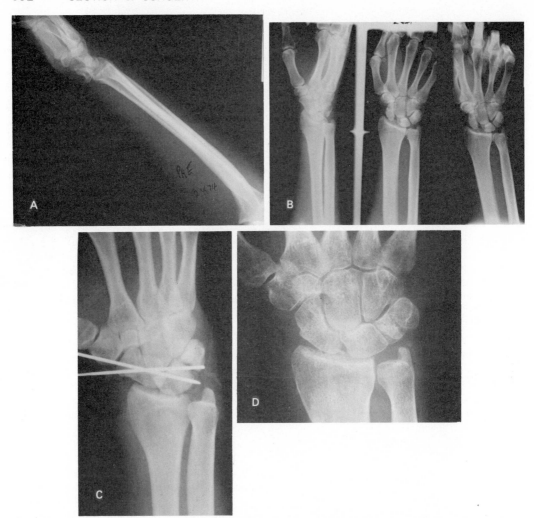

Figure 31.13.   Volar dislocation of lunate resulting from a fall on the outstretched hand. **(A)** X-ray film of injury. **(B)** After closed manipulation the lunate dislocation is completely reduced. There remains, however, rotatory subluxation of scaphoid. This is best demonstrated by widening between proximal pole of scaphoid and radial side of lunate. *Left*, oblique view; *center* posteroanterior view in pronation; *right*, anteroposterior view in supination. **(C)** Open reduction and internal fixation are usually required for rotatory subluxation of scaphoid. In this case, transverse Kirschner wires are placed between the scaphoid and the lunate. The dorsal wrist capsule had been avulsed from the radius and was reattached. The wrist was immobilized in a plaster cast for 6 weeks. Occasionally, rotatory subluxation may be reduced without operation by positioning the hand with the wrist in neutral flexion-extension and mild radial deviation. **(D)** One year after operation, intercarpal and radiocarpal alignment is maintained.

the replantation of limbs. Following the success in 1962 in replantation of an arm severed at the middle of the humerus, replantation of limbs and digits has been performed successfully in many centers throughout the world, aided by recent advances both in microsurgical techniques and in materials.

An amputated arm, hand, or portion of the hand should not be replanted if it has been severely crushed, subjected to severe heat or cold, or torn from its attachment with avulsion of major nerves and blood vessels. Replantation is also contraindicated if there has been mishandling of the amputated part or excessive delay in transit. The amputated part should be wrapped in sterile saline sponges or towels and placed in a plastic bag. The wrapped unit is then transported cooled in a bucket of ice. The amputation stump should be covered with sterile or clean dressings. Limbs have successfully been replanted many hours after

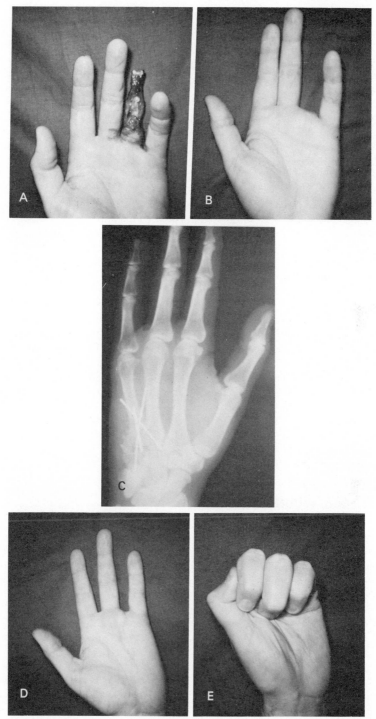

Figure 31.14.   Treatment of ring avulsion injury. **(A)** Two hours previously, this patient caught his ring on a hook and sustained an avulsion injury of the ring finger with amputation of the tip. **(B)** Primary treatment consisted of amputation of finger at site of avulsion. **(C)** Two months later, digital ray transfer was performed. The fourth metacarpal was removed to its base. Osteotomy of the fifth metacarpal was performed and it was transferred radially. Transferred metacarpal is held in place with multiple Kirschner wires. **(D)** After healing of metacarpal osteotomy and ray transfer, appearance of hand is considerably improved. **(E)** Ray transfer also closes the gap between middle and little fingers, resulting in improved hand function.

injury. Thus, although speed is desirable, a delay of up to several hours that is spent transporting a patient to a hospital prepared to perform replantation surgery is preferable to prompt replantation at an institution where the staff is inexperienced in microvascular techniques.

Whether a portion of a hand should be replanted even under optimal conditions depends to a great extent on the patient's needs and the extent of the injuries. A hand with an amputation of either the index finger or the little finger has such good appearance and function that the value of replantation of either of these fingers is questionable. The physician should consider whether it is advisable to replant the tip of a finger or thumb or to shorten the digit and to cover it with skin of normal sensation. In patients with amputations of more than one finger or clean amputation of the hand at the wrist, replantation should be attempted if the condition of both the patient and the amputated part is satisfactory.

The patient, his family, and medical personnel should understand that the success of a replantation does not depend solely on the viability of the replanted part. If a replanted limb or digit remains relatively insensitive, stiff, or immobile, it may ultimately require reamputation. In these circumstances the patient may find a prosthesis more functional. Nonetheless, a cleanly amputated part in a suitable patient should usually be replanted (Fig. 31.15). The potential advantages of a successful replantation justify the risk and large expenditure of time.

SPECIAL WOUNDS

Certain wounds of the hand require particular attention by the emergency physician. A laceration over a metacarpophalangeal joint should lead the physician to suspect a human bite. These bites are highly contaminated and should be left open. The patient should receive antibiotics and tetanus prophylaxis if indicated, and the wound should be well irrigated and allowed to heal by secondary intention.

Injuries due to injection of a foreign substance under pressure, such as injuries resulting from paint guns and grease guns, may appear innocuous on first examination, but can result in extensive contamination, vascular spasm, and ultimately necrosis. All such injuries should receive emergency treatment consisting of wide excision and thorough débridement. These patients should be admitted to the hospital for immediate surgical care, since the foreign material can extensively dissect soft-tissue planes, causing severe chemical irritation. If the injured finger appears blanched after extensive débridement, anticoagulants and cervical sympathetic blockade may restore the circulation to the contracted vessels.

Wringer injuries have become less common since the advent of the electric clothes dryer. A wringer injury may result in extensive deep soft-tissue damage that is not apparent on initial examination. Skin and subcutaneous tissue may be ripped from underlying fascia with resultant deep thrombosis and ecchymosis. The limb must be elevated and observed. Necrotic tissue is promptly débrided and appropriate skin grafts are applied.

Thermal burns due to either excessively low or high temperature or passage of electrical current require special treatment and close observation, and are discussed in detail in Chapter 28.

After a poisonous snakebite to the hand, the snake venom is activated by the body temperature and tissue pH. The activated venom hydrolyzes, destroys local tissues, and causes local bleeding due to the rupture of vessel walls. Within a short time, venom and partly hydrolyzed tissue circulate throughout the vascular system, causing hypotension, nausea, tachycardia, and eventually anuria. Hemoglobin, hematocrit, and platelet levels fall because of both massive hemorrhage in the area of the bite and intravascular cell destruction. Intravascular venom also causes a rapid decrease in fibrinogen levels. As local tissues are destroyed by hydrolysis, the osmotic pressure in the area of the bite rises. This causes increasing edema in the area of hemorrhage and results in progressive cyanosis and pain in the region of the bite.

In the past, one of the more popular methods of treating poisonous snakebites included the use of crosscuts over the wound, local suction, and antivenin. The value of this method of treatment has been questioned. The use of crosscuts over a snakebite has frequently caused considerable unnecessary damage to tendons and nerves that lie beneath the site of injury. Suction has added bacteria from the mouth to an open and edematous wound. Antivenin must be used in large quantities to be effective. Many patients are allergic to the horse serum from which the antivenin is derived, and may have a severe allergic reaction. All too often, this regimen of crosscuts, suction, and antivenin has been used with tragic consequences in patients who had been bitten by a nonpoisonous snake. For these reasons, many medical centers now recommend the following treatment for snakebites to the hand:

(1) Apply ice bags to the bite site.

(2) Compression dressings may be applied

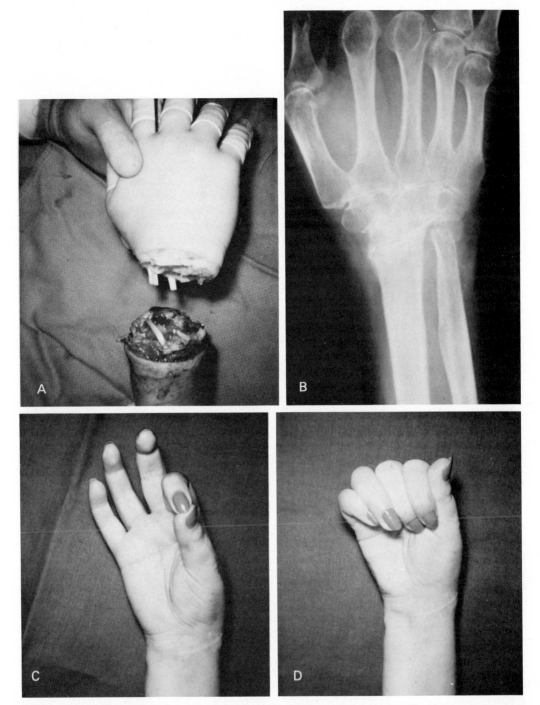

Figure 31.15. Replantation of amputated hand. **(A)** Two hours previously the hand had been amputated in a machine accident. It was transported in a plastic bag placed in an ice bucket. Replantation was performed with primary repair of nerves and tendons and resection of the proximal row of carpal bones. Two arteries and four veins were repaired. **(B)** Secondary reconstructive procedures included wrist arthrodesis, volar metacarpophalangeal capsulorrhaphy, intrinsic muscle release, and arthrodesis of metacarpophalangeal joint of thumb. **(C)** The patient regained good return of thenar muscle function and fair return of intrinsics. Pinprick sensibility was restored about entire hand, and two-point discrimination of 5 mm was present in several fingertips. **(D)** Extension and flexion of fingers and thumb permitted her to return to her occupation as hairdresser.

above and below the bite site to minimize spread of the venom in the soft tissues. Dressings should *not* be venous or arterial tourniquets.

(3) Closely monitor hemoglobin, hematocrit, platelet count, prothrombin time, plasma fibrinogen level, and vital signs. Central venous pressure and urinary output should be carefully checked and appropriately treated if abnormal.

(4) Administer intravenous fluids to maintain normal central venous pressure and 24-hour urinary output of 50 ml/hr.

(5) Give intravenous antibiotics, tetanus toxoid, and analgesics.

(6) Administer hydrocortisone sodium succinate, 1 gm intravenously, before operation.

Surgical treatment should consist of total débridement of the wound and fasciotomy. The wound should not be closed primarily. It may be closed after 5–7 days with a skin graft if necessary.

Many physicians now believe that antivenin is unnecessary and dangerous. They advise that neither antivenin nor crosscuts be used as first aid. Since definitive care of the poisonous snakebite can be performed only in the hospital, the best treatment that can be rendered as first aid is application of ice about the wound and transportation of the patient to the hospital as rapidly as possible.

INFECTIONS

Treatment of the infected hand depends on the causative organism and the location and extent of the infection. Considerable information can be obtained by meticulous history-taking. For example, an infection at the dorsum of the hand after a fight is probably due to the streptococci and spirochetes of the opponent's mouth, a puncture wound from a barnyard nail may harbor clostridia, and an infected finger lacerated in a hospital ward should arouse suspicion of penicillin-resistant staphylococci. In each case, the selection of antibiotics would vary (see Chapter 11). Persons with superficial skin infections, cellulitis without underlying abscess, paronychia, and intradermal abscesses may be treated as outpatients. If the patient has tender or enlarged axillary or epitrochlear nodes, the red streaks characteristic of lymphangitis, fever, or leukocytosis, he should be hospitalized. Felons, purulent tenosynovitis, deep space abscesses, joint infection, and osteomyelitis warrant prompt admission and operation.

On examination the position of the fingers and the location of swelling and redness must be accurately noted. Palpation must be gentle and slow, since the entire hand may be painful and the area of maximal tenderness may be masked by rough examination. The pattern of tenderness, redness, and heat will reveal the dome of an abscess better than the swollen area. For example, lymphedema at the dorsum of the hand may be more striking than palmar swelling with a midpalmar abscess, and a thenar space infection may cause more puffiness of the loose dorsal skin of the first web than of the firm structures that border the abscess. The examiner must not mistake the swelling of the loose dorsal areolar tissue for the site of infection.

In the treatment of infections, local block anesthesia is not recommended. If an anesthetic agent is injected in an area of potential lymphatic drainage, infection may spread, and if local anesthesia is induced about the base of a finger, severe vascular compromise may result. Intravenous lidocaine (Xylocaine) is never advised, since it requires exsanguination of the limb by compression, which may seed bacteria throughout the blood stream. Paronychia and small subcutaneous and intradermal abscesses may be opened and drained on an outpatient basis, with anesthesia achieved by ethyl chloride spray. Deeper infections require general anesthesia or interscalene block. A tourniquet (without rubber bandage exsanguination) is used during operation for all deep infections.

Common pyogenic infections of the hand include the following:

(1) Intradermal abscess or "infected blister." Symptoms include localized swelling and tenderness that often occurs at the fingertip. Motion of the fingers is painless and there is no proximal edema. The area should be anesthetized with ethyl chloride spray and the abscess incised in the emergency ward; the patient then should soak the area periodically at home.

(2) Subcutaneous abscess. Patients with a subcutaneous abscess have diffuse redness and tenderness of the hand and motion that is usually relatively painless at noncontiguous joints. The abscess is usually limited by fascial attachments. If the abscess occurs at the dorsum, there may be a large area of undermined skin requiring drainage.

(3) Shirt-stud or collar-button abscess. This is a subcutaneous abscess of the distal part of the palm that points both in the web and more proximally between the pretendinous bands. When these lesions are drained, pus must be evacuated from the dorsal web and proximal to the natatory ligaments of the palmar fascia into the distal palm.

(4) Paronychia. Early in its development, paronychia is a superficial abscess between the nail and the eponychium. If it is untreated, the infection may extend into deeper tissues and "run

around" the nail margins deep to the nailbed. In early cases, the eponychium should be elevated from the nail with a No. 11 scalpel blade after induction of anesthesia with ethyl chloride spray. A skin incision is rarely necessary. Petrolatum gauze is inserted between the nail and the eponychium for several days. In later cases with more severe infection around the entire nail margin, the patient should be hospitalized and the entire eponychium should be elevated with parallel longitudinal incisions under general anesthesia. If it is necessary, the nailbed should be elevated.

(5) Felon. A felon is an abscess in the pulp space of the fingertip. The tip is hot, exquisitely tender, and firm, and the finger is relatively unaffected more proximally. The fascial septa hold the pus in the fingertip under great pressure, and osteomyelitis of the distal phalanx may result. The patient should be admitted and treated under general anesthesia. All septa must be divided. A J-shaped incision at the dorsolateral side of the distal segment of the finger just anterior to the fingernail is adequate for exposure and drainage. The distal portion of the wound (anterior to the tip) may be closed at the end of the operation. The wound should be packed with gauze until it closes "from below."

(6) Tendon sheath infection. If the index, middle, or ring finger is involved, infection extends from the base of the distal phalanx to the distal palmar flexion crease. Infections of the thumb and little finger may extend into the radial or ulnar bursa and into the wrist. The four cardinal signs of tenosynovitis, according to Kanavel, include: (1) *tenderness* over the course of the sheath, limited to the sheath; (2) *symmetrical enlargement* of the volar side of the finger; (3) *pain on extension* of the fingertip; and (4) *partial flexion* of the finger at rest.

In patients with purulent flexor tenosynovitis, operation should be performed under general anesthesia. A dorsolateral incision is made at the side of the finger and a second incision is usually necessary in the palm. At least two of the flexor tendon pulleys should be left intact during incision and drainage of the tendon sheath. The wound is occasionally closed around a plastic catheter that is used for intermittent antibiotic irrigation for 3 or 4 days. With mild early flexor tenosynovitis, a 12-hour trial of splinting and intravenous antibiotics may be warranted.

(7) Infections of the radial and ulnar bursae. The radial and ulnar bursae are the proximal prolongations of the flexor tendon sheaths of the thumb and little fingers, respectively. A tendon sheath infection of either of these two digits may drain proximally and into the opposite side of the hand, forming a "horseshoe" abscess. Infections of the ulnar bursa may be drained through an ulnar incision. Those of the radial bursa frequently require an incision adjacent to the thenar eminence. In either case, an incision within the wrist is usually mandatory to drain the cul-de-sac of these bursae.

(8) Thenar space infection. The borders of the thenar space include the thenar muscles radially, the adductor pollicis deeply, flexor tendons of the index and middle fingers superficially, and a septum extending deep to the flexor tendons of the middle finger ulnarly. Distally, the infection may involve the first and second lumbrical canals and may extend to the dorsum of the first web. Fullness and tenderness of the radial half of the palm are noted.

Incisions for drainage should *not* parallel the first web. A dorsal longitudinal incision radial to the second metacarpal bone usually provides sufficient exposure to permit adequate irrigation and drainage of the thenar space. This incision allows access to the radial half of the palm over the first dorsal interosseus and adductor muscles. If necessary, a second incision may be made in the palm.

(9) Midpalmar space infection. The midpalmar space extends from the hypothenar muscles ulnarly to the septum of the flexor tendon of the middle finger radially. Deeply it is bound by the third, fourth, and fifth metacarpal bones and the palmar interosseus muscles and superficially by the tendons to the middle, ring, and little fingers and the third and fourth lumbrical muscles. Distally, midpalmar abscesses may extend into the fourth and fifth lumbrical canals. The infection causes fullness and tenderness of the ulnar side of the palm.

A curved midpalmar incision paralleling the flexion creases of the palm allows ready access to the midpalmar space. Great care should be taken to avoid injury to the flexor tendons and neurovascular bundles to the third and fourth webs.

(10) Joint infection. The most frequent joint infection in the hand involves the metacarpophalangeal joint after a bite received in a fight. Any small laceration over the metacarpophalangeal joint should be suspected of being the result of a tooth injury (particularly on Saturday nights). If the extensor tendon is lacerated, contamination of the joint should be assumed. The wound should be lavaged and left open. If an infection develops in the untreated patient, the joint should be opened, lavaged, and allowed to drain.

All hand infections require splinting. Gentle active or passive motion may be instituted 2 or 3 days after treatment, depending on the nature of the infection and injury. Complete range-of-motion exercises just once a day may be sufficient to prevent joint contractures.

Many of the more chronic and more severe infections of the hand, including osteomyelitis and tuberculosis, do not involve the emergency physician. Superficial infections that are not associated with abscess formation are rarely surgical problems.

THE STIFF AND SWOLLEN HAND

A stiff hand has little function. Stiffness often can be prevented by judicious and meticulous primary care of hand wounds, strict attention to surgical principles, careful application of dressings, and appropriate exercises after operation.

Treatment of the swollen hand should be directed toward maintaining joint mobility and rapid resolution of the edema. All constrictive dressings should be loosened. Circular casts should be either bivalved or removed and replaced with splints. A crushed or swollen hand in which there are neither fractures nor injured tendons should be immobilized with the wrist in mild dorsiflexion, the thumb in maximal abduction, the metacarpophalangeal joints in approximately 70 degrees of flexion, and the proximal interphalangeal joints in almost full extension. Although this is not the position of function, it is the position in which joint contractures are least likely to develop. When considerable edema and stiffness are feared after severe injuries, Kirschner wires may be used to fix the metacarpophalangeal joints of the fingers in flexion and the thumb in abduction.

The arm should be elevated several inches higher than the level of the heart. If there is no arterial insufficiency, we suspend the arm from an intravenous pole. A well-padded volar splint supports the wrist. A stockinette, with appropriate openings cut for the fingers and thumb, is placed over the splint and suspended from the pole. The value of oral enzymes in decreasing edema has not been well substantiated.

We do not use elastic bandages in the treatment of edema of the hand. These bandages may cause more harm than good since they interfere with venous drainage. Elastic bandages are difficult for a surgeon to apply properly; they are dangerous when applied by the patient. The rubberized elastic bandage has little place in the treatment of any injury of the hand.

Occasionally, severe intermittent edema may result from self-induced injury. The patient may apply a tourniquet around the wrist or forearm, for example. Such patients may not be malingerers, but rather they may be suffering from behavioral psychiatric disorders. This diagnosis must always be suspected when severe, otherwise inexplicable edema is limited proximally by a circumferential sulcus about the wrist or forearm. Edema often subsides rapidly if a heavily padded dressing is applied from the fingertips to the upper arm. Such a dressing prevents access of the patient to the limb. If the diagnosis of factitious lymphedema is established, the patient should be referred for psychiatric evaluation.

Any severe injury of the hand or forearm may result in edema of the soft tissues of the hand. Without prompt treatment, irreversible changes may develop rapidly about the median nerve and within the adductor pollicis and interosseus muscles of the fingers.

The median nerve lies directly beneath the transverse carpal ligament and overlies the flexor tendons of the fingers and thumb. The carpal tunnel is bound deeply by the carpal bones and the volar wrist ligaments. As edema develops, the synovium surrounding the flexor tendons swells and presses the median nerve tightly against the volar ligament, and an acute carpal tunnel syndrome develops. The patient will have paresthesia and hypesthesia in the thumb, index and middle fingers, and radial side of the ring finger. There will be tenderness proximal to the carpal canal, and percussion in this area will elicit a positive Tinel's sign in the sensory distribution of the nerve. Palmar flexion of the wrist for 1 minute will add to the compression of the median nerve and increase the paresthesia. This is known as Phalen's sign.

In these patients, carpal tunnel release is an emergency procedure that should be performed as soon as possible. A curved incision is made in the thenar crease and extended proximally to the ulnar side of the midline of the wrist and to the distal forearm. All dissection is performed ulnar to the midline to avoid injury to the palmar cutaneous branch of the median nerve. The median nerve is identified proximal to the carpal canal. With the nerve visualized, the transverse carpal ligament is transected. Epineurectomy is rarely necessary.

If the patient with a potentially stiff or swollen hand is treated and allowed to return home, he and his family should be urged to return to the emergency ward or to telephone if pain becomes more severe or if the fingers become pale or cold.

The physician's responsibility for the patient's care extends beyond the time that emergency treatment is rendered, and the patient must be aware that a physician is available and eager to be called if any problems develop.

Suggested Readings

Boyes JH: Operative technique in surgery of the hand, in American Academy of Orthopaedic Surgeons: *Instructional Course Lectures*, vol 9, Ann Arbor, Mich. JW Edwards, 1952, pp. 181–195

Boyes JH (Ed): *Bunnell's Surgery of the Hand*, ed 5. Philadelphia, JB Lippincott, 1970

Flatt AE: Minor hand injuries. *J Bone Joint Surg 37-B:*117–125, 1955

Flynn JE: *Hand Surgery*, ed 2. Baltimore, Williams & Wilkins, 1975

Grabb WE, Myers MB (Eds): *Skin Flaps.* Boston, Little, Brown, 1975

Milford L: The hand, in *Campbell's Operative Orthopaedics*, Crenshaw AH (Ed). ed 5. St. Louis, CV Mosby, 1971, pp. 138–411

Rank BK, Wakefield AR, Hueston JT: *Surgery of Repair as Applied to Hand Injuries*, ed 4. Baltimore, Williams & Wilkins, 1973

Seddon H: *Surgical Disorders of the Peripheral Nerves*, ed 2. Baltimore, Williams & Wilkins, 1975

Smith RJ: Intrinsic muscles of the fingers: Function, dysfunction, and surgical reconstruction, in American Academy of Orthopaedic Surgeons: *Instructional Course Lectures*, vol 24. St. Louis, CV Mosby, 1975, pp. 200–220

Symposium on Tendon Surgery in the Hand, Philadelphia, 1974. St. Louis, CV Mosby, 1975

Wynn Parry CB: *Rehabilitation of the Hand*, ed 3. London, Butterworths, 1973

CHAPTER 32

Pediatric Surgical Emergencies

SAMUEL H. KIM, M.D.

Surgical emergencies in pediatric patients include not only many problems found in adults but also disorders peculiar to infants and children. Surgical problems in the newborn and in older children will be discussed up to the time when the patient is transferred out of the emergency setting. Special aspects of trauma in the pediatric patient will also be discussed.

NONTRAUMATIC EMERGENCIES IN THE NEWBORN

General Considerations

When a newborn has a surgical disorder that requires prompt attention, certain precautions must be taken to ensure safe transport to the nearest treatment facility. The most important precaution is heat conservation. All too often in the past, an otherwise healthy newborn would arrive at a major referral center with a correctable surgical problem only to succumb from complications of hypothermia. Today, any hospital that cares for newborns should have the equipment to provide safe transport of the infant.

The first step is to wrap the baby when this is possible. However, these children often have to be observed closely without blankets, so isolettes or incubators are essential. Wrapping with plastic sheeting or placing covered hot water bottles next to the infant may be necessary in extreme situations. The newer incubators allow easy observation and access to the infant and have built-in monitoring equipment. The pulse rate, respiration rate, and temperature should be monitored. The temperature is easily measured by a rectal or cutaneous thermometer. When oxygen administration is necessary, to lessen the danger of retrolental fibroplasia one must remember not to give too high a concentration unnecessarily over a prolonged period.

A portable suction machine with catheters of appropriate size should always be available to keep the airway clear and sometimes to prevent secretions from accumulating in either the stomach or the pharynx. If an endotracheal tube is in place, suction is necessary for secretions.

A nasogastric tube is essential in any child with intestinal obstruction or vomiting. A No. 8 or No. 10 French feeding tube is much more effective than a smaller tube. Intermittent suction by machine or hand during transport minimizes the danger of aspiration.

If intravenous fluids are necessary before or during transport, a threaded plastic intravenous catheter or a cutdown catheter is less likely to become dislodged than a scalp-vein needle. Pediatric-sized intravenous tubing, burettes, and solutions should always be used. Fluids are best administered by means of a mechanical pump if available.

A check should always be made that vitamin K has been administered to the newborn in the delivery room. In the hurry associated with an unusual delivery, routine is often disrupted and vitamin K administration is overlooked. This could prove disastrous later.

Cutdown Technique

Cutdown is usually performed in the antecubital fossa or at the ankle. In the latter case the greater saphenous vein is dissected just anterior to and above the medial malleolus. After the limb is immobilized above and below the site of the incision, it is prepared with povidone-iodine (Betadine) and alcohol, and draped with sterile towels. In the arm, a transverse incision is made in the crease of the antecubital space over a visible vein. A fine hemostat is passed around the vein and the vessel is tied distally with a ligature of 4-0 or 5-0 silk. A second ligature is then passed around the vein proximally, and after a small incision is made into the vein, a 20- or 22-gauge plastic catheter is inserted and tied securely. The skin is closed around the catheter with interrupted 4–0 silk sutures; 4–0 or 5–0 chromic catgut and polyglycolic acid (Dexon) sutures have also been used. The ends of the silk ligatures used to tie the vein and the catheter should be left long and protruding through the closed incision so that when the skin sutures are removed the ligatures can also be removed entirely to prevent their future extrusion. An antibiotic dressing is then applied to the incision. The saphenous vein is isolated and cannulated with a similar technique.

Insertion of Arterial Lines

Arterial lines are commonly used for frequent blood sampling and for blood pressure monitoring. The most accessible and most commonly used artery is the umbilical artery. For less experienced medical staff, this provides the easiest insertion, but the technique is not without danger. The region of the umbilicus should be prepared carefully with povidone-iodine and alcohol, and the cord should then be cut behind the umbilical clamp or tie. A few 4–0 silk traction sutures through the remaining portion of the umbilical cord allow easier handling. The umbilical vein should be identified and ligated to prevent retrograde blood flow, and one of the umbilical arteries, usually located at 4 o'clock and 8 o'clock, should be dissected for a distance of 5–10 mm. A No. 3.5 or No. 5 French umbilical artery catheter is introduced into the artery until free retrograde flow of blood is noted. X-ray examination allows placement of the tip of this radiopaque catheter below the renal arteries. No attempt should be made to pass the catheter further because of the possibility of embolus to a mesenteric, renal, or iliac vessel. Some groups prefer the tip to lie at the diaphragm. The catheter is tied securely and flushed continuously by a mechanical pump with heparinized normal saline solution, 1 unit of sodium heparin per milliliter of saline. An antibiotic dressing is placed around the umbilicus, and the arterial line is removed after 96 hours.

Radial artery cannulation is preferred to umbilical catheterization. After satisfactory collateral flow from the ulnar artery is verified, the arm is immobilized with the wrist extended. Using sterile technique, the physician performs direct percutaneous puncture with a 22-gauge catheter and needle, pushing the needle through the vessel and then slowly pulling back until brisk retrograde flow is noted. The catheter is then advanced without the needle. If the catheter is accurately placed, retrograde flow should continue. If there is any question of its not being in the vessel, the catheter should be removed. Flushing solutions should not be injected.

In smaller patients, cutdown of the artery at the wrist with direct puncture of the vessel without any ligatures may be preferable. Whatever technique of radial artery cannulation is used, if discoloration or blanching of the hand or arm occurs, the catheter should be instantly removed.

Other sites used include the dorsalis pedis artery and the temporal artery.

Esophageal Atresia

The diagnosis of esophageal atresia should be suspected when a newborn (1) has excessive nasopharyngeal secretions, (2) is unable to handle secretions adequately, (3) has episodes of coughing or cyanosis, or (4) chokes, coughs, or has difficulty breathing when being fed. Polyhydramnios and prematurity are common in the history. Pneumonia revealed on a chest x-ray film suggests aspiration due to esophageal atresia, and lack of intestinal air below the diaphragm suggests esophageal atresia without fistula.

The diagnosis is made by passing a stiff No. 10 or No. 12 French nasogastric tube through either the nose or the mouth into the stomach. Smaller feeding catheters are not recommended since they will curl in the upper esophageal pouch, giving the impression that the catheter has entered the stomach. If the catheter stops before reaching the stomach, an x-ray study should be done. With the infant upright, 1–2 ml of water-soluble radiopaque dye (Hypaque) is injected through the catheter into the pouch and fluoroscopic examination is performed (Fig. 32.1). As soon as the diagnosis is confirmed, the dye is aspirated. The catheter is left in place, and intermittent suction is applied to keep the upper pouch from collecting secretions that may then spill into the tracheobronchial tree, causing pneumonia.

The infant is kept in a head-up position with sump suction through the nose from the blind pouch. The suction catheter can be constructed by making a hole in the side of a No. 10 French nasogastric tube and passing a No. 20 Intracath plastic catheter through the hole to the end of the tube, sealing the puncture site afterward (Fig. 32.2). The tip of the tube is placed in the pouch, and suction is applied to keep the pouch free of secretions. If pneumonia is present, appropriate antibiotics such as oxacillin and gentamicin should be administered. The infant is placed in an isolette with the head up. Oxygen is administered if necessary. Chest physical therapy and tracheal suction

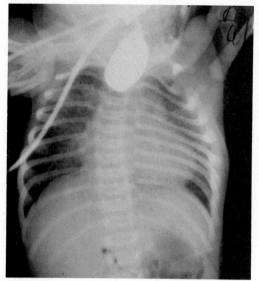

Figure 32.1. Esophageal atresia. Demonstration of blind upper pouch by injection of 1–2 ml of water-soluble dye through upper pouch sump catheter under fluoroscopic control.

aid in resolving the pneumonia. Intravenous fluids are usually not needed in the first 24 hours after birth, but if intravenous antibiotic administration is necessary, a scalp vein needle or 22- or 23-gauge catheter can be threaded into a vein (Hendren, 1964b).

Isolated Tracheoesophageal Fistula

The diagnosis of isolated tracheoesophageal fistula (H fistula) is usually made in older infants with recurrent pneumonitis. The patient usually has a history of difficulty with feedings, especially choking, and if the recurrent infections and feeding problems are serious, failure to thrive is apparent. A thin barium swallow with the infant in the prone position may reveal the fistula; normal x-ray films, however, do not rule out this condition. Endoscopic examination should be performed if symptoms persist.

Intestinal Obstruction

In the newborn, intestinal obstruction is suspected with the triad of green or bile-stained vom-

SUMP SUCTION IN ESOPHAGEAL ATRESIA

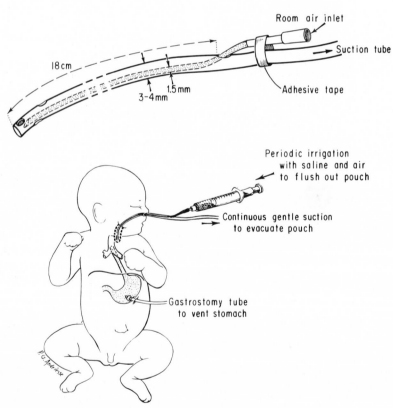

Figure 32.2. Simple but effective sump catheter made from No. 10 French infant feeding tube and 20-gauge polyethylene intravenous catheter.

itus, abdominal distention, and failure to pass meconium. There are exceptions to all three signs, however. If an infant has pyloric atresia, which is extremely rare, the vomitus will not be bile-stained. A patient with duodenal atresia will not have abdominal distention, but occasionally the examiner will see upper abdominal fullness and peristaltic waves caused by the hypertrophied, distended stomach and proximal part of the duodenum. Finally, depending on the type of obstruction and antenatal occurrence, normal green meconium may be passed in the presence of intestinal atresia. Polyhydramnios and prematurity may be part of the history in intestinal obstruction.

In all patients with intestinal obstruction, a nasogastric tube is essential. Aspiration should be carried out intermittently during transport to prevent vomiting or regurgitation; the syringe should not be left attached to the tube when aspiration is not being performed. If intravenous fluids are necessary, especially when peritonitis or sepsis is suspected, an intravenous line should be placed immediately. The type of fluid administered depends on the illness. A recommended maintenance solution is a 5% dextrose solution in 0.25% saline. Antibiotics can usually be given intravenously. If colloid is required, a 5% solution of normal human serum albumin (Albumisol) is administered.

Pyloric atresia is extremely rare. The diagnosis can usually be made within the first 24–48 hours after birth. Oral feeding is not tolerated, but the vomitus is not bile-stained. There is no abdominal distention, but there may be upper abdominal fullness. X-ray films of the abdomen show gastric outlet obstruction and no gas beyond that point. No further diagnostic studies are necessary.

In patients with *duodenal atresia,* a plain film of the abdomen confirms the diagnosis with the typical "double bubble" sign (Fig. 32.3). No further diagnostic studies are necessary.

If the plain film of the abdomen shows a few dilated loops, the diagnosis is *jejunal atresia* and no further x-ray studies are necessary. If there are many air-filled loops (Fig. 32.4), however, a barium study should be done. Usually, large and small intestine cannot be differentiated on the plain film in a newborn. A barium enema may reveal rare *colonic atresia* or a microcolon, which usually indicates *ileal atresia.* If the colon appears to be normal, however, meconium ileus or Hirschsprung's disease should be suspected. Large bowel present on the left side of the abdomen or displacement of the cecum from the right lower quadrant is diagnostic of intestinal malrotation with associated midgut volvulus.

Patients seen with *meconium ileus* have bile-stained vomitus, abdominal distention of moderate to severe degree, and occasionally a doughy

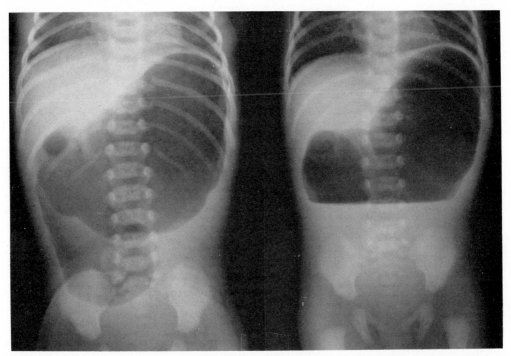

Figure 32.3. Duodenal atresia. The smaller second bubble on right side of abdomen represents dilated proximal duodenum. *Left,* kidney-ureter-bladder (KUB) film. *Right,* upright abdominal film.

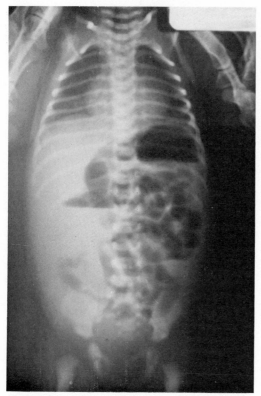

Figure 32.4.   Low intestinal obstruction. Small intestine cannot be differentiated from colon on plain film in newborn. Barium enema study should be done if peritonitis is not present.

feel to the abdomen. There may also be a mass-like effect. The family history may be significant for cystic fibrosis. A plain film of the abdomen will show multiple dilated loops of intestine and occasionally a mass with tiny bubbles of air (Fig. 32.5A). The latter, of course, is the dilated terminal ileum with the impacted abnormal meconium and trapped air bubbles. If abdominal calcification is present, antenatal *meconium peritonitis* has probably occurred. Intestinal atresia often complicates meconium peritonitis. Barium enema examination may reveal a microcolon or a normal colon. If obstruction is mechanical only, meglumine diatrizoate (Gastrografin) enemas (Fig. 32.5B) have been shown to relieve the obstruction and to avoid laparotomy (Noblett, 1969). Intravenous fluids should be administered during and after the study, and careful monitoring in the darkened fluoroscopy room should be carried out since hypovolemia can occur very easily because of the "hypertonicity" of the contrast medium. Laparotomy should be carried out in the infant with previous meconium peritonitis or signs of gan-

grene, or if instillations of meglumine diatrizoate are unsuccessful.

Hirschsprung's disease or *congenital megacolon* in our experience constitutes approximately one-third of newborn intestinal obstruction. The classic finding of a dilated segment and an associated narrow segment in the rectosigmoid and rectum is usually not seen in the routine barium enema examination (Fig. 32.6A). A careful barium study, however, often shows that the aganglionic segment is spastic and poorly distensible compared with the normal colon (Fig. 32.6B). An x-ray film obtained 24 hours after evacuation is equally important. If this shows retained barium beyond the lower part of the rectum, Hirschsprung's disease should be suspected. The abdomen is usually extremely distended. Introduction of a nasogastric tube often elicits a bile-stained aspirate. Digital examination of the rectum with the smallest finger may reveal that it is narrow. A sudden, explosive evacuation of liquid stool and fluid after withdrawal of the finger should suggest Hirschsprung's disease. Rectal biopsy is the most reliable diagnostic study, although rectal manometry and superficial submucosal punch biopsies of the rectum have recently been used with encouraging results. Early diagnosis is essential to prevent colitis, which is usually nonbacterial. We prefer a loop colostomy proximal to the aganglionic segment until a definitive pull-through procedure can be carried out at an older age.

In *meconium plug syndrome*, low intestinal obstruction results from a large plug of meconium. This entity can mimic Hirschsprung's disease, meconium ileus, or colonic atresia. A barium enema, however, usually causes evacuation of the plug and resolution of the obstruction. All these infants should be screened carefully for cystic fibrosis and Hirschsprung's disease, since the chance that one of these is present is 10–20%.

Intestinal malrotation with volvulus is usually catastrophic in the newborn or small infant. Often the child who has been feeding normally will stop feeding and will vomit bile-stained material. Abdominal distention develops. The passage of guaiac-positive stools is usually ominous, signifying vascular compromise of the intestine. A plain film of the abdomen usually shows pyloric or duodenal obstruction with little air present in the small intestine. If the child is seen rather late after vascular compromise, the intestine may be very dilated. A barium study is usually performed first to see whether the cecum is in the normal location. If there is any doubt about the diagnosis, an upper gastrointestinal series should be performed to see

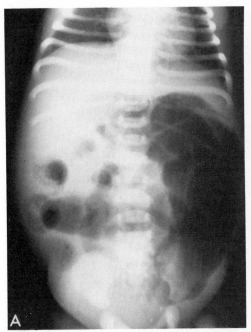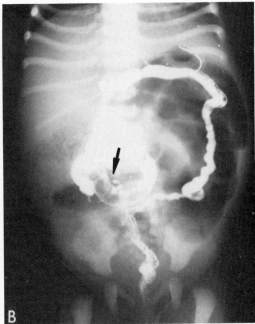

Figure 32.5.   Intestinal obstruction due to meconium ileus. **(A)** Plain film of abdomen. Note small bubbles of trapped air on right side. **(B)** Meglumine diatrizoate (Gastrografin) enema demonstrating abnormal meconium (*arrow*) in terminal ileum. Two or three washouts in 24 hours produced complete relief from intestinal obstruction. (Reproduced by permission, from *Surgical Clinics of North America*, Vol. 54, No. 3, © 1974, W. B. Saunders Co.)

whether the duodenum has a normal configuration and normal attachment at the ligament of Treitz. Once the diagnosis is made, the patient should be operated on immediately. If peritonitis is present, no contrast studies should be performed. After administration of colloid, other intravenous fluids, and antibiotics, the patient is taken to the operating room.

Stenosis of the small intestine may occur in a newborn or small infant. If the duodenum is narrowed, the abdomen may not be distended, although the child will intermittently vomit bile-stained material and food. An upper gastrointestinal series shows the partial obstruction that is often due to the "wind-sock" deformity of the duodenum. If the stenosis is distal in the gastrointestinal tract, a careful small-bowel follow-through may show the area of narrowing with proximal dilation.

Gastric Perforation

Perforation of the stomach leads to massive abdominal distention and respiratory distress (Fig. 32.7). There may be a history of perinatal distress followed by distention, lethargy, toxicity, and shock. To relieve the respiratory distress, needle aspiration with a 20- or 22-gauge needle should be performed first. A nasogastric tube, intravenous fluids including colloid, and antibiotics are essential preoperative measures.

Necrotizing Enterocolitis

Necrotizing enterocolitis is likely to develop in the premature newborn who has undergone severe stress and associated hypoxia. There is progressive abdominal distention and bile-stained vomitus. X-ray examination may reveal air within the intestinal wall (pneumatosis cystoides intestinalis), free air in the peritoneal cavity, or in the most seriously ill, air in the portal vein (Fig. 32.8). Immediate measures include insertion of a nasogastric tube, administration of broad-spectrum antibiotics, and administration of intravenous fluids including colloid. Transfusions may be necessary. Administration of neomycin or kanamycin by enema and through the nasogastric tube has recently had some beneficial effect on this highly lethal disease (Bell et al., 1973). After appropriate preoperative support, the infant with necrotic or perforated intestine should undergo laparotomy.

Omphalocele and Gastroschisis

The diagnosis of omphalocele and of gastroschisis is usually obvious (Fig. 32.9). The physician

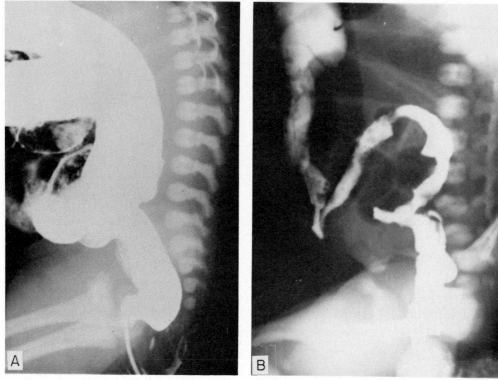

Figure 32.6. Hirschsprung's disease in newborn. **(A)** Normal-appearing barium enema. **(B)** Careful barium enema with only small amount of barium under fluoroscopy by experienced radiologist demonstrates clearly the abnormal, narrow, scalloped, aganglionic segment in same patient. (Reproduced by permission, from *Surgical Clinics of North America*, Vol. 54, No. 3, © 1974, W. B. Saunders Co.)

should be wary, however, of the occult or very small omphalocele involving the base of the umbilical cord. If the umbilical clamp or tie is placed too close to the abdominal wall, a small omphalocele will be ligated, and if intestine is present in it, intestinal obstruction, peritonitis from perforation, or a fistula may develop. In large omphaloceles, sterile warm saline dressings should be placed over the intact sac, and many layers of dry gauze should then be wrapped about the abdomen. Recently, placing a transparent plastic bag filled with warm saline solution over the lower part of the body and omphalocele has been useful in preserving the temperature of the infant and has helped prevent desiccation of the thin protective sac. A nasogastric tube is essential. Intravenous fluids and antibiotics are usually unnecessary during transport.

In gastroschisis or a ruptured omphalocele, blood and meconium are easily removed by gentle irrigation with warm saline solution. Warm saline dressings with a wrap-around sterile dressing or the plastic bag previously mentioned should then be used to protect the infant during transport. The

intestine is often matted and thickened, and appears violaceous. If the color of the intestine is extremely dark, derotation of the protruding malrotated midgut may be lifesaving. Antibiotics should be administered and a nasogastric tube should be inserted (Kim, 1976).

Omphalomesenteric Duct

Persistence of tissue or drainage of fluid at the umbilicus should suggest a communication with the gastrointestinal tract or urinary bladder. If only an umbilical granuloma is present, there will be no evidence of a sinus tract, and simple excision of the persistent umbilical tissue and cautery of the bleeding vessel with silver nitrate will be all the treatment necessary.

If an opening can be seen, passing a No. 3.5 or No. 5 French feeding tube and injecting water-soluble contrast material will demonstrate communication with either the small intestine or a urachal cyst. The infant with an omphalomesenteric duct should be admitted and operated on when the diagnosis is made to avoid intussusception or internal volvulus. The infant with a patent urachus should have an intravenous pyelogram and voiding cystourethrogram, and should undergo excision before infection occurs.

Imperforate Anus

In the newborn, imperforate anus is usually obvious on careful inspection of the perineum. Rarely, however, atresia or severe stenosis may exist several centimeters proximal to the anus with a normal external appearance. If a well-lubricated rectal thermometer cannot easily be passed several centimeters, imperforate anus should be suspected.

In the male infant the most common site for a fistula is along the median raphe from the anal dimple, forward across the perineum, and onto the midline of the scrotum (Fig. 32.10A). In the female infant the fistula usually occurs at the posterior rim of the vaginal introitus, the so-called fourchette fistula (Fig. 32.10B). If a fistula is present on the perineum, dilatation with a hemostatic forceps often allows normal passage of meconium until the infant is admitted for elective operation several months later. If the fistula is so small that it cannot be dilated or stretched easily, the infant

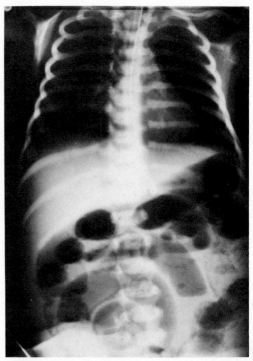

Figure 32.8. Necrotizing enterocolitis. Note air within intestinal wall (pneumatosis cystoides intestinalis) and within portal vein. (Reproduced by permission, from *Surgical Clinics of North America*, Vol. 54, No. 3, © 1974, W. B. Saunders Co.)

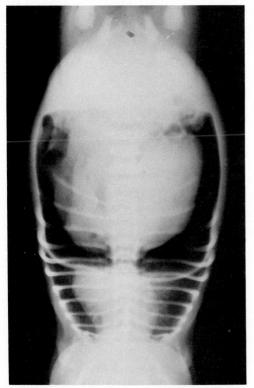

Figure 32.7. Gastric perforation with massive pneumoperitoneum. Initial lifesaving treatment consisted of immediate aspiration of air from peritoneal cavity.

should undergo a surgical procedure before intestinal obstruction becomes severe.

Sigmoid colostomy is performed if there is no evidence of a fistula. Pull-through procedures should not be performed in the newborn since there is a great danger of missing or tearing the important components of the levator muscles that are responsible for continence. A nasogastric tube is all that is necessary in transport, and is mandatory if the abdomen is distended.

Here a note of caution is necessary about the upside-down plain film of the abdomen. In the past, a marker was placed at the anal dimple and the distance was measured from the most distal rectosigmoid or rectal air to the marker. Depending on the distance, an abdominal or perineal exploration was performed. This film is often misleading, and no surgical decision should depend on it. A fistula usually means a perineal operation; no fistula means a colostomy (Hendren and Kim, 1974).

When the patient with a colostomy is about 1 year old, a definitive procedure is carried out. There is a high incidence of genitourinary anom-

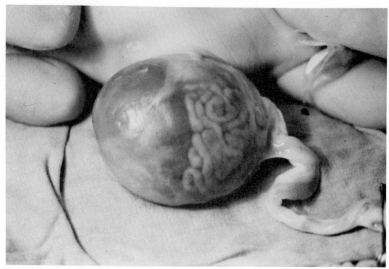

Figure 32.9.   Large omphalocele with intact sac. Note umbilical cord arising from sac and not from abdominal wall. The large sacs often contain liver as well as small and large intestine. (Reproduced by permission, from *Surgical Clinics of North America*, Vol. 56, No. 2, © 1976, W. B. Saunders Co.)

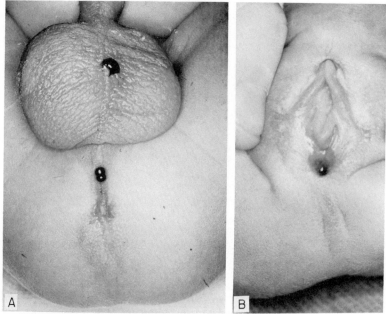

Figure 32.10.   Low imperforate anus. **(A)** Male with perineal fistula. **(B)** Female with posterior fourchette fistula. (Reproduced by permission, from *Surgical Clinics of North America*, Vol. 54, No. 3, © 1974, W. B. Saunders Co.)

alies, so all patients should have an intravenous pyelogram.

Respiratory Distress

An infant who has stridor in the newborn period should be evaluated immediately. Direct laryngoscopic examination should be familiar to all physicians who care for the newborn. It can be life-saving for an infant with airway obstruction. Anatomic obstructions such as a thyroglossal duct cyst at the base of the tongue, a pharyngeal duplication, a laryngocele (Fig. 32.11), or a subglottic web or tumor such as an hemangioma that is impinging on the trachea can be bypassed by endotracheal intubation, and the infant can then be transferred to a facility where the obstructing

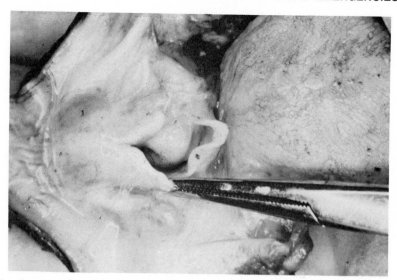

Figure 32.11.   Laryngocele causing severe respiratory distress and stridor in newborn. Direct laryngoscopy and insertion of endotracheal tube bypassing the obstruction would have been lifesaving.

lesion can be removed. Tracheotomy is rarely necessary as an emergency procedure in the newborn, although two infants with congenital subglottic stenosis with a pinpoint opening in whom even the smallest endotracheal tube could not be passed have undergone lifesaving tracheotomy at the Massachusetts General Hospital.

Proper pediatric laryngoscopes and plastic or Silastic endotracheal tubes of appropriate size should be immediately available in the delivery room and nursery.

When tracheotomy is indicated, it is preferable to perform it in the operating room. After induction of general anesthesia, a bronchoscope of the proper size is passed through the vocal cords and into the upper part of the trachea. Bronchoscopic examination is first carried out, if indicated, to rule out a foreign body; this is particularly appropriate in older infants. The end of the bronchoscope is then positioned in the middle of the trachea. Rolled towels are placed under the shoulders. By tilting the rigid bronchoscope, the examiner can lift the trachea into a superficial position in the neck (Fig. 32.12). While an anesthesiologist ventilates the patient through the bronchoscope, a transverse skin incision no more than 1.5–2.0 cm long is made over the third and fourth tracheal rings. The tracheal wall is reached rapidly because of the superficial position, but no portion is excised. A transverse incision is made between the rings. A proper-sized tracheotomy tube is introduced. A useful maneuver is to place 3–0 silk sutures around the third or fourth ring on either side of the trachea before making the incision into

the trachea. Should the tracheotomy tube become dislodged before a mature tract has formed, traction on these two silk sutures allows quick replacement of the tube or introduction of an oxygen-carrying catheter until the tube can be replaced. Tracheotomy over an endotracheal tube is a reasonable alternative, and is certainly easier and safer than tracheotomy in the absence of any type of intubation.

Diaphragmatic Hernia

The infant with a diaphragmatic hernia usually has severe respiratory distress immediately after birth (Fig. 32.13). Unexplained tachypnea, retractions, and cyanotic episodes in a very pale, pasty infant should suggest the diagnosis. The abdomen is often scaphoid since most if not all of the abdominal contents are displaced into the chest. Breath sounds may be unreliable in such a small patient, being readily transmitted from the unaffected side. The diagnosis is confirmed by chest x-ray examination.

Initial treatment includes 100% oxygen by face mask. A No. 8 or No. 10 French nasogastric tube is passed into the stomach to prevent vomiting and aspiration and to remove any swallowed air that could otherwise pass into the intestine. Intestinal distention will shift the mediastinum and further compress the unaffected lung. Nasopharyngeal and oral suction is essential to keep the airway cleared of secretions. Positioning the patient with the affected side down may prevent further mediastinal shift.

Endotracheal intubation should not be per-

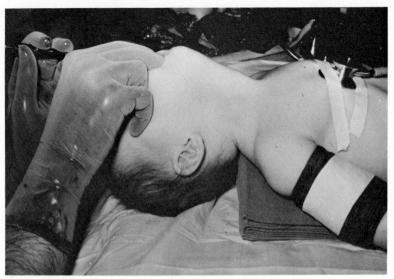

Figure 32.12.   Tracheotomy position. Anesthesia is provided through bronchoscope held by anesthesiologist. By tipping the bronchoscope, the examiner can bring the trachea to superficial position.

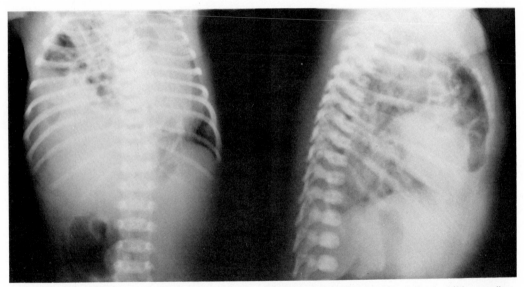

Figure 32.13.   Right-sided diaphragmatic hernia. Abdominal contents fill right side of chest, shifting mediastinum to left. Insertion of nasogastric tube will keep intestines decompressed and prevent further compromise of unaffected left lung. *Left,* anteroposterior chest film. *Right,* lateral film.

formed routinely, but someone experienced in intubation of infants should accompany the baby in transport. Positive-pressure ventilation should be avoided because of a high associated risk of pneumothorax on the unaffected side, which could be fatal.

Sudden deterioration in the already precarious condition of one of these infants indicates pneumothorax, and placing 22-gauge needles into each side of the chest may prove lifesaving. Although intravenous fluids are usually unnecessary during transport, if there is a waiting period before operation, intravenous fluid administration should be started. Sodium bicarbonate should be given to help combat severe respiratory and metabolic acidosis.

In the older infant whose diaphragmatic hernia is undetected as a newborn, the hernia is discovered as an incidental finding on a chest x-ray film obtained because of repeated episodes of upper respiratory tract infection, dysphagia, or the interesting finding of bowel sounds in the chest. Unlike in the newborn, an emergency operation is unnecessary, but the hernia should be repaired when found because of the possibility of volvulus.

Pneumothorax

In the newborn, pneumothorax is usually seen on a chest x-ray film taken for tachypnea, retractions, cyanotic episodes, stridor, or possible aspiration (Fig. 32.14). Treatment depends on the degree of collapse and the severity of symptoms. If a small degree of pneumothorax (10% or less) is present in an infant without acute distress, another chest film 4 hours later may show that the air has decreased or gone. If it is still present in a symptomatic infant, aspiration with a 22-gauge needle or Intracath is recommended. If pneumothorax progresses or if the infant becomes more symptomatic, a No. 10 or No. 12 French chest tube should be inserted in the third or fourth interspace in the anterior axillary line. The tube is removed after there has been full expansion for 24–48 hours with no evidence of air leakage. Tension pneumothorax requires immediate tube insertion.

In the older child the most common cause for pneumothorax is rupture of a congenital bleb of the lung. Insertion of a chest tube is indicated although rarely a small asymptomatic pneumothorax (Fig. 32.15) can be aspirated with a needle. The child should be observed in the hospital after needle aspiration. If a chest tube is inserted, it can be removed after there has been full expansion for 24–48 hours without evidence of air leakage, as in

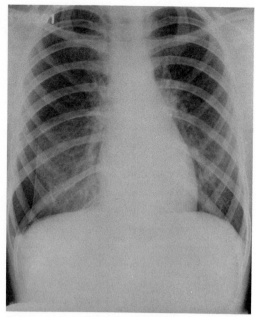

Figure 32.15.   Smaller pneumothorax in older child. Treatment depends on symptoms and severity of pneumothorax. A chest tube should be inserted if there is any doubt.

infants. If pneumothorax recurs on the same side, thoracotomy is necessary (Fig. 32.16).

Lobar Emphysema

A less common cause of serious respiratory distress is lobar emphysema (Hendren and McKee, 1966). This most commonly occurs in the infant beyond the newborn stage. Most of these children have repeated episodes of bronchiolitis, and in severe cases the presenting findings usually include hypoxia, tachypnea, retractions, and respiratory acidosis. Occasionally the patient is cyanotic. Chest x-ray films usually show an area of increased radiolucency that can be difficult to differentiate from pneumothorax, pulmonary cyst, or pneumatocele (Fig. 32.17). Using a bright light, however, the physician can often see attenuated vascular markings through the radiolucent area. Only rarely is more than one lobe affected. This lobe is overinflated, compressing the normal remaining lung. The left upper lobe and right middle lobe are the most frequently involved. The emphysema may be severe enough to cause not only compression of ipsilateral lobes but also mediastinal shift and compression of the opposite lung. Bronchography is generally not necessary; pulmonary scanning may be useful (Mauney and Sabiston, 1970).

In the severely ill, immediate endotracheal intubation is necessary with ventilatory support. In-

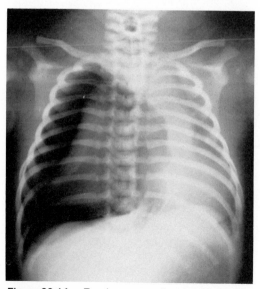

Figure 32.14.   Tension pneumothorax following tracheotomy. Immediate needle aspiration and tube thoracostomy were lifesaving.

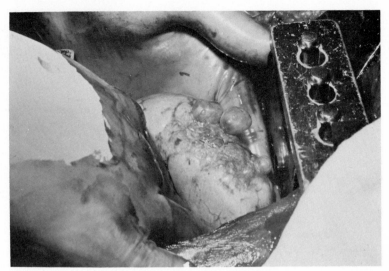

Figure 32.16.   Congenital apical blebs in patient with pneumothorax and persistent air leakage. At thoracotomy the blebs were resected, the area oversewn, and pleurodesis carried out.

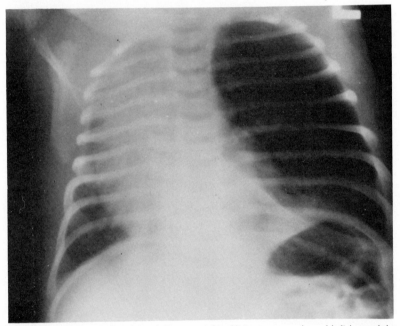

Figure 32.17.   Lobar emphysema involving left upper lobe. Note compression of left lower lobe and shift of mediastinum. Careful examination of plain chest x-ray film under bright light will reveal attenuated vascular markings in the hyperlucent area. This will differentiate lobar emphysema from pneumothorax.

travenous fluid administration should be started, and although ventilatory support may aid in reversing the respiratory acidosis, sodium bicarbonate is usually required. Immediate transfer and operation are necessary. In the less severely ill, endotracheal intubation will facilitate emergency care in transport.

With increased use of ventilatory support, more cases of lobar emphysema are evident. Most of the cases associated with ventilation will resolve when support is no longer necessary.

Gastrointestinal Hemorrhage

In the newborn, the onset of hematemesis and melena in a previously healthy infant should suggest hemorrhagic disease. Although it is routine to administer vitamin K to every newborn, this is occasionally forgotten and massive bleeding may ensue. Although the physician often thinks first of the ingestion of maternal blood, this does not usually cause the significant hematemesis and melena seen with vitamin K deficiency. While a blood sample is being drawn for clotting studies, typing, and crossmatching, 1 mg of vitamin K_1 oxide should be administered. This usually stops the bleeding before laboratory studies are completed.

In the older infant, massive upper gastrointestinal bleeding may come from several sources, such as a duodenal or gastric ulcer, esophageal varices, hiatal hernia, gastritis, and intestinal duplication. A nasogastric tube is passed to confirm the hematemesis and the extent of active bleeding. Intravenous fluid administration is started in a large vein, preferably the subclavian or jugular vein. Ringer's lactated solution or colloid is administered until blood is available. Lavage with iced saline is as useful in the infant or small child as in the adult, although a rapid temperature drop can occur in the smaller child. If hemorrhage persists, the child should undergo angiographic examination for further delineation of the bleeding site.

If the massive bleeding is lower gastrointestinal only, Meckel's diverticulum, intestinal duplication, congenital arteriovenous malformation, and rarely, ulcerative colitis should be considered. Causes of lesser amounts of bleeding include polyps, chronic intussusception, and intermittent volvulus due to malrotation.

Sigmoidoscopic examination should be carried out in all infants and children with rectal bleeding. If bleeding is active, angiography should be performed. A technetium scan may reveal a Meckel's diverticulum. Further contrast studies may also be useful, including a barium enema, upper gastrointestinal series, and small-bowel follow-through. Endoscopy with flexible pediatric equipment may also reveal an actively bleeding site, but the colon and stomach are the only easily accessible areas at present.

It has been our policy not to perform exploratory operation on the basis of one episode of massive bleeding without an obvious source. Should the child have a second major episode, however, even if the results of diagnostic studies are normal, exploratory laparotomy should be carried out.

Painful, bright-red, rectal bleeding in an infant most commonly is due to an anal fissure. Anoscopy or careful digital examination confirms the diagnosis. As in the adult, a sentinel pile often marks the fissure. Treatment is anal dilatation and administration of stool softeners. Unlike in the adult, operation is rarely necessary.

Abdominal Masses

Approximately 50% of abdominal masses in the newborn are in the genitourinary tract (Hendren, 1964a; Koop, 1973). Usually they occur in the flank or in the suprapubic area, although if they are very large, they may occupy most of the abdomen. An intravenous pyelogram is essential. If there is no function on the side of the mass, a unilateral multicystic kidney is statistically most likely. Hydronephrosis is another possibility. If bilateral masses are palpable and if there is delayed function seen on the intravenous pyelogram, infantile polycystic kidney disease, bilateral hydronephrosis, and megaureter syndrome are possibilities.

A suprapubic mass with bilateral flank masses should indicate the megaureter syndrome, in which the three masses palpable are the distended bladder and the hydronephrotic kidneys. Occasionally, the infant is asymptomatic, but more often has sepsis. The introduction of a No. 5 French feeding catheter into the bladder usually relieves the obstruction, but may also precipitate a postobstructive diuresis. An intravenous line should be inserted in these infants not only for administration of antibiotics but also for maintenance of hydration and administration of sodium bicarbonate, 20–40 mEq/liter, to treat metabolic acidosis. These infants have both a concentrating defect and an acidifying defect, so they produce urine continuously after the obstruction is relieved; they therefore require an intake to match the output. In addition, the inability to excrete excess acid products requires administration of alkali.

In the female infant, an imperforate hymen may lead to hydrocolpos and a suprapubic mass. A catheter introduced into the bladder will eliminate bladder distention. A cystogram and barium study may be useful to pinpoint the mass between the bladder and the rectum. Careful inspection of the vaginal introitus often shows a bulging membrane, and on rectal examination a tense anterior mass is felt. Aspiration through the hymen with a large-bore 18- to 19-gauge needle will reveal a thick, whitish, mucoid material. Hymenectomy corrects the problem.

Other possible masses in the suprapubic area include ovarian cyst, urachal cyst, and sacrococcygeal teratoma. An ovarian cyst in the newborn is usually palpated in the abdomen since the pelvis is too small to accommodate the mass. A urachal cyst may have a communication to the umbilicus;

in addition, compression of the dome of the bladder may be seen on a cystogram, and if the cyst is palpable, it may feel fixed to the anterior abdominal wall. In the case of a sacrococcygeal teratoma, a portion of the neoplasm is palpable on rectal examination in front of the coccyx or sacrum and behind the rectum. Occasionally the tumor is felt as a suprapubic or pelvic mass. Wilms' tumor is rarely seen in the newborn; if it is present, there is a palpable flank mass. Some function is visualized on the intravenous pyelogram.

Duplications of the gastrointestinal tract may be manifested by abdominal masses or intestinal obstruction. They are asymptomatic, and the involved area is usually apparent in gastrointestinal contrast studies. Surgical removal will avoid obstruction, gastrointestinal bleeding, perforation, and intussusception.

Other causes of abdominal masses in the newborn include hepatic tumors and cysts, subcapsular hematoma, retroperitoneal hematoma and teratoma, neural tumors, adrenal hemorrhage, and renal venous thrombosis.

NONTRAUMATIC EMERGENCIES IN INFANTS AND CHILDREN

Hernia

Hernias are a common surgical problem in children. *Umbilical hernias* rarely need surgical intervention. Approximately 95% of umbilical hernias close spontaneously by age 5 years. They rarely become incarcerated, and so although they are often prominent and therefore worrisome to the parents, reassurance and watchful waiting are usually indicated. If the hernia is still present by the time the child starts school, surgical repair should be carried out to prevent complications in adult life.

In contrast, all *inguinal hernias* should be corrected surgically. In newborns, inguinal hernias are often incarcerated (Fig. 32.18), but rarely is strangulation present. Applying gentle but firm pressure to the sac and simultaneously massaging the inguinal region at the level of the internal and external rings often reduces the hernia. If intestinal obstruction is not evident and if the hernia cannot be reduced, Trendelenburg's position and sedation with chloral hydrate or phenobarbital may cause spontaneous reduction. If the hernia cannot be reduced, emergency operation is necessary. If the intestine is obstructed, nasogastric suction and correction of dehydration and electrolyte imbalance are necessary.

Some infants have a fluid-containing sac that

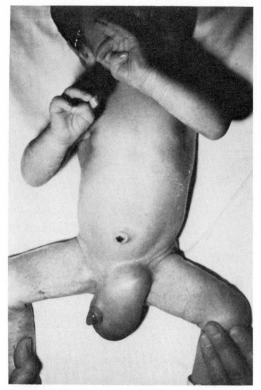

Figure 32.18.   Incarcerated left inguinal hernia. Note swelling in groin as well as in scrotum. Manual reduction can usually be carried out with sedation, elevation, ice packs, and gentle compression.

cannot be reduced. If there is no evidence of incarceration or hernia, the parents should observe the infant carefully to determine whether this is a hydrocele that may not need excision unless it becomes large or a communicating hydrocele in which the neck of the sac is so narrow that only fluid can go back and forth. If it is the latter, the parents will observe that the sac enlarges and diminishes in the course of 24 hours. A communicating hydrocele is a hernia, and it should be corrected surgically; this can be done electively rather than as an emergency procedure. A hydrocele in a newborn often disappears spontaneously, but if it persists for several months or if it enlarges, operation should be considered.

Inguinal hernias in the female are often only manifested by a sac at the level of the external ring. This is sometimes observable only if the patient is upright. Sometimes, especially in the infant, a movable lump is present in the inguinal region. This is not a lymph node but an incarcerated ovary. Repair should be carried out to prevent torsion and subsequent infarction of the ovary.

Femoral hernias are unusual in both male and female children. As in adults, careful examination reveals either a sac or a tender mass below the inguinal ligament medial to the femoral vessels. If a tender mass is present, immediate admission and surgical repair are indicated. If a sac is palpated, an elective procedure can be carried out.

Exploratory operation on the other side is recommended for all boys less than 2 years old with an inguinal hernia, unless the hernia is incarcerated. Patients more than 2 years old are considered individually, although if there is any question, exploration is carried out on the asymptomatic side. Both sides are explored in the female, regardless of age. In patients with a femoral hernia, both sides are usually explored, whether the patient is male or female.

Acute Scrotal Swelling

Several diseases can produce scrotal swelling. The most dangerous is *torsion of the testis*, since if it is not treated properly, testicular infarction will occur. *Scrotal cellulitis* is a streptococcal infection of the skin of the scrotum that sometimes spreads to the lower abdomen and the thigh. Both sides of the scrotum are symmetrically involved, and the skin is tender. A demarcation line can occasionally be seen. In such a case, the testes feel normal. Penicillin produces rapid resolution.

Torsion of the appendix of the testis or epididymis, if seen early, may be differentiated from testicular torsion by the presence of well-localized tenderness at the upper pole of the testis. If there is no testicular tenderness, treatment with bed rest, scrotal support, broad-spectrum antibiotics, and sitz baths is sufficient. *Epididymitis* is unusual until the teenage years unless it is associated with mumps. An *incarcerated hernia* produces swelling in the inguinal region as well as in the scrotum. There may be a history of intermittent swelling. Also, patients with an incarcerated hernia do not have erythema and edema of the scrotal wall. A *hydrocele* that appears acutely can be differentiated by transillumination and is not tender on palpation. Since 50% of patients with scrotal swelling have an antecedent history of trauma, a *hematoma* of the scrotum or tunica vaginalis is a possibility. Some discoloration of the skin on the traumatized side is usually present.

If the patient has scrotal erythema, edema, and tenderness with associated testicular retraction, the scrotum should be explored. If operation is carried out within 8–12 hours from the onset of symptoms, the testis can often be saved. Fixation of the opposite testis at operation is mandatory.

Appendicitis

Appendicitis is the most common abdominal surgical problem encountered in children. The classic triad of fever, abdominal pain, and vomiting should alert the clinician to this diagnosis. Appendicitis is often preceded by a viral upper respiratory tract infection, and early appendicitis is frequently missed during an epidemic of gastroenteritis. Although appendicitis is unusual in children less than 2 years old, when it is present there is usually generalized peritonitis because the patient is seen late.

Appendicitis mimics many disorders. The history is often not classic, and on physical examination only one finding is entirely reliable. Tenderness in the right lower quadrant at initial and subsequent examination without evidence of constipation, gastroenteritis, pelvic inflammatory disease, or recent ovulation should indicate appendicitis. The rectal examination is useful only if the inflamed appendix or some inflammatory process is palpable. Bowel sounds, rebound tenderness, cough tenderness, and the psoas sign are variable. In the very young, less cooperative patient, sedation without analgesia is often useful to detect tenderness. The white blood cell count may be within normal limits, but the differential usually shows some acute inflammatory response. Results of urinalysis are usually normal, but if the inflamed appendix is near the ureter, both red and white blood cells will be present in the urine. A plain film of the abdomen (Fig. 32.19) may show a fecalith, obliteration of the right psoas margin, obliteration of the right lateral peritoneal fat line, or scoliosis to the right.

If there is any question about the diagnosis, the child should be hospitalized and intravenous fluids should be administered. The child should receive nothing by mouth. He should be examined at intervals, preferably by the same observer. In the very sick child, fluid replacement is necessary. Through a peripheral intravenous line, Ringer's lactated solution of 5% dextrose in 0.25% saline solution is administered to rehydrate the patient. If vomiting is present, a nasogastric tube should be placed to empty the stomach and to prevent further vomiting and potential aspiration. In the presence of either perforation or peritonitis, colloids, antibiotics, and antipyretic agents should be administered. A central venous line and a Foley catheter are also useful monitoring devices.

Intussusception

In any infant or small child brought to an emergency ward with episodes of crampy abdom-

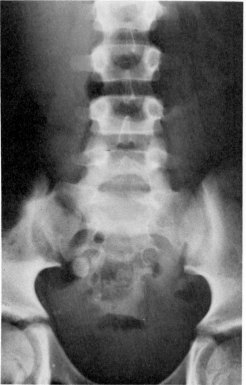

Figure 32.19.   Appendicolith in child with acute appendicitis. Note the radiopaque density in right lower quadrant.

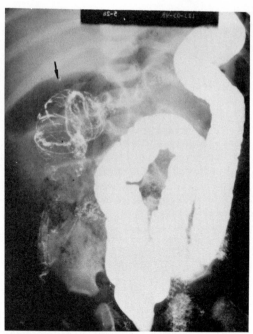

Figure 32.20.   Intussusception. Barium enema reduction should be carried out if there are no signs of peritoneal inflammation. Note "coiled spring" appearance of the intussusception (*arrow*). (Reproduced by permission, from *Surgical Clinics of North America*, Vol. 54, No. 3, © 1974, W. B. Saunders Co.)

inal pain alternating with periods of well-being, intussusception should be suspected. Classically, the disease occurs in children between 9 and 18 months old, but it can occur in 4- and 5-year-olds as well. Melena or passage of a currant-jelly stool should confirm the diagnosis. The abdomen may not be distended if the child is seen early. A tender mass is often difficult to palpate because the patient is frequently frightened and uncooperative. If a mass is present, it is usually in the right lower or right upper quadrant and less frequently in the left lower or left upper quadrant. Rectal examination should always be performed to check for blood in the stool, and rarely, the end of the intussusception may be palpated.

If there is no evidence of peritonitis, a barium enema examination is carried out. Plain films of the abdomen may be completely normal. A barium study should be performed regardless of the plain film if the clinical history warrants it (Fig. 32.20). The height of the barium column should be no more than 40 cm above the x-ray table. If the contrast study demonstrates an intussusception, it may be reduced with one or more barium

enemas. If no reflux or contrast material is seen in the terminal ileum, it must not be assumed that the intussusception has been reduced. If the child is not ill, however, careful observation in the hospital will reveal whether reduction has occurred. If an intussusception is successfully reduced by barium enema and then recurs, surgical exploration should be carried out. The physician should remember that although ileocolic intussusception is most common, ileoileal intussusception may also occur, and unless the barium enema refluxes easily into the small intestine, the obstruction may not be demonstrated.

If the patient has evidence of peritonitis, an intravenous line and a nasogastric tube are inserted, colloid and antibiotics are given, and the patient is taken to the operating room.

Pyloric Stenosis

A nasogastric tube should first be passed to check for residual gastric contents. Even in an infant who has recently vomited, there will be a significant amount of gastric contents in the presence of pyloric stenosis. If more than 2 ounces of fluid, mucus, and air are present, pyloric stenosis should be suspected. After the stomach has been emptied, palpation of the abdomen is easier and the chance of feeling the pyloric mass is greater. If no mass is palpable, a barium swallow is often diagnostic (Fig. 32.21). In a younger infant, only pylorospasm may be demonstrated; if vomiting persists, another study a week later often reveals pyloric stenosis. Once the diagnosis is made, a nasogastric tube is left in place to keep the stomach decompressed, intravenous fluids are administered to restore electrolyte balance and hydration, and an elective pyloromyotomy is carried out.

Foreign Bodies

A foreign body in the esophagus usually causes difficulty in swallowing. If obstruction is severe enough, the patient will even have difficulty in swallowing saliva. Radiopaque objects are obvious on plain chest films, and radiolucent objects can be visualized by means of a barium swallow. If the foreign body has been present for less than 24 hours, it can often be removed with a Foley catheter under fluoroscopic examination without anesthesia. An appropriate-sized Foley catheter is introduced through the nose into the stomach. The balloon is then inflated with radiopaque water-soluble contrast material so that it is snug in the

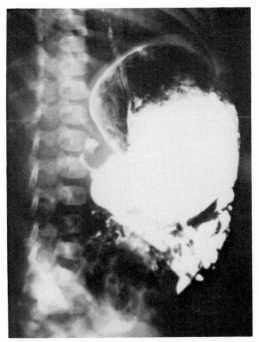

Figure 32.21. Pyloric stenosis. Delayed passage of barium through narrowed pylorus is associated with large stomach.

esophageal lumen. The balloon is then gently pulled up the esophagus and the foreign body is brought with it into the pharynx. If this technique is unsuccessful, general anesthesia with esophagoscopy should be carried out immediately.

A foreign body in the stomach or intestine is usually passed without surgical intervention. Even dangerous objects such as straight pins and open safety pins will traverse the gastrointestinal tract without incident. The progress of the foreign body should be followed with x-ray films, and all stools should be examined to search for it. If it is still in the stomach after 6 weeks, it can often be retrieved by gastroscopy. Any child with evidence of obstruction or possible perforation should undergo operation.

A foreign body in the airway can be obvious or subtle. In the obvious situation there is a history of eating with subsequent stridor or repeated episodes of coughing. Bronchoscopy with removal of the foreign body is necessary. Likewise, endoscopy is necessary if the chest x-ray film shows hyperinflation, atelectasis of one lung field, or a radiopaque foreign body such as a tooth or metal object (Fig. 32.22). However, some patients with an unknown or questionable history of aspiration who actually have a foreign body may have normal findings on physical examination and a normal chest x-ray film. The most commonly aspirated objects are food particles, particularly peanuts, and small plastic pieces that are radiolucent. If such a patient is untreated, the end result is bronchiectasis and pulmonary resection. Bronchoscopy to rule out the possibility of a foreign body in questionable cases should be available in all medical centers caring for infants and children. With the newer miniaturized fiberoptic bronchoscopes available today there is little morbidity. Pulmonary physical therapy and bronchodilators may be tried first if there is no evidence of obstruction or infection. If this is unsuccessful, bronchoscopy must be performed during the same hospitalization.

Urinary Tract Infection

All children, both male and female, should be examined for congenital abnormalities of the urinary tract after one documented urinary tract infection. After proper medical treatment (see Chapter 19, pages 433–434), an intravenous pyelogram and voiding cystourethrogram should be obtained. The latter study must be done after the patient has been free of infection for at least 6 weeks so that bladder edema and inflammation do not cause

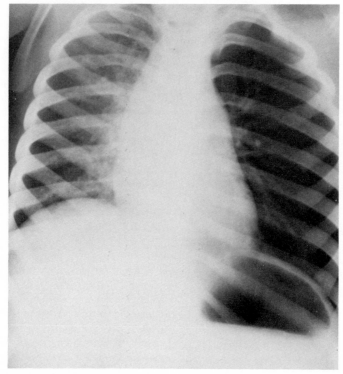

Figure 32.22.   Foreign body of tracheobronchial tree with hyperlucency of left lung. The foreign body could be on either side, depending on whether there is complete obstruction or a ball-valve effect. A normal chest x-ray film does not rule out a foreign body.

distortion. In children who have infection with normal x-ray findings, cystoscopy is recommended. The intravenous pyelogram and cystourethrogram will show the more severe abnormalities, but may not reveal the minor causes that are frequently diagnosed by cystoscopy.

Croup

When a child is admitted with stridor and respiratory distress secondary to acute epiglottitis or laryngotracheobronchitis, he should receive oxygen immediately. If the child is too young to tolerate separation from parents, the mother should be allowed to stay with and hold the child. The child should be sedated to alleviate anxiety, but not enough to aggravate the hypoxemia. Specimens should not be drawn for arterial blood-gas analysis in a child who is already hypoxemic, since this often does more harm than good. An intravenous line should be inserted for administration of antibiotics and maintenance fluids. Laryngoscopy should not be carried out in the emergency ward in a hypoxic child unless the child is moribund. If the child's condition does not improve within 1 or 2 hours, he should be taken to the operating room for direct laryngoscopy under general anesthesia. Under anesthesia, bronchoscopy, intubation, or rarely tracheotomy can be performed in a controlled situation. This protocol is by far the safest for the child.

Lye or Caustic Ingestion

In cases of obvious ingestion, although the history is sometimes only suggestive, most patients show evidence of burns in or around the mouth and in the pharynx. These patients must be admitted for further treatment. Some patients, however, have no obvious burns but a definite history of ingestion. They also should be admitted. Nothing should be given by mouth. *Vomiting should not be induced.* Intravenous fluid administration is started, and corticosteroids and broad-spectrum antibiotics are given immediately. Esophagoscopy should be performed within the first 24 hours to determine the extent of burn in the esophagus. If burns are confirmed in the esophagus, the patient should be treated with antibiotics and corticosteroids for a minimum of 10–14 days. A barium swallow should be performed during this time. If no esophageal burns are seen, therapy can be discontinued and the patient discharged from the hospital. The family should be screened to make sure that this is not a form of child abuse.

Staphylococcal Pneumonia and Empyema

Since the advent of methicillin and the other synthetic penicillins in 1962, the complications of staphylococcal pneumonia requiring surgical treatment have decreased remarkably. However, even today, patients with staphylococcal empyema are occasionally seen. If empyema is present, tube thoracotomy rather than needle aspiration is our choice for drainage. Pneumatoceles, often seen with acute infections, do not require chest tube drainage; they are temporary and respond to proper antibiotic management.

Neck Masses

Neck masses occur in patients of all ages. In the newborn the most common is *torticollis*. This is swelling from hematoma in the sternocleidomastoid muscle. Limitation of neck motion is variable. Treatment consists of weekly injections of triamcinolone directly into the hematoma and vigorous physical therapy. If treatment is undertaken early enough and if physical therapy is carried out regularly, surgical intervention for contracture is rarely necessary.

Cervical abscess is usually located in the lateral aspect of the neck just below the mastoid process. Since these abscesses are fairly deep, they are usually firm or hard and often nontender. Some degree of overlying erythema may be present. The margins of the abscess are usually not well defined. If febrile, the patient is hospitalized, with application of moist heat to the indurated area and intravenous antibiotics. If the patient is not febrile or ill, oral antibiotics and application of moist heat can be accomplished at home, with repeated office visits. When the abscess is ready for drainage, a central fluctuant area is usually defined, sometimes without the usual overlying skin changes. Incision and drainage should be carried out under general anesthesia. A cervical abscess rarely resolves without incision and drainage. The patient should be examined carefully after the induration has completely resolved to make sure that the condition is not an infected congenital cyst.

Branchial cleft cysts or *sinuses* occur on the anterior border of the sternocleidomastoid muscle and may be unilateral or bilateral. If a sinus is present, the drained fluid is usually clear or slightly cloudy unless infected. If a cyst is present, it may be movable unless it is inflamed. In the absence of inflammation, the cyst or sinus should be excised with its associated communication with the pharynx to prevent later infection. If an abscess is present, the lesion should first be drained, and when the inflammation has subsided, elective excision should be carried out.

A *thyroglossal duct cyst* or *sinus* usually occurs in the midline starting just above the thyroid cartilage. The cyst often moves with protrusion of the tongue. As with other congenital cysts and sinuses, early excision should be carried out before infection occurs. Thyroglossal cysts have a tract that communicates with the foramen cecum at the base of the tongue, traversing the midportion of the hyoid bone. All the tract should be removed; otherwise the incidence of recurrence is very high. The physician should remember that aberrant thyroid may also be a midline neck mass, and a thyroid scan should be done if there is any question.

Cystic hygromas may be present at birth or may become apparent suddenly. With trauma, sudden hemorrhage may occur, causing a bluish swelling. If a soft, fluctuant, cystic mass is present without recent hemorrhage or infection, the mass may be transilluminated. Other times a tender, erythematous infected area may appear. After infection is treated, excision should be carried out. A chest x-ray film should be taken before operation to make sure that the hygroma is not an extension from the mediastinum.

Tuberculous cervical lymphadenitis or *scrofula* is still seen today. A fluctuant, nontender, erythematous area in the posterior cervical or submandibular area should suggest this diagnosis. Antituberculous medications do not appear to be effective. If surgical drainage is carried out, a fistula may remain. To be safe, the area should be excised.

Wilms' Tumor

Approximately 400 new cases of Wilms' tumor occur in the United States every year (Koop et al., 1964). The mass is usually found incidentally, most often during an examination after minor trauma. In retrospect the patient often has not been well for the preceding several months, with low-grade fever, decreased appetite, increased fatiguability, pallor, and increased abdominal girth. The younger patient is commonly irritable and difficult to examine. The mass usually fills the flank area and can sometimes pass over the midline. Differentiation from the liver on the right side or the spleen on the left side is often difficult. An intravenous pyelogram usually shows renal function on the side of the mass, but distortion of the caliceal pattern. After the mass has been documented, repeated palpation should be avoided to prevent blood-borne dissemination of tumor cells. A simple sign painted on the abdomen or placed at the foot of the bed is usually sufficient to prevent unnecessary examinations. A cavogram of the inferior vena cava is essential to rule out tumor extension into the renal vein or inferior vena cava as far as the right atrium. An arteriogram is obtained to note the main blood vessels supplying the mass. A chest x-ray film is necessary to establish whether pulmonary metastases are present. Further evaluation of metastases should include bone scans, a liver scan, and bone marrow examination. The presence of metastatic disease, however, should not discourage aggressive combined treatment. Even in the patient with pulmonary metastases (stage IV), a combination of radical excision, chemotherapy, and radiotherapy can produce cure rates as high as 50%.

Constipation

In the newborn, delayed passage of meconium and signs of low intestinal obstruction usually indicate *Hirschsprung's disease.* The abdomen is distended, and rectal examination often reveals an empty ampulla. In the older patient the presenting symptom of Hirschsprung's disease is most often constipation, but is occasionally intermittent diarrhea. These children have sometimes been treated with suppositories and enemas since infancy. Physical examination reveals a distended abdomen and a poorly thriving child, usually with palpable loops of intestine containing feces. Rectal examination usually reveals an empty ampulla. Barium studies show the classic finding of a normal dilated colon narrowing to the spastic aganglionic segment. The level of colonic dilatation depends on the length of the aganglionic segment. The transitional area between normal and abnormal segments is usually in the distal sigmoid colon, but aganglionosis can occur as far proximally as the ileum. Rectal biopsy will confirm the diagnosis of Hirschsprung's disease and rule out other disorders.

Habit constipation can be differentiated from Hirschsprung's disease. This problem usually develops after infancy. The onset is sometimes correlated with a traumatic event. Patients often have overflow incontinence with resultant soilage, and some have urinary incontinence as well. On physical examination the abdomen is usually distended, with palpable feces in the large intestine. Rectal examination often reveals impaction down to the anus, with a remarkably large bolus of feces at the anus. After manual disimpaction, enemas are given to empty the colon and to allow it to return to a more normal caliber. Barium enema examination shows a colon that is dilated to the anus with no narrow area. Placing the patient on a strict program of mineral oil, stool softeners,

mild laxatives, suppositories or enemas, and toilet training if necessary is usually curative. If there is any question of Hirschsprung's disease, rectal biopsy should be performed.

Ectopic anus is a form of imperforate anus. In this situation the anus is located more anteriorly than is normal. These children are usually constipated since birth or shortly thereafter. On physical examination the abdomen may or may not be distended, but fecal material is usually palpable in the colon. Careful inspection of the perineum may reveal that the anus is anterior to its normal location. It may be apparent that the anus is not located centrally in the darker pigmented skin of the perianal area. In the female the distance from the posterior edge of the vaginal introitus to the anus may be too short. Rectal examination reveals dilatation down to the anus, as in habit constipation. In patients in whom the ectopic anus is not obvious, a program similar to that used to treat habit constipation should be tried first. The treatment for patients with obvious ectopic anus is posterior anoplasty.

TRAUMATIC EMERGENCIES

Any child who has been involved in an accident requires rapid general assessment of the nature and severity of the injuries, assignment of priorities, and efficient resuscitation. In general, one person should oversee management when a team is involved, this person usually being a general surgeon, emergency physician, or someone experienced in total care and priorities of care. Proper-sized oral airway and endotracheal tubes should be available with suitable laryngoscope blades in any emergency area where children are treated. Today there is no excuse for using oversized adult red rubber cuffed endotracheal tubes in pediatric patients, which can often result in complications that have a higher morbidity than the initial injury. A central venous line for administration of blood, colloid, or crystalloid solution, for rapid administration of medications, and for monitoring of central venous pressure is necessary since fluid overload occurs more quickly and insidiously the smaller the patient. Subclavian lines are used in patients 4 years of age and older with the technique used for adults. Smaller-gauge needles and catheters are used, depending on the size of the child. We prefer 22-gauge needles to locate the vein and 20-gauge catheters. In patients younger than 4 years or in whom subclavian vein cannulation has failed, venous cutdown is performed in the antecubital fossa over the basilic vein to allow central venous pressure monitoring through a long catheter. If the catheter is tunneled under the skin so that the cutaneous and venous openings are not adjacent to each other and if the arm is properly immobilized, infection can be avoided for up to a week. A central line has other advantages, including being nearer the central circulation for administration of medications and being more available to the anesthesiologist in the operating room. If cutdown is performed in the greater saphenous vein at the ankle, the line usually cannot be placed centrally, and if there is a major injury to the inferior vena cava or major branches, fluid administration will be useless.

Monitoring of arterial blood-gas levels is becoming routine in serious trauma cases. With the availability of 22- and 23-gauge plastic intravenous catheters, percutaneous catheterization of the radial artery at the wrist allows determination of pH and of the partial pressures of oxygen (Po_2) and carbon dioxide (Pco_2). Arterial lines should *not* be used even in an emergency for administration of hypertonic glucose solutions, calcium, or other medications. Spasm and thrombosis can easily occur, with loss of the extremity. Normal saline containing a very small amount of heparin administered by a continuous flow pump should be the flushing solution. If the line is flushed by hand, flushing should be extremely gentle, since it has been shown in the small infant that flushing a radial artery line with 1 ml of dilute dye produces retrograde flow into the carotid artery and cerebral circulation.

Nasogastric tubes should always be placed, especially in the patient with head, thoracic, or abdominal injury. This not only helps prevent vomiting but also allows assessment of injury to the esophagus and stomach. A Foley catheter inserted into the bladder is mandatory in the presence of shock or any abdominal injury, especially damage associated with a fractured pelvis. The patency of the urethra can be evaluated and hematuria noted; a cystogram can be obtained if a ruptured bladder is suspected. If there is any question of a disrupted urethra, no attempt should be made at urethral catheterization. A suprapubic catheter should be inserted directly into the bladder for drainage and to allow further study of the urethra.

Any superficial bleeding is stopped by direct pressure, and suspected fractures are splinted until radiologic evaluation is available.

Careful evaluation of the whole patient cannot be emphasized too strongly. The fractured extremity is not the life-threatening danger that an unsuspected perforated intestine is. Obvious damage to superficial tissues and extremities should be treated expeditiously, but the physician should keep in mind those injuries that are *less obvious* and that are often lethal when unrecognized. This includes not only intracranial injuries but also thoracic, abdominal, and spinal injuries.

Spleen

The spleen is the most commonly injured abdominal organ in children. Although damage is frequently associated with other major injuries, it can result from rather trivial or commonplace accidents such as falling or being tackled while playing football. These patients commonly have some evidence of hypovolemia; blood volume usually returns to normal with intravenous fluid replacement. There is often localized tenderness and spasm and sometimes bruising of the left upper abdominal quadrant or left costal margin. The patient may complain of pain in the left shoulder when sitting. Initial treatment includes administration of intravenous fluids, placement of a nasogastric tube, and monitoring of central venous pressure if possible. Blood is typed and crossmatched and the usual blood tests are performed. An abdominal x-ray film with the patient upright may show that the gastric bubble is displaced medially or that the folds of the stomach along the greater curvature are thicker than normal, representing blood that has dissected the gastrolienal ligament. Fractured ribs may be seen in teenagers, but are unusual in younger, smaller patients. If continued slow blood loss is indicated by a decreasing hematocrit, laparotomy should be considered; further diagnostic studies for other injuries can usually be carried out before laparotomy is necessary, however. If the findings are equivocal except for a slowly decreasing hematocrit, angiography or splenic scanning may be useful for demonstrating the splenic injury.

A child with a recent history of trauma who has pain in the left upper abdominal quadrant or in the left shoulder should undergo angiography to rule out the possibility of a subcapsular splenic hematoma, since such an injury may result in delayed rupture of the capsule and shock.

Liver

Treatment of hepatic injuries is always more urgent than treatment of splenic injuries. The management of shock is much more difficult, and these patients often have to be taken directly to the operating room. There is usually no time for evaluation of other injuries. Whereas splenic bleeding frequently stops because of clot formation, hepatic injuries continue to bleed because the enzymes released from liver damage have clot-lysing properties. At least two intravenous lines should be placed in the upper extremities or sub-clavian veins to bypass any inferior vena caval injury. A nasogastric tube is essential, and fresh blood should be obtained for transfusion as soon as possible. Fresh-frozen washed cells and 5% normal human serum albumin should be available to minimize the complications of massive whole blood transfusions. Despite the increased aware-ness of the urgency of hepatic injury and the better treatment now available, the mortality is still as high as 40% (Hendren and Kim, 1975).

Kidney

Next to splenic injuries, renal injuries are most common. An intravenous pyelogram should be obtained in any patient with hematuria. The most frequent renal injury is contusion. With mild ex-travasation, nonoperative management results in normal kidney function several weeks later. Sur-gical intervention is indicated only in the presence of continuous uncontrolled bleeding, increased ex-travasation of blood and urine, or absence of kidney function. If there is angiographic demon-stration of injury to the renal artery, exploration is necessary.

Lower Urinary Tract

Injuries of the bladder and urethra are unusual in the small child. If urethral injury is suspected or if a suitable-sized catheter cannot be inserted easily, there should be no further attempt to cath-eterize the patient. A full bladder should be con-firmed by bimanual abdominorectal examination, and an Intracath should then be introduced into the bladder through a suprapubic approach for drainage and for further diagnosis of urethral in-jury.

Pancreas

Acute injuries to the pancreas may lead to ful-minant findings of peritonitis associated with a rapid elevation in serum amylase and white blood cell count or to a chronic condition with eventual development of a pancreatic pseudocyst. Acute features also occur with perforation of the bile duct or intestine (Hartman and Greaney, 1964). The most common area injured in the pancreas is the body where it crosses the vertebral bodies. Initial treatment includes a nasogastric tube, Foley catheter, and an intravenous line for administra-tion of 5% dextrose in 0.25% saline or Ringer's lactated solution. There will be a need for 5% normal human serum albumin or salt-poor albu-min and intravenous antibiotics as well. A central venous line is useful to monitor administration of fluid and to prevent overloading the circulation. Occasionally, transfusion will be necessary. Ex-ploratory laparotomy should be carried out when the child's condition is stable to minimize the pancreatic enzyme damage in the peritoneal cav-ity.

In contrast, the child with a pseudocyst of the pancreas is often suffering from weight loss and general debility. The use of hyperalimentation for several days before exploration often not only prevents complications of operation but also speeds recovery.

Duodenum

Blunt trauma to the right upper abdominal quadrant can cause duodenal obstruction from submucosal hematoma. The patient has episodes of vomiting, and on examination the right upper quadrant is tender. An upper gastrointestinal series demonstrates the scalloped duodenum secondary to intramural hematoma. Hospitalization with bed rest, nasogastric suction, and intravenous fluids may allow resolution of the hematoma, but occa-sionally, laparotomy with evacuation of the extra-vasated blood is necessary.

Retroperitoneum

Retroperitoneal hematoma can occur from vas-cular injury. In most cases tamponade usually occurs. An angiogram may demonstrate the ret-roperitoneal bleeding. If this is the only injury, surgical exploration is not necessary unless bleed-ing continues. Treatment includes intravenous fluids with appropriate blood replacement, anti-biotics, and nasogastric suction.

Thorax

Serious thoracic injuries are much less common in children than in adults. Fractures of vertebral bodies as well as of ribs are infrequent, and serious mediastinal injuries are unusual. The most com-mon injury with blunt trauma is pulmonary con-tusion. In milder cases, humidified oxygen sup-plied by face mask or tent is all that is needed. In the presence of respiratory insufficiency, nasotra-cheal intubation and ventilatory support with pos-itive end-expiratory pressure allow rapid resolu-tion of the pulmonary injury.

Hemopneumothorax should be treated imme-diately by insertion of a proper-sized chest tube. If air leakage persists even with full expansion of the lung, a bronchial tear should be suspected. Bron-choscopy should be carried out to assess the injury.

Thoracotomy may be necessary to repair the laceration. Likewise, in the presence of continuous blood loss, thoracotomy should be performed for severe pulmonary injury or, more seriously, mediastinal injury.

Ruptured diaphragm is rare, but should be suspected in patients with increasing respiratory distress and an abnormal chest x-ray film. Immediate surgical repair is mandatory since respiratory distress will increase with herniation of abdominal contents into the chest. Usually the severity of the injury is extreme, so other injuries must be looked for before operation (Radhakrishna et al., 1969).

Suggested Readings

Bell MJ, Kosloske AM, Benton C, et al: Neonatal necrotizing enterocolitis: Prevention of perforation. *J Pediatr Surg* 8:601–605, 1973

Hartman SW, Greaney EM, Jr: Traumatic injuries to the biliary system in children. *Am J Surg 108:*150–156, 1964

Hendren WH: Abdominal masses in newborn infants. *Am J Surg 107:*502–510, 1964a

Hendren WH: Esophageal atresia and tracheo-esophageal fistula: Principles of management. *Clin Pediatr 3:*30–41, 1964b

Hendren WH, Kim SH: Abdominal surgical emergencies of the newborn. *Surg Clin North Am 54:*489–527, 1974

Hendren WH, Kim SH: Trauma of the spleen and liver in children. *Pediatr Clin North Am 22:*349–364, 1975

Hendren WH, McKee DM: Lobar emphysema of infancy. *J Pediatr Surg 1:*24–39, 1966

Kim SH: Omphalocele. *Surg Clin North Am 56:*361–371, 1976

Koop CE: Abdominal mass in the newborn infant. *N Engl J Med 289:*569–571, 1973

Koop CE, Hope JW, Abir E: Management of nephroblastoma (Wilms' tumor) and abdominal neuroblastoma. *CA 14:*178–186, 1964

Mauney FM, Jr, Sabiston DC, Jr: The role of pulmonary scanning in the diagnosis of congenital lobar emphysema. *Am Surg 36:*20–27, 1970

Noblett HR: Treatment of uncomplicated meconium ileus by Gastrografin enema: A preliminary report. *J Pediatr Surg 4:*190–197, 1969

Radhakrishna C, Dickinson SJ, Shaw A: Acute diaphragmatic hernia from blunt trauma in children. *J Pediatr Surg 4:*553–556, 1969

General References

Ravitch MM, Welch KJ, Benson CD, et al (Eds): *Pediatric Surgery*, ed 3. Chicago, Year Book, 1979

Rickham PP, Johnston JH: *Neonatal Surgery*. 2nd ed. New York, Butterworths, 1978

CHAPTER 33

Emergencies of the Ear, Facial Structures, and Upper Airway

ERNEST A. WEYMULLER, Jr., M.D.
RUFUS C. PARTLOW, Jr., M.D.

THE EAR

Terminology and Examination Technique

Hearing loss may be divided into two basic types—conductive and sensorineural. Conductive hearing loss is caused by lesions of the sound conduction mechanism, including the ear canal, eardrum, middle-ear space, and ossicular chain (Fig. 33.1). Sensorineural hearing loss results from defects of the cochlea or the central auditory pathways.

Simple clinical tests for the degree and type of hearing loss include the voice test, Rinne's test, and Weber's test.

In the *voice test*, each ear is tested separately for the minimal level of audible hearing while a noise box creates a masking noise in the untested ear. If a noise box is unavailable, the examiner can occlude the nontested ear canal with his finger, moving it gently to generate sufficient masking noise for testing at low voice levels. Hearing is roughly normal if the patient can hear a soft whisper in the tested ear. If the patient cannot hear the examiner's voice close to the ear at normal conversational levels, there is a significant hearing loss.

Rinne's test is performed with a tuning fork with a frequency of 512 cycles/sec. The fork is struck and the patient is asked to compare the degree of loudness with the fork in two positions. First the base is placed on the mastoid cortex behind the ear (bone conduction), and then the vibrating tines are placed 2–3 inches away from the ear (air conduction). In a person with normal hearing, air conduction is better than bone conduction (posi-

tive Rinne's test). A patient with sensorineural hearing loss also has a positive test. In the patient with a significant conductive hearing loss, bone conduction is greater than air conduction (negative Rinne's test). Rinne's test by itself is unreliable in a patient with total neural deafness in one ear. Such a patient will report conduction through bone as louder than conduction through air when the deaf ear is tested (false-negative Rinne's test). In this instance, when the base of the fork is on the bone, sound vibrations are transmitted through the skull and are heard in the opposite ear; the patient hears nothing in the deaf ear through air conduction, however. The examiner can distinguish this condition from conductive hearing loss by performing Weber's test.

Weber's test is performed by placing the vibrating tuning fork in the midline of the skull, usually on the forehead or on the middle incisor teeth. The patient is asked to which side of the head the sound travels. In a patient with normal hearing, or when hearing loss is symmetrical, sound is heard in the middle of the head. In a patient with unilateral conductive hearing loss, the sound is louder in the abnormal ear. In a patient with unilateral total neural deafness, the sound is heard in the normal ear.

Other tests used in examination of the ear include the fistula test and the position test.

The *fistula test* is performed by placing an olive-tipped rubber-bulb syringe in the ear canal of the affected ear. Sufficient pressure must be applied to prevent air leakage around the olive tip. The rubber bulb is squeezed, increasing air pressure in the ear canal. When a rubber bulb is not available, the examiner may occlude the ear canal with his

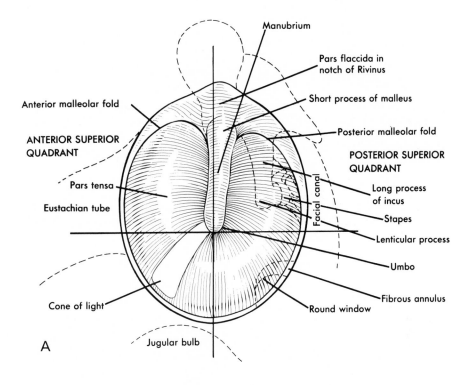

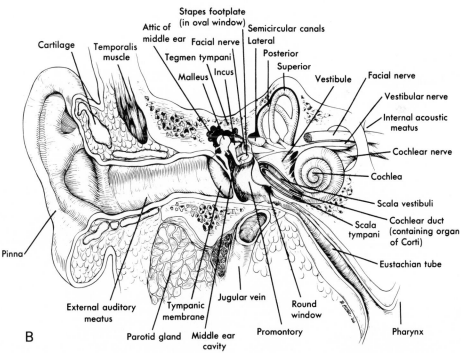

Figure 33.1.   **(A)** Major landmarks of eardrum (left ear). Long process of incus may be visualized through normal eardrum. **(B)** Basic anatomy of the ear. (Reproduced by permission, from Saunders WH, Paparella MM: *Atlas of Ear Surgery*, ed. 2. St. Louis, The C. V. Mosby Co., 1971).

finger and firmly pump the air column. In a positive fistula test, the patient's eyes deviate away from the affected ear, and sometimes his body sways in that direction. A positive fistula test suggests that inner ear membranes have been exposed by erosion of the bony wall.

In any patient with positional dizziness, the *position test* should be performed. The patient should be asked to sit on an examining table and then, in succession, to lie back with his head hanging straight over the edge, with his head to the right, and with his head to the left. The patient's eyes are observed and the direction, duration, and character of any nystagmus (rotatory, horizontal, or vertical) are recorded. It is also important to note any delay in onset and whether nystagmus can be fatigued to the point of disappearing on repeated testing.

Trauma

External Ear

Traumatic injury to the external ear usually results from being hit, torn, or bitten. On physical examination, a hematoma, laceration, or avulsion may be present. Abnormal contour of the external ear with a fluctuant swelling that may be discolored indicates hematoma. A laceration may be partial thickness or full thickness, and auricular cartilage may be exposed. All or part of the external ear may be avulsed.

Hematoma. If a hematoma is present, the ear canal and eardrum should be carefully examined. A clinical estimate of hearing should be established. After the surface of the ear is cleansed and the hair is shaved 1 inch around the ear, the hematoma may be aspirated with a large-bore needle (No. 15) and sterile technique. If this measure fails to eliminate the hematoma, a stab incision is made in the area of greatest fluctuance to evacuate the clot, and a small rubber drain is placed through the stab incision. A soft dressing of sterile cotton should be applied. The cotton, moistened with povidone-iodine (Betadine) solution, is applied in small enough portions to conform to all the convolutions of the external ear; the dressing is held in place with a wrap-around gauze head bandage. Dressings should be changed daily until the hematoma no longer reaccumulates, and the hematoma should be reaspirated if necessary. It is advisable to refer the patient to an otolaryngologist. Some controversy exists over the efficacy of systemic antibiotics. We recommend erythromycin, 250 mg every 6 hours for 5 days or longer if the hematoma persists.

Laceration and Avulsion. Careful closure of a laceration with standard soft-tissue techniques (see Chapter 29) should be sufficient treatment; cartilage does not hold sutures, and the edges should be apposed by sutures in the perichondrium. Sutures should be removed in 5–7 days. In the case of a patient with total or partial avulsion of the external ear, an otolaryngologist, plastic surgeon, or general surgeon should immediately be consulted. Any fragments of the ear should be placed in iced sterile saline solution as soon as possible. Small avulsed pieces (2 cm maximal diameter) may be débrided and reattached, or the small defect can be closed primarily by advancing the freshened edges of the ear wound. Total avulsion of the ear may be treated by various methods, including immediate reattachment or burying the ear cartilage in the postauricular soft tissues after it is dermabraded, with plans for later reconstruction. If the latter technique is used, the raw surface left by the avulsion should be covered with a sterile dressing.

Thermal Injuries. Thermal injuries of the external ear resulting from exposure to extreme heat or cold are usually obvious from the history. In a patient with a frostbitten ear, the pinna will be cold and pale; erythema and vesicles will appear when the ear is warmed. Most patients with significant facial burns have associated auricular burns. Depending on the depth of burn, there may be erythema, vesicles, or charring of the external ear.

A frostbitten ear should be rapidly rewarmed with sterile cotton soaked in water at a temperature of 100–108°F (37.8–42.2°C). Systemic analgesics such as meperidine hydrochloride (Demerol) may be administered for pain as the ear is warmed. Hair around the ear should be trimmed, but débridement with attendant rupturing of vesicles should be avoided. A topical antibacterial agent such as povidone-iodine should be applied. Silver nitrate solution (0.5%) is also an effective antiseptic agent. Oral antibiotics are indicated only if infection develops. The patient should be advised not to smoke because of the vasospastic effects of nicotine. When the ear is thawed, the patient should be hospitalized to allow continued sterile care for the ear.

First- to third-degree burns should be treated by the open method with mafenide acetate (Sulfamylon) cream. A doughnut pillow prevents pressure on the ear. A major complication is perichondritis, which may occur from 2–5 weeks after the burn, and the ear must be watched carefully during convalescence. Severe charring of the ear results in autoamputation.

Ear Canal

Laceration of the ear canal usually occurs in conjunction with other traumatic injuries of the ear. Any laceration involving cartilage or skin around the external acoustic meatus should be treated in the following manner. Blood should be suctioned from the ear canal, and the eardrum should be carefully inspected. Hearing should be tested with a tuning fork and whispered voice. In cases of major trauma, x-ray views should be obtained if fracture of the temporal bone is suspected.

The laceration should be treated by open packing with 0.5-inch iodoform gauze saturated with an antibiotic ointment such as aureomycin or bacitracin. The packing not only controls the bleeding but also averts such potential complications as stenosis of the ear canal and perichondritis. After emergency treatment the patient should be referred to an otolaryngologist. The packing should be left in for 2–3 weeks or until healing is complete.

Eardrum

Traumatic perforation of the eardrum usually occurs when a cotton-tipped applicator, bobby pin, or small stick inadvertently penetrates deeply into the ear canal and lacerates the drum. A slap to the ear and slag burns in welders can also cause traumatic perforation. The patient should be questioned about hearing loss, pain, and vertigo. All debris and blood should be removed from the ear canal with a small metal suction tip. Irrigation with water is contraindicated. When the eardrum is inspected, an irregular tear is usually visible; it may be actively bleeding. The hearing should be tested with tuning fork and voice tests. A patient with a perforated eardrum may have conductive or sensorineural hearing loss or both. The eyes should be observed for nystagmus, and the fistula test should be performed. The patient's balance should be tested by heel-toe walking and the station test (Romberg's test).

Emergency referral to an otolaryngologist is indicated in the case of vertigo, major hearing loss, or a positive fistula test. Ear drops should not be instilled. The patient can be treated with intramuscular prochlorperazine maleate (Compazine) for nausea and vomiting.

Temporal Bone

Temporal bone fracture may be an isolated injury, but is more often one of many fractures present in a person with severe multiple injuries. A conscious patient with only a fractured temporal bone may complain of pain, bloody discharge from the ear, decreased hearing, and vertigo. On physical examination, ecchymoses behind the ear and over the mastoid tip (Battle's sign) may be noted, as well as laceration of the ear canal or eardrum, nystagmus, and weakness or complete paralysis of the facial muscles. The patient may complain of vertigo, nausea, and vomiting. Tests may reveal conductive or sensorineural hearing loss or both.

Before treatment of temporal bone fracture is begun, the physician should first exclude other serious injuries, including fracture of the cervical spine, obstruction of the airway, or major trauma to the chest and abdomen. A patient with cerebrospinal fluid (CSF) otorrhea should be hospitalized and treated with application of a gauze dressing to absorb drainage and with administration of systemic antibiotics. An otolaryngologist should be consulted as soon as possible after injury to complete the evaluation of such a patient.

Pain or Discharge

Local Pain

External Otitis. This condition is manifested by 1–3 days of progressive itch, pain, and discharge, sometimes with diminished hearing. The patient should be questioned about trauma to, or a foreign body in, the ear canal. On physical examination, pressure on the tragus or auricular cartilage produces pain. The ear canal is erythematous and swollen; it may be filled with debris obscuring the eardrum. In more advanced cases, periauricular cellulitis and regional lymphadenopathy can be noted. Conductive hearing loss may occur. Often both ears are involved.

The keystone of therapy is removal of debris from the ear canal by means of a suction apparatus and a narrow metal suction tip. Examiners unfamiliar with the use of the head mirror (Fig. 33.2) can utilize a hand otoscope, suctioning through the speculum. If a foreign body is encountered, it should be removed by means of suction, a wire loop curette, or water irrigation. Any abscess in the ear canal should be incised for drainage. If the ear canal is of normal diameter, the patient may be treated with antibiotic drops, 3–4 drops four times a day for 10 days. If the ear canal is narrowed, a wick should be inserted to ensure adequate distribution of the antibiotic drops. A simple method is to insert a 2-inch strip of 0.25 inch iodoform gauze saturated with antibiotic drops by means of a small bayonet forceps. Systemic antibiotics are not indicated unless the patient has periauricular cellulitis or regional lymphadenitis;

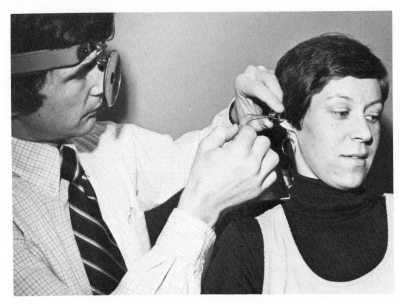

Figure 33.2.   Use of ear speculum and suction for examination and cleansing of ear. A head mirror or head light may be used.

penicillin is the usual drug of choice for an out-patient. A patient with severe perichondritis of the pinna should be hospitalized and treated with intravenous antibiotics. Since external otitis can be extremely painful, a moderately strong analgesic should be prescribed for 48–72 hours. For at least 1 month after treatment the patient should keep the affected ear protected from water during showering or hair washing by means of a cotton ball saturated with petrolatum. Simple external otitis with minimal edema of the ear canal usually does not require follow-up care. If a wick has been placed in the ear, the patient should remove it after 48 hours and continue using drops for a total of 10 days, at which time he should be seen by an otolaryngologist.

In an elderly diabetic patient, external otitis may be more severe. A well recognized entity, *malignant external otitis* must be considered if external otitis has failed to resolve after 1–2 weeks of routine care. The patient with malignant external otitis experiences severe pain below the ear canal and in the parotid region anterior to the tragus. Granulation tissue may be evident, usually in the inferior or anterior portion of the ear canal. Malignant external otitis is life-threatening, requiring immediate hospitalization and intensive antibiotic therapy with gentamicin and carbenicillin, since Pseudomonas is the usual infecting organism.

Otitis Media. Usually an upper respiratory tract infection precedes otitis media, but it may arise without previous illness. This disease occurs at any age, but is most common in children. Pain is usually constant, lasting from hours to days, and may be exacerbated by lying prone. The pain may clear after a sudden discharge of purulent material from the ear canal, signifying spontaneous rupture of the tympanic membrane.

A special form of otitis media, aerotitis occurs after sudden barometric pressure changes, especially in persons with nasal congestion from a cold, allergy, or upper respiratory tract infection. Usually the patient experiences severe pain on descent either in an airplane or during deep-sea diving.

In *acute otitis media* the landmarks of the eardrum are frequently distorted by erythema, thickening, and bulging of the drum. The skin of the ear canal can be macerated. Conductive hearing loss is usually present. If the tympanic membrane has perforated, a pulsating discharge may be seen.

The eardrum in a patient with *aerotitis* may be red, purple, or almost black if hemotympanum exists. As in acute otitis media, conductive hearing loss may or may not be significant. The appearance of red or yellowish bullous eruptions on the surface of the eardrum signifies *bullous myringitis.* When the bullae are ruptured, clear fluid is noted. *In serous otitis* the eardrum may vary in color from gray to blue to yellow. The drum may be retracted and air-fluid levels (bubbles) may be visualized behind it. Blood vessels on its surface may be dilated, giving the appearance of erythema.

In children less than 6 years old the antibiotic

of choice is amoxicillin, 125–250 mg every 8 hours orally for 10 days. In the penicillin-allergic patient a combination of erythromycin and sulfisoxazole (Gantrisin) with the dosage adjusted for age should be used. In older children and in adults, penicillin, 400,000 units four times a day orally for 10 days, is the drug of choice; in penicillin-allergic patients, erythromycin alone should be sufficient. Nasal decongestant agents in liquid or tablet form should be used for 2 weeks, and nasal drops should be administered three to four times a day for 10 days. Moderately strong systemic analgesic medications are often indicated for the first 2 or 3 days until infection subsides. There is some disagreement concerning the value of myringotomy in acute otitis media. Myringotomy of a bulging eardrum can relieve severe pain; a patient with only mild to moderate pain may not require this procedure. When myringotomy is necessary, the incision should be made in the anterior inferior quadrant of the eardrum to avoid the ossicles and the facial nerve (Fig. 33.3).

Chronic otitis media may be difficult to diagnose. Some patients have an intermittent foul-smelling discharge from the affected ear, vertigo, a progressive conductive hearing loss, or facial paralysis. Others are asymptomatic. The eardrum may be intact; the only evidence for the disease may be squamous debris or cholesteatoma in the pars flaccida of the eardrum. The diagnosis is made

easier when there is a chronic draining perforation of the drum. The patient with uncomplicated chronic otitis media should be referred to an otolaryngologist.

Complications of Acute and Chronic Otitis Media. *Mastoiditis* may occur 1–2 weeks after acute otitis media. The most common symptom is persistent discharge from the affected ear. Ordinarily, pain is not significant; when it is present, abscess formation should be suspected. On physical examination of a patient with mastoiditis secondary to acute otitis, a small perforation in the eardrum with purulent discharge can often be seen. Tenderness is elicited on palpation in the postauricular region and commonly over the mastoid tip, where the skin may be thickened. The patient may have a slightly elevated temperature, but frequently does not seem extremely ill. Severe pain and tenderness or systemic toxemia suggests any one of the complications of mastoidits. In a patient with manifestations of chronic otitis media such as chronic perforation, chronic drainage, or cholesteatoma, mastoiditis can occur at any time and can develop into any of several conditions mentioned in the following paragraph. In a patient with mastoiditis complicating chronic otitis media, a large perforation or a cholesteatoma may be apparent. There may or may not be foul-smelling drainage from the ear. Tenderness of the mastoid tip and hearing loss are sometimes present. The

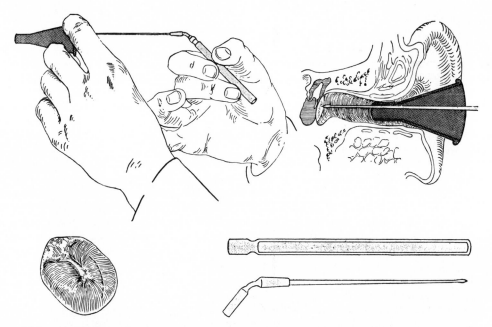

Figure 33.3.   Myringotomy. Illumination is provided by head light or mirror, and an anterior inferior incision is made in eardrum with sharp myringotomy knife. (Reproduced by permission, from Boies LR: *Fundamentals of Otolaryngology: A Textbook of Ear, Nose and Throat Diseases*, ed. 3. Philadelphia, W. B. Saunders Co., 1959.)

emergency physician should consult an otolaryngologist immediately. In the interim, x-ray views of the mastoid bone may be obtained.

Further complications of otitis media result from extension of the disease process to involve adjacent structures. All require immediate evaluation by an otolaryngologist. *Subperiosteal abscess*, an extension of infection within the mastoid bone to the mastoid tip (Bezold's abscess) or to the root of the zygomatic bone, produces pain, swelling, and tenderness in these areas. An *epidural abscess* occurring in either the middle or the posterior cranial fossa produces symptoms of localized headache, fever, and meningism. Signs of increased intracranial pressure may also be present. *Cerebellar* or *temporal lobe abscess* may develop following otitis media and may produce the typical signs of mass lesions in these areas. *Gradenigo's syndrome* is the result of an abscess or osteomyelitis at the apex of the petrous portion of the temporal bone, and consists of a chronically draining ear with ipsilateral abducens nerve palsy and pain behind the ipsilateral orbit. In *meningitis* following acute otitis media, the usual infecting organism is either a gram-positive coccus or *Hemophilus influenzae*. Meningitis is a rare complication of chronic otitis media; when it occurs, the agent is usually a gram-negative organism. Initial management should be directed at identifying the organism and treating the meningitis (see Chapter 11, pages 231–234). Once the meningitis is under control, the otologic disease should be treated. *Cavernous sinus thrombosis* is typified by spiking fever, obtundation, and increased intracranial pressure occurring in the course of acute or chronic otitis media. Treatment consists of controlling the septic process with intravenous antibiotics. An otolaryngologist should be consulted regarding early operation to drain the infected thrombus.

Tumor. Aural tumors can produce pain; usually a mass can be noted on examination. After the diagnosis is made, the patient should be referred to an otolaryngologist.

Referred Pain

Pain resulting from a distant pathologic process may be felt in the ear. The source of the pain may be a lesion of a tooth, the temporomandibular joint, the pharynx, or the neck; the pain of sinus conditions can likewise be felt in the ear. Uncommon sources of referred pain to the ear include lesions in the distribution of cranial nerves IX and X, such as those of the thyroid gland, chest, and abdomen. Some of the conditions in which pain is referred to the ear are detailed below; the remainder are treated in other sections of this chapter.

In the case of a *dental lesion*, the affected tooth may often be asymptomatic; instead, constant pain may be felt deep in the ear for days or weeks. Physical examination reveals a normal ear with no hearing loss; examination of the mouth often demonstrates a decaying tooth that is tender to pressure or percussion. Gingivitis or a dental abscess may be visible. These patients should be referred to a dentist.

The chief symptom of the *temporomandibular joint syndrome* is a sharp pain related to chewing. The patient may have a history of recent injury to the jaw, recent dental work, or long-standing malocclusion. Most patients with this syndrome are women between the ages of 20 and 40. Often the problem is a manifestation of emotional stress and is the result of constant clenching of the jaw muscles. On physical examination, malocclusion may be obvious. The physician may elicit tenderness over the temporomandibular joint, especially when the mouth is open, and swelling may be noted. Limited motion of the temporomandibular joint and crepitation may be demonstrated. Complications of this syndrome include chronic disability from pain and development of arthritic changes. The patient should be instructed to eat soft foods, apply heat locally, and take buffered aspirin, 2 tablets four times a day. If the symptoms are unrelieved, the patient should be referred to an oral surgeon or a dentist.

Acute Hearing Loss

Conductive Loss

Table 33.1 outlines the differential diagnosis of conductive and sensorineural hearing loss. Ear canal obstruction causing acute conductive hearing loss is discussed in the following section; other causes such as penetrating trauma and acute or chronic otitis media are discussed elsewhere in the chapter.

Obstruction of Ear Canal. A patient with obstruction of the ear by cerumen or a foreign body has diminished hearing and a sensation of fullness or pain in the affected ear. There may be discharge from the ear with associated external otitis. The physical examination will reveal the obstruction or external otitis or both. A foreign body may be obscured by infection. Treatment consists of removal of the obstruction and management of external otitis (see pages 727–728). Liquid dioctyl sodium sulfosuccinate (Colace), 10–20 drops in the ear canal for 15 minutes, often softens hardened cerumen. If the first few attempts to remove the obstruction are unsuccessful or if edema of the ear canal and hemorrhage are present, the patient should be referred to an otolaryngologist.

Table 33.1.
Acute hearing loss: differential diagnosis.

	Conductive	Sensorineural
Symptoms		
Hearing abnormality	Sudden sensation of blockage Hollow feeling in ear	Loss of hearing Fullness in ear Tinnitus Abnormal sensitivity to loud sounds
Pain	Often present	Uncommon
Vertigo	Infrequent	Often present
Related problems	Acute infection Trauma Obstruction of Eustachian tube Upper respiratory tract infection Allergy Trauma (penetrating or blunt) Skull fracture	Diabetes Arteriosclerotic occlusive disease Hyperlipidemia Ménière's disease Hypercoagulable state Trauma (labyrinthine concussion or temporal bone fracture)
Physical examination		
Ear canal	Occluded or infected	Normal
Ear drum	Infected or perforated	Normal
Hearing tests		
Voice test	Slight or moderate hearing loss	Decreased hearing or total hearing loss
Rinne's test	Negative in affected ear	Positive in affected ear or false-negative
Weber's test	Sound heard in affected ear	Sound may be heard in unaffected ear or midline
Laboratory tests to be ordered if indicated	Culture discharge if present Temporal bone x-ray film if blunt trauma Audiometric examination	Fasting blood glucose test Fluorescent treponemal antibody-absorption test for syphilis Serum cholesterol test Partial thromboplastin time Platelet count Temporal bone x-ray film if blunt trauma Bárány's caloric test Audiometric examination

Sensorineural Loss

Exertional Loss. An otologic emergency, the sudden onset of significant hearing loss after exertion is associated with a sensation of fullness in the ear and tinnitus; transient or persistent vertigo, nausea, and vomiting may occur. Frequently, the exertion involves activities such as lifting, pushing, or straining in such a way as to create an increase in CSF pressure that is transmitted through the cochlear aqueduct, causing rupture of the membranes of the oval and round windows. On physical examination the patient may have obvious dysequilibrium with nystagmus. On testing of hearing, a partial or total sensorineural hearing loss with a normal eardrum may be noted. The major complication is permanent total hearing loss in the affected ear. Patients with this condition should be evaluated by an otolaryngologist immediately for consideration of an urgent exploratory operation on the middle ear. Some advocate nonoperative treatment with hospitalization and 4–5 days of total bed rest.

Postoperative Loss. Any patient with recent operation on the ear who has a loss of hearing or vertigo should be referred immediately to his aural surgeon. Exploratory reoperation may be necessary, especially in a patient with a recent stapedectomy.

Other Causes. Patients with some or all of the typical signs and symptoms of sensorineural impairment described in Table 33.1 require early evaluation, including audiometric study by an otolaryngologist. Mechanisms of this hearing loss include trauma, infection, tumor, systemic disease, and ototoxic drugs; occasionally no mechanism can be identified.

Noise trauma resulting from any sound in excess of 100 decibels, especially explosive noise such as gunfire, may cause a temporary or permanent hearing loss. There is no treatment available except prevention by employing adequate sound protection.

Infectious processes can cause acute sensorineural hearing loss, such as that occurring during or after a viral upper respiratory tract infection. In children, unilateral deafness can be caused by the mumps virus. Another specific viral illness, herpes zoster oticus is manifested by painful herpetic lesions of the external ear, with occasional associated facial paralysis. Hearing loss and facial paralysis caused by herpesvirus are untreatable at present, although an involved eye should be protected. Sudden unilateral sensorineural hearing loss accompanied by severe vertigo can occur during bacterial otitis media and signifies invasion of the labyrinth. Since the labyrinthine fluid is in direct communication with the subarachnoid space, meningitis is a potential complication. Intensive antibiotic therapy is necessary, and myringotomy is also indicated.

Tumors of the temporal bone are an uncommon cause of sensorineural hearing loss. Tumors in this group include vestibular schwannoma, congenital cholesteatoma, glomus jugulare tumor, and other rare tumors such as leukemic infiltrates and metastatic lesions from the breast, kidney, and lung.

Sensorineural hearing loss may be one of the symptoms of *Ménière's disease*; others include tinnitus, aural pressure, and vertigo. These symptoms typically fluctuate in intensity and degree. There may be a hiatus of many years between attacks or they may recur often. Vertigo may be mild to severe; attacks usually last from 1–4 hours. Droperidol has been proved effective in the management of the severe nausea and vertigo of Ménière's disease; the dosage is 2.5 mg every 4–6 hours administered intramuscularly.

Sudden sensorineural hearing loss associated with *diabetes mellitus* probably reflects occlusion of small vessels (diabetic microangiopathy); anticoagulants such as heparin may be considered, and the underlying disease should be treated. *Degenerative diseases* such as multiple sclerosis, syphilis (tertiary and congenital), and collagen disease can cause sudden hearing loss. If syphilis is suspected, serologic studies including the fluorescent treponemal antibody-absorption test should be performed. This is one of the few forms of sensorineural hearing loss that responds to treatment. When the diagnosis is made, treatment with corticosteroids and penicillin should be initiated.

Toxic substances also cause sensorineural hearing loss. The most common toxins are certain antibiotic and diuretic medications, as listed in Table 33.2. Sudden hearing loss can also occur in adults without obvious cause. The physician should exclude all the previously mentioned conditions and an otolaryngologist should be consulted. At present, there is no well-defined treatment for this entity; vasodilators, anticoagulants, and high-dose corticosteroids have been used without statistically proved benefit.

Acute Vertigo

The diagnostic evaluation of patients with vertigo is a challenging problem. The differential diagnosis between peripheral vertigo (caused within the temporal bone) and central vertigo (caused within the central nervous system or cardiovascular system) is found in Table 33.3. Differentiation between the two major sources of vertigo often rests on subtle differences in history, clinical examination, and ancillary studies. If no diagnosis is readily apparent, the patient's symptoms should be treated and he should be referred for further evaluation to an internist, an otolaryngologist, or a neurologist, depending on the physician's general impression of the diagnosis.

Peripheral Vertigo

Peripheral vertigo can be caused by several conditions that have been mentioned, such as ex-

Table 33.2.
Toxic agents causing hearing loss.

Antibiotics (mostly aminoglycosides)
    Streptomycin D
    Gentamicin
    Neomycin sulfate
    Kanamycin sulfate
    Viomycin
    Chloramphenicol
Diuretics
    Ethacrynic acid
    Furosemide
Others
    Quinine
    Salicylates
    Nitrogen mustards
    Phenylbutazone
    Tetanus antitoxin (serum sickness – rare)

Table 33.3.
Peripheral and central vertigo: differential diagnosis.

Manifestation	Peripheral	Central
Hearing loss	Common, often unilateral, lasting minutes to hours (fluctuating)	Rare, may be unilateral, lasting days or weeks
Tinnitus	Common	Rare
Aural pressure or sense of fullness	Common	Rare
Ear pain	Possible	Rare
Nausea and vomiting	Common	Possible, degree of dizziness may not correlate with degree of nausea and vomiting
Spontaneous nystagmus	Common, usually horizontal and away from affected ear	Common, usually bizarre (direction changing, up-beating)
Other cranial neuropathy	Rare	Common
Papilledema	None	Possible
Change in consciousness	None	Possible
Decrease in vision	None (subjective blurring)	Possible, especially with basilar arterial insufficiency
Headache	Rare	Possible
Positional nystagmus	Common (rotatory or horizontal)	Possible (may be bizarre with vertical component)
Recurrence	Common	Possible, especially with basilar arterial insufficiency

ternal otitis, otitis media, serous otitis, Ménière's disease, and trauma. It can also occur following an ear operation, in which case the surgeon should be immediately consulted. Other conditions involving peripheral vertigo are discussed in the following sections.

Complications of Chronic Otitis Media. A patient with *labyrinthitis* usually has a sensation of light-headedness or vertigo. If labyrinthitis is severe, vertigo may be constant. On examination, the affected ear may have an obvious foul-smelling discharge, or a dry cholesteatoma may be noted. The patient may be nauseated and vomiting; nystagmus that is usually directed toward the affected ear may also be present.

Symptoms may be relieved by meclizine hydrochloride, 25 mg orally every 4–6 hours, or prochlorperazine maleate, 10–15 mg orally every 4–6 hours or 5–10 mg intramuscularly every 4–6 hours. If the ear is draining, antibiotic ear drops are indicated, 4 drops four times a day. Systemic antibiotics are probably not beneficial. The patient should be referred without delay to an otolaryngologist.

Erosion due to chronic infection or cholesteatoma that gradually exposes the membranes of the semicircular canal gives rise to a *labyrinthine fistula*. The patient may state that he becomes dizzy whenever he places his finger in the ear canal of the affected ear, and he may demonstrate dysequilibrium and nystagmus. The fistula test is often positive, and conductive hearing loss is frequently present. These patients should be referred immediately to an otolaryngologist.

A patient with *cerebellar abscess* related to chronic or acute otitis media has signs of a cerebellar lesion such as dysarthria, headache, and loss of coordinated movement on the side of the affected ear. Physical examination demonstrates ipsilateral muscular incoordination and increased ipsilateral tendon reflexes. Signs of increased intracranial pressure may be noted as well as abnormal patterns of nystagmus. These patients should be referred immediately for otologic and neurosurgical consultation.

Benign Positional Vertigo. A patient with this condition usually experiences 1- to 3-minute episodes of severe spinning vertigo commonly precipitated by movement of the head either to the side or backward. Occasionally the patient has had an infection of the upper respiratory tract or trauma to the head; more often these symptoms occur without prior illness. Physical examination will reveal normal findings with the exception of rotatory nystagmus on position testing. The diagnosis of benign positional vertigo is based on the position test and includes the following findings:

(1) Delay in the onset of nystagmus (5–10 seconds) when the patient is placed in the head-hanging position.

(2) Rotatory nystagmus, reproduced whenever the patient is placed in the stimulating position.

(3) Reverse of direction of nystagmus when the patient is brought upright.

(4) Fatigability of nystagmus after three or four repetitions of the position test.

The patient should be instructed to avoid positions that cause vertigo and situations in which a vertiginous attack would endanger him, such as driving or working on scaffolding or in other elevated areas. A trial course of meclizine hydrochloride, 25 mg every 6 hours, can be given; this occasionally provides symptomatic relief. The patient should be told that benign positional vertigo generally clears within 2–6 months. Patients with this problem should be referred to an otolaryngologist for complete evaluation.

Other causes. A patient with *vestibular neuritis* usually has been unsteady and dizzy for a few days to several weeks with no change in hearing. This type of vertigo may appear in epidemic form, and in this form is usually of viral origin. Physical examination reveals normal hearing and normal aural structures with occasional spontaneous nystagmus. Treatment is directed toward relief of symptoms, since this is a self-limiting disease.

In general, drugs that cause acute hearing loss (Table 33.2) can also cause *acute toxic vertigo* that is also manifested by ataxia. In the case of gentamicin, a vestibular toxic reaction usually occurs before hearing loss. Physical examination may reveal a hearing deficit, spontaneous nystagmus, Romberg's sign, and sometimes ataxia. The causative drug should be discontinued as soon as possible, since permanent hearing loss and ataxia may result. On the other hand, any of these drugs are used for life-threatening illnesses, and a decision to discontinue them must be based on the clinical status of the patient.

Vertigo can be caused by *acute syphilitic labyrinthitis* of secondary syphilis or by inflammation of the osseous labyrinth from congenital syphilis. The diagnosis is made by means of a positive serum test for syphilis. Treatment includes administration of penicillin and corticosteroids.

Central Vertigo

Central vertigo, as manifested by signs and symptoms listed in Table 33.3, can be caused by several neurovascular lesions or states. Some of these, such as epilepsy and migraine headache, are discussed elsewhere (see Chapter 15, pages 345–351); the remainder are treated as described in the following paragraphs.

Vertebrobasilar arterial insufficiency is often manifested by episodic attacks of vertigo. These attacks are usually associated with other symptoms, including visual "blackouts," dysarthria, headache, and muscular weakness, and the patient may become unconscious. On physical examination the ear appears normal, and there may be variable nystagmus. The patient may exhibit the stigmata of peripheral arterial disease. The diagnosis is usually made from the history and the general appearance of the patient, who should be referred to an internist or a neurologist.

In the *subclavian steal syndrome* the patient has a history of episodic vertigo and other symptoms of basilar arterial insufficiency, associated with cramping and tiredness in one arm. The patient may have a bruit over the subclavian artery and an occasional pulse deficit in the radial artery, especially with elevation of the affected arm. Patients with this syndrome should be referred to a vascular surgeon.

Usually a patient with a *cerebrovascular accident* has experienced a catastrophic onset of acute vertigo with nausea and vomiting, cerebellar ataxia, dysarthria, and dysphagia. Physical examination reveals cerebellar ataxia, bizarre nystagmus, and lower cranial nerve palsies. The patient should be hospitalized with supportive measures and a neurologist should be immediately consulted (see Chapter 15, pages 351–358).

A *tumor of the cerebellopontine angle* causes unilateral sensorineural hearing loss with episodic or constant dizziness and sometimes an associated unilateral facial palsy. Physical examination may confirm all these findings, and an absent corneal reflex on the side of the lesion may be noted. These patients should be referred to an otolaryngologist.

A patient with *acute demyelinating disease* may have vertigo associated with other symptoms of neurologic disorder such as diplopia, dysarthria, muscular weakness, and loss of bladder and bowel control. Bizarre nystagmus may be seen on physical examination. Such patients should be referred to a neurologist.

A *lowered effective blood volume* can cause dizziness. This is not true vertigo, but rather a lightheaded feeling. Among conditions causing this symptom are cardiac arrhythmias, anemia, and vasovagal attacks.

THE SINUSES AND FACE

Examination Technique

If a sinus condition is suspected, the physician should perform the following maneuvers. *Sinus transillumination* is performed in a darkened room with a narrow-beam light source such as a penlight. The penlight is placed under each supraorbital rim to evaluate the frontal sinuses and over the infraorbital rims to evaluate the maxillary sinuses. Light transmitted through the palate is viewed through the open mouth. One side is compared with the other for the amount of light transmitted (Fig. 33.4). If the pattern of light transmission is asymmetric, the test is considered positive. Although this test is helpful in diagnosis and in follow-up evaluation, sinus x-ray views provide more accurate information (Fig. 33.5).

Keeping in mind the exquisite tenderness of acute sinus disease, the examiner should gently *palpate the sinuses*. The maxillary antrum is best evaluated by palpation over the canine fossa (Fig. 33.6A); the frontal sinus is examined by placing the finger just deep to the suproaorbital rim (Fig. 33.6B).

Facial Pain

Sinustis

Sinusitis may occur as a complication of an acute upper respiratory tract infection or of allergic rhinitis. The pain is often described as steady pressure, and it may be severe. It may be experienced in the anterior part of the face, behind the orbits, or in the vertex or occiput of the skull. Typically, the pain is exacerbated by hanging the head down and is most pronounced in the afternoon or evening. Purulent nasal discharge may be associated.

Acute aerosinusitis occurs during flight in persons with an upper respiratory tract infection or allergic diathesis. Pre-existent local edema obstructs the sinus ostia, and painful hemorrhage into the sinus mucosa results from rapid pressure changes during descent.

The patient with sinusitis may have only a mildly elevated temperature. Localized swelling over the involved sinus may be visualized, and palpation of the anterior aspect of the maxillary antrum or of the floor of the frontal sinus may elicit tenderness. Intranasal examination may reveal purulent mucus draining from the sinus ostium, but the absence of discharge does not exclude sinusitis. During the intranasal examination the examiner should search for nasal polyps, a foreign body, or tumor as a possible cause for sinusitis. Because infection in the upper teeth can cause symptoms similar to those of maxillary si-

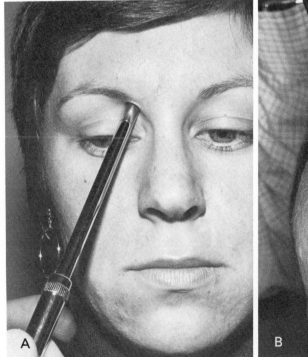 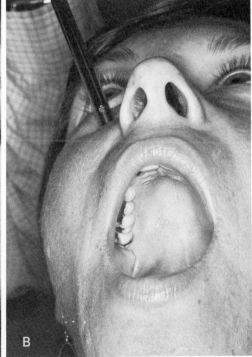

Figure 33.4. **(A)** Transillumination of frontal sinus. Light source is placed deep to supraorbital rim. **(B)** Transillumination of maxillary sinus. Light source is placed deep to infraorbital rim and light is viewed through palate. Totally darkened room is used.

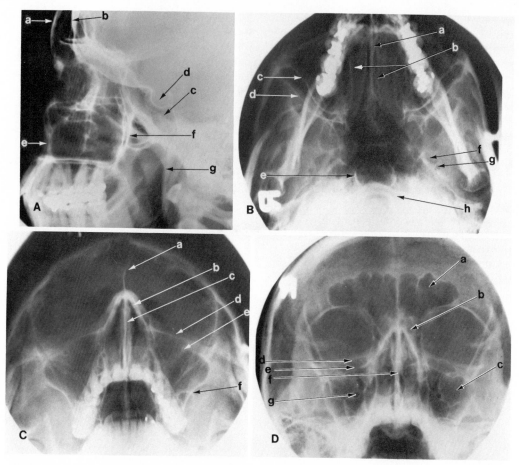

Figure 33.5. **(A)** Lateral x-ray view of normal sinuses. *a*, Frontal sinus—anterior wall; *b*, frontal sinus—posterior wall; *c*, sphenoid sinus; *d*, pituitary fossa; *e*, maxillary antrum—anterior wall; *f*, maxillary antrum—posterior wall; *g*, nasopharynx—posterior wall. **(B)** Basal x-ray view of normal sinuses. *a*, Nasal septum; *b*, nasal turbinates; *c*, antrum—posterior wall; *d*, orbit—lateral wall; *e*, wall of sphenoid sinus; *f*, foramen ovale; *g*, foramen spinosum; *h*, first cervical vertebra. **(C)** Waters' x-ray view of normal sinuses. *a*, Frontal sinus; *b*, nasal arch; *c*, nasal septum; *d*, orbital rim; *e*, infraorbital foramen; *f*, antrum—lateral wall. **(D)** Caldwell x-ray view of normal sinuses. *a*, Frontal sinus; *b*, ethmoid sinus; *c*, antral sinus; *d*, orbital rim; *e*, orbital floor; *f*, nasal septum; *g*, foramen rotundum.

nusitis, the mouth should be carefully examined and each tooth should be palpated. Transillumination of the sinuses may demonstrate a unilateral opacification, further aiding in diagnosis. Sinus x-ray films are indicated to determine the extent of disease and to establish a baseline for follow-up care.

Complications of Sinusitis. Occasionally seen in the emergency ward, these conditions all require immediate hospitalization under the care of an otolaryngologist. During the course of sinusitis (usually ethmoid), *orbital cellulitis* may develop. This complication is suggested by worsening pain in and behind the eye, with erythema and swelling of the upper and lower lids, proptosis, chemosis, and decreasing ocular mobility. Vision may dete-

riorate. The end stage of orbital cellulitis, an *orbital abscess* is suggested by a fixed eye and rapidly deteriorating vision. A patient with this condition should be referred to an otolaryngologist and an ophthalmologist for consideration of urgent decompression of the orbit via a transethmoidal approach. Uncommon in the antibiotic era, *osteomyelitis of the skull* usually occurs as a complication of frontal sinusitis. Typically, the patient has puffy swelling of the brow over the frontal sinus and a localized frontal headache. Treatment includes hospitalization with intensive antibiotic therapy. Operative drainage of the sinus and débridement of dead bone may also be necessary. When uncontrolled sinus disease extends to the central nervous system, *meningitis, epidural ab-*

scess, brain abcess, and *cavernous sinus thrombosis* can all occur.

In cases of uncomplicated sinusitis, emergency care consists of the following measures. If obvious purulent mucus is apparent in the nose, specimens for culture and sensitivity testing should be obtained. Sinus x-ray films should be ordered, and if a complication involving the eye is suggested, an ophthalmologist should be consulted. Local heat should be applied, and medications should be administered as follows:

(1) Antibiotics. In an adult, penicillin or erythromycin should be administered orally, 250 mg four times a day for 10 days. In a child who weighs less than 20 kg. oral amoxicillin should be prescribed, 20 mg/kg/day divided into 8-hour doses for 10 days. In a penicillin-allergic child, erythromycin and sulfisoxazole are administered in combination in appropriate doses for weight for 10 days.

(2) Decongestants. In an adult, any long-acting combination of antihistamines and decongestants is administered for 10–20 days. For a child, a similar medication in liquid form for 10–20 days is usually adequate.

(3) Nasal drops or spray. For an adult, oxymetazoline hydrochloride (Afrin) spray is prescribed,

to be applied in each nostril three times a day for a week. Phenylephrine hydrochloride (Neo-Synephrine) nasal drops (0.125% or 0.25%), 3 drops/day for a week, is sufficient for a child. The patient or the patient's parents should be warned that use of nasal drops for more than 1 week may cause rebound nasal swelling.

(4) Analgesics. Both adults and children may need moderately high doses of analgesic medications for the first 4 days of treatment.

Other Causes of Facial Pain

Acute unilateral facial pain in the absence of sinusitis suggests a pathologic process involving cranial nerve V. Neurologic disease such as tic douloureux or herpes zoster must be considered. If anesthesia is present in the area of pain, an exhaustive workup is indicated to exclude an occult neoplasm involving the affected branch of the trigeminal nerve.

Facial Swelling

Facial swelling may be produced by several conditions. Swelling caused by sinus disease has been discussed. The following sections detail other conditions that give rise to this symptom.

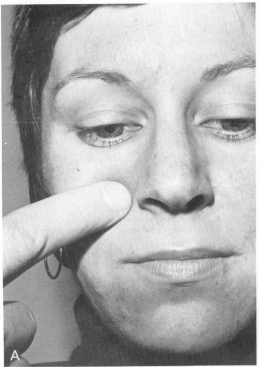 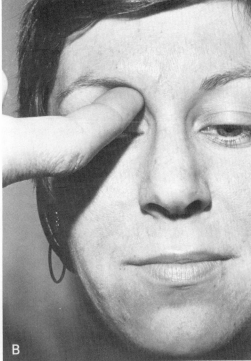

Figure 33.6. **(A)** Palpation of maxillary antrum. **(B)** Palpation deep to supraorbital rim to demonstrate tenderness of frontal sinus.

Allergic Reactions

A patient with facial swelling may have been exposed to a known allergen or may have been bitten by an insect. Facial swelling occurring with a generalized allergic reaction may involve varying degrees of edema of the eyelids, the conjunctivae, the oropharynx, and occasionally the larynx. The eyes may sometimes close completely, and the upper airway may become obstructed. In addition to airway obstruction, another potential complication of a generalized allergic reaction is anaphylactic shock.

If the swelling is due to an insect bite, the site will itch, but there are usually no systemic symptoms. In a child with swelling of one or both eyelids, sinusitis with periorbital cellulitis rather than an insect bite should be suspected, until the former is excluded.

Treatment depends on whether the swelling is due to a local bite or a generalized allergic reaction. In the former case, 1% hydrocortisone cream and an ice pack should be applied to the bite. Diphenhydramine hydrochloride (Benadryl) may be given intramuscularly or orally, adjusting the dosage for the patient's age. The adult dosage is 50 mg every 8 hours until the reaction subsides.

In the case of a systemic allergic reaction, initial treatment consists of administration of epinephrine (1:1000) intramuscularly or subcutaneously, 0.5 ml in an adult and an appropriately smaller dose in a child. In patients with anaphylactic shock, diphenhydramine hydrochloride and intravenous corticosteroids are suggested with ventilatory assistance and cardiac support as needed.

Angioneurotic Edema

A patient with this condition commonly has had recurrent edema of the face, pharynx, and larynx developing over a few hours and sometimes progressing to cause respiratory obstruction. Endotracheal intubation may be necessary until resolution of the edema, which occurs as a rule in 24–72 hours, thus obviating tracheotomy. The condition is related to a deficiency in the complement system, and some centers are experimentally treating it with androgens, fresh frozen plasma, and ϵ-aminocaproic acid. Definitive medical treatment is not yet available.

Tumors and Chronic Conditions

In the patient who has experienced progressive localized facial swelling over a period of weeks or months, a chronic infectious process or tumor must be suspected. If swelling is in the supraorbital region, frontal sinus mucocele is the most common causative lesion, but a malignant condition of the frontal or ethmoid sinus must be considered. In the infraorbital region and the cheek, fibrous dysplasia and malignant tumors of the maxilla are the two most common neoplasms. In the mandible, neoplastic swelling is usually related to a dental cyst or an odontogenic tumor, but fibrous dysplasia and malignant lesions may also occur.

Lesions in the Newborn

An infant up to 2 months old who exhibits swelling, erythema, and tenderness over the maxilla, and a high temperature may have osteomyelitis of the maxilla. The mother may have an infected nipple. On examination, swelling may extend to the medial canthus. In an advanced case, an abscess may be seen on the face, in the nose, or even on the palate, and pressure on the affected cheek may produce purulent discharge from the nose. Purulent material should be obtained for a Gram stain, culture, and sensitivity testing. High-dose intravenous antibiotics should be instituted and later adjusted according to the culture and sensitivity reports; the usual causative organism is a staphylococcus. The patient should be hospitalized under the care of a pediatrician and an otolaryngologist. No abscess should be drained until pointing is obvious.

Congenital facial lesions in a newborn may appear in several sites. A midline swelling of the nasal dorsum with or without a sinus tract suggests a dermoid cyst. Patients should be referred to an otolaryngologist for evaluation. Swelling in the region of the medial canthus suggests an encephalocele, a hemangioma, or a tumor of the lacrimal apparatus or sinuses. These infants should be evaluated by an otolaryngologist and an ophthalmologist. Swelling in the parotid region may represent hemangioma, branchial cyst, or rarer tumors. Such a lesion requires excision involving facial nerve dissection, and the patient should be referred to a head and neck surgeon.

Facial Paralysis

Terminology and Testing

Any lesion of the facial nerve (Fig. 33.7) from its nucleus in the brainstem to the motor endplate is considered *peripheral*. A peripheral lesion usually causes total unilateral facial paralysis, except when the lesion is distal to the branching of the nerve within the parotid gland. A lesion proximal to the facial nerve nucleus in the brainstem is considered *central*, and causes ipsilateral weakness

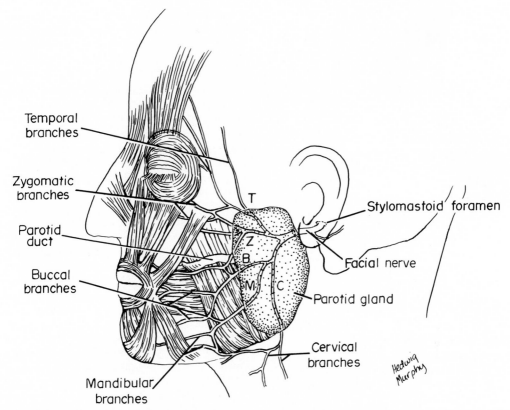

Figure 33.7. Extratemporal portion of facial nerve. Note exit at stylomastoid foramen, course through parotid gland, and relation to parotid duct.

in the lower two-thirds of the face. The forehead is usually unaffected because of its bilateral crossed motor innervation.

There are numerous methods of testing the function of the facial nerve, but they are usually not performed by the emergency physician. In the emergency ward, facial nerve weakness should be noted; the examiner should specify whether weakness is partial or complete, and whether it is evident in the upper, middle, or lower third of the face.

Common Disorders

Bell's Palsy. This condition is diagnosed after the treatable causes of facial weakness that are discussed in this section are excluded. The patient experiences progression of unilateral facial weakness over 1–3 days, often associated with facial numbness and pain around the mastoid tip. The patient may also experience ipsilateral facial pain. This condition may recur, and may involve both sides of the face. On examination, varying degrees of facial paralysis ranging from partial to complete are present. In a case of complete paralysis, Bell's

phenomenon will occur: when the patient is asked to close the eye on the affected side, it closes incompletely and the globe rotates upward. In addition, the patient cannot elevate the eyebrow, wiggle the nose, whistle, or smile on the affected side. The ear should be examined to exclude lesions that might explain the facial paralysis.

The affected eye should be protected from the drying effects of constant corneal exposure by placing methylcellulose drops in the eye every 2–4 hours and taping down the eyelid during sleep. The patient should be referred to an otolaryngologist for complete evaluation. Controversy exists regarding the benefits of corticosteroid therapy and of surgical decompression. At present, we believe that surgical decompression for acute Bell's palsy is unwarranted, and we recommend a short course of oral corticosteroids.

Trauma. Crushing injury or sharp penetrating trauma distal to the stylomastoid foramen may involve the main trunk or the branches of the facial nerve, depending on the location of the injury. When evaluating a patient with midfacial penetrating trauma, the examiner should also consider laceration of the parotid duct and parotid gland. A patient with acute penetrating midfacial trauma with associated facial paralysis is a candidate for immediate operative exploration with suture of the nerve ends and repair of the parotid duct if necessary. Vigorous bleeding should be controlled preoperatively by pressure rather than by blind clamping, since the latter may result in damage to the facial nerve.

Temporal bone fracture may cause paralysis of cranial nerve VII. If immediate facial paralysis results from a temporal bone fracture, operative decompression of the nerve should be considered in patients whose condition is stable enough to permit anesthesia. An otolaryngologist should assist in any decision involving operation, since the timing of operation depends on the results of facial nerve testing (electrical stimulation and salivary flow tests).

Other Common Causes. Partial or complete facial paralysis may develop during *acute otitis media*. A patient with this complication should immediately undergo myringotomy. Facial paralysis should lessen as the ear infection resolves after antibiotic therapy. Facial paralysis in a patient with *chronic otitis media* usually progresses slowly over a few days. It may be partial or complete when the patient comes to the emergency ward. The patient must be referred to an otolaryngologist for consideration of urgent operative decompression of the involved portion of the facial nerve. *Tuberculosis of the ear* causing chronic otitis media may produce facial paralysis and should be treated medically.

When *birth injury* resulting from prolonged labor or use of forceps causes complete facial paralysis, the infant should undergo surgical decompression of the nerve as soon as possible. Newborns are considered reasonable candidates for operation when they reach a weight of 4 kg. Other sources for neonatal facial paralysis include thalidomide injury and Treacher Collins' syndrome.

A patient with *herpes zoster oticus* (Ramsay Hunt's syndrome) has painful herpetic eruptions of the ear canal and auricle. Associated facial paralysis and occasional sensorineural hearing loss imply herpetic involvement of the ganglia of cranial nerves VII and VIII. There is no direct therapy for this problem; the only treatment is local skin care to prevent secondary infection, analgesia as indicated, and protection of the involved eye. The possible efficacy of acyclovir is yet to be determined. The patient should be referred to an otolaryngologist for follow-up care. Facial paralysis associated with facial pain is also consistent with a *malignant parotid tumor*. Frequently, this tumor can be palpated on physical examination. Patients should be referred to a head and neck surgeon.

Uncommon Disorders

Benign and malignant tumors of the temporal bone may cause paralysis of the facial nerve. A benign tumor of the vestibular nerve, *vestibular schwannoma* may be manifested initially by facial paralysis, but usually the patient's primary complaints are vertigo and sensorineural hearing loss. Patients in whom this lesion is suspected should be referred to an otolaryngologist for evaluation. Pulsatile tinnitus is the most prominent symptom in patients with a *glomus jugulare tumor*. Conductive hearing loss may be present, and facial paralysis may be a late symptom. Physical examination reveals a pulsatile reddish mass behind the eardrum. Cranial nerves IX, X, and XII may be involved; referral to an otolaryngologist is necessary. Other rare tumors of the temporal bone causing facial paralysis include *cholesteatoma, eosinophilic granuloma*, and *metastatic tumors*, most commonly from the breast, kidney, and lung. Radiologic examination reveals a lytic or blastic lesion of the temporal bone in this instance.

Disorders of the central nervous system such as multiple sclerosis and other demyelinating diseases, stroke, and arachnoiditis may be manifested by facial paralysis, but usually other signs and symptoms make the diagnosis apparent.

Melkersson-Rosenthal syndrome is a rare condition beginning with swelling of the lip or palate or both, followed by bilateral facial paralysis. A markedly fissured tongue may be noted. This condition is typified by spontaneous regression and recurrence; it may respond to a short course of corticosteroids tapered over 1 week.

SALIVARY GLANDS AND FLOOR OF MOUTH

Trauma

Parotid Gland

In the case of blunt injury to the parotid gland (Fig. 33.8), hematoma, swelling, and abrasions are obvious. The examiner should bimanually palpate the cheek and mandible for possible associated fractures (Fig 33.9A), and facial nerve function should be evaluated.

In an open injury, continuity of the parotid duct should be established. This duct is located along an imaginary line drawn from the tragus of the ear to the nasal vestibule. Continuity is examined by introducing a lacrimal probe into the oral opening

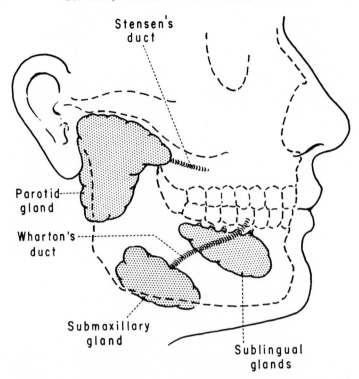

Figure 33.8. Location of major salivary glands and their ducts. (Reproduced by permission, from DeWeese DD, Saunders WH: *Textbook of Otolaryngology*, ed 4. St. Louis, The C. V. Mosby Co., 1973.)

of the parotid duct, which is adjacent to the second maxillary molar (Fig. 33.9B). Additional search should be made for associated facial fractures, dental injuries, and injuries to the major vessels of the upper neck.

In a victim of blunt trauma, the abraded skin should be thoroughly cleansed, débrided, and covered with antibiotic ointment and a sterile dressing. Cold compresses may reduce the swelling. Immediate total facial nerve paralysis suggests facial nerve avulsion at the stylomastoid foramen, and an exploratory operation should be performed. If delayed facial paralysis develops, the patient should be observed by an otolaryngologist, but operative exploration is not immediately indicated. Associated facial fractures should be managed as discussed in Chapter 29, pages 651–654.

An open injury involving the parotid gland requires hospitalization for careful cleansing of the wound and meticulous operative closure including suture of the parotid duct and facial nerve if these structures are injured.

Submaxillary Gland

Although this gland is rarely involved in trauma because of its protected location, its duct may be lacerated by intraoral trauma or by extensive dis-

location fractures of the jaw. Physical examination reveals the traumatic injury; anesthesia of the distal tongue resulting from lingual nerve injury may be associated.

An isolated laceration of the submaxillary duct may be treated expectantly since an intraoral fistula from the duct will probably develop spontaneously. In extensive injuries the entire gland may be removed without significant loss of salivary function.

Pain and Swelling

Obstruction of Salivary Ducts

Patients with infection associated with a salivary calculus experience acute pain and swelling of the involved gland; many previous episodes may be reported. On physical examination the gland is swollen and tender, and erythema of the overlying skin may be seen. Bimanual palpation sometimes demonstrates a calculus in the duct of the affected gland. By introducing a lacrimal probe into the punctum of the duct (Fig. 33.9B and D), the physician may experience the gritty sensation of a calculus. Probing may also produce either clear secretions or purulent secretions; the latter should be cultured.

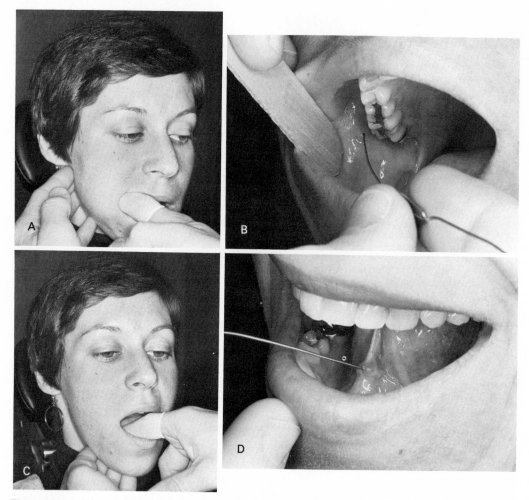

Figure 33.9.   **(A)** Bimanual examination of parotid region. **(B)** Lacrimal probe in parotid (Stensen's) duct. **(C)** Bimanual examination of floor of mouth and submaxillary region. **(D)** Lacrimal probe in right submaxillary (Wharton's) duct.

Patients with an infection should be treated with high doses of penicillin or erythromycin, analgesic medications, and hot soaks over the affected gland. Any obviously fluctuant area along the duct should be drained intraorally either by probing the duct or by direct incision and drainage. If the calculus is readily approachable intraorally, it should be excised under local anesthesia and the duct should be left open as a permanent fistula. Calculi deeper in the salivary ducts require more extensive operative procedures under the care of an otolaryngologist or oral surgeon.

Infection

Mumps. Acute painful swelling of one or more salivary glands associated with a low-grade fever and malaise is typical of mumps. Viral involvement of the pancreas, gonads, and rarely the brain or heart can occur. Usually the patient is 5–12

years old and has a classic "chipmunk" appearance due to bilateral parotid and sometimes submaxillary swelling. In an adult the gonads may be tender; signs of central nervous system involvement are rare. Treatment for mumps includes hydration and analgesic medications.

Acute Suppurative Parotitis. This condition usually occurs in elderly patients with severe general debility due to uncontrolled diabetes, dehydration, or cardiovascular disease. Progressive pain and swelling of the affected parotid gland occur over 1–3 days. On examination the parotid gland is swollen and tender. The patient is often dehydrated and exhibits signs of septicemia. Poor dental hygiene and oral dehydration are the usual underlying factors in this ascending infection of the parotid gland. Any discharge from the duct should be evaluated by Gram stain, cultures, and sensitivity testing, and the patient should be hospitalized with general supportive therapy including rehydration and control of any systemic condition such as cardiovascular instability or diabetes. Specific treatment of acute parotitis includes intravenous administration of an antibiotic such as a penicillinase-resistant penicillin. Incision and drainage of the infected parotid gland may be necessary. Acute suppurative parotitis signals a marked diminution of host defense mechanisms; this illness is often associated with terminal disease.

Ludwig's Angina. Patients with this condition have a history of progressive pain and swelling in the tongue and floor of the mouth with dysphagia and respiratory obstruction. The tongue and floor of the mouth have a "woody" feeling and are extremely tender. Often this condition develops after a dental infection or dental extraction. On inspection the tongue is swollen and displaced posteriorly and superiorly, sometimes obstructing the airway. An infected tooth or site of recent extraction may be noted. Lymphadenopathy is minimal, but the patient may have signs of sepsis.

This is a life-threatening illness because of potential airway obstruction, extension of the infection to the deep neck spaces and to the mediastinum, and generalized sepsis. The patient should be hospitalized, and specimens of oral secretions and blood should be cultured immediately. High-dose broad-spectrum antibiotics and high-dose corticosteroids should be administered intravenously. Tracheotomy is indicated in the presence of significant airway obstruction. Incision and drainage should be performed either intraorally or externally only if obvious pointing is visualized.

Dental Abscess. The patient complains of progressive pain localized to one tooth. The tooth is tender, and there may be associated edema of the gums and overlying facial tissues. The infection is treated by oral penicillin, analgesic medications, and local heat. A dentist should be consulted.

Tumors

Benign and malignant tumors may be manifested by salivary gland swelling. A discrete mass is usually palpable. Facial paralysis in association with a parotid neoplasm suggests an aggressive malignant process, and in this instance, early consultation should be obtained from a head and neck surgeon.

Rare Disorders

Salivary gland swelling may be related to tuberculosis, sarcoidosis, and Sjögren's syndrome. Another causative factor is toxic inflammation from ingestion of a heavy metal such as lead, copper, or mercury, or of a halogen such as bromide or iodide.

THE NOSE

Epistaxis

Causes

Epistaxis in children is almost invariably caused either by crusting and mucosal irritation during upper respiratory tract infection or by direct trauma. Some adults have recurrent epistaxis, usually from a small blood vessel or group of blood vessels located in the anterior portion of the septum.

Common causes of epistaxis include the following:

(1) Trauma: Epistaxis is due either to intranasal trauma from "nose picking" or to external trauma.

(2) Hypertension: Epistaxis may be difficult to manage until the hypertension is controlled.

(3) Upper respiratory tract infection: Bleeding is due to mucosal engorgement and subsequent crusting and irritation of the nasal mucosa.

(4) Foreign body: This is most commonly seen in children.

(5) Nasal polyps: Polyps may bleed in association with an acute allergic or infectious episode.

(6) Iatrogenic induction: Epistaxis may be precipitated by manipulation of the nose after fracture or after intranasal operation. In the latter case the emergency physician should contact the operating surgeon immediately.

(7) Abnormality of hemostasis: This condition is usually related to therapeutic use of sodium warfarin (Coumadin) and is more rarely associated with hemophilia, leukemic disorders, and hepatic or renal disease. The emergency physician should control bleeding with the most atraumatic method available. Treatment consists of gentle packing of the nose with either cotton soaked with epinephrine or petrolatum gauze saturated with antibiotic ointment. Cautery is contraindicated, since it usually forms an eschar, which, if it is detached, enlarges the area of bleeding.

Some rare causes of epistaxis include the following conditions and lesions: Benign *nasal tumors* infrequently bleed, but malignant tumors may cause unilateral bleeding. A tumor most commonly found in adolescent males, *nasopharyngeal angiofibroma* may be manifested by epistaxis and nasal obstruction; it should be kept in mind in the differential diagnosis of nosebleed in these patients. *Hereditary telangiectasia* (Rendu-Osler-Weber syndrome) is an autosomal dominant trait causing dilated thin-walled capillaries and venules throughout the body. This syndrome is characterized by recurrent nasal bleeding and telangiectasias of the lips and oral mucosa. Chronic diseases such as *Wegener's granulomatosis*, *lethal midline granuloma*, *tuberculosis*, and *syphilis* also cause epistaxis.

Treatment

In the management of epistaxis (Fig. 33.10), location of the specific bleeding point is of utmost importance. Adequate illumination and suction equipment are essential for precise management. The patient with active epistaxis is usually anxious and often needs reassurance. Sometimes mild sedation with an intramuscular narcotic or tranquilizer is helpful before examination and treatment. The blood pressure and pulse should be checked and recorded, and a blood sample should be drawn for hematocrit determination. If the patient's history suggests a blood dyscrasia, the physician should order the following tests: prothrombin time, partial thromboplastin time, platelet count, and bleeding time. The patient should be seated in a comfortable chair with a headrest, and should be given a basin to catch the blood.

The emergency physician and an assistant then evacuate clots with a metal suction tip and examine the nose by means of a nasal speculum and a head light or head mirror. The nasal examination should be orderly, and the nasal septum and the middle and inferior turbinates should be identified (Fig. 33.11). If the bleeding point is anterior, it can be cauterized. If it is posterior, it is important to decide which side of the nose is bleeding and whether the bleeding point is above or below the level of the middle turbinate.

Packing. After identification of an anterior bleeding point, the nose should be packed for 10 minutes with cotton gauze saturated with 4% cocaine or 2% tetracaine hydrochloride (Pontocaine). After removal of the packs, the nose will be moderately anesthetized and a silver nitrate stick can be employed for cauterization. If point cauteriza-

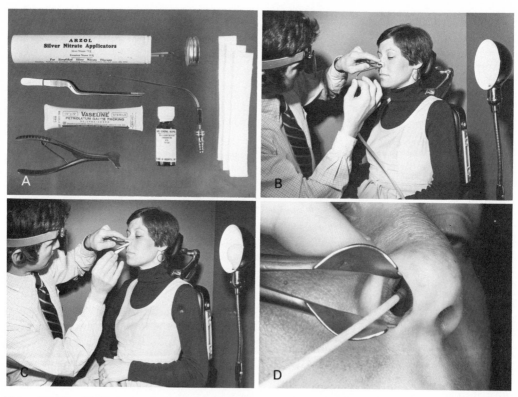

Figure 33.10. **(A)** Basic equipment for management of anterior epistaxis. *Counterclockwise from top left:* silver nitrate sticks, bayonet forceps, petrolatum gauze, nasal speculum, anesthetic solution, Frazier suction tip, compressed cotton strips for initial anesthesia. **(B)** Position of patient for nasal examination. Note position of nasal speculum. Suction apparatus may be used to remove mucus, foreign body, or blood. **(C)** Placement of compressed cotton packing for initial control of epistaxis, vasoconstriction, and anesthesia. Note position of bayonet forceps. **(D)** Application of silver nitrate to anterior nasal septum.

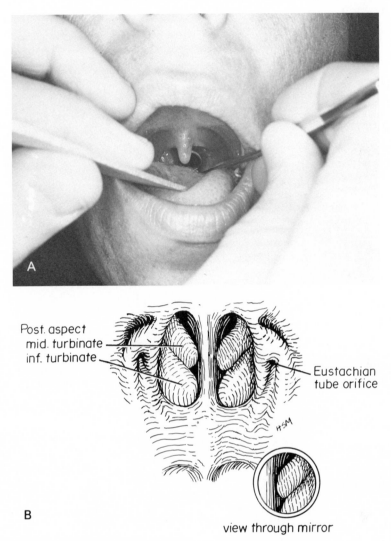

Figure 33.11. **(A)** Mirror examination of nasopharynx. Mirror must be warmed with water or alcohol lamp to prevent fogging. Tongue is depressed firmly and gently with tongue blade, and mirror is inserted behind and below free margin of soft palate; the patient is requested to breathe steadily and to say "uhn . . . uhn" to drop palate down. **(B)** Anatomy of nasopharynx. The posterior nasal septum is virtually always straight and is the best initial landmark. *Inset* demonstrates restricted field of view from nasopharyngeal mirror; the examiner must angle the mirror to visualize all areas.

tion fails to stop the bleeding, the nose should be packed with 0.5-inch petrolatum gauze saturated in antibiotic ointment. The packing is placed in the nose with a bayonet forceps (Fig. 33.12A) while the nares are held open with a nasal speculum. As it is inserted, the packing should be watched to ensure that it has passed posterior to the visualized bleeding point. The packing is then built up from the floor to the roof of the nose to fill the anterior chamber tightly (Fig. 33.12B), and is supported by a strip of tape underneath the nares. The patient should be given analgesics and

may be discharged. The packing is routinely removed after 3 days.

Posterior epistaxis is usually more severe and more difficult to control. The physician should note whether bleeding is from the upper half or lower half of the nose, since specific arterial ligation may be necessary if posterior packing fails to control bleeding. Occasionally, a well-placed full-depth anterior pack stops epistaxis from the posterior half of the nose, but it is often necessary to place a complete anteroposterior pack. The purpose of a posterior pack is to allow placement of

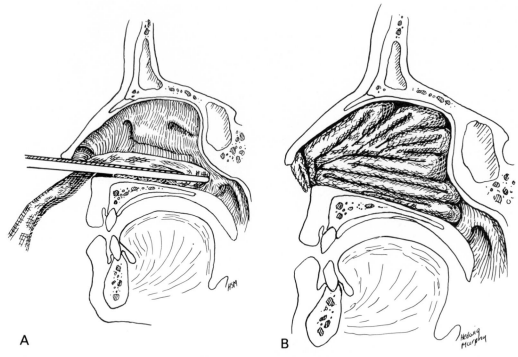

Figure 33.12. **(A)** Insertion of anterior nasal pack. Gauze is grasped with forceps 2–3 inches from end to prevent tip of gauze from slipping posteriorly. **(B)** Anterior nasal pack in place. Leading tip of pack does not protrude from choana. Pack is built up from floor of nose, then posterosuperiorly, and finally anterosuperiorly.

an extensive anterior pack that will not fall out through the posterior aspect of the nose and down the patient's throat.

Placement of a posterior pack is an uncomfortable experience for both patient and physician. If the patient has a normal blood pressure and pulse, meperidine hydrochloride or a similar narcotic analgesic should be administered and the nose should be anesthetized by means of packs of cotton gauze saturated with 4% cocaine or 2% tetracaine hydrochloride placed in the appropriate nostril and left in place for 10–15 minutes if feasible. Additional anesthesia may be obtained by performing a bilateral sphenopalatine ganglion block by injecting 1 ml of lidocaine (Xylocaine) with epinephrine (1:100,000) with a No. 21 needle (1.5-inch length) into the greater palatine foramen, which is located in the posterolateral aspect of the hard palate approximately 1 cm anterior to the posterior rim. One of the dangers of this procedure is insertion of the needle too deep into this area, thus penetrating the orbit. This complication can be avoided if the needle is prevented from passing any deeper than 2.5 cm by bending it to a 45-degree angle at this distance from its tip. Bilateral block provides much better anesthesia of the na-

sopharynx. Bleeding often stops on injection because of temporary tamponade of the internal maxillary artery, but it almost always resumes when the block wears off. Even with these efforts at anesthesia the patient will experience pain while the pack is placed.

A traditional posterior nasal pack consists of one or two pads of cotton gauze (4 × 4 inch) saturated with antibiotic ointment, rolled into a ball, and tightly tied in the middle with two pieces of 0 silk suture, each approximately 2 feet long. This pack is placed by passing a soft rubber catheter through the nostril on the affected side, retrieving the catheter tip from the pharynx by means of a Kelly clamp and tying two strands of the suture to it, and withdrawing the catheter through the nose, bringing out the two silk sutures. The physician should tell the patient to keep his mouth wide open and to pant with deep breaths during placement of the pack. Grasping the two nasal strands with a Kelly clamp, the physician steadily pulls them with his right hand and guides the pack behind the palate and into the nasopharynx (Fig. 33.13), employing moderate pressure with the index finger of the left hand. The uvula should be pushed free of the pack; otherwise it will become necrosed. When the posterior pack is in place, an anterior pack can be built up in the nose; a tight pack usually requires 3–6 feet of 0.5-inch petrolatum gauze. An assistant must maintain constant tension on the strings holding the posterior pack in place while the anterior pack is inserted. After the anterior pack is in place, the two free ends of the silk suture coming out the nares are tied over a dental roll. The ends dangling out the mouth should be taped loosely to the cheek, and are used to retrieve the pack after it has been in place for 4 days.

The patient with a posterior pack in place should be hospitalized with modified bed rest and a semisolid or liquid diet. Moderate doses of analgesics and barbiturates can be administered; obtundation should be avoided since hypoxia can

occur. Antibiotics should be administered to prevent sinusitis.

Arterial Ligation. When epistaxis is uncontrolled by cauterization or packing, arterial ligation is necessary. Bleeding in the upper portion of the nose can derive from the anterior and posterior ethmoid arteries that are part of the internal carotid system. These arteries usually bleed because of nasal trauma or hypertension. The main contributor to the blood supply of the lower half of the nose is the sphenopalatine branch of the internal maxillary artery and anteriorly the facial artery. Both these arteries are part of the external carotid system. The internal and external carotid systems are depicted in Figure 33.14. In the past, ligation of the external carotid artery was popular. Recent techniques for ligation of the internal max-

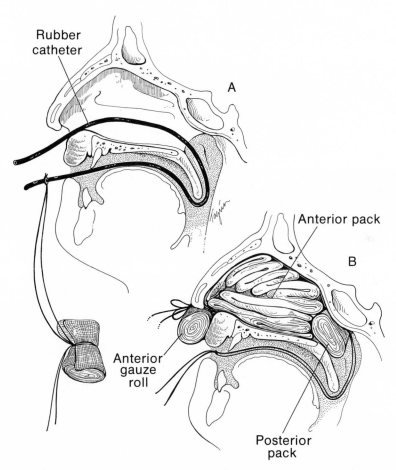

Figure 33.13. Insertion of posterior nasal pack. **(A)** Soft rubber catheter is in place with pack attached to it by silk suture material. **(B)** Pack has been guided into nasopharynx by means of digital manipulation and traction on suture material. Anterior pack is placed and suture material from the naris is tied in a bow around a gauze roll.

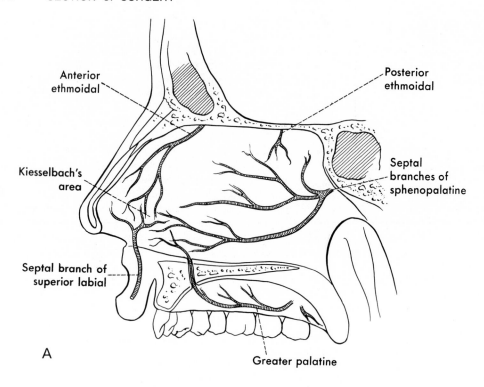

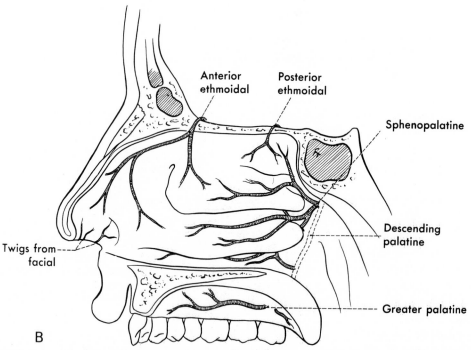

Figure 33.14. **(A)** Blood supply to nasal septum. Kiesselbach's area is most common site of epistaxis. Bleeding in this area can be controlled with cautery or nasal packing or both. **(B)** Blood supply to lateral nasal wall. The ethmoidal arteries are branches of internal carotid system; the others are branches of external carotid system. (Reproduced by permission, from Hollinshead WH: *Anatomy for Surgeons*, vol. 1. Hagerstown, Md, Hoeber-Harper, 1954.)

illary artery through the Caldwell-Luc approach and the anterior ethmoid artery through an external approach are more effective. A decision to perform arterial ligation should be made by an otolaryngologist.

Pain

Furuncle

This diagnosis can be suspected in a patient with a short history of inflammation and tenderness around the nasal tip with no specific causative factors. The physician may detect erythema, swelling, and tenderness in this area, and may see an obvious furuncle sometimes covered with dried pus within the nostril.

Treatment includes warm moist soaks, frequently applied, and intranasal antibiotic ointment. Systemic antibiotics specifically directed at resistant staphylococci should also be given. No attempt should be made at surgical drainage; since the facial veins that drain this area are valveless and communicate directly to the cavernous sinus, excessive manipulation of the infected area should be avoided to prevent septic thrombosis of the cavernous sinus.

Nasal Vestibulitis

A chronic recurrent problem, this may be a reflection of poor nasal hygiene, sinus infection, adenoid infection, or diabetes mellitus. On examination the tip of the nose is usually tender and sometimes inflamed. Folliculitis of the vibrissae can be visualized. Treatment consists of frequent cleansing of the nose with a dilute solution of hydrogen peroxide or soap and water with application of a local antibiotic ointment two or three times a day. The patient should be advised that this can be a chronic problem, and can be somewhat resistant to therapy. In a patient with no apparent underlying disease, a screening test for diabetes is recommended.

Uncommon Causes

Nasal pain may be caused by a herpes simplex infection or by herpes zoster of the maxillary nerve. Lupus vulgaris may produce pain, as may the gumma of tertiary syphilis. Primary syphilitic chancre of the nose is rare.

Trauma

Simple Fracture

The traumatic event causing fracture is usually obvious. All varieties of depression and lateral displacement of the nose can be seen with simple nasal fractures. In a more severe fracture, immediate swelling and ecchymosis are obvious, but in a milder fracture, displacement of the nose may occur without significant swelling. Fracture may be accompanied by epistaxis and deviation of the nasal septum. Careful examination of the nasal septum should be performed to exclude a septal hematoma, which is typified by soft, fluctuant swelling. Deviation of the nasal septum without hematoma should also be noted. The examiner should always search for CSF rhinorrhea and significant injury to the cervical spine or airway. Radiologic evaluation is not helpful in the management of a patient with a minor fracture. In the case of severe trauma, x-ray views should be taken to exclude accompanying fractures of other facial bones.

In the case of minor fractures and minimal swelling, reduction of the fracture may be immediate or it may be deferred from 4–7 days. Reduction should be deferred if there is significant soft-tissue edema. This procedure is indicated for cosmetic reasons and for functional improvement of the airway.

Nasal reduction is performed under local anesthesia in the emergency ward. The patient with stable vital signs should be sedated with intramuscular or intravenous meperidine hydrochloride. Both sides of the nose should be packed with gauze soaked in a 4% cocaine or a 2% tetracaine hydrochloride solution for 15–20 minutes. Since it is difficult to obtain anesthesia high in the nose, it is sometimes helpful to remove the initial anesthesia packs after 10 minutes and to replace them with a second set high in the vault of the nose. This may be supplemented with bilateral submucosal infiltration of lidocaine high in the nasal septum. An infraorbital nerve block (see Fig. 29.3) is accomplished by infiltration of 1% lidocaine with epinephrine (1:100,000), and field block anesthesia is gained by infiltration of these agents across the glabellar region and the base of the columella. When anesthesia is complete, reduction may be accomplished by means of a straight blunt elevator placed no further up in the nose than a line drawn between the medial canthi of the eyes. The level can be ascertained by laying the elevator on the side of the nose with the tip next to the medial canthus and grasping it at the level of the nares. If the grip is maintained at this point throughout the procedure, the elevator will not be inserted too far and will not endanger the cribriform plate. The fracture is then reduced by placing the elevator within the nasal cavity, gently raising the nasal framework anteriorly to disimpact the fragments, and manipulating the fractured nasal bone back into the midline. If significant epistaxis occurs, the nose may have to be packed, although epistaxis will often cease after approximately 10 minutes. Splinting a nasal fracture with plaster or a disposable nasal splint is helpful for the first week.

Septal Hematoma and Abscess

Hematoma of the septum is uncommon. It will be overlooked if intranasal examination is not performed in cases of nasal fracture. A soft widening of the nasal septum, septal hematoma should be treated after 1% lidocaine anesthesia by making a 1-inch incision in the inferior aspect of the hematoma for drainage. A small Penrose drain can be placed in the hematoma. An anterior pack of petrolatum gauze should be inserted in the nostril to compress the flaps of the hematoma, and the patient should be referred to an otolaryngologist.

An untreated septal hematoma may become infected, and painful swelling of the nose may appear several days after a nasal fracture. Since infection can destroy the nasal septal cartilage, producing a nasal saddle deformity, and since it can progress to septic thrombosis of the cavernous sinus, it should be treated by immediate incision and drainage with culture of the abscess. Until culture reports are available, penicillinase-resistant antistaphylococcal antibiotics are administered.

Acute Cerebrospinal Fluid Rhinorrhea

This condition is usually related to facial trauma, although it may be spontaneous. Trauma to the middle of the face that appears to have caused only a simple nasal fracture may have also caused a fracture of the cribriform plate that is signaled by CSF rhinorrhea. Massive trauma to the middle and upper face should make the physician suspect CSF leakage, even though it may not be readily apparent because of bleeding. CSF rhinorrhea can also occur via the Eustachian tube after a temporal bone fracture. In spontaneous rhinorrhea, the patient is aware of discharge of clear watery fluid with a salty taste usually from one nostril but sometimes from both. Leakage may be associated with the dependent head position.

On inspection, spontaneous rhinorrhea is evident as a clear, watery nasal discharge. In a patient with midfacial trauma, subcutaneous emphysema of the eyelids implies fracture of the ethmoid complex and should heighten suspicion of cribriform plate injury and associated CSF leakage.

Bloody nasal drainage can be tested by placing a drop on a white cloth; if CSF is mixed with the blood, a double ring will develop, a paler outer ring and a darker inner ring, since CSF diffuses more rapidly than blood and serum. The clear drainage from the nose should be tested for glucose content.

Patients with spontaneous CSF rhinorrhea should be hospitalized for thorough radiologic evaluation of the facial bones and fluorescein dye studies of the CSF to determine the location of the leak. Prophylactic administration of antibiotics is recommended, along with constant elevation of the patient's head. Traumatic CSF rhinorrhea often ceases when the fractures are reduced; this should be accomplished when the patient's general condition permits. An otolaryngologist and a neurosurgeon should be consulted.

Acutely Deviated Nasal Septum

The nasal septum may be displaced by blunt trauma from below or in front of the nose. While reducing a nasal fracture under local anesthesia, the physician may be able to shift the septum back into a midline position, but this is usually difficult. We recommend consulting an otolaryngologist for consideration of an immediate operative procedure to repair this injury.

Discharge and Obstruction

Common Cold

Ordinarily, a cold has four stages, a description of which follows:

(1) Prodrome: This is characterized by a hot, dry, or tickling intranasal sensation with a widely patent nose, lasting a few hours.

(2) Initiative: As the viral infection spreads from the portal of entry to affect the adjacent mucous membranes, the nose becomes obstructed, with associated sneezing and watery rhinorrhea. The patient may have a sore throat with a low-grade fever. This persists for 2–5 days.

(3) Secondary infection: After 3–5 days, bacterial superinfection may take place, heralded by increased mucopurulent nasal discharge and signs of systemic illness.

(4) Resolution: A mild cold clears in a few days; when bacterial superinfection occurs, resolution may take 5–10 days, depending on the effectiveness of therapy.

A patient with the first stages of a cold usually has a nasal discharge and a low-grade fever, with minimal clinical findings. Bacterial superinfection causes a rise in temperature, sinus tenderness, mucopurulent nasal discharge, erythema of the throat, and regional lymphadenopathy. The symptoms of allergic rhinitis, vasomotor rhinitis, and rhinitis medicamentosa may all be confused with those of the initial stages of a cold. These conditions are discussed in the following sections.

There is no specific therapy for a cold; symptomatic treatment should be adjusted to the age and general medical condition of the patient. Bed rest aids the resolution of systemic symptoms, and humidification of inspired air (50%) at 65°F (18.3°C) is recommended. Antihistamines and vasoconstrictive agents aid in relief of symptoms and may prevent the complications of sinusitis and otitis media. Nasal drops containing phenylephrine hydrochloride or oxymetazoline hydrochloride may be employed, but the patient should be warned not to use them beyond 1 week. Salicylates help reduce fever and associated malaise. Antibiotics should not be administered in the initial stages of a cold. If bacterial superinfection occurs, however, administration of penicillin or erythromycin for 7 days speeds recovery. Ascorbic acid has been recommended in the treatment of colds, but its value is debatable.

Allergic and Vasomotor Rhinitis

It is sometimes difficult to differentiate between these two forms of irritative nasal reaction.

Allergy. In the classic situation, a patient with this condition has nasal irritation, itch, and obstruction, with paroxysmal sneezing and copious watery rhinorrhea. Episodes are usually seasonal, being exacerbated in the spring or fall or both, whenever the pollen of allergenic plants is prevalent. The patient may have a strong family history of hay fever or asthma. On examination the patient may have a watery nasal discharge and pale, swollen nasal mucosa. Often the conjunctivae are red, associated with increased lacrimation. Auscultation of the chest may disclose wheezing breath sounds.

Similar, usually milder, symptoms may be due to perennial allergens, most commonly foods in children and inhalants, such as dust and molds, in adults. Common food allergens are milk, wheat, chocolate, eggs, fish, and citrus fruits. Common drugs that may produce an allergic reaction include salicylates, iodides, quinidine, sulfonamide compounds, and penicillins. Bacterial allergens include staphylococci, pneumococci, and streptococci.

In a patient with acute allergic rhinitis, the systemic antihistamine chlorpheniramine maleate, 4 mg every 6 hours, and dexamethasone sodium phosphate spray (Turbinaire Decadron Phosphate), one or two sprays three times a day, will usually control symptoms. The patient should be referred to an allergist or otolaryngologist for evaluation.

Vasomotor Rhinitis. The patient may complain of any combination of nasal obstruction, discharge, postnasal drip, sneezing, facial pain, malaise, and fatigue. Physical examination may reveal massive engorgement of the turbinates with watery discharge, or the nasal passages may be widely patent. In treating this condition the physician must remember that many factors may alter the patency of the nasal airway. One major factor is excessive tone of the parasympathetic nervous system caused by the following agents or states:

(1) psychologic disturbance, usually depression.

(2) endocrine disorder, which may be related to menstruation, pregnancy, or the use of oral contraceptives.

(3) hypotensive drugs, such as methyldopa, reserpine, guanethidine sulfate, and rauwolfia, which prevent peripheral release of adrenalin.

(4) physical changes, such as temperature and humidity fluctuations.

This condition is nonemergent, and the patient should be so informed and referred to an otolaryngologist for further workup. The emergency physician should question the patient regarding hypertensive medications and psychologic history, since referral to an internist or a psychiatrist might be more appropriate.

Rhinitis Medicamentosa

One of the most common causes of severe nasal obstruction is habitual use of nasal drops. Since the drops are effective for only a few minutes or hours with habitual use, they are applied more frequently. It is virtually impossible for the examiner to see beyond the tips of the inferior turbinates in these patients because of swelling. A patient with this condition should be referred to an otolaryngologist for a thorough nasal examination to exclude any underlying nasal problems and for therapy, including topical and systemic corticosteroid agents.

Foreign Bodies

A foreign body in the nose is a common problem among young children. Ordinarily, the child is brought in immediately after placing a foreign body in the nose. A child with a foul-smelling discharge from one nostril should be suspected of having a chronically impacted foreign body. In the acute case, the foreign body can usually be seen when the nose is inspected with a speculum and head light. If the examiner is unfamiliar with the use of these instruments and is uncomfortable performing intranasal manipulations, the patient should be referred to an otolaryngologist.

Most foreign bodies can be removed in the emergency ward, but if previous manipulations have caused swelling and bleeding, removal becomes more difficult, sometimes requiring general anesthesia. Solid objects may be removed in the emergency ward with a bayonet forceps or a metal (Frazier) suction tip shod with rubber tubing over the tip. Before removal, 0.5% or 1.0% phenylephrine hydrochloride drops should be instilled to shrink the nasal mucosa, and the patient should be instructed to blow out the foreign body if possible. The physician must avoid posterior displacement of the foreign body into the nasopharynx and thence into the upper part of the airway, causing obstruction.

Other Causes

Patients with *chronic granulomatous disease* may have a history of blood-tinged or clear nasal discharge, unilateral or bilateral nasal obstruction, and symptoms of sinusitis. Physical examination reveals granulomatous lesions in the nasal cavity and sometimes perforation of the nasal septum. In the advanced case, total destruction of the nose may take place, along with involvement of the palate and ear. The diseases included in this group are Wegener's granulomatosis (a triad involving the respiratory tract, the genitourinary tract, and generalized vasculitis) and lethal midline granuloma, a neoplasm of lymphoreticular cells that generally has a better prognosis than Wegener's granulomatosis. Clinical evaluation should include x-ray films of the nasal cavities, sinuses, and chest and renal function tests. A biopsy of the intranasal tissue aids in diagnosis. Wegener's granulomatosis is usually treated with corticosteroids and with cytotoxic and immunosuppressive drugs. Lethal midline granuloma is sometimes treated with local irradiation.

In a chronically ill and debilitated patient, especially one with uncontrolled diabetes, *fungal infections of the nose and sinuses* such as mucormycosis may cause nasal obstruction. Treatment consists of identification of the fungus and administration of appropriate systemic antifungal drugs, along with débridement of the nose and sinuses.

Syphilitic lesions rarely cause nasal discharge. Although acquired syphilis rarely affects the nose, gummata can occur in this area. Congenital syphilis also can cause nasal obstruction and discharge.

Obstruction

Nasal obstruction can result from swollen membranes due to such previously described conditions as the common cold, allergy, rhinitis medicamentosa, and chronic granulomatous disease. Traumatic events causing obstruction, such as acutely deviated septum, septal hematoma or abscess, and foreign body, have been discussed. Anatomic defects causing obstruction include deviated septum, intranasal scars, adenoid hypertrophy, nasal polyps, and tumors. Patients with the first two conditions should be referred to an otolaryngologist for repair of the septum or lysis of scar tissue.

Adenoid hypertrophy is probably the most common cause of nasal obstruction in children. The patient should be evaluated by an otolaryngologist. *Nasal polyps* resulting from allergic rhinosinusitis appear as boggy, grape-like intranasal masses and are almost always bilateral. In a child with nasal polyps, a workup for cystic fibrosis should be carried out. If nasal polyps are unilateral, the diagnosis of encephalocele should be considered. Dexamethasone sodium phosphate is often effective in shrinking polyps; two sprays are administered three times a day for 2–3 weeks. The patient should be referred to an otolaryngologist. Any form of epithelial or mesenchymal *tumor* can obstruct the nose. The tumors typically found in the nose include juvenile angiofibroma, olfactory neuroblastoma, lymphoepithelioma, and squamous cell carcinoma.

An unusual atrophic change of the nasal mucosa, *atrophic rhinitis* causes the patient to feel that he cannot breathe through the nose, although the nasal airway is widely patent. Physical examination reveals intranasal crusting and marked atrophy of the nasal mucosa. The patient may gain symptomatic relief by means of nasal irrigation with physiologic saline solution twice a day using a soft rubber bulb syringe. The patient should be referred to an otolaryngologist.

THE THROAT

Trauma

Oropharynx

Laceration. Treatment of lacerations of the lip and cheek is discussed in Chapter 29, pages 648–650. Most lacerations of the *tongue* can be closed loosely in one or two layers with absorbable suture material. Since the tongue is very vascular, questionably viable flaps of tissue should be preserved in hope that they will survive. Lacerations in the *floor of the mouth* may involve the lingual nerve or the submaxillary duct or both. The integrity of the submaxillary duct can be established by a lacrimal probe. Since the lingual nerve supplies sensation to the anterior portion of the tongue, simple testing of sensation can establish its continuity. Most of these lacerations, unless they are extensive, should not be sutured, because they will close better by granulation with less likelihood of abscess formation. If a laceration of the floor of the mouth is sutured, however, care should be taken not to suture through or around the duct or the nerve, and tight closure is contraindicated.

Most injuries of the *hard palate* occur in children who fall with a stick in the mouth. Small tears and flaps close well without operative intervention. The patient and family should be instructed to wash the mouth out with warm water or dilute hydrogen peroxide solution after each meal, and the wound should be closely observed until it has healed. Large tears and flaps should be closed under general anesthesia with absorbable suture material in a loose fashion to prevent abscess formation. Any penetrating wound in the region of the *tonsillar fossa* is potentially dangerous. There have been reports of internal carotid arterial thrombosis with hemiplegia and death following blunt trauma in this area. Optimal treatment for these patients is hospitalization for 48–72 hours. Careful neurologic evaluation and observation for the development of unilateral pupil dilation, hemiplegia, or obtundation is necessary. Signs of unilateral neurologic deterioration warrant arteriographic evaluation and appropriate vascular operation.

Burns. Thermal and chemical burns of the oropharynx, upper airway, and esophagus are treated in Chapter 22.

Larynx and Trachea

A moderate injury may result from a blow by a fist or hockey stick. Recently, use of motorcycles and snowmobiles has accounted for increasing numbers of "clothesline" injuries—direct trauma to the laryngotracheal complex caused by striking an unseen wire fence. Symptoms include varying degrees of hoarseness, airway obstruction, dysphonia, dysphagia, and localized pain and swelling. Significant laryngeal trauma is often overlooked in a patient with severe multiple injuries who has undergone early tracheotomy because of airway obstruction and whose other problems demand immediate attention.

On physical examination (Fig. 33.15A), a patient with a minor laryngeal injury is hoarse with no stridor and with moderate pain on swallowing or speaking. Examination of the neck may reveal either a normal laryngeal contour or perhaps a palpable fracture of the laryngeal cartilage. There may be tenderness and subcutaneous emphysema in the neck. Anteroposterior and lateral x-ray films of the neck should be requested (Fig. 33.15 B and C) and an otolaryngologist should be consulted. Signs of more significant injury include contusions or open lacerations of the neck, subcutaneous emphysema, progressive airway obstruction, loss of voice, and loss of laryngeal contour. Subcutaneous emphysema signifies air leakage, implying rupture of the laryngeal or tracheal cartilage and mucosal tears. Complete laryngotracheal transection can occur without an open wound on the neck.

A patient with a history of severe laryngotracheal trauma should be evaluated for the possibility of cervical spine injury and cervical esophageal tears. In an unconscious patient with multiple injuries including airway obstruction, careful evaluation of possible laryngeal injury is essential. At the time of initial tracheotomy the thyroid cartilage and cricoid cartilage should be closely examined. If there is any suggestion of significant laryngeal injury, an otolaryngologist should be consulted regarding the timing of endoscopy to assess the extent of injury and to determine whether it requires operative repair. The endoscopist should proceed with extreme caution so that loose fragments of cartilage are not detached from their blood supply.

In minor to moderate injuries, the patient must be observed over 48 hours for progressive airway obstruction. Hematoma, mucosal edema, vocal cord paralysis, and anatomic derangement all contribute to this complication. During observation, systemic corticosteroids should be administered, 20 mg of prednisone every 8 hours. The patient should be in a high-humidity atmosphere, and heavy sedation should be avoided. Progressive hoarseness and stridor warrant tracheotomy, performed preferably under local anesthesia, because endotracheal intubation may further traumatize the larynx. In severe laryngotracheal trauma, early tracheotomy is essential. Long-term complications of laryngotracheal injuries include total aphonia, permanent obstruction of the airway, aspiration pneumonia, and laryngotracheoesophageal fistula. Many of these difficult sequelae may be minimized or prevented by early recognition and proper management of these injuries.

In summary, emergency management of a patient with laryngotracheal trauma consists of the following measures:

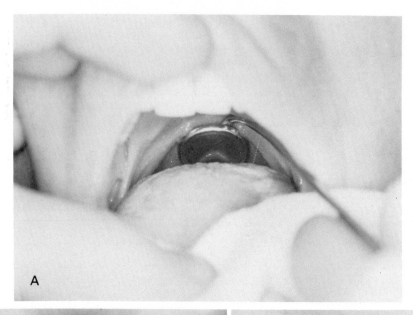

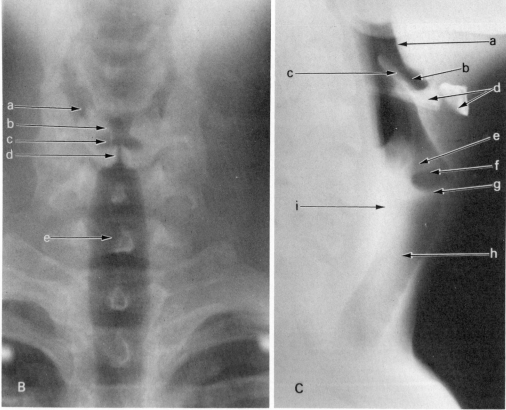

Figure 33.15. **(A)** Mirror examination of larynx. Mirror must be warmed with water or alcohol lamp to prevent fogging. Patient's tongue is held gently with gauze sponge and palate is depressed in posterosuperior direction by mirror (note that epiglottis is seen in mirror). **(B)** Anteroposterior soft-tissue x-ray view of normal airway during phonation (not a tomogram). *a*, Pyriform sinus; *b*, false cords; *c*, laryngeal ventricle; *d*, true cords; *e*, trachea. **(C)** Lateral soft-tissue x-ray view of normal airway. *a*, Base of tongue; *b*, vallecula; *c*, epiglottis; *d*, hyoid bone; *e*, area of false vocal cord; *f*, laryngeal ventricle; *g*, area of true vocal cord; *h*, trachea; *i*, retrocricoid area.

(1) Assure the patency of the airway, with tracheotomy if necessary.

(2) Protect the cervical spine.

(3) Request radiologic studies of the cervical spine and lateral and anteroposterior x-ray films of the neck.

(4) Consult an otolaryngologist as soon as possible.

(5) Administer antibiotics and corticosteroids.

(6) Avoid endoscopy or endotracheal intubation.

(7) Prescribe parenteral rather than oral nutrition.

(8) Perform corrective operation for laryngotracheal damage as early as the general status of the patient permits.

Cervical Esophagus

A patient with either a penetrating neck injury or a blunt neck injury may have a tear of the cervical esophagus. In cases of penetrating trauma, leakage of saliva into the wound suggests a hypopharyngeal or esophageal tear. If the patient is awake, this diagnosis may be confirmed by having him swallow water colored with methylene blue and observing the wound. A barium swallow with a small amount of barium can be performed to evaluate the possibility of a tracheoesophageal fistula. Endoscopic examination should be considered if the patient's condition is stable.

A patient with a suspected tear of the cervical esophagus should be hospitalized and oral alimentation should be discontinued. The wound should be treated with absorbent gauze dressings and prophylactic antibiotics should be instituted. If no other major structures of the neck are injured, and if a small tear less than 0.5 cm in length is noted on endoscopic examination, the lesion can be treated expectantly, since it will probably close spontaneously. Larger tears should be sutured during a transcervical exploratory operation, especially if the wound must be explored so that other structures can be repaired.

Acute Obstruction of the Airway

In most cases of acute obstruction, there is a clear-cut history suggesting foreign body, infection, or trauma. It is important to determine whether the patient has experienced stridor or hoarseness for a long period, since this implies a chronic infection, tumor, or other long-standing laryngeal problem.

In general, a patient with upper airway obstruction has stridor on inspiration. As obstruction progresses, suprasternal retraction, tachycardia, a panicky expression, and pallor develop. The immediate problem is hypoxia; a major complication is sudden cardiac arrest when hypoxia becomes extreme.

Tracheotomy

A physician treating a patient with acute upper airway obstruction should make every effort possible to secure an airway short of tracheotomy. A true emergency tracheotomy is a difficult and dangerous procedure, and endotracheal intubation is preferred if it is at all feasible. Three operative procedures can be utilized to obtain an airway: emergency cricothyrotomy, urgent tracheotomy, and elective tracheotomy.

Emergency Cricothyrotomy. This procedure is the fastest approach to the patient's airway. It is the procedure of choice when total and complete respiratory obstruction exists and if endotracheal intubation is impossible. Common indications for this procedure include foreign-body obstruction; facial or laryngotracheal trauma; inhalation, thermal, or caustic injury of the upper airway; angioneurotic edema; upper airway hemorrhage; epiglottitis; and croup.

The patient is placed supine with support under the shoulders and hyperextension of the neck. Usually anesthesia is either unnecessary or unavailable. The neck is palpated and the space between the thyroid and cricoid cartilages is identified. A skin incision, either vertical or horizontal, is made over the cricothyroid membrane, and the subcutaneous tissues are bluntly dissected to this level. A 1-cm horizontal incision is made between the cricoid and thyroid cartilages. Any flat instrument, such as the scalpel handle, is inserted in the incision and turned 90 degrees to hold the incision open. The incision can be kept open by the introduction of a small tube. As soon as the patient's condition is stable, this temporary airway should be replaced by a standard tracheotomy between the second and third tracheal rings.

Cricothyrotomy is an excellent method of securing an airway rapidly with minimal blood loss, but it risks significant damage to the laryngeal structures, the cricoid cartilage, the thyroid cartilage, and the vocal cords. This damage can result in chronic laryngeal stenosis with airway obstruction and hoarseness.

Emergency Tracheotomy. Emergency tracheotomy (Fig. 33.16) is performed on a patient with progressive airway obstruction in imminent danger of total obstruction. The physician must first consider endotracheal intubation; a decision for tracheotomy may be made if endotracheal intu-

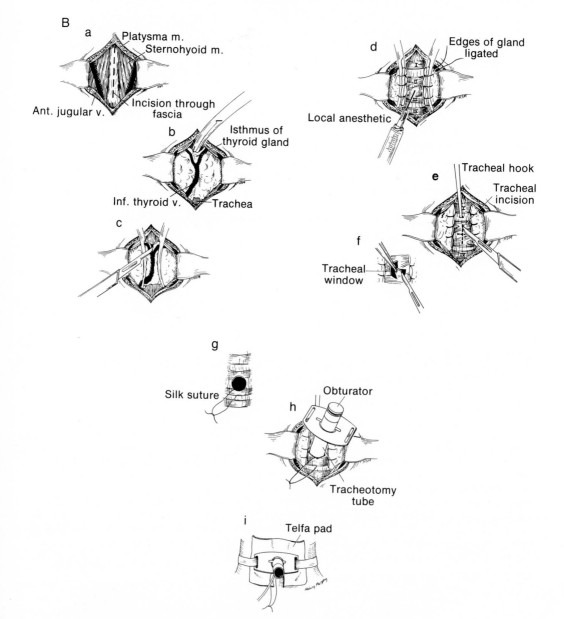

A

Common carotid a.
Ant. jugular v.
Isthmus of thyroid gland
Inf. thyroid v.

Hyoid bone
Thyroid cartilage
CRICOTHYROTOMY
Cricoid cartilage
Trachea
EMERGENCY TRACHEOTOMY

B

a
Platysma m.
Sternohyoid m.
Ant. jugular v.
Incision through fascia

b
Isthmus of thyroid gland
Inf. thyroid v.   Trachea

c

d
Edges of gland ligated
Local anesthetic

e
Tracheal hook
Tracheal incision

f
Tracheal window

g
Silk suture

h
Obturator
Tracheotomy tube

i
Telfa pad

bation equipment is unavailable or if distortion of the upper airway makes intubation unlikely to succeed. This procedure is often indicated in patients with obstructing tumors, traumatic injury, or infectious disease.

One or two experienced assistants facilitate this operation. The patient is placed supine with support under the shoulders if possible. Often the patient with respiratory obstruction is extremely apprehensive, agitated, and uncooperative; the operation may have to be performed with the patient in a semi-sitting position because total obstruction occurs when he lies down. This position increases the likelihood of an improper (high) placement of the tracheotomy. In an acutely obstructed infant, placement of an endotracheal tube or broncho-scope is essential before tracheotomy, since the trachea of an infant is extremely small and mobile, making it difficult to manage, especially during respiratory stridor.

The patient's neck is cleansed with an antiseptic solution and sterile drapes are applied if possible. The skin and subcutaneous tissues are infiltrated with 1% lidocaine with epinephrine (1:200,000). The surgeon palpates the thyroid and cricoid cartilages to avoid transection of the latter, and makes a vertical skin incision from just below the cricoid cartilage extending approximately 5 cm distally. A vertical incision is preferred since it directs dissection to the midline. The physician performs blunt dissection through the subcutaneous tissue and between the strap muscles, retracting them laterally and avoiding blood vessels wherever possible. Dissection should be performed beneath the full length of the incision so that a funnel-shaped wound is not created. The isthmus of the thyroid gland lies immediately beneath the strap muscles and is usually invested with numerous vessels. Although the thyroid gland often can be retracted inferiorly or superiorly without dividing it at the isthmus, division is necessary if the isthmus is

large, completely obstructing access to the trachea. The thyroid is divided by dissecting through the pretracheal fascia just above and below the isthmus and tunneling with a clamp in the anterior midline space between the thyroid and the trachea. Heavy clamps are then placed on either side of the isthmus and it is divided between them. Tracheotomy is completed before or after closing the two edges of the isthmus with a 2–0 chromic catgut purse-string suture.

The second and third tracheal rings should be identified and the tracheotomy should be performed through this area. Injection of 1–2 ml of 1% lidocaine into the tracheal lumen with a No. 25 needle minimizes coughing. The preferred method of fenestrating the trachea is partial excision of the anterior portions of the second and third or the third and fourth tracheal rings. The trachea is retracted superiorly by means of a tracheal hook inserted into the first or second interspace, a cruciate incision is made with a No. 15 knife blade with the intersection of the cuts at the interspace between the selected rings, and the resultant four corners of tracheal tissue are removed by ring punch-biopsy forceps or by sharp excision. Care must be taken to prevent aspiration of the small cartilaginous fragments. To minimize the danger of subsequent tracheal stenosis, no more than one-third of a tracheal ring should be excised.

A tracheotomy tube with a low-pressure cuff is then inserted with an obturator that is immediately removed after tube placement. The wound is lightly packed with petrolatum gauze, and the extremes of the incision are loosely closed around the tube with skin sutures. The tracheotomy tube is carefully secured with tapes tied around the neck, and a sterile dressing is applied to the tracheotomy wound.

A postoperative lateral x-ray film of the neck is advised to ensure proper positioning of the tracheotomy tube. Because pneumothorax can compli-

---

Figure 33.16. **(A)** Sites of incision for relief of airway obstruction. Major palpable landmarks are hyoid bone, notch of thyroid cartilage, and cricoid cartilage. Cricothyrotomy is performed by incision directly over cricothyroid membrane; vertical incision for emergency tracheotomy begins at or below cricoid cartilage. Potential for venous bleeding increases as dissection proceeds inferiorly, especially below thyroid isthmus. **(B)** Emergency tracheotomy. *a*, Skin and platysma are incised and the midline raphe is identified and incised. *b*, Thyroid gland is identified as strap muscles are retracted, tracheal fascia above and below thyroid isthmus is exposed if isthmus must be divided, and clamp is tunneled in midline between thyroid and trachea. *c*, Gland is divided between clamps. *d*, Free ends of thyroid gland are sutured and appropriate tracheal interspaces are infiltrated with local anesthetic. *e*, Tracheal hook is inserted to stabilize trachea, and cruciate incision is made. *f*, Circular opening is made just large enough to accommodate appropriate tracheotomy tube. *g*, Silk suture (2–0) with long ends is placed around lower tracheal ring to identify tracheal lumen should decannulation occur accidentally. *h*, Tracheotomy tube is inserted with obturator that is then replaced by inner cannula. *i*, Tube is secured, wound is loosely closed, and sterile dressing is applied. (Modified by permission, from Applebaum EL, Bruce DL: *Tracheal Intubation.* Philadelphia, W. B. Saunders Co., 1976.)

cate an emergency tracheotomy, especially in children in whom the apical pleura lies close to the trachea proximal to the clavicle, a postoperative chest x-ray film is also recommended.

Elective Tracheotomy. Elective tracheotomy is performed in the same fashion as emergency tracheotomy except that a transverse incision may be employed and an endotracheal tube is in place. There is also time for endoscopic examination to obtain specimens for culture and biopsy.

Postoperative Complications. Both immediate and late complications may arise after tracheotomy, as detailed in the following:

(1) Reflex apnea may occur as the patient's ventilatory status improves, since the central respiratory mechanism has been responding to hypoxia. Reflex apnea can be managed by mechanical ventilation until normal respiratory drive returns.

(2) Immediate surgical complications of tracheotomy include pneumothorax, bleeding from unrecognized vessels, and subcutaneous emphysema. Pneumothorax is corrected by insertion of chest tubes (see Chapter 22, pages 489–490). Bleeding can usually be controlled by packing the wound; if this fails, the wound should be explored to ligate the bleeding vessel. If the wound is packed too tightly, however, subcutaneous emphysema will result.

(3) The tracheotomy tube may become dislodged, usually because it is not well secured. If this happens in the first 48–72 hours, urgent reintubation or repeated tracheotomy may be required. After 3–4 days, the tube can be easily reinserted through the tracheotomy opening. The obturator should be taped to the patient's bed in case of this emergency.

(4) The tube may become occluded. To prevent accumulation of dried mucus crusts, the inner cannula is removed and cleansed with a pipe cleaner every 6 hours, after it is soaked in a hydrogen peroxide solution. Inspired air should be well humidified, since this also minimizes obstruction of the tube.

(5) Many of the long-term complications of tracheotomy can be prevented by an accurate and careful initial procedure. Postoperative stenosis of the trachea can result from excessive removal of cartilage, flaps of tracheal cartilage that fall into the lumen after the tube is removed, insertion of improperly sized tracheotomy tubes that curve into the anterior tracheal wall, and high-pressure tracheotomy cuffs. Infection at the tracheotomy site can cause late stenosis.

Infectious Disease

In general, management of the patient with acute infectious obstruction of the airway begins with evaluation of the cause of obstruction. One of the major diagnostic aids is the lateral x-ray view of the neck (Fig. 33.15C), which will demonstrate epiglottitis, retropharyngeal abscess, narrowing of the trachea from tracheitis, and laryngopyocele. The examiner should avoid instrumentation of the upper airway if possible, since gagging during introduction of a mirror may produce a sudden fatal respiratory arrest.

Acute Epiglottitis. This inflammatory condition is most common in children from 3–6 years old, but it can occur at any age. Symptoms include a rapidly progressing sore throat, painful swallowing, and dysphagia. Respiratory obstruction may arise within a few hours after the onset of symptoms. The patient leans forward to improve breathing, respirations are slow and stridorous, and the voice is muffled but not hoarse. The patient may be drooling because of painful swallowing.

Any effort to examine the intraoral structures may precipitate acute respiratory obstruction and should be avoided. A lateral x-ray film of the neck (Fig. 33.17) should confirm the diagnosis of acute epiglottitis without the need for intraoral examination.

Treatment consists of administration of high-dose corticosteroids, humidified oxygen, and antibiotics; ampicillin or chloramphenicol is preferred because of the possibility that *H. influenzae* is the infecting organism. In approximately 50% of cases, the disease is caused by a virus. Common bacterial organisms causing this problem include *H. influenzae*, staphylococcus, streptococcus, and pneumococcus. The patient should be closely observed; endotracheal intubation is indicated in any patient with signs of progressive obstruction or hypoxia.

Considerable debate exists over the necessity for tracheotomy in this situation. At present, most physicians prefer intensive medical therapy and intubation rather than tracheotomy. In the young child, treatment should be more aggressive and intubation should be performed at an earlier stage, preferably in the operating room under general anesthesia. The tube must be firmly secured in the young child to prevent accidental extubation. If tracheotomy is necessary, it should be performed with an endotracheal tube in place and with resection of a minimal amount of cartilage.

Croup. Formally termed acute laryngotracheo-

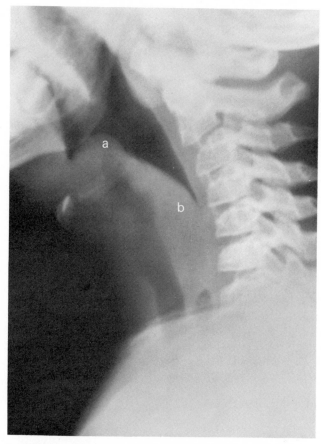

Figure 33.17. Lateral soft-tissue x-ray view of neck demonstrating epiglottitis. *a*, Edema of epiglottis; *b*, edema of arytenoid region and retrocricoid area.

bronchitis, croup is characterized by a barking cough and inspiratory-expiratory (biphasic) stridor. In temperate climates, attacks usually occur at night in the winter and spring. The typical patient is 6 months to 3 years old, and has had a mild upper respiratory tract infection for 1–3 days, often with a barking cough. Physical examination reveals the above symptoms and retractions, cyanosis, and tachycardia if obstruction has progressed.

In milder cases, the child is placed in a high-humidity atmosphere with oxygen (croup tent). Therapy also includes administration of ampicillin and corticosteroids, for example, dexamethasone, 1 mg/kg/day in four divided doses. In severe cases, 2.5% racemic epinephrine (microNEFRIN) has proved effective. This substance is diluted in sterile saline solution (1:4 or 1:8) and delivered by means of the nebulizer of an intermittent positive-pressure breathing apparatus. The treatment is repeated every 15 minutes for 1 hour; if this fails

to reverse the progress of obstruction, intubation and tracheotomy are advised.

Peritonsillar Abscess. Peritonsillar abscess usually occurs after a sore throat that has lasted 5–10 days. In many cases the patient has been treated with ineffective doses of penicillin or another antibiotic and begins to complain of increasing unilateral throat pain, dysphagia, trismus, and fever. The patient appears to be in acute pain, and has difficulty swallowing even saliva. Trismus may make examination of the mouth difficult, but once the patient opens his mouth, the physician may note a bulge in the superior pole of the tonsillar fossa, with displacement of the entire tonsil toward the midline. Edema of the tonsillar pillars and soft palate with displacement of the uvula away from the peritonsillar abscess may exist. Cervical lymphadenopathy and fever are often associated. This condition is frequently confused with peritonsillar cellulitis, and the examiner should determine whether there is true fluctuance in the superior pole of the tonsil, signifying an abscess. Aspiration with a large-bore needle should be performed prior to incision and drainage to prove the presence of purulent material, since aneurysmal swelling of the internal carotid artery can occur in this area.

If purulent material is present, incision across the superior pole will drain it. Penicillin should be administered intravenously, and the patient should be observed for development of respiratory obstruction. Untreated peritonsillar abscess often drains spontaneously, but the condition should be treated since deep neck infection, septic thrombosis of the internal jugular vein, and mediastinitis are potential complications. The patient should undergo tonsillectomy after the acute infection has resolved; we favor immediate tonsillectomy as definitive treatment for acute peritonsillar abscess.

Retropharyngeal Abscess. Unlike peritonsillar abscess, which is usually found in adults, retropharyngeal abscess most often occurs in children 3 years old or younger. Commonly there is a history of an upper respiratory tract infection that has worsened, with fever, tachycardia, drooling, dyspnea, stiff neck, and marked irritability. The patient appears ill on examination, holding the head rigidly and complaining of pain on moving the neck. Stridor is present in varying degrees. Oral examination demonstrates a bulge on the posterior pharyngeal wall, which should be confirmed by a lateral x-ray film of the neck (Fig. 33.18). In an adult, this condition results from a break in the mucosal surface of the pharynx caused by trauma, a foreign body, or rarely, osteomyelitis of the cervical spine.

The patient should be hospitalized for monitoring of respiratory status and administration of antibiotics. A drainage procedure should be performed under general anesthesia with the patient's head in a dependent position to prevent pooling of purulent material in the lower airway. An adenoidectomy is indicated at operation.

Laryngopyocele. Laryngocele, a herniation of the laryngeal ventricle, usually arises in patients whose profession involves creation of intensive pressures within the upper airway, for example, glassblowing or playing a wind instrument. A laryngocele can become infected during an upper respiratory tract infection, producing progressive hoarseness, thickening of the voice, and stridor. Speech and swallowing are painful. Indirect examination of the larynx with a mirror demonstrates unilateral edema and inflammatory changes. Anteroposterior and lateral views of the neck assist in making the diagnosis (Fig. 33.19).

Tracheotomy is mandatory, and is best performed with an endotracheal tube in place. If intubation is impossible, tracheotomy under local anesthesia may be extremely difficult; the patient may be reluctant to lie down to allow the procedure because of air hunger. After tracheotomy, the laryngopyocele should be drained externally by an otolaryngologist, and appropriate antibiotics should be given.

Foreign Bodies

Aspiration of foreign bodies occurs most frequently in young children. Some symptoms of respiratory obstruction caused by a foreign body are wheezing, coughing, stridor, salivation, and inability to swallow; the parents may or may not be aware of the cause. On examination the child may have signs of acute respiratory obstruction or he may be sitting quietly with wheezing audible only on auscultation. Examination should include inspection of the oral cavity and evaluation of the hypopharynx and larynx with a mirror if possible. Auscultation of the chest may demonstrate localized consolidation or obstruction. Anteroposterior and lateral x-ray views of the neck and chest may reveal a foreign body; fluoroscopic pulmonary examination may show mediastinal shift or air trapped in one lung, and bronchograms may be helpful.

The adult with a foreign body in the upper part of the airway can often describe it and identify its level reasonably accurately. Common lodging sites include the tonsil, the base of the tongue, the posterior pharyngeal wall, the vallecula, the larynx, and the cricopharyngeus muscle. A foreign body at the tonsil or at the base of the tongue can be seen on direct inspection; pharyngeal and laryngeal foreign bodies can be seen on examination with a mirror or can be located by means of anteroposterior and lateral films of the neck. A tracheobronchial foreign body may be outlined by chest x-ray film or fluoroscopic study.

Acute total obstruction of the airway may be managed by performing the Heimlich maneuver as detailed in Chapter 22, page 487. Cricothyrotomy is necessary if this fails to dislodge the object. Often, a patient with acute obstruction has died before arrival at the emergency ward; if he has survived, there is usually time for an orderly evaluation. No attempts should be made to remove a foreign body with the fingertips, since this may only move it distally. Once the object is located by history or radiologic evaluation, endoscopic removal is indicated. Occasionally, an object at the tonsil or base of the tongue may be removed directly with forceps.

Tumor

A patient with a laryngeal tumor has progressive respiratory obstruction over weeks to months, with

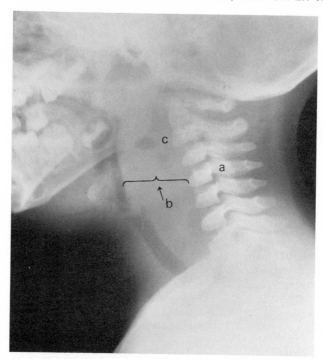

Figure 33.18.   Lateral soft-tissue x-ray view of neck demonstrating retropharyngeal abscess. *a*, Straightening of cervical spine; *b*, increase in distance between posterior pharyngeal wall and vertebral column; *c*, gas pocket within abscess.

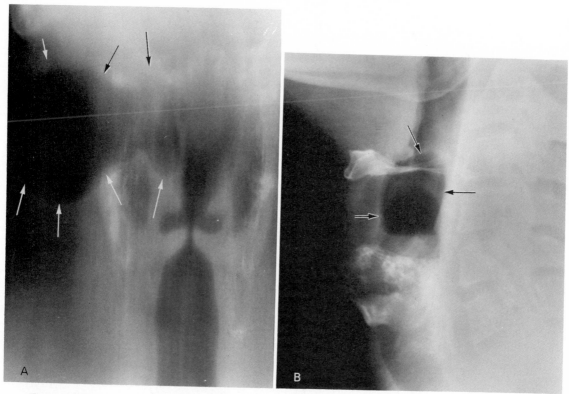

Figure 33.19.   Laryngocele. **(A)** Anterior tomographic view of neck. *Arrows* indicate margins of sac. **(B)** Lateral soft-tissue x-ray view. *Arrows* demarcate border of sac.

associated symptoms of dysphagia, hoarseness, and pain in the throat and the ear. Respiratory stridor may be evident, and the tumor may be visible on direct or mirror examination. Cervical lymphadenopathy may be apparent if the tumor has metastasized. Lateral x-ray views of the neck may show soft-tissue shadows in the airway. The patient should be referred to an otolaryngologist for urgent evaluation and for consideration of immediate tracheotomy if severe dyspnea exists.

Conditions in the Newborn

Incomplete development of the laryngeal cartilaginous framework (laryngomalacia) is the most common cause of noninfectious respiratory stridor in the neonatal period. The infant usually has no stridor when he is upright or prone, but it develops when he is supine. This phenomenon results from collapse of the supraglottic airway with negative inspiratory pressure. Since the condition disappears by the time the child is 1–2 years old as the cartilaginous structures harden, it is treated expectantly.

Many rare conditions cause stridor in the newborn. These include laryngeal papillomatosis, massive enlargement of the adenoids and tonsils, craniofacial anomalies, abnormalities of the aortic arch, and hemangiomas of the subglottic region. They all require the attention of a specialist.

Acute Sore Throat

Many of the conditions discussed in the following sections are indistinguishable on clinical grounds. In general, the more severe the symptoms and physical findings—erythema, edema, and exudate, for example—the more likely it is that the infecting organisms are group A β-hemolytic streptococci. Milder symptoms and findings suggest viral disease, although the possibility of streptococcal infection still exists.

Viral Infection

Coxsackie virus A, *adenoviruses*, and *the influenza and parainfluenza viruses* cause rhinitis, cough, and a mild sore throat with hoarseness and malaise. On physical examination the throat is mildly inflamed and erythematous, without exudate, although Coxsackie virus A may cause herpangina with pharyngeal vesicles or ulcers. There is a low-grade fever, and laboratory findings are consistent with viral infection. Treatment is directed toward symptomatic relief.

Patients with *herpetic infections of the oral mucosa* have severe pain. On physical examination, mucosal vesicles with an erythematous base and regional lymphadenopathy can be seen. Treatment includes narcotic analgesics if necessary and use of a dilute hydrogen peroxide mouthwash (3%) to maintain oral hygiene. Viscous lidocaine or triamcinolone acetonide in emollient dental paste (Kenalog in Orabase) may be applied to the lesions every 4 hours.

One of the manifestations of *infectious mononucleosis* is a sore throat. Others include fatigue, malaise, fever, dysphagia, and a diffuse rash. On physical examination the patient may exhibit pharyngotonsillitis with a gray exudate, marked cervical lymphadenopathy, fever, an enlarged liver or spleen, and rash. Laboratory findings include lymphocytosis with many atypical lymphocytes (up to 70%) and a positive test for mononucleosis. A culture of the throat exudate may show concomitant streptococcal infection. Emergency care consists of bed rest with a short course of corticosteroids, for example, prednisone, administered over 3 days in decreasing doses (60, 40, 20 mg). Penicillin should be given intravenously or intramuscularly along with analgesics and fluids.

Aphthous stomatitis, a condition of unknown cause, is manifested by a localized area of severe throat pain, and tends to recur. The patient will have a flat, well-demarcated mucosal ulcer up to 2 cm in diameter in the mouth or the pharynx without purulent exudate. The patient is afebrile, and laboratory findings are normal. The condition is treated in the same manner as herpetic lesions, with follow-up care until the lesion clears. If the lesion persists longer than 2–3 weeks, the physician should consider a diagnosis of chronic granulomatous disease, syphilis, or carcinoma.

Bacterial Infection

"Strep throat" caused by group A β-hemolytic streptococci is characterized by a rapid onset of sore throat and fever. Generalized rash, headache, nausea, and vomiting may be associated. When he appears in the emergency ward, the patient may have a fever, pharyngitis, or tonsillitis with exudate and regional lymphadenopathy. In the case of scarlet fever, the patient may have circumoral pallor, a strawberry-colored tongue, cutaneous rash, petechial rash of the palate, and an accentuated flexor crease of the elbow. Laboratory findings include granulocytosis and a throat culture positive for β-hemolytic streptococci. Therapy includes oral penicillin, 250 mg (400,000 units) three times a day for 10 days, or one injection of intramuscular benzathine penicillin G, 1.2 million units in adults, 600,000 units in children less than 6 years old, and 900,000 units in children from 6–9 years old.

Now reported only sporadically, *diphtheria* is typified by a mild to moderate slowly progressing sore throat, a mildly elevated temperature, anterior cervical lymphadenopathy, and progressive toxemia with nausea, vomiting, and headache. Physical examination discloses marked tachycardia, a temperature to 101°F (38.3°C), and an adherent gray membrane over the tonsils and the pharynx. The pharyngeal mucosa characteristically bleeds when it is rubbed with a culture swab and has a musty odor. Laboratory tests should include an immediate sputum smear for *Corynebacterium diphtheriae*. When the physician suspects diphtheria, he should isolate the patient and administer a skin test with diphtheria antitoxin to elicit an allergic reaction. If the skin test is negative, 20,000–30,000 units of diphtheria antitoxin should be administered intramuscularly as soon as possible. After all laboratory studies are done, penicillin should be administered.

The symptoms of *Vincent's angina* are a sore throat, painful gums, enlargement of the submaxillary and cervical lymph nodes, and a foul breath. The physician will detect a shaggy grayish membrane on the tonsils, palate, and gingivae that rubs off easily, with underlying bloody, granular, ulcerated tissue. The temperature is usually only minimally elevated. Gram stain reveals a mixed infection with fusiform bacilli and spirochetes. Therapy includes gargling with a 3% hydrogen peroxide solution and a 10-day course of penicillin, 250 mg four times a day.

Other Conditions

A *monilial pharyngeal inflammation* may be secondary to immunosuppression, leukemia, or an overgrowth after recent antibiotic or corticosteroid therapy. The pharyngeal mucosa exhibits erythema and white patches similar to curds of milk. Emergency care consists of nystatin (Mycostatin) oral suspension, 5 ml to be gargled and swallowed every 6 hours until 2 days after the last lesions disappear.

Bullous erythema multiforme is typified by a massive bullous eruption of the lips and the mucous membrane and the cutaneous lesions of erythema multiforme. The condition may be due either to an upper respiratory tract infection or to an allergic reaction to drugs. Although the illness is self-limited, systemic corticosteroids seem to hasten healing of the lesions.

Agranulocytosis and *acute leukemia* can both be manifested by acute sore throat and fever with pharyngeal exudate or membrane. The diagnosis is made by complete blood cell count and other signs of generalized disease, such as petechiae, ecchymoses, hepatosplenomegaly, and lymphadenopathy.

Thyroiditis may result in pain and tightness of the lower portion of the throat lasting for days to weeks. The pain may extend up the neck to the ear, and the patient will have fatigue and malaise. On examination the thyroid gland is tender and sometimes swollen. Laboratory findings include an elevated sedimentation rate and normal or elevated levels of triiodothyronine and thyroxine. The patient is treated with salicylates, 600 mg every 4 hours, local heat, and bed rest. He should be referred to an endocrinologist for the possibility of corticosteroid therapy.

THE NECK

Masses

For the purpose of differential diagnosis of neck masses, three areas may be defined (Fig. 33.20). Possible diagnoses for each area, divided into pediatric and adult age groups, are presented in Table 33.4. Any patient with a mass in the neck should be referred for thorough examination including indirect laryngoscopy and nasopharyngoscopy. Acutely infected lesions must be treated on an emergency basis.

Deep Infection

A deep neck infection is usually secondary to infection in one of three areas: a tooth, the pharynx, and the parotid gland. Often the patient has been taking antibiotics for tonsillitis or an infected dental extraction site. Signs of progression to deep infection include a high temperature, swelling and tenderness of the neck or the submaxillary space, trismus, pain on motion of the neck or tongue, and stridor. The physician should search for an obvious primary site of infection such as tonsillitis, peritonsillar abscess, infected tooth, dental extraction site, or parotitis. Antibiotics often mask obvious signs of sepsis.

In the submaxillary region, Ludwig's angina (see page 743) is the most common deep neck infection. Infection of the pharyngomaxillary space is commonly seen in children as an extension of tonsillitis or mastoid infection. Signs include trismus and swelling of the parotid region or the lateral pharyngeal wall or both. In the parotid space, signs of infection are swelling and marked tenderness over the parotid gland without trismus. The anterior part of the neck is usually infected after esophageal or hypopharyngeal trauma. Signs include tenderness along the sulcus between the sternocleidomastoid muscle and larynx, hoarseness, stridor, and dysphagia.

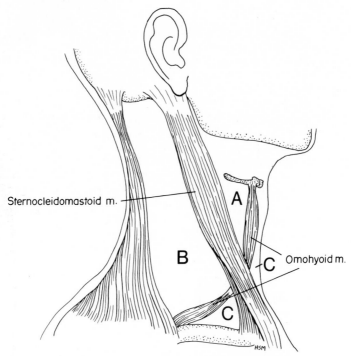

Figure 33.20.   Division of neck into three areas for differential diagnosis of neck masses (see Table 33.4).

Table 33.4.
Neck masses: possible diagnoses.

Zone[a]	Child	Adult
A	Branchial cyst Dermoid cyst Thyroglossal cyst Nonspecific lymphadenopathy Lymphoma Infectious disease (pharyngitis, dental abscess, tuberculosis, cat-scratch disease) Metastatic disease (rare)	Metastatic carcinoma from upper aerodigestive tract Primary tumor of parotid or submaxillary gland Inflammatory node (acute or chronic, including tuberculous) Zenker's diverticulum (rare) Laryngocele (rare) Carotid arterial aneurysm (rare) Chemodectoma (rare)
B	Infectious lymphadenopathy (pharynx, adenoids, scalp) Lymphoma Neurofibroma	Lymphoma Nasopharyngeal tumor Local skin infection Neurofibroma
C	Cystic hygroma Thyroid lesion Branchial cyst or sinus Lymphoma	Thyroid lesion Metastatic carcinoma (laryngeal, pulmonary, gastrointestinal) Aneurysm of the aorta or great vessels

[a]See Figure 33.20.

If the airway is compromised, intubation or emergency tracheotomy may be necessary. Anteroposterior and lateral x-ray films of the neck may aid in evaluation of the airway. Specimens should be taken from the primary site of infection for culture and from the blood if septicemia is apparent. Administration of fluid and high-dose antibiotics should begin and the patient should be hospitalized for intensive therapy and possible operative drainage. Antibiotics have decreased the incidence of customary infections, and at the same time have allowed the introduction of new pathogens. Streptococcus has given way to staphylococcus or mixed flora. Antibiotics should be selected to cover a wide range of pathogens, including penicillinase-producing staphylococcus and gram-negative organisms. The antibiotic regimen may be modified after results of culture and sensitivity tests. A short course of high-dose corticosteroids, such as prednisone, 60–80 mg/day for 3 days in an adult, may hasten the resolution of edema.

Trauma

Blunt Injury

Blunt trauma to the neck, especially the "clothesline" injury, can cause extensive damage to internal structures without breaking the skin. Potential injuries include complete laryngotracheal transection or lesser laryngeal fractures, esophageal tears, thrombotic occlusion of major vessels, contusion or stretching of the brachial plexus, and dislocation of the cervical spine.

On physical examination, abrasions and edema of the skin may make evaluation of the deeper structures more difficult. The contour of the laryngeal cartilage should be carefully palpated, and signs of disruption of the airway, such as hoarseness, stridor, hemoptysis, and subcutaneous emphysema, should be sought. Paraplegia or quadriplegia with sensory defects suggests trauma to the spinal cord, whereas hemiplegia, obtundation, or expanding hematoma suggests carotid injury. Treatment of blunt trauma to the neck is discussed on pages 753–755.

Penetrating Injury

High-velocity missiles and shot from a shotgun less than 20 feet away cause extensive tissue destruction. The wound is usually infected from foreign material such as particles of clothing, wadding, and shot. If the patient survives until arrival at the emergency ward, his life can probably be saved if hemorrhage can be controlled.

On examination the physician may observe either an ooze of dark blood suggesting venous laceration or a pulsatile flow of blood from a transected artery. A hematoma may be noted, which should be carefully observed for expansion or enlargement. The patient may be in hemorrhagic shock. Isolated neurologic defects can occur, reflecting injury to one or more nerves in the neck. Pulses should be palpated at the superficial temporal and carotid arteries to assist in diagnosis

of major vascular injury; the presence of pulses does not necessarily exclude the possibility of such an injury, however. An audible bruit also suggests significant vascular trauma.

As many as one-third of patients with a major vascular injury have no clinical evidence of it. Some physicians advise exploration of all transplatysmal injuries that are near vascular structures; we recommend this approach for injuries above the cricoid cartilage. However, we believe that injuries of the lower neck should be initially evaluated by means of arteriography. Patients with normal arteriographic results should be observed, and those with an obvious vascular lesion should undergo exploration with transthoracic proximal control of the bleeding vessels if necessary.

The first priority in the treatment of a penetrating injury is control of hemorrhage by compression of vessels against the cervical spine. Integrity of the airway must be assured, and the cervical spine should be immobilized until significant injury to it is excluded. Intravascular volume should be replaced by means of large-bore intravenous lines. The lines should not be placed distal to possible venous laceration.

Suggested Readings

Applebaum EL, Bruce DL: *Tracheal Intubation.* Philadelphia, WB Saunders, 1976

Ballenger JJ (Ed): *Diseases of the Nose, Throat, and Ear,* ed 11. Philadelphia, Lea & Febiger, 1969

Becker W, Buckingham RA, Holinger PH, et al: *Atlas of Otorhinolaryngology and Bronchoesophagology.* Philadelphia, WB Saunders, 1969

Boies LR: *Fundamentals of Otolaryngology: A Textbook of Ear, Nose and Throat Diseases,* ed 3. Philadelphia, WB Saunders, 1959

Bossy J: *Atlas of Neuroanatomy and Special Sense Organs.* Philadelphia, WB Saunders, 1970

Calcaterra TC, Holt GP: Carotid artery injuries. *Laryngoscope* 82:321–329, 1972

Chandler JR: Pathogenesis and treatment of facial paralysis due to malignant external otitis. *Ann Otol Rhinol Laryngol* 81:648–658, 1972

Converse JM, Kazanjian VH: *Surgical Treatment of Facial Injuries,* ed 3. Baltimore, Williams & Wilkins, 1974

DeWeese DD, Saunders WH: *Textbook of Otolaryngology,* ed 4. St. Louis, CV Mosby, 1973

Dowling JA, Foley FD, Moncrief JA: Chondritis in the burned ear. *Plast Reconstr Surg* 42:115–122, 1968

Ferguson CF, Kendig EL (Eds): *Pediatric Otolaryngology. Disorders of the Respiratory Tract in Children,* vol 2. Philadelphia, WB Saunders, 1972

Goodhill V, Harris I, Brockman SJ, et al: Sudden deafness and labyrinthine window ruptures. *Ann Otol Rhinol Laryngol* 82:2–12, 1973

Grant JCB: *Grant's Method of Anatomy: By Regions, Descriptive and Deductive,* ed 9. Baltimore, Williams & Wilkins, 1975

May M, West JW, Heeneman H, et al: Shotgun wounds to the

head and neck. *Arch Otolaryngol 98:*373–376, 1973

Montgomery WW: *Surgery of the Upper Respiratory System.* Philadelphia, Lea & Febiger, 1971 (vol 1), 1973 (vol 2)

Schuknecht HF: *Pathology of the Ear.* Cambridge, Harvard University Press, 1974

Sessions DG, Stallings JO, Mills WJ, Jr.: Frostbite of the ear. *Laryngoscope 81:*1223–1232, 1971

Shambaugh GE, Jr: *Surgery of the Ear.* ed 2. Philadelphia,

WB Saunders, 1967

Shanon E, Cohn D, Streifler M, et al: Penetrating injuries of the parapharyngeal space. *Arch Otolaryngol 96:*256–259, 1972

Valvassori GE (Ed): Symposium on radiology in otolaryngology. *Otolaryngol Clin North Am* 6 (no. 2), 1973

Wolfson RJ (Ed): Symposium on vertigo. *Otolaryngol Clin North Am* 6 (no. 1), 1973

CHAPTER 34

Ocular Emergencies

ALBERT R. FREDERICK, JR., M.D.
B. THOMAS HUTCHINSON, M.D.

Emergency ocular care, like combat surgery, may not always be optimal or definitive. There is often a confluence of serious problems that compete for attention and that require establishment of priorities. In addition, the instrumentation necessary to perform a detailed ophthalmic examination may not be available. In an ocular emergency, however, it is important to deliver the best care possible, since prompt, knowledgeable evaluation and treatment can drastically affect the patient's eventual ability to see; attention to the ocular status also can enable the physician to assess certain aspects of the patient's intracranial and general condition.

Limited space permits no more than a brief survey of emergency ocular conditions and their management. In each instance, the attending physician will have to assess his own competence in examination and treatment and to judge whether specialty or subspecialty consultation is necessary. The responsibility for discovering ocular injuries rests with the person who makes the initial evaluation; missed diagnoses frequently can be avoided by awareness of the spectrum of conditions affecting the eye and orbit. Readers desiring a fuller discussion of the topics covered are enthusiastically encouraged to read additional texts devoted to ocular emergencies.

EXAMINATION

Instrumentation

A minimum of equipment is required for competent examination by a nonophthalmic physician (Table 34.1).

Technique

Initial examination should include determination of visual acuity. For patients who cannot read the largest character on the vision chart, a notation of poor vision such as "finger counting at ____ ft," "hand motion," "light projection in ____ field," or "denies light perception" is preferred to "no vision." Confrontation field examination, status of orbits and lids, extraocular motor functions, anterior segments (conjunctiva, cornea, anterior chamber, iris, and pupil), media (lens and vitreous), and fundi (with mydriasis, when appropriate) should also be studied, and other specialized examinations as tonometry, exophthalmometry, and ophthalmodynamometry should be performed when indicated. Treatments to be avoided in specific situations are enumerated in Table 34.2.

After trauma, when the possibility of global rupture exists, examination must be performed under controlled conditions and with utmost care. Inadvertent pressure on a lacerated globe may result in expulsion of intraocular contents and loss of function of the eye. Necessary elements in examination of the eye and orbit after trauma are listed in Table 34.3. In some instances, as with irritating foreign bodies, the instillation of a topical anesthetic (proparacaine hydrochloride, 0.5%) increases patient cooperation. Children must be adequately restrained, and if an open wound of the eye is detected or suspected in either a child or an adult, evaluation must be made by an ophthalmologist with the patient under general anesthesia. If laceration of a lid is to be repaired in a young child under anesthesia it may be best to defer the remaining ocular examination until then. In lid and conjunctival lacerations, the physician must be aware of possible deeper penetration; the condition of the globe must be determined in the event of through-and-through laceration or puncture of the lid.

RAPID VISUAL LOSS

It is often difficult to evaluate visual loss occurring over the course of minutes to days. The

Table 34.1.
Required equipment for emergency ocular examination.

Vision chart
   Standard distance chart, preferably at 20 ft with adequately intense illumination of 100 footcandles, and near-card at 13 inches to be used with patient's reading glasses
Occluder and pinhole device (poor vision that improves significantly when patient looks through small-diameter perforation in occluder is usually due to refractive error)
Focal illuminator
Loupe or magnifying hood
Ophthalmoscope
Schiøtz tonometer
Lid retractors
Topical anesthetic (proparacaine hydrochloride, 0.5%)
Fluorescein (impregnated, sterile paper strips; do *not* use previously opened bottles of solution)
Mydriatic and cycloplegic drops (phenylephrine hydrochloride [Neo-Synephrine], 10%, and cyclopentolate hydrochloride, 1%)

physician should attempt to establish whether the loss occurred in one or both eyes by asking the patient whether he covered each eye alternately to determine which was involved. He should also establish the time span over which the loss occurred and the field in which the loss was noted; the patient may describe central blurring, distorted vision (metamorphopsia), the development of spots or "floaters," or the sensation of "a curtain coming down." Because of normally overlapping fields of vision, a visual deficit affecting one eye may be long-standing and unknown to the patient until something calls his attention to it; for example, he may close one eye to rub it or to aim a camera or gun. Assessment of the causes of this type of loss must be based on ophthalmoscopic examination. Except in patients with suspected intracranial injury or potential angle-closure glaucoma, there is seldom any reason not to dilate the pupils for adequate evaluation of the fundi, and both eyes should be examined comparatively. Alleged lack of light perception can be confirmed by absence of a consensual pupillary response when the suspected blind eye is stimulated with a bright light. Table 34.4 lists the more often encountered causes of acute visual loss.

Retinal Arterial Occlusion

Central, superior, or inferior visual field loss occurring painlessly and within minutes in an older patient suggests retinal arterial occlusion.

Funduscopic examination reveals a pale disc and a retinal change characterized by "milkiness," or loss of retinal transparency, due to intraretinal edema. This obscures details of the underlying choroidal vessels. Retinal change occurs in the distribution of the affected artery; if central vision is affected, a macular red spot is common. "Boxcar" segmentation of blood within vessels signifies stagnant blood. Occasionally at the bifurcation of a vessel or at the disc, an occluding embolic fragment can be identified. To be effective, treatment must enhance perfusion of the retinal arterioles immediately by decreasing the intraocular pressure or increasing the systemic arterial pressure or both. Intermittent massage, or ballottement of the globe, will soften the eye as well as offer an opportunity to dislodge an obstructing embolus at an arterial bifurcation by rapidly changing the intraocular-intravascular pressure-volume relationships. Exercising the patient will increase blood pressure, and having him breathe in a bag or breathe oxygen containing 5% carbon dioxide may encourage retinal arteriolar vasodilation. Intravenous administration of acetazolamide, 500 mg, and mannitol, 1.5 gm/kg of body weight, will aid in decreasing intraocular pressure; acute lowering can also be accomplished by paracentesis of the anterior chamber with a beveled incision through the peripheral cornea. However, few physicians who are not ophthalmologists are willing to attempt this maneuver.

Retinal Venous Occlusion

In central venous occlusion, vision becomes blurred less rapidly than in arterial occlusion, and the loss may be less profound. The disc margins are blurred, the veins are distended and tortuous, and retinal hemorrhages are present throughout the fundus (Table 34.5). Blockage occurs either within the nerve head or in the case of branch occlusion, at arteriovenous crossings where vessels share a common adventitia. Coincident open-angle glaucoma and hyperviscosity states such as polycythemia, leukemia, and macroglobulinemia should be ruled out. Treatment is controversial; anticoagulation sometimes is advised, but its usefulness is unproved. Frequently, an increase in retinal or systemic hemorrhage occurs following its institution; the gastrointestinal, genitourinary, and central nervous system may be affected.

Optic Neuritis

Loss of central acuity with a swollen, hemorrhagic optic disc and retrobulbar pain on movement of the globe suggests optic neuritis or papil-

Table 34.2.
Ocular emergencies and measures to avoid.

True emergencies (therapy should be instituted within *minutes*)
   Chemical burns of the cornea
   Central retinal arterial occlusion
Urgent situations (therapy should be instituted within 1 to several *hours*)
   Penetrating injuries of the globe
   Acute narrow-angle glaucoma (angle-closure)
   Pupillary block glaucoma (lens or vitreous incarcerated in pupil); lens in anterior chamber
   Orbital cellulitis/cavernous sinus thrombosis
   Corneal ulcer
   Gonococcal conjunctivitis
   Corneal foreign body
   Corneal abrasion
   Acute iritis and formation of synechiae
   Giant cell arteritis with acute ischemia of optic nerve
   Acute retinal tear with hemorrhage
   Acute retinal detachment
   Acute vitreous hemorrhage
   Descemetocele
   Hyphema
   Lid laceration
Semiurgent situations (therapy should be instituted within days whenever possible—or sometimes weeks)
   Optic neuritis
   Ocular tumor
   Exophthalmos
   Previously undiagnosed chronic simple glaucoma
   Old retinal detachment
   Strabismic or other remediable amblyopia
   Blow-out fracture of orbit
Measures to avoid
  1. Anesthetic ointments (too prolonged an effect; patient may inadvertently traumatize himself)
  2. Anesthetic drops or prescriptions to patient for outpatient use (patient may become addicted or may injure
     himself inadvertently; anesthetic delays or prevents corneal wound healing)
  3. Ointments of any kind:
    In the presence of penetrating trauma (ointment may gain access into the globe)
    When fundus examination will be required (view of fundus is mechanically obscured by ointment)
  4. Atropine for routine use (shorter-acting cycloplegics such as tropicamide or cyclopentolate are more
     desirable)
  5. Antibiotics if fungal overgrowth is a possibility, e.g., corneal abrasion from rosebush, corn husk, cow's tail
  6. Corticosteroids in any form if:
    Diagnosis is uncertain
    Fungal overgrowth or herpes simplex infection is likely

(From Paton D. Goldberg MF: *Injuries to the Eye, the Lids, and the Orbit.* Philadelphia, W. B. Saunders Company, 1968.)

litis. If no abnormality of the nerve head can be seen, the condition is called retrobulbar neuritis. Vision may be reduced only a few lines (to 20/30 or 20/40), or it may be profoundly depressed. There may be a history of previous episodes. Especially in patients between 20 and 40 years of age, multiple sclerosis may be the cause, and a detailed history in terms of episodic neurologic deficits is required. Attacks are self-limited, and vision usually improves. Although no proven therapy exists, some neuro-ophthalmologists recommend systemic administration of corticosteroids or adrenocorticotropic hormone. Toxic agents and intracranial lesions must be ruled out.

Vitreous Hemorrhage and Retinal Detachment

These conditions are properly considered together. A patient who reports light flashes followed by black spots, strands, or a "film" or who is aware of a "shadow" or "curtain" type of field defect must be examined to determine whether vitreous hemorrhage or retinal detachment or both are present. The most common ocular causes of vit-

Table 34.3.
Emergency ward procedure for evaluation of trauma affecting the orbit, lids, or eye.

1. Obtain history of previous eye disorders, type of chemical burn, or nature of injuring object, and history of tetanus immunization.
2. Render first aid in case of true emergency.
3. Determine visual acuity and screen visual fields by confrontation with test object.
4. Differentiate partly penetrating and completely penetrating (perforating) injuries of cornea and sclera. Use lid retractors. Note uveal, vitreal, or lenticular prolapse.
5. Note hemorrhages and infections of orbit, lids, or conjunctiva. Account for chemosis.
6. Investigate depth of all lid lacerations, noting fat in wound. Seek foreign bodies under lid; evert lid and sweep fornix with cotton swab after use of topical anesthetic.
7. Palpate orbital rim; feel for crepitus through lids; test facial and corneal sensation; auscultate for orbitocranial bruit.
8. Appraise real or apparent displacement of globe—anterior, posterior, or vertical. Use exophthalmometer.
9. Characterize diplopia by analysis of ocular ductions and versions; attempt forced duction test using forceps and topical anesthetic.
10. Record pupil shape, size, and reactions.
11. Inspect for hyphema, iridodonesis, and iridodialysis.
12. Examine cornea for opacities, ulcers, foreign bodies, rust rings, and abrasions (use fluorescein paper); avoid corticosteroid-containing medications.
13. Use loupe or slit lamp to detect foreign-body paths in cornea, iris, and lens.
14. Estimate comparative depths of anterior chambers for evaluation of intumescent cataract, displaced lens, and recessed chamber angle.
15. If traumatized globe is intact and cornea is undamaged, measure intraocular pressure with tonometer.
16. Ophthalmoscopic examination: Differentiate various types of intraocular hemorrhage. Record appearance of nerve head, macula, and retinal circulation. Visualize foreign bodies if possible.
17. Obtain x-ray films in all cases of possible retained foreign body in globe or orbit and whenever orbital fracture is conceivable.
18. Consider photographing all injuries.

(From Paton D, Goldberg MF: *Injuries to the Eye, the Lids, and the Orbit.* Philadelphia, W.B. Saunders Company, 1968.)

Table 34.4.
Common causes of rapid painless visual loss.

Vascular occlusion
  Central retinal artery
  Branch retinal artery (if macula is involved)
  Central or branch retinal vein
Optic neuritis
Vitreous hemorrhage
Retinal detachment
Macular hemorrhage or exudative macular detachment
Macular hole
Uveitis
Hysteria and malingering

reous hemorrhage are retinal tears, possibly with retinal detachment; posterior vitreous detachment; and neovascularization secondary to diabetes mellitus or old venous occlusion. Early referral of patients with vitreous hemorrhage is advised because of the high frequency of associated retinal tears or detachment. Such patients complain of sudden onset of floaters or black spots and variable visual loss, and examination shows loss of the red reflex.

A higher incidence of retinal detachment occurs among patients with myopia and in patients in whom cataracts have been removed. Detachment resulting from trauma constitutes a small percentage of cases. In the patient with a retinal tear or peripheral retinal detachment, subjective visual acuity may be normal until the detachment extends to the macula, and the field may be full. It is therefore necessary to perform careful ophthalmoscopic examination with a dilated pupil to establish whether either of these usually progressive but treatable conditions exists. If retinal detachment is present, the fundus appears gray and rippled or undulating, the retinal vessels are elevated and abnormally tortuous, and there is loss of the normal underlying choroidal pattern. If the macula is still attached, an ophthalmic emergency exists, since macular function may not be regained after its detachment even if the retina is reattached by operation. Prompt referral to an ophthalmologist for admission and bed rest is indicated until operation can be performed.

Since the entire retina can be scrutinized only by indirect ophthalmoscopic examination with scleral depression and since a significant pathologic condition can exist in an eye considered normal only after direct ophthalmoscopy, any patient with unexplained symptoms related to the posterior segment should be referred for ophthalmic evaluation.

Macular Disease

Painless, rapid, central visual loss, particularly in patients more than 50 years old, may be due to hemorrhagic or serous (exudative) macular disease. Usually, however, insidious loss of vision results from this degenerative process. Ophthalmoscopic examination reveals abnormal macular anatomy. In serous lesions, the foveal reflex is lost and the macular region of the retina is elevated. Yellow, drusen-like deposits are frequently seen in the opposite eye. In the past, these patients could not be treated. Patients with abnormal maculae with reduction of central vision should be referred to an ophthalmologist, since some types of macular lesions can now be successfully treated by laser photocoagulation. Nontraumatic macular hemorrhage may be seen in younger patients with myopia, hemorrhagic diathesis, or angioid streaks, or after marked exertion. Hemorrhagic detachment of the pigment epithelium presents as a grayish or reddish, solid-appearing lesion in the posterior pole. Blood may migrate into the subretinal space.

Posterior Uveitis

Inflammatory reaction of the posterior uveal tissues can result in hazy vision due to variable opacification of the vitreous by cells and proteinaceous outpouring. If the process is severe and if it directly affects the macula, useful central vision may be rapidly and irreparably lost. The fundus may be difficult to see, and thus the condition may be confused with vitreous hemorrhage. Yellowish-white patches in the choroid and retina are common. The cause of posterior uveitis often remains unknown even after exhaustive evaluation. Among the more common causes are toxoplasmosis and sarcoidosis. Histoplasmosis causes multifocal choroiditis that often produces a hemorrhagic lesion of the macula, but the vitreous remains clear. When the macula is threatened by inflammation, it may be justified, even in the absence of a specific cause, to begin therapy with high doses of prednisone, 100 mg/day initially, if no systemic or medical contraindication exists.

RED EYE

It is important to remember that the lids, conjunctivae, sclera, and uveal tract may become inflamed from diverse causes—physical and chem-

ical factors, trauma, viral and bacterial infections, iritis, glaucoma, and allergic reactions. Often the nonophthalmic physician and even the ophthalmologist cannot determine the exact diagnosis, especially if the pathophysiologic process is in an early stage; however, in most patients a provisional diagnosis can be made that eliminates other pathologic processes for which the therapy would be ineffectual or even harmful. The following differential diagnosis of the red eye is meant only as a screening aid. Signs and symptoms of different diseases often overlap, and may persist with or without the correct diagnosis and therapy. Patients with a red eye unresponsive to treatment in which vision is threatened should be referred to an ophthalmologist. Table 34.6 has been prepared to aid in the differential diagnosis.

Conjunctivitis

One of the more common ocular diagnoses made in emergency rooms is conjunctivitis. Bacterial conjunctivitis is often manifested by a gritty or poorly localized sensation of a foreign body, minimal to slight blurring of vision that should clear with blinking (caused by mucoid exudate on the corneal surface), and abnormal flow of tears. Exudate, variable lid edema, tearing, and conjunctival injection are the only positive findings in examination of the entire anterior segment. Specific attention should be paid to the cornea, anterior chamber, and pupil, since careful, complete examination may lead the physician from an incorrect diagnosis of conjunctivitis to a correct diagnosis of another disease of the anterior segment. A Gram stain and a culture of the exudate may be of value before therapy, especially in severe inflammation, since they may determine the causative organism and thereby indicate both diagnosis and treatment. A conjunctival scraping stained with Wright's or Giemsa may also be informative, since in bacterial conjunctivitis such a stain usually demonstrates polymorphonuclear neutrophils, whereas in viral inflammations, lymphocytes and monocytes predominate. In allergic conjunctivitis, scrapings are likely to reveal an increased number of eosinophils.

Most ophthalmologists do not culture specimens from patients with conjunctivitis unless initial therapy is unsuccessful. Use of a single antibiotic such as erythromycin ointment is recommended for topical therapy four times daily. If the infection persists or worsens on therapy, discontinue the antibiotic, and obtain appropriate cultures. Although some types of viral and allergic conjunctivitis are responsive to topical corticosteroids, the hazard of this medication is great enough to con-

Table 34.5.
Differential diagnosis of "blurred" optic nerve heads.

Condition	Vision	Visual Fields	Retinal Veins	Nerve Head Color	Retinal Hemorrhages	Peripapillary Retinal Edema	Vitreous Cells	Symmetry of Nerve Heads	Comments
Early papilledema	Normal	Normal (except blind spot enlargement)	Slightly distended; early loss of spontaneous pulsations	Pink	±	±	−	Often asymmetric	Headaches
Advanced papilledema	Normal or at times somewhat reduced	Normal (except blind spot enlargement)	Distended without spontaneous pulsations	Very pink to pale	+	+	−	Often symmetrical	6th nerve palsies additional clue to increased intracranial pressure
Hyperopia and physiologic variants	Normal	Normal	Normal	Normal	−	−	−	Often symmetrical	Fundus seen with + lens; central disc cupping usually present
Optic neuritis	Impaired	Central scotoma ± peripheral loss	Distended ± spontaneous pulsations	Pink	±	±	±	Usually unilateral	Precipitous onset; may have pain with ocular motility
Optic nerve tumor	Normal or markedly reduced	Normal or markedly reduced	Normal or distended	May be pigmented if disc tumor	±	±	−	Usually unilateral	May involve only the orbital or

				contains melanin; very pink to pale	—	—			intracranial optic nerve, and not the intraocular portion; primary nerve tumors are rarely observed on disc
Optic nerve avulsion	Blind eye	—	Sludged	Pale	±	—	±	Contralateral eye normal	Contrecoup or direct trauma
Hyalin bodies of nerve head	Normal	Normal or a variety of field cuts	Normal	Normal	— (very rarely +)	—	—	Often symmetrical; hyalin bodies sometimes seen at disc margins in one eye only	Often familial (examine parents and siblings)
Hypotonia of eye (after trauma)	Slightly impaired	Usually normal	Distended	Pink ±	±	Peripheral edema	—	Unilateral	Soft eye, commotio retinae
Central retinal venous occlusion	Slightly to markedly reduced	Usually full	Distended and show increased tortuosity	Hyperemic	+++	+	—	Asymmetric	Retinal hemorrhages usually extend to far periphery

(Modified from Paton D, Goldberg MF: *Injuries to the Eye, the Lids, and the Orbit.* Philadelphia, W.B. Saunders Company, 1968.)

Table 34.6.
Signs and symptoms in differential diagnosis of the red eye.

Symptom or Sign	Bulbar Perforation	Foreign Body	Conjunctivitis Bacterial	Conjunctivitis Viral	Conjunctivitis Allergic	Iritis	Acute Glaucoma	Corneal Ulcer Bacterial	Corneal Ulcer Herpes simplex	Spontaneous Subconjunctival Hemorrhage
Foreign-body sensation	+	++++	++	++	+	±		+++	+++	
Tearing	+	+++	++	+++	+++	++	+	+++	+++	
Sticky or matting lids			+++					++		
Photophobia	+	±		±		++++	+ to +++	+++	+++	
Pain	±	+++				++	++ to ++++	+ to ++	+	
Blurring of vision	+ to ++++	±	+			++	+++	Variable	Depends on location	
Halos							++++			
Rapid onset	++++	++++	±	±	+ to +++	±	+++		+	±
Conjunctival injection	±	++	+ to ++++	++	±	++	+ to +++	+++	+++	
Ciliary flush						+ to +++	++	++		
Corneal defect	Variable	Variable						++++	++++	
Exudate	±	±	+ to ++++		±	+	+	+++		
Pupil	Variable	Normal	Normal	Normal	Normal	Small	4–5 mm, fixed	Normal	Normal	Normal
Red reflex	Variable ↓	Normal	Normal	Normal	Normal	Usually ↓, may be ↑	→ → ↓	Variable	Normal	Normal
Intraocular pressure		Normal	Normal	Normal	Normal		↑ ← ← ←	Normal	Normal	Normal
Blepharospasm or squinting	±	+				+++	++	++	++	
Anterior chamber	Variable	Normal	Normal	Normal	Normal	Normal	Shallow	Normal	Normal	Normal
Lid edema	±	±	+ to ++++		+ to +++		++	++		

traindicate its use unless a specific diagnosis has been established.

Glaucoma

Glaucoma is characterized by elevation of intraocular pressure sufficient to damage the optic nerve. The diagnosis is established by determination of the elevated intraocular pressure with a tonometer in an eye with a nerve head that is either normal or cupped and atrophic.

In open-angle glaucoma, the trabecular meshwork is anatomically open to the flow of aqueous but has a reduced capacity for aqueous outflow. Rise of intraocular pressure in chronic open-angle glaucoma is usually slow, occurring over months or years; it causes no symptoms. This type of glaucoma may be detected with relative frequency in the emergency room, since it is present in more than 2% of the population who are more than 40 years of age.

Figure 34.1 depicts the normal eye, and Figure 34.2A shows the eye with angle-closure glaucoma. In this latter condition, the iris balloons forward into apposition with the trabeculum, and obstruction to aqueous flow develops abruptly, often causing symptoms that prompt the patient to seek emergency care. Generally a disease of the fifth and later decades, acute angle-closure glaucoma can also occur in younger persons with shallow anterior chambers. Physiologic mydriasis caused, for example, by a darkened environment or psychic stress and pharmacologic mydriasis caused by belladonna-like drugs can result in sudden obstruction to aqueous outflow. Only in the small or farsighted eye or in the eye in which the lens begins to swell will the space between the iris and the trabecular meshwork be narrow enough to be occluded with mydriasis.

The patient with angle-closure glaucoma may not recognize that the symptoms originate from the eye, and may present to an emergency ward with "tension headache," "sinusitis," or even "the flu." Acute angle-closure glaucoma may be either missed or diagnosed easily, depending on the astuteness of the emergency physician. The patient can usually document the onset of symptoms that include deep aching within the globe, decrease in visual acuity that is sometimes described as smoky or misty vision, and the classic symptom of red and blue halos around point sources of light.

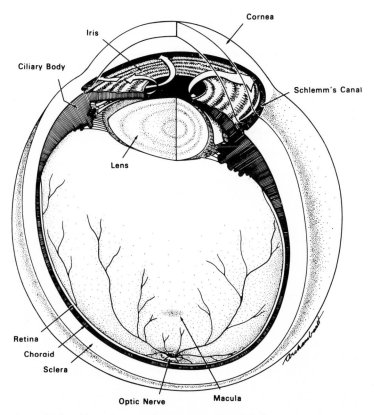

Figure 34.1. Normal eye; path of aqueous flow is indicated by *white arrows*.

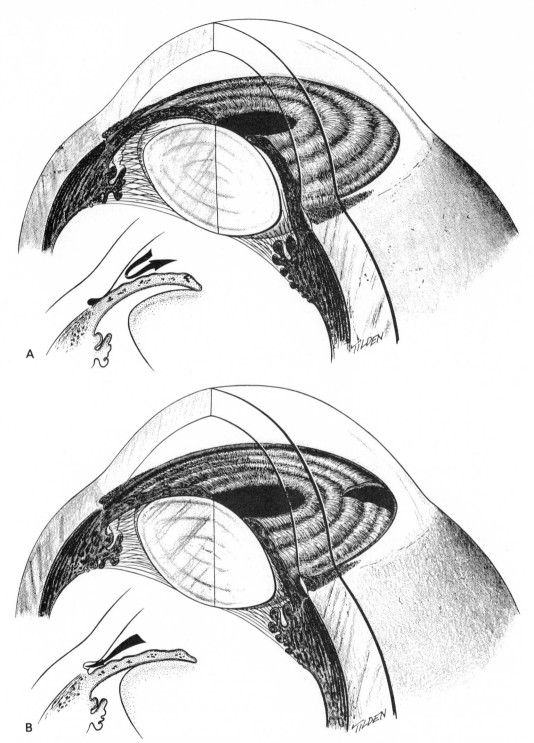

Figure 34.2. Angle-closure glaucoma. **(A)** Aqueous, secreted into posterior chamber behind iris, flows through pupil into anterior chamber, gaining access to outflow channels of Schlemm's canal. The pressure behind the iris is slightly higher than in the anterior chamber—the difference being sufficient to lift iris off anterior surface of lens. In an anatomically predisposed eye, this small pressure difference can cause iris to bow forward to block aqueous flow into Schlemm's canal, especially if iris becomes lax, as occurs when pupil dilates. Pressure elevation depends on amount of angle closure in circumference of drainage system. *Inset* shows anatomic closure of drainage system with iris bowed forward. **(B)** Effect of iridectomy. Aqueous can flow freely from posterior to anterior chamber via the iridectomy opening. The pressure differential is eliminated. The iris assumes flat contour on lens surface, and the threat of angle closure is minimal. *Inset* shows how iris drops away from outflow channels in absence of adhesions. Pupil may now be dilated without risk.

Additionally, the patient may be debilitated by the attack, and may experience nausea and vomiting.

Examination of the eye in acute glaucoma reveals a variably injected anterior segment. The cornea is usually slightly edematous, blurring the fine details of the stroma of the iris and reducing the intensity of the red reflex. The anterior chamber is shallow, with the iris approximating the peripheral endothelial surface of the cornea. The pupil is somewhat dilated, often slightly irregular, and fixed in position, even when stimulated by light. Whereas chronic glaucoma results in slowly progressive visual loss, acute glaucoma can rapidly destroy useful vision in hours to a few days, depending on the severity of the attack.

Initial therapy for acute angle-closure glaucoma includes 4% pilocarpine hydrochloride drops every 10–15 minutes; acetazolamide, 500 mg intravenously and 500 mg orally; and an osmotically active agent—either mannitol, 1.0–1.5 gm/kg intravenously, or glycerol, 1.0–1.5 gm/kg orally. This recommendation presupposes no medical contraindication to systemic osmotic therapy. A decrease in the intraocular pressure to a normal level, miosis, and clearing of the cornea indicate successful therapy. The patient should be referred immediately to an ophthalmologist.

Other types of acute glaucoma may simulate angle-closure glaucoma. A common acute secondary angle-closure type characterized by neovascularization of the anterior surface of the iris and trabeculum may occur in patients with diabetes and in patients whose ocular function is seriously compromised by central retinal arterial occlusion, central retinal vein occlusion, tumor, or long-standing retinal detachment. This and other forms of acute glaucoma usually require an ophthalmologist to make the definitive diagnosis. However, almost without exception, the aforementioned therapy will cause no harm and may be utilized as initial treatment by the nonophthalmic physician in managing an acute elevation of intraocular pressure.

Should there be reason to view the posterior segment, it is better to dilate the pupil than not to see the fundus. If the physician dilates the pupil but makes the diagnosis of angle-closure glaucoma induced by the mydriasis, the patient will have been served rather than harmed, since prompt therapy and either laser treatment to the iris or operation will result in a complete cure in almost all cases (Fig. 34.2B).

Acute Iritis

The causes of inflammation of the uveal tract are protean. Iritis, or iridocyclitis, refers to inflammation of the anterior uveal tract. Iritis is usually seen by the emergency physician as an acute, nonspecific inflammation of the anterior segment. Symptoms often progress over a few hours, and include photophobia, pain, and blurring of vision. Although iritis may be associated with glaucoma, the intraocular pressure in patients with iritis is usually low. The eye is more sensitive to light than it is in conjunctivitis and glaucoma. Vasodilation in the anterior segment usually involves both conjunctival vessels and deep vessels of the limbal episclera, and is manifested by a faint, deep pink to violet flush of the sclera close to the cornea. The pupil is usually small and round, and the cornea is usually clear; however, the red reflex can be reduced if protein and debris are circulating in the anterior chamber. Adhesions tend to form between the iris and the anterior lens capsule, a condition referred to as posterior synechia. If these adhesions are complete, iris bombé develops with forward displacement of the iris, and secondary angle-closure glaucoma occurs. This type of sterile intraocular inflammation is best treated by an ophthalmologist; detailed slit-lamp examination is necessary for both accurate diagnosis and follow-up care.

Cycloplegic-mydriatic drops are effective in the treatment of iritis; cycloplegia relieves the discomfort of ciliary muscle spasm and mydriasis helps to prevent posterior synechia. Corticosteroids reduce intraocular inflammation and may be administered either topically or, in severe cases, by injection beneath the superficial layer of the conjunctiva in Tenon's capsule. If secondary glaucoma develops, acetazolamide timolol maleate, and osmotic agents may be necessary. Pilocarpine hydrochloride is usually avoided in the treatment of glaucoma secondary to iritis, since the pupil tends to adhere to the anterior surface of the lens when constricted. Recurrent iritis is common, but these patients are seldom seen in the emergency ward, since they are aware that ophthalmologic care is needed.

Subconjunctival Hemorrhage

Bleeding beneath the conjunctiva may occur either spontaneously or after trauma to the globe. If trauma is the cause, perforation of the globe must be considered, especially if the intraocular pressure is low, if the anterior chamber is abnormally deep or shallow, or if the pupil is distorted. The cause of spontaneous subconjunctival hemorrhage may be obscure as precipitating events such as severe coughing or rubbing of the eye may not be recalled by the patient. Although infections caused by pneumococci or Hemophilus may be associated with subconjunctival hemorrhage, they are rare and are accompanied by other symptoms of conjunctivitis. Subconjunctival bleeding may be the presenting manifestation of systemic diseases such as hypertension and the bleeding diatheses. Spontaneous subconjunctival hemorrhage is almost always asymptomatic; it is painless and does not affect the globe or vision. It usually takes 10–14 days for complete resolution; no treatment is necessary except patient reassurance.

Corneal Bacterial Ulcer

A bacterial ulcer may develop after a corneal abrasion or injury by a foreign body, or it may occur with conjunctival or lid infections. Symptoms include irritation of the anterior segment and foreign-body sensation, mild photophobia, and tearing, often with exudate. The surface light reflex is irregular, and the ulcerated area is opaque, staining lightly with fluorescein. If long-standing or extensive, the ulcer may be associated with a sterile hypopyon, that is, a collection of white blood cells inferiorly in the anterior chamber. Scrapings for smears and cultures should be taken before therapy, since these infections are serious and may cause permanent corneal scarring or lead to loss of the globe from corneal perforation and endophthalmitis. Antibiotic therapy should be started immediately, while waiting for culture results, and as in patients with conjunctivitis, it should be broad spectrum and frequent. Cycloplegia is often effective in reducing ocular discomfort, and is indicated in patients with intraocular inflammation. Patients should be referred to an ophthalmologist for follow-up evaluation.

Herpetic Keratitis

Herpes simplex keratitis, most often a unilateral infection, produces foreign-body sensation, tearing, prominent injection of the perilimbal tissue, and if in the visual axis, blurring of vision. Sterile fluorescein solution should be instilled in the conjunctival sac of any patient with a red eye not obviously caused by bacterial infection or glaucoma. The corneal epithelial defect produced by the herpes simplex virus is characteristic, and when stained with fluorescein, its dendritic pattern is easily seen. Corneal sensation is also reduced, so testing of corneal sensitivity before applying topical anesthetics is suggested. Secondary iritis may be treated with cycloplegic agents. Topical corticosteroids in any form are absolutely contraindicated, since they may potentiate viral activity. Eyes have been lost from perforation due to herpes simplex infection and steroid therapy! The treatment of herpes simplex keratitis is specific; iododioxyuridine or other antiviral agents every 1–2 hours is often effective in reducing the duration of infection. Topical antibiotics are administered in addition to the antiviral agent. Since permanent corneal scarring can result from herpes simplex keratitis, patients should be referred to an ophthalmologist for follow-up care.

Dacryocystitis

Acute inflammation of the lacrimal sac usually produces pain as well as local swelling, tenderness, and inflammatory reaction around the inner canthus of the eye. There is likely to be mucoid or mucopurulent material in the conjunctival sac, and tearing usually occurs. In some patients, gentle pressure over the sac expresses pus from the lacrimal puncta. Although the lacrimal sac contains pus, it is best not to incise it unless it is pointing to the overlying skin. If symptoms suggest extension of inflammation into the sinuses, radiographs are warranted. Treatment includes topical and systemic administration of antibiotics after culture of any exudate, as well as hot compresses similar in temperature, frequency, and duration to those applied in any cutaneous or subcutaneous infection.

Mucoid exudate may often be expressed from the lacrimal sac in patients with blockage between the sac and the opening into the nasal cavity and without signs of inflammation other than a cystic lacrimal mass. These patients need not be treated for acute infection, but should be referred to an ophthalmologist.

Hordeolum (Stye)

The hordeolum represents the most common lesion of the lid, and is usually rcognizable even by the laity. This inflammatory mass may be cystic, and results from infection within Moll's glands or the glands of Zeis that secrete lubricating oils to the lashes and lid margins. The causative agent is often staphylococcal. Early styes may be distinguished only by erythema, slight edema, and localized tenderness of the skin adjacent to the lid margin; treatment with frequent hot compresses and topical antibiotics may prevent development of a mature hordeolum that might require surgical drainage. Fortunately, most inflammatory lesions of the lid are self-limited, and may be resolved with conservative therapy or drainage. Continuation of local therapy after drainage results in disappearance of inflammation, but granulation tissue or a cystic mass may persist and require excision.

Chalazion

Obstruction of a meibomian gland in either the upper or lower lid results in a nodular mass located within the tarsal plate and lid, in contrast with the marginal location of the hordeolum. The chalazion may be either a nontender lipogranuloma containing secreted material or an inflammatory mass. For chalazia with a superimposed bacterial infection, warm compresses usually suffice; unlike styes, chalazia rarely drain spontaneously. Continued application of compresses for 3–4 weeks may resolve the inflammatory process, but most often, incision and curettage in the conjunctival side of the lid are necessary.

Orbital Cellulitis

Cellulitis of the orbit is usually bacterial, and may be a dramatic inflammatory reaction with pain, fever, leukocytosis, global proptosis, limitation of extraocular movement, chemosis with congestion of the anterior segment, and even visual loss in severe cases. The condition may be especially serious in young patients. Although it may be caused by mucocele of the orbit or sinusitis, orbital cellulitis may also exist without other local sites of infection. Traumatic injury and sinus disease must be eliminated as possible causes. Hospitalization with ophthalmologic evaluation is indicated. Specimens should be cultured and systemic antibiotics should be administered; hot compresses may also be helpful. The cornea must be protected with frequent instillation of antibiotic ointment or even a temporary tarsorrhaphy.

NONPENETRATING INJURIES

Injury to the eye from blunt, nonpenetrating trauma may result in transient blurring of vision with minimal discomfort, or may lead to permanent, irreversible loss of vision with disorganization of the globe. It is far too easy for the non-ophthalmic physician to miss significant pathologic findings, since not all injuries are detectable on routine external examination and funduscopy. Hemorrhage, glaucoma, and rupture of the globe should be treated immediately by an ophthalmologist. Most other defects may be treated at the initial examination, with less immediate need for ophthalmic consultation. The following injuries may occur alone, or frequently in combination when trauma of moderate to severe force occurs.

Corneal Abrasion

Avulsion of the epithelium or cornea by a glancing blow may cause slight to moderate blurring of vision, severe foreign-body sensation, photophobia, and tearing. It is best recognized as a zone of bright-green staining after instillation of sterile fluorescein, but may be seen by direct examination with a flashlight, since the surface reflection of the cornea from the light is irregular and a shadow of the optical defect is cast on the iris. Much of the discomfort from larger abrasions is caused by exposure of free nerve endings at the corneal surface. In addition, ciliary muscle spasm occurs, and can be relieved by cycloplegics (homatropine hydrobromide, 0.5%, or scopolamine hydrobromide, 0.3%). Antibiotic drops are also often instilled. A firm double patch for 12–48 hours immobilizes the lid and allows more rapid epithelialization of the defect.

Recurrent corneal erosion is a possible sequela of corneal abrasion, and may occur weeks or months after some lesions, especially abrasions caused by some organic agents such as fingernails or small tree branches. Characterized by a sudden, sharp, foreign-body sensation similar to the initial injury, recurrent corneal erosion is classically noted on awakening. Examination soon after symptoms recur often reveals an irregular epithelial defect with ragged edges of loose epithelium. This is caused by nocturnal adherence of the corneal surface to the palpebral conjunctiva after inadequate reattachment of corneal epithelium to the underlying Bowman's membrane following the original injury. Since not all abrasions are followed by a second episode of erosion, prophylactic therapy is unwarranted without recurrent symptoms. Treatment is the same as for the initial injury, but in addition, an ophthalmic ointment should be applied nightly to keep the epithelial surface lubricated and to decrease the possibility of adherence to the overlying lid; this may be necessary for weeks to months. An hypertonic ointment containing 5% sodium chloride or an antibiotic ointment such as erythromycin should be prescribed; ointments containing corticosteroids must not be used as a secondary open-angle glaucoma may develop with chronic steroid therapy in individuals who are genetically predisposed to the disease.

Foreign Bodies

A foreign body on the conjunctival surface of the lid or on the cornea is one of the most common ocular complaints in an emergency room. The examining physician must consider the possibility of ocular penetration. Since single or multiple foreign bodies may be present, the entire anterior segment of the eye must be examined. Ocular discomfort occurs suddenly, and is usually localized under the upper lid, even if the foreign body is embedded in the cornea. Lessening of discomfort may mean that the foreign body has been washed out by tears or lid motion or both; however, irritation may persist because of an epithelial defect. A foreign body on the conjunctival surface of the lid can usually be removed with a moistened cotton-tipped applicator after topical anesthesia and lid eversion, while corneal foreign bodies can often be lifted out of the anterior stroma with a sharp instrument, the point of which is directed deep to the foreign body tangential to the corneal surface. A disposable 25-gauge needle on a syringe is suitable for this purpose.

Metallic foreign bodies containing iron may rust rapidly, leaving a rust ring in the cornea within a few hours. A small rust ring can be ignored if it is outside the visual axis, since it will eventually clear by itself, but the rust does delay re-epithelialization of the area. Rust can often be removed more easily a few days after injury when it has reacted with the corneal stroma. Large foreign bodies and rust rings in the visual axis should be removed by an ophthalmologist.

Tiny epithelial defects require only antibiotics with an optional patch, but if a foreign body has been removed from the cornea by instrumentation, the eye is usually more comfortable if it is treated with antibiotics, cycloplegics, and a patch overnight. If a foreign body is embedded deeply in the cornea, with the possibility of intraocular perforation, it is advisable to apply a sterile topical anesthetic, antibiotic drops, and a light sterile dressing and to refer the patient to an ophthalmologist for removal utilizing the operating microscope.

Chemical Injury

The types of solution that can harm the eye are too numerous to relate, and the reader is referred to the second edition of *Toxicology of the Eye* (Grant WM: Springfield, Illinois, Charles C Thomas, 1974), a required textbook for all emergency rooms. The transparency of the cornea, the integrity of the anterior segment, and even the survival of the eye after chemical injury to the globe are often directly related to the immediacy of treatment. Injuries to the globe caused by an acid, alkali, or other chemicals are true ocular emergencies, and the need for immediate irrigation of the anterior segment with water cannot be overemphasized. A search should *not* be made for a neutralizing solution initially, since the time that would be lost might prove disastrous. Industrial health units and emergency rooms should instruct nurses and paramedical personnel in the technique

of flushing the eye with water. A topical anesthetic makes flushing easier, but the eye should be irrigated first and the anesthetic obtained later for repeated irrigation. The physician should completely evert the lids to reveal the depths of the fornices in order to extract toxic solid material. The conjunctival sac should be tested for persistent acidic or alkaline residues. Alkaline and phenolic burns tend to be more severe than acidic burns, since the corneal stroma is rapidly penetrated. A hazy cornea early after an alkaline injury is ominous, and may indicate extensive corneal destruction and associated intraocular inflammation. Cycloplegics, antibiotics, and patches with appropriate systemic analgesia and sedation are useful early in therapy while ophthalmologic consultation is being obtained.

Radiation Injury

Radiation injury to the eye may occur without immediate symptoms. Ultraviolet energy from a sunlamp or a welder's arc, for example, may produce transient, painful keratitis with symptoms developing several hours after exposure. In such a case, intense foreign-body sensation, tearing, and blepharospasm occur, blepharospasm sometimes being so severe that a topical anesthetic must be instilled before examination. Examination of the anterior segment with fluorescein shows only diffuse corneal stippling indicating multiple epithelial defects. Local therapy consists of administration of a short-acting cycloplegic such as a 5% solution of homatropine hydrobromide, two to three times in the course of 12 hours, as well as topical antibiotics and double patches. Although topical anesthesia produces immediate transient relief of symptoms, anesthetic medication is not to be given to the patient for continued use. In addition to topical therapy, systemic support with oral analgesics and sedation is appropriate; it is required only for 12–18 hours, since the corneal epithelium recovers rapidly and the patient soon becomes asymptomatic.

Almost all ultraviolet wavelengths are absorbed by the cornea; however, this is not the case with infrared energy, which can cause cataracts. Levels of x-radiation used in the treatment of cutaneous epithelioma, for example, also present a hazard; when consistent with the goals of therapy, the eye should be completely protected from such radiation.

Thermal Injury

Thermal injuries to the eyes and adnexa are more commonly confined to the lid than are chemical injuries, because of the rapid blink reflex that protects the globe. Treatment should be directed toward minimizing scarring, since cicatricial defects of the lid commonly cause ocular exposure and may even be responsible for permanent visual loss. If a thermal burn of the conjunctiva does occur, antibiotics, cycloplegics, and corticosteroids are utilized to reduce inflammation and discomfort in the anterior portion of the eye. A patch is usually unnecessary, and may be contraindicated if the skin is severely burned.

Hyphema

Because the potential for continued or repeated bleeding into the anterior chamber after blunt, nonpenetrating injury is considerable and because the consequences are often severe, ophthalmologic consultation and follow-up care are usually indicated. Most ophthalmologists admit these patients to the hospital with bed rest, a patch, and sedation. Severe or recurrent bleeding may obstruct the outflow of aqueous and cause severe secondary glaucoma, which usually can be treated medically. However, operation is occasionally warranted when pressure elevation and discomfort are unresponsive to medical therapy. Another consequence of hyphema and (usually) elevated pressure is hematogenous staining of the cornea. A minimal amount of bleeding into the anterior chamber without layering in the inferior angle may be difficult to detect. Slit-lamp examination may reveal circulating red blood cells showing by flashlight only a diffuse haze that blurs the detail of the iris stroma. More commonly, hyphema is manifested by layering of blood anterior to the iris in the inferior angle; this can be seen with a flashlight.

Concomitant forms of ocular damage include corneal epithelial defects, tearing of the sphincter of the pupil, traumatic mydriasis with iridoplegia, partial or complete dislocation of the lens, vitreous hemorrhage, and retinal edema, hemorrhage, or detachment. In addition, filtration angle recession occurs in more than 80% of patients with traumatic hyphema; this condition can only be detected by gonioscopic examination, which allows visualization of the iridic root and trabecular meshwork. Since secondary glaucoma may result from the blood in the anterior chamber or the angle recession or both, tonometry is an important part of the initial examination. Elevated intraocular pressure due to hyphema may be treated with acetazolamide, 250–500 mg orally (intravenously if nausea is present), followed by divided doses up to 1 gm/day, and with osmotic agents, 1.0–1.5 gm/kg of either glycerine orally or mannitol intravenously. Topical therapy for glaucoma, as pilocarpine hydrochloride or an ophthalmic epinephrine solution, is usually ineffective. Oral administration of prednisone is advocated if there is evidence of retinal edema or hemorrhage in the macular region. Analgesia and sedation are useful supportive measures.

Loss of the normal topography of the anterior segment, a soft eye, and an excessively deep anterior chamber in an eye with extensive subconjunctival hemorrhage after blunt, nonpenetrating trauma should alert the physician to the possibility of posterior global rupture. As has been noted, this is more common in older patients with a relatively inelastic sclera. Rarely, rupture occurs at the limbus of the cornea and sclera, with dislocation of the lens into the subconjunctival space. A light, sterile dressing and protective shield should be placed over the injured eye, with immediate referral to an ophthalmologist. Since it is unusual for any useful vision to be retained in a traumatically ruptured eye, prognosis should be guarded.

Retinal Damage

Commotio retinae, or Berlin's edema, refers to retinal whitening after nonpenetrating trauma. This patchy pallor, which may last for hours or days, occurs not only at the site of impact but also posteriorly, opposite the site of impact. In the macula, the appearance is that of a "cherry-red spot," with foveal redness surrounded by posterior polar pallor due to loss of retinal transparency. Variable loss of vision occurs that may be transient or permanent. In some patients, macular holes develop. Crescentic ruptures of the choroid that are often concentric with the nerve head and that often go through the macula can also be seen after nonpenetrating traumatic injury; visual loss in this case is associated with serous exudation or hemorrhagic disorganization of the macular photoreceptors.

Retinal Detachment

Contusion of the globe may result in a variety of retinal tears, the most typical of which—dialyses—occur at the retinal periphery. An eye so injured often has a constellation of stigmata that usually can only be seen by indirect ophthalmoscopic examination, including avulsed vitreous base, peripheral chorioretinal degeneration and pigmentary changes, and vitreous hemorrhage. Detachment due to trauma usually develops soon after the injury (30% within 1 month and 80% within 2 years); however, the patient initially may not be aware of any change in vision. Funduscopic examination with an indirect ophthalmoscope is advised for all contused eyes soon after trauma to detect retinal breaks before detachment, if present, extends posteriorly.

Vitreous Hemorrhage

Vitreous hemorrhage may occur after contusion injuries of the globe, and usually results from torn retinal capillaries. It is important to rule out a retinal tear that may result in transection of larger vessels and cause considerable intravitreal bleeding, dimming the red reflex and obscuring details of the fundus. The same considerations apply as for patients with retinal detachment, and early ophthalmologic consultation should be sought.

Optic Nerve Damage

A direct blow to the eye can result in hemorrhage into the optic nerve anywhere along its path or occasionally in complete avulsion of the nerve. In addition, contusion necrosis of the optic nerve can occur because of orbital trauma, as in a gunshot wound. In injuries in which bleeding within the optic canal or nerve sheath is suspected, pressure necrosis of the nerve may be minimized by prompt unroofing of the canal, provided that vision was not entirely lost initially. The decision to operate requires immediate ophthalmologic and neurosurgical consultation.

Causes of post-traumatic visual loss are listed in Table 34.7.

PERFORATING INJURIES

Conjunctival Laceration

An opening in the conjunctiva may result from the eye being struck by a wire, branch, or other object. Its chief significance is that it may indicate a deeper laceration with entry into the globe itself. Because of bleeding within or beneath the conjunctiva, it may be difficult to determine whether the eye has been perforated. The eye may be soft, especially if the laceration is large enough to allow extrusion of intraocular contents, but normal intraocular pressure does not exclude a significant bulbar perforation. Leakage of vitreous gel, distorted topography, and an abnormally deep anterior chamber or a distorted pupil or both are other signs of possible perforation. Most conjunctival lacerations are small and do not require repair. If the laceration is large and if much of Tenon's capsule is exposed, the conjunctiva can be brought into apposition with 7–0 vicryl sutures, utilizing a 4% solution of cocaine as a topical anesthetic. If a scleral laceration cannot be excluded, an ophthal-

Table 34.7.
Differential diagnosis of post-traumatic loss of vision.

Lid swelling, blood, or foreign material covering cornea; corneal damage
Hyphema; vitreous hemorrhage
Traumatic cataract; luxation of lens
Central retinal arterial or venous occlusion (from markedly increased orbital pressure or embolus)
Traumatic retinal edema and hemorrhages of retina from direct or contrecoup blows
Retinal detachment
Avulsion of optic nerve by lateral orbital wall trauma or contrecoup blow to head
Indirect trauma to optic nerves or chiasm or both
Intracranial interruption of visual pathways (hemorrhage, foreign body)
Cortical blindness from hematoma, ischemia, or anoxia (patient may be unaware of blindness)
Acute congestive (angle-closure) glaucoma precipitated by emotional trauma of recent accident or from intumescent lens or other cause
Hysteria
Malingering

(From Paton D, Goldberg MF: *Injuries to the Eye, the Lids, and the Orbit*. Philadelphia, W. B. Saunders Company, 1968.)

mologist should explore the globe using general anesthesia.

Corneal Laceration

This lesion can be easily diagnosed if the anterior segment can be visualized, but if the lids swell after trauma, evaluation can be difficult. In such an instance, sedation, a topical anesthetic, and careful separation of the lids with retractors may prove useful. A flat anterior chamber due to apposition of the iris with the posterior surface of the cornea or a teardrop-shaped or peaked pupil due to incarceration of the iris in the corneal wound confirms the diagnosis. Repair utilizing an operating microscope should be performed as soon as possible, since delay causes swelling and distortion of the cut edges, makes watertight closure more difficult, and weakens the tissue so that sutures do not hold well. Débridement and repair should be undertaken only by an ophthalmologist.

Scleral Laceration

Some considerations relating to examination were introduced in the section on conjunctival laceration. It is imperative that the examiner neither apply pressure nor use ointments. Also, squeezing of the lids by the patient during examination may be extremely dangerous because of possible extrusion of ocular contents with the external pressure. Once scleral laceration is diagnosed, surgical exploration and repair should be planned without delay. A protective eye shield should be worn in the interim, and if necessary, hand restraints should be employed with children. Preoperative radiographs to exclude intraocular foreign bodies are necessary, as well as antibiotic therapy and tetanus prophylaxis. The long-term prognosis for such injuries can be improved by prompt, meticulous management, but is still guarded.

In many eyes with a scleral laceration, the underlying choroid and retina are also injured. When a penetrating injury is suspected, examination of the posterior segment by an ophthalmologist is necessary. The indirect ophthalmoscope offers not only the advantage of broader, more peripheral viewing but also stereoscopic visualization even when the clarity of the media is compromised. Of utmost importance is determination of the retinal status. When this layer has been lacerated, it must be repaired with the techniques employed in vitreoretinal surgery in order to reduce the risk of subsequent retinal detachment.

Ruptured Globe

The age of the patient may be consequential in severe, blunt, ocular trauma. In the older eye with a less elastic sclera, rupture occurs at the thinnest region, either beneath the rectus muscles, at the limbus, or where scleral ectasia exists. The younger eye might sustain filtration angle recession, retinal dialysis, or contrecoup retinal damage, possibly with choroidal tears. Awareness of the possibility of global rupture is necessary, as is early surgical attention with appropriate preoperative protection of the eye.

Intraocular Foreign Bodies

This type of injury occurs most commonly from the striking of steel-on-steel (for example, hammer and chisel) and the use of grinding wheels. It is surprising how little discomfort initially may occur. A red eye existing for several days or blurred vision (which may be due to a developing cataract, uveitis, endophthalmitis, or vitreous hemorrhage) may be the problem that ultimately prompts medical attention. The possibility of a foreign body must be considered when there is a perforation of the cornea or iris (best seen by slit-lamp examination), acute development of a cataract, or a focal intraocular inflammatory reaction. In the acute situation, if the foreign body is of moderate or large size, the anterior chamber may be shallow or flat, or the iris may be incarcerated in the wound. If the foreign body perforates the ciliary body, extensive vitreous hemorrhage may result.

Direct visualization of the foreign body is of utmost importance. Slit-lamp examination provides the best evaluation of the anterior segment, although gonioscopy may be required to rule out a small foreign body in the iridocorneal angle. After pharmacologic mydriasis, the vitreous and retina should be examined with an indirect ophthalmoscope. Early evaluation by this technique is imperative, since a developing cataract or dispersion of vitreous blood may cause subsequent opacification of the media. Most retained foreign bodies are found in the posterior segment of the globe. The examiner must attempt to determine whether there is a posterior exit wound. Radiographs and CAT scans are essential in the evaluation of intraocular foreign bodies, and should be obtained whenever one is suspected; survey films of the orbits and bone-free projections should be ordered whenever the possibility of a foreign body exists.

Although small, metallic foreign bodies seldom result in infection, systemic antibiotic therapy and tetanus prophylaxis should still be administered. The patient should be referred to an ophthalmologist for removal of a magnetic or nonmagnetic intraocular foreign body.

Sympathetic Ophthalmia

This tragic consequence of ocular trauma fortunately is much rarer than in the past. Sympathetic ophthalmia is bilateral granulomatous panuveitis that develops after unilateral penetrating ocular trauma. From 3 weeks to years after the injury, photophobia, redness, inflammatory reaction in the anterior and posterior segments, and variable visual loss develop in the uninjured eye. Sympathetic ocular disease is usually associated with bulbar lacerations and prolapse of uveal tissue with belated or neglected repair of such. Some believe infection may predispose to the disease. If an injured eye is enucleated within 10–14 days after trauma, almost complete protection is afforded, but enucleation after the onset of symptoms in the reacting or sympathizing eye usually is without therapeutic benefit. Sympathetic ophthalmia is believed to occur as an immunologic response; allergic reaction to an autologous uveal antigen is postulated.

Prompt attention to all ocular wounds and antibiotic and corticosteroid therapy contribute to a lowered incidence of sympathetic ophthalmia. When it is unlikely that vision in an injured eye can be salvaged, especially if the iris and ciliary body have been damaged, a decision regarding early enucleation must be made.

TRAUMA TO OCULAR ADNEXA

Lid Laceration

Consideration of lid lacerations involves both the functional and the cosmetic features of the injury. In addition, the examiner must be aware of the possibility of a deeper global laceration or blunt contusional damage, and these must be adequately excluded or treated. Possible orbital fractures must also be considered. The "harmless black eye" may be a sign of diverse, less conspicuous, but much more serious injuries.

To treat a lid laceration, the physician must determine whether (1) the canalicular or lacrimal drainage system has been lacerated, (2) the canthal tendons have been transected, (3) the lid margin is discontinuous, and (4) the levator muscle has been damaged. Impetuous repair of a complicated lid laceration in an emergency room can be extremely disfiguring; a well-planned procedure

even 24 hours later should be performed in a properly equipped operating facility. Command of the detailed anatomy of the lids and other adnexa and delicate instrumentation are prerequisites for success.

In lacerations of the canaliculi, reunion is best accomplished by end-to-end anastomosis with microscopic visualization. A stent is used to stabilize the cut ends, and silicone tubing is inserted to maintain the lumen.

If the horizontal dimension of the palpebral fissure is shortened or if the lid is abnormally lax, the physician must search for possible laceration of the canthal tensions. Prevention of ectropion after injury requires accurate approximation of sutures.

Commonly, lid lacerations involve vertical incisions through the margin; if repair is poor, the margin may be notched. The lid comprises two layers—the posterior conjunctival-tarsal plate and the anterior muscle-skin layer. An intact fibrous tarsus at the margin is necessary for stability. The technique of lid repair is illustrated in Figure 34.3. A laceration of the upper lid that has severed the

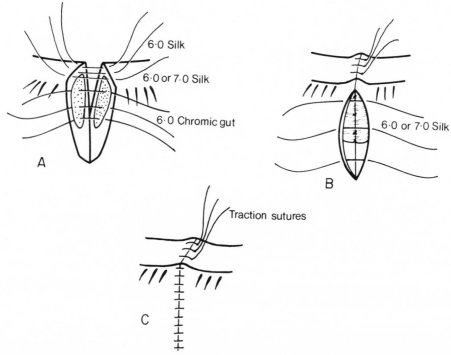

Figure 34.3. Method of closure of eyelid laceration involving margin. **(A)** Tarsus should be approximated by three 6–0 chromic catgut sutures after closure of lid margin with three 6–0 silk sutures, one in gray line and one each anteriorly and posteriorly. **(B)** Muscle and fascia anterior to tarsus are closed with interrupted 6–0 chromic catgut sutures to minimize wound tension, followed by skin closure with 6–0 or 7–0 silk sutures. **(C)** Sutures in lid margin are left long, as traction sutures. They are taped to brow or cheek opposite injured lid for 3 days to produce puckering of margin. (Modified from Beyer CK, Reeh MJ: Lid trauma. *Int Ophthalmol Clin* *14*:11–21, © 1974, Little, Brown).

levator aponeurosis must be repaired with a technique to reapproximate this layer to prevent ptosis.

Orbital Fracture

Orbital fracture must be considered when evaluating cranial injuries and possible ocular damage. Because of the often massive swelling that may result from facial trauma, a bony deformity may not be apparent on physical examination; radiographs must therefore be used (Table 34.8).

Of particular concern are blow-out fractures, in which the orbital floor is fractured with displacement of contents; fractures of the lateral wall, with avulsion of the lateral canthal tendon; involvement of the orbital roof, which may lead to leakage of cerebrospinal fluid and meningitis; and damage to the medial wall, resulting in a medial blow-out fracture with violation of the ethmoid sinus, orbital emphysema, and possible muscle entrapment. These patients should be cautioned against nose blowing, which may introduce bacteria and result in orbital infection.

Major or multiple fractures of the orbit may require coordinated attention of the ophthalmol-

ogist, neurosurgeon, otolaryngologist, and maxillofacial or plastic surgeon.

Orbital Floor Blow-out or Hydraulic Fracture

Blunt trauma usually caused by a fist or a ball against the lid and orbit can produce a particular kind of orbital fracture of which every examiner should be aware. An abrupt increase in intraorbital pressure occurs that is transmitted equally in all directions. The two most vulnerable sites for fracture are the lamina papyracea of the ethmoid sinus and the orbital floor. In the former case, incarceration of muscle is rare, but in the latter, entrapment of the inferior rectus or inferior oblique muscle in the bony defect results in restricted movement of the globe. Such involvement must be excluded by specific examination, since failure to do so may result in late enophthalmos and permanent oculomotor dysfunction. Lid and orbital edema and orbital hemorrhage may make the results of early physical examination inconclusive. A red glass should be utilized to test for limitation of upward and downward gaze as man-

Table 34.8.
Recommended radiographic projections in orbital trauma (exclusive of intraocular foreign bodies).

Projection	Technique	Remarks
Prone posteroanterior Caldwell (nose-forehead)	Canthomeatal line perpendicular to center of film and central ray angled 27° caudally to place petrous ridge at level of inferior orbital rim	Provides best view of frontal and ethmoid sinuses and orbital floor complex; orbital floor and paperplate fractures occur with almost equal incidence
Erect Waters'	Canthomeatal line angled upward at 45° and central ray horizontal; petrous ridge is at level of third molars	Shows facial arch fractures involving zygomatic arch, zygoma, inferior orbital rim, and nasal arch; fluid levels demonstrated
Prone, open mouth	Canthomeatal line angled upward 5° more than in erect Waters'	Complements erect Waters'
Base of skull		Shows base of skull and especially antra, with front walls commonly depressed toward back
Erect true lateral	Can be across the table face up	Shows emphysema and fluid levels
Right and left optic canal	Prone or reverse	Permits evaluation of optic canals and regional anatomy
Occipital	Center over face—canthomeatal line perpendicular to film and central ray 35° caudal	Shows facial area, including mandible
Anteroposterior and lateral tomography	Linear or pleuridirectional; 0.5 cm cuts; anteroposterior includes skin surface to external auditory canal; lateral, from skin surface to skin surface	May give best details of orbital floor or optic canal fracture; can be done only with excellent patient cooperation
"Jug-handle"		Provides submental vertex soft-tissue view of each zygomatic arch; complements Waters' view

(Courtesy of A. S. Macmillan, Jr., M.D.)

Table 34.9.
Priority for evaluation and treatment.

Condition	Emergency Ward Treatment by Nonophthalmic Physician		Referral to Ophthalmologist		
	Immediate	Routine	Hours	1–2 Days	Within 1 Week
Central retinal arterial occlusion	X		X		
Chemical burn	X		X	(X)	
Bulbar laceration	X		X		
Acute glaucoma		X	X		
Nonpenetrating foreign body		X		X	
Penetrating foreign body	X		X		
Iritis		X		X	
Corneal ulcer		X	X		
Conjunctivitis		X			X
Herpes simplex keratitis		X		X	
Traumatic hyphema	X		X		
Orbital cellulitis		X	X		
Retinal detachment, macula attached		X	X		
Retinal detachment, macula detached		X		X	
Intraocular (vitreous) hemorrhage		X		X	
Subconjunctival hemorrhage with trauma		X		X	
Optic neuritis		X		X	
Infected hordeolum and chalazion		X			X
Dacryocystitis		X			X

ifested by diplopia and to examine the patient for hypesthesia in the distribution of the infraorbital branch of the trigeminal nerve. A "forced duction test" may be useful in confirming the diagnosis; this is performed by grasping the insertions of the inferior and superior rectus muscles with forceps after instillation of a topical anesthetic and by noting the resistance to a full range of passive motion of the globe. This allows differentiation of muscle entrapment from muscular or neural paresis as the basis of limited movement. Expert interpretation of radiographs and occasionally tomography or CAT scans may be helpful. If the fracture results in entrapment of extraocular muscle, prognosis is improved by performing surgical correction within 2 weeks. The tissue is freed and a supportive silicone plate is inserted inferior to the periosteum on the orbital floor.

Table 34.9 has been prepared to indicate generally the urgency for evaluation and treatment of a variety of ocular problems. The question is frequently asked, "Which patients with eye signs or symptoms should be referred for ophthalmologic consultation?" In each case the answer relates to the severity of the problem and the interest and experience of the examining physician. Thus, the situation is not really unique in medicine, and it is the responsibility of each to know the limits of his competence.

Suggested Readings

Cox MS, Schepens CL, Freeman HM: Retinal detachment due to ocular contusion. *Arch Ophthalmol* 76:678–685, 1966.

Gombos GM: *Handbook of Ophthalmic Emergencies: A Guide for Emergencies in Ophthalmology.* Flushing, NY, Medical Examinations Publishing Co, 1973

Grant WM: *Toxicology of the Eye,* ed 2. Springfield, Ill, Charles C Thomas, 1974

Paton D, Goldberg MF: *Management of Ocular Injuries.* Philadelphia, WB Saunders, 1976

Walsh FB: Pathological-clinical correlations. I. Indirect trauma to the optic nerves and chiasm. II. Certain cerebral involvements associated with defective blood supply. *Invest Ophthalmol* 5:433–449, 1966

CHAPTER 35

Angiography: A Diagnostic and Therapeutic Aid in Emergencies

CHRISTOS A. ATHANASOULIS, M.D.
ARTHUR C. WALTMAN, M.D.

Emergency angiography is performed on the acutely ill or injured patient for diagnosis or therapy or both. Diagnostic angiography provides information about the nature of illness and the extent of injury. Therapeutic angiography provides the means for nonsurgical control of hemorrhage and for the treatment of ischemia.

Emergency Angiography Team

Emergency angiographic procedures call for utmost skill in their performance and expertise in interpretation of the findings. Around-the-clock availability of an expert angiography team is essential. At the Massachusetts General Hospital, such a team comprises a senior radiologist-angiographer, an assistant (fellow in training), a radiology technologist with special training in angiographic procedures, and a registered nurse. For emergencies during nonworking hours, the team can be alerted through a paging system and can be at the hospital within 30 minutes of the initial call. The initial call is made not when the need for emergency angiography is obvious and urgent, but as soon as information reaches the emergency ward about a patient with such illness or injury that might require emergency angiography. The vascular radiologist thus has an early opportunity to familiarize himself with the patient and that nature of the problem, to witness the initial assessment of the illness or injury, and in consultation with the physician in charge to advise about the optimal type of and time for an angiographic procedure.

Angiography Room

Once the decision is reached to perform an emergency angiographic procedure, the patient is transferred to the angiography room. Incomplete or "single-film" angiography attempted in the emergency ward by inexperienced personnel or in the emergency radiology department without the appropriate equipment is more hazardous than no angiography at all. The entire time that the patient is in the angiography room, intensive care continues with the assistance of medical or surgical staff who have escorted the patient. It is essential that the angiography room contains the appropriate x-ray equipment including 1000 mA 3/phase generators, television fluoroscopy and serial film changers with biplane filming capability. Reliable 105 mm cine cameras are now available and they are extremely valuable for rapid shot imaging of vessels in acutely injured patients. In addition to x-ray apparatus the angiography rooms are also equipped with appropriate accessories and supplies for patient monitoring and resuscitation (Fig. 35.1).

Methods of Angiography

No anesthesia is required. Mild sedation, however, may be necessary in some patients. Arteriography is carried out with catheters percutaneously introduced via either femoral artery. If no femoral arterial pulses are present, access can be gained either from an axillary artery or through translumbar puncture of the abdominal aorta. Access to the large veins of the abdomen and chest is also achieved percutaneously from either a femoral vein or an antecubital vein. Needles, flexible guide wires, and straight or preshaped angiographic catheters are available for these procedures.

The recent introduction of digital subtraction angiography (DSA) offers an additional means for

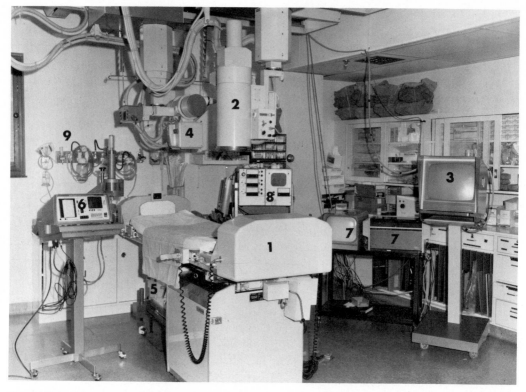

Figure 35.1.   The modern facility for emergency diagnostic and therapeutic vascular radiographic procedures. Room is equipped with x-ray and recording equipment and also with monitoring and resuscitation apparatus for continuous care of patient during vascular procedures: *(1)* radiographic table with cradle, *(2)* image intensifier, *(3)* television monitor, *(4)* overhead high-power x-ray tube, *(5)* multiple film changer, *(6)* pressure injector with electrocardiographic monitoring apparatus, *(7)* videotape recorder, *(8)* electrocardiographic pulse and pressure monitor and recorder, and *(9)* wall oxygen and suction apparatus.

rapid imaging of blood vessels. This modality is the product of angiographic x-ray equipment and computers combined. The signal emanating from the image intensifier is digitized and fed into the computer. Manipulation of the digitized signal is then possible. With the use of electronic subtraction and electronic enhancement of the subtracted image, blood vessels can be imaged after intravenous injections of radiographic contrast media. DSA has already proved clinically useful in the evaluation of carotid, renal, and peripheral arteries. The method is currently being evaluated for imaging of the aorta and branches in patients with trauma or acute ischemia. The obvious advantages over standard angiography with catheters are speed, reduced morbidity, and considerably reduced costs (Fig. 35.2).

The mortality directly related to angiography is negligible; the incidence of thrombosis at the site of catheter insertion is 0.2%.

Contraindications

Contraindications to emergency angiography are profound shock and uncontrollable torrential hemorrhage. In the first instance, angiography must be postponed until the patient is out of shock. In the second instance, the patient is taken directly to the operating room. However, immediate exploration does not preclude postoperative angiography if the surgical findings so warrant. For example, a patient with massive trauma to the abdomen and pelvis on exploration may be found to have no abdominal organ injuries but retroperitoneal hemorrhage from fractures of the bony pelvis. Angiography in this instance would follow exploration in order to determine the bleeding site and to control hemorrhage by nonsurgical means.

Known sensitivity to contrast media is only a relative contraindication, provided that emergency resuscitation equipment is available.

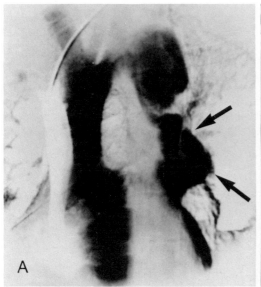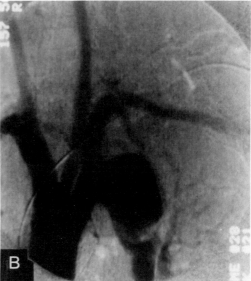

Figure 35.2.   Digital subtraction intravenous angiography in the evaluation of the thoracic aorta **(A)** *Arrows* point to a false aneurysm at the site of previous surgical repair of aortic coarctation. **(B)** Intravenous study of the aortic arch provides information about the anatomy of the brachiocephalic vessels.

CLINICAL CONDITIONS THAT MAY REQUIRE EMERGENCY ANGIOGRAPHY

An emergency diagnostic or therapeutic angiographic procedure should be considered when any of the conditions listed in Table 35.1 is suspected. Conditions pertaining to the heart, the head, and the central nervous system are dealt with elsewhere in the text, and will not be included in this discussion.

Trauma

The indications for angiography and the type of vascular procedure depend on the nature of the traumatic injury. With penetrating trauma and clinical symptoms limited to one organ or system, emergency angiography includes selective arteriography or venography, or both, of the particular organ. This is exemplified by the patient with a knife wound in the right upper quadrant of the abdomen or a penetrating wound in the flank associated with hematuria. In the first instance, abdominal aortography is complemented with selective hepatic arteriography, whereas in the second instance, selective renal arteriography or venography or both are performed.

Blunt trauma due to a motor vehicle accident or a fall is usually multiple, and the clinical symptoms may be obscured by associated head injuries. Angiography in these patients can be particularly helpful, because many anatomic areas or organs

Table 35.1.
Clinical conditions that may require emergency angiography.

Trauma
  Head trauma
  Trauma to chest, heart, and great vessels
  Abdominal trauma
  Fractures of bony pelvis with hemorrhage
  Trauma of extremities
Nontraumatic vascular conditions
  Acute myocardial infarction
  Pericardial effusion, cardiac tamponade, cardiac
    rupture
  Acute aortic dissection
  Ruptured aortic aneurysm
Ischemia
  Acute peripheral arterial occlusion
  Renal ischemia—acute renal failure
  Bowel ischemia
Hemorrhage
  Gastrointestinal hemorrhage
  Abdominal apoplexy
  Postoperative hemorrhage
  Hemorrhage of central nervous system
Acute pulmonary embolism

can be evaluated rapidly and multiple injuries of varying severity may be diagnosed. This is illustrated by the case of a patient who sustained injuries to the chest, abdomen, pelvis, and lower extremities during a motorcycle accident. With the same angiographic catheter and in rapid sequence,

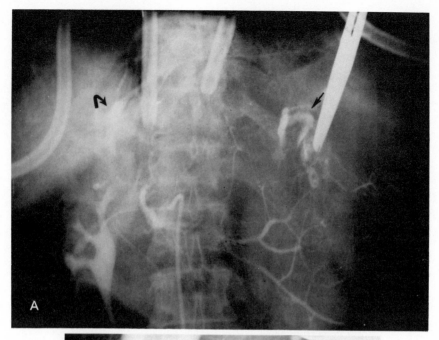

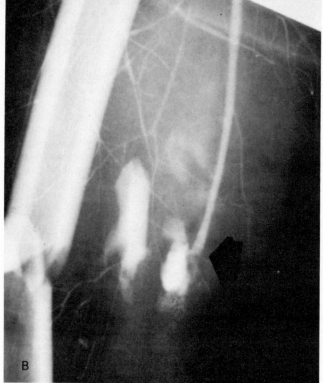

Figure 35.3.   Emergency angiography in patient with multiple trauma. **(A)** Celiac axis arteriogram. *Straight arrow* points to contrast medium extravasation in spleen secondary to splenic rupture. *Curved arrow* points to opacification of branches of portal vein, the result of a tear and arterioportal fistula in left lobe of liver. **(B)** Femoral arteriogram performed with same catheter as in **(A)** shows obstruction of superficial femoral artery (*arrow*) because of laceration from a bony fragment.

With this information the patient was taken to the operating room where he underwent splenectomy, repair of a tear of the left lobe of the liver, and femoral arterial reconstruction.

the thoracic aorta was studied for the presence of a traumatic tear; the abdominal aorta, liver, spleen, kidneys, and iliac and femoral arteries were studied for evidence of bleeding into the abdomen or pelvis; and the peripheral arteries were studied for traumatic occlusion (Fig. 35.3). The superior and inferior venae cavae and their tributaries also can be evaluated. Thus, listing the angiographic indications and findings according to anatomic areas or organs is only for purposes of discussion.

Trauma to the Great Vessels

Traumatic disruption of the thoracic aorta is the most important injury in this area. It is usually the result of automobile accidents. Due to rapid deceleration type of injuries, the thoracic aorta distal to the origin of the left subclavian artery is predominantly involved. Rupture of the thoracic aorta is found in 16% of victims of fatal automobile accidents. About 20% of those who sustain aortic rupture survive for more than 1 hour. If the entity is not properly diagnosed and treated, 60% die within 2 weeks of injury.

Early diagnosis of tear of the thoracic aorta is of paramount importance. If the chest radiograph of a patient involved in a vehicular accident shows widening of the mediastinum, aortography should be immediately performed. The value of computed tomography remains to be proven. DSA in the future may become the best imaging method for the evaluation of patients with suspected aortic tears.

The angiographic appearance may vary from irregularity of the aortic wall to a false aneurysm. Most common site of rupture is the aortic isthmus (45% in autopsy series followed by the supravalvar area [Fig. 35.4].

Abdominal Trauma

In patients with penetrating or blunt abdominal trauma, emergency angiography should be performed if injury to the liver, spleen, or kidneys is suspected.

Hepatic Trauma. Major avulsing lacerations of the liver may be associated with profound shock and hypovolemia requiring immediate surgical exploration; if bleeding continues after operation, hepatic angiography should be considered. In most patients, however, there is ample time for the angiographic procedure.

The purposes of angiography in patients with suspected hepatic injury are the following:

(1) to confirm or exclude a major laceration or hematoma of the liver;

(2) to determine precisely the segment or seg-

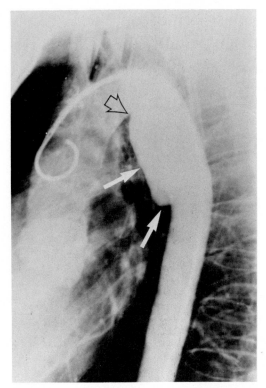

Figure 35.4. Traumatic tear of the thoracic aorta. *Arrows* point to disruption of the aortic wall and false aneurysm formation in patient with sudden deceleration injury to chest.

ments of the liver and the arterial branches involved in the injury;

(3) to diagnose underlying benign or malignant tumors that may be the cause of major bleeding incidental to minor trauma or that may aggravate hemorrhage initiated by trauma;

(4) to demonstrate the arterial anatomy and normal variations and to establish a vascular map before operation. The left hepatic artery may arise from the left gastric artery. The right hepatic artery may originate from the superior mesenteric artery. Crossclamping of the portal trunk, therefore, in these patients would not control all vascular inflow to the liver;

(5) to follow the course of an angiographically demonstrated lesion if the patient is not operated on. Radionuclide studies, computed body tomography and DSA also may be helpful in this instance;

(6) to diagnose and to locate complications of hepatic trauma such as traumatic aneurysms and hematobilia after medical or surgical management;

(7) to evaluate the presence of associated injuries in adjoining organs such as the right kidney;

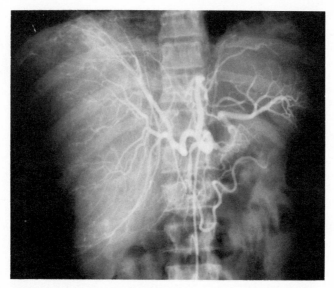

Figure 35.5.   Subcapsular hematoma of liver secondary to rupture of hepatocellular adenoma. Celiac axis arteriogram in a 29-year-old man with acute abdominal pain and decreasing hematocrit. The patient had been receiving long-term replacement therapy with anabolic corticosteroids following irradiation of a pituitary adenoma. Arteriogram shows splaying of branches of hepatic artery and medial displacement of opacified liver by large subcapsular hematoma. At operation it was found that the subcapsular hematoma was the result of a ruptured hepatocellular adenoma and carcinoma.

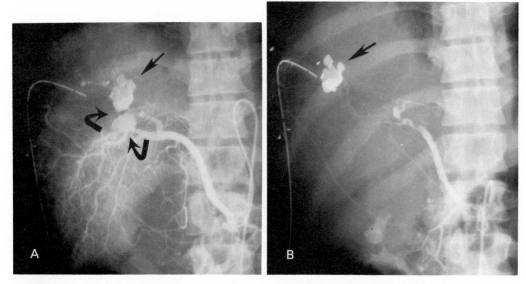

Figure 35.6.   Traumatic hematobilia treated with transcatheter embolization of right hepatic artery. Traumatic hematobilia in a 35-year-old man was the result of a bullet wound in the right upper abdominal quadrant. **(A)** Right hepatic arteriogram. Right hepatic artery originates from superior mesenteric artery. *Straight arrow* points to fragment of bullet. *Curved arrows* point to extravasation of contrast medium and a false aneurysm in right lobe of liver. **(B)** Right hepatic arteriogram with patient in oblique position following transcatheter embolization of hepatic artery with surgical gelatin. *Straight arrow* points to bullet fragment. There is no opacification of the false aneurysm. Blood supply to left lobe of liver was not compromised. The patient was discharged 8 days after the procedure. He has remained asymptomatic for a follow-up period of 6 months.

(8) to control hemorrhage with transcatheter embolization of hepatic arterial branches.

Depending on the nature and extent of hepatic injury, the angiographic findings may include any of the following:

(1) contusion—(a) straightening and elongation of the arterial branches, (b) delayed progress of the contrast medium column, (c) multiple punctate areas of contrast medium extravasation, (d) irregular heterogeneous hepatogram of one or more segments.

(2) intrahepatic hematoma—(a) arterial displacement, (b) small-artery occlusions, (c) extravasation of contrast medium, (d) defects during the capillary and venous phases of the hepatogram.

(3) capsular or deep tear of the liver—(a) subcapsular hematoma with hepatic displacement (Fig. 35.5), (b) extravasation of contrast medium (c) false aneurysm, (d) arterioportal fistula, (e) arteriobiliary fistula.

(4) hematobilia—one or several sites of contrast medium extravasation and opacification of adjoining biliary ducts (Fig. 35.6).

Tumor vascularity, arteriovenous shunting, and tumor stain are seen at angiography in patients with minor or major trauma and a coexistent tumor.

Splenic Trauma. Short of surgical exploration, there are presently two methods for the diagnosis of splenic rupture: radionuclide scanning and splenic arteriography. Ultrasound and computed tomography may be helpful in the detection of large subcapsular hematomas. In patients with multiple injuries requiring angiographic studies for diagnosis or therapy, splenic arteriography can confirm or exclude splenic rupture, and additional studies are not necessary. If splenic injury is suspected in a patient with single or minor injury to the left upper abdominal quadrant with or without fractures of the lower left ribs, a radionuclide scan should be obtained first. If the scan is unequivocably normal or reveals injury, further studies are unnecessary. If, however, findings are equivocal, the patient should undergo selective splenic arteriography.

The definitive angiographic findings of splenic rupture include the following:

(1) Gross or multifocal extravasation of contrast medium persisting into the capillary phase (Fig. 35.7). Visualization of small amounts of extravasated medium may be enhanced if arteriography is repeated after injection of 6–10 µg of epinephrine into the splenic artery.

(2) Direct intrasplenic arteriovenous communication.

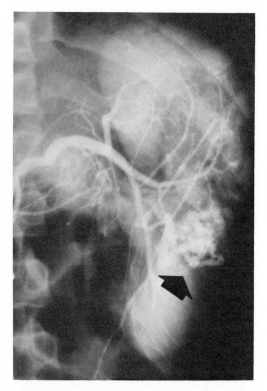

Figure 35.7. Splenic rupture. Splenic arteriogram in a 12-year-old boy who sustained severe injuries to the left upper abdominal quadrant during a fall. *Arrow* points to contrast medium extravasation within spleen. At operation a large splenic tear was found and the spleen was removed.

(3) Subcapsular hematoma.

(4) A wedge-shaped defect during the capillary phase with arterial displacement or occlusions secondary to a tear and intraparenchymal hemorrhage.

Displacement of the opacified spleen away from the lateral abdominal wall or the diaphragm, an irregular or mottled splenogram, and stretching of the splenic arterial branches—the so-called indirect signs of splenic rupture—are unreliable and should not be considered in the interpretation of the angiogram. A fluid- or gas-distended stomach may also produce such stretching of splenic arterial branches, especially those of the upper pole.

Renal Trauma. In 86% of renal injuries managed medically, recovery is complete and the intravenous pyelogram is normal 6 or more months after injury. As a result, the surgical approach to renal trauma has become less aggressive, as has renal angiography.

In all patients with hematuria after trauma or without hematuria but with suspected renal injury, an infusion intravenous pyelogram should be obtained. Emergency abdominal aortography and selective renal arteriography are performed if the pyelogram shows a nonfunctioning kidney. Arteriography is also performed when hematuria is massive or when it does not subside after several hours of bed rest and sedation (Fig. 35.8).

The objective of angiography in patients with suspected renal injury is to reveal any of the following conditions for appropriate management: (1) thrombotic occlusion of the renal artery; (2) false aneurysm; (3) arteriovenous fistula; (4) thrombosis of the renal vein; and (5) underlying renal disease such as tumor, hydronephrosis, ectopia, hypoplasia, or agenesis.

Control of Traumatic Bleeding with Angiographic Methods. In patients with multiple injuries and bleeding from the liver, spleen, or kidney, it may be desirable to avoid immediate surgical intervention for control of bleeding either because of the patient's poor general condition or because of associated severe neurologic injuries. If angiographic examination in such patients shows discrete extravasation of contrast medium, immediate control of bleeding may be achieved by positioning the angiographic catheter in the bleeding artery and obstructing blood flow with mechanical means. Blood flow may be obstructed either temporarily with balloon-tipped catheters or for a prolonged period by using particulate matter (surgical gelatin) for embolization of the bleeding artery (Fig. 35.6B). Therefore, splenectomy or nephrectomy for uncontrollable bleeding does not need to be performed on an emergency basis, and attention can be directed to the management of associated injuries. Further, transcatheter embolization can be selective with the tip of the angiographic catheter positioned in the bleeding branch. In patients with trauma and bleeding into the kidney, selective embolization often obviates nephrectomy. Massive bleeding into the liver, hematobilia, traumatic arteriovenous fistula, and retroperitoneal hemorrhage are other conditions that can be managed with angiographic methods.

Fractures of the Bony Pelvis with Hemorrhage

The mortality among patients with pelvic fractures varies from 9–27%. As many as 60% of these deaths result from massive extraperitoneal hem-

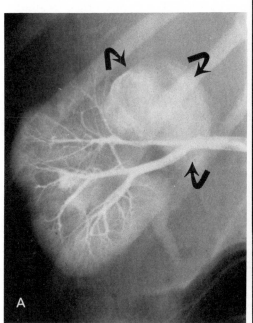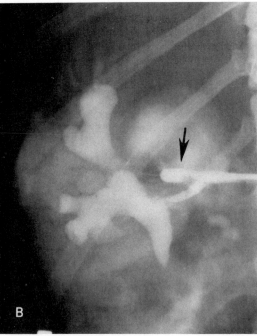

Figure 35.8. Kidney rupture with intrarenal hemorrhage. A 21-year-old woman had massive hematuria following an automobile injury. **(A)** Renal arteriogram shows contrast medium extravasation into large false aneurysm occupying upper pole of kidney (*arrows*). **(B)** Balloon catheter (*arrow*) has been percutaneously introduced into renal artery and inflated with radiopaque contrast medium. Injection of contrast medium proximal to balloon shows effective obstruction of blood flow and no opacification of false aneurysm. This allowed stabilization of patient's condition before transferral to the operating room for exploration and nephrectomy.

orrhage. Associated genitourinary and colorectal injuries are other serious complications, but hemorrhage that is usually concealed and that may become massive is the most difficult problem to manage.

The source of bleeding may be a transected iliac vein. In such patients, rapid recognition followed by surgical ligation is lifesaving. In most patients, however, bleeding arises from the arteries and venous plexuses lining the walls of the pelvis.

Control of bleeding has been attempted with ligation of both hypogastric arteries. However, most reports indicate that this procedure does not control hemorrhage because of the presence of collateral vessels. In addition, during surgical exploration the rate of bleeding may increase considerably since the tamponading effect of the peritoneum and of the hematoma itself is no longer present.

Angiographic methods have been employed to determine the site of arterial bleeding in patients with pelvic fractures and also to control hemorrhage. Arteriography in patients with fractures of the bony pelvis and an obvious large or increasing retroperitoneal hematoma displacing the urinary bladder, the ureters, or the kidneys can reveal the bleeding site by demonstrating contrast medium extravasation from branches of the hypogastric arteries, usually the obturator arteries. The internal pudendal, superior gluteal, and iliolumbar arteries have also been shown to be sources of hemorrhage, depending on the site of the major bony injury. Venography has been of limited usefulness in the evaluation of venous bleeding because there is no good method for visualization of all the pelvic veins.

Once the bleeding sites have been identified, hemorrhage can be controlled with selective catheterization of the bleeding arterial branches of the hypogastric arteries and obstruction of blood flow to these vessels. This has been achieved with balloon catheter occlusion and embolization with blood clots (Fig. 35.9). The preferred method is embolization with surgical gelatin (Gelfoam) introduced in the form of small (1 × 1 mm) plugs through the angiographic catheter.

Embolization of bleeding branches of the hypogastric arteries has two main advantages over surgical ligation. It produces distal rather than proximal occlusion, and it does not interfere with the tamponading effect of the intact peritoneum and already existing hematoma. In most patients treated with embolization, bleeding ceases. No serious complications are associated with this method.

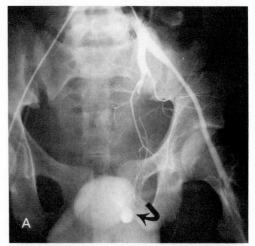
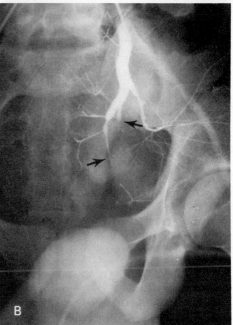

Figure 35.9. Pelvic fracture with hemorrhage—control of bleeding with embolization of branches of hypogastric artery. A patient with injuries to the bony pelvis following an automobile accident had a decreasing hematocrit. **(A)** Left hypogastric arteriogram. *Arrow* points to contrast medium extravasation from branches of left hypogastric artery. **(B)** Plugs of surgical gelatin were introduced through angiographic catheter, and branches of hypogastric artery were occluded (*arrows*). Repeated arteriogram shows no contrast medium extravasation.

The patient's condition became stabilized following the procedure. There was no evidence of subsequent hemorrhage, and the patient was discharged several days later.

When emergency angiography is performed for the diagnosis and control of bleeding from pelvic trauma, it can be extended to evaluate the abdominal organs as well. As mentioned earlier, if emergency operation is performed for suspected intra-abdominal injury and if a retroperitoneal hematoma is found originating from the pelvis, angiography can still be performed immediately after operation for embolization of the bleeding arteries.

Trauma of Extremities

Traumatic arterial injury may be manifested by either hemorrhage or arterial insufficiency. In both instances the therapeutic goal is to restore normal vascular anatomy. Early recognition and knowledge of the exact level of vascular injury are important.

Major limb ischemia may be concealed by generalized shock or vasoconstriction or both. If ischemia is suspected, the point of arterial obstruction may be difficult to determine clinically or with oscillometry. Further, major arteries may suffer lacerations that need repair, with no clinical evidence of arterial insufficiency. The indications, therefore, for angiography are as follows:

(1) pulse deficit, if the exact site of obstruction cannot be established clinically or with other laboratory techniques;

(2) suspected vascular injury because of proximity of the vessel to a wound or fracture in the absence of clinical evidence of arterial insufficiency (Fig. 35.10);

(3) suspected false aneurysm or arteriovenous fistula;

(4) large or enlarging hematoma of the wound site.

If no specific structural arterial lesion is seen during the course of arteriography, but diffuse arterial spasm of the examined limb is demonstrated, 1–2 mg of papaverine can be injected intra-arterially through the angiographic needle or catheter to combat the vasoconstriction. If necessary, this may be followed with intra-arterial infusion of papaverine, 0.1 mg/min for 8–12 hours.

Based on initial clinical experience with DSA, it seems reasonable to believe that this new imaging method will play an important role in the evaluation of patients with suspected injuries of peripheral arteries. With intravenous injections of contrast and the use of DSA, vessel injury can be compared and the outcome of surgery may be more easily evaluated (Fig. 35.11).

Peripheral phlebography may also be considered in patients with large or enlarging soft-tissue hematomas and normal arterial studies.

Nontraumatic Vascular Conditions

Patients with conditions other than trauma affecting the aorta and its major branches may benefit from emergency angiography. In this chapter, discussion will be limited to acute aortic dissection and ruptured aortic aneurysm.

Acute Aortic Dissection

In patients with clinical symptoms or signs raising the suspicion of acute aortic dissection, emergency aortography is indispensable for the following reasons:

(1) If acute aortic dissection is not diagnosed and not treated, it will be fatal in 75–90% of patients.

(2) Angiography is currently the only method that can establish or exclude the presence of aortic dissection. Computed tomography also has been used in the evaluation of patients with aortic dissection. However, after initial enthusiasm, and with more experience, it was concluded that computed tomography is not accurate in the diagnosis of aortic dissection.

(3) The surgical approach and the prognosis for each of the three types of dissection (DeBakey I, II, and III) are different, and it is with angiography that each type may be identified.

(4) Opacification of the false lumen during aortography or lack of opacification may be significant in selecting patients for medical vs. surgical treatment.

(5) Aortography provides information about extension of the dissection into the branches of the aorta. This information may become important during subsequent management, whether the treatment is surgical or medical.

Aortography should be rapidly and meticulously performed. Accurate diagnosis requires excellent film quality. The study should include the thoracic and abdominal aorta, and radiographs should be obtained in two planes at 90 degrees; therefore, biplane filming capability is essential.

The approach from either femoral artery has proved to be safe when the procedure is performed by an experienced angiographer. Use of an axillary or brachial artery is necessary if both femoral arterial pulses are absent. A combined approach via femoral and axillary arteries may be necessary if the catheter cannot be advanced into the ascending aorta from the retrograde femoral route. The venous approach to the study of dissections does not provide optimal opacification of the aorta and results are unreliable.

The angiographic signs of aortic dissection are

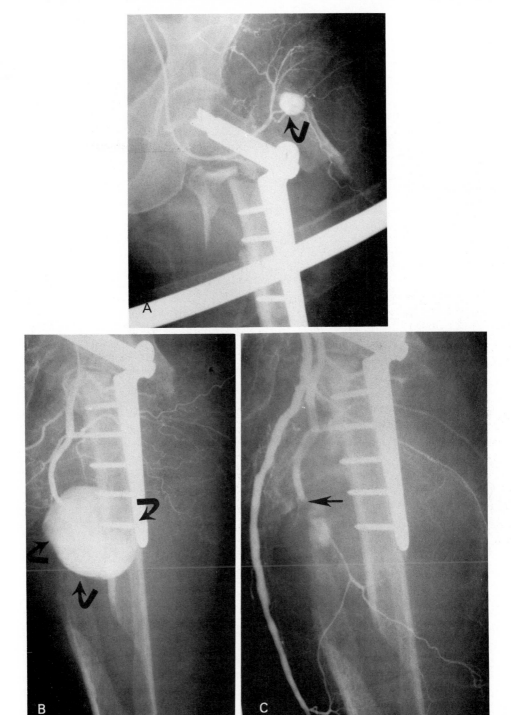

Figure 35.10. Hemorrhage resulting from fracture of a hip and femur—control of bleeding with transcatheter vessel occlusion. A 70-year-old woman sustained an intertrochanteric fracture of the femur. Following fixation the patient had an enlarging hematoma at the operative site and a decreasing hematocrit. **(A)** *Arrow* points to contrast medium extravasation from branch of lateral femoral circumflex artery. Embolization with surgical gelatin controlled the bleeding. The patient was discharged.

Nine months later, the patient sustained a fracture of the femoral shaft with an associated enlarging soft-tissue mass. **(B)** Arteriogram of profunda femoris artery. *Arrows* point to large false aneurysm, the result of a tear of this artery. **(C)** The false aneurysm has been obliterated following embolization of distal segment of profunda femoris artery (*arrow*) with surgical gelatin.

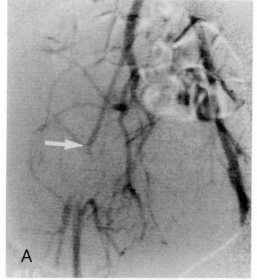

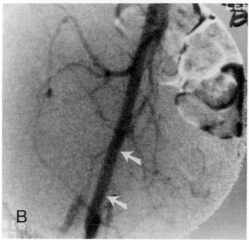

Figure 35.11. Peripheral vascular trauma evaluated with digital subtraction intravenous angiography. **(A)** *Arrow* points to occlusion of femoral artery the result of a fall injury in a 9-year-old boy. **(B)** Postoperative digital subtraction intravenous angiogram shows patent vein graft (*arrows*).

direct and indirect. The direct signs include:

(1) linear radiolucency coursing longitudinally along varying lengths of the opacified aorta, representing the torn or separated intima (Fig. 35.12);

(2) opacification of two channels;

(3) demonstration of points of entry or re-entry; The indirect signs include:

(1) compression of the true aortic lumen by the nonopacified false lumen;

(2) abnormal catheter position, with the catheter in the aortic arch lying along the inner wall rather than resting against the lateral wall;

(3) thickening of the aortic wall more than 6 mm;

(4) ulcer-like projection from the aortic lumen.

Extension of the dissection to involve major branches such as the celiac, superior mesenteric, renal, or iliac arteries is common in types I and IIIb. The lumen of an aortic branch may be compressed or occluded by the false lumen of the dissected aorta (Fig. 35.12). A branch may be supplied by both the true lumen and the false lumen or by the false lumen only.

Ruptured Aortic Aneurysm

Intraperitoneal rupture of an abdominal aortic aneurysm is usually rapidly fatal, not allowing for any diagnostic procedures. Fortunately, it is less common than rupture into the retroperitoneum, which initially is manifested by slow leakage. If available, computed tomography may be helpful in delineating the hematoma around the aneurysm. Use of angiography in the preoperative evaluation of these patients is controversial. It appears that if it is performed with expedience and safety, it may prove beneficial for the following reasons:

(1) Rupture may be into the intestine, the inferior vena cava, or the ureter, making the diagnosis difficult without aortography (Fig. 35.13).

(2) Preoperative knowledge of suprarenal extension of the aneurysm or involvement of the renal arteries is useful in planning the operative procedure.

(3) Associated aneurysms or occlusive disease of the outflow vessels to the lower extremities may be demonstrated by angiography.

Ischemia

Acute Peripheral Arterial Occlusion

Sudden cessation of major arterial flow to an extremity may be caused by thrombosis, embolism, trauma, or compression secondary to dissection. Trauma and dissections have been discussed. As in trauma patients, the goal of therapy in patients with an acute peripheral arterial occlusion is not only preservation of life and the limb but also restoration of blood flow and return of function.

Acute thrombosis of a major peripheral artery is commonly superimposed on atherosclerosis. Acute ischemia may also result from extrinsic compression, such as compression of the subclavian artery by a cervical rib or a fibrous band, and from hypotension of any cause in patients with

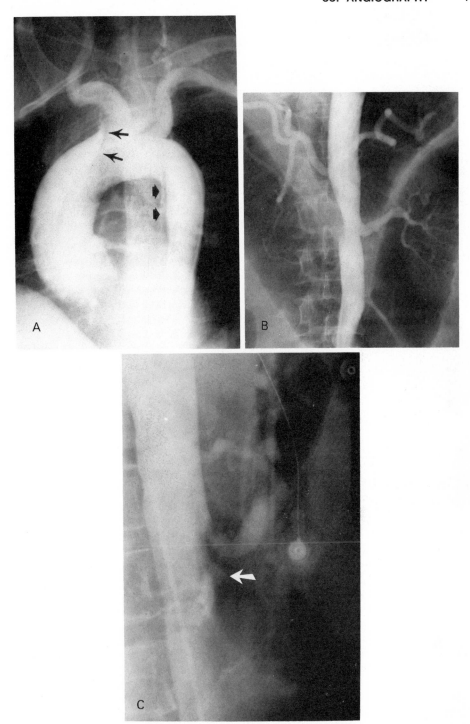

Figure 35.12. Aortic dissection extending into abdominal aorta. A 65-year-old hypertensive man was seen with acute chest pain radiating both anteriorly and posteriorly. **(A)** Thoracic aortogram. Dissection extends into ascending and descending thoracic aorta (*arrows*). **(B)** Abdominal aortogram, anteroposterior projection. Dissection has extended into abdominal aorta. There is no opacification of superior mesenteric and right renal arteries. **(C)** Abdominal aortogram, lateral projection. *Arrow* points to stump of superior mesenteric artery, which was occluded as result of extension of dissection in the abdominal aorta.

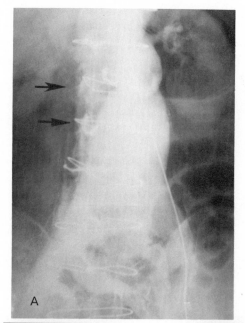

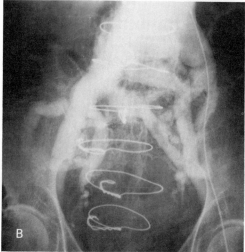

Figure 35.13. Abdominal aortic aneurysm with rupture into inferior vena cava. A 70-year-old man had a pulsatile abdominal mass and hematuria. **(A)** Abdominal aortogram shows large aneurysm of abdominal aorta with simultaneous opacification of inferior vena cava *(arrows)*. **(B)** Pelvic arteriogram. Contrast medium was injected at aortic bifurcation. There is opacification of iliac veins and of multiple venous tributaries.

At exploration, rupture of the aortic aneurysm was found with communication with the inferior vena cava.

underlying peripheral vascular disease. It may also be a complication of an arterial puncture performed for coronary, cerebral, or visceral arteriography or for physiologic monitoring. Preopera-

tive arteriography in such patients is necessary to determine the extent of the thrombotic process and the adequacy of distal runoff.

The clinical diagnosis of arterial embolism is usually inferred from a history of myocardial infarction, atrial fibrillation, proximal aneurysm, a recent cardiac or vascular operation, or endocarditis. The purpose of arteriography in patients with a suspected embolic arterial occlusion is to establish the site and extent of the occlusion, the degree of collateral circulation, and the distal vessel reconstitution. When embolism results in complete occlusion of an artery, the arteriographic appearance is fairly typical, the proximal end of the embolus forming a convex margin (Fig. 35.14).

More recently, there has been interest in the administration of low-dose regional thrombolytic enzymes in patients with acute vascular occlusion. Low-dose streptokinase (5000 units/hr) has been infused through the angiographic catheter for resolution of acute thrombus in the coronary, renal, or peripheral arteries. Of particular interest has been the resolution of thrombus and recanalization of acutely or subacutely occluded bypass grafts. The obvious advantage of regional over systemic thrombolysis is the avoidance of complications, such as bleeding, with the lower dose and the more rapid effect of the enzyme on the thrombus because of delivery through the catheter near the occluded vessel (Fig. 35.15).

Renal Ischemia—Acute Renal Failure

Sudden development of impaired renal function may be due to prerenal (circulatory inadequacy), postrenal (obstruction), or primary renal injury. An important step in the management of these patients is to diagnose reversible or specifically treatable causes of acute renal failure. In patients with primary renal injury, aortography and renal arteriography provide the means for early diagnosis in the following situations:

(1) Renal arterial embolism—approximately 10% of arterial emboli involve visceral organs, including the kidneys. Although the isotopic flow study will establish the presence or absence of blood flow into the kidney, it is with aortography and selective renal arteriography that proximal and distal occlusions can be appreciated and operability assessed.

(2) Renal arterial thrombosis—whether thrombosis is due to trauma, operation, or extension of a thrombotic process from the abdominal aorta, aortography has similar value and indications as in cases of renal arterial embolism.

(3) Renal failure in the immediate period after

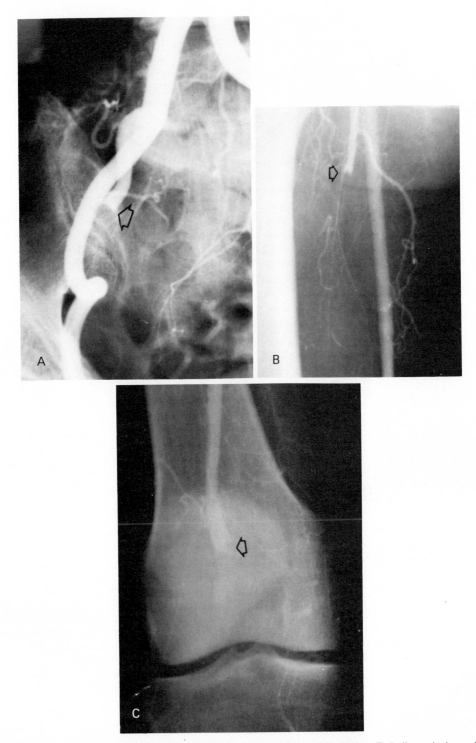

Figure 35.14. Multiple arterial embolic occlusions in patient with atrial fibrillation. Embolic occlusions of **(A)** the hypogastric artery, **(B)** the profunda femoris artery, and **(C)** the popliteal artery are indicated with *arrows*. The curvilinear defect of meniscus is characteristic of arterial emboli.

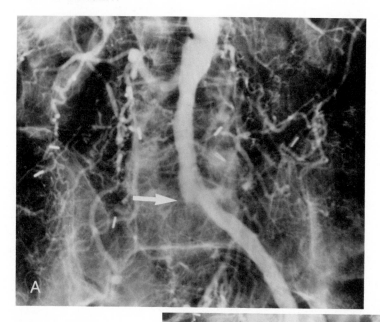

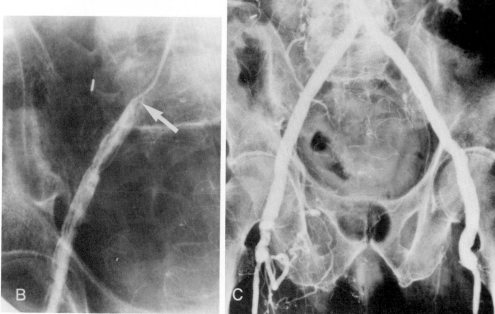

Figure 35.15. Regional thrombolysis with streptokinase. **(A)** *Arrow* points to occluded right limb of an aortobifemoral bypass graft. The occlusion was acute by clinical history. **(B)** A catheter has been positioned with the tip (*arrow*) in the occluded graft. Contrast injection shows partial resolution of thrombus after infusion through the arterial catheter of streptokinase at 2000 IU per minute for 40 minutes. **(C)** Thrombus completely resolved after additional intra-arterial infusion of streptokinase at 5000 IU per hour for 12 hours.

renal transplantation—this may be due to hyperacute rejection or thrombosis at the site of the anastomosis. Simple lumbar aortography or ipsilateral iliac arteriography can confirm or exclude the latter diagnosis.

(4) Atypical course for acute vasomotor ne-

phropathy—if acute renal parenchymal disease, vasculitis, cortical necrosis, or undiagnosed chronic renal parenchymal disease is suspected on clinical grounds, renal arteriography may be applied in conjunction with renal biopsy to avoid "sampling errors" of the biopsy if the disease process is not uniformly distributed throughout the kidney.

Bowel Ischemia

Three points need to be considered in the diagnosis and management of patients with suspected acute, extensive bowel ischemia:

(1) Early diagnosis on the basis of physical findings alone is difficult and often impossible. A high index of suspicion and emergency angiography are essential to confirm or to exclude its presence.

(2) Organic occlusions of the mesenteric artery must be differentiated from low-flow states (nonocclusive ischemia) because the treatment is different. This differentiation can be made only with angiography.

(3) No complex "superselective" arteriography is necessary to evaluate these patients. Abdominal aortography and selective superior mesenteric ar-

teriography are sufficient for diagnostic and therapeutic purposes.

Figure 35.16 shows a classification of bowel ischemia based on pathophysiology and clinical manifestations. The signs and symptoms that should alert the clinician to the possibility of acute bowel ischemia may be found in Chapter 23, pages 517–519. This discussion will be limited to the application of emergency angiography.

Occlusive Disease. Obstruction of the superior mesenteric artery resulting in acute bowel ischemia is evenly divided between acute thrombosis because of atheroma and embolism. Occasionally, dissection of the abdominal aorta that extends to involve the mesenteric artery may be the underlying cause. Intestinal infarction secondary to mesenteric venous obstruction accounts for less than 10% of acute occlusive ischemia.

As soon as the diagnosis of bowel ischemia is suspected and while initial measures for fluid replacement and restoration of normal cardiac func-

CLASSIFICATION OF BOWEL ISCHEMIA

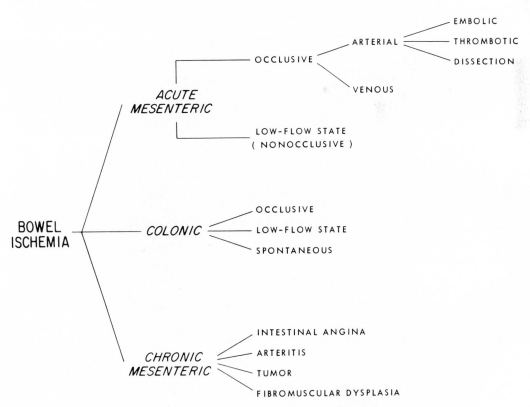

Figure 35.16.   Classification of bowel ischemia.

tion are being taken, plain films of the abdomen should be obtained, followed by mesenteric angiography. The plain films are useful in providing baseline information concerning the intestinal gas pattern and in excluding the presence of free intraperitoneal air from a perforated viscus. Angiography must be performed on an emergency basis. It takes approximately 6 hours from the onset of ischemia until infarction occurs.

Biplane abdominal aortography must be performed first to evaluate the origin of the mesenteric arteries in the lateral projection. If the diagnosis is not made at aortography, selective superior mesenteric arteriography is performed to establish the level of the occlusion, the presence of additional distal arterial occlusions, the degree and extent of collateral vessel development, and the patency of the mesenteric veins (Fig. 35.17).

Thrombosis more often involves the origin or proximal segment of the superior mesenteric artery, whereas emboli usually lodge at bifurcations and most often at the takeoff of the middle colic artery. Atheromatous lesions of the origins of the mesenteric arteries are extremely common in patients without symptoms of bowel ischemia. The clinical setting and the presence or absence of large collateral vessels during selective mesenteric arteriography should help determine the significance of a superior mesenteric arterial stenosis or occlusion. Midstream abdominal aortography may also demonstrate aortic dissection when this is the underlying cause for bowel ischemia. Infusion of streptokinase at low doses (5000 units/hr) in the superior mesenteric artery may have a role in the management of patients with embolism, when peritoneal signs are not present.

Low-Flow State. In this condition, otherwise referred to as nonocclusive bowel ischemia, ischemia may proceed to infarction without occlusion of major mesenteric arteries or veins. Experimental investigations and clinical observations suggest that profound mesenteric vasoconstriction may oc-

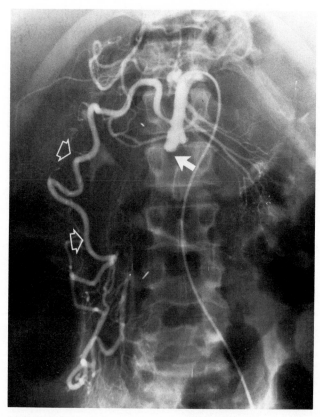

Figure 35.17.   Embolic occlusion of superior mesenteric artery in patient with myocardial infarction and mural thrombus. Superior mesenteric arteriogram shows complete occlusion of superior mesenteric artery distal to origin of first jejunal and middle colic arteries (*solid arrow*). The *open arrows* point to dilated middle and right colic arteries that serve as collateral pathways to the distal ileum and right colon.

cur because of diminished cardiac output. Hypovolemia is a prominent factor in the development of ischemic symptoms in these patients. Thus, the entity is seen in patients with recent myocardial infarction and congestive heart failure and in patients who have undergone a major thoracic or abdominal operation. Digitalis, which is a potent mesenteric vasoconstrictive agent, has been implicated as a contributing factor. The consistent process in all these clinical situations is decreased mesenteric blood flow.

Abdominal aortography in the anteroposterior and lateral projections shows that the origins and main trunks of the mesenteric arteries are patent. Selective mesenteric arteriography demonstrates vasoconstriction characterized by narrowings at the origins of the branches of the superior mesenteric artery, irregularities and spasm of the arcades,

and incomplete filling of intramural vessels. These changes may reverse after intra-arterial infusion of vasodilative drugs into the superior mesenteric artery; if they do not, the implication is that intestinal infarction has already occurred.

In view of the extremely high mortality and the increasing frequency of bowel ischemia secondary to low-flow states, a diagnostic and therapeutic approach has been developed consisting of mesenteric angiography as soon as the diagnosis of acute bowel ischemia is strongly suspected (Fig. 35.18). In the absence of organic large-vessel occlusions and in the presence of local or generalized mesenteric vasoconstriction, drug infusion into the mesenteric artery is started in an attempt to reverse vasoconstriction, promote bowel perfusion, and prevent further extension of the ischemic process or progression to infarction. Most clinical experi-

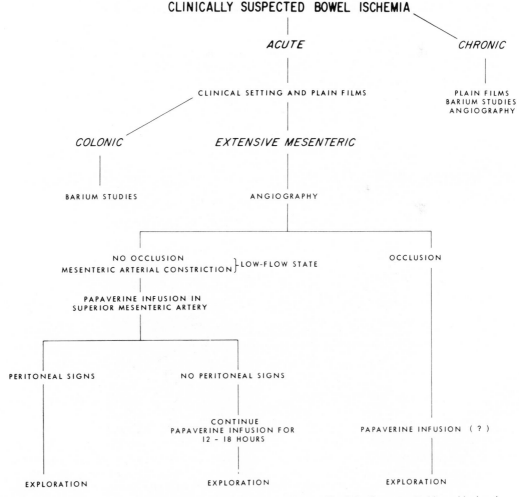

Figure 35.18. Sequence of radiologic procedures in patients with clinically suspected bowel ischemia.

ence has been with papaverine, 30–60 mg/hr for 12–18 hours. In the absence of any peritoneal signs, this seems to be a reasonable alternative to abdominal exploration. During infusion, measures are taken for adequate volume support, improvement of cardiac function, and control of sepsis. At the end of the infusion, abdominal exploration is commonly undertaken for resection of ischemic bowel segments.

Hemorrhage

The objectives of emergency angiography in the hemorrhaging patient are to determine the source of bleeding and to control the hemorrhage with nonsurgical means. The latter can be accomplished with infusions of vasoconstrictive drugs or with transcatheter embolization of the bleeding vessels.

Hemorrhage resulting from trauma and its angiographic control have already been discussed. The following will focus on the applications of angiography in gastrointestinal hemorrhage and in bleeding caused by neoplasia and inflammation.

Gastrointestinal Hemorrhage

Emergency angiography cannot and should not be applied to every patient with acute gastrointestinal hemorrhage. It should be reserved for those patients who continue to bleed despite conservative measures and in whom operative intervention is considered for control of the hemorrhage.

Upper Gastrointestinal Bleeding. *Determination of Bleeding Site.* The sources of massive gastrointestinal bleeding are about equally distributed among peptic ulcerations, gastric mucosal lesions, and ruptured esophageal varices. Gastric mucosal conditions include stress bleeding associated with major trauma, a surgical procedure, or sepsis.

After initial measures are taken for volume repletion, determination of the bleeding site is the next important step in patient management. Endoscopy is the method of choice. Angiography is performed only when endoscopy is difficult to perform or is inconclusive. Midstream abdominal aortography is performed in patients with a history of an abdominal aortic reconstructive procedure. The purpose is to detect an aortoenteric fistula. If there is no such history or suspicion, selective celiac axis arteriography is performed. If findings are normal, selective left gastric, gastroduodenal, splenic, or superior mesenteric arteriography follows. In 80–95% of patients with persistent red gastric aspirate on irrigation, arteriography demonstrates contrast medium extravasation at the bleeding site (Fig. 35.19).

In approximately 70% of patients with gastric mucosal hemorrhage, bleeding is shown at angiography to originate from the left gastric artery. It is therefore essential that this vessel be well opacified during an emergency angiographic examination. Celiac axis arteriography would not suffice if the catheter tip were placed and the contrast medium injected distal to the origin of the left gastric artery or if the left gastric artery did not originate from the celiac axis. The supraduodenal branch of the gastroduodenal artery is the site of extravasation in most patients with bleeding duodenal ulcers (Fig. 35.20).

If no arterial extravasation is seen with selective arterial catheterization and injection of contrast medium, if gastroesophageal varices are demonstrated during the venous phase, and if the gastric aspirate continues to be pink or red, ruptured gastroesophageal varices are assumed to be the source of hemorrhage. Therefore, the diagnosis of variceal bleeding by angiographic means is a diagnosis of exclusion. Contrast medium extravasation is rarely seen from a ruptured varix because by the time the medium reaches the veins it is diluted, and it cannot be visualized on serial radiographs unless bleeding is massive.

Control of Hemorrhage with Angiographic Methods. When the bleeding site has been determined with endoscopy or angiography, angiographic methods may be applied for the control of hemorrhage in those patients who continue to bleed despite conservative measures. The purpose is to prevent emergency operative intervention. Angiographic methods for the control of bleeding include infusion of vasopressin and occlusion of the bleeding vessel by means of embolization.

The best results from the infusion of vasopressin for control of bleeding from an arterial source are obtained with vasopressin infused directly into the bleeding artery. This is the left gastric artery in most patients with gastric mucosal hemorrhage and the gastroduodenal artery in patients with bleeding pyloroduodenal ulcers.

The step-by-step procedure includes the following:

(1) A baseline arteriogram is obtained to show contrast medium extravasation.

(2) Vasopressin, 0.2 unit/min for 20 minutes, is infused into the left gastric or the gastroduodenal artery with a constant infusion pump.

(3) The arteriogram is repeated. If extravasation persists, the infusion rate is increased to 0.4 unit/min and the arteriogram is repeated 20 minutes later. If bleeding is still seen angiographically, the chances are that it will not be controlled pharmacologically. Further increase of the infusion rate is not recommended.

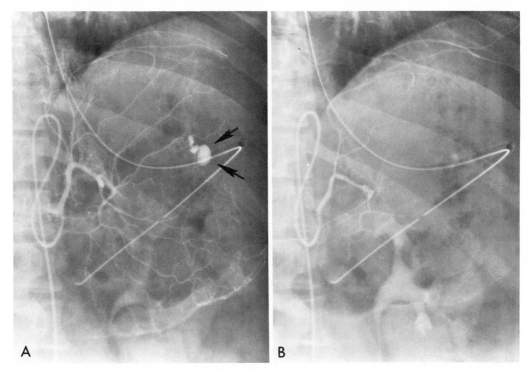

Figure 35.19. Stress bleeding in stomach controlled with infusion of vasopressin into left gastric artery. Upper gastrointestinal bleeding occurred in a patient with massive trauma and sepsis. **(A)** Left gastric arteriogram shows extravasation of contrast medium at bleeding site in stomach (*arrows*). **(B)** Left gastric arteriogram repeated 20 minutes after infusion of vasopressin at 0.2 unit/min shows constriction of branches of left gastric artery and no extravasation. Infusion was continued for 48 hours and bleeding was controlled. (Reproduced by permission, from *Radiol Clin North Am*, Vol. 14, No. 2, © 1976, W. B. Saunders Co.).

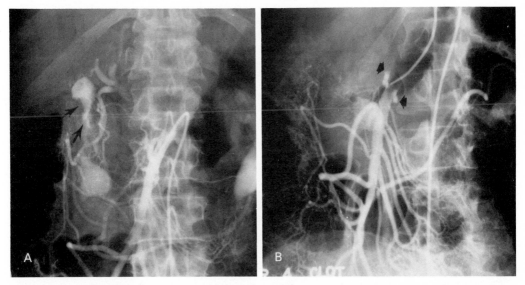

Figure 35.20. Bleeding from duodenal ulcer controlled with transcatheter embolization. A 60-year-old man had carcinoma of the colon metastatic to the liver and porta hepatis with upper gastrointestinal bleeding. Endoscopy showed a duodenal ulcer. An operative procedure with ligation of the right hepatic artery did not control the bleeding.

(A) Superior mesenteric arteriogram shows extravasation in duodenum (*arrows*) from branches of gastro-duodenal artery. **(B)** Following embolization of anterior and posterior branches of inferior pancreaticoduodenal artery, a repeated arteriogram shows no extravasation. *Arrows* point to occluded branches of inferior pancreaticoduodenal artery. There was no recurrent bleeding for 6 months after embolization.

(4) When the optimal infusion rate is established, the patient is transferred to an intensive care unit with the catheter in place, and infusion is continued for 24 hours.

(5) If there is no clinical evidence of bleeding, the infusion rate is decreased by half and infusion is continued for another 12–24 hours. At this point, 5% dextrose in water is substituted for vasopressin, and the catheter is removed a few hours later.

(6) If bleeding occurs at any time during infusion, the position of the catheter tip needs to be confirmed. Although this can be done with a portable radiograph, preferably the patient is transported to the angiographic suite for repeated arteriography.

When catheterization of the celiac axis branches is technically difficult or impossible, vasopressin may be infused in the celiac axis. Clinical, biochemical, and experimental data have shown that such infusions are not associated with hepatic ischemia.

With intra-arterial infusion of vasopressin, bleeding is controlled in 80% of patients with gastric mucosal hemorrhage and 50% of patients with bleeding duodenal ulcers. Recurrent bleeding occurs in 16% of patients with gastric mucosal hemorrhage. Angiography and vasopressin infusion may be repeated when bleeding recurs.

Complications of vasopressin infusion include reduction of urinary output (antidiuretic hormone effect) and occasionally, bradycardia and hypertension. Bowel ischemia and infarction should not occur as a result of vasopressin infusion if arteriography is performed to assess the degree of vasoconstriction produced with a given infusion rate.

Transcatheter arterial embolization may be considered in patients in whom intra-aterial infusion of vasopressin fails to control gastroduodenal hemorrhage from arterial sources. For this purpose, it is essential that the tip of the catheter be positioned in the left gastric artery, the gastroduodenal artery, or one of the branches. Absorbable surgical gelatin (Gelfoam) in the form of small plugs (1 × 1 mm) is the material currently used (Fig. 35.21). Double-lumen balloon catheters are desirable and are now applied during arterial embolization to prevent dislodgment of emboli and obstruction of vessels supplying adjacent organs.

The following guidelines should be observed during transcatheter arterial embolization in the gastrointestinal tract:

(1) Diffuse gastric mucosal hemorrhage is best treated with intra-arterial vasopressin and not with transcatheter embolization.

(2) A discrete bleeding point in the stomach supplied by a single arterial branch is amenable to control with embolization if superselective catheterization is possible.

(3) For bleeding duodenal ulcers, embolization may be considered as the primary mode of angiographic therapy. Collateral takeover from the pancreaticoduodenal branches of the superior mesenteric artery must be considered and excluded after embolization of the gastroduodenal artery.

(4) Intense inflammatory reaction surrounding a bleeding site associated with penetrating peptic ulcers or a pancreatic abscess may prevent the arteries from constricting in response to vasopressin. Embolization should be considered as an alternative.

(5) Skill, experience, and good judgment are important in the application of embolization for bleeding control.

Vasopressin infusion may be used for control of bleeding esophageal varices. Vasopressin infused in the superior mesenteric artery reduces portal pressure and may arrest bleeding from gastroesophageal varices. The infusion rate is 0.2 unit/min for 24–36 hours followed by 0.1 unit/min for an additional 24 hours.

This form of therapy has given way to low-dose intravenous administration of vasopressin. Similarities exist between mesenteric arterial and intravenous infusions of vasopressin regarding the effect on mesenteric blood flow and portal pressure reduction. Cardiac output reduction is no greater with intravenous administration than with mesenteric infusion of vasopressin—10–15% with both modes. The regimen for intravenous infusion of vasopressin is 0.3 unit/min for 24 hours followed by 0.2 unit/min for 24 hours followed by 0.1 unit/min for an additional 24 hours.

The efficacy of vasopressin infusion in controlling bleeding from ruptured varices depends on the patient's clinical status and the severity of the underlying hepatic disease. Bleeding is controlled in 90–95% of patients in Child's group A, 75% in group B, and 55% in group C.

In transhepatic occlusion of the coronary vein for control of bleeding esophageal varices, the portal venous system may be entered and the coronary vein selectively catheterized via the transhepatic route. The method is simple and the risk of intraperitoneal hemorrhage from the point of entry in the liver is negligible. The coronary vein may be occluded with balloon catheters, blood clots, or surgical gelatin.

At present, this procedure seems to be best indicated for patients with endoscopically proved bleeding varices who continue to bleed despite

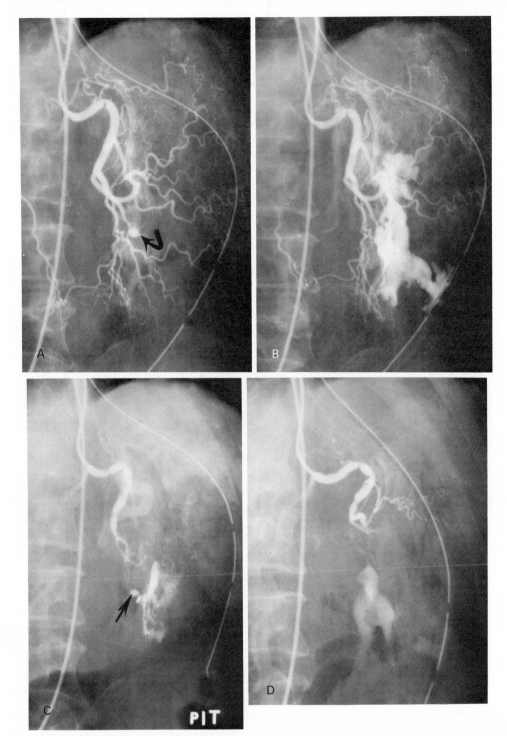

Figure 35.21. Bleeding gastric ulcer controlled with left gastric artery embolization. A 54-year-old woman, an alcoholic, had massive upper gastrointestinal bleeding. Endoscopy showed a bleeding ulcer of the lesser curvature.

   (A) Left gastric arteriogram shows contrast medium extravasation at bleeding site (*arrow*). **(B)** Massive extravasation of contrast medium is noted during late phase. **(C)** Left gastric arteriogram following infusion of vasopressin at 0.2 unit/min for 20 minutes in left gastric artery shows constriction of branches of left gastric artery and persistent extravasation (*arrow*). **(D)** The bleeding branch of left gastric artery was embolized with surgical gelatin. Repeated arteriogram shows no extravasation. The bleeding was clinically controlled and the patient was discharged.

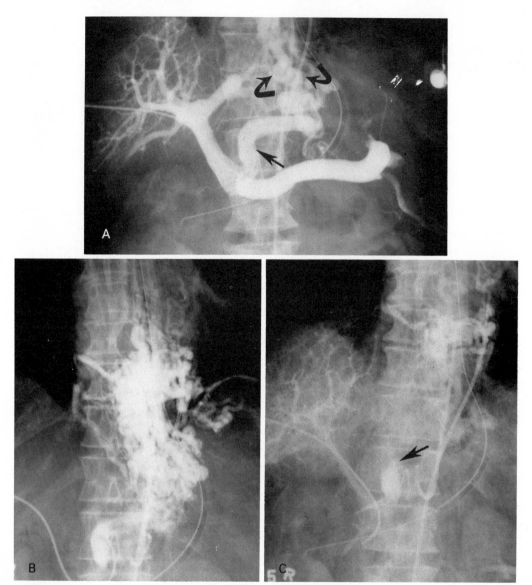

Figure 35.22.   Transhepatic obliteration of coronary vein and gastroesophageal varices for control of variceal bleeding. A 65-year-old man had cirrhosis of the liver, portal hypertension, and bleeding gastroesophageal varices. Conservative measures including infusions of vasopressin and placement of a Sengstaken-Blakemore tube had failed to control bleeding.

(A) Transhepatic catheterization of portal vein. Contrast medium was injected with tip of catheter in splenic vein. There is hepatofugal flow through an enlarged coronary vein (*straight arrow*). The coronary vein drains into massive gastroesophageal varices (*curved arrows*). (B) Selective coronary vein injection shows extent of gastric and esophageal varices. (C) Coronary vein was obliterated with injection of several plugs of surgical gelatin. Repeated study following embolization shows stump of coronary vein (*arrow*).

vasopressin infusion or balloon tamponade or both. Transhepatic occlusion of the coronary vein and varices could serve as an alternative to emergency transthoracic ligation of varices for the acute control of hemorrhage, therefore allowing for adequate preparation of the patient before an elective decompression shunt procedure is performed (Fig. 35.22).

Lower Gastrointestinal Bleeding. It was mentioned earlier that in patients with upper gastrointestinal bleeding, endoscopy should be performed to establish the source. However, in patients bleeding from a source distal to the ligament of Treitz, endoscopy is of limited value. Angiography is the procedure of choice for determination of the bleeding site. For best results, mesenteric arteriography including the superior and inferior mesenteric arteries should be performed on an emergency basis at the time of active bleeding so that the source can be identified with contrast medium extravasation.

Diverticular Hemorrhage. Bleeding diverticula demonstrated by angiography are more common in the right colon (75%). As a result, when bleeding colonic diverticulosis is suspected, a superior mesenteric arteriogram is obtained first. If this is normal, an inferior mesenteric arteriogram follows. If this too is normal, a celiac axis arteriogram is obtained to exclude a bleeding duodenal ulcer. If extravasation is demonstrated from a branch of the mesenteric arteries, vasopressin is infused in the superior or inferior mesenteric artery to control bleeding (Fig. 35.23). The infusion schedule is comparable with that described earlier for upper

gastrointestinal hemorrhage. With mesenteric arterial infusion of vasopressin, bleeding from colonic diverticulosis is controlled in 90–95% of patients. The management of patients subsequent to the acute control of hemorrhage is debatable. Approximately one-half of these patients have recurrent hemorrhage, at which time segmental colonic resection is carried out on the basis of the previous angiographic findings. Patients who do not bleed again and who do not undergo operation should have a barium enema examination or colonoscopy or both to exclude neoplasms and other lesions.

Colonic Angiodysplasia. Angiodysplasia of the cecum and ascending colon is a potential source of massive rectal bleeding in elderly patients. The lesion can be diagnosed by means of angiography based on the following findings (Fig. 35.24):

(1) Clusters of small arteries are seen during the arterial phase adjacent to the ileocecal valve or in the ascending colon.

(2) Contrast medium accumulates in vascular spaces.

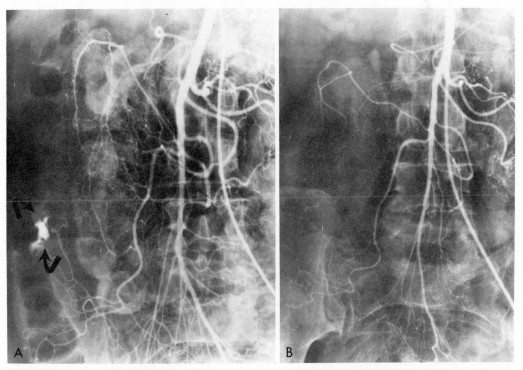

Figure 35.23. Bleeding from diverticulum of ascending colon controlled with intra-arterial infusion of vasopressin. A 59-year-old woman had massive rectal bleeding. **(A)** Superior mesenteric arteriogram shows extravasation of contrast medium (*arrows*) in ascending colon. **(B)** Superior mesenteric arteriogram following 20-minute infusion of vasopressin at 0.2 unit/min into superior mesenteric artery. There is constriction of branches of superior mesenteric artery and no extravasation. Infusion was continued for 48 hours and bleeding was clinically controlled. Subsequent barium enema showed diverticula of right and left colon. (Reproduced by permission, from *Radiol Clin North Am*, Vol. 14, No. 2, © 1976, W. B. Saunders Co.).

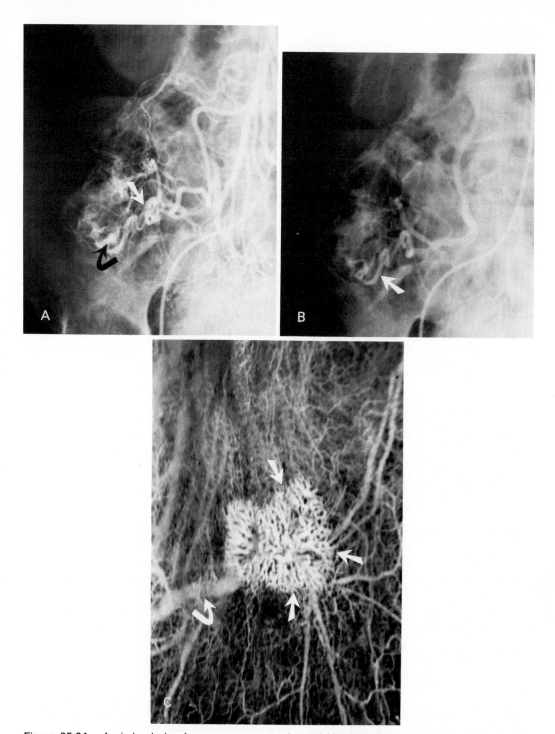

Figure 35.24. Angiodysplasia of cecum as source of rectal bleeding. A 60-year-old man had multiple episodes of rectal bleeding. Repeated barium studies and colonoscopy were unrevealing.

(A) Detailed view of cecum in superior mesenteric arteriogram. During arterial phase there is simultaneous opacification of an artery and a vein. *Curved arrow* points to vascular tuft in antemesenteric border of cecum. *Straight arrow* points to early draining vein. (B) In late phase of superior mesenteric arteriogram there is intense, persistent opacification of vein draining the lesion in the cecum (*arrow*). (C) Angiodysplasia of colon as seen under the dissecting microscope. Vessels of specimen have been injected with silicone rubber and tissues have been cleared with dehydration of specimen and immersion in methyl salicylate. *Straight arrows* point to several dilated vascular structures—mostly veins—that have assumed the typical appearance of angiodysplasia resembling a coral. *Curved arrow* points to a large draining vein in the submucosa.

(3) Early opacification of the veins drains the cecum or the ascending colon or both.

(4) Intense opacification of the draining veins persists late in the venous phase.

Contrast medium extravasation may be seen if bleeding is active at the time of arteriography. Hemorrhage may be temporarily arrested with infusion of vasopressin. The definitive therapy, however, is right colectomy.

Angiodysplasia can be neither seen nor palpated by the surgeon, and the pathologist has difficulty in identifying the lesion in resected specimens. Injection of the vessels of the specimen with sili-

cone rubber and examination of the clear specimen under the dissecting microscope have made it possible to identify angiodysplasia in patients in whom the lesions were diagnosed by angiographic examination. Histologic study reveals that the dilated vascular spaces correspond to thin-walled channels in the submucosa.

A higher incidence of bleeding from colonic angiodysplasia may occur among patients with aortic stenosis; however, a cause-and-effect relationship between these entities has not been established.

Intra-abdominal Hemorrhage. Hemorrhage into

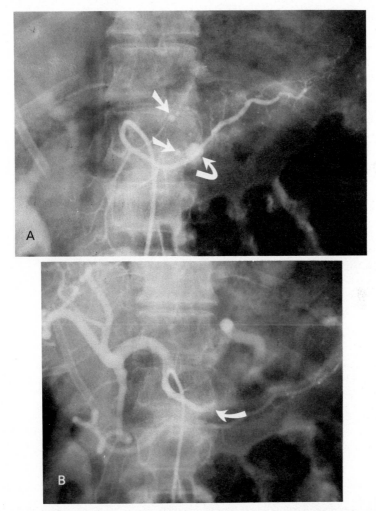

Figure 35.25. Retroperitoneal bleeding from ruptured aneurysm of transverse pancreatic artery—bleeding controlled with transcatheter embolization. A 57-year-old man had recurrent pancreatitis and a decreasing hematocrit. **(A)** Selective catheterization of dorsal pancreatic artery shows multiple small aneurysms (*straight arrows*), the result of pancreatitis, *Curved arrow* points to contrast medium extravasation secondary to rupture of one of these aneurysms. **(B)** The dorsal pancreatic artery was occluded with introduction through the angiographic catheter of surgical gelatin plugs. Repeated arteriogram shows occlusion (*arrow*) and no extravasation. Clinically the bleeding was controlled.

the peritoneal cavity or retroperitoneum unrelated to trauma may be due to a neoplasm, inflammation, or other condition affecting the vessels. If hemorrhage is massive, there is little time for diagnostic procedures before exploration. If, on the other hand, vital signs are maintained and the condition is stable after the initial episode, the patient may be evaluated with angiography so that the optimal operative procedure can be planned.

Tumors of the kidneys, liver, and retroperitoneum manifested by hemorrhage can be diagnosed with angiography, their local extent established, and the vascular supply defined. Hemorrhage may be controlled with balloon-tipped catheters or embolization so that the definitive surgical procedure can be performed under more favorable conditions rather than on an emergency basis.

Pancreatitis may at times be complicated by retroperitoneal hemorrhage resulting from erosion into surrounding vessels. The same diagnostic and therapeutic possibilities of angiography are applicable as with hemorrhage from tumors (Fig. 35.25).

Ruptured or "leaking" abdominal aortic aneurysms were previously discussed. Aneurysms of the splenic, hepatic, and renal arteries may also rupture. When they do, they may be diagnosed and their location determined with abdominal aor-tography. Transcatheter occlusion with embolization may be attempted either preoperatively or as definitive therapy.

Postoperative Bleeding

Hemorrhage into the abdominal cavity or gastrointestinal tract directly related to an operative procedure is uncommon. When it does not subside with conservative management, it may be controlled with infusion of vasopressin or transcatheter embolization. A second exploration can thus be prevented. In most instances, bleeding into the gastrointestinal tract secondary to a slipped ligature or as the result of biopsy or polypectomy via the colonoscope can be best controlled with selective infusion of vasopressin into the bleeding artery. Embolization, on the other hand, is the method of choice for the control of bleeding from the uterus, cervix, prostate gland, or bladder after a pelvic operation. The results are good with the exception of retroperitoneal bleeding after operation on the pancreas (Fig. 35.26).

Acute Pulmonary Embolism

Conditions that require emergency opacification of the inferior vena cava and pulmonary angiography for immediate and accurate diagnosis

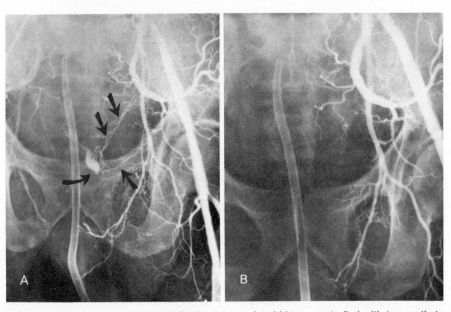

Figure 35.26. Bleeding in prostatic bed following transperineal biopsy controlled with transcatheter vessel occlusion. A 65-year-old man had an enlarged prostate gland. Transperineal biopsy was performed, followed by massive hematuria.

(A) Left common iliac arteriogram. *Curved arrow* points to extravasated contrast medium at bleeding site in prostatic bed. *Straight arrows* point to middle and superior vesical branches arising from left hypogastric artery.
(B) Left hypogastric arteriogram following embolization of vesical branches with surgical gelatin. There is no extravasation. Hematuria subsided subsequent to the procedure.

of pulmonary thromboembolism include the following:

(1) clinically suspected pulmonary embolism and an equivocal perfusion-ventilatory radionuclide study of the lungs;

(2) massive pulmonary embolism requiring thoracotomy and cardiopulmonary bypass for embolectomy;

(3) recurrent pulmonary embolism in patients on anticoagulant therapy requiring interruption of the inferior vena cava;

(4) specific contraindications to anticoagulant therapy;

(5) moderate or severe embolism in patients with associated cardiovascular problems.

To evaluate these patients, studies of the iliac veins and inferior vena cava are carried out initially. These provide anatomic information, especially if vena caval interruption is contemplated, and also provide information as to the presence of

thrombi in the inferior vena cava itself. If cavography reveals no thrombosis, selective right and left pulmonary arteriography is then performed. The diagnosis of pulmonary embolism is based on demonstration by angiography of either an intraluminal filling defect representing a thrombus or a vessel cutoff (Fig. 35.27).

Transvenous Filter Interruption of the Inferior Vena Cava

Indications for interruption of the inferior vena cava include the following:

(1) Pulmonary embolism proven angiographically in patients with contraindications to anticoagulants.

(2) Extensive venous thrombosis proven with leg venography and also in patients who cannot be treated with anticoagulants.

(3) Evidence of recurrent pulmonary embolism

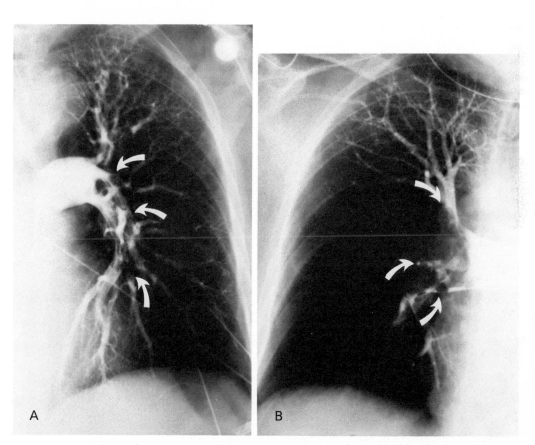

Figure 35.27. Angiography in diagnosis of pulmonary embolism. A 55-year-old woman had chest pain and shortness of breath after a pelvic operation. The lung scan showed perfusion defects. There had been a history of peptic ulcer with bleeding, and confirmation of pulmonary emboli became necessary.

(A) Left pulmonary arteriogram shows multiple intraluminal filling defects representing pulmonary emboli (*arrows*). **(B)** Right pulmonary arteriogram shows obstruction of branches to middle and lower lobes by large thrombus (*arrows*).

in patients already under treatment with antico-agulants.

The inferior vena cava may be interrupted either surgically with a clip or with a filter placed trans-venously. The ease of placement and the avoid-ance of general anesthesia have made the filter method a popular one especially among older patients with accompanying diseases such as can-cer, heart disease, etc. The Kimroy-Greenfield filter (Meditech, Inc., Watertown, MA) is currently the filter most commonly used for transvenous interruption of the IVC. It is usually introduced via the surgically exposed right internal jugular vein, although the femoral vein route may also be used if clot is peripheral thereto. It is best to perform the procedure in the angiography room because fluoroscopy is necessary for accurate po-sitioning of the filter in the infravenal segment of the inferior vena cava. With the Kimroy-Green-field filter, the incidence of recurrent pulmonary embolism is 2% and the incidence of inferior vena cava thrombosis distal to the filter is approxi-mately 10%.

Suggested Readings

Athanasoulis CA, Pfister RC, Greene RE, et al (Eds): *Interventional Radiology.* WB Saunders Co, Philadelphia, 1982

Athanasoulis CA, Baum S: Vascular disorders of the gut. Part III. Angiography, in Bockus HL, Berk JE, Haubrich WS, et al (Eds): *Gastroenterology*, ed 3, vol 4. Philadelphia, WB Saunders, 1976, pp. 329–358

Athanasoulis CA, Waltman AC, Baum S: Angiography of trauma, in Cave EF, Burke JF, Boyd RJ (Eds): *Trauma Management.* Chicago, Year Book, 1974, pp. 197–211

Athanasoulis CA, Baum S, Rösch J, et al: Mesenteric arterial infusions of vasopressin for hemorrhage from colonic diverticulosis. *Am J Surg 129:*212–216, 1975

Athanasoulis CA, Waltman AC, Novelline RA, et al: Angiography: Its contribution to the emergency management of gastrointestinal hemorrhage. *Radiol Clin North Am 14:*265–280, 1976

Baum S, Athanasoulis CA: Diagnostic studies in colonic affections. Part V. Angiography, in Bockus HL, Berk JE, Haubrich WS, et al (Eds): *Gastroenterology*, ed 3, vol 2. Philadelphia, WB Saunders, 1976, pp. 866–886

Baum S, Athanasoulis CA, Waltman AC, et al: Gastrointestinal hemorrhage. II. Angiographic diagnosis and control. *Adv Surg 7:*149–198, 1973

Freeark RJ: Role of angiography in the management of multiple injuries. *Surg Gynecol Obstet 128:*761–771, 1969

Hayashi K, Meaney TF, Zelch JV, et al: Aortographic analysis of aortic dissection. *Am J Roentgenol Radium Ther Nucl Med 122:*769–782, 1974

Hollenberg NK, Adams DF, Merrill JP, et al: Renal angiography in oliguria, in Abrams HL (Ed): *Angiography*, ed 2, vol 2. Boston, Little, Brown, 1971, pp. 887–914

Lunderquist A, Vang J: Transhepatic catheterization and obliteration of the coronary vein in patients with portal hypertension and esophageal varices. *N Engl J Med 291:*646–649, 1974

Meaney TF, Lalli AF, Alfidi RJ: *Complications and Legal Implications of Radiologic Special Procedures.* St. Louis, CV Mosby, 1973

Ring EJ, Athanasoulis C, Waltman AC, et al: Arteriographic management of hemorrhage following pelvic fracture. *Radiology 109:*65–70, 1973

White RI, Jr: *Fundamentals of Vascular Radiology.* Philadelphia, Lea & Febiger, 1976

ADMINISTRATION

CHAPTER 36

Emergency Medical Services

LENWORTH M. JACOBS, M.D.
BARBARA R. BENNETT, R.N., B.S.N.

Editor's Note: This chapter replaces two in the first edition which covered the internal workings and the external relationships of the Emergency Ward in 1975. During the interim between the two editions, the Boston Emergency Medical Services System has come of age. General considerations in the development of an EMSS are presented, in each case with a commentary on the "Boston Experience." The M.G.H. has been an integral part of this experience, having contributed the first Chairman of the Hospital Committee of the Conference of Boston Teaching Hospitals (1975–1979) and the first Medical Director of Medic IV, the EMSS for the metropolitan Boston region (1980–1982).

The following chapter explores the history of the development of emergency medical services (EMS) from a federal, state (Massachusetts), and local (Boston) perspective. The 15 EMS Components specified in P.L. 93–54, the Emergency Medical Series Systems Act of 1973, (Manpower, Training, Communications, Access to Care, Public Education/Information, Consumer Participation, Public Safety Agencies, Disaster Linkages, Facilities, Critical Care Units, Transportation, Evaluation, Patient Transfer Agreements, Mutual Aid, and Record Keeping) are discussed individually with highlighted examples of implementation from Massachusetts and Boston experiences.

INTRODUCTION AND HISTORY

Emergency Medical Services (EMS) is a multicomponent system designed to respond to a perceived or actual medical emergency. The manner in which EMS are delivered across the country has taken dramatic changes over the last two decades. War experiences, federal investigations, federal legislation, a "systems" planning approach, federal and private monies, local mandates have all contributed to making EMS systems what they are today.

Beginning with military history, statistics indicate that there has been a significant decrease in death rates beginning with World War I where the rate was 8%, to the World War II rate of 4.5%, to Korea's rate of 2.5%, to the Vietnam rate which was below 2% (Heaten, 1966). This decrease has been attributed to a system response to assessment, on-the-scene management, efficient evacuation and transportation, and coordination between field and definitive hospital-based services.

The statistics of civilian mortality and morbidity resulting from trauma have received significant scrutiny from presidents, federal agencies, and legislators. Accidental injuries totaling 52 million accounted for 107,000 deaths, 10 million temporarily disabling injuries, and 400,000 permanent injuries in 1965 (NAS-NRC, 1966). Motor vehicle accidents accounted for 49,000 deaths. In 1977, 650,000 injuries were reported as a result of trauma, with 104,000 deaths (National Safety Council, 1978). Trauma is the fourth leading cause of death in America; the first cause of death for persons between the ages of 1–37. For persons up to the age of 75, motor vehicle accidents are the leading mechanism of accidental death (DHEW, 1973). Therefore, highway safety became an important issue for the federal government. In 1966, the Governor's Highway Safety Act was signed by President Lyndon Johnson. Authority for promulgating this legislation was bestowed upon the Department of Transportation's Federal Highway Administration through its National Traffic Safety Agency (Sadler et al., 1977). Standard 11 of the Act addressed emergency medical services and made funds available through Department of Transportation (DOT) for: (1) purchase of ambulances; (2) communications equipment; (3) development of statewide EMS plans; (4) organization and administration of state programs; and (5) support of basic emergency medical technician (EMT) training (Public Law 85–564, 1966).

Also in 1966 appeared the publication of the report "Accidental Death and Disability: The Neglected Disease of Modern Society" by the National Academy of Sciences: National Research Council (NAS-NRC, 1966). This report outlined the magnitude of the trauma problem and outlined approximately 30 recommendations to mount a national effort to reduce trauma deaths and disability. The problems cited and recommendations proposed were:

(1) **Accident Prevention:** The report recommended a National Council on Accident Prevention so that there would be a consolidation of information, implementation, and formation of standards to address accident prevention.

(2) **Emergency First Aid and Medical Care:** The Report cited a gap between "knowledge" and "application" of first aid by citing inadequacies in first aid, triaging, communications, and transpor-

tation. NAS-NRC recommended training of the lay public in basic and advanced first aid along with a request for standardized texts, curricula, and programs for training police, fire, and ambulance attendants. Deficiencies in ambulance services were noted to include: (a) limited information regarding research towards improvement of ambulance services; (b) lack of data regarding current services; (c) diverse standards for vehicles, design and equipment; (d) inadequate community financial support; (e) inadequate training standards for attendants; (f) insufficient available data about the number of persons who die at the scene or en route to the hospital; (g) little or no certification standards for ambulance attendants; (h) few state ordinances regarding ambulance driving codes; (i) poor adaptation of helicopters for air rescue and transportation.

Some of the recommendations cited to answer these deficiencies were: (a) implementation of standards for ambulance design, construction, equipment, and regulations for conduct of ambulance services; (b) coordination of ambulance services with hospitals, health departments, and communications services; (c) piloting physician-staffed ambulances; (d) piloting of helicopter services in remote areas where hospital facilities were scarce; (e) designation of radio frequencies for ambulance-to-hospital and ambulance-to-dispatcher communications; (f) feasibility study for implementing a single nation-wide ambulance access number.

Other deficiencies noted were those in emergency departments including; being poorly equipped, inadequately staffed, lack of around-the-clock services, and a limited number of physicians trained in multiple emergency patient management. Strong recommendations were given to categorize hospitals as either an "Advanced First Aid Facility", a "Limited Emergency Facility", a "Major Emergency Facility", or a "Trauma Research Unit." The intent of such categorization was to determine the most appropriate hospital for a particular patient so that ambulance attendants would transport patients to hospitals that were equipped, staffed, and capable of managing them. Recommendations were made to inspect, categorize, and accredit emergency departments based on established criteria.

(3) **The Development of Trauma Registries:** Since trauma was identified as the neglected disease, recommendations were made to establish trauma registries in hospitals; to develop a national central registry; and to incorporate certain illnesses with other reportable diseases under Public Health Service control.

(4) **Hospital Trauma Committees:** A recommen-

dation centered on the need for establishing individual hospital trauma committees so that standards of care, training programs, emergency department supervision, research and follow-up studies, cardiopulmonary resuscitation (CPR) training, and evaluation of prehospital care would be addressed.

(5) **Convalescence, Disability, and Rehabilitation**: NAS-NRC recommended the conduct of studies to determine degrees of disability vis-a-vis the point at which productive work return would be indicated.

(6) **Medicolegal Problems**: The report discussed problems that end in courtrooms due to lay coroners' lack of familiarity with forensic pathology and recommends substitution of these coroners with physician medical examiners with pathology expertise.

(7) **Autopsy of Victim**: The report strongly recommended routine autopsies of accident victims to determine actual causes of death so as to guide future care rendered to accident victims.

(8) **Care of Casualties Under Conditions of Natural Disaster**: The lack of ability of the day-to-day emergency medical system to meet the needs of a multiple casualty disaster was cited as a deficiency. It was recommended that a center be designated to act as the educational and consultant authority to the lay public and medical profession.

(9) **Research in Trauma**: Not recognizing trauma as a significant health problem, and not having a defined federal or nonfederal mechanism to identify the problem, encourage research, or to enlist financial support, advice, and information were noted as significant deficiencies. Recommendations to correct this problem were rooted in establishing and financing specialized centers for clinical research in trauma, shock, medical emergencies, and war injuries to establish eventually a National Institute of Trauma.

Pilot EMS Projects

Probably as a result of recommendations made to the Department of Health, Education and Welfare (DHEW) by its Advisory Committee on Traffic Safety, chaired by Dr. Daniel Moynihan of MIT in 1968, five EMS demonstration projects were funded with 16 million dollars by the Health Services and Mental Health Administration of the DHEW. In 1972, these funded areas (the state of Arkansas, three-county area of Southern California, seven-county area of Northeast Florida, the state of Illinois, and a seven-county area of Ohio) were designated to develop various approaches to EMS systems and to serve as models for other communities and states.

Between 1966 and the awarding of funds for

pilot EMS projects, two national EMS conferences were held, one in 1969 and the other in 1972. As a result of these conferences, a number of advances occurred:

(1) The National Registry of Emergency Medical Technicians was established.

(2) The American Trauma Society was founded.

(3) Ambulance design criteria were developed.

(4) A plea to the President of the United States was made to support the improvement in EMS.

Other Funding Entities

Between 1970–1972, the Regional Medical Program provided funds totaling $10.8 million to local regional EMS planning groups (Sadler et al., 1977). The Robert Wood Johnson Foundation supported 44 grants between 1972–1977 in 32 states and Puerto Rico, totaling approximately $15 million to design emergency medical services systems (EMSS) using a regional approach to communications systems (Robert Wood Johnson Foundation, 1979).

Emergency Medical Services System Act

In 1972, a year of congressional hearings, a number of EMS-related bills were introduced, and there was some opposition from President Nixon towards the request being made for EMS funds (Nixon, 1973; US House of Representatives, 1972). However, in November of 1973, Senate Bill 2410 passed both the House and Senate and was signed into law by President Nixon (Public Law 93–154, 1973). Public Law 93–154 (EMSS Act of 1973) was later amended as Public Law 94–573 in 1976 and again in 1979 as Public Law 96–142 (1976, 1979). The sections of the grant were as follows:

Section 1202, Feasibility Projects.

Section 1203, Establishment and Initial Operations of a System.

Section 1204, Expansion and Improvement of Systems.

The Emergency Medical Services Systems portion of the Public Health Services Act is Title XII. Title VII of the same act is related to EMS Research (Section 1205) and is administered by the National Center for Health Services Research. Title VIII is related to training in EMS and is administered by the Bureau of Health Manpower, Division of Medicine of the Health Resources Administration (DHEW, 1975).

Administration of the EMSS Act from 1974–1981 was the responsibility of the Division of Emergency Medical Services of the DHEW, currently the Department of Health and Human Services (DHHS) (1975). This agency divided the states into approximately 300 regions geographically for the purpose of EMS planning and funding. The funding of EMS projects over the last 7 years was founded on specific classical principles: (1) the concept of organizing a system on a regional basis; (2) planning and implementing EMS as a "system" of care; (3) establishment of basic EMS by components integrated into a system (the mandatory basic components: manpower, training, communications, transportation, facilities, critical care units, disaster linkages, consumer information, consumer participation, public safety agencies, patient transfers, record keeping, evaluation, mutual aid, access to care); (4) seven critical-care clinical groups defined as requiring specialized subsystems within the total EMS system (DHEW, 1975): burns, spinal cord injuries, trauma, acute cardiac, poisonings, behavioral emergencies, high risk infants and mothers; (5) identification of two levels of EMSS (DHEW, 1975):

(a) *Basic life support* (BLS): "implementation of the 15 components of an EMS system to a level of capability which provides prehospital noninvasive emergency patient care designed to optimize the patient's chances of surviving the emergency situation. There should be universal access to and dispatch of national standard ambulances, with appropriate medical and communication equipment, operated by EMT-A's. Regional triage protocols should be used to direct patients to appropriately designated hospitals."

(b) *Advanced life support* (ALS): "implementation of the 15 components of an EMS system to a level of capability which provides both noninvasive and invasive emergency patient care designed to optimize the patient's chances of surviving the emergency situation. Services should include use of sophisticated transportation vehicles, a communications capability (two-way voice and/or telemetry) and staffing by EMT-P's providing on-site, prehospital mobile and hospital intensive care under medical control."

The Division of EMS of the DHHS under the direction of Dr. David Boyd, has affected almost every region of the country. The impact of this federal effort is impressive and dramatic, extending across the nation. Boyd reports that 98.4% of the nation's regions have received some sort of federal support related to EMS; five regions (1.6%) have received no funds; and 57 regions (18.9%) have received funding at all three levels (1202, 1203, 1204) (Boyd, 1981).

Current Status

The EMS program is now part of the Reconciliation Act of 1981, and is part of the Health Prevention Block Grant which is Public Law 97–35. The implications of this change center around a shift of responsibility from the federal government to state governments who will now have authority over the discretionary placement of funds among various other prevention programs, of which EMS is one. Table 36.1 demonstrates the amount of funds, purpose of funds, and awarding agencies for EMS funding from 1970–1981.

Considerable focus of the EMS planning effort was on prehospital services, including training and certification of EMTs and paramedics, vehicular standards for ambulances, and coordinated communications systems. Trauma care was obviously the reason for much of the elaborate national effort to improve EMS. However, the sudden medical illness patient is more frequently the recipient of these improved services. The deaths from ischemic heart disease far exceed those from trauma. Over 650,000 persons die each year from ischemic heart disease. Approximately 350,000 of these deaths occur outside of a hospital setting (American Heart Association, 1981). As discussion follows detailing the 15 EMS components and the 7 critical care categories, various areas of the country that have implemented systems to meet the needs of certain emergency patients will be identified.

Massachusetts Experience

The Massachusetts State Office of EMS under the State's Department of Public Health has been the lead agency for EMS planning, implementation, and technical assistance to regional, area and local health planners and providers. The scope of the EMS problem in the early 1970s in Massachusetts was similar to what was seen by the national perspective. Cardiovascular disease claimed 21,109 lives in 1975, and was the leading cause of death. Trauma, the third cause of death in Massachusetts in 1975, claimed 2310 lives (Kovar, 1980). After receiving initial regional medical program monies, Massachusetts received its first federal EMS Act monies totalling $1,888,891 in 1974 (Department of Health Services Delivery [DHSD], 1981). From 1974–1981, Massachusetts was awarded a total of $7,235,375 (DHSD, 1981). Table 36.2 compares the amounts of federal monies awarded to each of the six states in Region I (New England).

The change in the delivery of EMS in the city of Boston stands as a profound example of EMS development achieved through the efforts of persons committed to the goal and supported by various federal, state, city, and local agencies. As the description of the EMS components follows, various experiences of the Boston system will be described to define this change.

Table 36.1.
Monies expended towards EMSS (Emergency Medical Services Systems) development.

Year	Agency[a]	Purpose	Monies
1974–1981	EMS-HEW	EMS Systems	$244,702,000
1974–1980	EMS-NCHSR	EMS Research	$ 31,625,000
1974–1980	EMS-BHM-HRA	EMS Training	$ 33,099,000
1972	HSMHA	EMS Demos[a]	$ 16,000,000
1970–1972	RMP	EMS Systems	$ 10,800,000
1972–1977	RWJ	EMS Systems	$ 15,000,000
1967–1981	NHTS-DOT	EMS Standard 11	$173,709,070
1967–1981	NHTS-DOT	EMS Research	$ 8,000,000 (approximately)
Total			$532,935,070

[a] Key: EMS—Emergency Medical Services, HEW—Department of Health, Education and Welfare (Health & Human Services), NCHSR—National Center for Health Services Research, BHM-HRA—Bureau of Health Manpower-Health Resources Administration, HSMHA—Health Services Mental Health Administration, RMP—Regional Medical Program, RWJ—Robert Wood Johnson Foundation, NHTS-DOT—National Highway Traffic Safety-Department of Transportation, Demos—demonstration projects.

Table 36.2.
Title XII funds in region I.

Connecticut	$ 3,510,936
Maine	$ 4,573,504
Massachusetts	$ 7,235,375
New Hampshire	$ 3,586,678
Rhode Island	$ 1,250,000
Vermont	$ 2,296,000
Total Region I	$22,452,493

MANPOWER AND TRAINING

Introduction

The improvement in the organization and delivery of EMS has strengthened the links between those emergency care providers in the field, and the health professionals providing care within receiving hospitals. The planning processes used to organize EMS systems usually recognize not only those persons who provide direct patient care, but also those persons involved at the administrative level, i.e., officials of public safety agencies, hospital administrators, and EMS system planners and coordinators.

Over the last decade, a number of educational advances have resulted in establishing standards of training and certification for these EMS providers. Most profoundly, these advances are best defined in the areas of basic and advanced emergency medical technology, emergency nursing, emergency medicine, and specialty education for a number of varied disciplines focusing on the initial management of emergency patients.

The following section will define the role, education/training approaches and certification, for the members of the EMS manpower team. Additionally, examples taken from statewide as well as city of Boston experiences will highlight specific educational programs.

Basic Emergency Medical Technology

History and Curriculum

The manner in which ill and injured persons were treated and transported to emergency departments received considerable scrutiny by the authors of the document "Accidental Death and Disability: The Neglected Disease of Modern Society", by NAS-NRC (1966). This document stressed the need for improved handling of trauma victims at the scene and en route to hospitals. In this same year, the National Highway Safety Act provided the authorization for the DOT to administer funds for programs for the development of basic EMSS. These funds led to the development of a standard curriculum for the training of ambulance attendants. Prior to the development of the DOT curriculum, the Committee on Injuries of the American Academy of Orthopedic Surgeons were the leaders in offering training programs, beginning in 1964, for emergency care providers (Committee on Allied Health, 1971). In 1971, the text *Emergency Care and Transportation of the Sick and Injured*, by the American Academy of Orthopedic Surgeons was published. This text provided the standard for the educational material needed to educate an ambulance attendant, now called an EMT. A standard curriculum and text were used to further the educational level of those persons responsible for handling patients prior to hospital-based intervention.

The 81-hour DOT curriculum encompasses the principles of patient assessment, the techniques of patient management limited to noninvasive management, such as splinting, CPR, bandaging, ox-

Table 36.3.
EMT course design.

Lesson Number	Lesson	Hours
1	Introduction to emergency care training	3
2	Airway obstruction and respiratory arrest	3
3	Cardiac arrest	3
4	Mechanical aids to breathing/resuscitation	3
5	Bleeding shock: CPR practice	3
6	Practice: test/evaluation lessons 1–5	3
7	Wounds	3
8	Principles musculoskeletal care: fractures upper extremity	3
9	Fractures: pelvis, hip, lower extremity	3
10	Injuries of neck, face, spine	3
11	Injuries to eye, chest, abdomen, genitalia	3
12	Practice: test/evaluation lessons 7–11	3
13	Practice: test/evaluation lessons 7–11	2.5
14	Medical emergencies, part I	3
15	Medical emergencies, part II	2.5
16	Emergency childbirth	2.5
17	Environmental emergencies	3
18	Lifting and moving patients	3
19	Extrication techniques	3
20	Practice: test/evaluation lessons 14–19	3
21	Operations/driving/maintenance/records/communications	3
22	Responding to ambulance calls	2
23	Situational reviews	3
24	Final written examination	2
25	Final practice evaluation of skills	3
Total Classroom Hours		71.5
Emergency Department Observation		10
Total Course Hours		81.5

ygen administration, extrication, and transportation techniques. Table 36.3 illustrates the topics and hours of a basic EMT training program.

Approach To Training

Considerable coordination was needed to determine the approach to this new training endeavor. The DOT estimated that there were approximately 14,000 ambulance services nationally. These services were diversely operated by municipal departments such as police or fire, by volunteer groups, or by private companies, as well as a few municipally operated health departments.

The Massachusetts approach to implementing the newly available training standards serves as a descriptive example of a statewide coordinated effort that integrated the training of emergency medical technicians with the simultaneous implementation of other EMS components.

Other states, such as New York, Florida, Virginia, California, Illinois, and Washington, were pioneers in the early 1970s in the area of training prehospital providers (DHEW, 1975; Liberthsen et al., 1974; Grace and Chadbourn, 1969; Boyd et al., 1973). However, it was in August of 1973 that the Massachusetts Department of Public Health—Office of EMS conducted an ambulance service survey to launch their training of ambulance personnel (Office of EMS, 1974). Conducting such a survey prior to training should achieve the following objectives: (1) to determine the providers of ambulance service in a specific geographic area; (2) to estimate the number of persons providing prehospital care; (3) to identify the scope of ambulance service provided, i.e., number of transports; (4) to correlate survey results with the need for ambulance service based on size, geography, population and medical resources, and; (5) to set standards for training and to determine a phase-in requirement for services to meet such standards.

As the survey was underway, an effort was begun to pass legislation that would firmly establish the standards for training and certification of EMTs. In October 1973, the Massachusetts legislature enacted Massachusetts General Law 111C, an "act to Insure High Quality Emergency Care through Regulation of Ambulances and Ambulance Services." The previous standard of Advanced First Aid was replaced with the basic EMT Training Program as developed by the DOT.

To comply with this new training requirement, a phase-in process was defined that resulted in having all ambulance operators and attendants employed by an ambulance service, trained and certified at the end of three years. Federal EMS funds and a Division of EMT Training at the state office of EMS level have served, since 1973, as the basis for initiating and maintaining EMT standards.

Certification

As of May, 1981, 20,046 persons have been certified by the National Registry of EMTs in Massachusetts with 13,623 EMTs maintaining current certification (Registry, 1981).

The National Registry of EMTs is the leading certifying and testing agency in the country. Although other states have adopted their own certifying examinations, 29 states do recognize National Registry Certification as a basis for reciprocity. The Registry reports a total of 159,273 certified EMTs in the US and eight other countries. It is recognized that an EMT has a well defined role in an EMSS, and that the scope of his/her practice is relatively uniform throughout the nation.

Recertification for basic EMTs, certified by the National Registry, is a process completed every 2 years. The activities required for basic recertification include: (1) 20-hour refresher course; (2) certification in CPR yearly; (3) 48 hours continuing education; e.g., 15 hours in emergency department as an observer, attendance at continuing education conferences, and/or in-service training.

Advanced Emergency Medical Technology

History and Curriculum

As basic emergency medical technology flourished, a number of states proceeded directly towards training a technician who would manage patients using more sophisticated and advanced techniques. Other countries such as England, Ireland, and Russia were already involved in comprehensive, sophisticated methods of prehospital care utilizing mobile intensive care teams (Pantridge, 1970; Briggs et al., 1976; Scribner et al., 1974). Although California passed the Wedworth-Townsend Paramedic Act in July, 1974, other states were providing advanced prehospital care beyond the basic EMT level without accompanying authorizing legislation (Page, 1979).

The out-of-hospital cardiac arrest continues to be a topic of physician-sponsored research and the focus of training EMS personnel to meet the needs of such a patient group (Rockswald et al., 1979, Eisenberg et al., 1980, Copley et al., 1977; Crampton et al., 1975; Baum et al., 1974). Immediate intervention at the scene needed definition in terms of management and use of resources. The American Heart Association (1980) defined the problem and has updated its statistics in the recent 1980 Standards of Basic Cardiopulmonary Resuscitation (CPR) and Emergency Cardiac Care (ECC). It has been estimated that 60–70% of sudden deaths from any cause occur outside of the hospital (American Heart Association, 1980). Of these deaths, 54% occur as a result of ischemic heart disease (American Heart Association, 1980). As the trauma patient was the focus for improving *basic* emergency medical care, it is the sudden death cardiac patient who is the focus for providing *advanced* emergency medical care.

Advanced ambulance services were initiated in the late 1960s and early 1970s often as a result of a single interested physician leading the effort (Page, 1979). The programs that resulted, therefore, were developed and defined at a local level, and varied significantly from state to state. Beginning with Dr. Eugene Nagel's first advanced EMT training program in 1967, the growing numbers of courses over subsequent years have varied in length, skills taught, depth of academic basis, certification, and testing. However, it was not until 1977 that the DOT, Department of Labor, and the DHEW published The Emergency Medical Technician—Paramedic National Training Course. This course was developed with the University of Pittsburgh. As a result of this gap between the actual training and the setting of national curriculum standards, there is considerable controversy and confusion surrounding the definition of an advanced EMT, as well as defining in concrete terms the scope of the practice of paramedicine (Page, 1979; Romano et al., 1977; Lambrew, 1975).

According to the National Training Course Guide, the subject materials needed to train advanced EMTs can be found in the following modules:

(1) The Role of EMT-Paramedic;
(2) Human Systems and Patient Assessment;
(3) Shock and Fluid Therapy;
(4) Pharmacology;
(5) Respiratory Emergencies;
(6) Cardiovascular Emergencies;
(7) Central Nervous System;
(8) Soft Tissue Injuries;
(9) Musculoskeletal Emergencies;
(10) Medical Emergencies;
(11) Obstetric/GYN Emergencies;
(12) Pediatric/Neonatal Emergencies;

(13) Behavioral Emergencies;

(14) Rescue Techniques;

(15) Telemetry and Communications.

Since there exist various levels of advanced EMTs, the National Training Course suggests teaching specific modules for the various levels. The number and title of specific modules are used as a guide for identifying the level of education of the graduating EMT. For example: *EMT-Intravenous*: Modules 1, 2, 3; *EMT-Cardiac*: Modules 1, 2, 3, 4, 5, 6, 15; *EMT-Paramedic*: Modules 1–15.

Approach to Training

The city of Boston serves as an example of a health department's response to forming an advanced life support system by first training paramedics. With start-up funds awarded to the Department of Health and Hospitals (DHH) of the city of Boston by the State Office of EMS, the first paramedic training program following the detailed HEW-DOT-DOL Training Course was initiated.

The 15-module course provides the educator with fundamental objectives and corresponding curriculum content. The training course is flexible in terms of hours, certain skills, faculty designations, and testing. However, the foundation provided in the course materials serves as a national educational standard. The course can be adapted, because of its modular approach, to coincide in length with available funds, as well as with the clinical needs germane to the service's responding area.

Didactic classroom training accompanied by supervised rotations in appropriate hospital areas is required to refine those skills related to a particular level of training. The Boston City Hospital (BCH) and its neighboring Boston University Medical Center provide the needed clinical resources for skills practice. These areas include the operating room, emergency department, labor and delivery, the New England Regional Spinal Cord Injury Center, coronary care unit, and medical and surgical intensive care units. Supervision in these areas was provided by 3rd-year or above specialty residents. The 6-months of didactic sessions followed by a 3-month clinical rotation paved the way for a final 500-hour supervised field internship.

Field internships vary significantly from program to program. Examples include paramedic student supervision by experienced EMT-Ps; supervision by mobile intensive care nurses; or supervision by physicians. Judging the appropriate time needed for individual students to complete an internship is often based on: (1) hours in the field; (2) objective evaluation of performance; (3) performance of certain skills a number of times

previously determined. Supervision of paramedic students in Boston was performed by paramedic nurse educators and physicians in a pattern that permitted these field supervisors to respond to any one of two advanced life support (ALS) vehicles staffed by two paramedic students and one veteran paramedic. (Fig. 36.1) Table 36.4 illustrates the format for the year-long paramedic training program conducted at BCH.

Certification and Evaluation

Evaluation of advanced EMT training programs and their graduates is varied and lacks standard evaluative measures that are accepted nationwide. The National Registry of EMTs offers a written and practical examination that corresponds to the curriculum of the National Training Course for EMT-I and EMT-P levels. Of the 45 states that offer EMT-P training, the National Registry EMT-P exam is used as the state certification exam in 21 and the EMT-I exam is offered in 6 (Weigel, 1980). Other states either use state approved exams, or individual programs conduct their own testing procedures. The Registry reports 1039 registered paramedics with an additional 174 persons with provisional certification.

As the need for standardization emerges along with a realization that certification reciprocity from state to state is poorly defined, the evaluation of programs and the performance of their graduates are challenging priorities for this new profession.

The National Registry quotes an overall 80% pass rate on the practical portion of the examination, and a 50% pass rate on the written portion. In comparison, the first paramedic training program conducted at BCH instructed 16 students, of whom 15 passed the National Registry's examination (93%). Its second paramedic training program instructed 13 students, all of whom passed both portions of the examination (100%). The measured success of these training programs is attributable to:

(1) close adherence to the objectives and curriculum content of the National Training Course;

(2) an in-depth academic basis;

(3) dedicated course faculty instead of multiple lecturers;

(4) comprehensive selection process for students including written examination, personal interview, previous field experience, and job performance review;

(5) comprehensive clinical resources at a major teaching hospital;

(6) a comprehensive field internship including EMS physician or emergency nurse supervi-

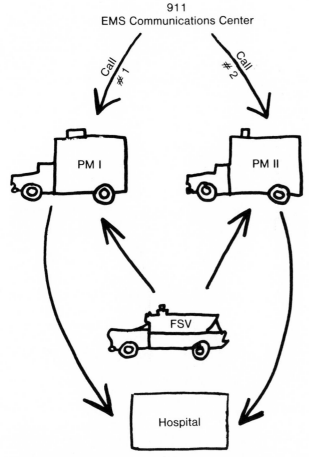

911
EMS Communications Center

Time Sequence

8:00 Call # 1 received
8:02 Dispatch PM I & FSV
8:30 Call # 2 received
8:32 Dispatch PM II & FSV

8:35 PM I leaves for hospital
8:46 PM I arrives hospital
8:55 PM II leaves for hospital
9:05 PM II arrives hospital

* Each paramedic unit has a crew of two paramedic students
  and one veteran paramedic.
* FSV = field services vehicle is staffed by one R.N. or M.D.
  paramedic intern field supervisor and one paramedic student.
* The advantage of this system is that once the patient is
  stabilized in the field and/or en route to the hospital,
  the FSV is free to respond to a second student-staffed
  unit.

Figure 36.1.   Boston City Hospital paramedic field internship design as part of paramedic training program.

sors, a total of 500 hours, conducted with a service that responds to an adequate number of emergency calls;

(7) full-time training schedule, and;

(8) close physician supervision.

Evaluation. The Center for the Study of Emergency Health Services at the University of Pennsylvania conducted a survey to identify the types of paramedic services operational in the US (Romano et al., 1978). Of the 310 services identified, 33% were operated by fire departments, 31% operated by a municipal service, 2% operated by police departments, 19% were hospital-based, and 14% were commercially owned. It was noted that the differences in service were not limited to the operating agency, but extended to the methods of training, certification requirements, and type of skills performed. This lack of standardization has made it extremely difficult to evaluate research statistics related to prehospital ALS. Cost-effectiveness and clinical outcome of patients managed with ALS techniques are the focus of studies now underway to address the controversy related to the need for prehospital ALS (Szczygiel et al., 1981; Eisenberg et al., 1979; Lauterbach et al., 1978).

The evaluation of prehospital ALS provided by advanced EMTs of various levels is in progress. Cayton et al. (1981) evaluated the use of clinical algorithms. Eisenberg et al. (1980) compared survival of patients defibrillated in the field by EMTs

Table 36.4.
Paramedic training program.

Module		Hours Boston City Hospital	Hours Recommended by National Training Course
1	Role/responsibilities of EMT-P	8	3
2	Human systems/patient assessment	24	10
3	Shock and fluid therapy	16	12
4	Pharmacology	16	9
5	Respiratory emergencies	16	27
6	Cardiovascular emergencies	81	48
7	Central nervous system	33	12
8	Soft tissue injuries	29	10
9	Musculoskeletal injuries	6	10
10	Medical emergencies	36	12
11	Obstetric/gynecologic emergencies	4	12
12	Pediatric emergencies	24	8
13	Behavioral emergencies	24	8
14	Rescue techniques	8	
15	Telecommunications	8	4
Total		333	185

Boston City Hospital Program Hours
Total didactic hours = 333
Total clinical hours = 320
Total classroom practice = 32
Intermittent ambulance = 143
Field internship = 500

Total Hours = 1328

trained in the recognition of ventricular fibrillation and countershock techniques with those patients receiving care by standard basic EMTs. The use of an esophageal obturator for airway control versus the use of an endotracheal tube is still under investigation (Berdeen, 1981). Reported cases of MAST device use have been reported by McSwain (1977) and Civetta (Kaplan et al., 1973). The use of bretylium tosylate for the treatment of ventricular fibrillation is also a topic of research (Koch-Weser, 1979; Hayes et al., 1978).

Training and certification of all levels of EMTs are activities that are monitored by most EMS systems. However, the method to determine the number of persons needed to meet the system's *actual,* instead of *perceived* need, is the present dilemma. The National Academy of Sciences in its follow-up report to its original 1966 report recommends addressing this dilemma:

(1) Determine a distribution of EMTs and advanced EMTs "on the basis of the expected frequency of life-threatening emergencies that require advanced care, the assumed capabilities of EMTs with various levels of training, and the relative cost of teaching and

maintaining skills and knowledge involved" (NAS-NRC, 1978).

(2) Coordinate the determination of numbers of EMTs needed by evaluating the effectiveness of advanced prehospital care that is rendered by following established written protocol and care provided by direct physician orders via telecommunications.

(3) Evaluate the performance of prehospital providers by direct-field observation instead of judging performance on the numbers of hours in service.

Table 36.5 shows the relation of population, ambulance services, and certified basic ambulance personnel per region in Massachusetts.

Recertification. Recertification of paramedics certified by the National Registry is a process which takes place every 2 years and includes: (1) 48 hours of refresher training, (2) 24 hours of continuing education, (3) certification in Advanced Cardiac Life Support (ACLS) by the American Heart Association, (4) medical director acknowledgement of satisfactory field performance and skill performance.

A unique process of recertification for paramed-

Table 36.5.
Massachusetts EMS regions: Numbers of EMTs by population.

Region	Population	Licensed Ambulance Services	Certified EMTs	Number Ambulance Operators/ Attendants
3	485,024	15	655	180
6	630,802	27	875	324
2	729,381	63	1864	756
1	777,592	35	1731	613
5	1,063,999	85	2206	1020
4	2,041,491	73	4567	875

ics certified in Massachusetts and employed by the DHH Ambulance Service includes: (1) attendance at 70% of weekly scheduled paramedic rounds, chaired by the medical director and two other medical control physicians. Rounds include case presentations from the previous week, which are presented by the paramedics and then discussed in an academic forum; (2) 12 hours of continuing education each year; (3) 24 hours of refresher training each year, and; (4) 100 multiple choice question examination each year: 80% pass required.

State of Advanced EMT Training

Forty-seven states plus the District of Columbia offer some form of advanced EMT training. Program length varies, yet the majority of programs do use the 15 module National Training Course as the curriculum. A number of programs offer an Associates Degree, e.g., programs in Miami, North Carolina, Ohio and Oregon (National Registry of EMTs, 1981). It is estimated that there are approximately 22,000 advanced EMTs in the US with over 50% of them located in five states (California, New York, Florida, Ohio, Illinois). The lack of a uniform certification system, however, remains a disturbing factor that prohibits program comparison, research credibility, and standardization within the profession.

Emergency Nursing

Definition

The Emergency Department Nurses Association (EDNA), the national organization that represents 11,000 of the estimated 60,000 emergency nurses in the United States defines emergency nursing practice as . . . "the nursing care of individuals of all ages with perceived physical and/or emotional alterations which are undiagnosed and may require prompt intervention. Emergency nursing care is unscheduled and most commonly occurs in a specific setting, i.e., an emergency department, a mobile unit, or a suicide prevention center. Thus the nursing care is episodic, primary, and acute in nature" (American Nurses Association, 1975). Derived from this is a definition of the responsibilities of an emergency nurse, including initial patient assessment and health history-taking, definition of treatment priorities, synthesis of information/data, and recognition and management of certain disorders including life-threatening emergencies.

Continuing Education Needs

As the number of patient visits to hospital emergency departments increases, and the education of prehospital providers advances, the demands on emergency nurses have expanded. The Massachusetts response to this demand was the development of the Critical Care Emergency Department Nurse Education Program (CEDNEP) as a comprehensive educational resource. In order to develop a continuing education program that would meet the majority of emergency nurses needs, the State Office of EMS and its designated Statewide Nurses Continuing Education Committee developed a questionnaire. In March of 1975, copies of the questionnaire were sent to head nurses of emergency departments in the state's 110 acute care hospitals. Over 400 of the estimated 1500 emergency department nurses responded. The results shown in Table 36.6 demonstrate strong interest in continuing education as well as refresher training interest, specifically in the areas of care related to patients who are critically ill.

An additional method used to evaluate the need for a continuing education program was to test nurses attending pilot CEDNEPs. During the first three pilot programs, 27 nurses were tested at the onset of the program, at the end, and at an interval of no less than 9 months after the program. The 100 multiple choice question examination was based on curriculum subject material. Table 36.7 shows certain clinical topics, pre- and post-scores related to these topics, plus the results of the questionnaire, which show a correlation between interest and a need for information. (Table 36.8)

Table 36.6.

Interest in continuing education expressed by Massachusetts emergency department registered nurses.

Workshops in Clinical Topics	Respondents Interested in Refresher[a]	Workshops in Manipulative Skills	Respondents Interested in Refresher[a]
Medical crises	86%	EKG interpretation	54%
Surgical crises	86%	Chest tube set-up	51%
Neurologic emergencies	82%	CVP insertion	47%
Electrocardiographic interpretation	80%	Ventilators	46%
Pediatric emergencies	79%	Hemorrhage control	38%
Emergency drugs	78%	Defibrillation	34%
Burn management	75%	X-ray	34%
Drug overdose	71%	Arterial puncture	31%
Eye emergencies	70%	Tourniquets	30%
Psychiatric crises	64%	Nasogastric tube	29%
Orthopedics/splinting	60%	CPR	23%
Obstetrics/gynecology	59%	Mechanical aids to breathing	20%
X-ray interpretation	59%	Intravenous insertion	20%
Neonatal crises	52%	Splinting	15%
Basic sciences	43%	Male catheters	10%
Dermatology	31%	Female catheters	2%

[a] % = percent of 210 registered nurse questionnaires received from survey conducted by the Office of Emergency Medical Services.

Table 36.7.

CEDNEP month-long pre- and post-test average scores/follow-up test scores.

Date	Number of Students	Pre-Test Average	Post-Test Average	Follow-up Average
April, 1975	7	50.7	75.7	79 (after 18 months)
September, 1975	12	61	95.7	85 (after 12 months)
January, 1976	8	57.4	91.2	89 (after 9 months)

Curriculum

The state office of EMS, through its Advisory Board, formed a Nurses Continuing Education Committee. The Committee had statewide representation from emergency departments and leading nursing organizations. The Committee advised the Office of EMS nursing staff in the development of a curriculum to form the basis of a continuing education program. Statewide objectives were established: (1) to make local hospitals aware of the need for continuing education so that hospitals would cosponsor educational programs in their area; (2) to orient physicians and nurses serving as course faculty to the educational needs of local nurses and to assist the faculty in the development of treatment protocols for nurses to follow, and (3) to conduct continuing education programs for emergency nurses that focus on the knowledge and techniques needed to provide appropriate care to patients with critical illnesses and injuries.

With these three objectives identified, area EMS committees, representing area hospitals, were utilized as the vehicle to plan and implement local programs. The CEDNEP program includes 97.5 hours of didactic sessions with 40 hours of clinical

experience. Twenty-four of the clinical hours are conducted in an emergency department, and 16 hours with an ambulance service.

Specific curriculum objectives are to: identify pathophysiological concepts related to illness/injury; differentiate between normal and abnormal data collected by assessment, radiology, and laboratory testing; identify the psychological and behavioral aspects of stress on the patient and family; conduct an assessment and physical examination of patients with specific clinical disorders; identify the presenting signs and symptoms of specific clinical disorders; evaluate outcomes of all nursing interventions; establish patient care priorities; identify teaching methods that meet patient family learning needs; construct a plan of nursing care.

Since the initial pilot CEDNEP in 1975, there have been 41 programs, and 892 graduates, as of April, 1981. Graduates receive 19.7 continuing education credits from the Massachusetts Nurses Association. Table 36.9 outlines topics and hours.

Emergency Department Nurses Association

As Massachusetts pursues the goal of programmatically meeting the educational needs of emergency nurses, the EDNA pursues the important role of identifying emergency nursing as a specialty. In so doing, EDNA has established a Core Curriculum containing, in modular form, the academic content of emergency nursing. EDNA has founded the Board of Certification for Emergency Nursing. Two certification examinations have been given, and there are now 2172 certified emergency nurses across the nation (1981). These nurses have successfully passed a 250 multiple choice question examination pertaining to the de-

fined knowledge related to emergency nursing. Of the total group applying for the examination in February of 1981, 88% were female, 39% were between the ages of 30–39, 65% were staff nurses, 87% were employed in emergency departments, 60% were employed in private hospitals, and 52% were also certified in ACLS.

Expanded Roles

Modern emergency nursing not only includes those professionals employed in emergency de-

Table 36.8.

Determination of correlation between interest and need for refresher training.

Clinical Areas on Test	3 Courses Pre-Test %	3 Courses Post-Test %	Questionnaire Respondents %
EKG interpretation	66	94	80
Medical emergencies	52	83	86
Burn management	39	80	75
Pharmacology	58	89	71
Surgical crises	59	76	86
CPR	59	92	23
Orthopedics/splinting	73	93	60
C.V.P. use	53	88	40

Table 36.9.

Critical care emergency department nurse education program clinical topics.

Topic	Hours	Topic	Hours
Overview of EMS	1	BLS certification	6
Role of the EMT and EMT-P	1	Cardiogenic shock	1
Role of the ED nurse	1	Quiz	1
Pre-course test	2	GYN emergencies	1
Anatomy/physiology review	6	CHF/pulmonary edema	1.5
Burn management	6	Fluids/electrolytes	1.5
X-ray principles	2	Pharmacology	1
Hypovolemic shock	1.5	Cardiac drugs	1.5
Head, neck, spinal cord	1.5	Vasoactive drugs	1
Clinical evaluation of multiple trauma victim	1.5	Respiratory failure	1
Psychological aspects of stress	3	Asthma and COPD	1
Thoracic trauma	1	Quiz	1
Quiz	1	Neurological emergencies	2
Eye emergencies	1	Conference RE clinical	1
Genitourinary trauma	1	Poisons	1
Abdominal trauma	1.5	Near-drowning	1
Peripheral vascular	1	Anaphylaxis	1
Facial trauma	1.5	DIC	2
Alcohol and other problems	1	Case studies	3
Arterial blood gases	2	Advanced life support	1
Blood and components	1.5	Drug abuse/overdose	1
Orthopedic injuries	1	Diabetic emergencies	1.5
Splinting	1	Tetanus prophylaxis	1
Cardiac anatomy/physiology	2	Quiz	1
Electrophysiology	1	CVP	1.5
Basics of EKG interpretation	1	Neurologic assessment	2
Dysrhythmias, part I	2	Medical legal aspects	1.5
Myocardial infarction	1	Triage principles	1
Pacemaker therapy	1	Post-course test	2
Dysrhythmias, part II	4		

partments, but has expanded recently to identify a specialized group of emergency nurses that are employed by air emergency services, providing both helicopter and fixed-wing transport. The newly formed organization called the American Society of Hospital-Based Emergency Air Medical Services is taking an active role in organizing and standardizing flight nursing within its group.

Physicians

Physician involvement in an emergency medical services system is necessary on a variety of fronts. The emergency department must be staffed by physicians. Prehospital ALS should be controlled and directed by physicians. The specialty systems (burns, poisons, spinal cord injuries, neonatal crises, acute cardiac, trauma, behavioral emergencies) must have physician consultants identified in each category. The EMS system as a whole should identify a medical director.

Emergency Medicine

The American Board of Emergency Medicine was approved by the American Board of Medical Specialties in September of 1979 (American College of Emergency Physicians, 1979). As of November, 1981, there are 461 diplomates of the Board across the United States (personal contact, 1982). Many events occurring during the last two decades have contributed to the emergence of this newest twenty-third specialty. Of particular significance has been the increasing utilization of the nation's emergency departments, and their changing functions as resources for the delivery of primary medical care. In 1978, there were 83 million visits to emergency facilities in the U.S.A. (American Hospital Association, 1979). This is an increase from 72.9 million in 1977. The "accident floor" concept has expanded to "emergency departments" with subsequent expansion in medical and nursing staffs, an extension of hours of function, an increase in services provided, and a modification of standards and criteria for optimum provision of care. With the development of federally funded EMS systems that have coordinated the prehospital and hospital components of EMS, there has been the growing need for physician leadership and direction (Committee on EMS, 1978).

The American College of Emergency Physicians (ACEP), representing 11,000 of the emergency physicians in the United States, defines emergency medicine specifically as follows . . . "encompasses the immediate decision making and action necessary to prevent death or any further disability for patients in health crises." Emergency medicine is practiced as patient-demanded and continuously accessible care. It is the time-dependent process of initial recognition, stabilization, evaluation, treatment, and disposition. The patient population is unrestricted and presents with a full spectrum of episodic, undifferentiated physical and behavioral conditions. Emergency medicine is primarily hospital-based, but with extensive prehospital responsibilities (1980).

Most traditional medical specialties deal with disease, illness, or injury affecting specific body systems; emergency medicine is defined by the *setting* in which the specialty is practiced, i.e., the emergency department, and also the *time interval* in which the medical event occurs. The practice of emergency medicine spans the entire range of body systems, the entire range of the traditional specialties, and includes all ages from pediatrics to geriatrics.

Emergency Department Staffing

The staffing of emergency departments by physicians varies and has undergone considerable change over the last two decades. As an example, Massachusetts reports a change in the trend of coverage in its 110 acute care hospitals for 1980. Eighty-four of these hospitals (76%) reported 17% full-time coverage by emergency physicians, and 40% reported a combination of full-time and part-time emergency physicians. Considering this as a total 57% of hospitals having emergency physician staffing, this is an increase in such coverage by 12% in 1978 and 11% in 1979. Of the reporting hospitals, 11% indicated a staffing pattern that rotates active medical staff members, some with, and some without "moonlighters." This is a 3% decline from this pattern as compared to 1978 and a 1.5% in 1979.

Resident staff coverage was reported in 13% of the reporting hospitals (Office of EMS, 1981). Larger, urban medical centers, such as found in Boston, are rendering emergency care services utilizing this resident staff coverage design.

Curriculum

A specialist in the medical profession practices within the scope of a particular field of medicine, and traditionally utilizes a unique core of knowledge, specific diagnostic/evaluative methods, management modalities, and decision-making processes. ACEP has defined this body of knowledge in the Core Content of Emergency Medicine (1979). Topics are found in Table 36.10. The extent of the role of the emergency physician is a defini-

Abdominal and gastrointestinal disorders
Cardiovascular disorders
Cutaneous problems
Disorders caused by antigens, foreign substances, biologic, chemical, physical agents
Hematopoietic disorders
Hormonal, metabolic, nutritional problems
Head and neck problems
Infancy and childhood disorders
Musculoskeletal problems
Nervous system disorders
Psychological problems
Thoracic and respiratory disorders
Urogenital problems
Emergency department administration
Emergency medical services
Physician, patient, manipulative, procedure skills

tional dilemma. The academic preparation of such a specialist is to teach assessment, evaluation, and stabilization of the acutely ill or injured person, and then triage the patient into the appropriate service or to a consulting traditional specialist. However, the term "specialist" connotes a definitive authority. This issue raises questions about the feasibility of a person being skilled to specialist level in a range of possible clinical problems that, to this date, have required intervention from a number of other medical and surgical specialties. As residency programs in emergency medicine develop, clarification of the role of this specialist will ensue. Since the first Emergency Medicine residency program in 1970 at the University of Cincinnati, there are as of December, 1981, 60 approved residency programs nationwide (American College of Emergency Physicians, 1979).

The Standards of Graduate Training in Emergency Medicine outline the requirements for such programs. For example, they state that programs must extend either 2 or 3 years, that 36 months of postgraduate training, and 24 months of a specific emergency medicine residency is essential (American College of Emergency Physicians, 1979). Various clinical rotations for emergency residents are shorter than for surgical or medical residents; 14% are 4 months or longer, whereas rotations in medical and surgical programs have 40% of their rotations longer than 4 months (Anwar, 1980). The directors of emergency medicine residencies are usually surgeons (51%) or medical physicians (34%) (Anwar, 1980).

Although emergency medicine grows as a specialty, the larger teaching hospitals and medical schools usually require that students rotate through the emergency departments. Specific curricula and learning objectives have been adopted, usually at the local level, and no standard curriculum exists.

Prehospital Medical Management

Regardless of which physician staffing pattern a particular hospital designs for its emergency department, the physician may be involved in the medical direction of advanced EMTs in the field via radio communications systems. The role of the physician in prehospital medical management is an important one. The physician can provide voice communication to advanced EMTs, can augment his understanding of the patient's problems utilizing telemetry, or can evaluate field performance by supervising out-of-hospital patient care as rendered by defined protocols (NAS-NRC, 1978).

Medical control is a phrase frequently associated with the ALS operations of an emergency medical services system. According to Boyd et al. (1979), "medical control provides the operational framework and justification for field paramedics and other physician extenders to provide emergency and critical care interventive treatments in out-of-hospital situations." The physician who provides the moment-to-moment communications to field personnel is termed the "on-line" medical director. The "off-line" medical director is that physician who is designated by the region's EMS entity as the person medically accountable for overall system operations (Boyd et al., 1979). The actual designs for implementation of medical control are discussed in *Facilities*. Medical direction may prove a less provocative term.

Physician Consultants to Specialty Systems

The third identified role for physicians relates to specialty systems. The Division of EMS of the DHHS identified seven critical care categories that require comprehensive planning, coordination, and identification of certain standards and criteria.

These standards and criteria would ensure a continuity of appropriately determined care from the onset of the event through rehabilitation. As an EMS system plans its specialty subsystems, the need for specialty physician involvement becomes apparent. Each specialty subsystem planning group must have a consultant identified. The responsibilities of these consulting specialists and their planning groups include:

(1) designing a system for prehospital, hospital,

and critical care of patients on a regional basis;

(2) categorizing hospitals who receive such patients to determine the level of care they are capable of providing;

(3) developing treatment and triage protocols for implementation during all phases of management;

(4) conducting educational programs for all providers within the subsystem, and;

(5) demonstrating subsystem compliance by conducting patient origin and tracer studies.

Special Programs for Initial Management Training

Two courses are available for instructing health providers in managing a critical patient during the first hour of the immediate medical event. They are the Advanced Trauma Life Support (ATLS) Program, sponsored by the American College of Surgeons (ACS), and the ACLS Program, sponsored by the American Heart Association.

Advanced Trauma Life Support Program

The ACS Committee on Trauma (1981) set forth specific standards for the care of trauma victims by physicians. These standards have been integrated into a teaching program designed for primary care and emergency physicians. The state of Nebraska first pioneered an ATLS Course through its Lincoln Medical Education Foundation in 1977. This foundation, along with the University of Nebraska Medical Center and the ACS Committee on Trauma refined the course curriculum and adopted it as the official program in 1979.

Standardization of practices and quality control and assurance are important objectives the ACS Committee on Trauma have established. In order to achieve these objectives, the following methods are used:

(1) Prior to conducting programs, all courses are approved by the ACS and individual chairmen of State Committees of Trauma.

(2) Distribution of all course materials, i.e., ATLS manuals, is done by only ATLS national faculty members, state chairmen, and others as authorized by state chairmen.

(3) Documentation of successful course completion is issued only by the ACS through national faculty members or state chairmen.

Two ATLS courses are available: one provider program and another for training instructors. Each program lasts 2½–3 days, and has a corresponding manual that contains curriculum materials for didactic instruction and skills performance. Specific to ATLS instructor courses is a portion of the program that is taught by an educator, usually a nonphysician, who conducts sessions on how to teach.

Curriculum. Topics of discussion in the ATLS curriculum include: initial assessment, upper airway management, shock, thoracic trauma, head trauma, spine and spinal cord trauma, extremity trauma, abdominal trauma.

Also included in the curriculum is discussion, demonstration, and practice related to the following skills: cricothyrotomy, venous cutdown, needle decompression, tube thoracostomy, Gardner-Wells tongs, spinal immobilization, pericardiocentesis, peritoneal lavage, upper airway management, I.V. shock therapy, pneumatic antishock garment use, extremity immobilization.

National ATLS faculty are primarily those who are designated by the ACS Trauma committee as Regional Chiefs. These physicians are responsible for monitoring instructor training programs being conducted by regional and/or state faculty candidates; assisting with other provider and instructor training courses; being available as an ATLS program consultant.

Regional faculty are those state chairmen of the ACS Committee on Trauma. State chairmen are responsible for planning, coordinating, and implementing ATLS programs in their state.

ATLS programs, once completed, are approved by the ACS and the ACEP for continuing medical education (CME) credit.

Advanced Cardiac Life Support Program

Training of persons in the techniques of basic CPR was a 1966 recommendation of the NAS-NRC Conference on CPR (NAS-NRC, 1966). The NAS-NRC and the American Heart Association cosponsored a National Conference to establish Standards for Cardiopulmonary Resuscitation (CPR) and Emergency Cardiac Care (ECC) in 1973. The actual standards were published with the following recommendations that relate to the delivery of emergency medical services:

(1) that both basic and advanced levels of certification in such training be a result of passing a nationally recognized written and practical examination derived from a standardized curriculum;

(2) that training programs in basic and ACLS integrate the manner in which access to an EMSS is achieved in the local area; and

(3) that promotion be encouraged of community-wide EMSS that are available to all people,

and that provide both prehospital and hospital based CPR and ECC (NAS-NRC Conference, 1980).

With the basic CPR training programs well underway across the US, the Nebraska American Heart Association designed the model for a training program in ACLS skills. As of 1975, ACLS courses have been conducted based on a standardized curriculum developed by a National ACLS faculty. Curriculum, teaching materials, testing, and certification are standard for both basic and advanced levels of cardiac care, and were updated as a result of a 1979 national American Heart Association conference.

The components of ACLS include: (1) basic cardiac life support; (2) ventilation and circulation supported by special techniques and adjunctive equipment; (3) monitoring and arrhythmia recognition; (4) intravenous route establishment; and (5) drug and defibrillation in the treatment of acute myocardial infarctions (American Heart Association, 1980).

The curriculum for ACLS training includes the principles and therapeutic practices necessary for managing an acute arrest victim. The curriculum, intended to be covered in an approximately 2-day course, includes both didactic and practical instruction, as follows:

Didactic Sessions	Practical Skills
Adjuncts for Airway and Breathing	Basic CPR
Adjuncts for Artificial Circulation	Airway Adjuncts Endotracheal Intubation
Cardiac Monitoring-Dysrhythmia Recognition	Static & Dynamic ECG Recognition
Useful and Essential Drugs	Central & Peripheral I.V. Lines
Defibrillation & Synchronized Cardioversion	Defibrillation
Intravenous Therapy	
Stabilization and Transport	

Specific guidelines and methods have been established to certify ACLS instructors by local American Heart Association chapters. Although not as strictly executed as by the ACS, instructors in ACLS must attend additional training sessions and be certified as ACLS instructors by affiliate ACLS faculty members. Once recognized by the American Heart Association as successfully completing an ACLS course, such recognition is valid for 2 years.

Conclusion

Both of these aforementioned training programs are being conducted for the purpose of standardizing and protocolizing the way in which acutely traumatized and acutely arrested victims are managed at the onset of the event. However, to maintain flexibility for incorporating new advanced and new concepts, as well as for providing some physician innovative individuality, both groups recognize the need for continuous revision of curricula and periodic updating of instructors.

First Responders

First responders are those persons who because of their occupation may be the first person responding to the scene of a medical emergency. The majority of these persons are police and fire department personnel. However, the definition is often extended to include lifeguards and persons from other public safety elements such as special police forces, e.g., state police. As a group, first responders have been identified as needing specific emergency care training. Such training would focus on the initial management required to meet the needs of emergency patients as well as specific details pertaining to how to access the local EMS system.

Establishing the legislation foundation for first responder training was the first step Massachusetts took in addressing this need. Massachusetts General Law, Chapter 111, Section 201 was enacted in 1974 and required all first responders to be trained to administer first aid and cardiopulmonary resuscitation. Additional legislation requires completion of a refresher course in CPR annually, and in first aid every 3 years (Office of EMS, 1976).

Curriculum

In response to its legislative authority to coordinate the provision of first responder training, the State OEMS promulgated regulations that defined minimum hours and topics for courses (Massachusetts Department of Public Health, 1978)

Emergency Medical Services System	0.5 hours
Patient Assessment & Actions at Scene	1.0 hours
Gaining Access & Emergency Rescue	1.5 hours

Medical Emergencies (heart attack, stroke, diabetic reactions, childbirth, allergic reactions, behavioral problems)	2.0 hours
Respiratory Emergencies (airway obstruction, head, neck, chest injuries, facial burns, and/or smoke inhalation, known respiratory emergencies, emphysema, bronchitis, asthma)	2.0 hours
Poisons	
Allergic Reactions	
Electrical Shock	
Drowning	
Bleeding Wounds and Shock	2.0 hours
Accidental Poisonings & Drug/Alcohol Abuse	1.0 hours
Thermal Injuries	1.0 hours
Head and Trunk Injuries	2.0 hours
Skeletal Injuries	2.0 hours
Examination	1.0 hours
Total	16.0 hours

Scope of Training

The number of police and fire departments in the state of Massachusetts is 723. An estimated number of first responders is 45,000. It is the responsibility of the Office of EMS to monitor and provide for first responder training for the citizens of the Commonwealth. Regional EMS entities assume responsibility at the regional level to ensure training of first responders.

ACCESS TO CARE

Description

A component of any health care system is the availability of the system to all persons. Whether health care be a right of all society or a privilege for those who can afford it, emergency medical services should be available whenever and wherever and to whomever needs it. "Access to care" is cited by DHHS as a necessary element for building the basic foundation of an emergency medical services system (EMS Program Guidelines, 1975). Synonymous with access to care is the provision of such care regardless of the recipient's ability to pay. This availability should extend from the prehospital care scene, through transport to the initial receiving hospital, and on through transport to a tertiary facility and/or a rehabilitative facility.

Coincident with providing access to EMS care for everyone, is the recommendation to all EMS entities to establish processes to monitor for any portion of the system that may be prohibiting access to any person or group of persons for any reason, be it political, social, or financial.

Experience

To legislate access to care for all persons probably stands as the most profound method to dictate such access. However, to enforce such legislation as well as to monitor the system for violations of the access principle is more difficult. Under the Governor's Highway Safety Act of 1966 is the requirement for state governors to administer highway safety programs including the delivery of emergency medical services. The US DOT, through its National Highway Safety Administration distributed a document entitled "Model Legislation for Emergency Medical Services" as part of the program to enact its legislation (DOT, 1978). This document serves as a model to all state, regional, and local EMS officials, for the formation of their own legislation related to their EMS programs. Section 3—Authority of (state agency) cites that an agency "should use all reasonable and lawful means to ensure that necessary emergency medical services are provided to all patients requiring such services without prior inquiry as to ability to pay." (DOT, 1978)

Along with these federal guidelines for providing access to care, the Joint Commission on Accreditation of Hospitals defines a standard for all hospitals to have a plan for the assessment, management, and or referral for all ill or injured persons. The provision of "essential life-saving measures" is also mentioned as a hospital standard (Joint Commission on Accreditation of Hospitals, 1980). The fact that court decisions have upheld the belief that hospitals should provide life-saving care to all persons regardless of their ability to pay, supports this societal conscience (Committee on Medical Services, 1980).

A problem that has surfaced as a result of EMS activities becoming more comprehensive and readily available to all persons, is to define how and who will ultimately pay for the services. It is estimated that 20–30% of a total EMS system's cost is for ambulance service operations. Personnel costs account for the largest cost expenditure for the system (NAS-NRC, 1978).

Third party reimbursement (Blue Cross/Blue Shield, Medicare, Medicaid, and coverage by insurance companies) as well as tax supported budgets are the two most popular methods for financially supporting EMS systems. The National Academy of Sciences reports that 20% of Blue Cross insured parties are not covered for emergency transportation, and 33% are covered for treatment of trauma-induced problems, but not for sudden illnesses (NAS-NRC, 1978). There is some degree of hesitation in revising third party buying policies that reflect the changing tides of EMS.

As quality EMS becomes more visible to the general public and demand increases, the financial reimbursement issues will have to be defined so as to maintain the operation of the system. Regionalization, cost-sharing, and an evaluation of economics vis-a-vis system efficiency are subjects for future EMS research. Once available to the public, however, EMS will be difficult to reduce or discontinue if funds become scarce. The public will demand the service and officials will have to determine the best method to pay for it so that it is accessible to all.

CONSUMER PARTICIPATION

Description

A growing management method for public and private planning groups is to involve the general consumer of the product in the policy-making related to the product. The DHHS also supports and recommends this method of consumer participation in its Program Guidelines for the development of EMSS (1974). Reasons cited for involving consumers in EMS planning groups are:

(1) linking health system agencies through consumers with EMS planning entitites;

(2) providing customer access to EMS policy planners to promote communications regarding general public needs, to promote involvement in planning, and to promote an exchange forum for policy implementation;

(3) providing consumers an avenue to register and discuss complaints regarding the general system or specific facets of the system.

It is further imperative that consumers be aware of problems related to financing the EMSS.

State Experience

The MGL 111C Ambulance Law mandates the formation and implementation of an Advisory Committee to the Office of Emergency Medical Services, the State EMS agency. The Law also mandates that three consumers be active members of the Advisory Committee (1973). Additionally, the Ambulance Law provides for a consumer grievance process that directs all grievances regarding ambulance service to the State Ambulance Regulation Program, the State Health Department's licensing branch specifically operating to inspect and licence ambulance services (1973).

COMMUNICATIONS

Modern telecommunications is an essential component of any EMS system. Communications, in a variety of forms, serves as a coordinating mechanism to link the many other EMS components with the patient. Elements of the communications framework include:

(1) *Public Access*: The telephone is the first link for the patient, family members, or bystander to access emergency medical services.

(2) *Triage and Ambulance Dispatch*: Trained EMS communicators receive and prioritize calls for medical assistance by obtaining information about the presenting problem, other pertinent medical information, and most importantly, the location of the incident. Once initially triaged, the dispatch of the closest ambulance is executed.

(3) *Hospital-to-Ambulance Communications*: Trained basic and advanced EMTs are then able to transmit clinical information and patient status to the physicians and nurses in the receiving hospital and can also obtain orders for medical intervention from the resource or associate hospital.

(4) *Telemetry*: The system is usually capable of transmitting an electrocardiographic signal from the patient in the field to an oscilloscope and strip chart recorder monitored by the physician in the Emergency Department.

(5) *Hospital-to-Hospital*: For purposes of consultation or during disaster operations it may be necessary for hospitals to intercommunicate, which is a coordinating function of comprehensive communications centers.

(6) *Record Keeping*: By means of a continuous tape recording of all communications traffic, a system is provided with an authentic record of the system's operations.

(7) *Medical Direction*: Medical direction of advanced EMTs is the critical element of extending the practice of medicine from the hospital to the prehospital setting. It is essential that the physician in the hospital be able to communicate with the advanced EMT in the field.

Federal Communications Commission

Two federal legislative acts, the Governor's Highway Safety Act of 1966 and the EMS Act of 1973, supported the concept of regional EMS Systems. Both Acts stressed the importance of a comprehensive communications system as the foundation of a multidisciplinary approach to EMS development (Public Law 93–154, 1973).

The new approach encouraged upgrading of equipment to meet national standards, provided more dedicated channels for EMS providers, and modern telephone radio crosslinkages for EMS users.

In 1974, the Federal Communications Commission (FCC) in Docket 19880 in the Federal Register, laid out the operational channels for EMS. These channels included 10 UHF radio channels for basic and advanced life support. Channels 1–8 were designated for medical voice and ECG telemetry communications between the hospitals and the prehospital services. Channels 9 and 10 were designated for intersystem dispatching and administrative radio traffic. One problem that surfaced was that UHF transmissions required different equipment than the pre-existing VHF, which EMS ambulance services and hospitals had previously purchased. To change to the UHF system was costly and redundant.

The continued use of VHF equipment and the use of UHF equipment by some led to incompatibility between EMS users. A second problem, radio interference, became apparent as more systems became operational within smaller geographic areas. Third, the increasing sophistication of the equipment also increased the cost of purchasing and maintaining the system.

Technical Approaches

In an attempt to provide coordinated regional EMS medical control communications, a number of technical approaches to telecommunications evolved: (1) Command and Control Systems, (2) Radio-Telephone Automatic Interconnect System, and (3) Mobile Relay System.

Command and Control System

This system utilizes a central multifaceted communications center with a control console which can interconnect ambulances, hospital physicians, and ambulance supervisory personnel on a routine minute-to-minute basis. It can also coordinate public safety agencies, such as police, fire, coast guard, and aerovac systems during a disaster.

This system requires a staff of trained communicators, preferably with medical triage training, on a 24-hour per day basis. The system has the responsibility and authority to assign priorities for ambulance dispatch, as well as ambulance-to-hospital communications. If there is a need for simultaneous emergency medical basic or advanced communications, the center can assign different frequencies to each user. The center can also coordinate telemetry from the advanced EMTs in the ambulance or the field to the hospital. The system used radio frequencies, microwave chan-

nels, and telephone lines, and relies on remote radios and base stations to link ambulances and hospitals.

The Command and Control System is complex and sophisticated, and requires a dedicated trained staff. It is expensive to purchase and maintain, and personnel requirements make it even more expensive to operate.

Kulp (1982) outlined the functions of a command and control system as:

(1) telephonic screening of medical emergency calls through the public access lines;

(2) dispatching of ambulance and rescue units;

(3) coordination of interagency EMS response in mutual aid;

(4) the as-needed assignment of medical control radio frequencies, particularly the UHF "MED" channels;

(5) the manual patching of radio to telephone and VHF to UHF to overcome incompatibilities in equipment;

(6) the coordination of implementing prehospital point-of-entry plans for appropriate patient transportation destination;

(7) direction and routing assistance for ambulance and rescue vehicles, including aircraft and marine medevac units;

(8) technical monitoring for assuring quality of ECG telemetry signals;

(9) hospital care capability status monitoring;

(10) multicasualty or disaster coordination, and;

(11) radiosystem testing.

Radio Telephone Automatic Interconnect System

The FCC notified its regulators to allow the UHF dedicated frequencies to be connected automatically to the public telephone network (Kulp, 1982). This is known as a Radio-Telephone Switch Station (RTSS). This system is particularly useful to cover a large geographic area. An EMS user can access the system by multifrequency UHF radio. The signal is then connected to the telephone network. The RTSS has the ability automatically to locate and select a free channel by means of an internal scanner.

The EMS user must have a dual-tone radio. Each hospital in the system has a special dedicated telephone line to a simple telephone in the Emergency Department. The EMS user can dial the hospital directly by means of the RTSS. The system has conference call capability in order that two hospitals (e.g., Resource and Associate Hospitals) or a hospital and a physician in an office can monitor the calls for medical direction.

The advantage of this system is that it does not require trained communications personnel, and is less expensive to operate than the Command and Control System. The disadvantages are that there is no call prioritization, thus the first user has sole operation of that frequency until the termination of the call. This makes it very difficult to deal with simultaneous ALS calls. The system is also controlled by the EMS user in the field, and the user has the ability to select the hospital to obtain medical direction, without direction from a third party. The system cannot interconnect UHF and VHF, and cannot be easily integrated into an area which has elements of both UHF and VHF radio frequencies in operation. The system is not designed to facilitate linkages to other public safety agencies. Consequently, another communications system would have to be in place to coordinate activities during a disaster. The system is part of the telephone network of a given area, and if the lines are overused, the EMS/ALS personnel could receive busy signals. The system is also subject to standard telephone outages secondary to storms or broken telephone lines.

Mobile Relay System

A mobile relay system is designed to cover large geographic areas. It is comprised of a UHF base station which receives a transmission from a mobile radio in an ambulance or other transmitting location, enhances and amplifies the signal, and transmits it automatically and simultaneously on a second frequency. The initial signal strength is about 30 watts of output power, and the amplified signal is 60 or more watts. The system can therefore dramatically increase the range of radio communications. The best location for the relay system would be the highest natural or man-made point in the given area. This system is simple and effective, but subject to the vagaries of the personnel using the system. There is no controlling authority to coordinate, assign, or prioritize frequencies or calls. The field EMS user is at liberty to select any hospital for medical control. However, a second EMS user can then begin to transmit, disrupting the prior radio traffic. The system is more useful where there are limited EMS radio traffic needs, and large geographic areas to cover. The system can be modified by connecting the mobile relay station via landline to a single hospital. An operator in the hospital can stop the amplifying ability of the relay station, and communicate directly with all parties on that frequency. Another modification adds another receiver to the mobile relay station, and requires another separate frequency

to achieve communications control. As the system is modified, it becomes more costly, more difficult to maintain, and requires dedicated personnel, thus defeating the original purpose of simplicity and cost effectiveness. Table 36.11 summarizes these approaches to EMS Communications.

Central Access

Public access to an emergency medical system is a critical element. The concept of a universal simple access number for emergencies originated in Europe. In 1937, Great Britain implemented a single, 3-digit number. Other European cities, such as Moscow and Stockholm, also have 3-digit numbers.

The incentive for the development of a single number in the United States was provided by the President's Commission on Law Enforcement in 1967 (Executive Office of the President of Telecommunications Policy, 1973). By 1979, 800 "911" systems had been developed across the country (Dayharsh et al., 1979). The 3-digit access number has the advantage of being universal, simple to remember, easy to dial, and in a number of locations, is toll free.

Decreasing the time needed to access emergency service agencies was the primary reason that 911 was implemented. Another advantage was that emergency medical, police, and fire services would be contacted by a single number. Trained communicators would be dealing with the public, and interservice cooperation, such as needed for a burned victim at a fire, or an injured person at the scene of a crime, could be more easily facilitated.

Slowly, 911 is being implemented nationwide. One of the reasons is that the Office of Telecommunications in Bulletin 73–1 (McCorkle et al., 1978), which outlined the adoption of 911 as a national toll-free emergency number, took a passive role in terms of providing information, advice and assistance to implement its mandate. The further implementation of 911 would be greatly enhanced by passage of federal legislation and by offering technical assistance to planners. Another reason for sluggish implementation is the overlap of municipal boundaries and 911 telephone catchment areas. A potential result is that a person living in one town may initiate a telephone link to 911 in another town causing delays. EMS providers, police, and fire services may have policies which prohibit crossing town lines without a formal request for mutal aid. The shunting of the request to the appropriate town is time-consuming and inefficient. This occurs in a statistically small number of cases, but could be a source of com-

Table 36.11.
Comparison of command and control, RTSS, mobile relay systems.

Topic	Command and Control	RTSS	Mobile Relay
Small metro area	Excellent: heavy call load metro	Fair: metro	Poor: metro area
Large rural area	Good: large geographic area	Good: large area	Excellent: large area
Centralized command	One site-trained communicator	Field personnel use automatic linkages, no CC	Minimal to none
Personnel	24 hour/day on-line personnel (5 persons = 1 full-time position)	Minimal uses automated equipment	Minimal
Consolidation of public safety agencies	Operator controlled, ability to handle simultaneous calls	Limited ability	Limited to nonexistent
Equipment costs	$25–35,000 = operator console $7000 = multifrequency base stations $3–6000 = hospital console	$20,000 = one station (each station handles only one call at a time)	
Flexibility	Excellent: operators responsible for channel assignments and equipment failure/repair protocols	Fair: automatic channel scanning	Fair to poor: requires modification for simultaneous call handling
Medical control	More conducive to protocol stability—reduces undisciplined network	Field personnel can select medical control hospital	Field personnel can select medical control hospital
Call prioritization	Excellent: can screen simultaneous calls, establish priorities	Limited: as first call locks system	Limited: would need modification
Disaster coordination	Excellent: link UHF, VHF	Limited: unable to link	Very limited
Training	Extensive: radio operator training	Minimal: operation is simple/automatic	Minimal
Operational costs	Expensive: personnel, land-line and multifrequency costs	Minimal: dedicated personnel needs small, use existing telephone network	Inexpensive: personnel needs minimal

plaint by the patient to the responsible system, especially if the delay and confusion results in morbidity and/or mortality.

Technological advances such as selective routing of 911 calls by an automatic system is available to minimize the mismatch problem. However, it can be expensive to implement, especially since the benefit is to a statistically small percent of the public. Other new technical developments are Automatic Location Identification, whereby the caller's address is automatically displayed to the 911 operator, thereby facilitating operator callback. This is useful if the caller is cut off, or if the ambulance attendant is unable to find someone at the stated location. This is more likely to be useful in the inner city, where perhaps an elderly caller may be reluctant to answer the door without verifying who is seeking entry.

Boston Experience

When designing an EMS communications system, it is necessary to determine the political, geographical, financial, and topographical influences (McCorkle et al., 1978). Planning an EMS communications system may mean designing a grass-roots system, overhauling a currently existing system, or even consolidating multiple system components into a new design. Essential to the planning process is compiling a list of the type of equipment that may already be in operation in base stations, communications centers, and mobile units. Once inventoried, the equipment pieces can be judged as to their compatability with the newly planned system.

The use of 911 as an access number to the three public safety agencies (police, fire, and ambulance) stands as the leading method to provide an immediate response to a call for help.

Whether 911 is implemented as the EMS access number, or another 7-digit number is used, a well publicized, easy-to-remember access number is the essential element of any EMS communications plan. The response to the call must then be well defined in terms of ambulance dispatch, BLS and ALS determination, coordination with other agencies, mutual aid, and a means to provide medical direction if required. Additional components of a communications plan include: (1) evaluation mechanisms, (2) back-up plans, (3) maintenance and service agreements, (4) adjustment, compliance, and modification policies. The following description of Boston's EMS Communications system serves as an example of a major city's response to its EMS needs.

The development and implementation of an EMS Communications Plan in Boston was achieved through the use of a written Memorandum of Understanding between the DHH Ambulance Service and the Conference of Boston Teaching Hospitals (COBTH). Essentially, this Memorandum outlined the relationship between the city's primary ambulance service (DHH) provider and the emergency receiving hospitals for a 2-year period. The Memorandum outlined a Boston EMS Communications Plan, the responsibilities of the seventeen teaching hospitals (members of the COBTH), the responsibilities of the Ambulance Service, the role of a Protocol Committee, and an Evaluation Committee. The Memorandum represented the collaborative relationship between prehospital and hospital providers that is needed to plan and execute an EMS communications plan that effects all EMS components.

As outlined in the Memorandum, the Boston EMS sytem has the following components:

(1) A UHF system that utilizes the 8 channels designated by the FCC for EMS use;

med one	463.000/468.000 MHz.
med two	463.025/468.025 MHz.
med three	463.050/468.050 MHz.
med four	463.075/468.075 MHz.
med five	463.100/468.100 MHz.
med six	463.125/468.125 MHz.
med seven	463.150/468.150 MHz.
med eight	463.175/468.175 MHz.

(McCorkle et al., 1978)

It also utilizes a 2-channel UHF ambulance dispatch system.

(2) It utilizes a Communications Coordinating Center (CCC) to coordinate ambulance dispatching, medical direction and consultation, and the interface with other public safety agencies, e.g., police and fire. The CCC was established in the main headquarters building of the Boston Police Department (BPD) in a room adjacent to the city's 911 answering terminals and the BPD dispatching center.

(3) It maintains the status regarding general hospital and specialty unit occupancy, monitors and administers transports according to an established point-of-entry plan, and coordinates transfers from outlying communities into Boston's tertiary facilities.

(4) It connects all Boston hospitals to the CCC via dedicated phone lines and telephone remote units installed in each hospital.

(5) It reorganized the use of radio channels for hospital paging systems so that overcrowded frequencies were decongested and systematized.

(6) It utilizes a staff of 5 EMTs at the CCC: two EMTs answering and screening EMS calls from the public (250–300 calls/24 hours), one EMT dispatcher, one C-MED operator, and one supervisor.

(7) It utilizes a Computer-Aided Ambulance Dispatching (CAD) system.

(8) It is capable of technical radio-telephone cross-banding and patching to coordinate disaster response among Boston public safety agencies.

(9) It manages EMS radio frequencies to provide coordinated voice and telemetry capabilities for hospital-to-hospital and hospital-to-ambulance communication.

(10) It is capable of expanding to outlying EMS communities within the region, as their local systems develop. Two outlying community hospitals are already implemented at the Boston C-MED console.

Financial Considerations

It was estimated that the Estimated Operating Cost for the EMS Communications System for Boston would be $86,600 annually. Therefore, for the 2-year term of the Memorandum, all 17 hospitals contributed to this operating cost as an example of cost-sharing between EMS providers so that not all costs were borne by the provider of ambulance service. Table 36.12 describes the actual costs over a 2-year period for purchasing certain equipment and operating an EMS Communications for a major US city.

PATIENT TRANSFER

Traditionally patients were transferred from smaller community or rural hospitals to larger

Table 36.12.
Department of Health and Hospitals Emergency Medical Services Communications Expenditures 1978 and 1979.

Fiscal Year	Type	Federal Funds	DHH Funds	Private Hospital Funds	Total
1978	Equipment	$200,000	$100,400	$29,000	$329,400
	Personnel		152,500	57,000	$209,500
	Maintenance		12,000		$ 12,000
	Telephone Lease		18,000		$ 18,000
Total		35%	50%	15%	$568,900
1979	Equipment	100,000	29,000	29,000	$158,000
	Personnel		202,000	57,000	$259,000
	Maintenance		15,000		$ 15,000
	Telephone Lease		21,000		$ 21,000
Total		22%	59%	19%	$453,000

Total Expenditure Cost 1978–1979 = $1,021,900

tertiary facilities by physician-to-physician contact. Although this practice continues, a more concrete, systematized, hospital-to-hospital approach is recommended. The reason is that it may be difficult to contact a particular physician in the receiving hospital to accept the emergency patient; the physician may not know the bed status in his/her receiving hospital; and the physician-to-physician type of transfer for a critically-ill or injured patient may take unwanted time.

An organized sustained approach for defining the manner in which a transfer can be efficiently executed is a component of an EMSS that can be implemented for an individual patient or for situations involving multiple patients. The manner in which patient transfer protocols can be formalized is to have hospitals represented on regional EMS committees, collaborate on the development of *transfer agreements* between each other or with hospitals from neighboring regions. Transfer agreements should contain:

(1) identification by name of the transferring facility and the receiving facility;

(2) identification of the clinical categories of patients that the receiving hospital is agreeing to accept. (e.g., trauma victims, burn victims, etc.)

(3) identification of the person at the receiving hospital to contact to initiate the transfer;

(4) signatures of both hospitals' chief executive officers as well as the physician chiefs of the particular clinical categories;

(5) identification of stabilization procedures to be performed prior to transport;

(6) identification of the particular ambulance service to contact to transport the patient.

Boston Experience

A number of Boston's teaching hospitals serve as receiving facilities for patients transferred from outlying community hospitals, from other New England states, as well as from areas across the nation and globe. A recent explosion in an aerosol plant in southeastern Massachusetts resulted in 12 patients being severely injured. Local hospitals were capable and equipped to handle a number of other injured persons, yet after stabilization of these 12 burn victims, transfer into Boston's burn facilities was indicated.

One phone call from the physician at the scene of the explosion to the Central Medical Emergency Direction (C-MED) center of Boston's EMS operational center initiated the transfer process. The following activities performed by the C-MED center systematically coordinated the transfer of all 12 patients to 6 hospitals in 2 hours and 10 minutes; (a) contact of all Boston hospitals to determine the number and location of burn beds; (b) Boston C-MED patching all hospitals in region of explosion (Region V) into Region IV (Boston) network; (c) Boston C-MED canvassing hospitals in neighboring regions for additional burn beds; (d) Boston C-MED coordinating hospital point-of-entry assignments for burn victim transfers by ground and air transport.

Transfer agreements and their accompanying

triage and treatment protocols recognize the importance of physician-to-physician contact and serve to formalize in writing predefined arrangements for expeditious transfer of a patient to comprehensive tertiary facilities.

MUTUAL AID

Traditionally, mutual aid refers to the ability of a certain community to call upon a neighboring community in times of stress, overextension, and/or during other predefined circumstances, e.g., if the need for heavy duty rescue equipment was needed in one town and is owned by another, e.g., Jaws of Life. Mutual aid is a phrase frequently used when referring to neighboring fire departments and their prearranged agreements to assist each other when needed.

As it relates to EMS, mutual aid connotes a slightly different arrangement as described by the EMS Program Guidelines of the DHHS:

"Each EMS system must provide for the establishment of appropriate arrangements with other EMS systems or similar entities serving neighboring areas for the provision of emergency medical services on a reciprocal basis where access to such services would be more appropriate and effective in terms of the services available, time, and distance (1974)."

Interpretation of this guideline may mean that if a patient borders two EMS regions that his request for ambulance service would generate a response from whichever of the two services may be the closest to him in terms of distance or time. Certain problems arise that make such arrangements difficult to execute. Town, county, or city lines are drawn so that there may be political and legal reasons that ambulances are unable to cross them. For example, in Boston, the DHH ambulance service is self-insured and only permits its vehicles to operate within the city's limits. Also, there may be a large *number* of neighboring services that would make such mutual aid arrangements on a day-to-day basis cumbersome, both in terms of communications and contact time.

The city of Boston, because of its sophisticated ambulance deployment plan and back-up arrangements with private ambulance companies does not have written mutual-aid agreements with other EMS regions. However, in times of disaster mutual aid does exist in Boston and has been activated on an incident-to-incident basis.

The problem of ambulances not being able to cross jurisdictional lines has been and probably will continue to be a stumbling block for EMS

planners to hurdle. Involvement of local political officials and ambulance service chiefs in EMS planning activites will help to publicize this issue and perhaps make a solution reachable.

PUBLIC SAFETY AGENCIES

Members of such public safety agencies as police departments, fire departments, special police forces, e.g., state police, and lifeguards, are often involved with the delivery of EMS. Some are first responders to the scene of accidents and/or sudden illnesses, some are trained and certified as EMTs, and some are performing dual functions as operators of ambulance services along with their primary profession.

Three specific roles of these public safety agencies as they relate to EMS are: (1) involvement in the planning and implementation of local and regional EMS systems; (2) integration of their services into day-to-day EMS operations as well as disaster operation; (3) continuous concentration on initial training and refresher training of public safety agency members as first responders, basic or advanced EMTs, or rescue personnel depending upon the design of the individual system.

Boston Experience

The DHH Ambulance Service central communications center is located immediately adjacent to the city of Boston 911 center and the Boston Police Communications/Dispatch Center. Because of the proximity, the coordination between public safety agencies during any EMS operation is enhanced. A summary of the Boston EMS system approach to public safety agency coordination includes the following: (a) geographic consolidation of Boston Police Department Communications Center, DHH Ambulance Operations Center, and the city 911 answering terminals; (b) hotlines with a VHF radio link from DHH Ambulance Operation Communications Center to the Boston Fire Department Central Alarm, the Coast Guard Search and Rescue Center, the Red Cross Headquarters, the Boston Emergency Operating Center at Boston City Hall, and the DHH Disaster Command Center at Boston City Hospital (the Resource Hospital for the Greater Metropolitan Boston Region); (c) direct telephone hotline links to the Massport Fire Department at Logan International Airport; (d) direct telephone hotline links to the Massachusetts Bay Transit Authority (MBTA) police, the police department that monitors the Boston extensive subway system; (e) direct hotline to the Boston Fire Department two Rescue Units that assist at the scene of vehicular accidents and other rescue incidents; (f) involvement of officials of all public safety agencies on regional executive, training, disaster, and communications EMS committees; (g) assistance from the DHH Ambulance Service physician and nursing staff in conducting basic and refresher training sessions for members of other public safety agencies.

RECORD KEEPING

Record keeping is a component of the EMSS directed toward standardization of data collection, and concerned with maintaining accurate files. "Record" refers to a standardized form that is completed by the EMS provider for each individual patient. To achieve a system of data collection within an EMSS necessitates collecting data from the time of the patient's initial contact with the system, e.g., call to 911, through the patient's last contact, e.g., hospital or rehabilitation center. A specific handbook, published by the Bureau of Medical Services—Division of EMS, outlines the specific areas where data is collected (DHEW, 1977): (1) general data—name, address, age, sex; (2) communications data; (3) transportation/intervention data, ambulance and personnel identification, dispatch and scene arrival; (4) emergency facility and Critical Care Unit data, patient evaluation, diagnosis, medical treatment, and patient disposition.

The information to be recorded must be understood and agreed upon by prehospital and hospital personnel. The prehospital run report should be completed following delivery of the patient to the hospital, and prior to the departure of the ambulance to another call. This report should become part of the patient's in-hospital record. The critical element is an accurate medical assessment and treatment record, which becomes the documentation of medical intervention and practice. It not only serves as the only record of the practice of medicine which was conducted by nonphysician extenders in the field, but is very important for hospital physicians as a record of the first few minutes of the patient's illness or traumatic event.

The purposes of coordinated record keeping include:

(1) *General Data:* These are used for patient identification and for crossreference of various records, e.g., ambulance run report with emergency department record; serves to define the EMSS needs in terms of numbers of patients who use the system; data will assist EMS planners and administrators to allocate funds and resources to meet the system's actual needs; serves to evaluate the system's utilization; serves to aid in redesigning or relocating system components, e.g., changing ambulance deployment plans to correspond with geographic areas with high demand.

(2) *Communications Data:* Such data serve to plot each patient on a time chart so that future time intervals can compare efficiency of the system's response.

(3) *Transportation/Intervention Data:* These data not only provide the times of dispatch, scene arrival and scene departure, but also serve to identify the vehicle and specific ambulance attendants who responded. This information is used to tabulate numbers of runs/attendant; to identify periods of delay, e.g., dispatch delay, departure from scene delay, etc.; to correlate certain skills performed in the field with geographic incidence, with individual attendants, with categorized clinical conditions; measures the incidence of certain conditions; to document intervention in the field in comparison with hospital-based intervention and to evaluate efficacy and appropriateness of care rendered; to monitor equipment used; to evaluate point-of-entry plan adherence; to summarize nontransport reasons, e.g., patient refusal.

(4) *Emergency Facility and Critical Care Unit Data:* These data can be cross-referenced with prehospital data to identify individual patients or certain patient tracer groups; to provide data to compare prehospital and hospital-based patient condition, assessment, and management; to provide statistics related to frequency of ambulance transports, types of patients received, incidence of patients received identified by geographic proximity to hospital, incidence of various grades of seriousness of patient conditions; to identify resources that require allocation to meet patient needs; to evaluate intervention by various members of health care team; to identify delays in treatment; to use for teaching and research projects.

The Division of EMS summarizes the purposes of collecting this data into three categories (DHEW, 1977): (1) management information, (2) process evaluations, (3) clinical impact studies.

A complete and accurate record is essential. The complete data set serves as a basis for evaluating the operation of the system, a record of the medical care given to the patient, and a legal document in the event of a medico-legal inquiry. It is also essential that the data be collected and recorded in a uniform and easily retrievable fashion.

Boston Experience

Prehospital Record

The DHH designed a medical run report which incorporated the standard demographic general data, the communications data, transportation and intervention data, and final disposition in the Emergency Department. The medical data are organized so that the physiologic vital signs are easily recorded and categorized into a trauma score based on Champion's Index of Severity (Champion et al., 1980). Figure 36.2 illustrates the DHH Trip Ticket. The information gained from the trauma score serves as the basis for transport of patients to trauma receiving facilities. It is also entered into the Trauma Registry and forms the initial evaluative instrument for assessing the quality of management of the trauma victim. This information is then transmitted to trauma center physicians and surgeons in order to gain insight into management of the patient from the initial injury through the discharge or demise of the patient.

The medical information recorded on the prehospital report is only as accurate as the technician examining the patient and recording the information. A study undertaken in Boston demonstrates an 81.8% correlation between EMT diagnosis and physician diagnosis (Jacobs et al., 1981). This type of research and evaluation demonstrates the areas of weakness in assessment and diagnosis of the system and is transmitted to the training areas of the department for corrective therapy in the form of lectures and on-scene supervision.

A portion of the ambulance run report is designed for completion by hospital personnel. Included in this information is the patient's final diagnosis and disposition. The copy of the run report that contains the hospital information is returned to the DHH Ambulance Service for analysis.

Communications Data

Boston's CAD system generates a daily summary of the ambulance service activities including times (call receipt, dispatch, arrival on scene, departure from scene, arrival at hospital) incident location, receiving hospitals, and dispatch clinical codes. Of particular interest is that each incident is recorded by the census tract where the incident occurs.

These census tracts are defined geographic areas bounded by easily located street addresses which contain a given number of people. Information is gathered from these tracts by the US Census Bureau, and these data not only contain socioeconomic information, but also mortality data in disease-specific cohorts. The ambulance service, therefore, can generate data on the incidence of emergencies by specific disease and relate this to information generated by census tract. Public health preventive implications can be derived from such data.

The CAD system is the basis for the provision of quarterly reports to the members of the COBTH. Each hospital can analyze data that pertain to their hospital, e.g., number of patients received, geographic origin of patients by census tract. This type of comprehensive data collection is not only useful to monitor the medical and operational performance of the ambulance service, but serves as a planning tool for the hospitals.

Additionally, all telephonic and radio transmissions of the ambulance service are tape-recorded. These recordings are stored and can be retrieved for retrospective investigation as well as for training purposes. Table 36.13 contains a sample of information that can be tabulated from CAD-generated data.

Emergency Department Data

A comprehensive emergency department record contains general patient identification (name, age, sex, etc.), mode of transport, triage data and assessment information, physician history, physical examination, diagnosis, management plan, investigative results, final disposition, and intervention received. Follow-up information, e.g., clinic appointment, at-home instructions, is also useful to record.

A defined objective of the DHH Ambulance Service is to correlate prehospital and hospital data pertaining to each patient managed by paramedics. Approximately 45 patients per week are managed by paramedics and transported to any one of 12 Boston hospitals (DHH, 1980). The method used to follow-up on each ALS transported patient includes:

(1) A paramedic nurse educator reviews each ALS run report for completeness, accuracy, compliance with protocols.

(2) Each ALS run report data is recorded in a daily log book (name, unit, paramedic, ID numbers, patient, clinical problem, age, sex, intervention given, receiving hospital).

(3) Bimonthly, each receiving hospital is sent a list of ALS patients transported to their facility as well as follow-up forms to be completed by the

BOSTON DEPARTMENT OF HEALTH AND HOSPITALS

EMERGENCY MEDICAL SERVICES — AMBULANCE

ADMISSION NUMBER

PATIENT I.D. # (MEDICAL RECORD #) | DATE / / | DAY -96- | No. 710884-8

CC # | DISPATCH TIME

SCENE ARRIVAL TIME: | SCENE DEPARTURE TIME:

AMBULANCE DISPATCHED TO: STREET AND NUMBER | SECTION

MILEAGE AT SCENE | MILEAGE AT HOSPITAL

DISPATCH PRIORITY | NATURE | SPECIAL DIRECTIONS:

☐ HOME ☐ BUSINESS ☐ STREET/HIGHWAY | HOSPITAL ARRIVAL TIME

SOCIAL SECURITY NUMBER | D.O.B. | SEX | RACE

PATIENT NAME | PHONE

ADDRESS STREET & NO. | CITY | ZIP

NEXT OF KIN NAME | RELATIONSHIP | PHONE

ADDRESS STREET & NO. | CITY | ZIP

MEDICAL COVERAGE: VERIFIED BY HOSPITAL ☐ YES ☐ NO

CHECK:

MEDICARE_____ MEDICAID/WELFARE_____

INSURANCE_____ (COMPANY)_____

IND. ACC._____ SELF PAY_____ OTHER_____

FINANCIAL CLASS NUMBERS:

COMMENTS-PATIENT'S CHIEF COMPLAINT-HISTORY-CHANGE IN PATIENT STATUS

NO PATIENT TRANSPORTED — REASON

CANCELLED BY: ☐ OPERATIONS ☐ POLICE ☐ FIRE

PATIENT TRANSPORTED BY: ☐ POLICE ☐ OTHER AMB ☐ FIRE ☐ ALS

REFERRED TO: ☐ POLICE ☐ MED. EXAMINER ☐ PRIV. AMB ☐ ALS

MISCELLANEOUS: ☐ PATIENT LEFT SCENE ☐ PATIENT REFUSAL

☐ INCORRECT ADDRESS ☐ NO VISIBLE INCIDENT ☐ MVA/FIRE - NO INJURIES

ALSO RESPONDING: ☐ POLICE ☐ DHH AMB ☐ SPECIAL SERVICES UNIT

☐ FIRE ☐ M.D. ☐ OTHER AMB ☐ SENIOR EMT ☐ PARAMEDICS

PHYSICAL EXAM

NEURO STATUS			SKIN CONDITION
EYE OPENING:	☐ SPONTANEOUS ☐ TO VOICE	☐ TO PAIN ☐ NONE	☐ NORMAL ☐ COOL
VERBAL RESPONSE:	☐ ORIENTED ☐ CONFUSED ☐ INAPPROPRIATE	☐ INCOMPREHENSIBLE ☐ NONE	☐ HOT ☐ PALE ☐ FLUSHED
MOTOR RESPONSE:	☐ OBEDIENCE ☐ PURPOSEFUL ☐ WITHDRAWAL	☐ FLEXION ☐ EXTENSION ☐ NONE	☐ CYANOTIC ☐ DIAPHORETIC

VITAL SIGNS: ☐ UNABLE TO OBTAIN ☐ NOT ATTEMPTED

REASON:

TIME	BP	PULSE	CAPIL RETURN	RESPIRATIONS RATE/EFFORT

ALLERGIES: ☐ NONE ☐ UNKNOWN

CURRENT MEDS: ☐ NONE ☐ UNKNOWN

BROUGHT WITH PATIENT: ☐ YES ☐ NO

SUSPECTED DIAGNOSIS: ☐ CHRONIC ☐ ACUTE

☐ MAJOR TRAUMA ☐ ACUTE MEDICAL ☐ CARDIAC ARREST

☐ MINOR TRAUMA ☐ MINOR MEDICAL ☐ CARDIAC DISORDER

☐ SOFT TISSUE INJ. ☐ OB-GYN ☐ SHOCK

☐ BURNS ☐ ETOH ☐ SEIZURES ☐ NEURO

☐ ORTHO ☐ OD/POISON ☐ PSYCH ☐ NEONATE

EMERGENCY CARE: ☐ CPR ☐ EXTRICATION

☐ BLEEDING CONTROL ☐ BANDAGING ☐ HEAT/COLD APPLIED

☐ SPLINT ☐ TRACTION APPLIED ☐ BACK/NECK IMMOBIL.

☐ O2/VENTILATION RATE_____ ROUTE_____

AIRWAY: ☐ CLEARED ☐ ORAL SIZE_____ ☐ ESOPHAGEAL

☐ NASOPHARYNGEAL ☐ ENDOTRACHEAL SIZE_____

MAST ☐ LEGS + ABDO ☐ LEGS ☐ N/G TUBE

TRANSPORT POSITION:

PATIENT TRANSPORTED TO:_____ HOSPITAL

TRANSPORT PRIORITY:_____ ☐ AMBULANCE DECISION ☐ PATIENT DECISION

MEDICAL CONSULT: ☐ DIRECT ☐ C-MED CHANNEL _____

_____ MD/RN _____ HOSPITAL

HOSPITAL NOTIFIED ENROUTE: ☐ YES ☐ NO

☐ C-MED RADIO ☐ OPERATIONS DISPATCHER

PARAMEDIC/ADVANCED LIFE SUPPORT

TIME	FLUID/DRUG	RATE/DOSE	ROUTE (SPECIFY IV SITE)

TOTAL VOLUME FLUIDS INFUSED: MLS

EKG ☐ MONITOR ☐ TELEMETRY

COUNTER. SHOCK Time #1 _____ Time #2 _____

W-S #1 _____ W-S #2 _____

UNIT: SIGNATURES OF ATTENDANTS:

_____ / _____ NAME REGISTRY # _____ / _____ NAME REGISTRY # _____ / _____ NAME REGISTRY #

MEDICAL RECORDS

Figure 36.2. Department of Health & Hospitals ambulance service run report.

receiving hospital physicians. Information recorded on these forms includes final diagnosis, laboratory and x-ray results, final disposition, and comments pertaining to prehospital care.

(4) Two hospitals have designed their own ALS patient follow-up form that serves two purposes. When a paramedic team admits a patient to the emergency department, they are requested to com-

Table 36.13.
Data from Computer Aided Dispatch System (CAD), Department of Health & Hospitals, Division of Emergency Medical Services, 1974–1980.

Year	Number of Calls to 911	Responses by DHH Ambulances	Patients Transported by DHH Ambulances
1974	62,205	31,662	18,427
1975	65,101	35,879	22,231
1976	60,197	36,222	22,818
1977	62,984	44,892	30,444
1978	73,842	49,696	33,006
1979	77,056	49,802 (BLS)	31,989 (BLS)
		4,547 (ALS)	1,442 (ALS)
		54,349 (total)	33,431 (total)
1980	69,449	54,021 (BLS)	31,416 (BLS)
		5,361 (ALS)	1,780 (ALS)
		59,382 (total)	33,196 (total)

plete a specific section of the follow-up form that asks their comments about the manner in which they were received at the hospital, e.g., physician or nurse prepared to accept patient. The rest of the form is then completed by the physician attending the patient, and then a copy is returned to the DHH Ambulance Service. This method not only provides information for the receiving hospital in terms of its relationship with prehospital providers, but also gives the Ambulance Service the needed clinical information to trace each ALS patient through the entire EMS system.

(5) The paramedic nurse educator records final diagnosis and final disposition in daily ALS log book for each patient.

ALS follow-up information achieves a number of objectives:

(1) It tracks each ALS patient through entire EMS system.

(2) It maintains count of patients by hospital, clinical category, sex, age and geography.

(3) It maintains count of skills performed by each paramedic for purposes of education and refresher training.

(4) It provides clinical data for weekly paramedic rounds, clinical conferences, and research projects.

Correlation of All Data Elements

Evaluation of the EMS system performance is a worthwhile use of mounds of data that are generated on a daily basis from a system the size of Boston. With the assistance of a professional statistics company, the COBTH designed a study that examined this data in detail. Ten thousand consecutive calls to 911 for medical assistance were collected, coded, programmed, and analyzed from the time the call was received through in-hospital

patient management. Table 36.14 shows a sample of the information the study yielded.

Cooperation between prehospital and hospital-based services is essential to coordinate a record-keeping system that produces purposeful and usable data. Once issues such as patient confidentiality and unwillingness to share information with other hospitals are solved, meaningful analyses can assist the EMS system providers to evaluate performance and augment the system as necessary.

DISASTER LINKAGES

During devastating disasters an EMSS is activated to its maximum potential. However, to respond to a disaster situation that has generated multiple injuries and/or casualties, the EMSS as it operates on a day-to-day basis is usually not sufficient. Therefore, a predefined plan for disaster situations is recommended. Such a plan would be designed for incidents resulting from: (a) *natural disasters*: hurricanes, snow storms, volcano eruptions, etc.; (b) *national emergencies*: nuclear accidents, bombings, terrorist attacks, etc.; (c) *mass casualties*: aviation accidents, extensive fires, mining accidents, building collapses, etc.

An effective disaster plan cannot be constructed in isolation. A number of agencies have a role in a regional disaster operation, including (a) public safety agencies, i.e., police and fire; (b) civil defense operations; (c) public health agencies; (d) ambulance services, i.e., air, ground, sea rescue; (e) hospitals and specialty care centers; (f) Red Cross; (g) public governmental officials and departments; (h) disaster relief groups; (i) specialized groups, i.e., airport fire department; (j) Coast Guard and National Guard; (k) nuclear power plant safety personnel; (l) volunteer groups.

The role of the EMSS in disaster operations is

Table 36.14.
Data analyzed from City of Boston's EMS ambulance operation.

Frequency axis (top to bottom): 1100 +, 1000 +, 900 +, 800 +, 700 +, 600 +, 500 +, 400 +, 300 +, 200 +, 100 +

Horizontal axis (Dispatcher Defined Nature Code): 2 3 4 6 7 8 9 11 12 13 14 15 16 20 22 23 24 25 26 27 28 30 31 32 42 43 44 50

Dispatcher Defined Nature Code

01 Allergic reaction	08 Ingestion	14 SOB-respiratory	23 Possible injury	28 Person down	43 Unknown
02 Anxiety reaction	09 Illness unknown	15 Serious illness	24 Minor injury	30 Shooting	44 Assist another unit
03 Cardiac-chest pain	11 Minor illness	16 Seizure	25 Serious injury	31 Stabbing	50 Other or combination
04 Cardiac arrest	12 OB/GYN	20 Assault	26 Motor vehicle accident	32 Suicide	
06 Diabetic reaction	13 Psychiatric	22 Fire	27 Pedestrian struck	42 Unconscious person	

two-fold: (1) to coordinate and execute its activities in cooperation with other disaster participants, and (2) to render appropriate medical care to victims. Although prevention is a necessary deterrent for many disaster situations, when they do occur, it is the *number* of affected persons that defines the magnitude of the situation. Depending upon the routine capability of the individual EMSS, a disaster is usually defined by the inability of the regular system to cope with a certain number of victims.

Disaster Preparedness

Most EMSS planning groups are composed of individuals who are in positions to contribute to a regionwide disaster plan. Ambulance services and hospitals, because of their intrinsic roles in disaster operations, should be key planners, but may not necessarily be the lead agency for planning. Disaster plans and drills are requirements for accreditation by the Joint Commission on Accreditation of Hospitals and for federal EMS funding (DHEW, 1975).

Certain elements of disaster preparedness must be addressed in a written disaster plan, including:

(1) *Definition*: the definition of a disaster for a specific area, usually dependent upon the number of victims or type of incident, may be represented by degree or stages of disaster alert.

(2) *Notification*: identification of who can activate the disaster plan, manner in which disaster situation is confirmed.

(3) *Personnel*: defined methods for mobilizing additional personnel above and beyond those on-duty at the specific time.

(4) *Equipment*: location and inventory of special disaster supplies, methods for checking equipment on a routine periodic basis, methods for getting equipment to scene of disaster if needed.

(5) *Proceed-Out Teams*: identification of those persons (usually identified by the position, e.g., surgeon-on-call) who may need to be brought to scene and method of transportation.

(6) *Communications*: identification of communications plan, e.g., use of certain frequencies for radio transmissions; location of communications disaster coordinating center.

(7) *Triage*: identification of triage scheme, e.g., levels of injury severity, persons authorized to conduct triage, location of triage staging areas and equipment.

(8) *Victim Identification*: identification of the manner in which victims are identified, e.g., tags, tape, pen markings.

(9) *Personnel Identification*: identification of disaster personnel is necessary for coordination, organization, and security. Identification methods may vary, e.g., uniforms, badges, special headgear.

(10) *Authority/Leadership*: identification of who is in charge during certain specific disaster situations.

(11) *Point-of-Entry*: identification of those medical facilities capable of accepting accident victims for definitive treatment as well as determining method of hospital notification and number of available beds.

(12) *Decontamination*: identification of those facilities capable of decontamination and protocols for securing incident scene, on scene management, transport, and in-hospital management.

(13) *Transportation*: identification of transport services, including air, ground, and sea rescue units.

(14) *Media Operations*: specific plans for media intercommunications with disaster officials.

Most hospitals have an internal disaster plan that outlines the responsibilities of individuals as well as departments. However, hospitals and ambulance services must have their responsibilities clarified in the overall community response to a crisis with multiple casualties.

Boston Experience

The universal Boston Disaster Plan is frequently tested for purposes of: (1) identifying areas that need refinement or redefinition; (2) familiarizing new personnel with the plan; (3) refreshing and retraining veteran disaster participants; and (4) highlighting areas of possible disagreement among planners in order to reach workable solutions. Boston not only has disaster drills but has had a number of true disasters: Blizzard of 1978 (5 days of crippling snow that severely impeded transportation), two simultaneous hotel fires (March, 1979 with 73 victims), Courthouse bombing (April, 1976 with 20 victims) (Jacobs et al., 1979), and the DC-10 plane accident (January, 1982 with 39 injured persons and an additional 170 passengers requiring assistance from the aircraft). The Disaster Plan for the DHH (Boston City Hospital and the Ambulance Service) includes the following components to illustrate an approach to disaster preparedness:

(1) *Definition*: Three phases: *Administrative Alert*: designated personnel are alerted by the Ambulance Communications Center staff that a potential disaster exists; *Phase I*: after confirmation of the disaster situation, the hospitals are notified to mobilize their own internal disaster plans; *Phase*

II: off-duty personnel are summoned and specific disaster victim receiving and admission areas in hospitals are designated.

(2) *Notification*: The senior person on duty at the Communications Center is responsible for activating the phases of the disaster plan in consultation with the Medical Director of EMS.

(3) *Personnel*: The communications staff initiates the telephonic summoning of additional personnel and alerts other public safety agencies.

(4) *Equipment*: The ambulance supply station maintains an inventory of equipment used only during disaster situations. The materials are stored in light weight locker trunks for transport to the scene by supply center aides.

(5) *Proceed-Out Teams*: All Boston receiving hospitals have designated Proceed-Out Teams that are notified by the Ambulance Operations Communications Center. Transport to the scene is done by the BPD or Ambulance Service supervisory personnel. A proceed-out kit (contents determined by the COBTH's Disaster Committee) is present in each emergency department for the physician to bring to the scene.

(6) *Communications*: The Ambulance Service Operations Communications Center and supervisor execute the appropriate communications design to link all disaster participants. A group paging system is in operation that will notify Ambulance Service supervisory staff and the Medical Director simultaneously of any incident that necessitates more than a three ambulance response. The Communications Center is usually designated as the Disaster Coordinating Center for the purposes of:

(a) facilitating and coordinating hospital to field communications;

(b) serving as focal point for decision-making in regard to mobilization of resources;

(c) serving as receiving center for information from disaster scene;

(d) coordinating multiple agency responses to disaster scene;

(e) canvassing all hospitals for available routine and specialty care beds;

(f) coordinating with Boston City Hospital (Resource Hospital) Disaster Coordinating Center;

(7) *Triage*: A specific triage staging area is set up at the scene. The most senior medical person on scene, initially usually a DHH paramedic, is designated as the triage officer to (a) triage victims according to injury severity and (b) coordinate responding medical resources (Nissan and Elder, 1971). Four groups of patients are identified (Nis-

san and Elder, 1971; Ballinger et al., 1973; Miller and Cantrell, 1975)

Class I: severely wounded requiring immediate treatment, stabilization, and transportation.

Class II: urgent, less serious requiring minimal stabilization, transportation to hospital for definitive care.

Class III: walking wounded.

Class IV: dead or so severely injured that preventing death is unlikely.

(8) *Victim Identification*: specific disaster tags are brought to the scene with other disaster equipment and completed by the triage team.

(9) *Personnel Identification*: all ambulance personnel are required to wear DHH uniforms. Responding physicians have medical disaster officer badges.

(10) *Authority/Leadership*: the EMSS Medical Director has overall leadership authority for the *medical* services rendered at the scene. Coordination with other authorities is essential, e.g., airport safety officials.

(11) *Point-of-Entry*: since the Communications Center has all the information regarding the proximity and bed status of receiving hospitals, the Communications Center personnel direct the transporting units to specific hospitals.

(12) *Decontamination*: the special problems of the potential or actual radiation-exposed person require specific protocols for care at the scene, transportation, and eventual decontamination (Richter et al., 1980). Specific hospitals in Boston with decontamination facilities have been identified.

(13) *Transportation*: DHH Ambulance Service has primary responsibility for ground transportation services. Air rescue is accomplished by Coast Guard and/or State Police helicopters. The Coast Guard is equipped to handle sea rescues. Additional private ambulance services are contacted for back-up ambulance ground transport.

(14) *Media Operations*: public relations officials at area hospitals act as liaisons with media representatives as well as with members of victims' families.

Periodic planned and announced drills will test the disaster plans and help to educate disaster participants (Jenkins, 1978). Disaster preparedness is an essential component of the EMSS response to multiple victim incidents.

FACILITIES AND CRITICAL CARE UNITS

Considerable monies from both federal and private sources awarded to EMS planning agencies are paid for improvements in prehospital medical care, e.g., training, communications equipment, and ambulances. Although not as visible in terms of purchase and procurement of equipment, the changing role of hospitals in this new EMS system spanned a different type of revision. Organizing existing hospitals into a coordinated system to respond to the changing prehospital practices was a challenging portion of most EMS grant applications. With little or no funding for hardware and building, hospitals were asked to expand and improve services, participate in provision of medical care outside the hospital setting, and generally respond to an increase in patient visits. Three specific areas highlight the involvement of hospitals in the sculpturing of EMS systems; (1) categorization; (2) EMS system configuration; and (3) designation of responsibilities within the system (Committee on Emergency Medical Services, 1980; NAS-NRC, 1978; Boyd et al., 1975; Hoffer, 1979; Boyd, 1976).

Generally, the number of emergency departments and critical care units must meet the demand of the system for the types of patients within the system.

Categorization

Categorization is a term that often generates confusion, dispute, criticism, and fear among medical and administrative groups (Collins, 1973; Klippel, 1975; Tell, 1975; Hampton, 1975). However alarming, categorization does have a fundamental theoretic basis so that once accomplished, categorization will alter the point-of-entry and transfer patterns of patients to particular hospitals. Categorization is a process that utilizes certain criteria to measure the capability of a hospital to manage emergency patients. The belief that the closest hospital to the incident should be the receiving hospital is negated as a belief when discussing categorization. Once categorization is achieved, it may be determined that the closest hospital is the most appropriate receiving hospital, but this determination is based on capability and not geographic proximity.

The first criteria used to categorize emergency facilities were published in 1971 by the American Medical Association (AMA) under the title "Guidelines for the Categorization of Hospital Emergency Capabilities." The term *Horizontal Categorization* refers to the use of these or similar criteria to determine the general, overall capability of a hospital to manage emergency patients (Boyd,

1976). Once evaluated, each categorizing facility could be labeled *Comprehensive, Major, General,* or *Basic* (AMA Commission on EMS, 1981).

The AMA and its Commission on EMS have revised their guidelines to meet a different need in the categorization scheme. This need was to determine the capability of a hospital to manage specific emergent conditions. *Vertical Categorization* results in defining a particular capability to manage patients usually from the seven critical care groups: acute cardiac, burns, trauma, spinal cord, behavioral, neonatal/perinatal/pediatric, poisons. The newest AMA guidelines describe specific criteria that can be determined as either *Essential* or *Desirable* for one of the levels of capability for each clinical category. The three levels are:

I. *Level One*: capable of managing all types of medical emergencies definitively, including the use of complex and specialized services.

II. *Level Two*: capable of managing all types of medical emergencies in the emergency department and intensive care units; may not necessarily have specific specialized services.

III. *Level Three*: capable of rendering *initial* care to emergency patients; may have certain physicians on-call; should have firm transfer plans for specialty patients.

Categorization is a Law in Illinois (Public Act 76–1858). In most states, it is a voluntary process that hospitals agree to as part of the EMS planning effort. The benefit of categorization is presumably reflected in improved patient outcomes. To base improved outcomes solely on the capability of the receiving hospital is a research hypothesis not fully documented. The Committee on EMS-Assembly of Life Sciences in two of its documents cite a need for categorization because of the following:

"A major cause of inadequate hospital care, particularly in suburban and urban areas, is the delivery of patients to the nearest hospital rather than to a more qualified predesignated hospital capable of caring for the patients' injuries. There is little question but that hospitals with extensive experience with critically injured patients (trauma centers) provide better care for such patients than hospitals receiving them only occasionally" (NAS-NCR, 1978).

"Despite the tremendous growth and increasing sophistication of prehospital EMS systems in the last decade, which have brought more and more acutely ill and injured patients to hospital emergency departments, these departments still vary widely in their ability to provide adequate care for such patients. Studies continue to show that patients die or suffer avoidable disability as a result of inadequacies in emergency department care" (Committee on EMS, 1980).

Some studies and investigations do discuss mortality of trauma and cardiac patients once hospitalized, but do not prove that the mortality is a result exclusively of "inadequacies in emergency department care" (Foley et al., 1977; West et al., 1979; Mather et al., 1976).

Certain studies comparing mortality statistics before categorization and facilities designations were done with statistics after such processes were achieved (Otten, 1976; Cowley et al., 1973; Boyd, 1977). Although mortality rates dropped after "systems" were implemented, contributions to these reductions are difficult to attribute wholly to the system vis-a-vis considering such variables as increased prevention programs, more seat belt use, reduced traffic speeds, and improved prehospital care.

Categorization purports that care capability based on predefined criteria identifies which hospital(s) is better suited to care for a particular patient. Hospitals could conceivably augment their capabilities to achieve the criteria; yet how these capabilities, e.g., personnel, equipment, and in-hospital services, are organized in a plan to manage the patient may be lacking.

The landmark study by Luft et al. (1979) served to establish that the number of times a certain operative procedure is performed is a determinant reflected in mortality rates. Categorization criteria usually do not take into account this premise that if you treat certain types of patients more frequently, you do so more effectively than those who treat the same problems less frequently.

EMS System Configuration

The whole categorization process is useless unless the public and transport services know the conclusions of the categorization process. A point-of-entry plan that outlines the particular hospitals that are better staffed and equipped to manage certain patients is essential for the full implementation of the categorization process.

The manner in which patient flow through an EMS system from the original onset of the emergency through rehabilitation is dependent upon how the system is configured (Boyd, 1980) and the resources that are available within the EMS region.

Designation of Responsibilities

Once the resources within the region have been identified and categorized, the responsibilities for these resources can be designated. Usually these responsibilities are defined by the role the hospitals have in providing medical direction to para-

medics or advanced EMTs in the field, e.g., *resource hospital*: usually one per region; having on-line medical direction responsibilities; monitors ALS communications of any other hospital in the field; *associate hospital:* capable of providing on-line medical direction to advanced EMTs or paramedics within a certain area of the total region, but does not have responsibility for overall region; *receiving hospital*: receives emergency patients from transport services but does not participate in on-line medical direction.

Additional responsibilities for specialty care centers are also identified within the total region. If certain specialty centers are unavailable in one region, plans must be made to interact with neighboring regions. The description of sample systems are discussed below to illustrate the categorization, configuration, and designation processes.

Trauma

Boyd (1980) describes three configurations of national trauma systems. The criteria used for categorizing facilities within all of these configurations are available through the ACS document (1979), entitled "Hospital Resources for Optimal Care of the Injured Patient." These criteria utilize vertical categorization to determine hospital capabilities to manage injured persons at any one of three levels:

Level One: "Comprehensive hospital that has made a substantial commitment in both money and personnel to manage the care of the seriously injured";
Level Two: "Should have a serious commitment to trauma but may not have the availability of staff specialists at all times. This level institution may well handle the largest volume of trauma in a geographic area";
Level Three: "Should have a commitment to excellence in initial trauma care and should use established protocols" (ACS, 1980).

Boyd's trauma system configurations include a "Y" model for a rural-metropolitan area, an "X" model for an urban-suburban area, and a "Y'" model for a wilderness-metropolitan area. Some specific characteristics of these configurations include:
"Y" (rural-metropolitan area) (Fig. 36.3):
(a) 85% of the trauma patients can be managed at local (L) or areawide (A) trauma facilities;
(b) 10% of the trauma patients from local facilities and 5% of trauma patients from areawide facilities may require transfer to the more capable regional center (R);
(c) certain patients requiring specialized care, e.g., a burn center, may need to be transferred outside the region;

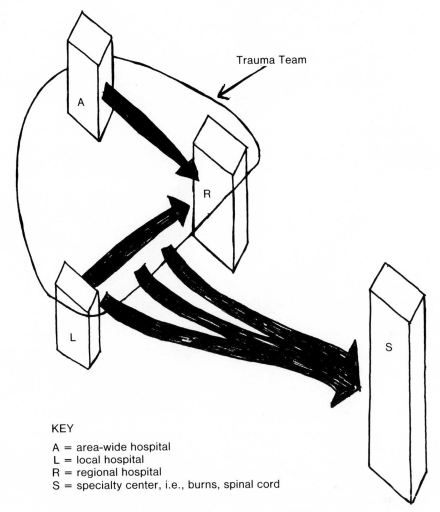

KEY
A = area-wide hospital
L = local hospital
R = regional hospital
S = specialty center, i.e., burns, spinal cord

Figure 36.3. Trauma system "Y" model (metropolitan-rural).

(d) may employ a special mobile trauma team (doctors, nurses) to stabilize patients at initial local receiving facilities.

"Y" (wilderness/metropolitan area) (Fig. 36.4):
(a) local trauma facilities (L) are within region;
(b) regional trauma facilities (R) are located outside this area and should receive transfers from local facilities; severe and critical patients would be in this transfer group of patients;
(c) uses trauma team.

"X" (urban/suburban area) (Fig. 36.5):
(a) has a defined number of areawide (A) and regionwide (R) trauma facilities;
(b) may transport less than 10% of trauma patients directly to areawide centers (A) instead of nearest hospital;
(c) may transport 5% of trauma patients to re-

gional (R) facilities; these patients may be transported directly to regional (R) facilities or may be transferred from initial receiving facilities;
(d) very few patients may need transfer to certain specialty centers outside the region;
(e) because of extensive capability within the region, local facilities (L) for trauma care are not designated.

The ACS (1979) suggests that managing 1000 trauma patients per year will contribute to a trauma center effectiveness, both clinically and fiscally.

Burns

The American Burn Association is actively involved in assisting health care systems define the

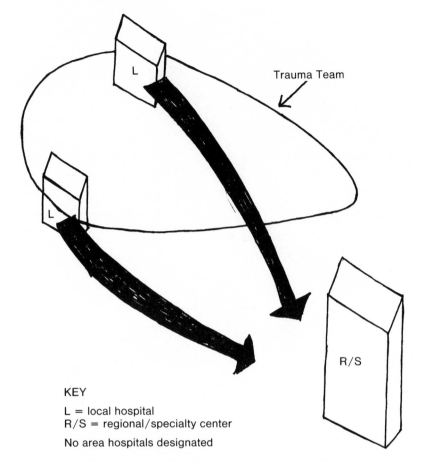

Figure 36.4.   Trauma system "Y" model (wilderness-metropolitan).

criteria for hospital-based capabilities, in a vertical categorization scheme, needed to care for burn victims. A major document first published in April, 1976, entitled "Specific Optimal Criteria for Hospital Resources for Care of Patients with Burn Injury" emphasizes the need for sophisticated treatment for the critically burned patient (American Burn Association, 1976).

The care of the burn patient can be achieved in one or more of four treatment settings: (1) burn center or hospital-based burn unit; (2) hospital with special expertise and a burn program; (3) hospital emergency department; (4) at the scene and during transportation. In order to identify the most appropriate treatment setting for burn patients, the American Burn Association has defined certain terms to categorize injuries based on the severity of the burn. Utilization of these terms will lead to standardization for easier identification and designation of appropriate facilities for the treatment of various kinds of burn injuries.

Once these definitions and treatment settings

have been accepted or adapted to local standards, state or regional committees designated to design the system can progress to categorizing their available hospital facilities using the Association guidelines. These guidelines outline the necessary resources of personnel, equipment, service specialties, and back-up capabilities that all three settings should consider essential or desirable for management of the burn victim. A part of determining capability is determining the severity of the burn. The American Burn Association suggests three levels of severity: major, moderate, and minor (Fig. 36.6). Edlich et al. (1978) have suggested modifying the ABA "minor burn" to include:

(1) Less than 5% BSA—second degree; less than 1%—third degree—involving eyes, ears, hands, feet or perineum, caused by short contact with heat or chemicals.

(2) Less than 15% BSA adults—second degree; less than 10% BSA children—second degree; less than 2% BSA—third degree.

The configurations of burn systems that utilize

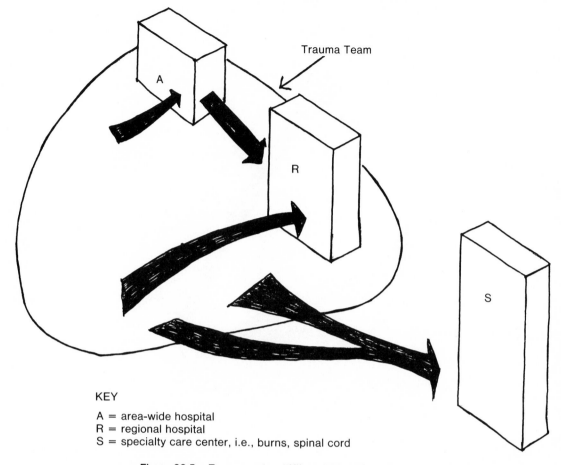

Trauma Team

KEY

A = area-wide hospital
R = regional hospital
S = specialty care center, i.e., burns, spinal cord

Figure 36.5. Trauma system "X" model (urban-surburban).

MAJOR BURN

More than 25% BSA (adult)—second degree
More than 20% BSA (children)—second degree

More than 10% BSA—third degree

Burns involving hands, face, eyes, ears, feet, perineum, inhalation—electrical-complicated burns, burns due to major trauma or high risk patients

MODERATE BURN

15–25% BSA (adult)—second degree
10–20% BSA (children)—second degree

Less than 10% BSA—third degree

MINOR BURN

Less than 15% BSA (adult)—second degree
Less than 10% BSA (children)—second degree

Less than 2% BSA—third degree

Figure 36.6. American Burn Association burn severity classes.

categorization, along with a certain number of facilities, and designation of responsibilities are similarly based on trauma systems models:

"Y" (urban-rural) (Fig. 36.7):
specialty burn facility within region—may receive burn victims initially;
local (L) and areawide (A) trauma facilities capable of managing burn victims.

"X" (urban/suburban) (Fig. 36.8):
specialty burn facility within region;
areawide (A) trauma centers capable of managing burn victims;
may transfer patients to burn facility from areawide facilities;
no need for transport to local (L) facilities because of numbers of areawide centers (A);
specialty burn center may receive burn victims directly.

"Y'" (wilderness/urban) (Fig. 36.9):
specialized burn facility is outside region;
local trauma facility (L) may need to stabilize victims, then transfer to center outside the region.

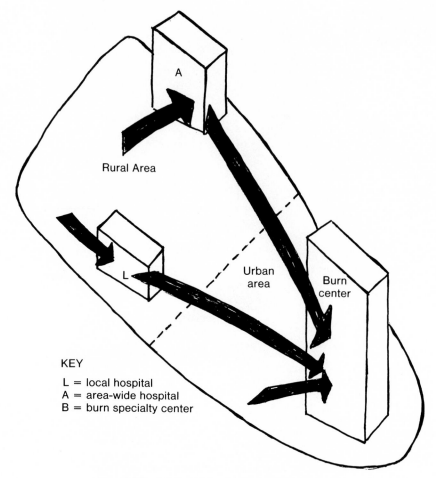

Figure 36.7. Burn system ''Y'' model (urban-rural).

One major concern of most health system planning agencies is to determine the number of burn beds needed in a specific EMS region. Edlich et al. (1981) suggested the following calculation to reach such a determination:

(1) total the number of moderate and major burns per year in the region;

(2) total the number of hospital days spent by the total number of burn patients per year in the region;

(3) determine the average daily census by dividing the figure determined in (2) by 365;

(4) divide the number determined in (3), the average daily census, by 80% (suggested occupancy rate).

Example:

(1) 100 patients/year

(2) 3640 patient-days/year

(3) 3640 ÷ 365 = 9.9

(4) 9.9 ÷ 0.8 = 12.3 or 13 burn beds

The determination of a burn system configuration is therefore based on predefined criteria for handling three levels of burn severity into a system that can designate emergency and in-hospital capabilities for burn centers, burn programs, and initial receiving facilities.

Poisons

Facilities categorization, system configuration, and designation of responsibilities as part of planning and implementing a poison system place considerable emphasis on specialized poison information control centers. Micik in San Diego (1979), Rumack in Denver (1978), and Lovejoy in Massachusetts (1979) have pioneered model poison systems. The American Association of Poison Control Programs (AAPCP) has made available "Standards for Poison Control Programs." Although this document is not a comprehensive vertical categorization tool that outlines specific criteria, the document does list general capabilities of a regional information center, including staff, education, data collection, and criteria for com-

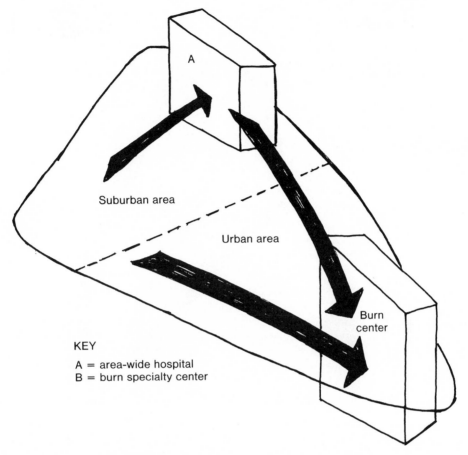

KEY

A = area-wide hospital
B = burn specialty center

Figure 36.8. Burn system "X" model (urban-surburban).

prehensive treatment centers. The AAPCP recommends that a single regional poison system
should be designed to meet the needs of no less
than 1 million people and no more than 10 million.

The system configurations of a poison system
are modeled after the EMS-DHHS trauma system
models. Micik (1981) describes the "X" model and
the "Y" model with each having the following
characteristics:

"X" Model (Fig. 36.10):
one poison information center in the region
receives all calls from the public;
concentrated training, data collection, and evaluation at one center;
local (L) and areawide (A) facilities for managing poisoned patients.

"Y" Model (Fig. 36.11):
one regional poison information control center
and one or more satellite centers;
calls from the public are received at all centers
within region (regional and satellite);
each center is involved in training, data collection, and evaluation;

local (L) and areawide (A) facilities for managing poisoned patients.

As in other systems such as burns and trauma
programs, a system of patient identification based
on severity has been introduced (Baker et al., 1974;
Tobiasen et al., 1981; Rimel et al., 1979; Micik et
al., 1979 a and b).

Level One (also termed Class III): little to moderate toxicity, requires assessment, treatment, 24-
hour out-of-hospital monitoring.

Level Two (also termed Class II): mild to moderate toxicity, may require prehospital assessment,
decontamination, emesis, and monitoring, hospital
care for definitive management, monitoring and
evaluation.

Level Three (also termed Class I): severe toxicity,
critically ill—may require specialized management, e.g., dialysis, hemoperfusion; require prehospital ALS assessment and management; hospitalization required for resuscitation, decontamination, and specialized medical care.

Responsibilities of facilities within a poison system are categorized according to the facilities des-

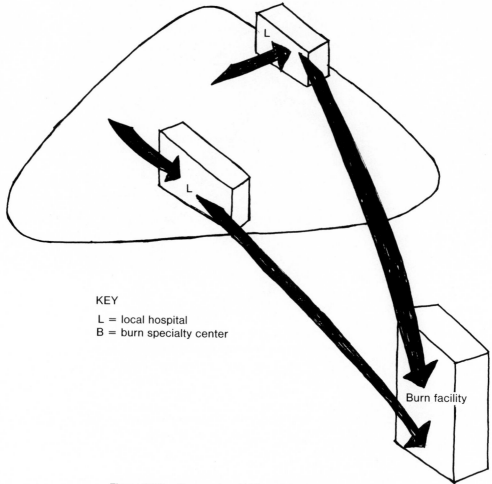

Figure 36.9.   Burn system "Y'" model (wilderness-urban).

KEY

L = local hospital
B = burn specialty center

Burn facility

ignation within the system (Micik, 1979 a and b). The local (L) treatment centers are responsible for initial evaluation and management, yet should consult with their regional center for transfer advice. The areawide (A) facilities have the same responsibilities, yet because of their increased capability, may admit the patient for either routine or intensive care. The satellite facilities (S) have the same responsibilities as the areawide facilities, yet also provide information and management advice to general public callers. The satellite centers have additional functions in the areas of evaluation, education for public and staff, as well as providing consultation to medical personnel. The regional poison information control center has all the responsibilities of the satellite centers, but is also capable of providing specialized care.

Certain common elements of a system approach are necessary to implement in any of these specialty care systems; they include:

(1) a regional planning group familiar with re-

gional resources;
(2) agreed-upon criteria for categorization of facilities;
(3) agreed-upon system configuration that designates responsibilities of various facilities;
(4) participation, education, and coordination with prehospital providers;
(5) public education of system design and capabilities;
(6) transfer agreements between facilities;
(7) adequate communications and transportation system to meet specialty systems needs;
(8) specific protocols for prehospital medical direction of advanced EMTs and Paramedics;
(9) methods for systems monitoring and evaluation; and
(10) fiscal management strategies.

MEDICAL CONTROL

Medical control is a phrase frequently used in EMS systems to describe the method whereby

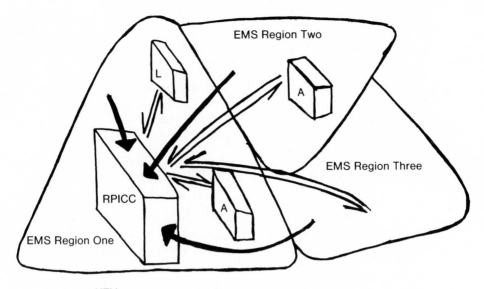

Figure 36.10. Poison system "X" model (one poison center).

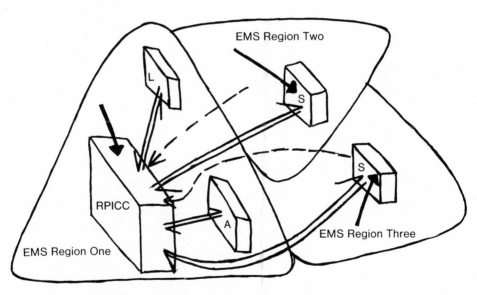

Figure 36.11. Poison system "Y" model (regional & satellite centers).

physicians manage directly and indirectly the performance of prehospital ALS. Although EMS systems have proliferated, the issues surrounding medical control are unresolved (Committee on EMS, 1981). Before discussing the unresolved dilemmas, a discussion of the meaning of medical control is essential.

The basic component of medical control is the physician who communicates with advanced EMTs in the field and who provides the actual voice *Medical Direction*. The other elements of medical control relate to the manner in which the Emergency Medical System is configured to respond to prehospital medical emergencies. These include an identifiable *Medical Director*, who is a physician and who is responsible for the *Medical Accountability* of the entire prehospital medical practice; *Treatment Protocols* which are the medically acceptable standards of medical practice in a particular geographic area; *Point-of-Entry* protocols which define particular hospital(s) where patients are taken; and the *Communications System* which is used to link the hospital personnel to the advanced EMTs in the field. All these elements are important to build a foundation for a physician-directed prehospital ALS system that utilizes the practice of medicine in the field.

The legislative process relative to the practice of medicine in the prehospital setting by nonphysicians in many states has not been clearly delineated by statute. Thirty states have some form of law identifying various titles for these providers (Page, 1979). There is little conformity or universality in the training and roles of these providers. Although the physician may have the right to delegate certain aspects of the practice of medicine to his/her surrogate, the physician does remain medically and legally accountable for the actions of that surrogate even in the event of inadvertent errors. This clear line of accountability leads to the need for total clarity in operational instructions for the prehospital personnel, and also the necessity for careful and accurate recording of all prehospital management ordered by physicians and executed by prehospital personnel.

With the inception of this new method of bringing emergency assistance to the victim, criteria have been established by the Division of EMS of the DHHS. They are:

(1) Effective region/area emergency medical planning with designation of a resource/base, associate/receiving hospital, and critical care centers with operational protocols and communications linkages with emergency medical systems personnel.

(2) Utilization of regional/areawide protocols adopted by the EMSS in which the ALS team participates from the scene of the incident, to the appropriate level of definitive care within the area. These protocols should be in accordance with pre-existing treatment, triage, and transfer protocols.

(3) Technological adaptations and innovations which support the system and its operations e.g., telecommunications, telemetry, MAST trousers, etc.

(4) Enabling legislative authority to provide accountable prehospital advanced life support services by nonphysician EMS personnel (Boyd et al., 1979).

The definition of on-line and off-line medical directors is also essential for adequate definition of medical control. Boyd and Lambrew (1979) have described an "on-line medical director" and an "off-line medical director." The on-line director is the physician at the resource or base hospital who is giving medical direction to the advanced EMTs in the field. This physician is practicing medicine and ordering therapy based on assessment data provided him through someone else's examination. For this reason, the physician is medically and legally accountable for the actions of the advanced EMTs whom he/she directs in the field. There are a number of models for on-line medical direction. They range from a two-tiered medical model involving senior medical/surgical residents in the emergency department providing direction via base console with attending faculty physicians monitoring these transmissions with the use of portable radios, to emergency physicians situated in emergency departments who provide total medical direction, to nurses in coronary care units or emergency departments who provide medical direction based on previously determined medical protocols or standing orders.

The administrative off-line medical director is that physician who is responsible for the entire operation of the prehospital system. He/she is also responsible for the appropriateness of the ALS practiced by the on-line medical director and the advanced EMTs in the field. This administrative off-line medical director may also be one of the physicians who gives on-line direction.

For organized medical control, the facilities categorization, systems configuration, and designation of responsibilities are essential efforts that must be accomplished as previously described.

Treatment protocols are essential. The resource hospital and any associate hospitals giving on-line medical direction to the advanced EMTs in the field are responsible for developing medical guidelines for the prehospital practice of paramedicine. Determination of these guidelines clarifies for both the physicians and the advanced EMTs the method and sequential management plan for any accident victim or ill person. That the physician still has the opportunity to individualize the management of a particular patient is important. However, all operating personnel who have an understanding of the general medical approach to clinical problems including the use of available drugs will increase their confidence in the system by increasing their familiarity with its management philosophies.

These protocols, developed by physician specialists from the community, can then be widely disseminated to all the receiving hospitals. This allows any physician whose patient may be treated in the prehospital phase to have input into, and a sound understanding of, the manner in which his/her patient will be managed in the event the system is accessed.

Of paramount importance for medical and legal stability of the prehospital ALS system is that the development of the guidelines for the practice of medicine by nonphysicians in the field be done by respected physician experts. The on-line medical director can be partially supported by his/her collegial specialists.

Although protocols stand as the most desirable type of medical direction, they still are tools for physicians who are actually communicating with the paramedics or advanced EMTs via radio. The second type of medical direction which may be used is the performance of prehospital ALS by standing orders. These standing orders, developed by the physician and his/her associates, guide advanced EMTs when they perform medical intervention based on whatever management is outlined for a particular medical or surgical problem. The obvious fault in this system is that it is often difficult to record every task which is performed during a difficult resuscitation effort in an uncontrolled prehospital setting and with minimal assistance. Therefore, the actual intervention can be easily performed yet not recorded or even sometimes not communicated to the awaiting hospital staff.

A responsibility of the system medical director is to establish a mechanism whereby regular and systematic review of all ALS transports can be conducted. This evaluation serves a management information purpose, as well as a research purpose.

Either physicians or specially trained ALS nurse coordinators can review each transport on a daily basis for adherence to protocols, completeness of charting, and accuracy of information. Various record-keeping practices are available in order to keep track of the utilization of ALS units, frequency of clinical problems, and the frequency of specific ALS interventions.

An additional evaluation tool, other than monitoring run reports and tracking patients through the various management phases, is to conduct case review sessions with the physicians and advanced EMTs who provide the on-line direction and the on-line field operations. Using unusual, challenging, poorly or well managed cases for these review sessions provides an excellent forum for continuing education and exchange of information from both professional perspectives.

In conclusion, the Subcommittee on Medical Control did agree on three basic functions of any medical control design (Committee on EMS, 1981): "(1) to assure that field personnel have immediately available expert direction for emergency care at whatever level they are capable of providing; (2) to assure a continuing high quality of field performance; and (3) to provide the means for on-going medical audit of both field performance and of the medical control itself."

Unresolved Issues of Medical Control

There are a number of various medical control arrangements; yet the efficacy of each is not well established. A common belief in most systems, however, is that the EMS system must be physician-directed and the prehospital medical care must be physician-managed. Some of the unresolved issues of medical control include (Committee on EMS, 1981):

(a) implementing medical control at the local level based on federal and/or state guidelines or regulations that may make implementation difficult;
(b) providing medical directors with precise authority;
(c) deciding whether medical control is needed in situations where patients present with immediate life-threatening emergencies that require immediate intervention;
(d) defining the various programmatic and legal responsibilities of all members of the medical control team;
(e) establishing the need for telemetry.

In an effort to examine some of these issues, a brief telephone survey was conducted recently to assess the state-of-the-art of national ALS systems. Officials in regional or state EMS offices were contacted and asked to respond to questions relating to the various aspects of medical control: medical direction provider, point-of-entry plan (categorization and triage protocols), prehospital treatment protocols, communications system (use of telemetry, central dispatch, UHF, or VHF), cooperation model (assignment of a resource hospital), evaluation mechanism of the prehospital treatment, and accessory components to the ALS system, such as helicopter service.

At present, ALS systems in the US are still developing and those that have been in operation for some time are continuing to upgrade and modify their systems of operation. Those in existence have developed as adjuncts of other community agencies (such as the fire department); in response to a perceived community need (such as volunteer or private ambulance services); as a branch of the community health care provider (such as a private or municipal hospital); or a combination of these. Consequently, there is great variance among systems in each state, and from state to state. However, some general descriptions have been drawn from the survey.

Twenty-six states were surveyed, 11 of which yielded information about ALS systems statewide; the remaining 16 systems (two systems in one state were surveyed) described specific metropolitan sites or regional areas in the state. Twenty-five of the 27 areas (93%) had advanced EMTs, EMTs trained beyond the 81 hours of basic emergency medical technology. Twenty-three (92%) had paramedic systems, and 6 of the 23 (26%) indicated they had both paramedic and other advanced EMTs operating in their systems. Other than the recognized title of paramedic referring to the fully trained prehospital health professional, advanced EMT meant anything from EMT-IV, EMT-Advanced, EMT-Intermediate, to EMT-II. It was clear, however, that the word "paramedic" universally meant someone who is trained to the 15-module DOT level or its equivalent. Size of the systems ranged from 10–500 advanced EMTs per system. Of those respondents describing systems throughout their state, some indicated that ALS systems were operational in only parts of their state, such as in the two or three major cities, or in ¼ to ½ of the state. Others indicated the advanced EMTs operated throughout the state. Length of time the systems had been in existence varied also, although the average and most frequent number of years systems have been operating is 6. The oldest system surveyed began 11 years ago, and many states already having advanced EMTs indicated that more systems will be implemented shortly.

Communications systems varied among the 25 metropolitan, regional, and statewide systems surveyed. A majority (56%) have a central dispatch system; just 40% used UHF exclusively, although an additional 24% used UHF in some parts of the state. The remaining 36% use only VHF, or in some rural areas, telephone contact and UHF are used. A majority (56%) have telemetry capabilities, but not all of those which have telemetry systems have a central dispatch system.

The delivery of medical direction to advanced EMTs treating patients in the field also varies from system to system, throughout a state as well as nationwide. Ten (40%) provide medical direction by a physician stationed in the emergency department; another six (24%) provide medical direction through a physician in the emergency department with standing orders used in cases where radio contact cannot be established (e.g., mountainous areas), or in some systems where advanced EMTs may begin treatment before contacting the physician providing medical direction. In one state, in the mountainous areas where radio contact is not always possible, advanced EMTs receive medical direction from a nurse who accompanies them on their transports. Only two (8%) of the systems surveyed (each serving a metropolitan area) operate solely on standing orders. In addition, in one state having both paramedic and other advanced EMT level (EMT-IV) personnel, only the paramedics have medical direction from a physician in the emergency department; the EMT-IV persons operate from standing protocols only. The seven (28%) remaining areas and states surveyed provide a combination of approaches for medical direction: nurses in the emergency department or coronary care unit; physicians in the emergency department or on portable radios; paramedics, nurses, or physicians assistants providing medical direction from the emergency department.

Of the 25 states, regions, or cities having advanced EMTs, 72% have resource hospitals through which medical direction is provided. Forty percent (40%) of those have just one resource hospital, while another 32% provide medical direction through more than one hospital. The rest (20%) have no designated resource hospital, or have only designated resource hospitals in some parts of the state (8%). Written prehospital clinical protocols are provided by 76%, while 48% provide written point-of-entry plans.

Prehospital care is monitored in 72% of the areas surveyed, but the person responsible for monitoring and the kind of monitoring varies greatly from system to system. Medical directors, training coordinators (physicians or nurses), medical advisory committees (consisting of various specialists such as cardiologists, pediatricians, as well as emergency physicians), committees comprised of the resource hospital staff, or regional or state EMS staff, are some of the monitoring organizations used. The format of the monitoring varies from weekly, bimonthly, or monthly meetings with the advanced EMTs, to review of the trip sheets and recordings of the ambulance transports, to a combination of the two.

As stated previously, 64% of the respondents indicated that medical direction is provided by a physician in the emergency department in all or most instances, while all except two of the remaining 9 statewide, regional, or metropolitan systems described have medical direction provided by a health care professional (a nurse, paramedic, physicians assistant, or an MD on a portable radio).

When asked if they felt medical direction in the field delayed patient transport and thus decreased the efficacy of treatment, 23 out of 25 (92%) of the respondents indicated no. Some explained further: (1) having back-up standing orders in case of radio contact difficulty eliminates delay; medical direction by radio is immediate; (2) even if transport is delayed, the quality of care is increased and therefore the patient benefits; (3) paramedics need medical control; (4) advanced EMTs, particularly EMT-IV persons (and other advanced EMT levels of the future) need medical control.

Sixty-eight percent of the areas provide accessory prehospital care through helicopter systems. However, the provider may not be the same as the provider for the ALS system, e.g., in a metropolitan area served by an ALS system operated by fire and private ambulance, the helicopter service is run by a private physician from a private hospital. Medical direction for the helicopter service is provided either by the resource or receiving hospital, or by a physician on board the helicopter. In only one instance does the helicopter staff (in this instance, an RN/EMT or RN paramedic team) operate on standing orders. Helicopter staff usually includes a nurse, a physician, a nurse/physician team, or an EMT or paramedic teamed with a physician or nurse. Three of the 17 helicopter systems staff their service with only an EMT or a paramedic.

Although several differences were evident among the advanced EMT systems, some general descriptions can be applied. (1) Most states have ALS systems, and many more than one level of advanced EMT operating. (2) Central dispatch, telemetry, and partial or total use of UHF is common. (3) Over two-thirds of the systems require direct physician involvement for medical direction, and use standing orders only when radio contact is impossible. This is particularly true in rural or mountainous areas served by advanced EMTs. (4) Almost all (92%) of the respondents indicated that medical direction in the field is needed and/or strengthens quality of treatment provided by advanced EMTs. (5) Almost three-quarters of the systems monitor the prehospital treatment; however, the mechanisms used and frequency of monitoring vary greatly. (6) Still in the developing stage is the designation of resource hospitals (40% have them now). Nearly one-third have several hospitals providing medical direction, and over one-quarter do not yet have a hospital designated to provide medical direction or have designated resource hospitals only in parts of their state. (7) Written triage (point-of-entry) protocols are provided in less than one-half of the systems, while three-quarters do provide written prehospital clinical protocols. (8) Many of the areas having advanced EMT systems also have helicopter systems, but rarely are they staffed by advanced EMTs, and often they are operated by a different agency from the main ground transport agency.

Discussion

The concept of medical control as compared to medical direction is an important consideration for modern EMS systems. Providing medical direction, the process of giving orders from a hospital to an advanced EMT in a remote location, is only one element of a medical control design that needs to be in place for monitoring and guiding the entire delivery of prehospital ALS. Two questions arise that when answered will provide needed data to support the medical control concepts. What are the results related to the accuracy of assessment and appropriateness of intervention, and is the practice of prehospital ALS the practice of medicine? If so, how should physicians maintain their control to ensure quality and patient protection?

Pozen et al. analyzed the electrocardiographic interpretations given by paramedics vis-a-vis those determined by physicians in 288 cardiac patients. He reported that 35% of all arrhythmias were misclassified by paramedics and 35% of the potentially life-threatening arrhythmias were also misclassified. Correct treatment was rendered in 74% of the cases. He concluded that more rigorous medical direction was needed to improve this assessment rate.

Briggs and Chamberlain (1976) in Brighton,

England reported 94% agreement between paramedic and physicians in ECG interpretation. The paramedics administered intravenous medication to 212 patients at their own discretion doing so by standing protocol. Of the 212 patients, 52% (111) responded wholly or partially to the medication. There was no statement regarding adverse effects.

Eisenberg et al. (1980) reported excellent results in patient outcome as a result of EMTs trained in defibrillation technique for the out-of-hospital victim in ventricular fibrillation. Of 54 patients, 10 were resuscitated and discharged from the hospital. Such intervention was performed based on protocols without medical on-line direction.

More research and evaluation needs to be conducted to review not only the final results in terms of mortality, but also in terms of error rate related to the administration of medication, and the possible negative effects that such an error produces. If the practice of paramedicine is the practice of medicine, it is most likely not immune to iatrogeny resulting from misassessment, misdiagnosis, or even mismanagement.

Due to obvious need for quality medical care and due to the mounting public awareness of health care in an age of available legal recourse, there are methods that can be implemented to reduce instability and to promote excellence. They are: established written triage protocols; established written treatment protocols; thorough record keeping of patient assessment data, interventions and responses to treatment; the identification of the physician who is responsible for patient care; standardization of advanced EMT training programs; and adherence to certification and recertification standards for those prehospital and hospital-based personnel involved in operation of the system.

Medical Control and the Legal Implication

Page (1981) describes some of the legal issues surrounding medical control and cites the lack of legal precedents. A certain trend was noticed in one large EMS area where medical control was weak and often nonexistent. There was an increase in the number of filed lawsuits relating to prehospital care.

Boston Experience

Facilities and critical care units are numerous in the city of Boston. With three major medical schools and 17 teaching hospitals, Boston has been acclaimed as a medically enriched center of service, science, education, and research. The organization of its EMS system is strongly based in the cooperative effort that was undertaken to categorize and designate facilities. The COBTH and its EMS subcommittee launched the categorization process in 1975 with the development of a care capability questionnaire. This questionnaire included the essential and desirable criteria for designating hospitals and their emergency departments as Level I, II, or III for care of patients in each of the 7 critical care categories. The questionnaire was completed voluntarily by all Conference hospitals. Site visit teams comprised of Conference members (physicians, nurses, administrators) were designated to visit hospitals other than their own. The purpose of the scheduled visits was to compare the answers on the completed questionnaires with on-site conversations, observations, and a review of pertinent written protcols, procedures, and staff schedules.

Figures 36.12 represents the final point-of-entry plan for the emergency facilities receiving patients in the Boston EMS system. The plan was implemented by the DHH Ambulance Service after final endorsement by COBTH members.

After completion of the categorization process, the Boston EMS system became the major EMS provider within a larger geographical area, called Region IV. The region has 35 hospitals with emergency departments, and a population of 2,107,746. The designation process of resource and associate hospitals began with an application process sponsored by the regional EMS entity, the Regional Emergency Medical Services Advisory Council (REMSAC). Each applying facility completed this process by offering documentation to support the fact that they met certain criteria relating to staffing, equipment, support services, in-hospital capabilities, education and research activities. After site visits to all applying facilities, the REMSAC Medical Services Committee endorsed the Boston City Hospital as the Resource Hospital.

The responsibilities of the BCH as the regional Resource Hospital include: (1) providing on-line medical direction to paramedics in the City of Boston; (2) providing off-line medical direction; (3) providing guidance and consultation to other agencies within the region; (4) contributing to education and research; (5) developing a complete manual of prehospital treatment protocols that serve as the prototype for the region; (6) operating the central communications center for City of Boston EMS operations (C-MED serves as the regional coordinating center for disasters and specialty bed updates) and (7) participating in regional planning, evaluation, and system revisions.

HOSPITAL POINT-OF-ENTRY PLAN

Hospital	Major Trauma	Acute Med.	Pediatric Emerg.	Behavioral Emerg.	Poison Emerg.	Burns	Neonatal Crises
Boston Emergency Medial Center: Boston City Hospital and University Hospital	IA	IA	IA	IA	IA	IB	IA
Brigham & Women's Hospital	IA	IA	III	IB	IA	IA	IA
Beth Israel Hospital	IA	IA	III	IA	IA	IB	IB
Carney Hospital	IB	IB	IB	IB	IB	II	III
Children's Hospital Medical Center			IA	IA	IA	IB	IA
Faulkner Hospital	II	IB	III	IB	IB	II	III
Massachusetts Eye & Ear Infirmary	IA for isolated Eye and ENT Injuries						
Massachusetts General Hospital	IA	IA	IA	IA	IA	IA	IA
New England Medical Center	IB	IA	IA	IA	IA	II	IA
St. Elizabeth's Hospital	IB	IA	IB	IA	IA	II	IB

St. Margaret's Hospital does have IA capability for neonatal patients

KEY:
IA = Stabilize, admit, and provide extended definitive care
IB = Stabilize, admit, and provide definitive care: not as much capability as IA
II = Stabilize only and transfer patient to another facility
III = No Capability

Figure 36.12.   City of Boston point-of-entry plan.

Trauma

Extensive planning and coordination as part of a Region IV EMS activity contributed to the eventual designation of three trauma centers in Boston. An application process sponsored by REMSAC was followed by site inspections by surgeons of the ACS Verification Program (1980). The three trauma centers are:

I. *Boston Emergency Medical Center:*
Boston City Hospital Trauma Center
University Hospital (New England Regional Spinal Cord Injury Center)
New England Medical Center (Pediatric Trauma)

II. *Massachusetts General Hospital/Massachusetts Eye & Ear Infirmary*

III. *Longwood Medical Complex:*
Brigham and Women's Hospital
Children's Hospital Medical Center
Beth Israel Hospital

Poisons

The Massachusetts Poison Control System serves as an example of a statewide approach to organizing a system of care. The State Poison Center is located at the Children's Hospital Medical Center and receives all calls for poison information from a state population of 5,737,037 persons. The system includes 98 hospitals that are *Member Hospitals*, all of which are acute care facilities and also provide support for the center. The Massachusetts Poison Control System also has *Consortium Institutions* (BCH, the Children's Hospital Medical Center, the Massachusetts College of Pharmacy and Allied Health Sciences, Tufts New England Medical Center, and University of Massachusetts Medical School) that provide continuing support to the system's operation.

The center also has defined procedures for obtaining information regarding unusual poisonings from such institutions as the Arnold Arboretum, the Occupational Medicine Division of the Harvard School of Public Health, and the Chemistry Department of the Massachusetts Institute of Technology.

The Center, staffed by physicians, nurses, and pharmacists, responds to an average of 180 cases per day (65,000 cases yearly). The staff achieves the following responsibilities: (1) provides information to the public and health professionals; (2) gathers and records data; (3) distributes educational materials, and; (4) educates on-site nursing, pharmacy, medical and paramedic students. The staff is supported by a team of medical toxicologists and poison specialists who also respond to physician inquiries from across the state concerning poisoned patient management.

The Massachusetts Poison Information System (1981) is involved in a number of programs as part of its overall role in the system. These programs include:

(1) *Professional Education:* weekly toxicology seminars; monthly continuing education sessions; conferences in various member hospitals; clinical symposia; training programs for students, both formally at the College of Pharmacy and at the Poison Center.

(2) *Public Education:* available brochures and telephone stickers; prevention campaigns; media involvement; designation of a satellite public education committee for Western Massachusetts.

(3) *Professional Update:* distribution of *Clinical Toxicology Review* to all member hospitals, 100 poison centers in USA and Canada, and private subscribers.

(4) *Prevention:* involvement in the Massachusetts Statewide Children's Injury Prevention Program (a federal Maternal and Child Health grant) studying the Poison System, comparing public awareness of poisons in a state with a poison system and one without; and studying poison-generated emergency department visits whether the visitor had accessed the poison system or not.

General Considerations

Boston, the Region, and the State of Massachusetts have implemented other subsystems including spinal cord care and neonatology care. Statistically, the Boston area and its EMS system respond to a significant number of emergencies. In 1981, the DHH ambulance service received 66,439 calls to its 911 number for medical assistance; ambulances responded to 65,885 of these calls with 10% of the calls receiving a two-tiered BLS and ALS response. The number of calls represents the actual number of calls received. The number of patients transported in 1981 was 29,807. The difference between calls received and actual transports is attributed to multiple calls for the same incident, false calls, calls for incidents that had no medical consequences, e.g., an MVA with no one injured, etc. The BCH received 31% of these transports; the Massachusetts General Hospital 15%; the New England Medical Center 11%; the Carney 9%; the Brigham and Women's 8%; with the remaining 26% received by 13 other facilities.

As part of a patient tracking feasibility study, a professional evaluation organization examined a sample of approximately three thousand transported patients. The study collected the following representative data:

Sex: 44.4% female   55.6% male
Race: 68.5% white   26.5% black   5% other
Age: 40% between
       ages 17–35

Additional information is available regarding ALS patients transported between December 1978 and February 1980 in that 28.8% of the patients were trauma patients, and 71.2% were medical patients (27.3% cardiac symptoms, 10% cardiac arrest).

The configuration of the Boston EMS specialty system is represented in Figure 36.13. The practice of medical control in the city of Boston is strict and follows the recommendations of the federal EMS Program. Twenty-five paramedics are employed by the DHH Ambulance Service. All of these paramedics were trained at the BCH and are certified by the National Registry of EMT-P. Prior to practicing paramedicine in the field, they must successfully complete an oral examination given by the Medical Director of EMS of the city of Boston. Medical control is conducted in the following fashion:

(1) When ALS intervention is required in the field by paramedics they contact CMED and request a channel assignment for medical direction.

(2) C-MED engages a patch with the medical or

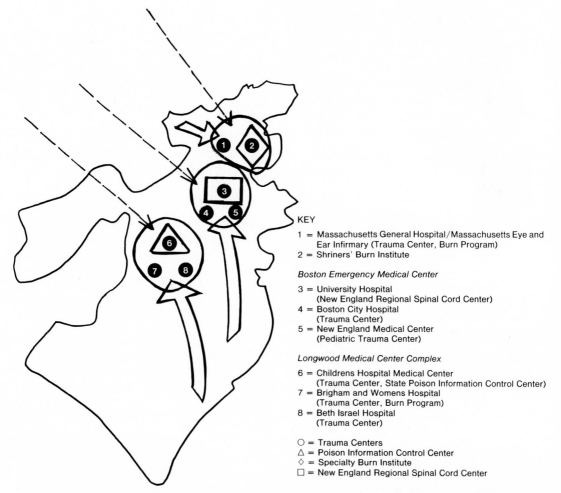

KEY

1 = Massachusetts General Hospital/Massachusetts Eye and
    Ear Infirmary (Trauma Center, Burn Program)
2 = Shriners' Burn Institute

Boston Emergency Medical Center

3 = University Hospital
    (New England Regional Spinal Cord Center)
4 = Boston City Hospital
    (Trauma Center)
5 = New England Medical Center
    (Pediatric Trauma Center)

Longwood Medical Center Complex

6 = Childrens Hospital Medical Center
    (Trauma Center, State Poison Information Control Center)
7 = Brigham and Womens Hospital
    (Trauma Center, Burn Program)
8 = Beth Israel Hospital
    (Trauma Center)

○ = Trauma Centers
△ = Poison Information Control Center
◇ = Specialty Burn Institute
□ = New England Regional Spinal Cord Center

Figure 36.13. City of Boston specialty system design (Trauma Centers, Poison Center, Burn Institute, New England Spinal Cord Injury Center).

surgical senior resident at the BCH (resource hospital) *and* with an attending faculty physician. The resident utilizes a regular radio-telemetry console in the emergency department. The attending physician utilizes a long-range portable radio. No ALS intervention is allowed without both physicians acknowledging the fact that they are on-line and ready for radio transmissions from the paramedics.

(3) There is a set of established protocols for clinical management of all patients in the field. These protocols have been mounted on the wall in the Emergency Department at the BCH. There is *one* standing protocol in the Boston EMS system. If the paramedics assess a patient in cardiopulmonary arrest, they are permitted to initiate an intravenous line, insert an endotracheal tube, defibrillate if the patient is in ventricular fibrillation,

and administer the first dose of sodium bicarbonate. All other interventions must be ordered by the physician.

(4) If the patient is transported to another hospital other than BCH, a channel is assigned to the paramedics in order for them to provide a notification to the receiving hospital.

(5) The BCH as the resource hospital is the only hospital permitted to provide medical direction to paramedics in the field.

(6) All ALS-treated patient run reports are reviewed daily by the paramedic nurse educator.

(7) Weekly paramedic rounds are held to review the previous week transports.

(8) The COBTH serves as a forum for discussion of any problems that may occur as part of the operations of the ALS system in the city of Boston.

PUBLIC INFORMATION AND EDUCATION

It is necessary that the general public know how to access the EMSS. Also important for the public to know is the type of services that are available, what to do while waiting for trained medical assistance to arrive, and when and for what reasons ambulance services are indicated. Public information and education programs are aimed at meeting these needs.

Considerable focus has been given to training the citizenry in CPR. It would seem that this focus is a result of the statistics related to out-of-hospital deaths due to cardiovascular reasons:

(a) 650,000 persons die annually of ischemic heart disease;

(b) 350,000 persons die annually of ischemic heart disease *outside of the hospital*;

(c) 1,000,000 persons died in 1978 of cardiovascular disease (American Heart Association, 1981).

In an attempt to reduce these rates, CPR programs have flourished across the nation. A Gallup poll has estimated that 12 million persons had received CPR training with an additional 60–80 million anticipating such training (Gallup Poll, 1977). However, there are a number of other health care issues, especially those that are related to emergency health care, that could be a part of a public education endeavor. The aforementioned 7 critical care categories that make up the majority of patients requiring emergency medical services, could also be the topic for public education programs. Because of its greater incidence, heart disease clearly stands as the area of education requiring a concentrated public education pursuit.

Acute Cardiac CPR Training

A number of researchers report improved survival of out-of-hospital cardiac arrest victims when the victims have received CPR (Thompson et al., 1970; Guzy et al., 1979). Eisenberg et al. (1980) in additional studies cite other variables that enhance survival, e.g., length of time from collapse to treatment with CPR and defibrillation. It has been demonstrated that it is almost impossible to compare outcome statistics from various EMS programs (Eisenberg et al., 1980b). For example, Eisenberg et al. (1980b) report a patient discharge rate of 23% for 595 patients who received "attempted resuscitation out-of-hospital." Eliastam et al. (1977) report a 3.5% discharge rate for 198 "attempted resuscitations." One major difference is that Eisenberg's group were patients demonstrating ventricular fibrillation only, while

Eliastam's group made no differentiation between various heart rhythms. The Brighton, England experience demonstrated a zero survival rate for 47 out of 207 patients with circulatory arrest and who were in asystole (Briggs et al., 1976). The significance of the studies stands amidst a precise definition of variables, categories of patients, outcome measures, research methodologies, and cross-referenced variables. In the majority of studies, an important factor contributing to survival appears to be the initiation of CPR as soon as possible.

Training Approaches

Seattle reports having trained more than one-third of its 500,000 citizens (Thompson et al., 1970). McElroy (1980) refers to this approach in training as the "saturation model." He suggests additional approaches including training the families of *high-risk persons*, training *civil servants*, training *school-aged children*, and training a combination of persons related to high-risk groups with the saturation model (McElroy, 1980). Inherent in training any group is to stress access the local EMS system, prevention of heart attacks, as well as the actual technique of cardiopulmonary resuscitation. The American Heart Association and the American Red Cross are leaders in promoting and organizing CPR training programs. Still to be determined and recommended to training agencies are such considerations as:

(1) how to retrain previously trained persons and is it necessary to do so?

(2) how to disseminate information regarding changes in techniques to previously trained persons?

(3) is there a better way to reach a larger audience?

(4) how do training programs reach the elderly, handicapped, non-English speaking and/or uninterested public?

Other EMS Public Education Needs

Trauma

Television viewers have been instructed how to prevent house fires as well as how to act when one occurs as part of an American Burn Association campaign. The use of seat belts in cars and a reduction of the speed limit to 55 mph are attempts to reduce highway injuries. Bumper stickers, car inspection stickers, and daily newscasts are all reminders to the public, in what can be considered education, to *prevent* death from trauma. To reduce death from trauma is a strikingly more challenging educational endeavor to lay educators than reducing death from coronary artery disease, since prevention of the incident does not rely on the medical community and its research expertise. It relies on *pure* prevention of physical, not physiological circumstances.

The course of events required to prevent trauma deaths is plagued by public disagreements and discrepancies. Despite the fact that 4082 deaths and 350,000 injuries in 1977 were a result of motorcycle accidents, 24 states either weakened or repealed their helmet laws between 1976–1978 (Watson et al., 1980). Studying this time period "implied that the mortality rate among unhelmeted riders is almost twice as high as that among helmeted riders." Alcohol sales remain a thriving national industry despite the following statistics: one-half of the drivers involved in fatal motor vehicle accidents had been drinking (Zuska, 1981); in 66% of fatal motorcycle accidents, the cyclist had a positive blood alcohol concentration (Baker et al., 1977); in 1345 fatal aviation accidents, 20.7% of the pilots had some evidence of alcohol and/or drugs (Lacefield et al., 1975); and a reported 50% of all fatal falls were connected with alcohol consumption (Haberman and Baden, 1978). In an era of political assassinations and other gun-induced fatalities, gun control remains a public and legislative dispute. Socioeconomic factors, i.e., poverty, unemployment, housing deficiencies, drug-induced crime, are contributors to the trauma statistics. Educational programs aimed at reducing trauma deaths take on a different cultural and societal slant that CPR educators do not necessarily have to face in light of the trauma problem genesis.

Neonatal Crises

There has been a decrease in the neonatal mortality rate in the US. In 1950, the mortality rate was 20/1000 births, in comparison to 11.6/1000 in 1975 (Lee et al., 1980). Three-fourths of the decline during this 25-year period occurred between 1965–1975 (Lee et al., 1980). Factors contributing to neonatal mortality were grouped into those affecting birthweight distribution, i.e., socioeconomics, parity, and medical complications (Dott and Fort, 1975; DHEW, 1972a and b); and those that affect birthweight-specific mortality rates, i.e., immediate perinatal care (Schlesinger, 1973; Stanley and Alberman, 1978; Kitchen et al., 1978); sex (DHEW, 1972 a, b, and c), and the relationship of the birthweight to the birth-gestation (Eberhart et al., 1964; Lubchenko et al., 1972). Race was considered to be a factor affecting both categories (DHEW, 1972c).

Lee et al. (1980) summarize their analysis of neonatal mortality by saying:

"Thus, although the evidence is indirect, and although it is impossible to rule out the contribution of factors as yet unspecified, the most plausible explanation for the demographic trends we have noted is the steady improvement in perinatal medical care which has made for greater infant survival at a given birthweight."

Some focus has been given the educational needs of this group as they relate to emergency medical services. A subject of most prenatal classes for expectant mothers is a description of the way in which to access the local EMS system when delivery seems imminent. Encouragement of professional perinatal care appears to have been a positive method to aid in the reduction of neonatal mortality.

Poisons

Accidents are the leading cause of death for children. Included in this category are accidental ingestions and other forms of poisonings. An estimated 5 million poisonings occur annually in the United States (Micik, 1979). Of these poisonings, approximately 80–85% are treatable outside of a hospital (Micik, 1979). In order to achieve such treatment, certain essential components of a Poison Control System that relate to public education should be implemented.

(1) There should be citywide, regionwide, or statewide publication and distribution of the Poison Control Center (PCC) access number.

(2) There should be a link between the central EMS access number, e.g., 911 and the PCC number.

(3) There should be consumer awareness campaigns related to potentially damaging products and methods for preventing poisonings and overdoses as a result of exposure to such products.

(4) There should be poison prevention programs for parents, children, schools, and other local groups.

Boston Experience

Various public education and information practices have been implemented as part of the Boston EMS system, including: (1) CPR training of the general public, sponsored by the DHH Ambulance Service; EMTs certified as BLS instructors teach Heartsaver (simple 3–4 hour program), and BLS CPR programs for local clubs, businesses, schools and social organizations; (2) The DHH Ambulance Service nursing and paramedic staffs participate in local high school "career days" and health education classes to describe EMS system components, EMS system access, and career opportunities; (3) 911, the EMS system access number, is imprinted on all city of Boston ambulances; (4) 911 is printed in Boston telephone books as the emergency access number; (5) All major television news shows, special feature programs, and evening magazine-time programs have featured the ambulance service: its capabilities, access, and instructions regarding how to respond to a medical emergency; (6) The Massachusetts Poison Information Control Center sponsors prevention weeks with concentrated public announcements regarding prevention, access, and treatment. Ipecac is provided free of charge. Telephone stickers with Poison Information Control Center telephone number are distributed statewide; (7) 911 telephone stickers are distributed citywide; (8) Discharge instructions for patients seen in local emergency departments include a description of EMS system access for future need; (9) Neighborhood health centers are stocked with informational brochures regarding the role of the EMS system and a description of EMS providers, e.g., EMTs and paramedics.

Public education can be provided by well planned and organized programs. A more stable and concrete awareness of emergency medical services will be established with time and person-to-person exchange of information. As aware as the public is of police and fire services, so will they be of EMS as the system matures and sustains its function among needed protective services.

TRANSPORTATION

The transportation of the sick and injured was one of the primary concerns of the original investigators who outlined the inadequacies in EMS (NAC-NRC, 1966). Ambulances were largely of the station-wagon or hearse-type vehicles in which patient management and CPR were difficult to execute. The changes in transportation are probably the most visible alterations that have occurred in the last two decades of EMS systems improvements.

Transportation is an EMS component receiving significant emphasis during original planning efforts of many EMS systems since transport of the victim from the scene to the hospital was a fundamental prerequisite to other components. Elements of this component are defined by the Division of EMS of the DHHS (DHEW, 1975) which divides the requirements into basic and advanced ground units and all other types.

BLS Ground Units:

(1) They should have radio equipment suitable for dispatch and medical consultation.

(2) They should meet the DOT General Services Administration KKK-A-1822 specifications.

(3) They should be equipped according to the ACS recommendations.

(4) They should be staffed by at least two EMTs.

(5) They should be located in a place conducive to a response time of no more than 30 minutes in rural areas 95% of the time.

(6) They should utilize a tiered response of vehicles.

ALS Ground Units:

(1) They should meet all six BLS unit elements.

(2) They should be staffed by at least two EMTs trained at ALS levels.

(3) They should have communications ability for telemetry.

Other transport units include: (1) helicopters, (2) fixed wing aircraft, (3) water rescue units, (4) snow rescue units.

Transportation Standards

The federal GSA-KKK-1822 specifications were adopted January 2, 1974 and revised in 1975 and 1980. The standards expressed a new thinking relative to design and technology and more importantly, allowed for a larger patient compartment with adequate room for the cot, attendants, supplies, oxygen, suction, and communications equipment. The ACS first developed a list of Essential Equipment for Ambulances in 1961. The fourth revision in 1981 addresses basic equipment items, i.e., suction, oxygen apparatus, bandaging supplies, etc. Various revisions have added items such as pneumatic garments. Other essential supplies include obstetrical kit, poison kit, splints, spinal immobilization boards, bag-mask ventilation units. Certain equipment necessary for ALS is mentioned and includes tracheal intubation and intravenous equipment, drugs, electrocardioscope, and defibrillator. Additional rescue equipment is also listed (ACS, 1981).

The performance of CPR in a moving ambulance continues to be a controversy centering on proficiency, protection for the attendant, and performance without interruption. French ambulances have centered the patient cot in the middle of the vehicle as an attempt to provide better access (1979). Practitioners in the field have recommended amendments to these specifications to optimize CPR performance (Rolandelli, 1981).

Guidelines for air ambulances were published by the DOT (DOT-HS-805–703) February, 1981. These guidelines were developed by the Commission on Emergency Medical Services of the AMA, the National Highway Traffic Safety Administration, and the DOT. The standards for air transport are voluntary recommendations that will probably serve as the national standard (George, 1982).

Deployment

Corresponding with an adequate number of transport vehicles is a defined deployment plan. This type of plan is designed to: (1) determine the appropriate number of ambulances needed for a particular area; (2) determine the most appropriate geographic satellite locations for the ambulances in order to achieve a given response time and a balanced work load for each unit.

Each city, town, and region has its own financial, political, and geographic restraints which determine the absolute number of ambulances available. The challenge to the EMS operator is how to use these resources best to achieve an acceptable short response time, and how to maintain skill proficiency by ambulance attendants. Deployment plans obviously need to include the manner in which the EMS system will respond to medical emergencies. Inter-agency cooperation between police, fire, and EMS services is usually indicated. Frequently, the first responders may be employed by a different service from the service that will actually transport the patient. Fire and police services traditionally have more personnel and equipment geographically interspersed throughout communities. Therefore, if EMS prehospital providers are other than police or fire, these two agencies may participate in the system as first-tier responders. Copass (1981) reports a tiered response in Seattle achieving a response time of 1.9 minutes for the neighborhood engine company, followed by the district car with a 3.5-minute response time with the MEDIC unit averaging a 7.5-minute response time.

Deployment plans may be constrained by a number of factors some of which can be alleviated and some which are permanently constraining such as:

(1) jurisdictional boundaries, e.g., town lines that differ from EMS boundaries,

(2) inadequate garaging facilities,

(3) financial limitations,

(4) difficult geographic access, e.g. mountainous areas,

(5) barriers to travel, e.g., cemeteries, rivers, parks,

(6) uneven distribution of workload,

(7) having an adequate maintenance and supply system which can respond to multiple satellite locations of vehicles.

Maintenance

An emergency ambulance has two separate areas which need to be kept in excellent working condition for optimal functioning of the units. The *Automotive Component* has to be maintained frequently and preventively so that the unit can always respond immediately. For example, the brakes are severely taxed and require inspection and replacement more frequently than on conventional vehicles. The *Patient Care Compartment* also needs to be continually stocked and maintained to ensure that all medical equipment and supplies are present and functioning at all times. Preventive maintenance schedules vary according to the type and frequency of usage of the vehicles. A busy municipal ambulance service performing in high traffic density on numerous calls per shift will require a more rigorous schedule than an infrequently used unit which travels great distances per call.

Helicopters

Helicopter medical transport systems have become a part of comprehensive EMS systems. There are major benefits of a helicopter system.

(1) Helicopters provide a faster response time in areas where EMS primary response is not well developed.

(2) Helicopters provide service to inaccessible areas, either due to poor or absent road conditions, or weather conditions.

(3) Helicopters provide delivery of trained medical personnel to initiate therapy on the scene.

(4) Helicopters provide smoother transportation of the patient in some instances.

(5) Helicopters provide rapid transportation to definitive specialty care facilities.

There are approximately 25 hospital-based helicopter programs in operation in the US. The apparent *key* benefit of helicopter services in emergency medical care is the rapidity with which they deliver medical care to patients and the rapidity with which a patient can be delivered to definitive care.

The successful application of the helicopter service applied to the civilian population was first reported by Foster (1969) and Frey (1969). The potential demand for helicopter systems for use in emergency transportation was further described by Turner and Ellington (1970). Roberts et al.

(1970) reported data regarding the benefits of helicopter services:

"The assessment of specific medical benefits of this project is documented by patients who arrived alive who otherwise would have been dead on arrival by the usual means of conveyance. Fifty patients were studied and, of the total, 13 patients were in this category—they were either not breathing, had voluminous secretions, cardiac arrest, or were in profound shock; 6 of these patients, including 4 from the accident scenes and 2 from the community hospitals, survived and were discharged."

This study reported a survival rate of 12% of 50 patients who otherwise would have died according to the authors. The success rate was also greater with patients taken directly from the accident scene than from those transferred secondarily from other hospitals. The Pennsylvania DOT (1972) reported their experience with helicopter emergency care systems and concluded that 2 of 47 severely injured patients are saved by such a system. Since 1972, the US DOT has officially recognized the efficacy of helicopter emergency care systems. A study conducted at Brooke Army Medical Center in 1973 (Moylan and Pruitt, 1973) concluded:

"Increasing use of aeromedical transportation will improve the delivery of coordinated medical care to critically ill patients and permit maximum utilization of special medical units."

McCombs (1978) outlined the role of the flight nurse; Mayer (1978) summarized some of the safety factors of helicopter landing and takeoff; Drury (1978) and Johnson (1975) reported general overviews to the process and implementation of helicopter evacuation; Felix (1976) reported on seven metropolitan aeromedical services and noted that such a patient care service was both economically feasible and improved emergency health care delivery; Burke (1978) presented a systems analysis of aeromedical evacuation; and Oxer (1977) outlined some of the medical considerations of the air-evacuated patient with respect to the different types of craft. Johnson (1977) reported on aeromedical disease, gastrointestinal disease, eye injuries, orthopaedic injuries, urologic injuries, and pregnancy. Arp (1969) was the first to report the extension of helicopter emergency care to the neonate, and his study has been followed by a number of recent reports confirming his findings. Reddick (1978) extended the concept of helicopter emergency care to the treatment of patients with decompression sickness.

One of the most successful helicopter emergency care systems in the nation is an integral part of the University of Maryland Trauma Center, and has been functioning now for 10 years. A recent study from this system reports experience with 1056 severely injured patients to the Trauma Center (Cowley, 1973).

Boston Experience

Massachusetts passed in 1973 an Ambulance Law (MGL 111C) which outlines the specific training and certification requirements for ambulance attendants as well as very specific vehicular standards and equipment requirements for five classes of ambulances. The Ambulance Regulation Program of the State Department of Public Health is responsible for administering this law by inspecting and licensing all ambulance services in the State of Massachusetts.

The Boston DHH owns and operates the EMS transport system for the city. The permanent population of Boston is approximately 600,000 and is estimated to increase to 1,200,000 during the day with the influx of students and working persons. Ambulance transportation is designed in a two-tiered response pattern. The city has 10 BLS ambulances and 3 ALS ambulances. DHH ambulance service is responsible for all emergency transportation through the 911 central access number. Private ambulance companies in the city transport patients from hospital to hospital and other scheduled non-urgent transports. A number of private companies provide back-up to the DHH service during peak times. While functioning as an emergency ambulance, the private companies must comply with departmental policy and follow DHH regulations regarding congruency with the point-of-entry plan for patient delivery. All communications are managed by the DHH Communications Division which ensures a uniform controlled operating system. The DHH ambulance service does not compete for any hospital to hospital, or hospital to nursing home transports. Because of this arrangement, there is a cooperative coordinated working system between private and municipal ambulance services.

Boston Ambulance Deployment

Traditionally, and dating back to 1890 when horse-drawn ambulances were stationed at the BCH, all municipal ambulances were centrally located at the BCH. In 1975, the city of Boston made the decision to decentralize the ambulance service and located emergency vehicles at strategic locations throughout the city. These locations include hospitals, police stations, fire stations, and neighborhood health centers. Each location has a dedicated telephone line to the ambulance operations center in crew quarters. In 1977, the decision was made to develop a scientific method for ambulance deployment. Larson of the Massachusetts Institute of Technology (Larson and Brandeau, 1978) developed a Hypercube Queueing Model to aid the Department in placing its vehicles in a computer-determined location to minimize response time and equalize work loads on each unit, thereby preventing skill decay. The city of Boston has 147 census tracts which are not only the basis for geographic location of ambulances, but allow the EMS planners to make use of all the medical and socioeconomic data available from the US Bureau of Census. These census tracts form the matrix for the ambulance location model.

The Hypercube program allows the user to determine the system configuration which is optimal for the particular system. The objectives selected were: (1) a response time of 4–6 minutes, (2) relative equality of work among the units.

The Hypercube Model is a computer program that inputs historical ambulance data. This data includes: the number and time of the call, travel time to the scene, average ambulance speed maintained, time spent on scene, travel time to the hospital, time spent at the hospital, and the time taken to return to the satellite. The EMS provider then locates a given number of ambulances at strategic locations throughout the city, and the program indicates the predicted response time and percentage of work each ambulance will perform. One problem which has to be overcome in using a simulated computer model of a city is that there are a number of barriers to travel. For example, in Boston there are reservations, parks, cemeteries, rivers, the Boston Harbor, and an area around the expressway where there are no streets. A special barriers program was developed to compensate for these geographical areas. Thus, if the call was such that an ambulance had to travel around one of these locations the computer automatically recalculates response time taking into consideration additional time to negotiate the barrier.

Figure 36.14 shows the number of ambulances that the Hypercube Model projected would be needed to achieve a given response time depending on a call level of 51,418 per year. Figure 36.15 shows the actual response time for DHH ambulances in the city of Boston and Figure 36.16 depicts the actual location of ambulances throughout the city. The economic implications of this type of planning became apparent in that by geographically relocating ambulances, better response times can be achieved which is reflected in a need for fewer vehicles. In Boston, personnel and equipment needed to operate one ambulance 24 hours/day, 365 days/year, costs approximately $175,000/year.

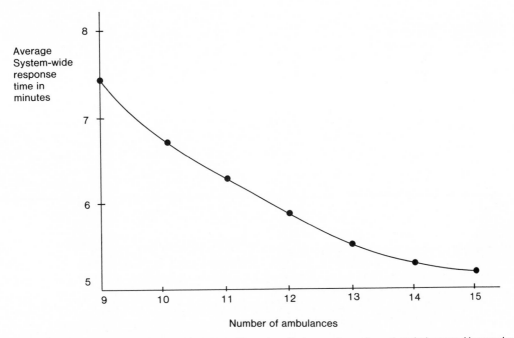

Figure 36.14. Average system-wide response times in minutes and number of ambulances: Hypercube queuing model based on 51,418 calls/year.

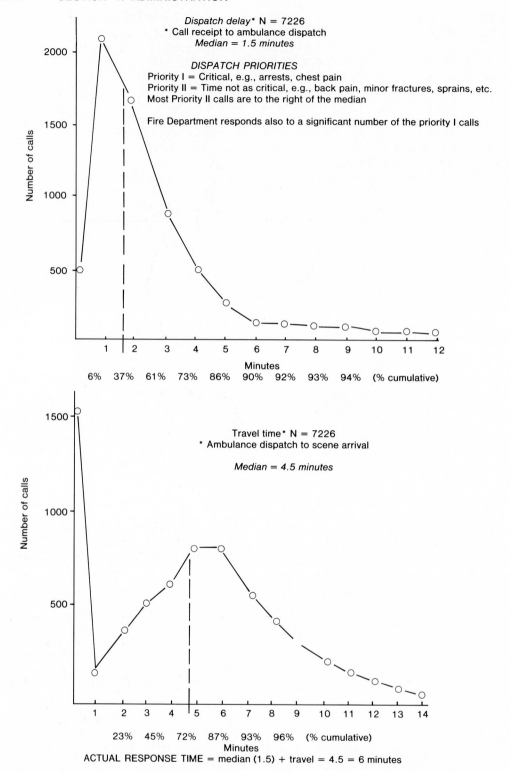

Figure 36.15. Response time for DHH ambulances, dispatch delay and travel time = response time.

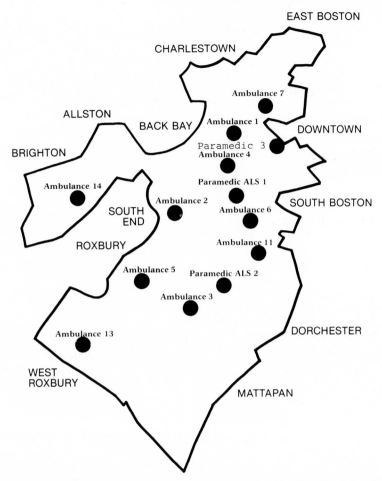

Figure 36.16. Deployment map of City of Boston, Department of Health & Hospital ambulances.

EVALUATION

The traditional placement of evaluation at the end of most discussions regarding EMS should in no way reflect its lack of importance. Throughout the discussion of the other EMS components there has been reference to a number of evaluative and investigative studies. EMS in this decade of its renaissance is now primed for concentrated evaluation and research.

A significant amount of evaluation being performed in EMS systems is related to compliance set forth by federal guidelines (Mayer, 1981; Committee on EMS, 1978). For example, federal guidelines suggest for funding purposes that the request include a chart for manpower that includes the total projected need, the current numbers of persons working, and the percent of the actual manpower need that has been met for all members of the EMS personnel team (DHEW, 1975). This type of evaluation must also reflect the geographic

elements that would contribute to a projected outcome that may differ from other systems.

The National Academy of Science has summarized the evaluation/research necessities (Committee on EMS, 1978):

Standards for Quality Assessment and Assurance:

(a) The NAS cautions EMS evaluators to evaluate performance based on explicit less vague standards than those that express such nebulous adjectives as "appropriate." The standards should be specific and able to be measured in concrete terms.

(b) An additional recommendation is that all standards be agreed upon by experts in the area and should not be the standards of an individual. The standards should also be decided as part of a total research/evaluation design.

(c) The standards that are agreed upon should significantly relate to patient outcomes.

(d) Various evaluation standards may need to be defined that represent evaluation of the entire EMS system. A diversity in standards development is necessary to measure each unique component or individual element.

(e) The definition of standards serves two purposes: to measure the degree of change that has resulted from various modifications or innovations that have been implemented, and to generate a needs assessment plan.

(f) The standards that are developed should pertain to those variables in the system that if needed can effect a change within the system.

(g) A suggestion is made that the evaluation of the EMS system be a plan that is agreed upon by all members of the team, including providers, consumers, and public officials.

(h) An evaluation plan should not only measure the system's compliance with achieved needs, but also with unmet needs.

Research Designs for Evaluation:

The research plan should be so constructed that it evaluates individual system elements as well as the entire system as a whole. Such evaluation methodologies may include: the use of control groups, multivariate analyses, logistic models for hypotheses testing.

Routine Data Collection Systems

NAS suggests that the data that is collected from routine system's operations be accurate, comprehensive, analytically significant, and collected in a way that is not burdensome. A uniform reporting system that correlates prehospital and hospital-generated data is suggested.

Organizational Entity for EMS Quality Assessment and Assurance

The NAC-NRS Committee on EMS agrees that the responsibility for quality assessment and assurance rests with the overall EMS entity as well as the individual facilities that provide actual service. The importance of conducting evaluative research is to effect change if the conclusions of the research so indicate. Therefore, the coordination of the research with those who are able to effect such change is essential to the evaluation process.

There are many individual EMS elements as well as components and subsystems that can be evaluated as part of a comprehensive EMS system. Cost effectiveness, impact on survival, and usefulness to the public health are key issues that require definitive analysis. Massachusetts, as other states, is now facing the impact of reduced federal support for EMS programs. As a federal cut for public health services results in $3.1 million being reduced to $2 million, EMS along with other programs such as high blood pressure detection, are being reduced (Boston Globe, 1982).

Such impacts as the prevention of mortality and morbidity from the mandatory Massachusetts re-

quirement that all children under 5 years of age who are traveling in a motor vehicle be wearing a seat belt or otherwise secured and fastened into a child passenger restraint device will need to be measured. The last two decades of EMS systems development and implementation will have to lead to systematic and comprehensive evaluation that will answer the routinely asked questions, "how much does it cost, does the public need it, and what impact does it have on the system as a whole?"

Suggested Readings

Introduction to Emergency Medical Services

American Heart Association: Standards of cardiopulmonary resuscitation (CPR) and emergency cardiac care (ECC). *JAMA 244*:453–509, 1981

Boyd D: *The Conceptual Development of Emergency Medical Services (EMS) Systems in the United States.* Emergency Medical Services 11(1): 1923; 11(2): 26–35, 1982

Department of Health, Education and Welfare: *Emergency Medical Services Program Guidelines*, Public Health Service, Health Services Administration, Bureau of Medical Services, Division of Emergency Medical Services, DHEW Publication HSA 75-2013, February, 1975

Department of Health, Education and Welfare: *Vital Statistics of the United States.* National Center for Health Statistics, Public Health Service Health Resources Administration, pp. 441–443, 1973

Department of Health and Human Services: *Profile of EMS Systems Development by State and Designated EMS Region for DHHS, PHS, DHSD: Region 1.* August 19, 1981

Heaton LD: Army Medical Service activities in Viet Nam. *Milit Med 131*:646–654, 1966

Rovar EB (Ed): *Major Health Problems in Massachusetts: A Handbook for Statewide and Local Policy Makers.* Boston, Public Health Association, 1980

National Academy of Sciences-National Research Council: *Accidental Death and Disability: The Neglected Disease of Modern Society.* Division of Medical Sciences, Washington, DC, 1966

National Safety Council, *Accident Facts.* Chicago, 1978

Nixon RM: *Veto Message on Emergency Medical Services Systems Development Act S-920-7,* Washington, DC, August 2, 1973

Public Law 89-564: *Highway Safety Act of 1966.* Law of the 89th Congress, Washington, DC, 1966

Public Law 93-154: *Emergency Medical Services System Act of 1973.* Law of the 93rd Congress, Washington, DC, 1973

Public Law 94-573: *Emergency Medical Services Amendments of 1976.* Law of the 94th Congress, Washington, DC, 1976

Public Law 96-142: *Emergency Medical Services Amendments of 1979.* Law of the 96th Congress, Washington, DC, 1979

Robert Wood Johnson Foundation: *A Review of Emergency Medical Services and Recommended Foundation Initiative.* 1979

Sadler A, Sadler B, Webb S: *Emergency Medical Care: The Neglected Public Service.* Cambridge, Ballinger Publishing Co., 1977.

US House of Representatives: Hearings of the Subcommittee

on Public Health and the Environment, Committee on Interstate and Foreign Commerce, Washington, DC, June 13–15, 1972

Manpower and Training

American Board of Emergency Medicine: Personal contact, January, 1982

American College of Emergency Physicians: Emergency medicine receives specialty recognition. *JACEP 8*:96–97, 1979

American College of Surgeons: *Advanced Trauma Life Support Course*. Committee on Trauma, Instruction Manual, 1981

American College of Emergency Physicians: Standards of graduate training in emergency medicine. Graduate Undergraduate Education Committee. *JACEP 8*:432–433, 1979

American Heart Association: *Standards and guidelines for cardiopulmonary resuscitation (CPR) and emergency cardiac care* (ECC). *JAMA 244*:453–454, 1980

American Hospital Association: *Hospital statistics*. 152 and 196–197, 1979

American Nurses Association: *Standards of emergency nursing practice*. Division of Medical Surgical Nursing Practice and the Emergency Department Nurses Association, Kansas City, Missouri, 1975

Anwar RAH: Trends in residency training: Focus on emergency medicine. *Ann Emerg Med 9*:60–71, 1980

Baum RS, Alvarez H, Cobb LA: Survival after resuscitation from out-of-hospital ventricular fibrillation. *Circulation 50*:1231–1235, 1974

Berdeen TN: One-year experience with tracheo-esophageal airway. *Ann Emerg Med 10*:25–27, 1981

Briggs RS, Brown PM, Crabb ME, et al: The Brighton resuscitation ambulances: A continuing experiment in pre-hospital care by ambulance staff. *Br J Med 2*:1161–1165, 1976

Boyd DR, Maine KD, Flashner B: A symposium on the Illinois Trauma Program. A systems approach to the care of the critically injured. *J Trauma 13*:275–284, 1973

Boyd D, Micik S, Lambrew C, et al: Medical control and accountability of emergency medical services (EMS) systems. *Transac Vehic Technol VT-28*:249–261, 1979

Cayten CG, Staroscik R, Walker K, et al: Impact of pre-hospital cardiac algorithms on ventricular fibrillation survival rates. *Ann Emerg Med 10*:432–436, 1981

Committee on Allied Health: *Emergency Care and Transportation of the Sick and Injured*. Chicago, American Academy of Orthopedic Surgeons, 1971

Crampton RS, Aldrich RF, Gascho JA, et al: Reduction of pre-hospital ambulance and community coronary death rates by the community-wide emergency medical care system. *Am J Med 58*:151–165, 1975

Copley DP, Mantle JA, Rogers J, et al: Improved outcome from pre-hospital cardio-pulmonary collapse with resuscitation by bystanders. *Circulation 56*:901–905, 1977

Department of Transportation: *National Training Course of EMT-P*. Department of Labor, Division of Health, Education, and Welfare, Washington, DC.

Eisenberg M, Bergner L, Hallstrom A: Paramedic programs and out-of-hospital cardiac arrest: Factors associated with successful resuscitation. *Am J Public Health 69*:39–42, 1979

Eisenberg MS, Copass MK, Hallstrom A, et al: Management of out-of-hospital cardiac arrests: failure of basic emergency medical technician services. *JAMA 243*:1049–1051, 1980

Eisenberg M, Copass M, Hallstrom A, et al: Treatment of out-of-hospital cardiac arrests with rapid defibrillation by emer-

gency medical technicians. *N Engl J Med 302*:1379–1383, 1980

Grace WJ, Chadbourn JA: The mobile coronary care unit. *Dis Chest 55*:452–455, 1969

Haynes RE, Copass MK, Chinn TL, et al: Randomized comparison of bretylium and lidocaine in resuscitation of patients from out-of-hospital ventricular fibrillation. *Circulation 58*:(suppl 2) 177, 1978

Kaplan BC, Civetta JM, Nagel EL, et al: The military anti-shock trouser in civilian pre-hospital emergency care. *J Trauma 13*:843–848, 1973

Koch-Weser J: Drug therapy: Bretylium. *N Engl J Med 300*:473–477, 1979

Lambrew C: The paramedic: The problem of defining a role. *J Emerg Nurs 1*:15–16, 1975

Lauterbach SA, Spadafora M, Levy R: Evaluation of cardiac arrest managed by paramedics. *JACEP 7*:355–357, 1978

Liberthsen RR, Nagel EL, Hirschman JC, et al: Pre-hospital ventricular defibrillation. Prognosis and follow-up course. *N Engl J Med 291*:317–321, 1974

Massachusetts Department of Public Health: *Proposed Regulations for the Training of Certain Police Officers, Fire Fighters, and Lifeguards, known as First Responders, in First Aid, Including Cardiopulmonary Resuscitation*, 1978

Massachusetts General Law 111C: An Act to Insure High Quality Emergency Medical Care Through Regulation of Ambulances and Ambulance Services, 1973

McSwain NE: Pneumatic trousers and the management of shock. *J. Trauma 2*:719–724, 1977

National Academy of Sciences-National Research Council: Cardiopulmonary Resuscitation: Statement by the Ad Hoc Committee on Cardiopulmonary Resuscitation of the Division of Medical Sciences. *JAMA 198*:372–379, 1966

National Research Council-National Academy of Sciences: Committee on Emergency Medical Services, Assembly of Life Sciences: Emergency Medical Services at Midpassage, 1978

National Registry of EMTs: *EMT-Paramedic sites in the USA & territories*. 1981

Office of Emergency Medical Services: Grant Application, March, 1981. Massachusetts Department of Public Health, Chapter 1, Overview, p. III-A: 26.

Office of Emergency Medical Services: *Massachusetts Emergency Medical Transport Services. Initial Data—1973 Ambulance Service Survey*. Massachusetts Department of Public Health, 1974

Office of Emergency Medical Services: *Notice Concerning the Massachusetts First Responder Law*. Massachusetts Department of Public Health, 1976

Page J: *Paramedics: An Illustrated History of Paramedics in Their First Decade in the USA*. NJ, Backdraft Publications, 1979

Pantridge JF: The effect of early therapy on the hospital mortality from acute myocardial infarction. *Quart J Med 39*:621–622, 1970

Registry. The Newsletter of the National Registry of EMTs, vol 13, no. 2. July, 1981

Rockswold G, Sharma B, Ruiz E, et al: Follow-up of 514 consecutive patients with cardiopulmonary arrest outside the hospital. *JACEP 8*:216–220, 1979

Romano T, Cayten CG, Eisenberg BA, et al: A nationwide paramedic clearinghouse. *Emerg Med Serv 6*:41–42, 1977

Romano T, Eisenberg S, Fernandez-Caballero C, et al: Paramedic services: Nationwide distribution and management structure. *JACEP 7*:99–102, 1978

Scribner R, Raithaus L, Ivanov P: Emergency Medical Service in the Soviet Union. *J Trauma 14*:447–452, 1974

Szczygiel M, Wright R, Wagner E, et al: Prognostic indicators of ultimate long-term survival following advanced life support. *Ann Emerg Med 10*:566–570, 1981

Access to Care

Committee on Medical Services: The Emergency Department: a Regional Medical Resource. Assembly of Life Sciences, National Academy Press. Washington, DC 1980
Department of Transportation: Model Legislation for Emergency Medical Services. National Highway Traffic Safety Administration, Washington, DC, DOT-HS 803–238, 1978

Consumer Participation

Massachusetts General Law 111C, Chapter 948, Section 7, 1973
Massachusetts General Law 111C, Chapter 948, Section 8, 1973

Communications

Dayharsh TI, Yung TJ, Hunter DK, et al: Update on the national emergency number 911. *Transac Vehic Technol VT-28*:292–97, 1979
Executive Office of the President of Telecommunications Policy: The emergency telephone number: A handbook for community planning. Washington, DC, 2205–0003, 1973
Kulp, R: Radio system design considerations affecting medical control and EMS resource coordination. *Emerg Med Serv Quart 1*:No. 2, 1982
McCorkle J, Nagel E, Penterman D, et al: *Basic Telecommunications for Emergency Medical Services*. Cambridge, Ballinger Publishing Co., 1978

Record Keeping

Champion H, Sacco W, Hannan DS, et al: Assessment of injury severity: The Triage Index. *Crit Care Med 8*:201–208, 1980
Department of Health, Education and Welfare: *EMS Handbook for Patient Record Keeping and List of Minimum Data*. Public Health Services Administration, Bureau of Medical Services, Division of Emergency Medical Services. DHEW Publ. No. HSA-77-2034, 1977
Department of Health & Hospitals: *Statistical Report for 1980*. Division of Emergency Medical Services, Advanced Life Support Transports, 1980
Jacobs L, Luise J, Eisenscher J: Congruency in physician-EMT assessment. *Ann Emerg Med 10*:205–208, 1981

Disaster Linkages

Gann DS, Nagel EL, Stafford JD, et al: Mass casualty management. In: *The management of trauma*. Zuidema GD, Rutherford RB, Ballinger WF II (Eds). Chapter 27, 3rd ed., Philadelphia, Saunders Co., 1979
Jacobs L, Ramp J, Breay J: An emergency medical system approach to disaster planning. *J Trauma 19*:157–162, 1979
Jenkins AL, Disaster planning. In: *Emergency Department Organization and Management*, Chapter 15, St. Louis, The Mosby Co., pp. 243–261, 1978
Miller R, Cantrell J: *Textbook of Basic Emergency Medicine*, St. Louis, Mosby Co., 1975
Nissan S, Elder R: Organization of surgical care of mass casualties. *J Trauma 11*:974–978, 1971

Richter L, Berk H, Larkham N, et al: A systems approach to the management of radiation accidents. *Ann Emerg Med 9*:303–309, 1980

Facilities and Critical Care Units

American Burn Association: *Specific Optimal Criteria for Hospital Resources for Care of Patients with Burn Injury*. April, 1976
American College of Surgeons: Committee on Trauma, Appendix A to hospital resources development. Bulletin *65(2): 28–33*, 1980
American College of Surgeons: Committee on Trauma, Hospital resources for optimal care of the injured patient. Bulletin *64(8)*:43–48, 1979
American College of Surgeons: *Verification Program for Hospitals*. 65(10):23–27, 1980
American Medical Association: *Provisional Guidelines for the Optimal Categorization of Hospital Emergency Capabilities*. Commission on Emergency Medical Services, 1981
Baker SP, O'Neil B, Haddon W, et al: The injury severity score: A method for describing patients with multiple injuries and evaluating emergency care. *J Trauma 14*:187–196, 1974
Boyd D: Efforts to improve emergency medical services. The Illinois experience. *JACEP 6*:209–220, 1977
Boyd D: Emergency medical services systems development: A national initiative. *Transac Vehic Technol VT-25*:No. 4, 1976
Boyd D: Trauma—A controllable disease in the 1980s. *J Trauma 20*:14–23, 1980
Boyd D, Pizzano W, Murchie P: Categorizing hospital capabilities. *Emerg Med Serv 4*:24–29, 1975
Collins J: Categorization of emergency capabilities. *Hosp JAHA 47*:69–72, 1973
Committee on Emergency Medical Services: Assembly of Life Sciences, *The Emergency Department: A Regional Medical Resource*, Washington, DC, National Academy Press, 1980
Committee on Emergency Medical Services: Medical Control in Emergency Medical Services Systems. Subcommittee on Medical Control, Assembly of Life Sciences, National Research Council, Washington, DC, National Academy Press, 1981
Cowley RA, Hudson F, Scanlan E, et al: An economical and proved helicopter program for transporting the emergency critically ill and injured patient in Maryland. *J Trauma 13*:1029–1038, 1973
Edlich RF, Larkham N, O'Hanlan JT, et al: Modification of the American Burn Association injury severity scoring system. *JACEP 7*:226–228, 1978
Edlich RF, Rodeheaver GT, Halfacre SE, et al: Systems conceptualization of burn care on a regional basis: *Topics in Emergency Medicine 3(3)*:7–15, 1981
Foley RW, Harris LS, Pilcher DB: Abdominal injuries in automobile accidents: A review of cases of fatally injured patients. *J Trauma 8*:611–615, 1977
Hoffer E: Massachusetts Department of Public Health: Emergency medical services, 1979. *New Engl J Med 301*:1118–1121, 1979
Lovejoy FH, Caplan DL, Rowland T, et al: A statewide plan for care of the poisoned patient: The Massachusetts poison control system. *N Engl J Med 300*:363–365, 1979
Luft HS, Bunker JP, Enthoven AC: Should operations be regionalized? *N Engl J Med 301*:1364–1369, 1979
Massachusetts Poison Control System Annual Report, July 1, 1980–June 30, 1981. Boston, MA, 1981
Mather HG, Morgan DC, Pearson NC, et al: Myocardial infarc-

tion: A comparison between home and hospital care for patients. *Br J Med 1:*925–928, 1976

Micik S: Developing Regional Poison Systems, Technical Manual Prepared for DHEW, 232–78–0173, 1979a

Micik S: Emergency Medical Service Systems and Poison Control, *Topics in Emergency Medicine: Poisonings and Overdose. 1(3):*129–137, 1979

Micik S: Medical control of EMS poison systems. In: *Medical Control in Emergency Medical Services Systems,* Subcommittee on Medical Control, Committee on EMS, Assembly of Life Sciences, National Research Council. Washington, DC, National Academy Press, 1981

Otten J: Impact of regionalization of trauma care in region 1B Illinois (1972–1976). Presented at DHEW National EMS Evaluation Symposium, New Orleans, January, 1976

Page J: Legal issues in medical control. In: *Medical Control in Emergency Medical Services Systems,* Committee on Emergency Medical Services, Subcommittee on Medical Control, Assembly of Life Sciences, National Research Council, Washington, DC, National Academy Press, 1981

Pozen MW, D'Agostino RP, Sytkowski PA, et al: Effectiveness of a pre-hospital medical control system—an analysis of the emergency room physician and paramedic intervention. *Circulation 63:*442–447, 1981

Public Act 76–1858: *Categorization Law.* State of Illinois.

Rimel, R, Rimel J, Rimel J, et al: An injury severity scale for comprehensive management of central nervous system trauma. *JACEP 8:*64–67, 1979

Rumack BH: Regionalization of poison centers—A rational role model. *Clin Toxicol 12:*367–375, 1978

Sacco W, Champion H, Carnazzo A: Trauma score. *Current Concepts in Trauma Care. 4(1):*9–11, 1981

Tell R: Categorization: A community based approach. *JACEP 4:*152–155, 1975

Tobiasen JM, Hiebert JM, Sacco WJ, et al: Burn injury severity scoring systems. *Current Concepts in Trauma Care, 4(1):*5–8, 1981

West JG, Trunkey DD, Lim RL: Systems of trauma care—Study of two counties. *Arch Surg 114:*455–460, 1979

Public Information and Education

American Heart Association: *Heart Facts 1981.* Dallas, American Heart Association, 1981

Baker SP, Fisher RS: Alcohol and motorcycle fatalities. *AJPH 67:*246–249, 1977

Briggs RS, Brown PM, Crabb ME, et al: The Brighton resuscitation ambulances: A continuing experiment in pre-hospital care by ambulance staff. *Br Med J* [Pract Obs], 1161–1165, 1976

Department of Health, Education and Welfare: National Center for Health Statistics: Weight at Birth and Survival of the Newborn by Age of Mother and Total Birth Order. DHEW Vital and Health Statistics, No. 51, Series 21. HSM 72–1055, Washington, DC 1972a

Department of Health, Education and Welfare: National Center for Health Statistics: A Study of Infant Mortality from Linked Records, By Birthweight, Period of Gestation and Other Variables. Vital and Health Statistics, No. 12, Series 20. HSM 72–1055, Washington, DC, 1972b

Department of Health, Education and Welfare: National Center for Health Statistics: A Study of Infant Mortality from Linked Records, Comparison of Neonatal Mortality from Two Cohort Studies. Vital and Health Statistics, No. 13, Series 20. HSM 72–1056, Washington, DC 1972c

Dott AB, Fort AT: The effect of maternal demographic factors in infant mortality rates. Summary of the Louisiana infant mortality study. *Am J Obstet Gynecol 123:*847–753, 1975

Eisenberg MS, Bergner L, Hearne T: Out-of-hospital cardiac arrest: A review of major studies and a proposed uniform reporting system. *AJPH 70:*236–240, 1980d

Eliastam M, Duralde T, Martinez F, et al: Cardiac arrest in the emergency medical service system: Guidelines for resuscitation. *JACEP 6:*525–529, 1977

Erhardt CL, Joshi GB, Nelson FG, et al: Influence of weight and gestation on perinatal and neonatal mortality by ethnic group. *Am J Public Health 54:*1841–1855,1964

Gallup Poll: *CPR Lifesaving Techniques.* Princeton, New Jersey, 1977

Guzy PM, Pearce ML, Greenfield S, et al: Citizen cardiopulmonary resuscitation during out-of-hospital emergency in metropolitan Los Angeles. *Clin Res 27(1):*79–80, 1979

Haberman PW, Baden MM: *Alcohol, Other Drugs, and Violent Death,* New York, Oxford University Press, 1978

Kitchen WH, Ryan MM, Richards A, et al: A longitudinal study of very low-birthweight infants. I. Study design and mortality rates. *Devel Med Child Neurol 20:*605–618, 1978

Lacefield DJ, Roberts PA, Blossom SW: Toxicological findings in fatal civilian aviation accidents, fiscal years 1968–1975. *Aviat Space Environ Med 46:*1030–1033, 1975

Lee KS, Paneth N, Gartner LM, et al: Neo-natal mortality: An analysis of the recent improvement in the United States, *AJPH 70:*15–21, 1980

Lubechenko LO, Searls DT, Brazie JV: Neonatal mortality rate: Relationship to birthweight and gestation age. *J Pediatr 81:*814–822, 1972

McElroy CR: Citizen CPR: The role of the lay person in pre-hospital care. *Topics in Emerg Med 2(4):*37–45, 1980

Schlesinger ER: Neonatal intensive care: planning for services and outcomes following care. *J Pediatrics 82:*916–929, 1973

Stanley FG, Alberman ED: Infants of very low birthweight. I. Perinatal factors affecting survival. *Devel Med Child Neurol 20:*300–312, 1978

Thompson RG, Hallstrom AP, Cobb LA: Bystander initiated cardiopulmonary resuscitation in the management of ventricular fibrillation. *Ann Intern Med 90:*737–740, 1970

Watson GS, Zador PL, Wilks A: The repeal of helmet use laws and increased motorcyclist mortality in the U.S., 1975–1978. *Am J Public Health 70:*579–585, 1980

Zuska J: Wounds Without a Cause. Bulletin of the American College of Surgeons, Trauma Without a Cause. *66(10):*5–10, 1981

Transportation

American College of Surgeons: Committee on Trauma, *Essential equipment for ambulances. 66(6):*17–21 1981

Arp LS: An emergency air ground transport system for newborn infants with respiratory distress syndrome. *PA Med 72:*74–76, 1969

Burke JB: Systems analysis of an aeromedical evacuation mission. *Aviat Space Environ Med 49:*637–640, 1978

Copass M: The Urban Experience in Medical Control: Medical Control in Seattle. Medical Control in Emergency Medical Services, Subcommittee on Medical Control, Committee on EMS, Assembly on Life Sciences, National Research Council, National Academy Press, Washington, DC, 1981

Department of Transportation: Air Ambulance Guidelines DOT HS 805–703, February, 1981

Department of Transportation: State of Pennsylvania, 1972

Drury LR: Evacuation and care of the trauma patient. *Heart Lung 7:*249–253, 1978

Federal Specification—Ambulance—Emergency Medical Care Vehicle. USGSA Jan. 2, 1974. KKK-A-1822

Felix WR: Metropolitan aeromedical service: State of the art. *J Trauma 16*:873–881, 1976

Foster J: Helicopters make sense in medical care. *Modern Hospital 112*:79–82, 1969

Frey CF, Huelke DF, Gikas PW: Resuscitation and survival of motor vehicle accidents. *J Trauma 9*:292–310, 1969

George JE (Ed): Emergency Medical Technician Bulletin. 6:1, Winter, 1982

Johnson A: Treatise on aeromedical evacuation: I. Administration and some medical considerations. *Aviat Space Environ Med 48*:456–549, 1977

Larson R, Brandeau M: Implementing the hypercube queueing model to plan ambulance districts in Boston. Cambridge, MA, 1978

Mayer G: Helicopter safety during emergency rescue. *J Emerg Med* 11, 1978

McCombs CM: An ambulance service: New horizons for emergency nursing. *J Emerg Med* 21, 1978

Moylan JA, Pruitt BA: Aeromedical transportation. *JAMA 224*:1271–1273, 1973

Oxer HF: Carriage by air of the seriously ill. *Med J Aust 1*:537–540, 1977

Reddick EJ: Movement by helicopter of patients with decompression sickness. *Aviat Space Environ Med 49*:1229–1230, 1978

Roberts S, Bailey C, Vandermade JR, et al: Medicopter: An airborne intensive care unit. *Ann Surg 172*:325–333, 1970

Turner HS, Ellington HV: Use of the helicopter as an emergency vehicle in the civilian environment: Results of a survey-questionnaire. *Aerospace Med 41*:135–138, 1970

Evaluation

Boston Globe, January 18, 1982

Commonwealth of Massachusetts. An Act Requiring the Use of Child Passenger Restraints in Certain Motor Vehicles, 1981

Mayer J: A Method for the geographical evaluation of EMS performance. *Am J Public Health 71*:841–843, 1981

CHAPTER 37

Emergency Ward Triage

M. B. MAUGHAN, R.N.
PETER L. GROSS, M.D.
SUSAN SCHMIEDEL FOX, R.N.

Editor's note: This chapter and the next emphasize the role of the nurse in the Emergency Ward. This role has been redefined and highlighted in the evolution of emergency medical services systems. The nurse's participation in the Boston EMSS was described in Chapter 36. In the teaching hospital mode where primary medical coverage is provided by rotating residents, the stability resulting from full-time nursing participation is essential.

Some of the most crucial decisions affecting emergency patient care are often made within the first moments of admission, and each emergency department should have a system for expeditiously evaluating patients as to need and best place for treatment. At the Massachusetts General Hospital, a triage system staffed by registered nurses performs this initial screening, the role having been transferred from physicians to nurses in the course of several years, coincident with increases in the total number of emergency ward patients. The term triage derives from the French *trier* (to sort out) and referred originally to the disposition of the injured in disasters and military situations. In the emergency ward, the triage nurse evaluates the nature and seriousness of each patient's complaint and effects a disposition for care based on this assessment. A senior resident physician is ultimately responsible for triage decisions, but being relieved of full-time triage responsibility, he can use his skills in teaching, supervision, and direct patient care.

ROLE OF THE TRIAGE NURSE

The role of the triage nurse encompasses more than directing patient traffic; as the first health professional to interview patients, the triage nurse also informs the patient about emergency ward procedures. There is an essential public relations aspect to this role; setting the proper tone and establishing rapport may greatly improve hospital-patient relations and allay patients' anxiety. In addition to utilizing crisis-intervention skills, the triage nurse may start treatment of minor injuries, such as application of splints or ice packs, or may begin the diagnostic workup by ordering pertinent laboratory or radiologic studies. The triage nurse also serves as liaison between the administration, specialty services, families, clinics, and community organizations. In a system in which the medical staff is composed primarily of residents on rotational assignment, continuity provided by nurse triage is unusually valuable.

Each hospital must tailor its triage system to its needs. The system must be responsive to such variables as physical layout, patient volume, physician coverage, and the availability of ancillary services such as walk-in medical and specialty clinics. In larger emergency departments, the triage system has an increased number of patient care options available to the triage nurse.

At the Massachusetts General Hospital, approximately 250 patients arrive at the emergency ward each day. During the hours of highest patient census (7 a.m. to 11 p.m.), two nurses are assigned to triage and a nursing assistant is available for recording vital signs and assisting the triage nurse or resident physician with patient examinations. In addition, for 10 hours each day, a registered nurse certified by the American Nurses Association as a nurse practitioner works under the supervision of the resident physician in the care of patients with minor illness.

During peak arrival time—10 a.m. to 3 p.m.—the triage nurse has the valuable option of referring nonemergent patients directly to services outside the emergency ward, including a walk-in screening clinic for nonacute, noncritical illness, which provides services from 9 a.m. to 9 p.m. each day, and several specialty clinics, including dermatology, gynecology, and oral surgery. This relieves the patient load in the emergency ward and allows more rapid service for true emergencies.

PATIENT CATEGORIZATION

The triage area is centrally located near the emergency ward entrance and the registration desk. From this vantage point the triage nurse can see both ambulatory and stretcher arrivals. With the primary goal of identifying the critically ill, the triage nurse interviews and may briefly examine all patients except those who are in extremis. It should be emphasized that the goal of triage is not diagnosis but determination of the need for treatment and the best place for a patient to receive it. In assessing patients, the triage nurse must determine the seriousness of illness and therefore the level of urgency: acute, critical (level I); acute, noncritical (level II); and nonacute (level III). The possible assignments that may result are outlined in Table 37.1.

Past experience in emergency ward nursing helps the triage nurse recognize and assess critical illness. Whereas the patient in extremis presents no problem of assessment, other seriously ill patients may not have an obvious need for acute care. If the assignment is difficult, the nurse always chooses the more serious level; it is understood that a certain percentage of patients assigned to level I may be discharged from the emergency ward. Occasional disagreements over assignments are common in any triage system. Assignments should be firm until evaluation is sufficient to indicate the need for transfer or discharge unless a patient's condition is rapidly deteriorating. Changes in triage decisions are made only between the responsible physicians. Although feedback is important in the triage nurse's continuing education, disagreement over triage assignments hinders the efficiency of patient evaluation and treatment. Triage decisions are best discussed at staff review meetings.

Level I includes seriously ill patients, such as those with major trauma, myocardial infarction or cardiac arrest, burns, shock, ingestion of poison, stroke, seizure, or respiratory distress. The disposition in these cases is usually straightforward and requires little or no interview. Patients in critical or potentially critical condition are immediately assigned to a separate section of the emergency

Table 37.1.
Triage assignment by degree and type of illness.

Level I: Acute, critical illness with major service assignment
  Surgery (trauma, burns, vascular disease, abdominal pain, gastrointestinal bleeding)
  Medicine (cardiac arrest, ingestion, respiratory distress, shock, sepsis, coronary disease, coma)
  Orthopaedics (trauma, fracture)
  Pediatrics (respiratory distress, ingestion, trauma)
  Neuromedicine (stroke, seizure)
  Specialty services on call
    Neurosurgery (head trauma, spinal cord injury)
    Psychiatry (acute psychosis, suicide attempt)

Level II: Acute, noncritical illness with minor service assignment
  Direct physician assignment
    Minor medicine (urinary tract infection, upper respiratory tract infection, gastroenteritis, minor gynecologic
      disorder, minor trauma, venereal disease, rash)
    Minor surgery (laceration, abscess, cellulitis, minor trauma)
    Orthopaedics (fracture, back strain, joint problem)
    Pediatrics (minor illness)
    Psychiatry (anxiety state, chronic psychosis, drug abuse)
    Oral surgery (dental problem, facial fracture)
  Triage nurse evaluation before assignment to physician or nurse practitioner
    Laboratory studies
    X-ray films

Level III: Nonacute illness
  Walk-in clinic (chronic complaints)
  Specialty clinics (by appointmentt)

ward. The triage nurse locates a room for the patient and notifies the appropriate house officer personally or by way of an intercom system. A master assignment list and chart markers that are color-coded by service allow the nurse to rapidly determine the patient load, responsible service group, and assigned physician.

Level II patients, who are treated in a separate section of the emergency ward, appear less acutely ill during the initial interview. An important aspect in evaluating their condition is continued surveillance for critical problems that are not immediately apparent.

The triage nurse may perform a brief physical examination specific to the presenting complaint, including vital signs (orthostatic, neurologic, and measurement of paradox when indicated), observation, palpation, percussion, and auscultation. The order and extent of examination depends on the type and severity of the patient's problem. Assimilating this material, the triage nurse makes an initial assessment and formulates a plan of action to include: (1) initiation of treatment (splints, ice pack, and so on), (2) further diagnostic data collection (laboratory studies, x-ray films), (3) patient education, and (4) disposition.

The triage nurse may choose either immediate evaluation by a physician or nurse practitioner or radiologic and laboratory studies before referral to one of these staff. If the patient's complaints are dysuria and frequency, for example, the triage nurse may order a urinalysis and urinary culture while awaiting physician evaluation. In the febrile patient, a complaint of abdominal pain requires determination of vital signs, a complete blood cell count, and perhaps urinalysis. By the time the physician's or nurse practitioner's examination is complete, the laboratory data usually are available to supplement those findings. The triage nurse works near the senior resident physician's desk so that questions about diagnostic studies can be answered.

Many centers allow triage nurses to order radiologic studies. In emergency departments where patients with minor trauma constitute a large part of the noncritical load, traffic flow can be greatly facilitated by directing some patients to the radiology department before they are evaluated by a physician. X-ray studies most commonly involve a contusion of an extremity or the differential diagnosis of a fracture or sprain, but films of the lumbosacral spine and chest x-ray films can be ordered as well. Having taken the history and examined the injury, the triage nurse can easily fill out an x-ray requisition describing the problem

and pinpointing the area in question. Current information from the radiology department as to special views is helpful for the triage nurse, as is the availability of a senior resident physician for consultation.

Many persons use the emergency ward in place of a family physician. Patients with nonacute or noncritical complaints are assigned to level III by the triage nurse. These patients come to the hospital expecting evaluation, and they should be seen, no matter how minor or chronic the complaint. The emergency ward, however, may not be the most appropriate place for treatment; referral of these patients to screening or specialty clinics greatly reduces congestion in the emergency ward, laboratories, and radiology department. At the Massachusetts General Hospital, the Walk-in Clinic is the main portal of entry to the ambulatory care system, treating some patients on a short-term basis and starting evaluation of other patients before referral to a primary care or specialty clinic.

Whereas patients with critical illness require immediate assignment, those with acute but noncritical illness and those with nonacute illness require a more extensive triage evaluation. In these cases, interviewing and history-taking skills are extremely important. The triage nurse must maintain a nonjudgmental, supportive manner while determining the patient's complaint. The triage nurses are oriented to consider the most serious or life-threatening consequence that could possibly evolve from each specific presenting complaint, and to obtain a history accordingly. Brief notes of the interview are transcribed in the record, including the chief complaint, duration of illness, associated symptoms, pertinent past medical history, medications, allergies, and any results of tests that have been ordered from the triage area. Tables 37.2 to 37.6 list some common primary symptoms and provide guidelines for questioning the patient.

ORIENTATION AND CONTINUING EDUCATION

Experience in emergency nursing is essential for those seeking triage positions. At the Massachusetts General Hospital, triage nurse candidates have had 9 months to 1 year of experience in the hospital's emergency ward.

Before orientation, the nurse is given study assignments in anatomy and physiology, physical assessment techniques, the recognition of major disease mechanisms and interpretation of presenting symptoms, and familiarization with the triage manual. The formal orientation program consists of a minimum of 80 hours of didactic and practical

Table 37.2.
Chest complaints: guidelines for screening questions.

Primary Symptom	Characteristics of Primary Symptom	Associated Symptoms	History
Chest pain	Character Duration and frequency Location and radiation Intensity Aggravating factors Alleviating factors	Shortness of breath Sweating Nausea and vomiting Palpitation Fainting Fever and chills Cough and sputum Hemoptysis Calf tenderness Weight loss	Cardiac disease Pulmonary disease Gastrointestinal disease Gallbladder disease Hypertension Diabetes Medications Trauma
Cough	Duration and frequency	Sputum production and character Chest pain Fever and chills Shortness of breath Upper respiratory illness Hoarseness Weight loss Calf tenderness Night sweats Wheezing Hemoptysis	Cardiac disease Pulmonary disease Smoking Medications

Shortness of breath	Duration and frequency
	Limitation of activity
	Aggravating factors
	   Stairs
	   Supine position
		Pain
		Cough and sputum
		Fever and chills
		Leg edema
		Calf tenderness
		Weight changes
		Wheezing
		Tingling of toes and fingers
			Cardiac disease
			Pulmonary disease
			Gastrointestinal disease
			Smoking
			Medications

Palpitation	Duration and frequency
	Previous history
	Character
	   Skipped beat
	   Pounding
		Weakness
		Dizziness
		Fainting
		Chest pain
		Nervousness
		Loss of consciousness
		Seizure
		Shortness of breath
			Cardiac disease
			Hypertension
			Stroke
			Thyroid disease
			Anxiety
			Medications

sessions. The program is closely supervised by the unit teacher. During the orientation period, 2 other nurses are scheduled to perform triage, relieving the trainee of any staffing responsibility. This gives him or her the opportunity to develop history-taking and physical assessment skills without the pressure of providing back-up. As the new triage nurse develops and becomes more comfortable with the role, speed is a natural byproduct. On completion of the formal program, the nurse is assigned with an experienced triage nurse who assumes the role of preceptor. The availability of the nurse practitioner and resident physician for consultation is invaluable during this time of transition.

Continuing education opportunities specifically for the triage nurse include: (1) a tour of the local police, fire, and emergency medical services communication coordinating center with detailed explanation of proper medical control radio operation; (2) observation of emergency medical technicians and paramedics as they treat patients en route to the hospital; and (3) in-hospital specialty clinic observation. These experiences help the triage nurse understand both hospital and community communication and resources.

Other training opportunities within the hospital include workshops on improving communication, interviewing skills, guidelines for common presenting complaints, crisis intervention, how to deal

Table 37.3.
Gastrointestinal complaints: guidelines for screening questions.

Primary Symptom	Characteristics of Primary Symptom	Associated Symptoms	History
Abdominal pain	Character Duration and frequency Location and radiation Intensity Aggravating factors Alleviating factors	Nausea and vomiting Diarrhea Fever and chills Hematemesis or melena Jaundice Weight loss Vaginal discharge Menstrual disorder Dysuria	Gastrointestinal bleeding Gallbladder disease Pelvic, gynecologic disease Cardiac disease Hypertension Diabetes Medications Trauma Previous operation

Nausea and vomiting	Character
	  Blood
	  Bile
	Duration and frequency
	Aggravating factors
	Alleviating factors
		Abdominal pain
		Diarrhea
		Hematemesis or melena
		Jaundice
		Fever and chills
		Trouble swallowing
		Belching
			Gastrointestinal disease
			  Hiatal hernia
			  Ulcer
			  Hemorrhage
			  Diverticulosis
			  Colitis
			Gallbladder disease
			Gastrointestinal operation
			Recent change in diet
			Affected acquaintances with
			  common food source
			Medications

Diarrhea	Character Duration and frequency Aggravating factors Alleviating factors	Abdominal pain Nausea and vomiting Hematemesis or melena Rectal bleeding Fever and chills Weight loss Jaundice	Recent change in diet Affected acquaintances with common food source Colitis Diverticulosis Diabetes Recent travel Medications

with the abusive patient, rape victim counseling, documentation using a modified Weed's Problem-Oriented Medical Record System, and physical assessment skills. They are presented by staff nurses, the psychiatric nurse specialist, the nurse practitioner, and the unit teacher. Medical staff conferences on episodic minor illness are held weekly. Specialists in the fields of medicine, surgery, ophthalmology, otolaryngology, dermatology, gynecology, neurology, radiology, orthopaedics, and oral surgery discuss patient problems, including salient points of history, unique physical findings, pertinent diagnostic studies, the most recent modes of therapy, and patient/family education.

DOCUMENTATION

The triage nurse's interaction is documented in the emergency department record. This documentation is in one of three forms:

(1) **Major emergency**—**Level I medical or surgical emergencies** requiring immediate interven-

tion have only the briefest notation as to the problem. Patient care is the first priority, routine administrative procedures are pared to a minimum, and processing and physician intervention are accelerated (see Case 1 in Appendix 1).

(2) **Referral**—Many patients are referred by staff physicians or from other hospitals. The appropriate resident physician accepts the referral, completes a designated form (Fig. 37.1) and alerts both the triage nurse and the administrative staff of the impending arrival. If the triage nurse finds that the written information accurately reflects the patient's status, "referral" is written on the patient's record and the triage nurse's name is indicated (see case 2 in Appendix 1). If the information is incomplete, the triage nurse should provide further documentation.

(3) **Problem-oriented notation**—The triage nurse may use a modification of the Weed System of Problem-Oriented Medical Notation, the SOAP note (Subjective data, Objective data, Assessment, and Plan). The patient's chief complaint is the problem from which the triage nurse proceeds to

Table 37.4.
Neurologic complaints: guidelines for screening questions.

Primary Symptom	Characteristics of Primary Symptom	Associated Symptoms	History

Dizziness	Duration and frequency
	Quality
	  Vertigo
	  Light-headedness
	Aggravating factors
	Alleviating factors
		Blurred vision
		Diplopia
		Tinnitus
		Motor weakness
		Palpitation
		Chest pain
		Syncope
		Seizure
		Shortness of breath
		Headache
			Central nervous system
			  disease
			Ear problems
			Cardiac disease
			Hypertension
			Medications
			Trauma

Headache	Onset Duration and frequency Intensity Location	Blurred vision Visual field cuts Motor weakness Syncope Seizure Neck muscle spasm Anxiety Sinus congestion	Central nervous system disease Stroke Migraine Hypertension Diabetes Medications Seizure Trauma
Motor weakness	Onset Location Duration	Sensory changes Headache Nausea and vomiting Dizziness Syncope Seizure Visual disturbances	Central nervous system disease Stroke Seizure Migraine Hypertension Trauma
Loss of consciousness	Duration Circumstances	Seizure Dizziness Nausea and vomiting Sweating Palpitation Chest pain Headache Motor weakness Trouble speaking	Head injury Seizure Diabetes Hypertension Cardiac disease Central nervous system disease Medications Trauma

formulate an initial plan with appropriate disposition as the outcome (see Cases 3–11 in Appendix 1). The subjective data may be a sign (left facial drooping, jaundice), a symptom (dizziness, sore throat, abdominal pain), a proved diagnosis (breast cancer with metastasis to the spine, pernicious anemia), or an abnormal finding (hematocrit of 22%, "spot on the lung" on a chest x-ray film). After the triage nurse's initial plan for disposition, a workable data base can be obtained—patient profile, history, physical examination, laboratory findings—from which a complete problem list can be formulated.

PATIENT EDUCATION

The triage nurse is in the ideal position to initiate the patient education process. The most efficient means, considering the time element, is to provide the patient and family with written material specific to the episodic problem. Triage staff have developed a series of pamphlets on wound care, head injury, back pain, and other topics. Appendix 2 includes material on back pain, some of which can be demonstrated to the patient.

Early patient education that is reinforced throughout the patient's emergency ward visit ver-

Table 37.5.
Musculoskeletal complaints: guidelines for screening questions.

Primary Complaint	Characteristics of Primary Complaint	Associated Symptoms	History
Sprain, strain, question of fracture	Area affected Duration Nature of trauma Pain	Sensory changes Weakness Ecchymosis Swelling Range-of-motion limitation	Previous injury to similar area
Low back pain	Character Duration Radiation Nature of trauma Aggravating factors Alleviating factors	Weakness Paresthesias Bowel or bladder problems	Back injury Degenerative joint disease Arthritis Urinary tract problems Vascular disease Medications

Table 37.6.
Minor illness and infection: guidelines for screening questions.

Illness or Infection	Characteristics of Primary Symptom	Associated Symptoms	History
Upper respiratory tract infection	Duration Intensity	Fever Myalgias Sore throat Swollen glands Pleuritic pain Cough and sputum Shortness of breath Malaise Headache	Streptococcal infection
Urinary tract infection	Duration Initial or recurrent episode	Dysuria Frequency Nocturia Urgency Incontinence Retention Flank pain Fever and chills	Past urinary tract infection Pyelonephritis Calculi Diabetes
Venereal disease	Duration	Vaginal or penile discharge Dysuria Rash, skin lesions Penile lesions Sore throat Abdominal pain Arthritis	Exposure to gonorrhea Exposure to syphilis Past infections and treatment

Hepatitis	Duration	Malaise
		Nausea and vomiting
		Fever
		Jaundice
		Dark urine
		Light stools
		Loss of taste for cigarettes
			Exposure
			  Needles
			  Infectious hepatitis
			  Seafood
			  Drugs
			Past hepatitis
			Medications
			Transfusions

MASSACHUSETTS GENERAL HOSPITAL

Admission to: ☐ MGH ☑ BM
_____

Adm. Date   **6/18/82**   Unit No. **949-07-17**
Prev. Adm.: ☐ OPD ☐ X-RAY ☐ MGH ☑ BM ☐ PH

NAME
    JANE HUDSON

ADDRESS
    55 MAIN ST.
    BOSTON, MASS.

PREV. ADDRESS
    76 LIBERTY ST.
    HUBBARD, OHIO

REFERRING DR. *MICHAEL LEAHY*

ADDRESS *M.G.H. (X 3326) please page*
    when patient arrives.

TEL. NO.

ADM. DIAG.
56 y∘ Insulin Dependent Diabetic (42u NPH
    this AM)
c/o L flank pain, dysuria, temp. 103°
c̄ rigor. Urine 4+/kg. Awake,
alert.
Allergic to Penicillin — edema

MGH DR.   *ROBERT WOOD*

ADMIT TO PH
        ⊙BM
        GH

House Officer   *MARLENE SMITH*
taking referral

Figure 37.1.   Emergency ward referral form.

bally, by written material, and by practical example has been shown to decrease the rate of recidivism.

APPENDIX 1

The following examples illustrate the type of chart documentation utilized by triage nurses at the Massachusetts General Hospital. These notations are made during the initial patient interview in less severely ill patients or at the time of patient assignment or referral for those more acutely ill.

Case 1

Unknown white male
Chief complaint (CC): multiple trauma
Surgical emergency
Trauma I

P. McNally, R.N.

Case 2

56-year-old female
CC: left flank pain
Referral

P. McNally, R.N.

Case 3

23-year-old male
CC: Back pain (Workmen's Compensation)
S: Sudden onset sharp, "like lightning", low back pain 1 hour PTA while lifting 75-pound block of ice. Pain greater on ⓡ. Extends down ⓡ post./lat. leg to foot. Denies numbness, tingling, weakness of extremities. Denies bowel, bladder problems. Pain aggravated in sitting position. No previous hx. of same. PMH: ō Meds: ō Allergies: NKA
O: Appears extremely uncomfortable c̄ any movement. Favoring ⓡ side. ō bony vertebral tenderness. Tender ⓡ lumbar paravertebral muscle c̄ 3+/4+ spasm.
A: Low back sprain. Possible disc herniation.
P: L-S spine x-ray. Orthopedics.

P. McNally, R.N.

Case 4

26-year-old female
CC: Abdominal pain
S: Gradual onset of achy periumbilical pain over 8-hour period—now constant in RLQ. ō fever, chills. C/O nausea s̄ vomiting. Anorexic. Loose BM × 2 (lt. bn. s̄ blood). Nl. BM this a.m. ō urinary sx. LMP 25d PTA. On time—light. PMP's on time—WNL. Uses foam for BC—relations regularly. C/O sl. increase in vaginal discharge—lt. yellow, odorless. PMH: Ⓛ ectopic 3 yrs. PTA. Meds: ō Allergies: NKA
O: In NAD, but moving very slowly and deliberately. Flushed. T 99 $\frac{8}{po.}$ Orthostatic vital signs stable.
A: Possible surgical abdomen.
P: Rectal temperature, urinalysis (clean voided) c̄ specs available for C & S and review by physician. Gravindex. CBC c̄ diff. and sed. rate. Extra red top tube. Minor medicine.

P. McNally, R.N.

Case 5

32-year-old female
CC: ⓡ Wrist injury
S: Tripped on carpet edge 2 hours PTA. Attempted to break fall c̄ arm outstretched, wrist

dorsiflexed. C/O ®️ wrist pain. Denies other trauma/pain. PMH: ō Meds: BCP's Allergies: NKA

O: Atraumatic in appearance. Radial pulse intact c̄ brisk capillary filling. Elbow θ, radius, ulna θ to palp. ⊕ Snuffbox tenderness. Hand θ. Sensation intact grossly.

A: Possible fracture.

P: Splint, ice, elevation, ®️ wrist x-ray c̄ navicular views. Hand service.

P. McNally, R.N.

Case 6

51-year-old male

CC: Hematemesis

S: Vomited 1 quart BRB in transit. Hx. of esophageal varices.

O: Pale, anxious. Pulse 130, thready.

A: GI bleed

P: Trauma Room II. Surgery.

P. McNally, R.N.

Case 7

21-year-old female

CC: MVA—neck pain

S: Front-seat passenger (wearing belt and harness) of stationary car struck from behind by another vehicle presents C/O ®️ neck pain. Onset of pain 12 hours p̄ accident. Denies radiation to or numbness, tingling, weakness of extremities. ō previous neck problems. Otherwise well. PHM: ō Meds: ō Allergies: NKA

O: In NAD. Holding head purposefully. Turns whole body to see periphery. ō bony vertebral tenderness, but tender ®️ trapezius c̄ 2+/4+ spasm palpable. Grasps = bilat. ō sensory deficit grossly.

A: Neck strain/sprain.

P: Soft collar. C-spine films. Minor medicine.

P. McNally, R.N.

Case 8

38-year-old male

CC: ®️ Abdominal pain

S: Awakened at 4 a.m. c̄ ®️ flank pain radiating to ®️ testicle. Colicky. C/O nausea s̄ vomiting. Denies diarrhea, constipation. Last BM yest.—nl. Denies dysuria, hematuria, urinary frequency, fever, chills. PMH: HTN, gout, bursitis. Meds: Hydroclorothiazide. Allergies: NKA

O: Pale, unable to assume a comfortable position. Vital signs stable. ®️ CVA tenderness. Urine—clear, yellow, 4+ heme by dipstick.

A: Possible renal calculus.

P: Urinalysis and culture sent. Strain all urine. Minor medicine.

P. McNally, R.N.

Case 9

25-year-old male

CC: Bilat. foot pain

S: Jumped 5 feet off truck bed onto cement. Landed flat on feet. C/O bilat. heel pain. Denies back pain. Denies any other trauma/pain. PMH: ō Meds: Tetracycline (acne) Allergies: NKA

O: Arrived via ambulance on stretcher. Atraumatic in appearance. Calcaneous tender bilat. Knees, ankles, feet otherwise θ. ō spinal tenderness to palpation.

A: Possible fractured calcaneus. Does not appear to have related lumbar involvement.

P: Bilat. calcaneus films. Minor medicine.

P. McNally, R.N.

Case 10

54-year-old male

CC: Chest pain

S: Substernal pressing chest pain c̄ diff. breath × 1½ hours.

O: Ashen, diaphoretic. Pulse irregularly irregular.

A: R/O MI

P: Rm. 7. Major medicine.

P. McNally, R.N.

Case 11

22-year-old female

CC: Ⓛ Ankle injury

S: Came down onto inverted Ⓛ foot from basketball rebound 1 hour PTA. C/O Ⓛ lat. ankle pain. PMH: ō Meds: ō Allergies: Penicillin (rash)

O: Knee θ. 3+/4+ soft-tissue swelling c̄ ecchymosis over Ⓛ lat. malleolus. Dorsalis pedis pulse intact. Tenderness ant. & inf. to Ⓛ lat. malleolus and over 4th and 5th metatarsals.

P: Wheelchair, elevation, ice. Ⓛ ankle and foot films. Orthopedics. Patient teaching regarding allergy. Medic Alert application given.

P. McNally, R.N.

Abbreviations used in Appendix 1 include: CC = chief complaint; PTA = prior to arrival; ®️ = right; post. = posterior; lat. = lateral; hx. = history; PMH = past medical history; ō = no or none; c̄ = with; Meds = medications; NKA = no known allergies; L-S = lumbosacral; RLQ = right lower quadrant; C/O = complains of; s̄ = without; BM = bowel movement; lt. bn. = light

Treatment for Acute Low Back Strain/Sprain

1

COMPLETE BEDREST
ON A FIRM MATTRESS
WITH HEAT TO YOUR LOWER BACK
FOR ___ DAYS.

COMPLETE BEDREST THIS MEANS THAT YOU LEAVE THE BED TO GO TO THE BATHROOM ONLY.

ON A FIRM MATTRESS IF YOU DON'T HAVE A FIRM MATTRESS, ASK A FRIEND (NOT YOU) TO PUT A BEDBOARD, A 1/2 TO 1 INCH THICK PIECE OF PLYWOOD, OR AN OLD DOOR BETWEEN THE MATTRESS AND THE BOX SPRINGS. TO BE MOST EFFECTIVE, THE MATTRESS AND BEDBOARD CHOSEN SHOULD BE THE SAME SIZE.

DO NOT LIE ON THE FLOOR! THE MOVEMENT INVOLVED GETTING DOWN TO THE FLOOR AND GETTING UP FROM THE FLOOR WILL AGGRAVATE YOUR PAIN.

DO NOT USE A WATERBED.. IT DOES NOT SUPPORT YOUR BACK IN PROPER ALIGNMENT.

WITH HEAT TO YOUR LOWER BACK THE MOST CONVENIENT SOURCE OF HEAT IS AN ELECTRIC HEATING PAD SET ON "LOW". NEVER APPLY LINAMENTS WHEN USING A HEATING PAD — THE COMBINATION COULD RESULT IN A BURN.

THE OTHER OPTIONS ARE:

- A HOT WATER BOTTLE WRAPPED IN A TOWEL.

- A HYDROCOLLATOR OR OTHER MOIST HEAT PACK.

- HOT, WET TOWELS (AFTER WETTING THE TOWEL, OPEN IT AND HOLD IT UP UNTIL ALL THE STEAM IS GONE. THEN, WRING IT OUT AND APPLY IT TO YOUR BACK.. IF THERE'S STEAM IN THE TOWEL, IT COULD BURN YOUR SKIN!).

THESE LAST THREE SOURCES OF HEAT ARE INCON- VENIENT. THEY ARE MESSY, COOL QUICKLY, AND INCREASE THE RISK OF BURNS.

2

FOLLOW THESE DIRECTIONS SHOWING
THE PROPER WAY TO GET INTO BED,
POSITIONS OF REST, AND
THE PROPER WAY TO GET OUT OF BED.

THE PROPER WAY TO GET INTO BED

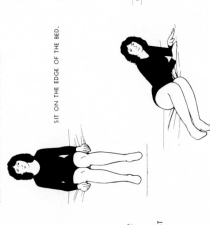

SIT ON THE EDGE OF THE BED.

BEGIN TO LIE ON YOUR SIDE BY FIRST RESTING ON YOUR ELBOW AND SLOWLY RAISING YOUR LEGS. DO NOT TWIST YOUR BACK.

CONTINUE TO LIE DOWN SO THAT YOU END UP ON YOUR SIDE WITH KNEES BENT TOWARD YOUR CHEST (THE "FETAL POSITION").

HOW TO TURN IN BED

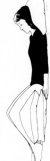

"ROLL LIKE A LOG".. WHEN YOU ROLL OVER, YOUR SHOULDERS, HIPS, AND KNEES SHOULD ALL MOVE AT THE SAME TIME. DO NOT TWIST YOUR BACK.

POSITIONS OF REST

YOUR KNEES MUST BE ALWAYS BE BENT. NEVER LIE ON YOUR STOMACH!

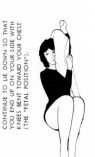

LIE ON YOUR BACK WITH A SMALL PILLOW UNDER YOUR HEAD AND 2–3 PILLOWS UNDER YOUR KNEES.

IF YOU DON'T HAVE PILLOWS, FOLD BLANKETS AND PUT THEM INTO PILLOW CASES.

OR

LIE ON EITHER SIDE WITH YOUR KNEES DRAWN UP (THE "FETAL POSITION"). YOU MAY USE A SMALL PILLOW UNDER YOUR HEAD.

THE PROPER WAY TO GET OUT OF BED

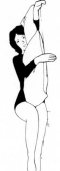

RETURN TO THE "FETAL POSITION"

PUSH YOURSELF UP SLOWLY, KEEPING YOUR LEGS TOGETHER, LOWER THEM OFF THE BED.

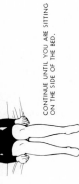

CONTINUE UNTIL YOU ARE SITTING ON THE SIDE OF THE BED.

Treatment for Acute Low Back Strain/Sprain

3

DO NOT TAKE HOT BATHS.

IT IS DIFFICULT TO GET INTO THE TUB WHEN YOU HAVE BACK PAIN.

IN ORDER TO COVER THE PAINFUL AREA WITH WARM WATER, YOU HAVE TO GET INTO AN AWKWARD AND OFTEN PAINFUL POSITION.

EVEN IF YOU BEGIN TO FEEL BETTER WHILE RESTING IN THE TUB, YOU STILL HAVE TO GET OUT—POSSIBLY CAUSING MUSCLE SPASM AND THUS, MORE PAIN.

4

TAKE A SHOWER SEVERAL TIMES A DAY

STAND IN THE SHOWER SO THE WARM WATER HITS THE PAINFUL AREA. DO NOT BEND FORWARD OR SIDE TO SIDE TO "WORK IT OUT".

IF YOU DON'T HAVE A SHOWER, YOU COULD INVEST IN A "SHAMPOO HOSE ATTACHMENT" SO THAT YOU COULD DIRECT THE WARM WATER OVER THE AREA OF PAIN.

PLAN TO SPREAD THE SHOWERS OUT OVER THE DAY.

RETURN TO BED AND CONTINUE THE LOCAL DRY HEAT (i.e. ELECTRIC HEATING PAD ON "LOW").

5

AVOID SITTING

WHEN YOU SIT, YOUR BACK MUSCLES ARE DOING ALL THE WORK IN SUPPORTING YOU—THUS AGGRAVATING YOUR DISCOMFORT.

6

FOR A RARE CHANGE YOU MAY STAND OR WALK IN PLACE.

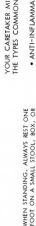

WHEN STANDING, ALWAYS REST ONE FOOT ON A SMALL STOOL, BOX, OR PILE OF BOOKS (4–6 INCHES HIGH). TRANSFER WEIGHT FROM ONE FOOT TO THE OTHER REGULARLY. ELEVATING ONE FOOT IMPROVES YOUR POSTURE AND TAKES SOME OF THE PRESSURE OFF YOUR BACK MUSCLES.

YOU MAY EAT SOME OF YOUR MEALS STANDING. PLACE THE FOOD ON A COUNTER AT CHEST LEVEL (THIS WILL HELP PREVENT YOU FROM BENDING FORWARD) AND STAND WITH ONE FOOT RESTING ON A STOOL.

YOUR CARETAKER MIGHT PRESCRIBE MEDICATIONS. THE TYPES COMMONLY PRESCRIBED ARE:

- ANTI-INFLAMMATORIES (ASPIRIN, MOTRIN).
- PAIN MEDICATIONS (TYLENOL, DARVON, CODEINE).
- MUSCLE RELAXANTS (VALIUM, ROBAXIN).

IF ANY OF THESE DRUGS ARE PRESCRIBED, FURTHER INFORMATION, SPECIFIC TO EACH DRUG, WILL BE PROVIDED FOR YOU.

Acute Low Back Strain/Sprain
INITIAL THERAPY

ACUTE LOW BACK STRAIN/SPRAIN IS AN OVERUSE OR MINOR INJURY OF EITHER THE TENDONS OR LIGAMENTS OF THE SPINAL COLUMN WITH MUSCLE SPASM (AN INVOLUNTARY TIGHTENING/CONTRACTION OF A MUSCLE) AS THE RESULT. THE ACUTE TYPE USUALLY FOLLOWS AN INJURY OR TRIVIAL STRAIN, IS OF RELATIVELY SHORT DURATION, AND RESPONDS WELL TO TREATMENT.

OUR GOAL WHEN DEVELOPING THIS PAMPHLET WAS TO HELP YOU THROUGH THIS EPISODE OF ACUTE LOW BACK STRAIN. THERE ARE NUMEROUS PUBLICATIONS AVAILABLE FOR YOUR REHABILITATION PHASE. YOUR CARETAKER MAY RECOMMEND ONE OR MORE OF THESE.

Catherine Feher-Wood, R.N., C.A.N.P.
M.B. Maughan, R.N., C.A.N.P., C.E.N.

MASSACHUSETTS
GENERAL HOSPITAL

brown; nl. = normal; sx. = symptoms; LMP = last menstrual period; d = days; PMP's = prior menstrual periods; WNL = within normal limit; BC = birth control; sl. = slight; (L) = left; NAD = no acute distress; T = temperature; po = by mouth; specs = specimens; C&S = culture and stain; CBS = complete blood count; diff. = differential; sed. = sedimentation; BCP's = birth control pills; palp. = palpation; BRB = bright red blood; GI = gastrointestinal; MVA = motor vehicle accident; p = after; bilat. = bilateral; C-spine = cervical spine; yest. = yesterday; HTN = hypertension; CVA = costovertebral angle; diff. = difficult; irreg. = irregular; R/O = rule out; MI = myocardial infarction; ant. = anterior; inf. = inferior.

Suggested Readings

Albin SL, Wassertheil-Smollar S, Jacobson S, et al: Evaluation of emergency room triage performed by nurses. *Am J Public Health* 65:1063–1068, 1975

Budassi, SA, Barber, JM: *Emergency Nursing: Principles and Practice.* St. Louis, CV Mosby Co, 1981

Estrada, EG: Advanced triage by an RN. *J Emerg Nurs* 5:8–11, 1979

Estrada, EG: Symposium on emergency nursing. Triage systems. *Nurs Clin North Am* 16:13–24, 1981

Jackson EB, Seeno E: The screening nurse. *Hospitals 45* (no. 11):66–73, 1971

Mazur W: *Problem-Oriented System.* Garden Grove, CA, Trainex Corporation, 1974

Mills, J, Webster AL, Wofsy, CB, et al: Effectiveness of nurse triage in the emergency department of an urban county hospital. *JACEP* 5:877–882, 1976

Slater RR: The triage nurse. *Hospitals 44* (no. 23);50–52, 1970

Slater RR: Triage nurse in the emergency department. *Am J Nurs* 70:127–129, 1970

Walker K, Hurst JW, Woody MF: *Applying the Problem Oriented System.* New York, Medcom Press, 1973

Weed, LL: *Medical Records, Medical Education and Patient Care.* Cleveland, Case Western Reserve University, 1971

Weed LL: *Your Health Care and How to Manage It.* Essex Junction, VT, Essex Publishing Co, 1975

Weinerman ER, Rutzen SR, Pearson DA: Effects of medical "triage" in a hospital emergency service. *Public Health Rep* 80:389–399, 1965

Willis, DT: A study of nursing triage. *J Emerg Nurs* 5:8–11, 1979

CHAPTER 38

Emergency Ward Nursing

VIRGINIA TRITSCHLER, R.N., B.S.
GERRI A. WITTROCK, R.N., B.S.N., M.S.N.
RUTH M. FARRISEY, R.N., BSc., M.P.H.

Emergency ward nurses at the Massachusetts General Hospital are members of the Department of Nursing (Fig. 38.1). The philosophy, functions, objectives, and standards of the department are observed in the development of standards of nursing practice specific to the emergency ward. In like manner, the quality assurance commitment of the department is carried out, appropriately modified, by the emergency ward nursing staff.

The emergency ward specific standards of nursing practice are congruent with the American Nurses' Association Standards of Emergency Nursing written in collaboration with the Emergency Department Nurses Association, and can be stated as follows:

General statement:

Irrespective of the intensity of the emergency, quality standards of nursing practice shall be encouraged and fostered at all times.

Recognizing the great variation in the intensity of patients' needs, the emergency ward nursing staff and its leaders shall:

—assess the intensity of patient need

—establish nursing care priorities

—assign nursing personnel, to the extent possible, according to their optimal clinical competences to deal with the existing unit situation.

Standards:

The emergency ward nursing personnel shall:

—take such life-saving and life-sustaining measures as may be required, initiating resuscitative procedures, and so on

—inform the patient of the nurse's plan of care and such physician's plans of care as can be communicated at the time

—assist physicians and trauma and resuscitation teams in the care of patients

—perform required emergency ward admitting procedures (take vital signs, obtain an electrocardiogram when indicated, acquire needed specimens, and prepare patient for necessary x-ray films and other procedures)

—maintain optimal privacy and provide for dignified care and emotional support for patients

—coordinate the activity of nursing professionals and nonprofessionals to afford safe and effective nursing service throughout the unit

—provide a physically safe environment according to the patient's needs

—assure continuity of patient care upon:

(a) transfer to another unit of the hospital, through appropriate communication to the receiving unit

(b) discharge, through simple instructions to patient and family or through referral to a community agency for continuity of nursing care

—keep family or friends informed of the patient's condition

—be constantly aware of, and practice according to, legal guidelines in an emergency ward setting, especially with regard to:

> Medical examiner cases
> Maternal death
> Death on arrival (DOA) practices
> Reportable disease regulations
> Child abuse regulations
> Rape protocols

—write concise, factual, unabbreviated nursing notes; record all medications given; and record all vital sign and other test results, signing all with full name and initials of nursing licensure.

NURSING LEADERSHIP

The Associate Director, Department of Nursing, Ambulatory Care Division, assumes overall responsibility for the nursing component of patient care and administration in the emergency ward/overnight ward, as well as in many clinics and hospital-associated neighborhood health centers, and provides direction (in particular, higher level interdepartmental planning) and administration in the context of the institution at large. The Associate Director attends a monthly emergency ward staff meeting, the meetings of the emergency

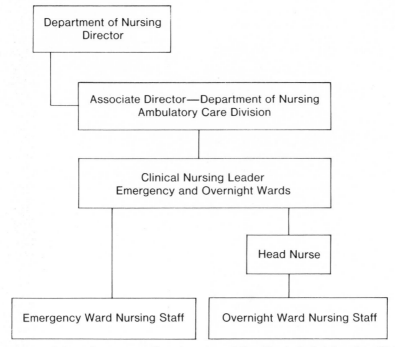

Figure 38.1. Schematic representation of nursing relationships in Ambulatory Care Division.

ward/overnight ward executive committee, and a variety of community-wide emergency ward and disaster planning committees, and is a resource and a problem solver, as well as being the liaison with the Director of the Department of Nursing.

Responsible to the Associate Director of Nursing, Ambulatory Care Division, is the on-site leader of the emergency ward, who is called the clinical nursing leader. He or she is the local spokesperson for the Department of Nursing, and is assisted in this assignment by several registered nurses with emergency ward experience and unit charge responsibility of considerable depth. Many opportunities for unit and department committee work are offered and encouraged. The head nurse of the associated overnight ward is a well-prepared medical/surgical nursing clinician.

The clinical nursing leader is, ex officio, the chairman of the emergency ward/overnight ward nursing practice committee, the leader of the local nursing quality assurance program, the nursing spokesperson on the cross-discipline emergency ward/overnight ward executive committee and the overall emergency ward/overnight ward committee. Responsibilities also include participation in several Department of Nursing and ambulatory nursing committees, as well as in several community-wide committees dealing with emergency medical affairs, community disaster planning, ad-

vanced continuing educational programs for emergency ward nurses, and so on.

The clinical nursing leader is an active participant in the development and periodic revision of the *Emergency-Overnight Ward Policy Manual* prepared by the emergency ward/overnight ward committee to meet the needs of the units as well as to meet Joint Commission for Accreditation of Hospitals and hospital licensure requirements. This role is most succinctly stated as follows: the clinical nursing leader has primary responsibility for the clinical and administrative aspects of emergency ward nursing; evaluates professional and nonprofessional nursing performance; conducts audits of nursing practice; recruits, selects, schedules, assigns, and supervises nurses in the emergency ward/overnight ward; prepares quality assurance studies and nursing practice and procedural changes; participates in the periodic cross-discipline evaluation of the total program of the emergency ward/overnight ward; and functions as the on-site nursing spokesperson in cross-discipline planning activities.

The emergency ward/overnight ward is served by a psychiatric nurse clinician who has had extensive emergency ward experience. This clinician is responsible directly to the Associate Director of Nursing, Ambulatory Care Division, and the Chairman of Psychiatric Nursing. The role involves direct patient service (especially crisis intervention), indirect coordination of some crisis work (particularly with an active rape victim service), in-service teaching, liaison activities with a large psychiatric residency service, and support of and counsel with the emergency ward/overnight ward nursing staff.

A unit teacher, who is also a certified adult nurse practitioner, assists in the orientation of all new personnel, prepares or assists in the preparation of all in-service education programs developed to meet the needs and interests of the staff, analyzes and evaluates staff strengths and weaknesses with the clinical nursing leader and the psychiatric nurse clinician, and assists in planning.

NURSING STAFF DEVELOPMENT

At the Massachusetts General Hospital, at least 2 years of full-time experience in intensive nursing care or previous emergency ward experience or a combination of the two provide the best background before emergency ward assignment. Such experience helps the nurse cope with the stressful situations encountered in a busy emergency department and to have a stronger grasp on the need to assess situations quickly and to set priorities. Successful completion of a written examination on commonly used emergency medications, certification in cardiopulmonary resuscitation, and Basic Life Support certification are also desirable qualifications in beginning emergency ward staff nurses. The personal qualities of stability, staying-power under tension, maturity of judgment, and sense of personal concern for those served are also of great importance, but are difficult to identify in recruitment and selection.

As individual nurses are appointed to the staff, a copy of the generic description of the post to which they have been appointed and a statement of the expectations and goals held of each nursing staff member are included with their letter of appointment. These documents are used in succeeding weeks and months by the unit teacher and clinical nursing leader in performance appraisal and monitoring of progress.

Orientation

Orientation of new staff must take into consideration the new nurses' previous experience and whatever may be known of their personal maturity, so that flexible planning of orientation and acclimatization to the pace of the emergency ward may be arranged. The unit teacher, assisted by experienced staff members and with ongoing input from the clinical nursing leader carries out the orientation program. Staff participation in orientation acknowledges their strengths and expertise, allows the new nurses to learn variations in practice, and helps the staff develop insights into the building of nursing staff strength and esprit. A written, individualized orientation plan assists all participants to follow the program of the new staff members and prevents omission of vital portions of the program. The length of the orientation period varies with the individual's speed of learning and skill acquisition, and the simultaneous availability of worshops produced by the Staff Education Department on intravenous therapy, cardiopulmonary care, life support, and life assisting services of various kinds. Registered nurses must successfully complete an intravenous therapy workshop to be certified to mix intravenous medication solutions and to administer selected and approved intravenous bolus medications.

Newcomers to the hospital are required to take part in a staff education department orientation program during the first 3 weeks. Orientation to triage and charge nurse functions in the emergency ward may not take place for 3–6 months after arrival.

In-Service Education/Professional Education

Ongoing education is essential for successful emergency nursing practice. The hospital has a liberal tuition benefit program which staff members use in the acquisition of bachelor's and master's degrees. The staff education department offers programs in management, geriatrics, and many other topics relevant to nursing. The Emergency Department Nurses Association, via its local chapters, provides steady opportunities for enrichment, as does the Office of Emergency Medical Services (operating within the Massachusetts State Department of Public Health). At the Massachusetts General Hospital, the following in-service education programs, planned and executed by staff members with expertise and teaching ability, have proved popular and are repeated regularly for new staff:

Physical Assessment Skills and the Recording of Such Findings
Crisis Intervention by Nursing Personnel
Rape Counseling by Nursing Personnel
Alcoholism as a Health Problem
Nursing Intervention in Burn Care
How to Write for Publication
Pediatric Need Awareness in the Emergency Department Setting

Early Recognition of Child Battering/Abuse
In addition to these formal learning opportunities, human resources are recognized (for example, there are informal conferences and information-sharing by physicians, nurses from other departments, special therapists, and patient care representatives), and conference opportunities are offered regularly.

The systems of prehospital service that have developed approximately in the last 15 years have expanded the necessity for the emergency ward nurse to think beyond the immediate hospital setting. In addition to their in-hospital awareness, they need to understand the work and capabilities of emergency medical technicians and more highly trained paramedics as they work in the community and transport patients to the hospital. For this reason, emergency ward nurses at the Massachusetts General Hospital spend 8–16 hours riding the ambulances with the emergency medical technicians and paramedics of the public ambulance services in Boston. The triage nurse is responsible for receiving radio communication from emergency medical technicians and paramedics planning to transport patients; he or she records the information on a preprinted note pad, and assigns the patient to a specific service and treatment area based on the radio communication and additional information obtained when the patient enters the unit. The triage nurse records any observations and treatments reported to have been initiated by the field team in the patient's medical record and ascertains that the physician caring for the patient has all necessary initial information.

PATIENT ASSESSMENT

Assessment of the patient's condition is a continuous process that starts with admission and continues unabated until discharge or transfer to another unit. The challenge presented to the nursing staff is to assess patients correctly in a limited time frame. Patients entering an emergency department and those who accompany them are usually anxious, frightened, and uncertain—this state of uneasiness may be expressed by anger, hostility, defensiveness, or resistance. Difficulty in communication is often seen.

Primary nursing in a modified form is practiced in the emergency ward of the Massachusetts General Hospital. Adequacy of nursing staff, the number of patients in the unit, and the intensity of their needs all affect primary nursing. Nursing assignments are made in such a way as to foster primary nursing practice. They are variably effective, because of shift changes, meal breaks, in-service education breaks, and the speed with which the care process takes place. Nurses are encouraged to wear name badges that also contain their title, such as staff nurse, nurse practitioner, or unit teacher, and to introduce themselves to all patients arriving in their area.

Triage

The triage nurse assesses all patients on admission in whom it is possible to determine needs by interview or by observation, and assigns them to the most appropriate service and treatment area (see Chapter 37).

A family nurse practitioner (a registered nurse with additional preparation in history-taking, physical assessment, diagnosis, and early therapy), who is certified by the American Nurses Association, works in the triage and minor medical areas of the emergency ward. This practitioner, following approved clinical practice guidelines and in concert with physician consultants provides direct care, assists the triage nurse, and provides nursing service continuity in this area. The family nurse practitioner is of particular value: (1) in developing the assessment skills of the triage nurse, (2) in delivering quality nursing care and teaching to a significant segment of the patients assigned to the minor medical unit, and (3) in providing continuity of patient care in an area otherwise staffed by physicians and nurses on rotation.

The psychiatric nurse clinician is also of great assistance to the triage nurse. He or she functions as a resource, as a person skilled in crisis intervention, as a liaison and caretaker between the emergency and acute psychiatry units (which are physically separate from each other) and as a consultant and assistant in caring for grieving families and patients with acute psychiatric or behavioral problems.

EFFECTIVE COMMUNICATION

Communication in a large and busy emergency department is a major challenge. The numbers of staff, the various shifts, the variability of patient census (by virtue of both numbers and intensity of need), and the problems of communication across disciplines and across services are all factors affecting successful communication.

Staff meetings are held regularly and minutes are promply prepared and posted for those unable to attend; this appears to be the best method for keeping nursing personnel informed. Opportunities to allow the staff to express ideas and criticisms, to participate in problem-solving, and to play a part in the planning of new or revised services cannot be overemphasized. A centrally located notebook available to the nursing staff containing current memos and an opportunity to write comments is also helpful.

The most frequent mode of communication—verbal—is expedient; however, every effort must be made to encourage written documentation. Written communication via the patient's record is essential for doctor-to-nurse, nurse-to-doctor, and nurse-to-nurse exchange of information. Patients in an emergency department frequently tell one staff member information not given to another—verbal communications may be forgotten or simply not passed on. The practice of recording relevant information must be emphasized. At the Massachusetts General Hospital, the nursing staff is encouraged to use the problem-oriented method of recording information, separating subjective and objective observations, and clearly stating nursing assessment, plan of care proposed, and nursing actions taken. The use of flow sheets in major trauma and cardiac arrest situations enables the nurse to document quickly and to have all pertinent data on a single, readily readable sheet (Fig. 38.2). Staff are encouraged to develop teaching manuals for new procedures and for the nursing use of monitoring devices and new equipment. In like manner, staff are expected to identify problems, study them, document findings, and prepare statements of suggested methods of solution. Participation in quality assurance exercises is also expected.

STAFF SCHEDULING

Scheduling in the emergency ward takes into account the flow of patients by hour of the day and day of the week, and requires a keen awareness of variables introduced by holidays, civic celebrations, and the general makeup of the case load (adults, children, usual number of house admissions daily, and usual numbers seen in the several individual treatment areas). Additionally, it must take careful note of the strengths and weaknesses of staff members, the stage of their development in emergency department nursing, and their expressed wishes regarding time arrangements and area assignments. Staff complements are arranged in the most balanced pattern possible.

The heaviest patient flow at the Massachusetts General Hospital occurs daily from 10 a.m. to 10 p.m.; there is some predictability of numbers of patients admitted per shift; however, it has never successfully been proved that one day's care load tended, in any predictable manner, to be more acutely ill than that of another day.

Although the normal Department of Nursing shifts are observed (7:00 a.m. to 3:30 p.m., 3:00 p.m. to 11:30 p.m.; 11:00 p.m. to 7:30 a.m.), a 10:00 a.m. to 7:00 p.m. shift has been found useful to cover meal hours and to meet peak hours of patient intake. In addition, experiments with four 10-hour days/week, which have been requested by individual staff members, have allowed shift patterns such as the following: 8:00 a.m. to 6:30 p.m.; 10:00 a.m. to 9:00 p.m.; 1:00 p.m. to 11:30 p.m.; 3:00 p.m. to 1:30 a.m.; 11:00 p.m. to 9:00 a.m.

Within the bounds of safe and balanced staffing patterns, considerable effort is expended to meet the requests of individuals who (1) require specific hours available for additional education or to tend to family needs, or who (2) desire assignment to a particular shift versus a rotational assignment, or who (3) are subject to limited public transportation or carpooling arrangements, and so on. Creative staffing patterns consistent with appropriate departmental coverage have been found to be beneficial to the department as well as to the individual nurse.

Alternating weekends off are planned, and 11 holidays are allowed per year. Scheduling on Thanksgiving, Christmas, and New Year's Day is carefully rotated, and individual choices are honored as far as possible for other holidays. Schedules are prepared 6 weeks at a time, and insofar as possible adhere to a master time plan established each year. Records of time plans and times actually worked are maintained for at least 2 years.

The principal scheduler is the clinical nursing leader. The schedule of the adjacent overnight ward is prepared by the head nurse of that unit; and the combined plans are studied to identify areas of thin staffing that may call for overtime. In such a case, staff are recruited by requesting volunteers rather than by assigning specific individuals. The one exception is the specification by the leadership of the nurse "in charge."

We currently do not have a formal "on-call" roster of nurses for either the emergency ward or the overnight ward. Considerable volunteering for extra duty takes place, and it is understood that in the event of a disaster of sufficient magnitude, staff would be called from their homes.

TREATMENT ROOM AND SUPPLY ORGANIZATION

The emergency ward nurse plays an active part in arranging basic treatment rooms and modifying the setup of special-purpose rooms. The clinical nursing leader must have knowledge of available equipment and sources of secondary supply, and

Onset Time _____   Name: _____

Unit No. _____ Age: _____

	Time/Dosage				
1. Defibrillation					
2. Medications					
Sodium bicarbonate					
Epinephrine					
Lidocaine					
Calcium chloride					
Atropine					
Bretylium tosylate					
Procainamide					
Dextrose 50					
Naloxone					
3. IV mixes					
Lidocaine, 2 gm/250 ml D_5W					
Isoproterenol, 2 mg/250 ml D_5W					
Levarterenol, 4 mg/250 ml D_5W					
Bretylium, 2 gm/250 ml D_5W					
Procainamide, 2 gm/250 ml D_5W					
Dopamine, 500 mg/250 ml D_5W					
Sodium nitroprusside, 50 mg/500 ml D_5W					
Epinephrine, 2 mg/250 ml D_5W					
CVP mix, 250 ml D_5W					
4. Other					
Blood gases					
Pacemaker (type)					
Open cardiac massage					

Figure 38.2.   Cardiac arrest flow sheet.

must periodically review set-ups with staff and physicians who use the rooms daily.

At the Massachusetts General Hospital, nurses plan set-ups and arrange for all room modifications; however, periodic stocking is performed throughout the day by trained unit assistants. It is the responsibility of the nurse assigned to a given treatment area on any particular shift to ascertain that each treatment room is fully supplied and to monitor supply use. Tables 38.1–38.5 list supplies appropriate to various settings in the emergency ward.

Table 38.1.
Basic equipment in all adult treatment rooms.

Outlets (one set for each bed)	Blood culture bottles (4)
Oxygen (2), one with bubble-jet, one with adapter for venturi mask, respirator, or positive-pressure mask	Pegboard
	Central venous pressure catheters (24-inch, 16-inch, 8-inch)
Suction (2), one with catheter for nasopharyngeal suction, one adaptable for gastric or thoracic suction	Arterial blood-gas set (plastic bag containing alcohol sponge, needles, glass syringe with cap and heparin, which becomes unit in which ice is placed and specimen is sent to laboratory)
Holder for catheters (1)—a cylindrical metal container (4- to 6-inch diameter, 12- to 15-inch length) attached to wall to hold 14- and 16-gauge suction catheters and tonsil-tip suction device	Airways
	Sputum traps
	Y-connectors (sterile)
Sphygmomanometer	Stopcocks (3-way) with catheter plugs
Dextrose in water solution (5%), 3 bottles (500 ml)	Scalp-vein needles (19-, 21-, and 23-gauge)
Intravenous supplies	Oxygen supplies (mask and nasal prongs)
Administration sets (3)	Urinary catheterization tray with No. 16 Foley catheter (5 ml) and urinometer
Microdrip administration sets (3)	Gloves (sterile and rectal)
Arm boards (3)	Adapters (Y-adapters, 5-in-1 adapters)
Bedpan (1), urinals (3 or 4), emesis basins (4 to 6), with metal holder behind door for both bedpan and urinals to save shelf space	Clamps (Hunt, Hoffman, butterfly)
	Bandages and applicators
	Tongue blades
Cups for dentures and for specimens of stool and sputum	Cotton-tip applicators
	Gauze pads
Guaiac kits	Tape
Blood specimen kits (8) placed in an emesis basin and tied with a tourniquet	Band-Aids
	Lubricating gel (Lubafax)
Tubes—plain red top (3), lavender (1), blue (2), gray (1)	Antiseptic supplies
	Alcohol preparation (solution and pads)
Needles (15- and 20-gauge)	Iodine solution
Intravenous catheters (14-, 16-, and 18-gauge)	Povidone-iodine (spray and ointment)
Syringe (50-ml Luer-lok)	Bed linen, pads (incontinence and sanitary)
Vacutainer for blood samples	Shopping bags for patients' clothing, with adhesive labels
Alcohol preparation pads	
Povidone-iodine (Efodine) ointment	

The nurses' role in the development of the emergency ward medicine closet has also been significant. Nursing personnel are the principal users of this area, and are the persons responsible for drug security in all units of the hospital. Thus, the emergency ward medicine closet was designed with strong nursing input regarding space, organization, room for more than one person to work at the same time, visibility of drugs, drug and narcotic security, and easy maintenance.

The medicine closet has tilted shelves with movable dividers to accommodate changes in the quantities of drugs and pharmaceuticals. Intravenous solutions are kept on movable carts within the unit to facilitate restocking. There is adequate counter space and optimal lighting, and all surfaces (counter, shelves, walls, ceiling, and floor) are easily washable. Shelf, counter, and sink arrangements allow for quick acquisition of emergency drugs while intravenous fluids, and medications are being prepared, and medications are arranged to facilitate the counting of narcotics on each shift.

In addition to the central medicine closet, two other medical supply units are maintained in closets designed for their purposes—one in the overnight ward and one in an area of the emergency ward designated as the Pediatric Episodic Care Unit.

Emergency drugs regularly needed in the two major trauma rooms and in the four-bed cardiac care room are stored in closed areas within the rooms. These drugs are also stored on the mobile emergency cart.

Resource materials provided to the physician and nursing staffs include an intravenous drug compatibility chart that was organized by the hospital pharmacists and that is posted prominently in cardiac treatment and cardiac arrest rooms; an approved list of intravenous medications, citing maximum dosage, common dosage, possible side effects, and special considerations, prepared by the

Table 38.2.
Equipment in cardiac arrest rooms.

Basic equipment as in all treatment rooms on wall-
    mounted pegboard or within easy reach
Specific equipment and supplies
    Cardiac monitor
    Defibrillator (monitor-synchronized with internal
        paddles)
    Ambu bag (100% oxygen)
    Respirator (Bird), wall-mounted
    Cardiac arrest board on bed
    Intravenous solutions (prepared for use and fitted
        with tubing and stopcocks)
        Dextrose in water (5%)
        Isoproterenol hydrochloride
        Lidocaine hydrochloride
        Levarterenol bitartrate
    Endotracheal tubes (sizes 7, 8, 9, 10) with stylet,
        syringe, and clamp
    Cardiac scalpel
    Nasogastric tubes (sizes 14, 18)
    Sutures (0 silk with straight needle)
    Pediatric feeding tubes
    Subclavian intravenous set
    Thoracotomy set with chest tubes and under-water
        suction device such as pleurovac
    Pacing kit (transthoracic curved bipolar pacing wire
        with adapter)
        Cordis semi-floating bipolar transvenous tempo-
        rary wire, cardiac needle, alligator clamp, ster-
        ile towel, 12-ml syringe
    Cardiac arrest flow sheet (Fig. 38.2)

clinical nursing leader and approved for use by
the pharmacy committee; an intravenous mixture
handbook assembled by the hospital's intravenous
team; and a conversion table for intravenous medications that is posted in every room (Table 38.6).

Optimally, every major emergency department
should have a full-time (40 hours/week) registered
pharmacist to perform the following duties:

—Facilitate the issuance of "starter doses" of
prescribed drugs.

—Improve and expand the pharmacologic
knowledge of the physician and nursing staffs.

—Maintain the medicine closet in an optimum
but economical inventory, taking into account the
usage patterns of drugs.

—Consider ways to maximize cost-effectiveness
in drug use, to prevent undue waste, to provide
unit dose packaging, and to process appropriate
charges for direct patient billing.

—Assist in the preparation of printed teaching
material for patients and families for drugs most
frequently prescribed.

—Assist in the identification of drugs brought
in by patients and families as possible causes of
toxicity and overdose.

—Increase familiarity with emergency drug
therapy patterns, consider the compatibilities and
reactions of these drugs, and advise physicians and
nurses accordingly.

—Serve as a liaison with the central pharmacy
and chief pharmacist in matters calling for changes
and modifications in unit practice.

DISASTER PREPAREDNESS

Familiarity with the hospital's disaster plan is
essential for the clinical nursing leader, the over-

Table 38.3.
Equipment on mobile emergency cart.

Pegboard attached to cart
    Stopcocks (3-way)
    Blades (Nos. 11, 15)
    Sutures (0 silk with straight needle)
    Endotracheal tubes (6, 7, 8)
    Syringes (50-ml)
    Cardiac scalpel
    Craefoord clamps (2)
    Scissors, hemostats (sterile)
    Pacing kit (Table 38.2)
Work surface
    Tray
        Laryngoscope with blades (4-inch straight, 5-
            inch straight, 5-inch curved, 6-inch curved)
        Endotracheal tubes (sizes 7, 8, 9, 10) with stylet,
            syringe (10-ml), and clamp
        McGill forceps
        Tonsil-tip suction catheter
        Mouth spreader
        Airway (No. 5)
        Lubafax
        Stylet
        Naso-oral airways
        Central venous pressure mix—water-soluble vi-
            tamins (Berocca-C)[a] and heparin in 250 ml 5%
            dextrose in water
        Medication (intravenous) labels
Drawers
    Medications—bronchodilators, antidysrhythmics,
        anticholinergics, vasopressors, β-receptor
        stimulators, β-receptor blocking agents, corti-
        costeroids, catecholamines, diuretics, alkalini-
        zing agents, narcotic antagonists, anticonvul-
        sants, cholinergic drugs
    Syringes (10-ml)
Shelves
    Medtronic pacemakers (2)
    Cutdown set (2)
    Subclavian intravenous set
    Thoracotomy set
    Blood pressure pump
    Extension cord
    Ambu bag (100% oxygen)
    Medications (back-up)

[a] For color identification only.

Table 38.4.

Major trauma room equipment.

Basic equipment as in all treatment rooms on wall-
  mounted pegboard or within easy reach
Specific equipment and supplies
  Intubating equipment (adult and pediatric)
    Ambu bag (100% oxygen)
    Emergency drugs (sodium bicarbonate, epineph-
      rine, atropine, calcium chloride, isoproterenol)
  Bronchoscopy equipment (adult and pediatric)
  Tracheotomy sets with tubes (all sizes)
  Closed thoracotomy sets (3) with tubes (all sizes)
    and suction sets
  Thoracotomy set
  G-suits or MAST trousers (5)
  Burr hole set
  Ventricular tap set
  Obstetric kit
  Esophageal varices set with tubes
    (Sengstaken-Blakemore, Linton)
  Cervical immobilization equipment
    Sandbags
    Collars (soft felt, four-poster, Philadelphia)
  Intravenous solutions
    Mannitol
    Ringer's lactate
    Physiologic saline/5% dextrose in water (1:1)
    Physiologic saline
  Suture kits with all common types of suture mate-
    rials
  Surgical preparation kits with razor and sponges in
    tray
  Subclavian intravenous sets
  Cardiac monitoring units
  Defibrillators with internal paddles
  Autotransfusion kits (2)—Sorenson
  Burn equipment
    Sterile sheets and towels
    Bandages (Kerlix)
    Sterile basins with sponges
    Antibacterial soapless skin cleanser (pHisoHex)
    Sterile physiologic saline solution
    Silver nitrate solution
    Silver sulfadiazine (Silvadene) cream
    Xeroform gauze
  Heat lamps
  Blood warmers
  Volume ventilator
  Craafoord clamps (2)
  Blood infusion pumps
  Gastric tubes (assorted)

Table 38.5.

Equipment in travel emergency box.[a]

Tackle box with two levels
  Lower level
    Endotracheal tubes (Nos. 32–38)
    Laryngoscope with straight and curved blades
    Ambu bag
    McGill forceps
    Spinal needles (Nos. 18, 20)
    Scalpel handle (No. 3)
    Scalpel blades (Nos. 10, 11, 15)
    Syringes (50 ml, 12 ml, 6 ml)
    5% dextrose in water solution (250 ml)
    Intravenous set (pediatric)
    Tape
    Tongue blades (padded)
    Airways (adult and pediatric)
    Lubricating gel
    Tourniquets
    Polymyxin B—bacitracin-neomycin (Neosporin)
      ointment
    Scalp-vein needles (19-, 21-, and 25-gauge)
  Upper level
    Syringes
    Needles (Nos. 19, 20)
    Angiographic catheters (2 each, Nos. 14, 16,
      18)
    Alcohol sponges
    Ammonia for inhalation
    Calcium chloride, 2 single-dose syringes (Bris-
      toject)
    Epinephrine, 2 single-dose syringes
    Lidocaine, 2 single-dose syringes
    50% dextrose in water, 2 vials
    Sodium bicarbonate, 2 single-dose syringes
    Sodium chloride for injection, 1 vial
    Water for injection, 1 vial
    Aminophylline, 2 ampules
    Phenytoin (Dilantin sodium), 2 vials
    Furosemide (Lasix), 3 ampules
    Naloxone hydrochloride (Narcan), 2 ampules
    Diazepam (Valium), 3 ampules
    Isoproterenol hydrochloride (Isuprel), 2 ampules
    Epinephrine, 3 ampules
    Atropine, 3 ampules
    Bretylium tosylate, 2 ampules
Additional items in pediatric emergency box
  Calcium gluconate (pediatric), 2 ampules
  Blood pressure cuff (child size)
  Suction catheters
  Feeding tubes (pediatric)
  Endotracheal tubes (2.5-5.0 cm instead of adult
    sizes)

[a] The "travel box" is used when a proceed-out
team is sent to a disaster situation outside the hospital
and when an emergency ward team responds to an
emergency call in certain areas of the hospital.

night ward head nurse, and all experienced nurses
who are regularly assigned as charge nurses.

  Emergency ward charge nurses are likely to
receive first notice of a disaster from the emergency ward administrator. A list of recommended
procedures for disaster preparation is readily avail-

Table 38.6.
Conversion table for intravenous medications.

Agent	Dosage (microdrops)
Lidocaine/procainamide/bretylium tosylate (2 gm/250 ml 5% dextrose in water)	15 gtt/min = 2 mg/min 30 gtt/min = 4 mg/min
Epinephrine (2 mg/250 ml 5% dextrose in water)	15 gtt/min = 2 μg/min 30 gtt/min = 4 μg/min
Isoproterenol hydrochloride (2 mg/250 ml 5% dextrose in water)	15 gtt/min = 2 μg/min 30 gtt/min = 4 μg/min
Levarterenol bitartrate (4 mg/250 ml 5% dextrose in water)	15 gtt/min = 4 μg/min 30 gtt/min = 8 μg/min 45 gtt/min = 12 μg/min 60 gtt/min = 16 μg/min
Dopamine (400 mg/200 ml 5% dextrose in water)	15 gtt/min = 500 μg/min 30 gtt/min = 1000 μg/min
Nitroglycerine (50 mg/250 ml 5% dextrose in water)	15 gtt/min = 50 μg/min 30 gtt/min = 100 μg/min 45 gtt/min = 150 μg/min 60 gtt/min = 200 μg/min
Phenylephrine hydrochloride (10 mg/250 ml 5% dextrose in water)	15 gtt/min = 10 μg/min 30 gtt/min = 20 μg/min 45 gtt/min = 30 μg/min 60 gtt/min = 40 μg/min
Sodium nitroprusside (50 mg/250 ml 5% dextrose in water)	15 gtt/min = 50 μg/min 30 gtt/min = 100 μg/min 45 gtt/min = 150 μg/min 60 gtt/min = 200 μg/min

able for charge nurses to follow. It is expected that they will:

—Notify selected members of the Department of Nursing at the hospital or at home.

—Notify the Radiology Department, requesting unexposed chest plates for stretchers, as well as a delay in all but emergency x-ray studies.

—Decide which treatment areas are likely to be most in demand in light of available information.

—Assign a nurse to proceed with evacuation of the area most likely to be needed or to plan for an alternative site.

—Assign an appropriate number of nurses to prepare for and be responsible for the reception of patients to designated areas, calling for additional nursing help via stipulated available nursing channels.

—Assign a second nurse to the triage area, and assign the primary triage nurse (1) to familiarize herself with disaster preparation in progress and (2) to be prepared to receive the first patients.

—Call upon the overnight ward staff to assist in the emergency ward or to prepare to evacuate the overnight ward or both, as information indicates.

—Appoint non-nursing personnel (secretaries) to assist any anxious family members to appropriate waiting areas.

—Consult with physicians and administrators regarding the expeditious disposition of waiting patients with minor problems.

—Report the status of emergency ward readiness to the senior nurse in the hospital.

—Proceed to acquire back-up supplies and additional equipment as required in each special treatment area.

REFERENCES PROVIDED AT NURSES STATION

The following is a list of printed material located at the nurses' station in the emergency ward:

(1) *Massachusetts General Hospital Nursing Policy Manual*

(2) *Emergency Ward/Overnight Ward Policy Manual*

(3) *Philosophy, Functions, Objectives, Standards of the Department of Nursing, Massachusetts General Hospital Ambulatory Care Division*

(4) *Approved Nurse Practitioner Clinical Practice Guidelines*

(5) *Ambulatory Care Division Nursing Procedure Manual*

(6) *Massachusetts General Hospital Disaster Plan*

(7) *Orientation to Emergency Department Manual*

(8) *Massachusetts General Hospital Nursing Procedure Manual*

(9) *Massachusetts General Hospital Pediatric Procedure Manual*

(10) *Massachusetts General Hospital Manual of Safety Policies*

(11) *Massachusetts General Hospital Triage Manual*

(12) A library of emergency, medical, and nursing texts as requested by the staff.

(13) Notebooks, minutes, tables of organization, and informational materials, including:

"Drug of the Week"

Emergency ward conference notes and summaries

Emergency ward/overnight ward executive committee minutes

Tables of organization

—Hospital

—Department of Nursing

—Ambulatory Care Division

Minutes of all departmental and unit nursing committees

Information regarding equipment in use in the emergency ward

Toxicology readings

Reading materials associated with in-service and staff education programs

Staff Education Department offerings

Emergency ward conference notes and tapes

Current emergency department and nursing periodicals

Summary of audits of nursing practice

OVERNIGHT WARD

At the Massachusetts General Hospital, emergency ward patients who need further observations, tests, or treatment for a period ranging from a few hours to 72 hours may be admitted to the adjacent overnight ward.

The overnight ward head nurse is charged with the day-to-day operation of this unit, including the planning of time, the performance evaluation of staff, coordination with other disciplines and auxiliary help, and the orientation and continuing education of the overnight ward staff.

The in-service education program for this staff is carefully planned.

The nursing skills necessary in this unit are a mixture of in-patient nursing skills and basic support nursing. Nurses must develop a beginning nursing care plan and arrange for the most expeditious schedule of required tests and procedures, realizing that the patient's short stay requires the setting of teaching priorities to provide the most nursing service in a limited time. Apparently stable patients in the overnight ward frequently become acutely ill and necessitate more intensive nursing care. Overnight ward nurses may be called to assist in the emergency ward when a crisis of staffing or patient care develops.

Selected Readings

Budassi G, Barber J: *Emergency Nursing Principles and Practice.* St. Louis, CV Mosby Co., 1981

American Nurses Association: *Standards of Emergency Practice,* Kansas City, 1975

Culbertson V, Anderson R: *Pharmacist Involvement in Emergency Room Services, Contemporary Pharmacy Practice,* 4, no. 3, Summer, 1981

Davis K: *Human Behavior at Work.* New York, McGraw-Hill Book Co., 1972

Eckert CE (Ed): *Emergency Room Care.* Boston, Little Brown Co., 1981

Sproul CW, Mellanney PJ (Eds): *Emergency Care.* St. Louis, CV Mosby Co., 1974

Stephenson HE, Jr (Ed): *Immediate Care of the Acutely Ill and Injured.* St. Louis, CV Mosby Co., 1974

Warner CG: *Emergency Care—Assessment and Intervention.* St. Louis, CV Mosby Co., 1978

CHAPTER 39

Medicolegal Considerations in Emergency Care

JAMES M. VACCARINO, J.D.

Increasing emphasis on the legal aspects of health care delivery necessitates an explanation of such aspects to the emergency practitioner. Two specific areas will be considered: the concept of liability and general practical considerations of a legal or quasi-legal nature.

LIABILITY

Factors Precipitating Malpractice Suits

Medical malpractice suits are increasing at an unprecedented rate, particularly in the hospital setting. Most claims are based on the following three factors, either alone or in combination: an unsatisfactory relationship between the physician and the patient, a poor result, and a bill that the patient considers excessive. A malpractice claim may be legitimate, as in cases of demonstrable negligence, or it may be frivolous; whatever the precipitating event, it constitutes failure to meet the patient's expectations of health care services.

Physician-Patient Relationship

Kindness, consideration, and sensitivity to the patient as a human being rather than awareness only of his disease process sets the stage for a good relationship between the patient and the physician. The patient who respects his physician rarely misconstrues or mistrusts the physician's actions. Conversely, an abrasive, insensitive, and alienating personality breeds mistrust, misconceptions, and a lack of confidence. The 1823 *Guide for Practising Physicians* notes: "He who does not understand the art to acquire the confidence and esteem of his patient . . . will make but a sorry progress, should his knowledge be ever so profound." It is apparent that lack of rapport between patient and physician may easily give rise to a malpractice claim, regard-less of whether such a claim has a foundation in fact.

Poor Result

On occasion, a poor result may be due to negligence on the part of the physician, the classic example being a retained surgical instrument after operation. However, a patient may bring suit on the grounds of a poor result because of a misconception that the physician promised a specific outcome that was not achieved. This often occurs if the physician does not fully inform the patient or if he too casually discusses a procedure that he may consider routine. A minor stitch infection, for example, might be grounds for a suit if the patient did not understand that it was a natural complication and that all precautions had been taken to prevent it. A patient may also sue if he is discharged from the emergency ward before his complaint has been completely relieved. Patients must be educated to understand that the emergency ward provides initial treatment only and that discharge from the emergency ward is always a matter of judgment. It should be emphasized that although poor results may range from actual negligence to trivial risks ordinarily accompanying treatment, all such injuries can become grounds for malpractice suits under certain circumstances.

"Excessive" Charges

Current hospital costs are admittedly high, but defensibly so. The patient demands quality care, and this is not an inexpensive commodity. Problems may arise from the patient's mistaken belief that his insurance covers all hospital charges, which in general is untrue. Before hospitalization or treatment in the emergency ward, the patient should be informed as to the extent of his insurance coverage if possible. This does not solve the problem of high costs, but it does make the patient aware that he is partly liable for hospital charges.

Avoiding Malpractice Claims

The primary principle in avoiding claims is to develop rapport with the patient. An effort to understand the patient's fears and desires will result in a relationship of confidence and trust. The patient of a humble and compassionate physician usually does not criticize his judgment.

Rapport is especially necessary in the emergency setting, since patients are often considerably apprehensive because of their illness or because of their concept of the emergency ward environment. In apprehensive patients, the potential for misunderstanding is dramatically increased. The inconvenience of a long waiting period, for example, can be magnified to the point where the patient is convinced that he has been ignored. A waiting patient should be reassured with a quiet voice, an understanding manner, and an unhurried attitude of sincere interest.

Medical records should be meticulously maintained. If a plaintiff is to prevail in an action for malpractice, he must demonstrate that standards of care have been violated. The only documentation of care is the medical record. It must accurately reflect the care that the patient received. As a general rule, the plaintiff's attorney examines these records before commencement of the claim, and if it is clearly indicated that the physician took a risk that was reasonable under the circumstances, the claim may be averted. On the other hand, an absence of detail about an injury or an ambiguous entry may imply an attempt to conceal the facts, which could prove to be critical in a subsequent legal action.

If the physician has justifiably departed from the usual treatment in a specific case, he should note his thought process in the medical record. Weed states that: "In the objective, interpretive and plan sections of the progress notes, the physician has a chance to reveal exactly why he took a given course of action, exactly what he chose to neglect, exactly what his priorities were as his load grew in size, and most important why he may have deviated from the usual criteria for the management of a specific problem . . ." In addition, although it may be argued that missing a diagnosis implies negligence, demonstration from the record that acceptable and reasonable standards of medical practice were utilized in arriving at the diagnosis usually refutes the argument.

The record should never include inappropriate or subjective commentary or unnecessary descriptions containing words such as "inadvertently" or "erroneously." Misinterpretation of such terms may often have overwhelming effects. On occasion, physicians under great pressure in the emergency ward unnecessarily criticize the clinical expertise of physicians who had previously attended the patient elsewhere. Such a use of the medical record is unwarranted and should be condemned.

Hospital administrative personnel should be made aware of potential claims by means of an effective reporting mechanism. Potential claims may be surmised from letters of complaint, failure to pay bills, or verbal expressions of discontent at the time of treatment. Physicians and other staff should report personal errors or problems to the hospital administration without fear of recrimination. The administrative staff can review the circumstances and give counsel on how to handle the situation.

Admittedly these steps are simple, but they are effective in their simplicity. Physicians and other hospital personnel must always remember to assure the patient that his best interests are being served.

GENERAL LEGAL CONSIDERATIONS

Many practical legal problems are encountered daily in the emergency ward. In many instances, local statutory law or regulatory policy determines the solution to a particular problem. Before being confronted with the types of situation discussed, the health care provider should acquaint himself with local policy. In the absence of a specific regulation, common sense often provides a satisfactory solution.

Informed Consent

It is a basic legal and moral tenet that a patient should be fully informed of a proposed procedure, the alternatives, and the risks of each before he assents. In a true medical emergency, lifesaving measures may be started even though the physician risks suit for a technical battery, that is, the touching of another's person without his consent. The same reasoning applies in an emergency if the patient is a minor and if no parent is available for consent. It is helpful if the patient has reached the age of reason and authorizes the physician to proceed, but this is not absolutely necessary. Common sense dictates the justifiability of undertaking therapy without parental consent in such cases rather than delaying treatment.

If the patient is incapable of giving consent and if a threat to his life or health is not imminent, consent should be obtained from the next of kin. If the next of kin cannot be contacted, an effort should be made to obtain judicial appointment of a guardian before starting treatment.

Leaving Against Advice

Another point causing concern in the medical community is the refusal of a patient to give consent to medical treatment and his desire to leave the hospital against advice. This situation is often encountered in the emergency ward when a patient who has waited a long time for treatment becomes irate and wants to leave. It may also occur when a patient clearly in need of medical treatment decides for other reasons that he no longer wishes to be in the hospital. As long as the patient is capable of understanding the nature of his acts, he should be free to refuse treatment or to leave the hospital against advice. It would be inappropriate to force the patient to be treated or to restrain him from leaving the hospital against his will. Differences in interpretation naturally exist as to a given patient's ability to understand the nature of his acts. Some physicians believe that any patient refusing a lifesaving operation must be incapable of such understanding. That conclusion is illogical, and the patient's refusal cannot be the sole evidence of his incompetence.

It is important that the medical record clearly set forth the circumstances of the case and the actions taken by the physician and the patient. A signed form of discharge "against medical advice" is helpful, but if the patient refuses to execute such a document, his request to leave should still be honored.

Child Abuse

In situations of suspected child abuse, the physician is entirely justified in refusing to release a child to anyone before reporting the case to the local authorities. The reason for this is that the physician cannot determine who inflicted the injury and he might be inadvertently releasing the child to the abuser. In the absence of clear evidence as to the origin of the injury, the physician should always seek legal assistance before releasing the patient.

Police Cases

The police are frequently present in the emergency ward. Not only do they bring patients into the hospital but they also commonly visit the emergency ward to obtain information regarding a patient's status or treatment. The police may request copies of the patient's medical record, blood samples for alcohol testing after automobile accidents, weapons or drugs brought in by the patient, or the patient's clothing or other personal property. Although it is reasonable to cooperate as much as possible, health care providers should always maintain a certain amount of discretion— not, however, to the extent of acting as a legal guardian and refusing to release any information. If the police request a copy of the medical record, they should be referred to the medical record administrator. Likewise, if they desire release of personal property, the patient's consent should be secured if it is possible. In both cases, the police have greater rights if the patient is under arrest than if he is merely under suspicion. In cases of requests for blood samples or for results of specific tests, the physician should consult with the hospital's legal advisors.

Psychiatric Patients

Care of the psychiatric patient can be a problem because of uncertainty as to the patient's mental capability to give an informed consent. Whenever a patient is obviously in danger of harming himself or those around him, care should be taken to protect everyone. In most states, legislation allows temporary commitment of such a patient to an appropriate facility for observation. In the absence of such legislation, it is reasonable to consider restraint if it is indicated. The decision must be made whether personnel should restrain the patient and risk a lawsuit for either false imprisonment or battery or whether they should do nothing and risk that the patient or others might be injured and sue on the grounds of negligence. Usually a patient may not be restrained except on the orders of a physician, but if the situation warrants, the patient should be restrained without such orders, on the premise that such an action is in the best interest of the patient.

Concealed Weapons

A routine examination may uncover concealed weapons or drugs. In most cases involving weapons a security officer or a police officer should be summoned if possible. If such an officer is unavailable, emergency ward personnel should exercise the utmost discretion and judgment in their actions. Emergency ward personnel should likewise use discretion in removing drugs from the patient.

Rape

Victims of rape are often evaluated in the emergency ward. It is essential that the examining physician limit his role to assessment of the medical condition of the patient. Attention should be paid to every aspect of the physical condition and findings should be carefully recorded. The patient may wish to relieve her tension by narrating the events of the attack. Although this is psychologically desirable for the patient, the medical record should not detail such a narration. A simple sentence noting the patient's allegation of sexual assault is sufficient. The physician who sets forth the patient's story in detail can be established as a witness to testimony that may conflict with subsequent statements. Since the defense against a claim of rape is often based on inconsistencies in testimony, the physician may have to testify personally and may be "caught in the middle."

Telephone Advice

It is important to give advice over the telephone in most cases. A physician cannot be assured that the information he has received is complete; to draw conclusions from such data is legally indefensible and, more importantly, is not in the best interest of the patient. It is best to ask the patient to come to the hospital or to dispatch an ambulance to him if this is indicated. The only exception might be in the case of a life-threatening emergency, such as ingestion of a known toxic material. In this instance it is reasonable to give therapeutic advice to the patient or to those with him while they wait for the ambulance.

Requests for Information

All requests by patients and others for information, such as copies of the medical record, recorded opinions in workmen's compensation cases, and test results, should be forwarded to the medical record administrator, who assures that appropriate authorizations have been submitted and that patient propriety is maintained. This procedure should be followed for all requests, whether oral or written, from any source. Such

Table 39.1.
Massachusetts Department of Public Health list of reportable diseases.

Reportable to Local Board of Health	Ophthalmia neonatorum
Actinomycosis	Plague
Animal bite	Poliomyelitis
Anthrax	Psittacosis
Brucellosis (undulant fever)	Rabies, human
Chickenpox (varicella)	Rickettsialpox
Cholera	Rocky Mountain spotted fever
Diarrhea of the newborn	Salmonellosis (except typhi and paratyphi)
Diphtheria	Salmonellosis: typhi and paratyphi (typhoid and
Dysentery	paratyphoid fevers)
Amebic	Smallpox (variola)
Bacillary (shigellosis)	Smallpox vaccination reactions
Encephalitis (specify if known)	Generalized vaccinia
Food poisoning	Eczema vaccinatum
Botulism	Streptococcal infections (including erysipelas,
Mushrooms and other poisonous vegetable	scarlet fever, streptococcal sore throat, etc.)
and animal products	Tetanus
Mineral or organic poisons such as arsenic,	Trachoma
lead, etc.	Trichinosis
Staphylococcal	Tuberculosis
German measles (rubella)	Tularemia
Glanders	Typhus fever (including Brill's disease)
Hepatitis, viral (includes infectious and serum	Whooping cough (pertussis)
hepatitis)	Yellow fever
Impetigo of the newborn	
Leprosy	*Reportable Directly to State Department of*
Leptospirosis (including Weil's disease)	*Public Health*
Lymphocytic choriomeningitis	Acquired Immune Deficiency Syndrome (AIDS)
Malaria	Chancroid
Measles (rubeola)	Gonorrhea
Meningitis (B. influenzal, meningococcal, pneu-	Granuloma inguinale
mococcal, streptococcal, and other forms)	Lymphogranuloma venereum
Mumps	Syphilis

requests can come from investigative agencies such as the Federal Bureau of Investigation, from administration agencies such as the Industrial Accident Board, from the press, from a friend or relative of the patient, or from the patient himself. Many hospitals have public relations officers and clearly formulated guidelines concerning release of information to the news media.

Reportable Injuries and Diseases

The types of injury and communicable disease that must be reported to the authorities vary with the state and locality. A similar variation exists in the types of case that must be reported to the medical examiner (coroner). Emergency ward administrators should be aware of statutory and regulatory requirements in their area. Reportable injuries and diseases in the Commonwealth of Massachusetts are listed in Table 39.1.

CONCLUSIONS

The best rule to follow in situations with legal ramifications is to exercise reasonable judgment and common sense. The law is not as concerned with the rightness or wrongness of a particular act as it is with its defensibility under the circumstances, as judged by practitioners who have faced the same or similar circumstances. It is impossible to chronicle all the situations with legal aspects and to suggest all solutions. It has been my intention rather to give the reader a proper perspective of the law relative to daily practice in the emergency ward.

Suggested References

Lobstein JFD: *A General Guide for Practising Physicians in the Examination of the Sick with An Appendix of Medical Formulae.* Philadelphia, Lewis D. Belair, 1823
Weed LL: Quality control and the medical record. *Arch Intern Med 127:* 101–105, 1971

CHAPTER 40

The Emergency Ward: A Human Focus

ISABELLA TIGHE, M.B.A.

Many studies have been performed describing why patients go to emergency wards. Although *ways to monitor care* have been described, no study has ever reported on the *quality of caring* in the emergency setting. The emergency ward is designed to deal quickly and efficiently with the saving of life, the palliation of pain, and the curing of disease by drawing on the knowledge of its personnel and the advances of contemporary technology. But what about the basic attitudes of humaneness, compassion, and understanding, and the role that they play in providing effective emergency care? Too often we are concerned with the life and breath and not with the heart and feelings.

The late Dr. Francis Weld Peabody, Professor of Medicine at Harvard Medical School, once said, "The secret of the care of the patient is in caring for the patient." Although these words were originally directed to the medical student in an effort to emphasize the emotional needs of the patient, they have become increasingly relevant to all persons involved in the delivery of health care. Today, many hospitals have become so large and, to the patient, so confusing and alienating that the responsibility for caring for the patient now rests on all hospital personnel. As the contacts of the patient within the hospital system have grown increasingly complex, in many instances the patient's feelings of isolation have intensified and opportunities to redress grievances and to pursue explanations or reassurance have diminished in the press for greater diagnostic and therapeutic potency, efficiency, and lower cost.

No area in the hospital is more likely to witness patient frustration than the emergency ward. It is there that the patient may get his first—and possibly his only—view of what the hospital is really like. When faced with complaints such as long waits, incorrect billings, the poor attitude of personnel, and "rotten" care, many staff members quickly defend the situation by explaining how busy they are, that they are providing a high quality of medical care, and that half the patients seen in the emergency ward should not be there anyway! However, if a patient has come to the hospital thinking that he needs emergency care and if he must wait a long time before he is helped, is it any wonder that anger mounts to the point where he leaves, taking with him a poor impression of the hospital that he willingly shares with all who will listen? Is it so difficult for a member of the staff to take the time to soothe the patient's growing irritation by a kind word of explanation?

It is unfortunate that many of the impressions that patients may have about hospitals are developed long before they need medical treatment. Situation television programs, for example, have furnished large audiences with mistaken notions of how health care is and should be administered, and are the standard against which some persons judge the health care delivery system.

In response to these problems and in an effort to humanize and to personalize the hospital environment, to provide "pathways for the uninitiated", and to improve the continuum of patient care, the Massachusetts General Hospital established the Patient Care Representative Office. Representatives serve as liaisons between the health care consumer and the institution, responding to the problems, requests, and complaints of patients and their families. The patient care representative is valuable in several ways. By delivering assistance and direction to patients and families, the representative becomes a warm and human focus in what otherwise may seem a hostile and confusing environment. By calling attention to systematized poor practice and by identifying patterns of complaints and requests, the representative acts on each patient's behalf to effect change. Objectives of the position include the following:

(1) Provision of emotional support to patients.

(2) Utilization of the existent resources of the institution to reduce the patient's feelings of isolation and to alleviate the dehumanizing effect of a hospital stay.

(3) Introduction of needed changes into the pattern of health care delivery in an effort to improve the quality of care, identification of problems in interdepartmental communication, and expedition of their resolution.

(4) "Defusion" of anger and reduction of "hospital-as-adversary" feelings, with the consequence of diminished lawsuits and claims against the hospital.

(5) Enhancement of the hospital's public image by increasing patient satisfaction.

There are three patient care representatives and a secretary in the Patient Care Representative Office. The representatives have the authority to deal with all referrals. They consult with staff in all departments of the hospital and see patients on every service. Floor personnel are encouraged to handle any problems that they believe they can manage themselves. In cases of referral, the patient care representative may not always see the patient, but may ask the help of a staff member outside the office who can best address or resolve the particular issue. The Patient Care Representative Office first provides backup for the resolution of the individual problem; it then applies the experience gained from this process to the resolution of recurrent patterns of complaints and requests.

Patient needs and dissatisfactions are communicated to the patient care representatives by:

(1) Telephone calls—the staff is available 24 hours a day, 7 days a week through the use of a portable signal device (Beeper) during non-office hours.

(2) Office visits.

(3) Patient contacts during floor visits either by the patient care representative or by a member of the Volunteer Patient Care Committee.

(4) Letters, which can be mailed either to the Patient Care Representative Office or to the general director of the hospital and subsequently referred to the office.

(5) Referrals from staff—since hospital personnel are the primary source of referrals, they participate in regular training sessions designed to make them aware of the patient's expectations and anxieties.

(6) Referrals from relatives or friends.

In any discussion about the human focus in the emergency ward, the problem of sudden death must be mentioned. Families must be supported and given time to recover somewhat from the shock of losing a loved one. It is important that the family have the opportunity to speak with the physician and to know that everything possible was done for the patient.

Good quality care must be coupled with warmth and kindness. Emergency wards are frightening places for most patients. We must learn to deliver care with a smile, with efficiency, and with politeness. Let us take time to see our patients not as statistics but as human beings with emotions such as our own. Let us pause to hold the hand of one in pain, to take a few moments with one who is anxious, to understand and care and to communicate that caring to the patient, thereby allaying his anxiety and relieving his isolation.

SECTION 5

Illustrated Techniques

Original drawings by Edith Tagrin

ILLUSTRATED TECHNIQUES

This section, "Illustrated Techniques," is designed to provide a visual and instructive aid to the placement of the more common "invasive" devices, including life-saving airway tubes, monitoring lines, and diagnostic or therapeutic catheters. Some of these techniques may differ from written accounts in previous chapters; when they do, it is to offer an alternative method or to emphasize recognized differences in styles of management. The following seventeen emergency procedures are illustrated:

1. OROTRACHEAL INTUBATION
2. NASOTRACHEAL INTUBATION
3. CRICOTHYROTOMY
4. SUBCLAVIAN VEIN CATHETER PLACEMENT
5. INTERNAL JUGULAR VEIN CATHETERIZATION
6. SAPHENOUS VEIN CUTDOWN
7. INSERTION OF TRANSVENOUS VENTRICULAR PACING ELECTRODE
8. PERICARDIOCENTESIS
9. THORACENTESIS
10. CHEST TUBE INSERTION
11. LUMBAR PUNCTURE
12. PERITONEAL LAVAGE
13. PERCUTANEOUS SUPRAPUBIC CYSTOTOMY
14. CULDOCENTESIS
15. SHOULDER—INJECTION FOR BURSITIS
16. ARTHROCENTESIS—KNEE
17. ARTHROCENTESIS—ANKLE

1. OROTRACHEAL INTUBATION

DAVID J. CULLEN, M.D.

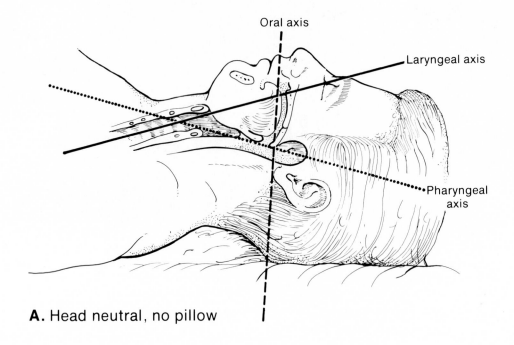

A. Head neutral, no pillow

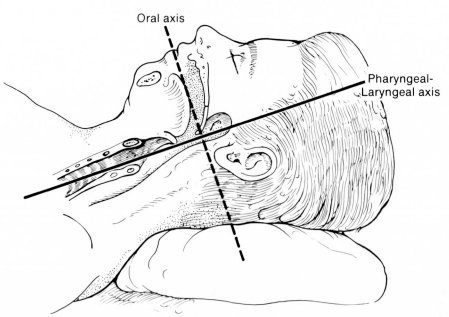

B. Head neutral, pillow under head

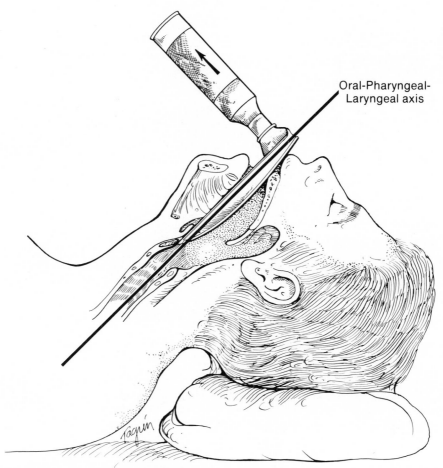

Oral-Pharyngeal-Laryngeal axis

C. Head extended, pillow under head

(A–C) When the head is supported by a pillow or blanket and is placed in the "sniff" position, the oral, pharyngeal and laryngeal axes merge toward one plane. Deviations from this position cause the axes to diverge, which makes intubation more difficult.

The sniff position with the head hyperextended affords a straight-line view to the vocal cords. A curved-blade (Macintosh) laryngoscope is placed in the mouth from the right side, sweeping the tongue to the left. The blade is inserted anteriorly into the vallecula; anterior force lifts the epiglottis and opens the view to the vocal cords. If a straight blade (Miller or Foregger) is used, it is inserted to just beyond the tip of the epiglottis. With lifting of the epiglottis the cords can be seen directly.

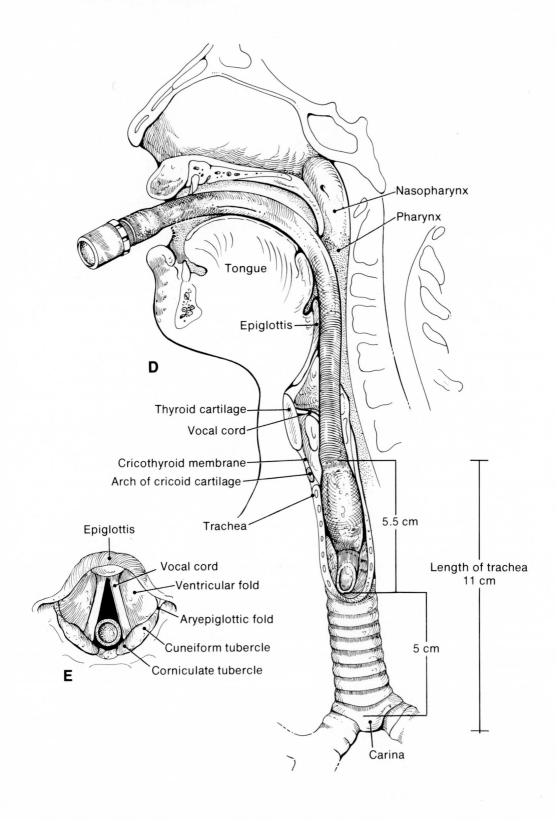

Nasopharynx

Pharynx

Tongue

Epiglottis

D

Thyroid cartilage

Vocal cord

Cricothyroid membrane

Arch of cricoid cartilage

Trachea

5.5 cm

Length of trachea
11 cm

Epiglottis

Vocal cord

Ventricular fold

Aryepiglottic fold

Cuneiform tubercle

Corniculate tubercle

E

5 cm

Carina

(D–E) Technical considerations: (1) The laryngoscope is not to be used as a level to pry the glottis open. After insertion, the entire blade and handle are lifted anteriorly to pull the jaw in a vector toward the operator's eyes. (2) Tubes with a slight curve at the tip are easier to direct into the trachea, particularly when a curved blade is used. Some tracheas angle anteriorly and a curved tube fits the angulation well. (3) For emergency intubation, a stiff tube will best resist kinking or bending as the tube is inserted into the trachea. (4) Use of a stylet will result in a fixed curve and a stiff tube at the tube's entry into the trachea. Once the tip of the tube is just beyond the vocal cords, the stylet should be removed to prevent trauma to the larynx and trachea. (5) On viewing the glottis, the physician usually sees a dark hole bordered by the two vocal cords, which appear pearl-gray. (6) Once the tube tip is through the cords, the tube should be inserted until the proximal end of the cuff is just beyond the cords. This will locate the tip of the tube in the middle part of the trachea. Since the trachea in adults is approximately 11 cm long and since the proximal end of the cuff is about 5 cm from the tip of the tube, intubation of the right mainstem bronchus can be avoided. (7) The two most serious errors in intubation are: (a) intubating the esophagus instead of the trachea, and (b) inserting the endotracheal tube into the right mainstem bronchus. When the esophagus has been intubated, a characteristic gurgling sound is emitted with each positive-pressure breath, the chest wall does not rise, and the abdomen increases in size. If any doubt exists, the patient should be auscultated over the stomach while being ventilated. If the right mainstem bronchus has been intubated, breath sounds may be absent on the left side, but this is not always reliable. Pulmonary compliance will be low, but in a patient requiring emergency intubation, compliance may be decreased already. The tube's location should be ensured either by chest x-ray examination or by direct visualization of the cuff just beyond the vocal cords.

2. NASOENDOTRACHEAL INTUBATION

DAVID J. CULLEN, M.D.

PREINTUBATION ASSESSMENT

Determine whether nasotracheal intubation is even possible or desirable when compared to the need for orotracheal intubation. Check for patency of the nares and, if possible, obtain information from the patient concerning previous difficulties in breathing through the nose.

If movement of the neck is not contraindicated (due to possible cervical spine injury), check for neck mobility by flexing and extending the head in order to determine optimal position for intubation.

INDICATIONS FOR NASOTRACHEAL INTUBATION

Nasotracheal intubation is indicated:

when airway obstruction actually is present or is likely to occur;

when airway protection from aspiration cannot be guaranteed;

when full exposure of the mouth for repair of intraoral injuries or restorative work is needed;

when anatomic abnormalities, trauma, diseases of the upper airway, or inexperience of the operator make direct laryngoscopy difficult, dangerous, or impossible;

when, in the opinion of some observers, long-term intubation and ventilation are anticipated, a nasotracheal tube is usually more stable and fixed, there is less chance of the tube kinking, and there is greater comfort to the awake patient.

AWAKE VS. ANESTHETIZED NASOTRACHEAL INTUBATION

When direct laryngoscopy or positive pressure ventilation after induction of anesthesia may be hazardous, awake nasotracheal intubation is particularly valuable. Otherwise, when anesthesia can be induced safely by mask, direct nasotracheal intubation can proceed blindly after induction of anesthesia or under direct vision after proper intubating conditions have been achieved. However, *in the emergency ward, awake blind nasal intubation is the most useful approach to securing the airway.*

PROCEDURE

Topically anesthetize the nasal mucosa with no more than 5 ml of 4% cocaine. This provides local anesthesia to the nose and nasopharynx and minimizes the possibility of epistaxis. If the patient does not have a full stomach (unlikely in an emergency ward), complete topical anesthesia of the tongue, pharynx, glottis, and vocal cords may be accomplished with topical lidocaine. However,

most patients must be assumed to have a full stomach or will be unconscious enough so that additional anesthesia to areas other than just the nasal mucosa is contraindicated.

The nostril chosen for intubation usually depends on anatomic and pathologic considerations. Check which nostril is more patent.

Obviously, the nasotracheal tube size will depend on the size and sex of the patient. A 7-mm internal diameter tube for most women and an 8-mm tube for most men, each with a large-volume, low-pressure cuff, is usually appropriate.

(A–B) After introducing a well lubricated nasotracheal tube into the chosen nostril using gentle but persistent pressure, place the head in the sniff position to align the epiglottis with the pharynx and trachea. Of greatest importance in the spontaneously breathing patient is the character of breath sounds which are used to guide the tube toward the glottis. If these sounds diminish, the tube is deviating away from the glottis; if the breath sounds increase in loudness and clarity, the tube is moving closer to the glottic opening.

When the tube is well positioned near the glottis, wait until inspiration, then quickly advance the tube with the incoming breath since the vocal cord opening is widest during that time. If airway reflexes are still present, the cords will attempt to close when the tube touches the glottis, hence the need for swift insertion while the cords are patent. Patients frequently cough violently once the tube is actually in the trachea and confirmation of tube location begins by hearing tubular breath sounds and feeling air movement with each exhalation through the tube. Further confirmation of the tube location can be made by listening for bilateral breath sounds.

Obtain a portable chest x-ray to confirm introtracheal location definitely and to ensure that the tube has not been inserted beyond the trachea into the right mainstem bronchus.

PROBLEMS OF AWAKE NASOTRACHEAL INTUBATION

(C–D) If the tube impinges the neck anteriorly because the tube's curvature is excessive, inspection of the neck will demonstrate this. The tube needs to be more posterior in relation to the glottis which can be accomplished by further flexing the head, and gently pushing the glottis posteriorly.

(E–F) If the tube passes posteriorly into the esophagus because the tube curvature is insufficient to move anteriorly into the glottic opening, hyperextend the head.

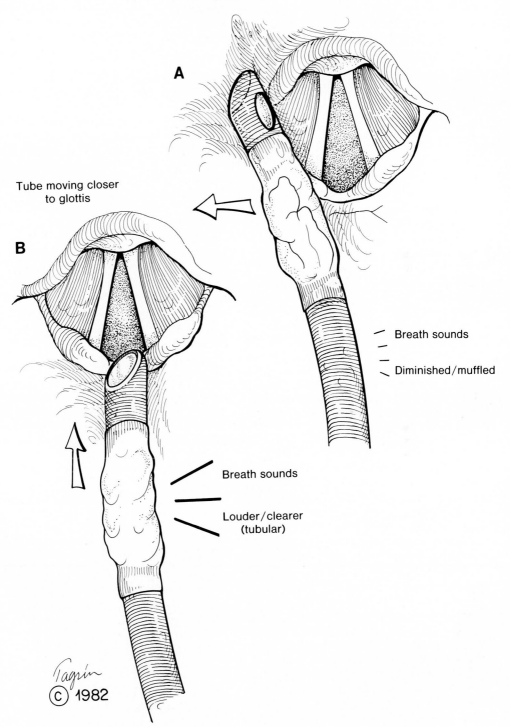

Tube deviating away
from glottis

A

Tube moving closer
to glottis

B

Breath sounds

Diminished/muffled

Breath sounds

Louder/clearer
(tubular)

© 1982

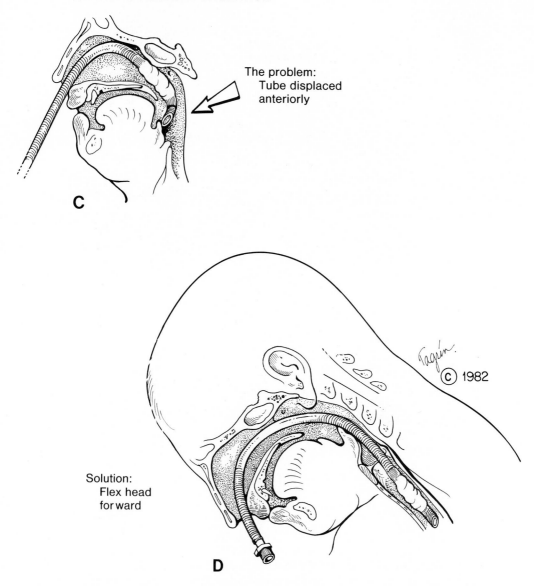

The problem:
Tube displaced
anteriorly

C

Solution:
Flex head
forward

© 1982

D

(G–I) If the tube is laterally displaced into the pyriform sinus which can be detected by seeing the neck bulge with movement of the tube, withdraw slightly and turn the tube toward the midline.

A variety of other techniques may be necessary to ensure placement of a nasotracheal tube in particularly difficult subjects, usually requiring an experienced operator. However, one can try tubes with greater or lesser curvatures, or attempt to insert a smaller tube than expected if the glottic opening is also smaller than anticipated. Obviously a stylette, useful in orotracheal intubation, cannot be used to obtain the desired tube curvature when the endotracheal tube is passed nasally.

If the patient is hypoxic, oxygen can be administered temporarily through the nasotracheal tube during the intubation process even though the tube still resides in the posterior pharynx. In the comatose patient with some degree of airway obstruction, the tube usually relieves such obstruction and allows oxygenation with spontaneous ventilation before placing the tube in the trachea.

COMPLICATIONS

Certain complications are specific to nasotracheal intubation (in addition to many of the same complications common to oral tracheal intubation).

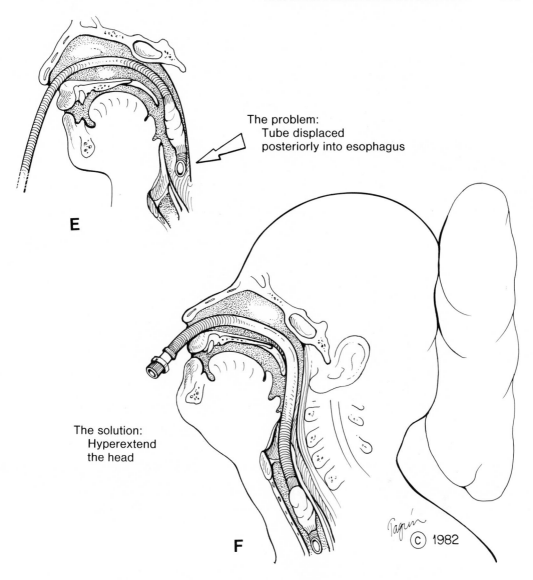

The problem:
Tube displaced
posteriorly into esophagus

E

The solution:
Hyperextend
the head

F

C 1982

Nasotracheal intubation may cause epistaxis which can be a severe problem particularly in the anticoagulated patient or the patient who develops a coagulopathy. Anterior and even posterior packing may be necessary as much blood may be lost.

The nasopharyngeal mucosa may be perforated to create a false passage, particularly if excessive force is used to advance the tube through the nasal pharynx. This usually can be detected if breath sounds are lost before the tube is inserted into the pharynx and further passage of the tube must cease.

Damage to the adenoids and/or tonsils may occur, particularly in children, even if care is used to advance the tube. A well lubricated tube passed gently usually avoids this problem.

Long-term complications include:
1. necrosis of the nasal cartilage if the tube is incorrectly fixed in position;
2. obstruction of the Eustachian tube which may impair hearing;
3. maxillary sinusitis because drainage of the sinus is prevented by the presence of the tube;
4. meningitis in patients with a cerebrospinal fluid leak via a fracture of the cribriform plate.

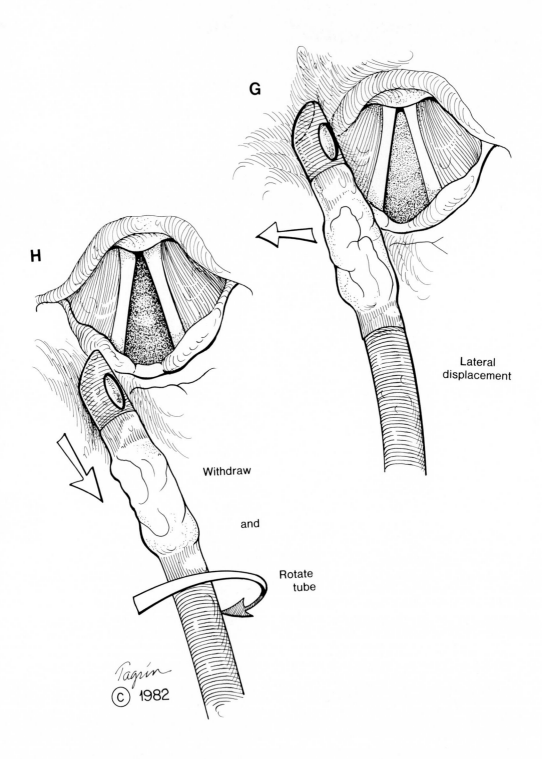

G

Lateral
displacement

H

Withdraw

and

Rotate
tube

Tagrin
© 1982

I

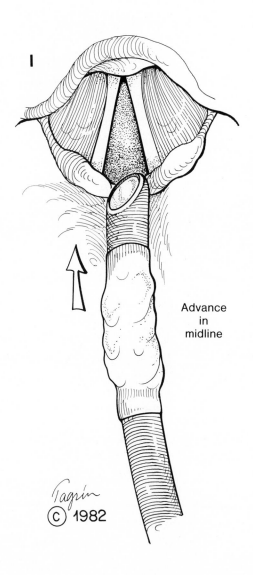

Advance
in
midline

© 1982

3. CRICOTHYROTOMY

ASHBY C. MONCURE, M.D.

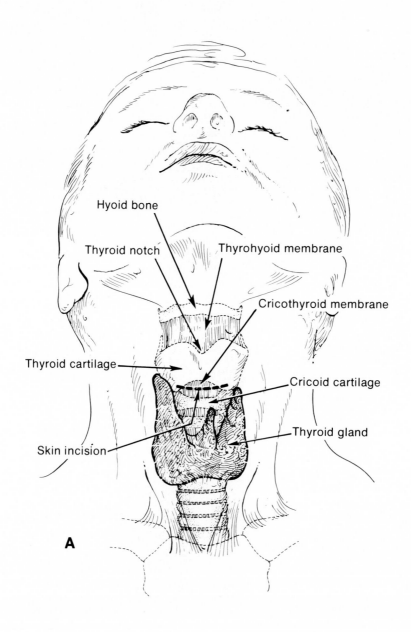

- Hyoid bone
- Thyroid notch
- Thyrohyoid membrane
- Cricothyroid membrane
- Thyroid cartilage
- Cricoid cartilage
- Thyroid gland
- Skin incision

A

Control of the airway usually can be gained by insertion of an endotracheal tube via the oropharynx or nasopharynx. Occasionally a bronchoscope can be utilized to achieve control quickly. If neither of these methods can be accomplished promptly, the obstructed airway is best managed by an incision through the cricothyroid membrane.

(A) With the patient's neck extended. the depression between the thyroid cartilage and the cricoid cartilage in the anterior midline is identified and a 2-cm transverse incision is made, centered in the anterior midline. The thumb and index finger are used to spread the wound apart in order to identify the cricothyroid membrane, which is incised horizontally on the cephalad edge of the cricoid cartilage.

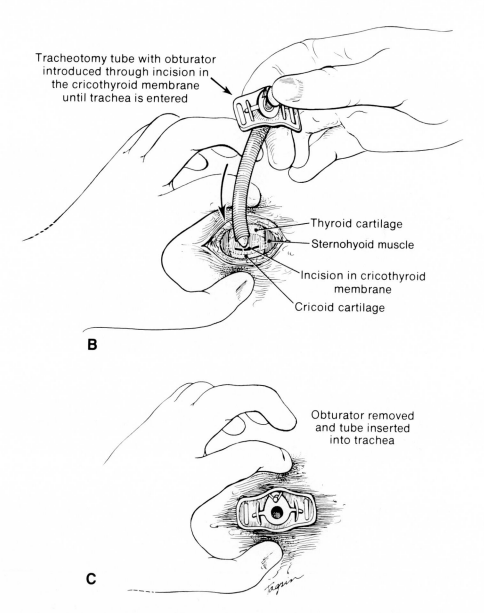

Tracheotomy tube with obturator introduced through incision in the cricothyroid membrane until trachea is entered

Thyroid cartilage

Sternohyoid muscle

Incision in cricothyroid membrane

Cricoid cartilage

B

Obturator removed and tube inserted into trachea

C

(B) A No. 3 or No. 4 silver tracheotomy tube with an indwelling obturator is inserted into the trachea. **(C)** The obturator is removed and endotracheal ventilation and suction are carried out without use of an inner cannula. Thereafter, tracheal intubation via the oropharynx can again be attempted, and if efforts are unsuccessful, conventional tracheotomy can be carried out.

4. SUBCLAVIAN VEIN CATHETER PLACEMENT

RITA COLLEY, R.N.
HERBERT FREUND, M.D.
JOSEF E. FISCHER, M.D.

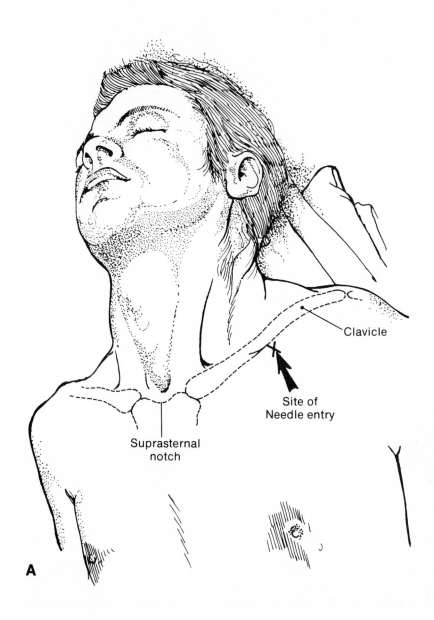

(A) The patient is placed in Trendelenburg's position to increase venous pressure. A towel roll under the cervicothoracic vertebrae allows the pa- tient's shoulders to drop back and the clavicles to rise.

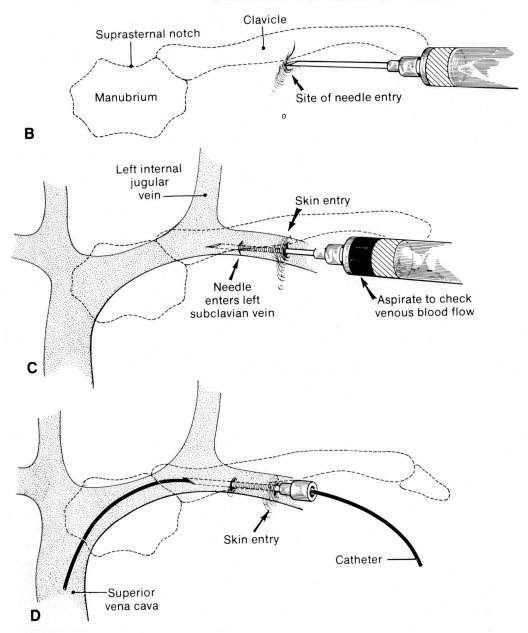

(B) After the skin surface is prepared with acetone and scrubbed with 2% iodine solution, the skin and underlying tissue are infiltrated with lidocaine (Xylocaine). Lidocaine is infiltrated along the needle track and the subclavian vein is located with the 22-gauge needle used for infiltration of the local anesthetic. The skin is then punctured with a 14-gauge needle along the middle third of the clavicle beneath the bony prominence. After puncture, aspiration should be constant to determine venous entry. **(C)** The needle is advanced to enter the subclavian vein. Entry is verified by aspiration of free-flowing blood into the syringe. **(D)** The bevel of the needle is turned caudad. The patient is told to take a deep breath and to hold it. After 2–3 seconds, the syringe is removed and a 16-gauge Intracath is inserted through the needle and advanced into the superior vena cava. The patient may then breathe normally again. The purpose of having the patient hold his breath is to prevent air embolism.

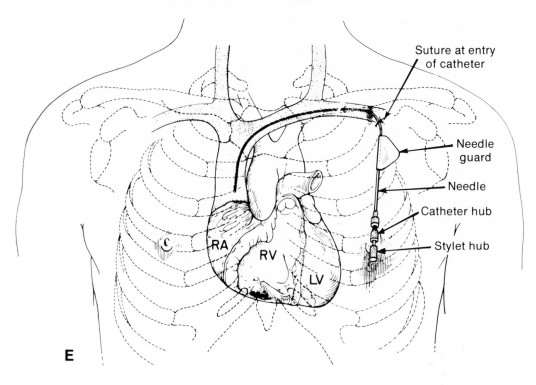

Suture at entry of catheter

Needle guard

Needle

Catheter hub

Stylet hub

RA

RV

LV

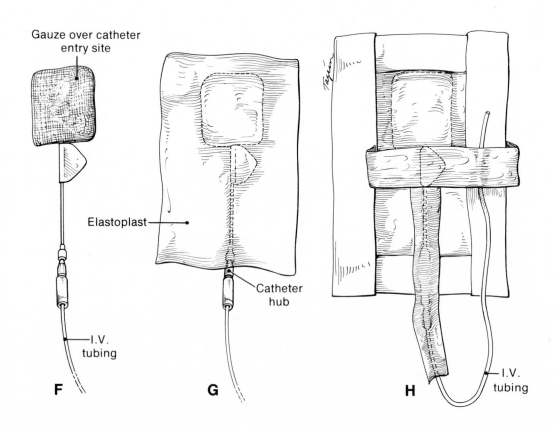

Gauze over catheter entry site

Elastoplast

Catheter hub

I.V. tubing

I.V. tubing

F

G

H

(E) The needle is pulled back over the catheter and locked into the catheter hub with a twisting motion. A needle guard is then clipped over the needle. After a single suture is placed at the insertion side to immobilize the catheter, the stylet is withdrawn, again with maintenance of the Valsalva maneuver while the catheter is open to air.

(F) Intravenous tubing is joined to the catheter hub and locked in with a twisting motion. Iodophor ointment is then placed on the catheter insertion site, and the site is covered with small gauze sponges. (G) After the larger area of skin around the puncture site and the needle is treated with tincture of benzoin, occlusive dressing (Elastoplast) is applied. The bandage comes *half-way* down the catheter hub; this allows the intravenous tubing to be changed without destroying the occlusive quality of the dressing. (H) One-inch ad-

hesive tape secures all sides of the dressing and all intravenous tubing junctions. It also anchors the intravenous tubing to the dressing.

Beware of possible complications from subclavian catheter placement: pneumothorax, hemothorax, hydrothorax, inadvertent arterial puncture, air embolus, catheter embolus, brachial plexus injury, hemorrhage, and cardiac irritability. To avoid complications, obtain a chest x-ray film after placement, withdraw the catheter tip from the atrium if necessary, apply appropriate direct pressure if an artery has been entered, have the patient perform the Valsalva maneuver when the catheter is open to air, give transfusions or vitamin K if necessary before catheterization, and observe the patient carefully for signs and symptoms of clinical deterioration.

5. INTERNAL JUGULAR VEIN CATHETERIZATION

CHARLES J. McCABE, M.D.

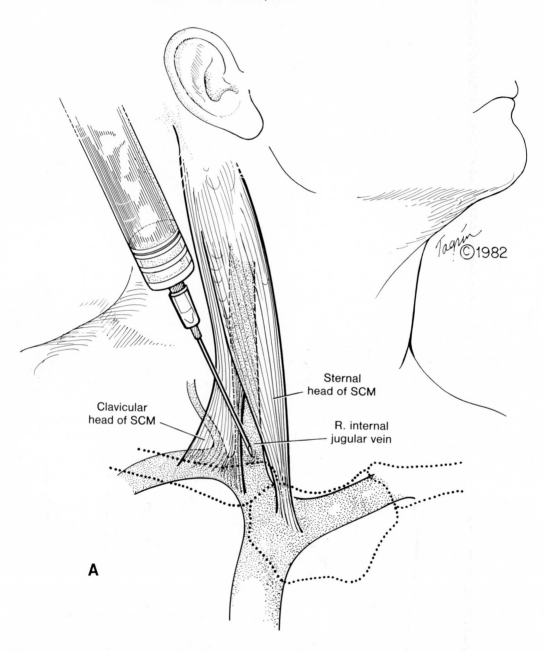

Sternal head of SCM

Clavicular head of SCM

R. internal jugular vein

©1982

A

(A) The approach to the internal jugular vein is between the sternal and clavicular heads of the sternocleidomastoid muscle. The patient is placed in 30° of Trendelenburg's position in order to distend the vein. Sterile prepping and draping of the area is performed. The apex of the triangle between the two heads of the sternocleidomastoid muscle is used for the insertion of the needle. The carotid pulse is palpated and the head turned to the opposite side. The needle is directed lateral to the pulse, aiming at the ipsilateral nipple at a 30° angle to the horizontal. The initial location of the vein is done with an 18-gauge needle.

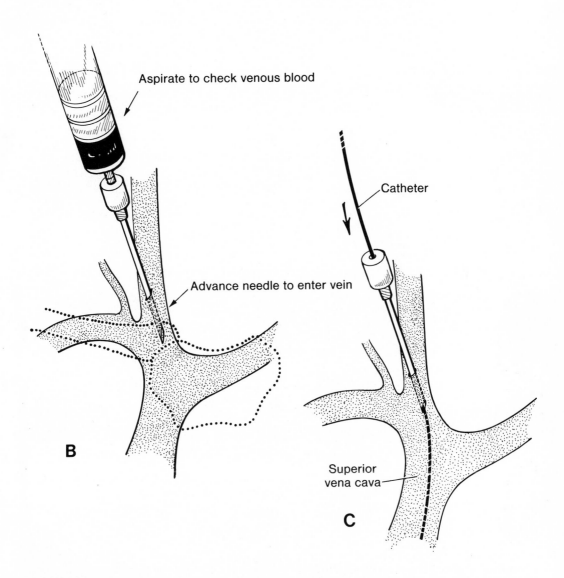

(B) Once the vein is located, the larger gauge needle then is inserted in the same direction as the smaller needle. The vein is entered and the venous blood is aspirated.

(C) Once good flow of venous blood is obtained, the syringe is removed and the patient is instructed to hold his/her breath. The catheter is inserted through the needle into the superior vena cava. If the catheter does not thread easily, the entire needle and catheter is removed as one piece to prevent sheering of the catheter. Another attempt is made.

6. SAPHENOUS VEIN CUTDOWN

CHARLES J. McCABE, M.D.

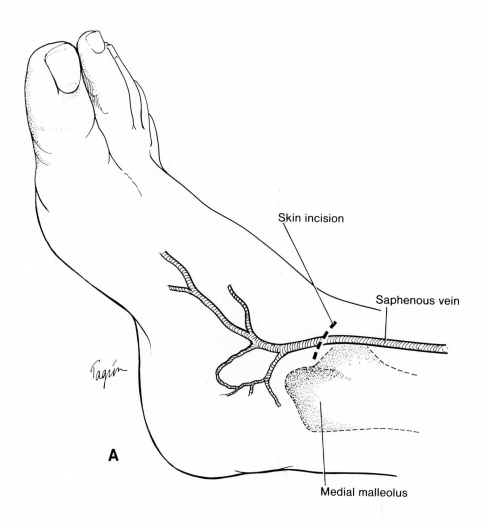

(A) The saphenous vein is located anteriorly and superiorly to the medial malleolus. After anesthetizing the skin, a 1½- to 2-cm transverse incision is made.

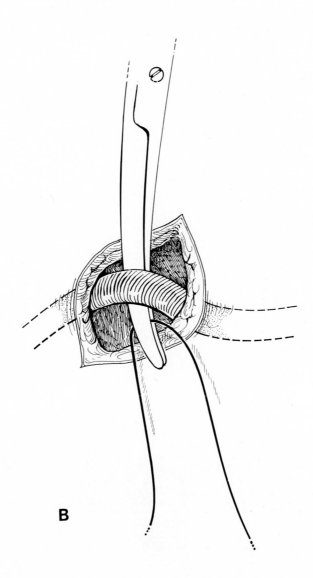

B

(B) The saphenous vein is located using blunt dissection with a curved hemostat. The vein is isolated by passing silk ligatures proximally and distally.

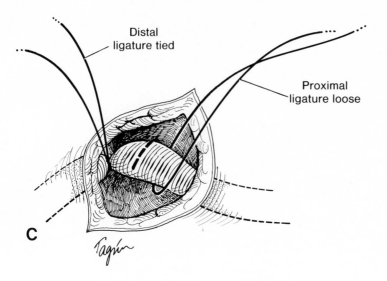

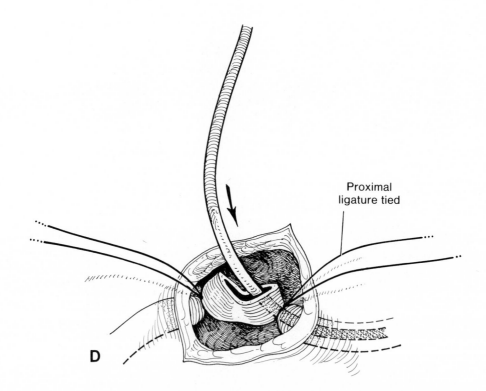

(C) The distal ligature is tied. A small incision is made in the anterior wall of the vein and the proximal ligature is used to control venous bleeding.

(D) The catheter is inserted through the incision in the vein. The proximal ligature is tied and the catheter is connected to the intravenous solution. The skin incision is closed and a sterile dressing applied.

7. INSERTION OF TRANSVENOUS VENTRICULAR PACING ELECTRODE

PETER C. BLOCK, M.D.

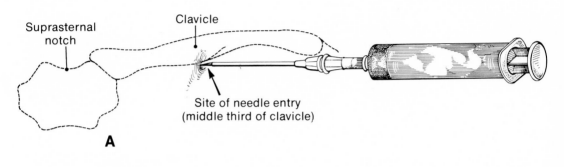

Suprasternal notch

Clavicle

Site of needle entry
(middle third of clavicle)

A

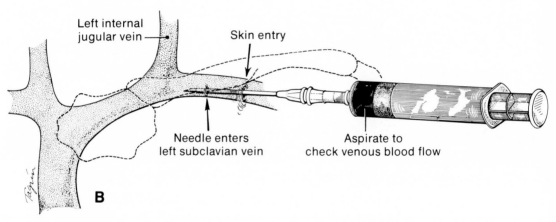

Left internal jugular vein

Skin entry

Needle enters
left subclavian vein

Aspirate to
check venous blood flow

B

The skin over the left subclavian vein should be prepared and draped with standard surgical technique. The left subclavian vein is preferred because of the natural "loop" of the pacing electrode, which facilitates passage across the tricuspid valve.

(A) With a No. 14 Angiocath, subclavian puncture is performed where the vein passes near the inferior clavicular surface along the middle third of the clavicle. **(B)** Venous blood should be aspirated to ensure proper placement of the cannula tip in the subclavian vein.

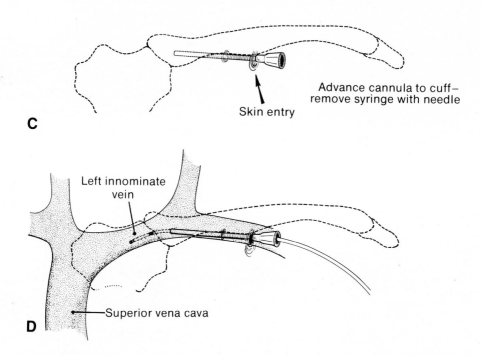

C

Skin entry

Advance cannula to cuff—
remove syringe with needle

D

Left innominate
vein

Superior vena cava

(C) The cannula is advanced slightly to maintain proper intravascular position, and the needle is removed. **(D)** The temporary pacing electrode is introduced through the cannula into the subclavian vein. Insertion of the electrode with the curved tip directed *inferiorly* facilitates passage into the left innominate vein and avoids cephalad passage into the internal jugular vein, which may occur if the tip is directed superiorly. The electrode is advanced approximately 15 cm. Electrocardiographic monitoring is then begun by attaching connected alligator clips to the proximal electrode terminal and to the V lead of the electrocardiograph.

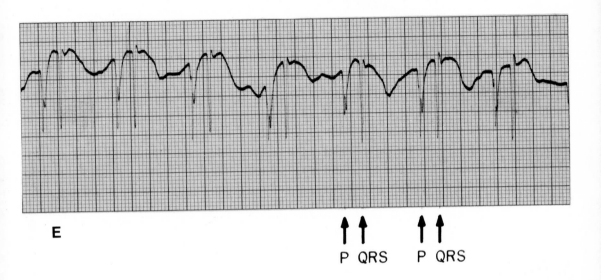

E

↑↑ ↑↑
P QRS P QRS

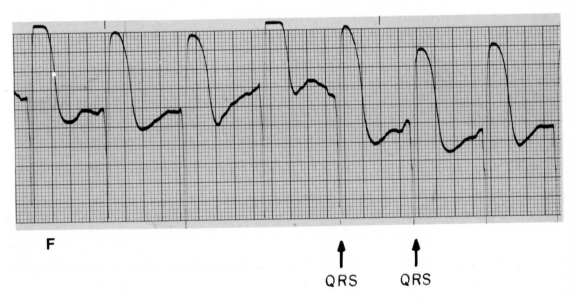

F

↑   ↑
QRS   QRS

(E) The V lead is monitored as the electrode is advanced into the right atrium, where the intra-atrial recording shows large spiked P waves.

(F) The electrode then is advanced across the tricuspid valve into the right ventricle, where the intraventricular recording shows its characteristic wide stylus displacement. One or two ventricular premature beats usually occur when the electrode tip first touches the right ventricular endocardium.

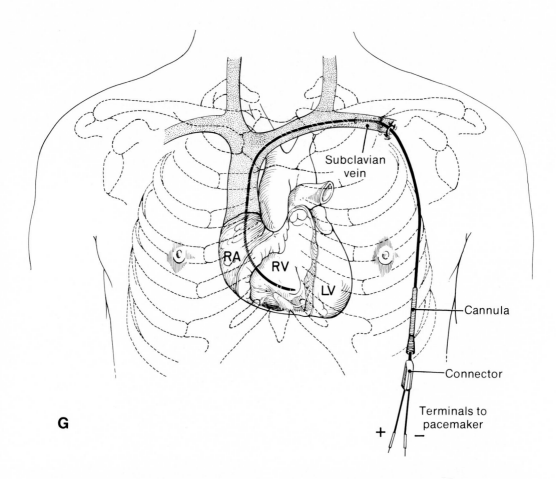

G

(G) At this point, the alligator clips are removed and the connector to the pacemaker is attached at the proximal end of the electrode. Pacing is begun and the threshold for pacing is determined. The threshold should preferably be less than 2 mA, but in emergency situations higher thresholds are acceptable. An ideal threshold is less than 1 mA. The cannula in the subclavian vein is carefully removed over the electrode without dislodging the electrode tip from the right ventricle and the electrode anchored to the skin at the insertion site with 3–0 silk.

The entire procedure must be performed under sterile conditions so that the electrode is not contaminated during insertion. A sterile dressing is applied at the end of the procedure to maintain sterility as long as possible.

8. PERICARDIOCENTESIS

A. JOHN ERDMAN III, M.D.

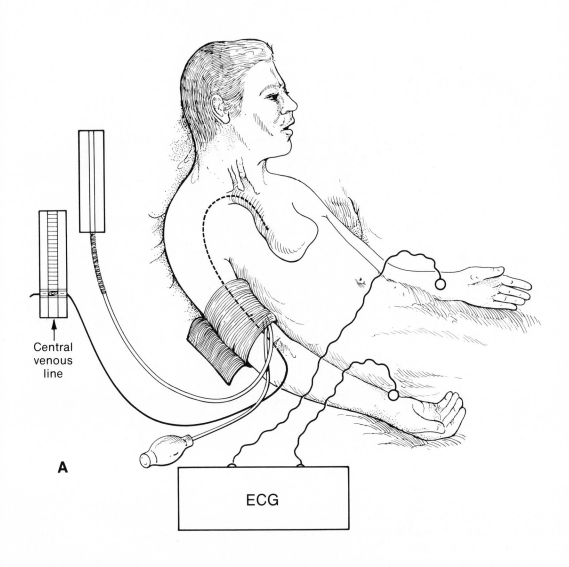

(A) The patient should be semi-recumbent. The electrocardiogram, systemic blood pressure and central venous pressure are followed. Continuous intra-arterial monitoring is extremely helpful.

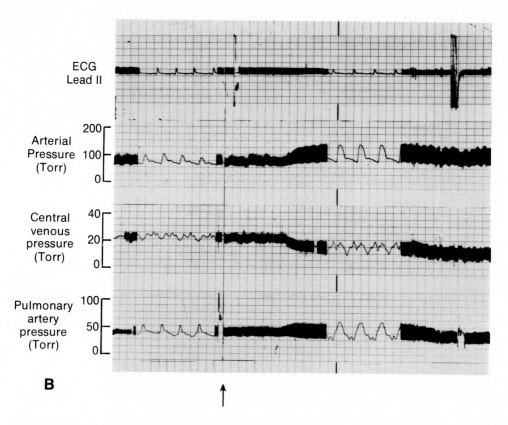

ECG
Lead II

Arterial
Pressure
(Torr)

200
100
0

Central
venous
pressure
(Torr)

40
20
0

Pulmonary
artery
pressure
(Torr)

100
50
0

B

↑

(B) Hemodynamic tracings of a patient with acute pericardial tamponade. Before drainage the central venous pressure is 25 mm Hg and the aortic pressure is 100/70 with marked pulsus paradoxus. At the *arrow* the needle is inserted into the pericardial space. A brief current of injury is obtained on the electrocardiogram, but fluid is then withdrawn. First the venous pressure falls and then the arterial pressure begins to rise. Simultaneously, the pulmonary arterial pressure falls, the pulsus paradoxus disappears, and hemodynamic stability is restored.

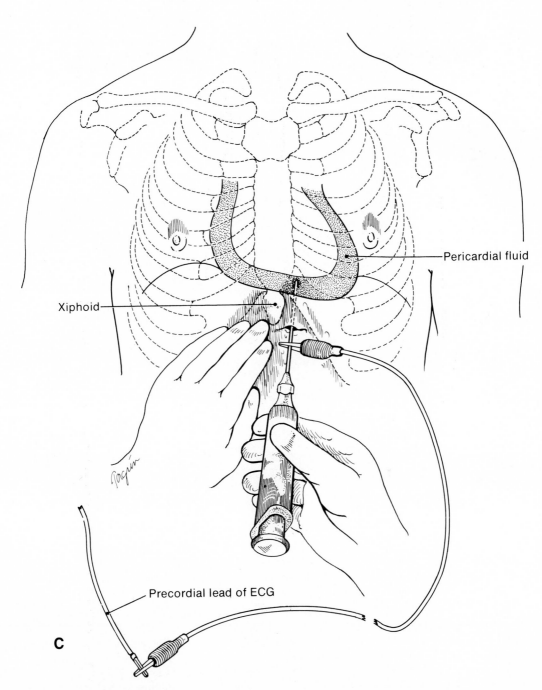

(C) Local anesthesia is obtained with 1% lido-caine (Xylocaine). General anesthesia should not be used in a patient with pericardial tamponade because it may precipitate profound hypotension. An 18-gauge spinal needle is insinuated beneath the xiphoid process, with continuous monitoring of the electrocardiogram through sterile alligator clips attached to the needle and to the precordial lead. The needle is advanced almost parallel with the skin and directed cephalad until either a current of injury is obtained on the tracing or blood or other fluid is aspirated with the syringe.

9. THORACENTESIS

EARLE W. WILKINS, JR., M.D.

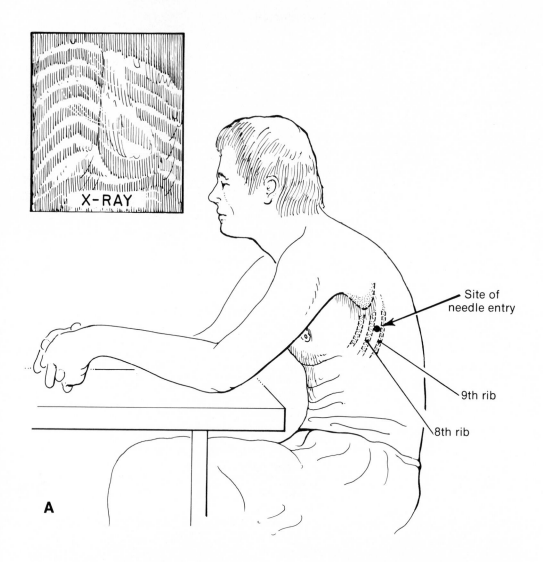

This technique of thoracentesis is offered as an alternative to that described in Chapter 22.

(A) The patient is comfortably seated with arms held forward and forearms resting on a movable table. A chest x-ray film is at hand to permit identification of the proper side and rib level for aspiration. The site for entry is selected below the meniscus of fluid level and well above the diaphragm, and the skin and proposed tract for the thoracentesis needle are infiltrated with 1% lidocaine (Xylocaine) without epinephrine.

(B) The sterile No. 14 intracath needle is inserted close to the lower rib (here shown as the 9th) to avoid laceration of the intercostal artery.

(C) The needle is advanced so that the entire bevel is just within the parietal pleura. (D) The plastic catheter is then guided, within its plastic covering, through the needle into the pleural fluid. (E) The needle is withdrawn, which minimizes the likelihood of laceration of the visceral pleura as fluid is aspirated and the lung expands. The collar of the catheter is attached to a three-way stopcock and 50-ml syringe for aspiration. A vacuum bottle of the type used for blood donation may be employed alternatively.

938

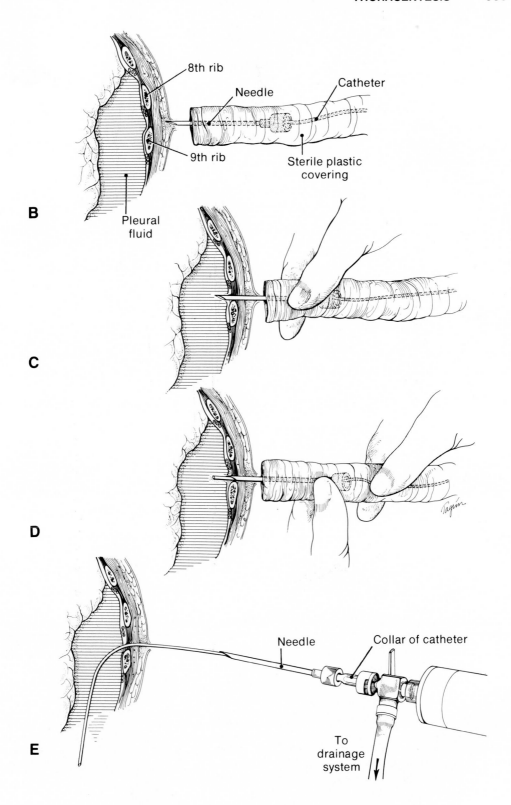

10. CHEST TUBE INSERTION

CHARLES J. McCABE, M.D.

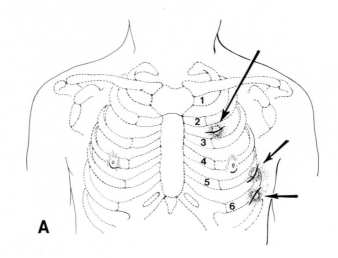

A

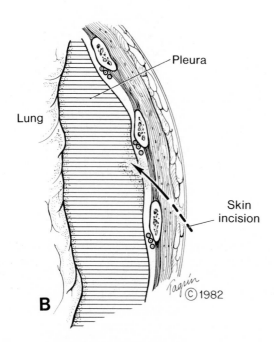

B

(**A**) The site of insertion is usually the 2nd intercostal space at the midclavicular line or the midaxillary line in the 5th or 6th interspace. A linear incision is made over the area of insertion after local anesthesia with 1% lidocaine (Xylocaine). Liberal use of lidocaine is recommended to provide anesthesia to the pleural level.

(**B**) The skin incision is made 2–3 cm below the interspace through which the chest tube will be inserted. This allows for a skin and subcutaneous flap to develop with insertion. The neurovascular bundle that runs along the under surface of the rib is avoided.

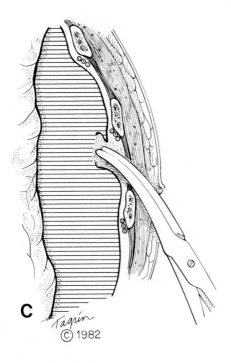

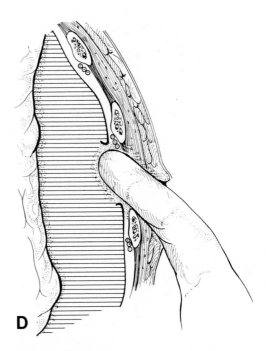

(C) A Kelly clamp is used to spread the subcutaneous tissue and muscle fibers to allow penetration of the intercostal muscle.

(D) Once the intercostal muscles have been spread, the digit is inserted through the intercostal space and muscle so that no damage to the underlying lung will occur. This will allow digital exploration of a limited portion of the pleural space.

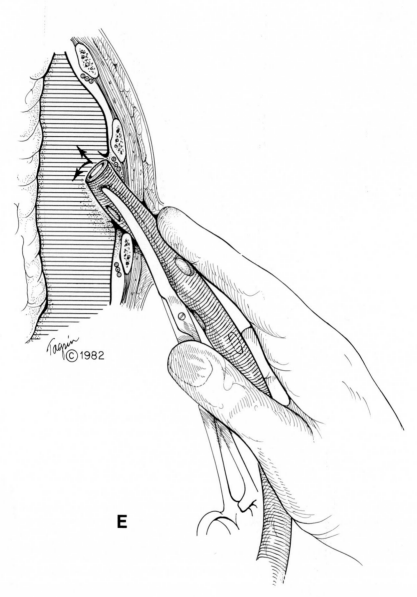

E

(E) After an adequate tract is made using the digit, the chest tube is inserted through the created tract. The chest tube is threaded superiorly or inferiorly. The chest tube should be inserted approximately 2–3 cm beyond the last hole in the catheter. The tube is secured to the chest wall with sutures and connected to the drainage device.

11. LUMBAR PUNCTURE

AMY A. PRUITT, M.D.

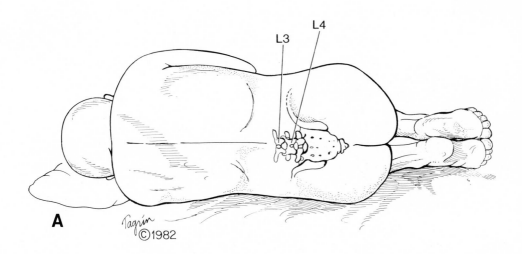

L3 L4

A

Tagrin
©1982

(**A-B**) Positioning the Patient. Whenever possible, place the patient on his side with the knees and hips flexed, the back perpendicular to the bed. For a right-handed physician, it is more convenient to have the patient on his left side while for a left-handed physician the patient is best positioned on his right side.

Place one hand on the iliac crest. A vertical line dropped from this landmark will cross the 4th lumbar vertebra. Use the other hand to feel the interspace just above this level. This will be the L3–4 interspace. If this space cannot be used, L2–3 and L4–5 are acceptable.

Wash the patient's back with iodine-soaked sponges alternating with alcohol soaked- sponges, moving in concentric circles outward from the puncture site.

Put on sterile gloves and drape the patient with a sterile drape.

(**C**) Introduction of the needle. Inject local an-

943

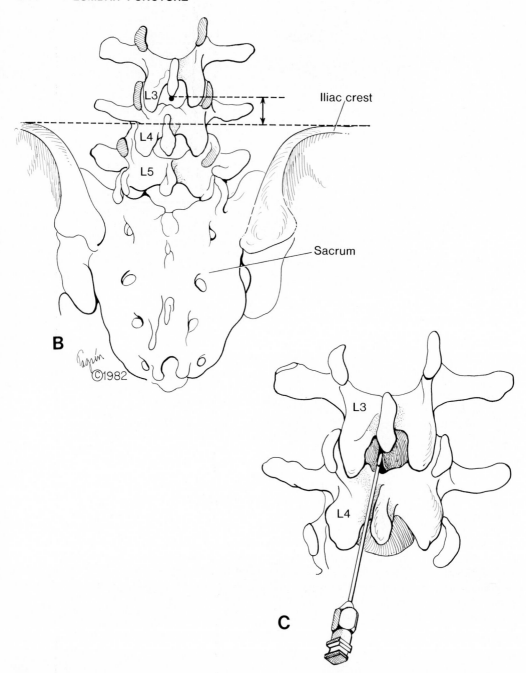

esthetic into the skin at the proposed site. Raise a skin wheal with a slow intradermal injection of 0.2 ml of anesthetic followed by a further 0.5 ml into the deeper layers of the skin. There is no need to change needles for this procedure, nor to anesthetize deeper layers of muscle.

Introduce a 20-gauge lumbar puncture needle with the stylet in place. The needle should be directed slightly cephalad (roughly toward the umbilicus) with the bevel parallel to the long axis of the patient's spine. The needle then will spread rather than cut the fibers of the ligamentum flavum.

Advance the needle slowly until the "give" of the ligamentum flavum is felt as the needle enters the subdural space. At this point, advance the needle in 2-mm steps removing the stylet between each step to check for CSF flow. If bone is encountered, withdraw the needle slowly and realign. Often the give of the ligamentum flavum is not distinct. Therefore, the stylet should be removed frequently to check for CSF return.

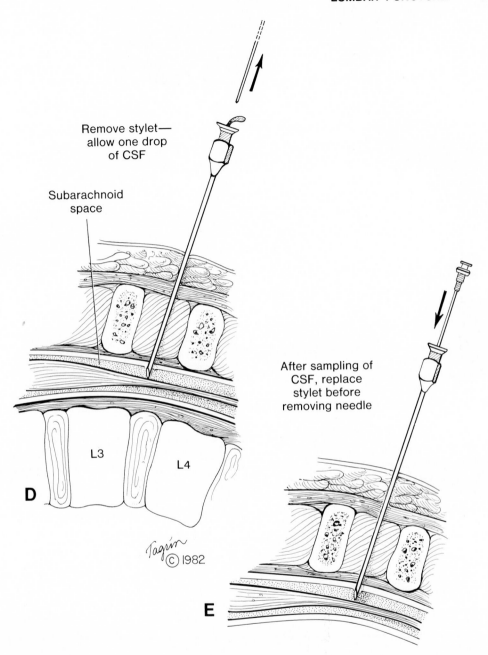

Remove stylet—
allow one drop
of CSF

Subarachnoid
space

L3

L4

D

Tagrin © 1982

After sampling of
CSF, replace
stylet before
removing needle

E

(D) When the needle is in the subarachnoid space, one drop of CSF should be allowed to flow out. Then turn the bevel perpendicular to the long axis of the spine and replace the stylet.

Allow the patient to relax as much as possible, extending legs and hips slightly from the maximally flexed position. Remove the stylet, attach the manometer and measure pressure. There should be good respiratory variation of the fluid level in the manometer.

Collect fluid in at least three sterile tubes. Tube #1 should be sent for protein and glucose (2–3 ml), tube #2 for culture and sensitivities (2 ml) and tube #3 for cell count (2 ml).

(E) After all specimens are collected, replace stylet, and remove the needle. Press on the area of the puncture to prevent local bleeding and put a small bandage over the site. The patient should be instructed to lie down for 2–4 hours after the puncture.

12. PERITONEAL LAVAGE

ASHBY C. MONCURE, M.D.

After initial resuscitation, patients suspected of having blunt abdominal trauma who have equivocal physical findings or an altered state of consciousness may be more accurately evaluated by means of peritoneal lavage. If the patient has had a previous lower abdominal operation or disease process, peritoneal lavage is best managed by placing the catheter under direct vision through a small infraumbilical midline incision. If this is not the case, the catheter may be placed percutaneously.

If no blood is recovered, lavage with a balanced salt solution is then performed, the results being considered abnormal if frank blood is recovered in the lavage fluid, if the red blood cell count is more than $100,000/mm^3$, if the white blood cell count is more than $500/mm^3$, or if high concentrations of amylase, bile, or bacteria are present in the fluid.

(A) The abdominal wall is prepared as a sterile field, and in the lower abdominal midline, one-third of the way between the umbilicus and the pubic bone, a small puncture wound is made with a No. 15 blade after infiltration with 1% lidocaine (Xylocaine). (B) A peritoneal dialysis catheter with an indwelling stylet (Trocath, McGaw Laboratories) is placed through the puncture wound, and is advanced to the linea alba, where resistance is encountered.

(C) The stylet tip is forced into the peritoneal cavity with a twisting motion; the depth of penetration is controlled by grasping the catheter with the thumb and index finger of the nondominant hand. (D) The stylet is withdrawn. (E) The catheter is advanced into the right or left pelvic gutter and is attached to an IV set with injection site for intravenous solution administration (McGaw Laboratories).

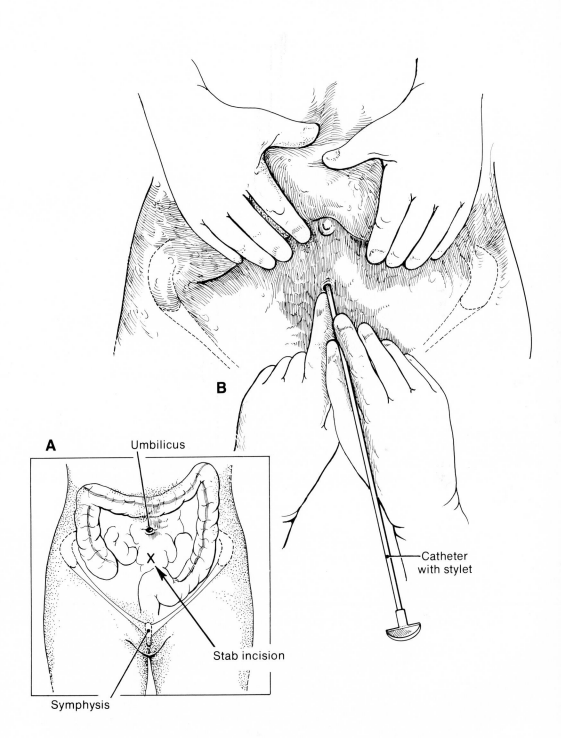

A

Umbilicus

Stab incision

Symphysis

B

Catheter
with stylet

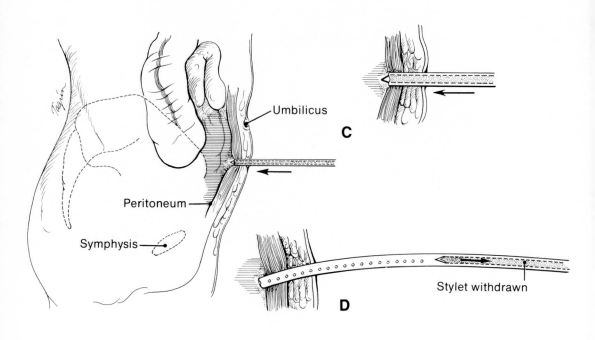

Umbilicus

Peritoneum

Symphysis

C

Stylet withdrawn

D

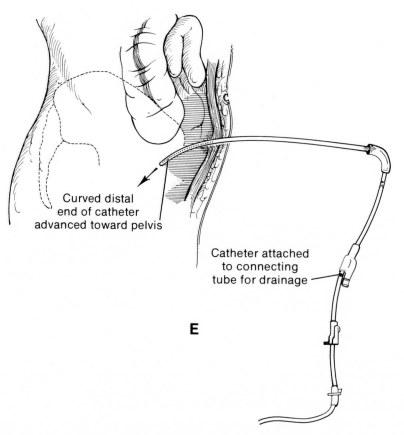

Curved distal
end of catheter
advanced toward pelvis

Catheter attached
to connecting
tube for drainage

E

13. PERCUTANEOUS SUPRAPUBIC CYSTOTOMY

ERIC J. SACKNOFF, M.D.

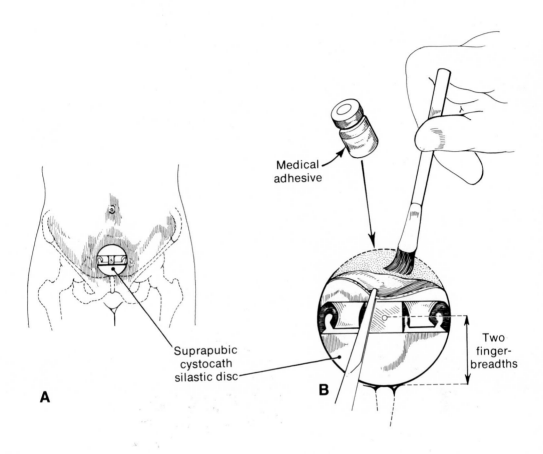

Medical adhesive

Suprapubic cystocath silastic disc

Two finger-breadths

A

B

Indications

Acute epididymitis (severe)

Acute prostatitis (severe)

Acute urethritis (severe)

Urethral stricture

Urethral rupture

Urinary retention

Contraindications

Previous pelvic and lower abdominal bowel surgery

Bladder neoplasm

Previous transpubic vascular procedure

Previous pelvic radiation therapy

Pelvic sepsis

(**A**) After the lower part of the abdomen is prepared with iodine and alcohol, the skin is anesthetized in the midline two fingerbreadths above the pubic symphysis. The location where the Silastic disc will be affixed is shown. (**B**) The skin is brushed with medical adhesive provided in the Cystocath kit, and the Silastic disc is then applied in the midline.

(**C**) Puncture of the skin surface with a No. 15 scalpel blade allows easy passage of the trocar and

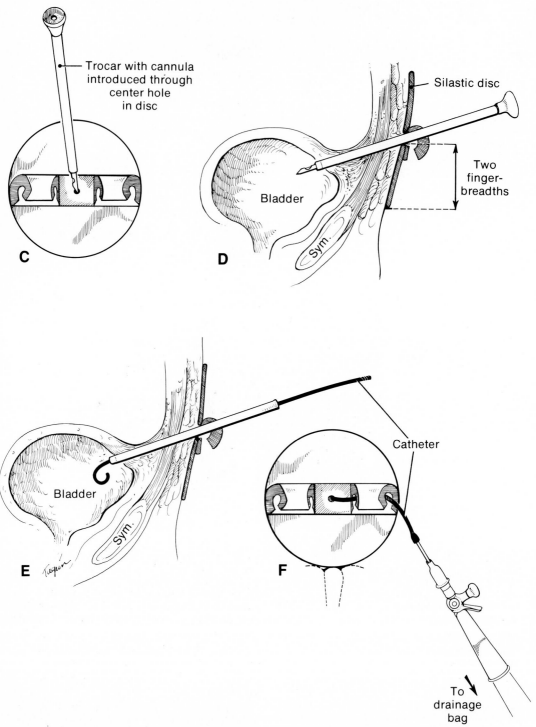

Trocar with cannula introduced through center hole in disc

C

Silastic disc

Bladder

Sym.

Two finger-breadths

D

Bladder

Sym.

Tripin

E

Catheter

F

To drainage bag

cannula through the skin and subcutaneous tissue. (**D**) At two fingerbreadths above the pubic symphysis in the midline, the trocar should be inserted in a direction slightly less than perpendicular to the skin so that the point is always directed inferiorly (*never* superiorly) to avoid entering the peritoneal cavity.

(**E**) After the bladder is entered, the trocar is removed and a Silastic No. 8 French catheter is introduced through the cannula. (**F**) Once the catheter is in the bladder, the cannula is removed. The catheter is then secured to the disc and attached to the three-way adapter and drainage system.

14. CULDOCENTESIS

DAVID S. CHAPIN, M.D.

Indications
    Suspected ectopic pregnancy
    Suspected pelvic abscess
Contraindications
    Markedly retroverted uterus
    Obvious cul-de-sac

Instruments
    Speculum
    Tenaculum
    20-cc syringe
    20- or 22-gauge spinal needle

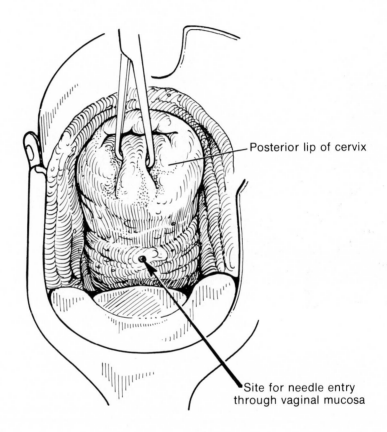

Posterior lip of cervix

Site for needle entry
through vaginal mucosa

A

(A–B) With the patient in the lithotomy position, the speculum is inserted, the cervix is visualized, and bulging of the cul-de-sac is noted. The vaginal apex is swabbed with antiseptic solution. If desired, 1% lidocaine (Xylocaine) may be used to anesthetize the puncture site, although this step is usually unnecessary. The posterior lip of the cervix is grasped with the tenaculum and elevated. The needle, mounted on the syringe, is inserted through the mucosa into the cul-de-sac. Withdrawal of pus or blood on aspiration suggests the presumptive diagnosis. If no fluid can be aspirated, the cul-de-sac is empty but the presumptive diagnosis is not ruled out.

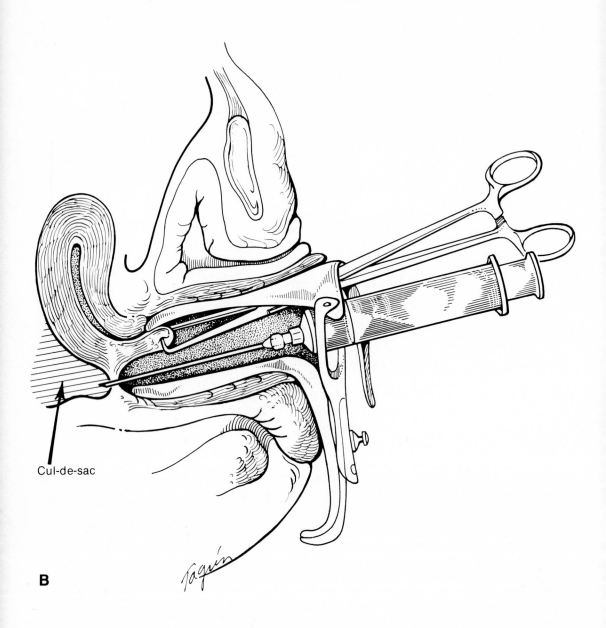

Cul-de-sac

B

15. SHOULDER—INJECTION FOR BURSITIS

BERTRAM ZARINS, M.D.

CARTER R. ROWE, M.D.

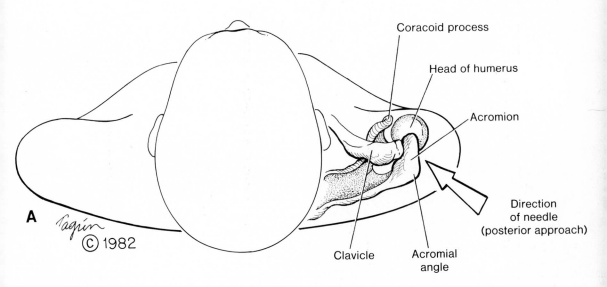

Coracoid process

Head of humerus

Acromion

Direction of needle (posterior approach)

A

© 1982

Clavicle

Acromial angle

The most common cause of acute "bursitis" of the shoulder is calcific tendinitis involving the rotator cuff. If injected, steroid should be instilled into the overlying bursa rather than the tendon itself. Anterior-posterior and axillary roentgenograms should be taken prior to steroid injection. Roentgenograms are evaluated for the presence of possible calcium deposition in the rotator cuff.

Injection into the subacromial bursa is carried out with the patient in a seated position and under sterile conditions. The posterolateral approach is the easiest and least painful (A). Palpate the spine of the scapula posteriorly, acromial angle, and acromion process; locate a "soft spot" 1 cm below the acromial angle and anesthetize the skin with local anesthesia. Instruct the patient to relax the muscles so the humerus drops downward. Pass a 22-gauge needle underneath the acromion near the acromial angle into the space between the acromion and the rotator cuff. Angle the needle slightly upward and anteriorly (B). Instill 5–10 cc of 1% lidocaine into the bursa. When local anesthesia has been achieved, puncture multiple holes into the bursa with the tip of the needle if this is not too painful. Leaving the needle in place, switch syringes to one containing a steroid solution, such as Triamcinolone Acetonide 40 mg, and instill the solution into the bursa. Avoid infiltrating the skin or subcutaneous tissues with steroid solution.

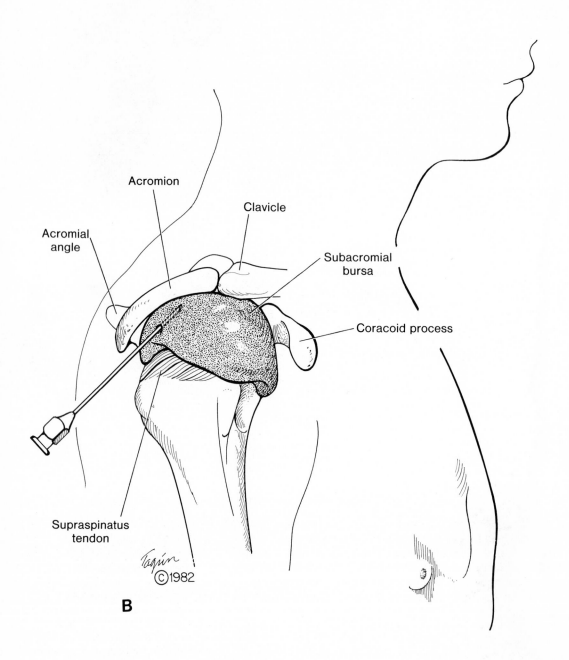

Acromion

Clavicle

Acromial
angle

Subacromial
bursa

Coracoid process

Supraspinatus
tendon

©1982

B

16. ARTHROCENTESIS—KNEE

BERTRAM ZARINS, M.D.

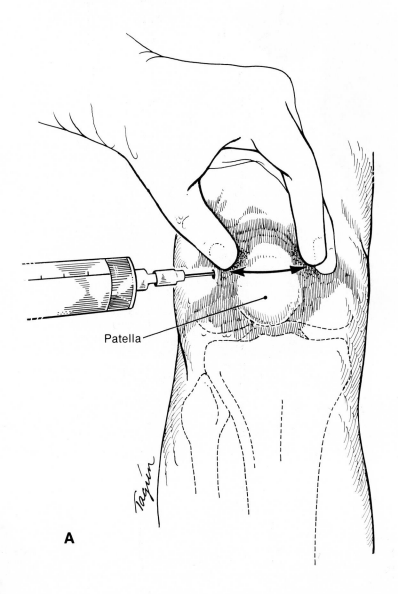

Patella

A

(**A**) Arthrocentesis of the knee is performed with the patient's knee extended and the quadriceps muscles and patella relaxed so that the patella can be moved mediolaterally. With sterile technique and adequate local anesthesia, a large-bore needle (15- to 19-gauge) attached to a 50-cc syringe is introduced into the joint space at a point just lateral to the patella near its upper pole. The needle is inserted parallel to the posterior (articular) surface of the patella. A lateral approach is easier than a medial one, but both are satisfactory.

(**B**) Insertion of the needle just behind the patella avoids the suprapatellar and infrapatellar fat pads. If there is excess fluid in the knee, the needle can be inserted just above the patella into the suprapatellar bursa.

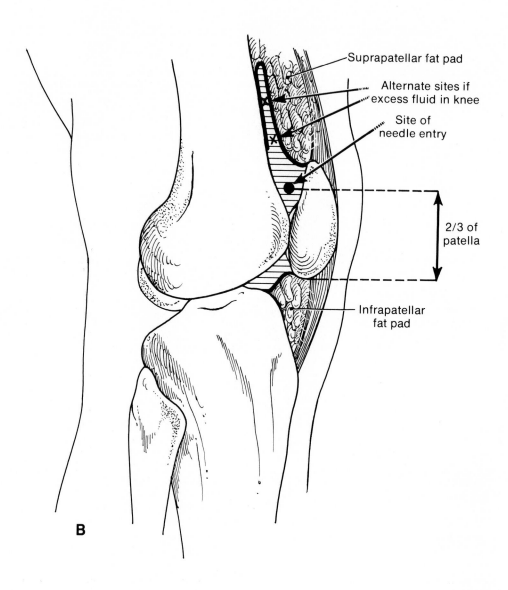

Suprapatellar fat pad

Alternate sites if
excess fluid in knee

Site of
needle entry

2/3 of
patella

Infrapatellar
fat pad

B

17. ARTHROCENTESIS—ANKLE

BERTRAM ZARINS, M.D.

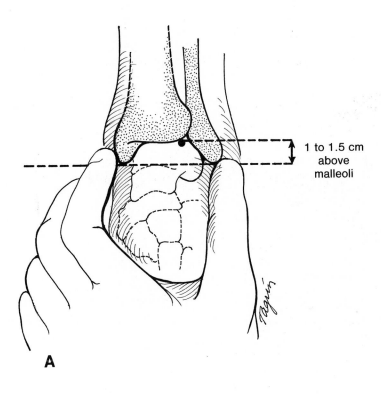

1 to 1.5 cm
above
malleoli

A

Arthrocentesis of the ankle is performed using sterile technique from the anterior approach. (**A**) Palpate the medial and lateral malleoli with the thumb and index finger. The joint space is located 1–1½ cm above the line joining the tips of the malleoli. (**B**) Palpate the dorsalis pedis artery and choose a puncture site anywhere on the anterior aspect of the ankle, avoiding the dorsalis pedis artery. (**C**) The needle should enter the joint parallel to the articular surface of the distal tibia; this is at approximately a right angle to the shaft of the tibia.

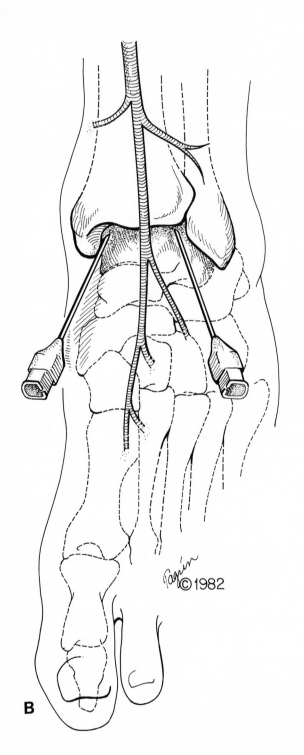

B

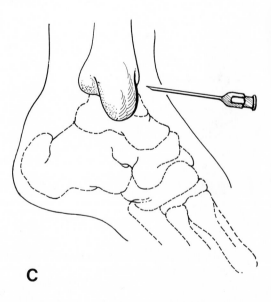

C

Index